# The Basic Science
## of Oncology

# Notice

Medicine is an ever-changing science. As new research and clinical experience broaden our knowledge, changes in treatment and drug therapy are required. The authors and the publisher of this work have checked with sources believed to be reliable in their efforts to provide information that is complete and generally in accord with the standards accepted at the time of publication. However, in view of the possibility of human error or changes in medical sciences, neither the authors nor the publisher nor any other party who has been involved in the preparation or publication of this work warrants that the information contained herein is in every respect accurate or complete, and they disclaim all responsibility for any errors or omissions or for the results obtained from use of the information contained in this work. Readers are encouraged to confirm the information contained herein with other sources. For example and in particular, readers are advised to check the product information sheet included in the package of each drug they plan to administer to be certain that the information contained in this work is accurate and that changes have not been made in the recommended dose or in the contraindications for administration. This recommendation is of particular importance in connection with new or infrequently used drugs.

# The Basic Science of Oncology

## Fourth Edition

### Edited by

**Ian F. Tannock,** MD, PhD, FRCPC

Daniel E. Bergsagel Professor, Department of Medical Oncology and Hematology
Princess Margaret Hospital/University Health Network
Senior Scientist, Division of Experimental Therapeutics
Ontario Cancer Institute/Princess Margaret Hospital
Professor of Medicine and Medical Biophysics
University of Toronto
Toronto, Ontario, Canada

**Richard P. Hill,** PhD

Senior Scientist, Division of Experimental Therapeutics
Ontario Cancer Institute/Princess Margaret Hospital
Professor of Medical Biophysics
University of Toronto
Toronto, Ontario, Canada

**Robert G. Bristow,** MD, PhD, FRCPC

Clinician-Scientist (Radiation Oncology) Radiation Medicine Program
Princess Margaret Hospital/University Health Network
Senior Scientist, Division of Experimental Therapeutics
Ontario Cancer Institute/Princess Margaret Hospital
Assistant Professor of Medical Biophysics
University of Toronto
Toronto, Ontario, Canada

**Lea Harrington,** PhD

Senior Scientist, Division of Cellular and Molecular Biology
Ontario Cancer Institute/Princess Margaret Hospital
Associate Professor of Medical Biophysics
University of Toronto
Toronto, Ontario, Canada

**McGraw-Hill**
**Medical Publishing Division**

New York   Chicago   San Francisco   Lisbon   London   Madrid   Mexico City   Milan
New Delhi   San Juan   Seoul   Singapore   Sydney   Toronto

**The Basic Science of Oncology, Fourth Edition**

1 2 3 4 5 6 7 8 9 0 QPD/QPD 0 9 8 7 6 5

ISBN: 0-07-138774-9

This book was set in New Baskerville by Matrix Publishing Services.
The editors were Marc Strauss and Michelle Watt.
The production supervisor was Richard Ruzycka.
Project management was provided by Chernow Editorial Services, Inc.
Quebecor World was printer and binder.

This book is printed on acid-free paper.

Library of Congress Cataloging-in-Publication Data
The basic science of oncology / edited by Ian F. Tannock . . . [et al.].—4th ed.
    p. ; cm.
  Includes bibliographical references and index.
  ISBN 0-07-138774-9
  1. Cancer. 2. Oncology. I. Tannock, Ian.
  [DNLM: 1. Neoplasms. QZ 200 B3115 2004]
RC261.B37 2004
616.99′4—dc22
                                                        2004044833

# Contents

Color plates appear between pages 274 and 275.

# Contributors

**Cheryl H. Arrowsmith, PhD**
Chief Scientist, Structural Genomics Consortium—
  Toronto
Senior Scientist
Ontario Cancer Institute/Princess Margaret Hospital
Professor
Department of Medical Biophysics and Banting and
  Best Department of Medical Research
University of Toronto
Toronto, Ontario, Canada
carrow@uhnres.utoronto.ca


**Nancy N. Berg-Brown, PhD**
Lecturer, Division of Science
Medicine Hat College
Medicine Hat, Alberta, Canada
nbrown@mhc.ab.ca


**Neil L. Berinstein, MD, FRCPC**
Medical Oncologist
Department of Medical Oncology
Toronto-Sunnybrook Regional Cancer Centre
Assistant Vice-President, Oncology
Director, Aventis Pasteur Cancer Vaccine Program
Professor of Medicine
University of Toronto
Toronto, Ontario, Canada
Neil.berinstein@aventis.com


**Michael J. Boyer, MBBS, PhD**
Director, Medical Oncology Department
Royal Prince Alfred Hospital
Sydney, New South Wales, Australia
michael.boyer@cs.nsw.gov.au


**Robert G. Bristow, MD, PhD, FRCPC**
Clinician-Scientist (Radiation Oncology) Radiation
  Medicine Program
Princess Margaret Hospital/University Health
  Network
Senior Scientist, Division of Experimental
  Therapeutics
Ontario Cancer Institute/Princess Margaret Hospital
Assistant Professor of Medical Biophysics
University of Toronto
Toronto, Ontario, Canada
rob_bristow@rmp.uhn.on.ca


**Susan P.C. Cole, PhD, FRSC**
Canada Research Chair in Cancer Biology
Cancer Research Laboratories
Professor of Pathology & Molecular Medicine and
  Pharmacology & Toxicology
Queen's University
Kingston, Ontario, Canada
coles@post.queensu.ca


**Jeffrey C.H. Donovan, MD, PhD**
Resident, Division of Dermatology
Department of Medicine
University of Toronto
Toronto, Ontario, Canada
Jeffrey_c_h_Donovan@yahoo.ca


**Daniel Dumont, PhD**
Director of Molecular and Cellular Biology
Sunnybrook and Women's Research Institute
Professor, Department of Medical Biophysics
University of Toronto
Toronto, Ontario, Canada
dan.dumont@swri.ca

**Steven Gallinger, MD, FRCSC**
Faculty, Department of Surgery
Mount Sinai Hospital/University Health Network
Professor of Surgery
University of Toronto
Toronto, Ontario, Canada
sgallinger@mtsinai.on.ca

**Denis M. Grant, PhD**
Professor and Chair, Department of Pharmacology,
   Faculty of Medicine
Associate Dean for Research
Leslie Dan Faculty of Pharmacy
Director, Institute for Drug Research
University of Toronto
Toronto, Ontario, Canada
denis.grant@utoronto.ca

**Razqallah Hakem, PhD**
Senior Scientist, Division of Cellular and Molecular
   Biology
Ontario Cancer Institute/Princess Margaret Hospital
Associate Professor, Medical Biophysics
University of Toronto
Toronto, Ontario, Canada
rhakem@uhnres.utoronto.ca

**Patricia A. Harper, PhD**
Senior Scientist, Program in Developmental Biology
Department of Clinical Pharmacology
Hospital for Sick Children
Associate Professor of Pharmacology
University of Toronto
Toronto, Ontario, Canada
pharper@sickkids.ca

**Lea Harrington, PhD**
Senior Scientist, Division of Cellular and Molecular
   Biology
Ontario Cancer Institute/Princess Margaret Hospital
Associate Professor of Medical Biophysics
University of Toronto
Toronto, Ontario, Canada
leah@uhnres.utoronto.ca

**Richard P. Hill, PhD**
Senior Scientist, Division of Experimental
   Therapeutics
Ontario Cancer Institute/Princess Margaret Hospital
Professor of Medical Biophysics
University of Toronto
Toronto, Ontario, Canada
hill@uhnres.utoronto.ca

**David C. Hodgson, MD, MPH, FRCPC**
Radiation Oncologist, Radiation Medicine Program
Princess Margaret Hospital/University Health
   Network
Assistant Professor of Radiation Oncology
University of Toronto
Toronto, Ontario, Canada
David.hodgson@uhn.on.ca

**Suzanne Kamel-Reid, PhD**
Scientist, Department of Pathology
University Health Network
Division of Molecular and Cellular Biology
Ontario Cancer Institute/Princess Margaret Hospital
Professor of Laboratory Medicine and Pathobiology &
   Medical Biophysics
University of Toronto
Toronto, Ontario, Canada
s.kamel.reid@utoronto.ca

**Rama Khokha, PhD**
Senior Scientist, Division of Experimental
   Therapeutics
Ontario Cancer Institute/Princess Margaret Hospital
Professor of Medical Biophysics
University of Toronto
Toronto, Ontario, Canada
rkhokha@uhnres.utoronto.ca

**Melanie A. McGill**
PhD Student (with Dr. McGlade)
Arthur and Sonia Labatt Brain Tumour Research
   Centre
Hospital for Sick Children and Department of
   Medical Biophysics
University of Toronto
Toronto, Ontario, Canada
mcgillma@sickkids.ca

**C. Jane McGlade, PhD**
Senior Scientist
Program in Cell Biology and the Arthur and Sonia
   Labatt Brain Tumour Research Centre
Hospital for Sick Children
Professor of Medical Biophysics
University of Toronto
Toronto, Ontario, Canada
jmcglade@sickkids.ca

**John McLaughlin, PhD**
Leader, Prosserman Centre for Health Research
Head, Program in Epidemiology and Biostatistics
Samuel Lunenfeld Research Institute at Mount Sinai
  Hospital
Associate Professor, Department of Public Health
  Sciences
University of Toronto
Toronto, Ontario, Canada
jmclaugh@mshri.on.ca

**Malcolm J. Moore, MD, FRCPC**
Ho Chair in Prostate Cancer Research
Active Staff, Department of Medical Oncology &
  Hematology
Director, Drug Development Program
Princess Margaret Hospital/University Health
  Network
Professor of Medicine and Pharmacology
University of Toronto
Toronto, Ontario, Canada
Malcolm.moore@uhn.on.ca

**Leigh Murphy, PhD**
Chair, Breast Cancer Research Group at the
  University of Manitoba
Senior Scientist, Manitoba Institute for Cell Biology
Professor of Biochemistry and Medical Genetics
University of Manitoba
Winnipeg, Manitoba, Canada
lcmurph@cc.umanitoba.ca

**Linh T. Nguyen, PhD**
Research Fellow, Immunology and Immunogenetics
Joslin Diabetes Center
Boston, Massachusetts, USA
linh.nguyen@joslin.harvard.edu

**Pamela S. Ohashi, PhD**
Senior Scientist, Division of Cellular and Molecular
  Biology
Ontario Cancer Institute/Princess Margaret
  Hospital/University Health Network
Professor, Department of Medical Biophysics and
  Immunology
University of Toronto
Toronto, Ontario, Canada
pohashi@uhnres.utoronto.ca

**Allan B. Okey, PhD**
Professor, Department of Pharmacology
University of Toronto
Toronto, Ontario, Canada
allan.okey@utoronto.ca

**Sara Oster**
Graduate Student (with Dr. Penn)
Division of Cellular and Molecular Biology
Ontario Cancer Institute/Princess Margaret Hospital
Department of Medical Biophysics
University of Toronto
Toronto, Ontario, Canada
Sara.oster@uhnres.utoronto.ca

**Linda Penn, PhD**
Senior Scientist, Division of Cellular and Molecular
  Biology
Ontario Cancer Institute/Princess Margaret Hospital
Professor of Medical Biophysics
University of Toronto
Toronto, Ontario, Canada
lpenn@uhnres.utoronto.ca

**Jason Read, PhD**
Postdoctoral Fellow
The Prostate Centre at Vancouver General Hospital
Vancouver, British Columbia, Canada
jread@vanhosp.bc.ca

**Patricia P. Reis, PhD**
Post-Doctoral Fellow, Division of Cellular and
  Molecular Biology
Ontario Cancer Institute/Princess Margaret Hospital
University of Toronto
Toronto, Ontario, Canada
preis@uhnres.utoronto.ca

**Paul Rennie, PhD**
Director, Laboratory Research
The Prostate Centre at Vancouver General Hospital
Professor, Departments of Surgery, Pathology and
  Laboratory Medicine
University of British Columbia
Adjunct Professor, Department of Biology
University of Victoria
Vancouver, British Columbia, Canada
prennie@interchange.ubc.ca

**Christopher D. Richardson, PhD**
Senior Scientist, Division of Molecular and Structural
  Biology
Ontario Cancer Institute/Princess Margaret Hospital
Professor, Department of Medical Biophysics
University of Toronto
Toronto, Ontario, Canada
chrisr@uhnres.utoronto.ca

**Michael D. Sherar, PhD**
Vice President, London Regional Cancer Program
London Health Sciences Centre
Professor of Oncology
University of Western Ontario
London, Ontario, Canada
Senior Scientist, Division of Medical Biophysics
Ontario Cancer Institute/Princess Margaret Hospital
Adjunct Professor of Medical Biophysics
University of Toronto
Toronto, Ontario, Canada
sherar@uhnres.utoronto.ca

**Lillian L. Siu, MD, FRCPC**
Active Staff, Department of Medical Oncology &
  Hematology and Drug Development Program
Princess Margaret Hospital/University Health Network
Associate Professor
University of Toronto
Toronto, Ontario, Canada
Lillian.siu@uhn.on.ca

**Joyce Slingerland, MD, PhD, FRCPC**
Director, Braman Breast Cancer Institute
Division of Hematology/Oncology
Sylvester Comprehensive Cancer Center
Professor
University of Miami School of Medicine
Miami, Florida, USA
jslingerland@med.miami.edu

**Jeremy A. Squire, PhD**
J.C. Boileau Grant Chair in Oncologic Pathology
Division of Cellular and Molecular Biology
Ontario Cancer Institute/Princess Margaret Hospital
Professor of Laboratory Medicine and Pathobiology
  and Medical Biophysics
University of Toronto
Toronto, Ontario, Canada
jeremy.squire@utoronto.ca

**Vuk Stambolic, PhD**
Canada Research Chair in Cellular Signaling
Scientist, Division of Experimental Therapeutics
Ontario Cancer Institute/Princess Margaret Hospital
Assistant Professor of Medical Biophysics
University of Toronto
Toronto, Ontario, Canada
vuks@uhnres.utoronto.ca

**Celina Sturk**
Graduate Student (with Dr. Dumont)
Sunnybrook and Women's Research Institute
Department of Medical Biophysics
University of Toronto
Toronto, Ontario, Canada
celina.sturk@swri.ca

**Ian F. Tannock, MD, PhD, FRCPC**
Daniel E. Bergsagel Professor, Department of Medical
  Oncology and Hematology
Princess Margaret Hospital/University Health Network
Senior Scientist, Division of Experimental
  Therapeutics
Ontario Cancer Institute/Princess Margaret Hospital
Professor of Medicine and Medical Biophysics
University of Toronto
Toronto, Ontario, Canada
ian.tannock@uhn.on.ca

**Evelyn Voura, PhD**
Post-Doctoral Fellow, Laboratory of Cellular
  Biophysics
Rockefeller University
New York, New York, USA
vourae@rockefeller.edu

# Preface

Not surprisingly, given the tremendous advances in our understanding of cancer since the third edition of the *Basic Science of Oncology* was published, this new edition of the book incorporates many changes. Two new editors (Drs. Bristow and Harrington) have brought expertise in molecular studies and have made major contributions to the revisions incorporated in the new edition. Although the format has remained the same, molecular advances in the respective fields have been added where possible.

The editors have brought together experts in various fields to convey the latest advances at a level we believe is suitable for fellows, residents, nurses, medical students, graduate students, and senior undergraduates who are interested in the biology of cancer. For those who wish to delve into these topics in greater depth, references are included at the end of each chapter that may be used as a springboard to more in-depth study. We believe that the book will be useful as a teaching aid and as a broad introduction for those interested in the study and treatment of cancer.

Ian F. Tannock, MD, PhD, FRCPC
Richard P. Hill, PhD
Robert G. Bristow, MD, PhD, FRCPC
Lea Harrington, PhD

# The Basic Science
## of Oncology

# 1

# Introduction to Cancer Biology

*Lea Harrington, Robert G. Bristow, Richard P. Hill, and Ian F. Tannock*

---

1.1 PERSPECTIVE

1.2 THE FUTURE OF ONCOLOGY

---

## 1.1 PERSPECTIVE

Although awareness of cancer has increased in modern times, it is not a modern disease. Malignant tumors were described in pictures and in writings from many ancient civilizations, and bone cancers (osteosarcomas) have been diagnosed in Egyptian mummies. Cancer occurs in all known species of higher animals. Early cultures attributed the cause of cancer to various gods, and this belief was held until the Middle Ages. Hippocrates, however, described cancer as an imbalance between the black humor (from the spleen) and the three bodily humors: blood, phlegm, and bile. Although incorrect, the theory was the first (~400 B.C.) to attribute the origin of cancer to natural causes. The suggestion that cancer might be an inherited or environmental disease appeared later: writings from the Middle Ages made reference to "cancer houses," "cancer families," and "cancer villages."

One of the first scientific enquiries into the cause of cancer dates from 1775, when Sir Percival Pott, an English physician, carried out an epidemiological study. At that time young boys were used as chimney sweeps in London because they were small enough to climb inside the chimneys. Pott observed that young men in their twenties who had been chimney sweeps as boys had a high rate of death due to cancer of the scrotum. He suggested that the causative agent might be chimney soot (now known to be tar) and recommended frequent washing and changing of clothing that trapped the soot so as to reduce exposure to the carcinogen.

Not only did Pott's study identify a putative carcinogenic agent, but it also demonstrated that a cancer may develop many years after exposure to the causative agent—that is, that there can be an extended latent period. Later epidemiological studies have identified major environmental causes of cancer, such as tobacco smoke and various occupational exposures. Such studies raise the possibility of prevention through changes in lifestyle and diet, as has already happened through decreased rates of smoking in some western countries.

Pott's deductions about the origin of scrotal cancer in chimney sweeps, and other epidemiological studies relating cancer to environmental or hereditary causes, were made with little knowledge of the biological properties of tumors. Advances in understanding of biological properties followed the development of the microscope: microscopic examination of tumors allowed Virchow, the eminent nineteenth-century pathologist, to declare that "every cell is born from another cell." This is also true of cells in normal tissues, but only in tumors do cells continue to accumulate beyond what is required for normal growth or replacement of cells in renewing tissues, such as the bone marrow, skin, and intestine. Thus, cancer was established as a cellular disease, where there was loss of normal control of cell proliferation.

Recently, the most important advances in knowledge about the biology of cancer have come from increased understanding of molecular genetics. Many of these advances were dependent on prior information from epidemiological studies. Studies of relatively inbred populations, such as the Mormons in Utah, have shown that many types of cancer depend on relatedness—that is, on the sharing of genes. Studies of families that have a high incidence of cancer have assisted in the identification of genetic defects that can lead to malignancy, such as mutations of the retinoblastoma gene (*Rb*) in children with that disease, of the *p53* gene in the Li-Fraumeni syndrome, and of the *BRCA1* and *BRCA2* genes, which are associated with familial breast and ovarian cancer. Studies of cancer incidence in families that have inherited genetically based defects in DNA repair have also demonstrated the involvement of DNA repair genes in preventing malignancy. Cancer has been established as a genetic disease.

The rapid evolution of techniques of molecular biology has led to the characterization, cloning, and sequencing of a variety of genes where mutation or changes in expression can lead to malignant transformation. The current model for cancer development envisions cells undergoing a series of genetic mutations and/or alterations, brought about in various ways, which result in their inability to respond normally to intracellular and/or extracellular signals that control proliferation, differentiation, and, ultimately, death. The number of required genetic alterations varies from as little as two to at least six for different types of cancer, and it is likely that further changes occur during progression to increased malignancy. These genetic alterations may arise directly or indirectly from such factors as inherited gene mutations, chemical- or radiation-induced DNA damage and genetic instability, incorporation of certain viruses into the cell, or random errors during DNA synthesis. It is becoming clear that specific types of cancers often display specific types of genetic changes, so that the old clinical concept that cancer is "many different diseases" is being borne out by genetic analysis.

While clinical observation has divided tumor development into a number of discrete categories of increasing severity (benign, malignant, metastatic), the underlying biology is better conceptualized as a process of many small changes similar to evolution. Thus, genetic changes that can affect the cell's growth potential may occur, and cells with such changes are selected for (or against) by the conditions that they are exposed to at that particular time. Increasing knowledge of signal-transduction pathways in cells has demonstrated that many aspects of cellular function, including proliferation and death, are controlled by a balance of positive and negative signals received from inside and outside the cell. Thus, lack of ability or increased ability to respond to a specific signal may allow the cell to proliferate in the face of other signals that would normally prevent such proliferation.

Investigations of interactions between cells in tissues and of extracellular factors that control cell growth and differentiation have also made major advances. We now understand many of the mechanisms responsible for the development of the new (and often poorly formed) vascular network in tumors (*angiogenesis*) necessary for their growth and that many features of the extracellular environment in tumors (such as poor oxygenation) can cause changes in gene expression that enhance the development of more aggressive phenotypes. These investigations are leading to a better understanding of how and why cancer cells can spread from the primary tumor to grow at other sites in the body (*metastasize*), a feature of a malignant cancer that makes it particularly difficult to treat successfully.

Until recently cancer treatment has depended on relatively nonspecific approaches that either spare normal tissues because therapy can be localized to the tumor mass (surgery and radiotherapy), or use drugs, which are selective for proliferating cells rather than cancer cells per se (chemotherapy). Major efforts are now directed to developing treatments that take advantage of the new knowledge of molecular properties of cancer, and which aim to counter the molecular abnormalities that lead to disordered growth. Ongoing genetic changes, however, give rise to subpopulations of cells that evolve varied mechanisms of resistance, both for traditional treatments and for those that modify the molecular properties of cells, and these cells may survive and repopulate the tumor. The genetic instability of cancer cells and the resulting heterogeneity of the phenotype of cells within an individual tumor pose a major challenge to the development of more effective treatments.

## 1.2 THE FUTURE OF ONCOLOGY

Since the publication of the third edition of *The Basic Science of Oncology*, the human genome has been sequenced and there has been a watershed in our understanding of the molecular basis of cancer. New drugs based on these advances have led to improved outcome for patients with cancer. For example, patients with chronic myelogenous leukemia can now be treated more successfully using a specific, competitive inhibitor (imatinib) of the nucleotide binding site of the Bcr-Abl protein kinase, the protein that is aberrantly expressed as a result of the Philadelphia chromosome translocation. Trastuzumab is a monoclonal antibody that recognizes the HER2/neu receptor that is expressed on the tumor cells of some patients with aggressive breast cancer, and treatment with this agent has been shown to improve quality and duration of survival. A monoclonal antibody (bevacizumab) that inhibits the receptor for vascular endothelial growth factor (VEGF), important in the process of angiogenesis can improve survival for patients with colorectal cancer. Traditional methods have also undergone substantial improvement in the last few years. New methods for delivery of radiation have allowed higher doses to be delivered to the tumor with lower doses delivered to normal tissue, improving local control of primary tumors such as prostate cancer, and new combinations of radiation with surgery and chemotherapy are also improving patient survival. On the horizon, is the possibility of vaccines against specific papilloma viruses that predispose to cervical cancer, a disease that, although declining in incidence in western countries, is one of the leading causes of cancer death in women in other parts of the world.

Techniques such as DNA microarrays are allowing the rapid analysis of expression of very large numbers of genes in tumors and normal tissues, and researchers are gaining an appreciation for the great molecular complexity that leads to cancer in humans. Cancers that present with the same spectrum of symptoms and clinical manifestations are being categorized at the molecular level into individual subtypes that can be used to predict prognosis and response to specific therapies. In breast cancer, for example, early studies suggest the possibility that the expression profile of thousands of genes expressed in the tumor sample may replace the traditional factors of stage and histological grade as the best predictor of a woman's prognosis and response to treatment. The classification of such "footprints" for individual cancers is rapidly increasing our understanding of tumor biology and is guiding the development of new types of treatment. The era following the sequence determination of the human genome is a time of exponential learning with respect to our ability to understand the many different types of human cancer. In the future it is likely that treatment strategies will be decided largely on the basis of the genetic footprint of a cancer, rather than on its histopathological type.

# 2

# Cancer Epidemiology

*John McLaughlin and Steven Gallinger*

## 2.1 INTRODUCTION

Epidemiology is the study of the distribution and determinants of disease in human populations. The subject is concerned with explaining why different populations or groups are at different risks for different diseases, which in turn can support inferences at the individual level, such as why a particular patient developed their disease at a specific time.

The purpose of this chapter is to introduce the principles, concepts, and methods that are central to cancer epidemiology. Other chapters give detailed accounts of specific etiological associations, and no attempt is made here to provide a comprehensive description of the epidemiology of all cancers. Rather, the general principles used in the epidemiological study of cancer are described, and the epidemiology of colorectal cancer is summarized to illustrate these principles and their application.

### 2.1.1 The Scope of Epidemiology

In addition to being the focus for those concerned with population health, epidemiology is also of concern to clinicians, clinical researchers, and laboratory scientists. Clinicians must advise patients about cancer risks associated with their lifestyle and with medical procedures or treatments. Clinicians also need to understand how data describing such risks are generated in order to assess the quantitative importance of the risks described and to appraise critically the credibility of reports of cancer risk.

Epidemiology contributes to the work of basic and clinical researchers through the description of the distribution of cancer and the identification of groups at different risks of developing cancer. This provides information that is required to test hypotheses concerning the causes of cancer. Laboratory and clinical sciences contribute to epidemiological studies by developing improved methods of measuring exposure to potential carcinogens or the biological consequences of such exposure. Some of the most striking examples of progress in understanding the causes of cancer have come from such collaborative work, where biomarkers of exposure or biologic effect were applied in studies of human populations. Research that has defined the role of genetic factors in colorectal cancer is an example of this collaboration (see Sec. 2.3).

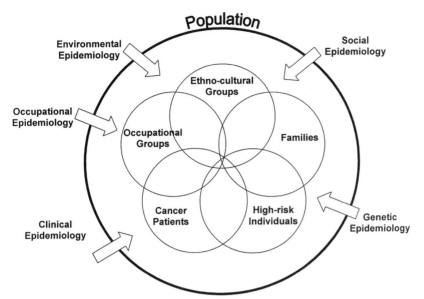

**Figure 2.1.** Types of epidemiological research and the subgroups within populations that are under investigation.

An important application of epidemiologic findings is in the planning and evaluation of cancer control strategies, including those of primary prevention and early detection. Epidemiologic methods can be applied to study determinants of a wide range of outcomes and possible causes of disease. Indeed, methodologies developed for epidemiological research have been applied increasingly in studies of cells and in animal models to study the role of molecular and genetic factors in cancer development. Simultaneously, the methods have been applied in studies of behavioral and psychosocial factors in clinical and societal settings. Although the scope of cancer epidemiology is broad, a primary concern is the search for causes of cancer that may enable the identification of populations where risk can be reduced, and, ultimately, the prevention of cancer in the population.

### 2.1.2 General Approach

There are two phases in the general approach taken by cancer epidemiologists. First, *descriptive epidemiology* provides an indication of how frequently cancer occurs in terms of rates, risks, and the number of cases. Second, *analytic epidemiology* is used to study the determinants of cancer, whereby comparisons of cancer risks are made between subgroups of the population.

It is in the identification of causes of serious illness that epidemiology has made its greatest contribution. One unique contribution of cancer epidemiology is its ability to study cancer etiology directly in human populations. To achieve this, epidemiology employs predominantly *observational* rather than *experimental* research methods, in part because it is unethical to intentionally expose people to carcinogens. There are potential limitations of observational research, such that

epidemiologists must carefully consider the design, methods, and interpretation of their studies.

Analytic epidemiologic studies search for causes of cancer by determining whether a particular trait or exposure is associated with the risk of developing the outcome of interest. Traditionally, the associations considered in epidemiologic studies were between readily identifiable states, such as potential risk factors measured by questionnaire, and a clearly defined outcome, such as cancer.

Specialized subdisciplines have evolved that focus on particular subgroups of the overall population, some examples of which are shown in Figure 2.1. In *occupational epidemiology* the effects of workplace exposures on workers are studied, while the outcomes of patients are studied in *clinical epidemiology*. The focus is on families or higher risk individuals in *genetic epidemiology*, which is concerned with the determinants of disease in families, and on inherited causes of cancer in populations. Other subdisciplines focus on particular sets of determinants, such as in *nutritional* or *environmental epidemiology*, or on particular methods of measurement, such as in *molecular epidemiology*, which incorporates molecular and cellular measurements of exposures and underlying biological processes. Each branch of epidemiology shares a common set of methods and basic principles.

## 2.2 METHODS OF EPIDEMIOLOGICAL INVESTIGATION

To study the causes of adverse outcomes in people, specialized research methods have been developed to enable scientifically valid, ethically acceptable, and cost-effective studies. To describe patterns of disease and risk factors in groups of people, epidemiology relies heavily on statistical and probabilistic methods. The reliance on observational rather than experimental methods has placed emphasis on the use of cohort and case-control designs, and on the need to control for the impact of chance variation and potential biases. These specialized methods are illustrated in Sec. 2.3 with examples related to colorectal cancer.

### 2.2.1 Epidemiologic Measures

To describe the health experience of a population, the most basic measure of disease *frequency* is a simple count of the total number of cases. The number of cases in the population is particularly relevant for planning health services as it relates directly to caseload. In counting cancer cases, a distinction is made between incidence and prevalence. *Incidence* refers to the number of new events, such as deaths or newly diagnosed cases that occurred in a defined population within a specified period of time. *Prevalence* is defined as the number of people with a given disease (or other condition), both newly and previously diagnosed, in a defined population at a designated time.

*Rates* are often a more meaningful measure of disease burden because disease frequency is then considered in relation to the size of the population and the length of time during which the events occurred. By accounting for differences in population size and duration of observation, rates are measures of disease frequency that can be used to make comparisons between populations or their subsets. An *incidence rate* is calculated by:

$$\text{Incidence Rate} = \frac{\text{(the number of new cases over the period of observation)}}{\text{(the total amount of person-time observed)}},$$

where the denominator is the sum of the lengths of follow-up for all persons in the study. Rates are often calculated to provide estimates of risk, where *risk* is defined as an individual's probability of suffering an adverse event (i.e., new case or death) in a specified time interval. If the period of observation is constant for all individuals, the risk of new disease can be summarized as a simple *incidence proportion*, which is sometimes referred to as *cumulative incidence*:

$$\text{Incidence Proportion} = \frac{\text{(the number of new cases over the period of observation)}}{\text{(the total number of people at the beginning of the interval)}}.$$

The patterns and trends of disease are usually summarized by annual rates, which fix the length of observation at 1 year for each member of the population. Annual rates thereby provide estimates of risk (i.e., incidence proportion) during a one-year period.

The relationship between incidence, incidence rate, and risk can be seen in the summary of the worldwide burden of all types of cancer (Table 2.1). It was estimated that in the year 2000, there were 5.3 million incident cancer cases among men and 4.7 million among women, which translates to annual incidence rates of 202 and 158 per 100,000 males and females, respectively. Considered as risk estimates, these rates indicate that in a one-year period approximately 2 per 1000 in the worldwide population will develop cancer.

Given that cancer rates vary substantially with age, the validity of comparisons between populations is made possible by calculating *age-standardized rates*, which account for differences in age distribution as well as population size. The populations of more developed countries are older on average than in less developed countries, thus the incidence rates shown in Table 2.1 are age-standardized to an average worldwide age distribution. Table 2.1 demonstrates that more cancer cases occurred in less developed countries among both men and women; however, after accounting for differences in population size and age, the risk was almost twice as high in more developed countries than in less developed countries.

**Table 2.1.** Worldwide Incidence and Prevalence of All Types of Cancer Combined (Excluding Non-melanoma Skin Cancer), by Level of Economic Development

| Location | Number of Incident Cases in 2000 (in Thousands) | | Age-standardized Incidence Rate per Year* (per 100,000) | | Number of Prevalent Cases in 2000 (in Thousands) | |
|---|---|---|---|---|---|---|
| | Male | Female | Male | Female | Male | Female |
| More developed nations | 2504 | 2176 | 301 | 218 | 5984 | 6448 |
| Less developed nations | 2814 | 2562 | 154 | 128 | 4264 | 5710 |
| World (total) | 5318 | 4738 | 202 | 158 | 10,248 | 12,159 |

*Age standardized to the World Standard Population.

*Source*: Adapted from Ferlay et al. (2001).

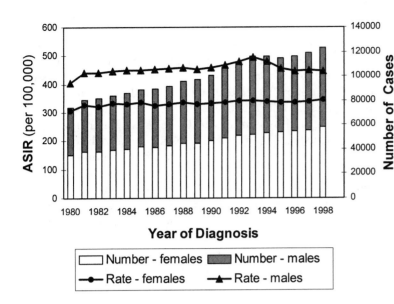

**Figure 2.2.** Age-standardized incidence rates (ASIR per 100,000) and the number of incident cases in Canada, for all types of cancer combined, by year and gender (figures exclude non-melanoma skin cancer; rates standardized to the 1991 Canadian census population). (Adapted from the National Cancer Institute of Canada, 2002.)

Figure 2.2 presents trends in these measures of disease frequency in Canada. Among Canadian males and females, the number of incident cases for all cancers combined (excluding non-melanoma skin cancer) increased from 74,000 in 1980 to 123,000 in 1998, while age-standardized incidence rates remained more stable. Given the stability of the rates, this change in the number of cancer cases can be attributed largely to an increase in, and aging of, the population.

The relative contribution to the number of new cases by changes in population size, age distribution, and disease risk is depicted in Figure 2.3. For Canadian men, over three decades the major determinants of the increase in incidence were the increasing age of the

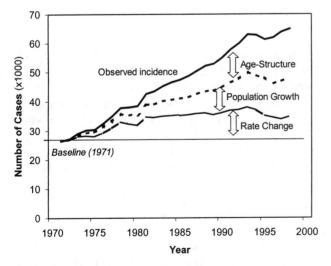

**Figure 2.3.** Trend in the number of incident cancer cases among males in Canada, showing the relative contribution of changes in rates, population growth, and aging of the population. (Adapted from National Cancer Institute of Canada, 2002.)

population and the increase in population size. The patterns for women are similar. Many countries have aging populations similar to Canada, and will face this pattern of continuously increasing cancer caseloads.

Prevalence is a function of both the incidence and duration of a disease or trait. Thus, for cancers with a favorable prognosis (i.e., high survival rate), prevalence is much higher than incidence, whereas prevalence can be much lower for cancers with poor prognosis. Examples of prevalence rates are the number of individuals surviving with cancer at a point in time per 100,000 in the population, and the proportion of individuals in a population who smoke at a point in time. Cancer prevalence can be estimated under various assumptions about how long the disease continues to impact individuals. In estimates for the world in 2000, there were over 10 million male and 12 million female prevalent cancer cases (Table 2.1); these estimates included incident cases in 2000, plus cancer cases within the previous five years in which the patient was alive in 2000. While such numbers provide an important indication of disease burden, studies of disease etiology generally focus on incidence rather than prevalence as the measure of disease frequency because it is not affected by what happens after diagnosis.

The above measures are used in descriptive epidemiology to depict the frequency of cancer in terms of person (e.g., age and sex), place (e.g., geographic distribution), and time (e.g., trends); however, additional measures are required to detect associations. Analytic epidemiologic studies search for disease determinants by comparing an observed course of events in a group with particular traits to the level expected if the traits were not present. The ratio of the observed (O) to expected (E) frequency is a convenient summary measure of the strength of the association between the disease risk and the traits that distinguish the groups. If the ratio has a value of 1.0, this indicates that the observed and expected frequencies or risks are equal, and that there is no association.

This ratio of O over E directly measures *relative risk* in the situation where both the numerator and denominator are risks, such as when two proportions are compared. Other estimates of *relative risk,* including ratios of rates (e.g., rate ratio) and counts (e.g., standardized mortality ratios), have similar interpretations even though the outcomes are measured on different scales. For example, in Figure 2.2 the relative risk estimate of 1.4, obtained by taking the ratio of age-standardized incidence rates for Canadian males and females in 1990, indicates that cancer risk was 1.4 times greater for males than females.

### 2.2.2 Generation and Testing of Hypotheses about Cancer Causation

The epidemiologic approach is an iterative process whereby hypotheses are first developed to explain patterns of disease risk, and these are then tested in specific studies. The *generation of hypotheses* can be based on ideas about the causes of cancer that arise from several sources. Astute observations by clinicians have frequently drawn attention to possible etiological associations. Examples include scrotal cancer, which was noted by Sir Percival Pott in 1775 to be common in chimney sweeps, the association of lung cancer and smoking, and clear-cell vaginal carcinoma in the daughters of mothers exposed to diethylstilbestrol.

Other hypotheses may be developed from epidemiological data collected for purely descriptive purposes. For example, descriptions of the geographic distribution of malignant melanoma led to the observation that the frequency of the disease was associated with latitude and to the hypothesis that the disease might be caused by exposure to the ultraviolet components of sunlight (see Chap. 3, Sec. 3.5.5).

For disease processes where little is known about the determinants, hypotheses are sometimes generated in exploratory studies conducted to generate leads requiring further investigation. In such exploratory studies, populations or groups at high and low risk for a particular cancer may be contrasted, in the first instance, for as many attributes as it is feasible to examine. Such exercises, while necessary and important in the preliminary search for the causes of cancer, must be interpreted carefully and it should be recognized that their role is to generate hypotheses.

*Hypothesis testing* is then performed by comparing cancer risks for groups that differ in their level of exposure to a suspected causal factor, to determine the extent to which exposure and risk of disease are associated. This can be accomplished, first, by specifying a null hypothesis: for example, that there is no association, such that the true relative risk due to exposure is 1.0. A statistical test can then be applied to assess whether the relative risk estimated from the data differs significantly from 1.0, or in other words, whether the null hypothesis can be rejected. When testing for statistical significance, a distinction can be made between the test of a specific a priori hypothesis as opposed to exploratory analyses of numerous potential risk factors, because the latter could give rise to a statistical association by chance alone (e.g., due to multiple comparisons). If a statistical association is found, the final step of epidemiologic research then involves its interpretation, by taking into consideration the potential for biases given the study design, and by considering the criteria used in causal inference (see Sec. 2.2.9).

### 2.2.3 Cohort Studies

In cohort studies, subsets of a given population are defined on the basis of whether individuals are exposed to a factor suspected of increasing or decreasing the risk of cancer. These subsets are followed forward in time and observed in order to detect the development of cancer. After a period of time sufficient for a number of cancers to develop, cancer risks in the exposed and nonexposed groups are then compared and the relative risk due to exposure can then be calculated directly. For example, in a prospective cohort study of 47,700 male health professionals, Giovannucci et al. (1995) demonstrated that colorectal cancer risk was 2.5 times higher among those in the lowest quintile of physical activity, when compared to the highest quintile (Table 2.2). While the ratio of risks shown in Table 2.2 is appropriate for demonstrating the concept of the cohort design, it is more accurate to account for differences in the length of follow-up for each cohort member, as is accomplished by comparing disease rates. In this example, Giovannucci et al. reported colorectal cancer rates of 11 per 10,000 person-years (55 cases over 51,660 person-years) in the low quintile, and 4.3 per 10,000 (23/53,544) in the high quintile, thus the *rate ratio* and *risk ratio* were identical [relative risk (*RR*) = 2.5].

Randomized controlled trials can be viewed as cohort studies that are experimental (i.e., risk factor is randomly assigned) rather than observational. Randomized trials provide the strongest possible evidence about etiological relationships, but can be applied only rarely in cancer epidemiology as carcinogenic exposures cannot be imposed on individuals. Randomized trials have the advantage that the exposure under investigation can be allocated randomly, and the process of ran-

**Table 2.2.** A Cohort Study of the Relationship Between Physical Activity and the Risk of Developing Colorectal Cancer Among Men, Extracted from the Health Professionals Study Which Followed 47,700 Men from 1986 to 1992, Showing the Estimation of Relative Risk

|  | Diseased (Developed Colorectal Cancer) | Not Diseased (Remainder in the Cohort) | Total |
|---|---|---|---|
| Exposed | | | |
| (Low Quintile of Physical Activity) | 55 (a) | 9337 (b) | a + b = 9392 |
| Not Exposed | | | |
| (Top Quintile of Physical Activity) | 23 (c) | 9602 (d) | c + d = 9625 |
| Disease risk among exposed = $a/(a + b)$ = 55/9392 | | | = 0.59 percent |
| Disease risk among those not exposed = $c/(c + d)$ = 23/9625 | | | = 0.24 percent |
| Risk Ratio $= \dfrac{a/(a + b)}{c/(c + d)}$ | | | = 2.5 |

*Source*: Adapted from Giovannucci et al. (1995).

domization should, on average, make the groups that will be compared similar at the start of the study (Chap. 22, Sec. 22.4.3). Ethical considerations limit the use of randomized trials to the investigation of exposures that may be protective against cancer, such as trials that examine the influence of dietary modification, vitamin supplements, cancer screening, and other possible means of reducing cancer risk (e.g., drug trials).

In prospective cohort studies, the investigator measures exposures to potential risk factors at a point in time, and then arranges for regular surveillance for outcome detection in the same way as in an experimental trial. The inability to control the allocation of exposure in an observational cohort study means that the results may be open to more than one interpretation. Exposure to many potential causes of cancer, such as occupation, cigarette smoking, and diet is self-selected. Thus the finding of an association with cancer risk may mean either that these factors are related causally to the development of cancer, or alternatively, that some other attribute both determined the lifestyle and influenced independently the risk of cancer. For example, it was at one time argued that a genetic factor influenced both the risk of lung cancer and the decision to smoke cigarettes. Studies in identical twins, discordant for smoking habits, later showed that this hypothesis was incorrect, and that smoking, rather than genetic makeup, was the major determinant of lung cancer risk; however, data from the original cohort studies were open to both interpretations.

Cohort studies can also be conducted retrospectively. A historical cohort study is possible if the exposure status can be determined retrospectively for members of the population, sufficient time has elapsed after exposure, and cancer has occurred in some subjects. It is not possible with this approach to arrange for the population to be examined with a predetermined frequency, as can be done in experimental trials or prospective observational cohort studies. This is a shortcoming when investigation is required to detect the presence of disease; however, many types of cancer will become evident even when not sought deliberately, and in these circumstances, the historical approach can give valid estimates of risk and relative risk.

The major advantage of cohort studies is that they address directly the etiological sequence of cause preceding effect. When carried out prospectively, it is feasible to measure exposure accurately, to characterize baseline cancer risk, and to follow the population for the development of multiple outcomes, including cancer. Cohort studies are efficient for studying rare exposures because they can be designed to incorporate the most informative individuals by including all who were exposed, but only a subset of the remainder.

A limitation of the cohort design is that because most human cancers occur infrequently, these studies often need very large numbers of subjects to have a good chance of finding an increase in risk associated with a particular exposure. Table 2.3 shows the required number of subjects according to the incidence of cancer in the nonexposed group and the magnitude of the relative risk that the investigator aims to detect. If a specific type of cancer occurred at a rate of 1/10,000 in the nonexposed group during the course of the study and an investigator wished to determine that a tripling of risk (i.e., a relative risk of 3) was not due to chance variation, then there would need to be 67,000 individuals in the nonexposed group and an equal number in the ex-

**Table 2.3.** Sample Sizes Required in Cohort Studies, by Level of Detectable Relative Risk and for Varying Levels of Baseline Risk in the Nonexposed Group*

| Relative Risk | Number of Events Required in Nonexposed Group | Number of Subjects Required in Nonexposed Group for Various Levels of Baseline Cancer Risk | | |
|---|---|---|---|---|
| | | If Risk = 1/10,000 | If Risk = 1/1000 | If Risk = 1/100 |
| 2 | 20.0 | 200,000 | 20,000 | 2000 |
| 3 | 6.7 | 67,000 | 6700 | 670 |
| 4 | 3.7 | 37,000 | 3700 | 370 |
| 5 | 2.5 | 25,000 | 2500 | 250 |
| 10 | 0.92 | 9200 | 920 | 92 |

*Table lists the number in each of the comparison groups obtained by dividing the required number of events (second column) by the baseline risk. Estimates are based on the selection of two groups (exposed and nonexposed) of equal size, and standard statistical parameters (alpha probability = 5 percent, beta probability = 20 percent).

*Source*: Adapted from Breslow and Day (1987).

posed group. Table 2.3 also shows how sample-size requirements decline with increasing relative risk and as the outcome becomes more common. The prevalence of exposure, which affects the relative sizes of exposed and nonexposed groups, is another important determinant of the required size of a cohort study (Breslow and Day, 1987). The rarity of cancer creates the need for most cohort studies to be large, time-consuming, and expensive, which has motivated the development of the more economical case-control design for the investigation of etiological relationships.

### 2.2.4 Case-Control Studies

Whereas a cohort study follows individuals from exposure to the development of disease, a case-control study begins with diseased individuals (cases) or individuals who are not diseased (controls), and then assesses their previous exposures. This design makes optimal use of the most informative individuals, who in the situation of a rare disease are the "cases," whereas the controls are a representative sample of unaffected individuals drawn from the population that gave rise to the cases.

The case-control design has been applied frequently to study cancer incidence but it has wide-ranging applications. In a typical etiological study, the source population is everyone living in a particular community, and a case series could include all newly diagnosed patients with a certain cancer in that population over a specified period of time. Alternatively, if the source population is a series of cancer patients, then the case definition might be the occurrence of an adverse outcome, such as recurrence of disease. Cases may be drawn from

several sources, including hospital diagnostic indices, cancer registry files, or the practices of one or more physicians. Controls may be selected from hospitals, outpatient facilities, or the general population using random-sampling techniques. In designing a case-control study, careful consideration must be given to the selection of cases and appropriate controls because there are many ways of introducing bias into the assessment of the relationship between exposure and disease (see Sec. 2.2.7).

The measurement of exposure in case-control studies can be based on personal recall, available information from medical records or other databases, or biological specimens. In etiological studies, questionnaires are often used to assess factors such as environmental exposures, occupational history, diet, or personal habits (e.g., smoking). In addition, the exposure assessment can be enhanced by referring to existing records or databases, as may be possible for medical history or workplace exposures. Other factors, such as prior exposure to viruses or the influence of some aspect of the individual's phenotype or genotype, may be assessed by direct examination or biomarkers.

Data analysis in case-control studies usually involves testing the null hypothesis that there is no difference in exposure frequency between cases and controls by estimating an odds ratio and assessing whether it differs significantly from 1.0. Odds ratios provide valid estimates of relative risk when the outcome is uncommon (e.g., present in less than 15 to 20 percent of the population), which holds true for the incidence of cancer. Furthermore, with appropriate methods of sampling and analysis, case-control studies that compare rates rather than risks (or proportions) can provide valid es-

**Table 2.4.** A Case-Control Study of the Association Between a Polymorphism in the Growth Hormone Gene (GH1) and Colorectal Cancer Risk Among Native Hawaiians, Where 75 Cases and 88 Controls Were Classified According to Genotypes Associated with Higher (Active Form = TT) or Lower (Variant Forms = TA or AA) Levels of Circulating Growth Hormone

|  | Cases (With Colorectal Cancer) | Controls (Unaffected in the Population) |
|---|---|---|
| Exposed (with lower GH level— TA or AA) | 48 ($a$) (64 percent) | 74 ($b$) (84 percent) |
| Not Exposed (with active form—TT) | 27 ($c$) (36 percent) | 14 ($d$) (16 percent) |
| Total | $a + c = 75$ | $b + d = 88$ |
| Odds of exposure: | $a/c = 48/27 = 1.8$ | $b/d = 74/14 = 5.3$ |
| Odds ratio = $a/c \div b/d = 1.8/5.3 = 0.3$ | | |

*Source*: Adapted from LeMarchand et al. (2002).

timates regardless of the rarity of the outcome. As an example, in a case-control study of colorectal cancer in Hawaii, Le Marchand et al. (2002) demonstrated that the odds of having a genetic variant (polymorphism) that results in reduced levels of circulating growth hormone was lower among cases than controls (Table 2.4). Given the rarity of this cancer in the population, the odds ratio may be interpreted in terms of relative risk by saying that colorectal cancer risk among Native Hawaiians who carried the polymorphism was 0.3 times that of those who did not carry it.

To detect a given level of cancer risk, case-control studies can be performed more quickly and involve fewer subjects than can cohort studies. For example, under the conditions described in the previous section, which required a cohort study to be based on 134,000 individuals ($RR = 3$, prevalence of exposure = 50 percent, baseline risk = 1/10,000), a case-control study would require only 33 cases and 132 controls for a total of 165 individuals (Breslow and Day, 1987, p. 219). The case-control design achieves this increased efficiency by focusing on the most informative individuals (i.e., all of the cases in the population), but only a small random sample of the large number of healthy individuals (controls). Case-control studies are particularly useful in the investigation of diseases that are rare or those that have a long interval between exposure and the development of disease. This applies to the incidence of almost all types of human cancer.

A limitation of the case-control design is that exposure must often be measured by the recollection of the subjects and there is frequently no means available to check the accuracy of this information. Also, there are many types of potential bias (see Sec. 2.2.7) in the se-

lection of subjects and in the measurement of exposure that are often easier to avoid or detect in cohort than in case-control research. Despite these disadvantages, case-control studies are frequently the most efficient or only feasible means of assessing, in human populations, the validity of new claims about the determinants of cancer risk.

### 2.2.5 Other Designs

Several additional designs for epidemiological research, such as ecological studies, cross-sectional studies, surveys, case series, and case reports, make a smaller contribution due to their inherent limitations. In contrast, hybrid designs that are specialized applications of the two basic designs can provide a strong basis for inference. One hybrid design is where a case-control study is undertaken within a cohort. If the cost of measuring exposure on all cohort members is prohibitively expensive (e.g., laboratory analysis of biomarkers in stored specimens), cost-effectiveness can be enhanced by measuring exposure for selected individuals, including the individuals who develop the cancer (cases) and a random sample of other cohort members who do not develop cancer (controls). Specialized applications of the standard designs are also used in genetic epidemiology, such as in a cohort study where, instead of being selected from the general population as in more traditional studies, the cohort is selected from family members. By comparing disease risk in families that differ in their genetic traits, while accounting for measured differences in environmental exposures, it is possible in genetic epidemiology to detect the relative contribution of both genetic and environmental risk factors to disease risk (Khoury et al., 1993).

### 2.2.6 Measurement Error and Random Error

In common with other forms of scientific inquiry, the results of epidemiologic studies can be distorted by features in their design and conduct. The sources of distortion are random error, bias, and confounding; an understanding of the origins and effects of these factors will help in the interpretation of epidemiologic data.

*Measurement error* may occur through the random misclassification of subjects, according to either exposure or disease status. Exposure status is often determined by asking subjects about events that took place many years earlier, and some inaccuracies in the classification of exposure are inevitable. The determination of disease status, even when based on histologic material, is also subject to error; thus, some incorrectly classified diseased and nondiseased individuals may be included in a study. Strategies used to minimize measurement error include the careful development, pretesting and validation of questionnaires, and the use of independent assessments of disease status. Even under ideal circumstances, some measurement error will remain and the impact of this error must be accounted for.

*Random error* is a deviation between an observed value and a true value that arises only by chance. The concept of random error, or chance variation, is important in epidemiology because it is central to the statistical analysis of data, such as in the assessment of whether or not an observed association (e.g., an increase in estimates of relative risk) may have arisen by chance. This can be accomplished by testing for statistical significance, whereby a $p$ value is calculated to determine whether the null hypothesis can be rejected. Confidence intervals for an estimate of relative risk or an odds ratio provide further information as they indicate the range of values with which the data are consistent.

### 2.2.7 Types of Bias in Epidemiological Studies

A study is biased if deficiencies in measurement, design, data collection, analysis or interpretation lead to results or conclusions that systematically deviate from the truth. In contrast to random error, which is likely to conceal true associations, *bias* distorts the truth by giving rise to results that either systematically overestimate or underestimate associations. Thus, biases can create associations where none exist, or magnify or diminish associations that are genuine.

A full discussion of bias is beyond the scope of this chapter and details should be sought in standard epidemiologic texts (e.g., Breslow and Day, 1987; Elwood 1998; Rothman and Greenland, 1998). Some types of

**Table 2.5.** Examples of Specific Types of Bias and Their Basic Features

| Type of Bias | Features |
|---|---|
| Selection bias | |
| Length bias | If exposure is related to survival, its frequency differs systematically between prevalent and incident cases |
| Response bias | Those who respond are systematically different from those who choose not to |
| Berkson's bias | Hospital admission rates differ systematically according to exposure and outcome |
| Information bias | |
| Recall bias | Ability to remember past events differs systematically between subjects |
| Measurement bias | Systematic error due to inaccurate measurement |

bias are of concern in every research design, while certain designs are susceptible to particular types of bias. These are demonstrated in the following examples, and are listed in Table 2.5.

Bias can be classified according to whether it arose from the *selection* of subjects or from the *information* that was collected. *Selection bias* may occur if there are systematic differences in traits between those selected for study and those who were not.

*Length (prevalence-incidence) bias* is a form of selection bias that refers to a distortion of an etiological association that would arise if prevalent cases were used, and exposure was related to survival after diagnosis. In this situation, an artifact may appear because long-term survivors would be more likely to have the exposure. Recognition of the potential impact of this bias is the reason that incident cases are usually preferred for etiological studies. A related form of length bias is important in clinical studies, when survival affects the exposure classification. For example, a report that carriers of cancer susceptibility alleles (e.g., BRCA1 mutations) have higher survival rates after cancer diagnoses (Rubin et al., 1996), might be biased if carrier status was more likely to be determined among survivors. A prospective cohort design that focused on incident cases would overcome the potential bias.

*Response bias* occurs if those who participate in a study differ from those who do not, and this occurs systematically, such that the response rate is itself associated with either the exposure or outcome of interest. For example, if individuals who chose not to respond to a questionnaire were more likely to have had the exposure of interest (e.g., smoking), and if the proportion of nonresponders differed between the two groups being compared (e.g., cases vs. controls), then an estimate of relative risk could be biased.

*Lead-time bias* occurs if the follow-up of two groups does not begin at comparable times, such as when one group is selectively identified earlier in the natural history of the disease. For example, survival rates for patients with screen-detected disease may appear longer because they were detected earlier (see Chap. 22, Sec. 22.2.4).

*Berkson's bias* is a type of selection bias that can arise in a case-control study of hospitalized individuals if differential rates of admission apply to those with cancer who were exposed to a putative risk factor, in contrast to those who had no such exposure. For example, a case-control study of lung cancer could underestimate the adverse effect of smoking in the population if it compared lung cancer cases to hospitalized controls because smoking is associated with many reasons for hospitalization (i.e., smoking prevalence among controls would be higher than the true value in the population). To overcome this potential bias in hospital-based studies, population-based designs are preferred for many epidemiologic studies.

*Information bias* is defined as a distortion of study results due to differential accuracy of information relating to exposure or outcome between the comparison groups. Information bias is of concern in all research designs (including experiments), but is particularly important in observational studies due to difficulties in the historical assessment of multifaceted environments.

*Recall bias* is a form of information bias that is of particular concern in case-control studies that arises because diseased subjects are more likely to think about and recall previous exposure than nondiseased controls. In genetic epidemiology there may be bias in information about illnesses in other family members because family members who are themselves diseased are more likely to know about disease in other members of the family than are those who are not diseased.

*Measurement bias* is systematic error that occurs if measurements are made inaccurately. The usual effect on study results is to conceal or reduce the magnitude of true associations rather than to give rise to associations that are spurious. For example, if there was random misclassification of smokers and nonsmokers, then a study of whether smoking was associated with lung cancer would result in an underestimation of the relative risk due to smoking.

## 2.2.8 Confounding and Effect Modification

*Confounding* is defined as a distortion of the effect of an exposure on risk that arises because of an association with other factors that affect risk (Last, 2001). A confounding variable must be both related to the risk of disease under study and associated with the exposure of interest (without being a consequence of exposure). Confounding is similar to bias in that it can produce spurious associations or mask associations that are real. A distinction is made because bias is an issue related to study design or appropriate interpretation, whereas confounding is an issue of alternative explanations for a study result.

Alcohol ingestion is an example of a confounder when the risk of esophageal cancer following exposure to cigarettes is under investigation. Both alcohol ingestion and smoking are risk factors for this disease; in addition, smokers are more likely to consume alcohol than are nonsmokers. Thus, confounding leads to uncertainty as to how much risk is due directly to smoking and how much is attributable to associated alcohol use.

Confounding can be dealt with either in the design or in the analysis of a study. This is in contrast to other sources of bias, which can be averted only in the design or conduct of the study. In the design, confounding can be controlled by comparing cases to matched controls who are alike with respect to the confounder, as this ensures that a difference in the exposure of interest is not due to confounding. In the statistical analysis of an etiologic study, confounding can be controlled for by stratifying the data according to the potential confounder, and then examining whether exposure frequency differs between cases and controls in these subsets. In the above example, the effect of smoking on esophageal cancer risk could be distinguished from the effect of alcohol by examining the association between smoking and risk separately for groups defined according to alcohol consumption.

*Effect modification*, which is sometimes referred to as *interaction*, occurs when the effect of a putative causal factor differs according to the level of another factor (Last, 2001). For example, age modifies the effect of exposure to ionizing radiation on risk of breast cancer, as the risk per unit dose varies with the age at which the exposure occurred (Howe and McLaughlin, 1996). In the esophageal cancer example, effect modification would be indicated if the relative risk for smoking differed between categories of alcohol consumption. Epidemiologic studies often collect information on numerous potential risk factors that would result in many potential combinations. Thus an unfocused search for statistical interactions would be subject to artifact due to spurious associations from multiple significance testing. Accordingly, the search for effect modifiers in a statistical analysis should be restricted to variables for which a biological or theoretical model can first be justified.

## 2.2.9 Causal Inference

Inference about whether an observed epidemiologic association is causal can be aided by following a logical framework that involves a critical appraisal of the results from an individual study, and then evaluating this in the context of other evidence. Important components of causal inference are outlined here, whereas more detailed reviews can be found in epidemiological texts (e.g., Elwood 1998; Rothman and Greenland, 1998).

*Temporality*   The need for an exposure to precede disease is an indisputable requirement. This requirement is met in cohort studies, but the retrospective assessment of exposure in case-control studies makes the assessment of temporality more difficult. Temporal patterns may also be examined in terms of how relationships change over time, such as in assessing whether relative risk varies with the period of exposure; however, the long latency in the development of most cancers often makes this difficult to assess accurately.

*Strength of Association*   A stronger association between an exposure and cancer risk is more likely to be causal than a weaker association. Even if a strong association was affected by modest levels of bias or confounding, there is still likely to be an association after accounting for these factors. Thus, the magnitude of the relative risk or odds ratio is a rough indication of whether the observed relationship is causally important.

*Consistency*   Strong support for a causal relationship comes from consistency with other studies, as associations between an exposure and outcome that are demonstrated repeatedly, by different investigators using different research methods, are more likely to be causal than those where different methods generated different results. The inability to replicate results does not rule out a causal role because some studies may be better designed and some effects may arise only under certain circumstances; however, this finding signifies the need for discrepant studies to be carefully critiqued.

*Gradient of Effect*   If successively increasing levels of exposure are accompanied by related increases (or decreases) in risk, this effect strengthens a causal interpretation. For example, with increasing amount smoked, there is an increase in carcinogen dose, in biological damage, and, consequently, a greater chance that cancer will develop. This concept can also apply to genetic exposures, such as the polymorphism shown in Table 2.4, where the investigator could go further to assess whether risk decreased monotonically with the number of A alleles present (TT, AT vs. AA).

*Biological Plausibility*   Associations are more likely to be causal between exposure and disease if they agree with present knowledge about the biology of the target cells and tissues, and the biological effects of the ex-

posure. However, the absence of supporting biological information may arise from an incomplete state of knowledge.

*Specificity*   If an association is present between a single exposure and a single disease, this association may support a causal interpretation; however, this outcome seldom occurs in cancer studies. Cancer has many causal pathways, and most major causes of disease have a wide range of effects. Thus, specificity contributes to causal reasoning only when it is present, whereas its absence is of little importance (e.g., many diseases are associated with cigarette smoking).

## 2.3 OVERVIEW OF THE EPIDEMIOLOGY OF COLORECTAL CANCER

The epidemiology of colorectal cancer (CRC), is described in this section as an example that demonstrates the links between descriptive and analytical epidemiological approaches. This review begins with population-based statistics that describe cancer patterns nationally and internationally in terms of person, place, and time, which have implications regarding disease burden and underlying disease determinants. The implications of these patterns of disease are then examined with regard to the development of various strategies for colorectal cancer control.

### 2.3.1 Sources of Data and Descriptive Epidemiology

Cancer incidence data are available in many countries from registries that monitor cancer occurrence in defined populations. The primary resource for international comparisons of incidence data is prepared by the International Agency for Research on Cancer (Ferlay, 2001; www.depdb.iarc.fr/globocan/GLOBOframe.htm), and includes data from cancer registries in various regions around the world. In the United States, an important source of data is the Surveillance, Epidemiology, and End Results (SEER) program, which maintains cancer registries covering approximately 10 percent of the population. Incidence, mortality, and survival data from the SEER program are published regularly in detailed statistical reports (Ries et al., 2000) and at a Web site (seer.cancer.gov). In Canada, one of the few countries with total coverage of its population by a national cancer registry, an overview of cancer incidence, mortality, and survival data is published annually by the National Cancer Institute of Canada (NCIC, 2004; www.ncic.cancer.ca) and more detailed reports are published periodically (e.g., the Public Health Agency of Canada at www.phac_aspc.gc.ca/ccdpc_cpcmc/index.html and by Statistics Canada at www.statscan.ca).

Among the 10 million incident cancer cases estimated for the world in 2000 (Table 2.1), the five most frequent types were cancers of the breast, cervix, colon-rectum, lung, and stomach among females, and cancers of the lung, stomach, colon-rectum, prostate, and liver among males (Fig. 2.4). For both sexes combined, these types of cancer accounted for 57% of all cancers. Colorectal cancer can thus be seen as one of the most frequent and serious cancers internationally. An estimated 945,000 new cases were diagnosed worldwide in 2000, placing CRC third in terms of incidence, after lung cancer and breast cancer, and accounting for 9.4% of all cancers (Ferlay, 2001).

While cancer is a major concern in all nations, the relative importance of particular types of cancer is highly variable, arising as a result of the combined effects of differences in population size, age structure, detection, reporting, and underlying etiological factors. For CRC, incidence rates vary widely internationally, with high-risk areas including the United States, Canada, Europe, and Australia, whereas incidence rates are low in Central and South America, Asia, and Africa. The international variation seen in Figure 2.5 indicates that incidence rates for CRC in high-risk regions (e.g., United States) can be up to five times greater than in low-risk countries such as India. Colorectal cancer occurs frequently in both men and women, although Figure 2.5 also shows that in higher-risk countries, the age standardized incidence rates are 30 to 40 percent higher among men than women.

The potential modifiability or preventability of cancer can be suggested by variation in cancer rates over

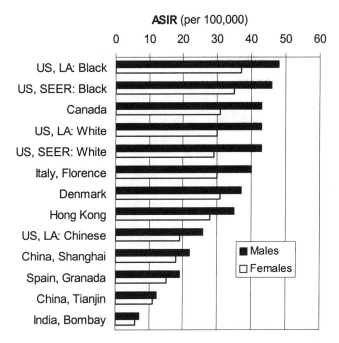

**Figure 2.5.** International variation in the annual age-standardized incidence rate (ASIR per 100,000) for colorectal cancer, by gender. (For 1988–1992; standardized to the world standard population; US-SEER, US Surveillance, Epidemiology and End Results Registry; US-LA, Los Angeles Registry. *Data source* = Ferlay et al., 2001.)

time. Time trends in incidence rates for the five most frequently diagnosed cancers in Canada are shown in Figure 2.6. Lung cancer incidence rates in men increased steadily until the mid-1980s, and then began to decline, whereas in women the rates are now about half as high as in men, but they continue to increase steadily. These lung cancer patterns follow, with a lag of about 20 years, the historical patterns of tobacco use among both men and women. Breast cancer incidence rates among women increased slightly but steadily over the past three decades. The change in prostate cancer incidence rates over time can be attributed partly to detection of occult cancer through use of a screening test based on serum levels of prostate specific antigen. Trends in incidence for CRC have been quite similar for men and women, with men having consistently higher rates than women. Colorectal incidence rates in Canada rose slightly but steadily from 1970 up to the mid-1980s, and then began to decline, with the rate of decline being slightly greater for women than men. The patterns depicted in Figure 2.6 for Canada are similar to those seen in the United States (Ries et al., 2000).

The variation in cancer risk with age is depicted by age-specific patterns in Figure 2.7 for the leading types of cancer in Canada. Colorectal cancer remains relatively rare until the fifth decade, when rates begin to increase rapidly from less than 5 per 100,000 before the

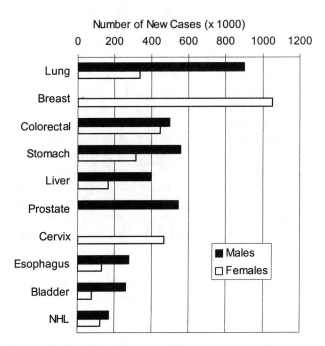

**Figure 2.4.** Number of incident cases for the ten most common types of cancer worldwide, estimated for 2000, by gender. NHL, Non-Hodgkin's lymphoma. (*Data source*: Ferlay et al., 2001, and Parkin, 2001.)

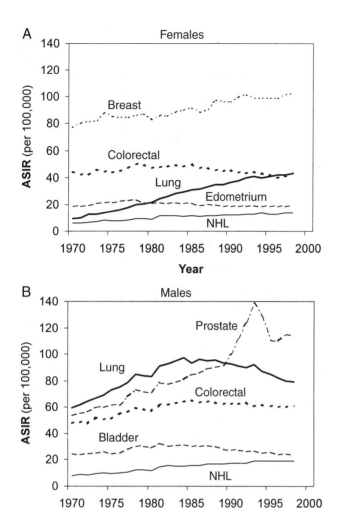

**Figure 2.6.** Trends in age-standardized incidence rates (ASIR per 100,000) for the leading types of cancer in Canada, by sex. (Standardized to the 1991 Canadian population; adapted from National Cancer Institute of Canada, 2002.) NHL, Non-Hodgkin's lymphoma.

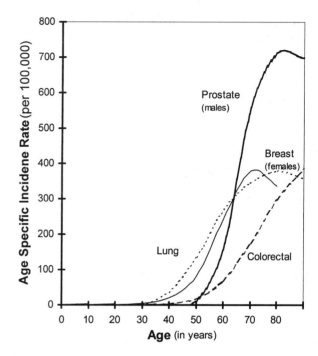

**Figure 2.7.** Relationship between age and cancer incidence rates in Canada for four types of cancer. (Adapted from National Cancer Institute of Canada, 2002.)

age of 40 to 300 per 100,000 or more after age 70. A cumulative measure that combines the effects of these age-specific incidence rates is the lifetime probability of developing cancer, which for CRC is about 6% for men and women in both Canada (NCIC, 2002) and the United States (SEER, 1999). A further implication of these age-specific patterns relates to the underlying biological model of how cancer develops. In particular, the shape of these age-incidence curves was noted almost 50 years ago to be consistent with a multistage model of carcinogenesis (Armitage and Doll, 1954), which was postulated subsequently to involve distinct mutational events (Knudson, 1973) and then applied specifically to the development of bowel cancer (Vogelstein et al., 1988; Luebeck and Moolgavkar, 2002; see Chap. 11, Sec. 11.1.2).

In cancer surveillance systems, CRC is a general grouping for cancers occurring in the colon (70 percent of cases), rectum (27 percent) and anus (3 percent), with most (90 percent) being adenocarcinomas (McLaughlin et al., 1995). While there are some differences in the descriptive epidemiology of CRC according to site, gender, and histology, the similarities are more striking, thus all types of CRC are often regarded as a single entity for some research purposes. However, some specific patterns are noteworthy because of their implications for cancer control programs.

Cancers occurring in the distal colon (descending and sigmoid colon) have particular relevance to cancer control because it is in this region that endoscopic screening procedures can detect and remove lesions before they become cancerous. Figure 2.8 shows that cancers of the distal colon occur more frequently among men than women, and that the incidence rates among men have been stable, whereas they have declined gradually among women. One possible explanation that warrants further investigation is that risk factor exposures changed over time and differed between men and women. For these patterns to be related to screening, the effectiveness or use of screening by men would have to be less than for women, an hypothesis to be explored in future studies.

The analysis of risk in migrant populations provides a descriptive epidemiological approach for identifying the relative contribution of genetic and environmental factors to cancer etiology. For example, if groups mi-

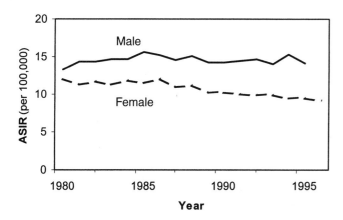

**Figure 2.8.** Age-standardized incidence rates (ASIR per 100,000) for cancer of the distal colon in Canada, by gender. (Standardized to the 1991 Canadian population; adapted from the National Cancer Incidence in Canada, 2001.)

grate from low-risk to high-risk countries, and disease rates increase to match that of the new host country, this suggests that factors in the new environment influenced risk (because the genetic profile remained constant). In the late 1950s, age-adjusted CRC mortality rates were five times higher in the United States than in Japan, whereas rates among those of Japanese ancestry living in the United States were similar to American White rates (Miller et al., 1996). In Japan in recent years, colon cancer incidence and mortality rates have risen dramatically, coming close to the levels seen in the United States (Ferlay et al., 2001). In this situation, both the migrant pattern and the time trend are consistent with cancer rates being influenced by environmental factors and, have been attributed in part to a westernization of diet and lifestyle.

Figure 2.9 demonstrates a gradient in the migrant effect, as CRC mortality rates among men from Southern Europe increased with longer duration of residence in Australia. In particular, after 30 years of residence in Australia, the CRC risk of men born in Southern Europe compared to those born in Australia rose from be-

ing significantly lower (age- and sex-adjusted $RR = 0.4$ within nine years of immigration) to being similar ($RR = 0.9$ after thirty years). In contrast, immigrants from the British Isles and Eastern Europe had rates that were not significantly different from those of Australia-born men. Such migrant studies provide strong evidence for the importance of environmental factors because, for many types of cancer, groups of migrants who move from one country to another eventually acquire the cancer incidence of the country to which they moved. The implication of migrant studies is that the international variation in cancer rates, can be only minimally affected by genetic differences between populations of each country, but instead is due to some feature of life in those countries, and consequently that cancer risks are modifiable.

### 2.3.2 Analytical Epidemiology

Numerous observational studies have identified a wide range of factors associated with an increased risk of developing CRC (Table 2.6), including a family history of CRC, a personal history of adenomatous polyps in the colon, the presence of inflammatory bowel disease, and lifestyle elements such as diet and low levels of exercise. The dietary factors that have been most consistently associated with an increased risk are low levels of vegetable intake and high levels of red meat or alcohol consumption. There has been less consistency between studies of other factors, although smoking at a young age and low levels of dietary fiber intake have been classified as possible risk factors (World Cancer Research Fund, 1997). In addition, as arose from the descriptive epidemiology, age and sex (male) are known to be associated with an increased risk. Observational studies consistently demonstrated that the use of aspirin and other nonsteroidal anti-inflammatory drugs (Greenberg and Baron, 1996), the use of hormone replacement therapy (Potter, 1995), and higher levels of folate and selenium intake (Giovannucci et al., 1998) were associated with decreased risks of developing CRC. Pro-

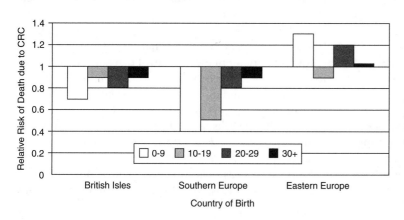

**Figure 2.9.** Relative risk of death due to colorectal cancer among immigrants to Australia compared to Australia-born men, by country of birth and years of residence in Australia. (Adapted from McCredie et al., 1999.)

**Table 2.6.** Risk Factors for Colorectal Cancer (CRC)

| Factor | Higher Risk Group | Lower Risk Group | Relative Risk Estimate |
|---|---|---|---|
| Demographic factors | | | |
| Age | Older | Younger | 10-20 |
| Country of residence | North America, Western Europe | Asia, Africa | 4-7 |
| Sex | Male | Female | 1.2-1.5 |
| Environmental and lifestyle factors | | | |
| Physical activity | Low quintile | High quintile | 1.5-3 |
| Dietary intake of vegetables | Low quintile | High quintile | 1.5-3 |
| Dietary intake of red meat | High quintile | Low quintile | 0.8-3 |
| Alcohol intake | High quintile | Low quintile | 0.8-3 |
| NSAID (nonsteroidal anti-inflammatory drug) use | Non-user | NSAID user | 1.5-3 |
| HRT use (hormone replacement therapy) | Non-user | HRT user | 1.2-2 |
| Genetic and personal history factors | | | |
| Family history | CRC among first-degree relatives | No family history | 2-5 |
| Carrier of a mutation associated with high risk | Carrier of a mutation in *MSH2*, *MLH1*, or *APC* | Noncarrier | 30-50 |

tective effects have been confirmed recently in randomized trials for hormone replacement therapy (Women's Health Initiative, 2002), and for the prevention of polyps by aspirin (Baron et al., 2003) and calcium (Wallace et al., 2004).

The contribution of genetic factors to the development of CRC was recognized many years ago in analyses that detected increased risks associated with a family history of cancer and early age at onset. One early study in Utah reported a higher number of CRC deaths (3.9 percent) among first-degree relatives of patients with CRC, compared to sex- and age-matched controls (1.2 percent) (Woolf, 1958). Numerous studies consistently detected similar two- to three-fold increased risks in first-degree relatives of CRC cases, despite the use of different designs and reference to distinct populations. For example, in prospective cohort studies of 119,000 American men and women in which 315 CRC cases occurred during follow-up, 10 percent reported having a history of CRC among first-degree relatives, which gave rise to an overall relative risk of 2.0 (Fuchs et al., 1994). Risk increased further with the number of relatives affected, and when CRC occurred at an earlier age, such that age of onset was, on average, about ten years earlier for individuals with an affected first-degree relative as compared to people with sporadic disease.

### 2.3.3 Molecular and Genetic Epidemiology

Following the identification of familial aggregation in a disease process, the next phase of genetic epidemiological research is to characterize the genetic mechanism. *Segregation analysis* of pedigree data examines whether the observed pattern of inheriting the phenotype (e.g., CRC) is as expected under a particular Mendelian model (e.g., dominant, recessive, mixed), and whether this is likely due to single or multiple genes. Pedigree analyses of families in which multiple members had developed CRC determined that the cancer susceptibility followed an autosomal dominant pattern of inheritance (Bailey-Wilson et al., 1986). Segregation analysis also enables the estimation of parameters that are useful in clinical genetics, including gene frequency (a prevalence estimate) and penetrance (a cumulative incidence estimate). For example, even before a specific cancer-predisposition gene had been discovered, such pedigree analyses estimated that 75 percent of gene carriers would develop CRC during their lifetime (Bailey-Wilson et al., 1986), which is similar to estimates reported recently among known mutation carriers (Green et al., 2002).

Studies of the association between adenomatous colorectal polyps and risk of CRC contributed substantially

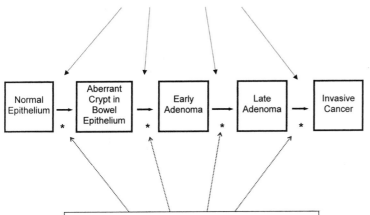

**Figure 2.10.** A conceptual model of carcinogenesis applied to colorectal cancer, where disease occurrence and progression is influenced by exogenous and endogenous factors.

to the characterization of the underlying pathogenesis of CRC. It is now well established that CRC occurs as a result of a complex multistage process that involves transition from normal epithelium to benign adenomatous polyps and then further to carcinoma, where the progression through these stages is influenced by interactions between numerous exogenous and endogenous factors (Fig. 2.10). Vogelstein and others proposed models of the underlying molecular basis of this progression whereby the neoplastic phenotype occurs as a result of alterations in multiple genes that control cell growth and differentiation (Vogelstein et al., 1988; Fearon and Vogelstein, 1990). In recent years, many molecular-genetic events involved in this process have been identified, such that the model of colorectal tumorigenesis is one of the most convincing paradigms of the role of mutational genetic events in human cancer (see Chap. 11, Sec. 11.1.2).

Research on the role of adenomatous polyps as risk factors for CRC found particularly strong associations in two separate genetic syndromes that were characterized initially in terms of phenotype and patterns of inheritance. Familial adenomatous polyposis (FAP) is a syndrome characterized by the development of hundreds or thousands of adenomatous polyps. Although FAP is rare (present in less than 1 percent of CRC cases), it is important because almost 100 percent of affected individuals will develop cancer (Herrera, 1990).

Most cases of FAP are now known to be due to mutations in the adenomatous polyposis coli (*APC*) gene, such that both clinical screening and genetic testing can be offered to family members. Hereditary non-polyposis colorectal cancer (HNPCC) is another type of CRC that runs in families. It is an autosomal dominant condition now known to be caused by mutation of one of several DNA mismatch repair genes (e.g., *MSH2, MLH1, MSH6*) (Peltomaki and Vasen, 1997; see Chap. 5, Sec. 5.4.2), although risk may also be modified by environmental factors (Mitchell et al., 2002). Although colonic polyps also occur in HNPCC, they occur less frequently than in FAP and are more dispersed, such that HNPCC is difficult to detect on the basis of polyps alone; however, in both syndromes, families have an increased incidence of CRC and earlier age of cancer onset. Hereditary non-polyposis colorectal cancer is more common than FAP, accounting for about 3 percent of all CRC Boland (1998), but is not quite as strongly predictive, with a lifetime risk of developing CRC of 70 percent among carriers of mutations in mismatch repair genes (Table 2.7). Interestingly, recent studies of penetrance indicate that lifetime CRC risk is greater for men than women in HNPCC families; however, for women in these families the risk of developing endometrial cancer is greater than for CRC (Green et al., 2002).

Compared to those who have no history of CRC in their family, a thirty- to fifty-fold increased risk is seen

**Table 2.7.** Lifetime Risk of Developing Colorectal Cancer (CRC) According to Family History

| Family History | Lifetime CRC Risk |
| --- | --- |
| No family history of CRC | 2 percent |
| One affected first-degree relative | 6 to 8 percent |
| One affected first-degree relative under age 45 | 10 percent |
| Two affected first-degree relatives | 17 percent |
| Mutation carrier within an HNPCC family | 70 percent |
| Mutation carrier within an FAP family | 100 percent |

*Abbreviations*: FAP, familial adenomatous polyposis; HNPCC, hereditary non-polyposis colorectal cancer.

*Source*: Houlston et al. (1990).

among carriers of mutations in known CRC-related genes, whereas a three- to five-fold increase in risk occurs among those with one first-degree relative with CRC (Table 2.7). Thus, as compared to individuals who have a recognizable pattern of inheritance (e.g., FAP, HNPCC), patients with other forms of familial CRC have more modest relative risks, but still contribute substantially to the burden of disease because they occur much more frequently (Fig. 2.11), accounting for approximately 15 percent of all CRC cases (Woolf, 1958; Fuchs et al., 1994).

After establishing that there is genetic transmission of disease risk by pedigree analysis, *genetic linkage analysis* is an important next step in the identification of the biological mechanisms of disease transmission. Linkage analysis is a genetic epidemiological method that provides statistical proof of genetic control in a disease process, by measuring DNA markers scattered throughout the genome and testing whether one or more of these are statistically associated with disease susceptibility. Linkage analysis also assists in gene discovery by iden-

tifying chromosomal regions where the responsible gene is likely to be found. The final specification of the gene involved and its mechanism of action must rely on other molecular-biological approaches; however, linkage analysis complements these methods and has often provided evidence of a genetic mechanism for a complex disease prior to the discovery of the gene. To succeed, linkage analysis relies on data from large, high-risk families, and tests whether the inheritance of two or more alleles or traits follows a pattern that suggests they are linked (i.e., the null hypothesis is that alleles are transmitted independently, suggesting that they are not in similar chromosomal regions). The strength of evidence for linkage between loci is represented by a log odds (LOD) score, whereby a value of three or more is considered to be strong evidence (a LOD score of 3 refers to 1000:1 odds in favor of linkage) (Khoury et al., 1993).

Genetic linkage analysis was used to identify a region on chromosome 2 that is closely associated with risk of CRC: this made possible the discovery of *MSH2* as a gene involved in HNPCC. Peltomaki et al. (1993) examined two large families with a strong history of CRC using microsatellite markers with repeating sequences throughout the genome (see Chap. 4, Sec. 4.3.9) and found LOD scores of six or more in a specific region of chromosome 2. This indicated the existence of a gene predisposing to CRC in this region, and subsequently, fine mapping and positional cloning identified one of the major CRC genes, *MSH2*, at this location. Furthermore, this level of statistical support for linkage has important practical implications because the clear demonstration of genetic determination of risk can be used in genetic counseling to inform decisions related to cancer prevention.

With the discovery of genes involved in CRC susceptibility, it became possible to offer genetic testing to individuals with a strong family history to distinguish between carriers and noncarriers. However, the process

**Figure 2.11.** Variation in attributable fraction as a function of exposure prevalence and the strength of association between exposure and disease (as indicated by relative risk lines for every 10% change in prevalence, which show that much of the potential attributable risk is achievable even for modest associations).

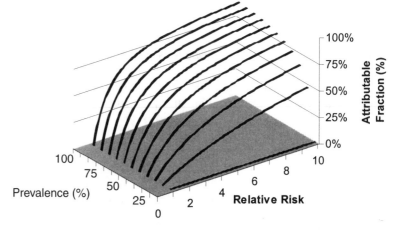

of detecting mutation carriers is complex and time consuming, in part because of the large size of the genes and the wide distribution of variants across the gene (Mitchell et al., 2002). Thus, molecular-genetic features of CRC have been studied in order to identify alternative strategies for detecting susceptibility in molecular epidemiological studies that have relied on case-control rather than family-based designs. Such studies characterized the frequency and mechanisms of specific mutations, and demonstrated the complex interactions between genes.

Analyses of DNA from colorectal tumors detected correlations between mutations in DNA mismatch repair genes and defects in microsatellite regions (repeating sequences throughout the genome), wherein widespread somatic mutations are indicative of an overall instability in the genome. Bapat et al. (1999) observed a high level of microsatellite instability (MSI-high) in 89 percent (16/18) versus 5 percent (1/21) of tumors from carriers and noncarriers of MLH1 or MSH2 mutations, respectively. A further analysis examined whether MSI was associated with the level of MLH1 and MSH2 protein expression, using an immunohistochemical assay in which monoclonal antibodies detected the proteins in the nucleus of tumor cells. Marcus et al. (1999) reported that the normal proteins were present in all ($n = 34$) MS-stable tumors but rarely in MSI-high tumors (1/38), which indicated that the immunohistochemical approach had excellent test characteristics (i.e., sensitivity and specificity were greater than 95 percent) (see Chap. 22, Sec. 22.2.1). Thus, even though these were small studies in terms of the numbers of tumors compared, they could detect statistically significant relationships because the associations were very strong. Larger studies have since been performed that more precisely demonstrated the high degree of correlation between the MSI and immunohistochemistry results (Lindor et al., 2002). These have clinical relevance, as the standard initial screening procedure when HNPCC is suspected is now an analysis of colorectal tumors first by one of the screening tests, such as in a set of international criteria known as the Bethesda Guidelines for testing MSI (Boland et al., 1998).

Molecular epidemiological studies have increasingly examined the impact of common genetic variants on the incidence of CRC. It is likely that weakly penetrant alleles of multiple genes will explain many of the intermediate-risk familial CRC cases, and indeed, natural genetic variability in humans probably contributes to some of the observed variability in all disease susceptibility. Polymorphisms (frequent but weakly penetrant variation in DNA sequences) are widespread throughout the genome. In addition to the example provided in Table 2.4, considerable research is under way to iden-

tify whether CRC susceptibility is due to polymorphisms in APC, mismatch repair genes (Houlston and Tomlinson, 2001), genes which control metabolism, and other pathways (de Jong et al., 2002). The direct effect on CRC risk is likely to be small for polymorphisms in genes involved in metabolic processes; however, they may modify the effects of environmental exposures, such as has been reported for cytochrome P450 (CYP) 1A2 and N-acetyltransferase (NAT2). Kiyohara (2000) reported that when both CYP1A2 and NAT2 were in a variant form, the risk associated with meat consumption was increased 2.8-fold (see also Chap. 3, Sec. 3.2.3).

Additional applications of molecular epidemiological studies include comparisons of subgroups of cases to identify phenotype-genotype correlations, such as the report by Bisgaard et al. (2002), which identified differences in clinical and pathologic features according to whether the patients were carriers of a known susceptibility gene or had a strong family history. Clinical outcomes have also been studied, such as in the report by Gryfe et al. (2000), which demonstrated that patients whose tumors had a high frequency of MSI had relatively favorable survival and low recurrence rates. Another research trend is that molecular-genetic profiles of CRC are being reported in increasing detail, again on relatively small numbers of cases, as modern, high-throughput analytic techniques are implemented. For example, Zou et al. (2002) employed microarrays (see Chap. 4, Sec. 4.4) to compare the level of expression for thousands of genes between colorectal tumors and normal colon tissue, and found differences among approximately 250 genes. In this way numerous candidate genes and pathways can be identified and targeted for further investigation.

### 2.3.4 Implications for Control of Colorectal Cancer

Numerous implications for cancer control programs arise from the epidemiologic observations described above. The possibility that CRC risk is modifiable and that it can be prevented is supported by the variation in risk over time, between nations, and between migrant and native populations. In the search for determinants of the variation in incidence, several risk factors have been identified consistently, thereby providing direction for the development of prevention programs. The ability to detect premalignant or early lesions in the bowel (e.g., by fecal occult blood test, endoscopy, or imaging) makes it feasible to mount screening or early detection programs. While the decline in incidence among women for cancer in specific regions of the bowel may suggest a beneficial impact of screening, the absence of such a decline among men raises questions for further research on gender differences in both incidence and utilization of screening. The observed tendency for CRC to aggregate in families, and the identification of genes (e.g., *APC, MSH2, MLH1*) that confer greatly elevated risks among mutation carriers, indicate that there are high-risk subgroups of the population for which targeted cancer control activities may be particularly beneficial. Advances in the understanding of the biology of colorectal tumors enabled the introduction of screening tests to detect abnormalities in a tumor's phenotype (MSI) or in protein expression (immunohistochemistry), so that comprehensive genetic testing can focus on those who are most at risk for HNPCC. Finally, with adenomatous polyps being an intermediate stage in the multistep process of carcinogenesis, an alternative approach for CRC control would be to prevent the development of polyps, such as by chemopreventive agents that are being evaluated in randomized trials.

Epidemiological features that enhance the potential impact of a cancer control strategy include a high prevalence in the population, and a strong association between exposure and disease as indicated by the relative risk. The combined effect of these two parameters is represented by the *attributable fraction* (*AF*, sometimes referred to as attributable risk or etiological fraction), which is the proportion of disease in the population that likely arose due to a given exposure (Last, 2001). It is calculated by:

$$AF = \frac{\text{prevalence} \times [RR - 1]}{1 + (\text{prevalence} \times [RR - 1])}.$$

Figure 2.11 shows that *AF* increases with both prevalence and relative risk, although the rate of change diminishes for *RR* greater than four for all levels of prevalence greater than 20 percent, and that for rare exposures to have a substantial *AF*, the *RR* must be very large.

The above concept is further illustrated by two hypothetical scenarios related to risk factors for CRC. First, consider a common genetic trait or risk factor that has a weak association with incidence of CRC (prevalence = 25 percent; *RR* = 1.4), such as has been reported for a polymorphic form of glutathione-*s*-tranferase (GST-T1), a gene involved in procarcinogen metabolism (de Jong et al., 2002). For GST-T1, the attributable fraction would be 9 percent. In contrast, for a rare genetic factor that is a much stronger determinant of CRC risk (prevalence = 1 per 1000; *RR* = 30), such as has been reported for *MSH2* (Mitchell et al., 2002), the attributable fraction is 3 percent. Thus, due to their higher prevalence, factors which confer only a modest increase in risk can account for as much or more disease in the population than strongly penetrant genetic factors.

Additional requirements for cancer control strategies to have an impact on risk in the population include that the disease must be serious, which is clearly true for CRC, the exposure status must be modifiable, and it must be possible to apply the intervention in a way that is sustainable and acceptable to individuals. Given that genetic endowment is not modifiable, considerable prevention research has examined the potential impact of population-wide lifestyle and behavioral interventions. Platz et al. (2000) used statistical models to estimate that 70 percent of CRC cases among American men could be prevented if they could be brought into low-risk categories of six lifestyle-related risk factors: obesity, physical activity, folic acid intake, red meat consumption, alcohol consumption, and tobacco use. Whereas these estimates are useful indicators of the potential impact of population-based prevention programs, such targets are often difficult to achieve. While randomized trials are ongoing for certain chemoprevention strategies, trials of nutritional interventions have not reported significant protective effects, such as in a trial of antioxidant vitamins C, E, and beta carotene (Greenberg et al., 1994). One recently reported trial found a reduction in CRC risk associated with selenium (*RR* = 0.5), but this was not statistically significant and the study was limited by its small sample size (Duffield-Lillico et al., 2002).

There is stronger evidence of effectiveness for interventions that aim to reduce CRC risk through screening and early detection programs, by strategies that apply both to whole populations and to high-risk subpopulations. Following the demonstration of effectiveness, a final phase of evaluation is the consideration of cost effectiveness. Ramsey et al. (2001) performed simulations of a high-risk strategy that started with screening for MSI among CRC patients, followed by genetic testing for HNPCC among those with high levels of MSI, genetic testing for siblings and children of patients who were carriers, and lifelong colorectal cancer screening for all carriers. These statistical models examined cost-per-life-year-gained under various scenarios, and demonstrated that such a program of screening based on patients with newly diagnosed CRC for HNPCC could be cost effective, especially if the benefits to their immediate relatives were considered.

It is clear that CRC can be prevented among high-risk individuals, defined according to polyp history or genetic testing, but the high-risk state is rare, which limits the potential impact of this approach on the incidence and mortality rate in the population. In contrast, for a population-based intervention the extent of the benefit to an individual may be unknown or small, yet there is still potential for this benefit to have a detectable impact at the population level. Ultimately, the greatest benefits will arise from a balanced approach that employs both population-based strategies and those directed to individuals at high risk; thus there is a continuing need for research that identifies the optimal way to reduce the health burden of CRC.

## 2.4 SUMMARY

The epidemiological approach involves the study of cancer patterns and determinants in human populations using specialized research methods that rely largely on observational rather than experimental designs. Methods employed in the design, conduct, and analysis of epidemiological studies aim to overcome potential biases and confounding, to account for random error, and to deal with the multiple factors that may contribute to risk. While interpreting and applying research findings, the quality of individual studies and the combined evidence must be carefully critiqued in order to assess whether an association is valid, causal, and important.

Recently, the epidemiological approach has been applied increasingly in studies that have clinical, genetic, molecular, and other components. Historically, epidemiology made its greatest contribution in the identification of risk factors that formed the basis of primary prevention and early detection programs, before the underlying biological mechanisms were fully understood (e.g., smoking cessation and lung cancer). Complete knowledge of causal mechanisms is, therefore, not required to achieve health benefits, and continuing recognition of this fact is important as new interventions are sought to reduce the burden of cancer. Nevertheless, the inclusion in recent epidemiological studies of measurements at the molecular and cellular levels has resulted in considerable advancement in our understanding of cancer etiology and progression. Great opportunities remain for molecular and genetic epidemiological research to contribute further to discoveries of new risk factors, gene-environment interactions, biological mechanisms, and causal pathways.

In modern epidemiology it is now possible to make observations at many levels—from the molecule and cell through to people and groups of people—and one of the challenges is in determining the relative importance of inferences drawn at each level of reference. Nevertheless, cancer epidemiology will continue to have its greatest impact and focus on the detection and measurement of disease determinants, so that groups of people can be identified who differ in their risk, which in turn can provide direction to cancer control programs. In doing so, it will remain necessary to examine the relative merits of determinants and interventions that act at the level of populations, high-risk groups, individuals, and patients. The integration of research findings across all of these levels of reference will enable the development of soundly based and well-balanced cancer control strategies to reduce the cancer burden.

## REFERENCES

Armitage P and Doll R: The age distribution of cancer and a multi-stage theory of carcinogenesis. *Br J Cancer* 1954; 8:1–15.

Bailey-Wilson J, Elston R, Schuelke G, et al: Segregation analysis of hereditary nonpolyposis colorectal cancer. *Genetic Epidemiol* 1986; 3:27–38.

Bapat B, Madlensky L, Temple L, et al: Family history characteristics, tumor microsatellite instability and germline MSH2 and MLH1 mutations in hereditary colorectal cancer. *Hum Genet* 1999; 104:167–176.

Baron JA, Cole BF, Sandler RS et al. A randomized trial of aspirin to prevent colorectal adenomas. *N Engl J Med* 2003; 348:891–899.

Bisgaard ML, Jager AC, Myrhoj T, et al: Hereditary nonpolyposis colorectal cancer: phenotype-genotype correlation between patients with and without identified mutations. *Hum Mutat* 2002; 20:20–27.

Boland C, Thibodeau S, Hamilton S, et al: A National Cancer Institute Workshop on microsatellite instability for cancer detection and familial predisposition: development of international criteria for the determination of microsatellite instability in colorectal cancer. *Cancer Res* 1998; 58;5248–5257.

Boland CR. Hereditary nonpolyposis colorectal cancer. In Vogelstein B, Kinzler K. eds. *The Genetic Basis of Human Cancer.* New York; McGraw-Hill, 1998; 333–346.

Breslow N, Day N: *Statistical Methods in Cancer Research:* Vol II. *The Design and Analysis of Cohort Studies.* Lyon, France: International Agency for Research on Cancer; 1987.

de Jong M, Nolte I, Meerman G, et al: Low-penetrance genes and their involvement in colorectal cancer susceptibility. *Cancer Epidemiol Biomarkers Prev* 2002; 11:1332–1352.

Duffield-Lillico AJ, Reid ME, Turnbull BW, et al: Baseline characteristics and the effect of selenium supplementation on cancer incidence in a randomized clinical trial: a summary report of the Nutritional Prevention of Cancer Trial. *Cancer Epidemiol Biomarkers Prev* 2002; 11:630–639.

Elwood M: *Critical Appraisal of Epidemiological Studies and Clinical Trials.* London: Oxford University Press; 1998.

Fearon ER, Vogelstein B: A genetic model for colorectal tumorigenesis. *Cell* 1990;759–767.

Ferlay J, Bray F, Pisani P, Parkin DM: *GLOBOCAN 2000; Cancer Incidence, Mortality and Prevalence Worldwide.* Lyon, France: International Agency for Research on Cancer; 2001. (Available at www.dep_iarc.fr/globocan/globocan.html.)

Fuchs C, Giovannucci E, Colditz G, et al: A prospective study of family history and the risk of colorectal cancer. *N Engl J Med* 1994; 331:1669–1674.

Giovannucci E, Ascherio A, Rimm EB, et al: Physical activity, obesity and risk for colon cancer and adenoma in men. *Ann Int Med* 1995; 122:327–334.

Giovannucci E, Stampfer MJ, Colditz GA, et al.: Multivitamin use, folate and colon cancer in the Nurses' Health Study. *Ann Int Med* 1998; 129:517–524.

Green J, O'Driscoll M, Barnes A, et al: Impact of gender and parent of origin on the phenotypic expression of Hereditary Nonpolyposis Colorectal Cancer in a large Newfoundland kindred with a common MSH2 mutation. *Dis Colon Rectum* 2002; 45:1223–1232.

Greenberg E, Baron J: Aspirin and other nonsteroidal anti-inflammatory drugs as cancer-preventing agents. *IARC Sci Publ* 1996; 139:91–98.

Greenberg ER, Baron JA, Tosteson TD, et al: A clinical trial of antioxidant vitamins to prevent colorectal adenoma. Polyp Prevention Study Group. *N Engl J Med* 1994; 331:141–147.

Gryfe R, Kim H, Hsieh E, et al: Tumor microsatellite instability and clinical outcome in young patients with colorectal cancer. *N Engl J Med* 2000; 342:69–77.

Herrera L, ed: *Familial Adenomatous Polyposis.* New York: Alan R. Liss; 1990.

Houlston R, Murday V, Harocopos C, et al: Screening and genetic counselling for relatives of patients with colorectal cancer in a family cancer clinic. *Br Med J* 1990; 301:366–368.

Houlston RS, Tomlinson IP: Polymorphisms and colorectal cancer risk. *Gastroenterology* 2001; 121:282–301.

Howe GR, McLaughlin JR: Breast cancer mortality between 1950 and 1987 following exposure to fractionated dose rate ionizing radiation in the Canadian Fluoroscopy Study and a comparison with breast cancer mortality in the Atomic Bomb Survivors Study. *Radiat Res* 1996; 145:694–707.

Khoury MJ, Beaty TH, Cohen BH: *Fundamentals of Genetic Epidemiology.* New York: Oxford University Press; 1993.

Kiyohara C. Genetic polymorphism of enzymes involved in xenobiotic metabolism and the risk of colorectal cancer. *J Epidemiol* 2000; 10:349–360.

Knudson AG Jr: Mutation and human cancer. *Adv Cancer Res* 1973; 17:317–352.

Last JM, ed: *A Dictionary of Epidemiology.* New York: Oxford University Press; 2001.

Le Marchand L, Donlon T, Seifried A, et al: Association of a common polymorphism in the human GH1 gene with colorectal neoplasia. *J Natl Cancer Inst* 2002; 94:454–460.

Lindor N, Burgart L, Leontovich O, et al: Immunohistochemistry versus microsatellite instability testing in phenotyping colorectal tumors. *J Clin Oncol* 2002; 20:1043–1048.

Luebeck EG, Moolgavkar SH: Multistage carcinogenesis and the incidence of colorectal cancer. *Proc Natl Acad Sci* 2002; 99:15095–15100.

Marcus V, Madlensky L, Gryfe R, et al: Immunohistochemistry for hMLH1 and hMSH2: a practical test for DNA mismatch repair-deficient tumors. *Am J Surg Pathol* 1999; 23:1248–1255.

McCredie M, Williams S, Coates M: Cancer mortality in migrants from the British Isles and Continental Europe to New South Wales, Australia, 1975–1995. *Int J Cancer* 1999; 83:179–185.

McLaughlin J, Sloan M, Janovjak D: *Cancer Survival in Ontario.* Toronto: Ontario Cancer Treatment and Research Foundation; 1995.

Miller BA, Kolonel LN, Bernstein L, Young JL Jr: *Racial/ethnic Patterns of Cancer in the United States, 1988–1992* (NIH Publ. No. 96-4104). Bethesda, MD; National Cancer Institute; 1996.

Mitchell R, Farrington S, Dunlop M, Campbell H: Mismatch repair genes hMLH1 and hMSH2 and colorectal cancer: a HuGE review. *Am J Epidemiol* 2002; 156:886–902.

National Cancer Institute of Canada (NCIC): *Canadian Cancer Statistics—2002.* Toronto: NCIC; 2002.

National Cancer Institute of Canada (NCIC): *Canadian Cancer Statistics—2001.* Toronto: NCIC; 2001:61–71.

Parkin DM: Global cancer statistics in the year 2000. *Lancet Oncol* 2001; 2:533–543.

Peltomaki P, Vasen H: Mutations predisposing to HNPCC: database and results of a collaborative study. The International Collaborative Group on HNPCC. *Gastroenterology* 1997; 113:1146–1158.

Platz E, Willett W, Colditz G, et al: Proportion of colon cancer risk that might be preventable in a cohort of middle-aged US men. *Cancer Causes Control* 2000; 11:579–588.

Potter J: Hormones and colon cancer. *J Natl Cancer Inst* 1995; 87:1039–1040.

Ramsey SD, Clarke L, Etzioni R, et al: Cost-effectiveness of microsatellite instability screening as a method for detecting hereditary nonpolyposis colorectal cancer. *Ann Intern Med* 2001; 135:577–588.

Ries LAG, Wingo PA, Miller DS, et al: The Annual Report to the Nation on the Status of Cancer, 1973–1997. *Cancer* 2000; 88:2398–2424.

Rothman KJ, Greenland S: *Modern Epidemiology.* Philadelphia: Lippincott-Raven; 1998.

Rubin S, Benjamin I, Behbakht K, et al: Clinical and pathological features of ovarian cancer in women with germ-line mutations of BRCA1. *N Eng J Med* 1996; 335:1413–1416.

SEER—Surveillance, Epidemiology, and End Results: *DEVCAN: Probability of Developing or Dying from Cancer Software,* Version 4.1. Bethesda, MD: National Cancer Institute; 1999. (Available at http://seer.cancer.gov.)

Vogelstein B, Fearon E, Hamilton S, et al: Genetic alterations during colorectal tumor development. *N Engl J Med* 1988; 319:525–532.

Wallace K, Baron JA, Cole BF et al. Effect of calcium supplementation on the risk of large bowel polyps. *J Natl Cancer Inst* 2004; 96:921–925.

Women's Health Initiative: Risks and benefits of estrogen plus progestin in healthy postmenopausal women: principal results from the Women's Health Initiative Randomized Controlled Trial. *JAMA* 2002; 288:321–333.

Woolf C: A genetic study of carcinoma of the large intestine. *Am J Hum Genet* 1958; 10:42–47.

World Cancer Research Fund: *Food, Nutrition and the Prevention of Cancer: a Global Perspective.* Washington, D.C.; American Institute for Cancer Research; 1997.

Zou T, Selaru F, Xu Y, et al: Application of cDNA microarrays to generate a molecular taxonomy capable of distinguishing between colon cancer and normal colon. *Oncogene* 2002; 21:4855–4862.

# 3

# Chemical and Radiation Carcinogenesis

*Allan B. Okey, Patricia A. Harper, Denis M. Grant, and Richard P. Hill*

## 3.1 INTRODUCTION

Many factors, including exposure to viruses, xenobiotic ("foreign") chemicals, and radiation contribute to cancer causation (Yuspa, 2000). This chapter discusses mechanisms by which chemicals and radiation may cause cancer and how knowledge of these mechanisms might be exploited to improve human health through prevention or intervention. That chemicals can cause cancer has been known at least since Percival Pott's observation in 1775 that scrotal cancer was linked to soot exposure in English chimney sweeps. In 1918, Yamagiwa and Ichikawa produced tumors by repeated painting of coal tar on the skin of rabbits. This breakthrough provided the foundation for the isolation, identification, synthesis, and biological testing of chemical carcinogens. Most chemicals that were identified as carcinogens in early research are by-products of industrial pro-

cesses (Fig. 3.1). For example, benzo[*a*]pyrene (BP) and related polycyclic aromatic hydrocarbons (PAHs) arise from partial combustion of petroleum or tobacco; benzidine and other aromatic amines were present in the workplace, as was vinyl chloride. Other chemical carcinogens are present in foodstuffs or in the environment. Examples include aflatoxin B1, a potent liver carcinogen formed by molds that contaminate improperly stored grains, and 2-amino-3-methylimidazo[4,5-*f*]quinoline (IQ), a heterocyclic amine derived from amino acids during high-temperature cooking. However, it has been estimated that chemical pollution accounts for less than 1% of human cancer (Ames and Gold, 1998).

Both ultraviolet (UV) and ionizing radiation are environmental carcinogens. Skin cancer is prevalent in people with high levels of sun exposure. Recognition of the role of UV radiation in the induction of this dis-

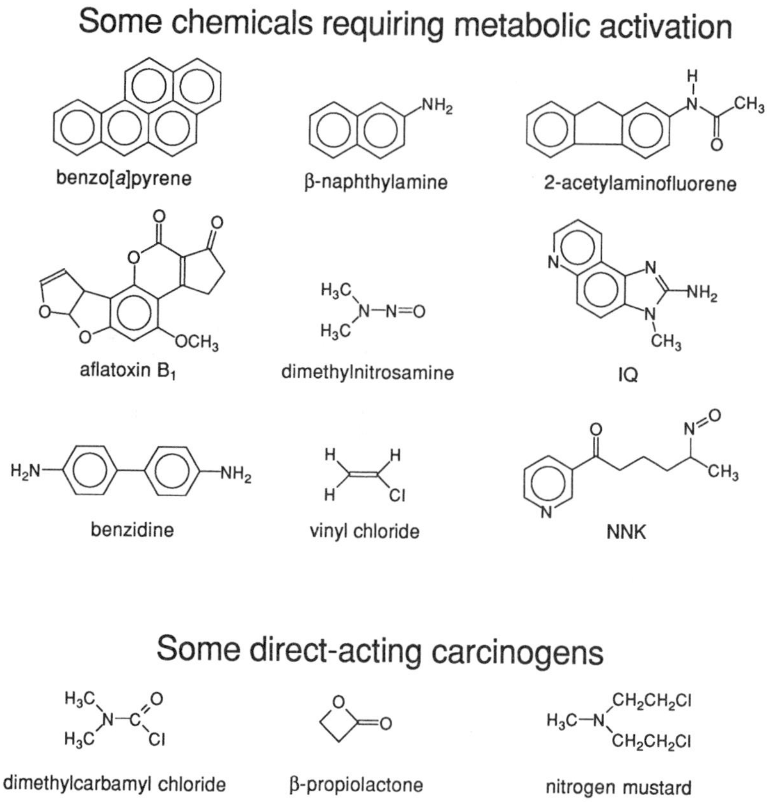

## Some chemicals requiring metabolic activation

**Figure 3.1.** Structures of some established chemical carcinogens that require metabolic activation (*top*) or act directly (*bottom*). IQ, 2-amino-3-methylimidazo[4,5-*f*]quinoline; NNK, 4-(methyl-nitrosamino)-1-(3-pyridyl)-1-butanone.

benzo[*a*]pyrene  β-naphthylamine  2-acetylaminofluorene

aflatoxin B$_1$  dimethylnitrosamine  IQ

benzidine  vinyl chloride  NNK

## Some direct-acting carcinogens

dimethylcarbamyl chloride  β-propiolactone  nitrogen mustard

ease and the degradation of the ozone layer, which absorbs UV in sunlight, has led to promotion of reduced levels of sun exposure and more extensive use of sunscreen preparations. Studies of populations exposed to high levels of ionizing radiation (e.g., medical x-rays, atomic weapons, radon in houses) have shown an increased risk of cancer and have led to acceptable levels of environmental radiation exposure being set for people working with radiation.

## 3.2 BIOLOGICAL PROCESSES IN CHEMICAL CARCINOGENESIS

### 3.2.1 Multistep Carcinogenesis

Early experiments led to a multistep model that divided the carcinogenic process into three stages: (1) initiation, (2) promotion, and (3) progression. However, it is clear that this process does not always compartmentalize neatly into these three classic stages, and that multiple sequential mutations are required in order to convert a normal cell into a malignant cell (Bertram, 2001; Knudson, 2001). In humans, this sequence of mutations has been established for several malignancies (see Chap. 2.3.3 and Fig. 2.10 and Chap. 11, Sec. 11.1.2) and, for example, in studies on colorectal malignancies alterations in at least four genes on different chromosomes must occur (Fearon and Vogelstein, 1992). Whether these mutations must be acquired in a partic-

ular temporal sequence remains uncertain. Nevertheless the classic model of initiation, promotion, and progression remains valuable as a conceptual framework for understanding carcinogenesis.

*Initiation*  An initiated cell is one in which a chemical carcinogen has interacted with DNA to produce a mutation, often a single base alteration, in the genome. At least three cellular functions are important in initiation, namely carcinogen metabolism, DNA repair, and cell proliferation. Metabolism may activate or inactivate the chemical carcinogen, DNA repair may either correct or introduce an altered base into the genome, and cell proliferation is necessary to permanently embed the change in the genome. Initiation is irreversible, but not all initiated cells will go on to establish a tumor, because many will die by apoptosis (see Chap. 10). An initiated cell is not a tumor cell because it has not yet acquired autonomy of growth. The DNA alteration may remain undetected throughout the life of the organism unless further events stimulate development of a tumor.

*Tumor Promotion*  There is no single unifying mechanism to explain the activities of the various tumor-promoting agents; however, in general, tumor promotion can be viewed as the clonal expansion of an initiated cell via altered gene expression that gives the cell a selective growth advantage. Tumor promoters cause cells to proliferate but not to terminally differentiate, resulting in proliferation of preneoplastic cells and the formation of benign lesions such as papillomas, nodules, or polyps. Many of these lesions will regress, but a few cells may acquire additional mutations and progress to a malignant neoplasm. The effects of a tumor promoter are illustrated by studies in mouse skin (Fig. 3.2). A single low dose of an initiating agent such as BP, applied directly to the skin, usually does not give rise to a tumor or other visible abnormality. When low doses of BP are followed by repeated doses of a promoting agent (e.g., croton oil), a large number of papillomas form and ultimately carcinomas develop. No tumors develop if only the promoting agent is applied or if the promoting agent is applied before the initiator. Tumors can still be induced, however, if the application of the promoting agent is delayed for several months after the initiator, but only when the intensity of the promoter exceeds a certain threshold. Examples of tumor-promoting agents are shown in Figure 3.3. The diterpene phorbol ester, tetradecanoyl phorbol acetate (TPA), the active component in croton oil, is a potent tumor promoter in mouse skin. Phenobarbital, certain chlorinated hydrocarbons such as 2,3,7,8-tetrachlorodibenzo-*p*-dioxin, and the peroxisome proliferator Wy-14,643 are effective promoters of rodent liver carcinogenesis. Unlike initiators, most promoters do not bind covalently to DNA and usually do not cause mutations or show genotoxicity in a variety of short-term tests (see Sec. 3.3.1).

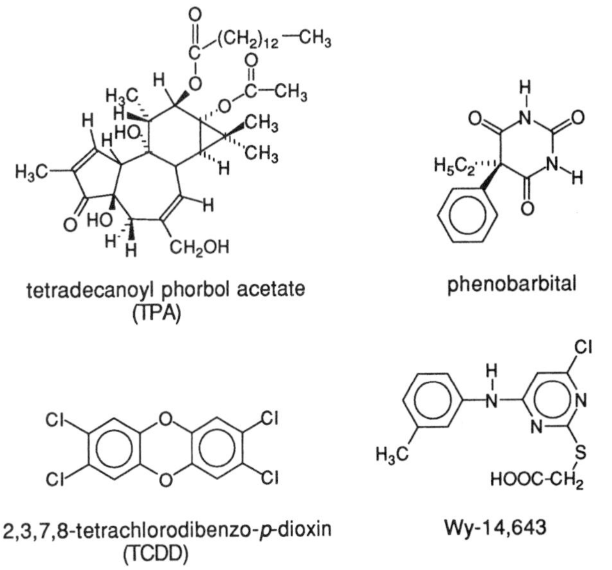

**Figure 3.3.** Chemical structures of some known promoting agents.

*Tumor Progression* Tumor progression describes the process whereby tumors acquire the ability to grow, invade local tissue, and establish distant metastases. Increased genetic instability and karyotypic alterations are hallmarks of progression (see Chap. 5, Sec. 5.2 and Chap. 11, Sec. 11.1). Inherited or acquired mutations in genes such as *p53*, *Rb*, or DNA mismatch repair genes (e.g., *MLH1* or *MSH2*) can increase the rates of mutation in other genes (creating a mutator phenotype), thereby accelerating accumulation of further mutations that are essential for development of clinical cancers. Chemicals that damage DNA and act as initiators thus can spur progression of tumors by increasing the mutation rate in key genes.

### 3.2.2 Metabolism of Carcinogens

Genotoxic carcinogens have a wide diversity of chemical structures (Fig. 3.1), but all of them are electrophilic (i.e., they attract electrons) either directly or after enzymatic conversion (Fig. 3.4). Reactive electrophiles interact readily with negatively charged, electron-rich groups on biological molecules such as proteins and nucleic acids, forming covalent adducts. Covalent adducts with bases in DNA, if not enzymatically repaired prior to the next cycle of DNA replication, may lead to errors in DNA replication and hence to fixation of the DNA damage. The majority of genotoxic carcinogens require enzymatic bioactivation in order to damage DNA. These reactions are catalyzed by enzymes whose physiologic role is to convert toxic lipophilic compounds into water-soluble metabolites that can be more efficiently excreted in urine or bile. They have evolved

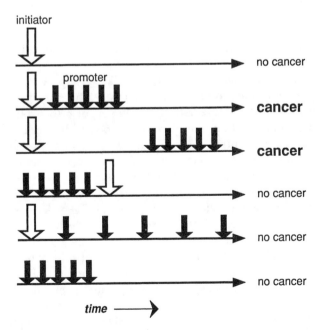

**Figure 3.2.** Outcome of various sequences of experimental exposure to initiating agents and promoting agents in mouse skin.

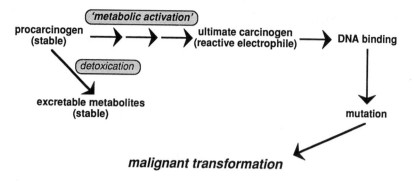

**Figure 3.4.** A general scheme illustrating the competition between pathways of procarcinogen detoxication and metabolic activation to reactive, DNA-binding electrophiles.

both multiplicity and catalytic promiscuity to ensure that potentially harmful environmental chemicals will undergo biotransformation and inactivation. However, carcinogens possess structures that lead to their inadvertent biotransformation to electrophiles, with the potential to react with DNA. Because biotransformation can produce many metabolites from a single chemical via multiple competing pathways, the effect of carcinogen exposure in a particular individual will depend on competing activation and detoxication pathways, which may be influenced by both genetic and environmental factors (Guengerich, 2000).

Drug-metabolizing enzymes are classed as phase I or phase II. Phase I enzymes (such as mono-oxygenases, oxidases, reductases, dehydrogenases, and esterases) introduce or unmask functional groups on the parent substrate. The most important phase I enzyme system is the cytochrome P450 mono-oxygenase (CYP) superfamily, consisting of several membrane-bound hemoproteins that catalyze the oxidation of carbon, nitrogen, and sulfur atoms in diverse chemicals to produce hydroxylated metabolites. Oxidation by P450 enzymes can produce either unstable electrophiles (such as epoxides) or stable hydroxylated compounds that may serve as substrates for further conjugation by transferase enzymes. Loss of chemical leaving groups can then yield electrophilic products. Table 3.1 lists some human isoforms

of cytochrome P450 implicated in pathways of carcinogen activation. Formation or unmasking of hydroxyl groups on chemicals may also be mediated by peroxidases, flavin-dependent mono-oxygenases, aldehyde and amine oxidases, and various esterases.

Phase II enzymes usually detoxify reactive metabolites. They include the UDP-glucuronosyltransferases, sulfotransferases, methyltransferases, glutathione *S*-transferases, and acetyltransferases that catalyze the conjugation of bulky, often water-soluble substituents onto hydroxyl groups on chemical molecules so that their products can be excreted. However, the transferases may also contribute to activation of carcinogens because the products formed are unstable and can break down spontaneously into DNA-reactive electrophiles. For example, glutathione *S*-transferases can activate certain dihaloethanes (Guengerich, 2000).

With a few exceptions, both directly acting carcinogens and those requiring prior metabolic activation interact ultimately with DNA by three general types of reaction chemistry. These reactions involve transfer of (1) an alkyl group, (2) an arylamine group, or (3) an aralkyl group, as shown in Figure 3.5. These chemical processes are described briefly below and in more detail by Dipple (1995).

Alkylating agents can add an alkyl group (e.g., R-$CH_2^+$) to electron-rich sites in DNA. This process is most commonly mediated by isoforms of cytochrome P450 in a reaction that involves loss of a hydrogen ion. For small *N*-nitroso compounds (e.g., dimethylnitrosamine; Fig. 3.6), which may be found in certain foods, beverages, cosmetics, and rubber products, cytochrome P450-mediated metabolism produces a carbonium ion, which is the ultimate alkylating agent. Larger *N*-nitroso compounds such as the tobacco-smoke–derived NNK (Fig. 3.1) are activated primarily by other P450 isoforms such as CYP2A13. Aflatoxin B1 (AFB1) also is metabolized by cytochrome P450 isoforms (including CYP1A2 and CYP3A4) to yield a reactive epoxide metabolite.

Aromatic amines and amides—as well as aminoazo dyes, nitroaromatics, and heterocyclic amine food-pyrolysis products—interact with DNA subsequent to formation of highly electrophilic arylnitrenium ions (Ar-

**Table 3.1.** Major Cytochrome P450 Enzymes Involved in Carcinogen Activation or Detoxification and Key Carcinogens that They Metabolize

| | |
|---|---|
| CYP1A1 | benzo[a]pyrene; 6-nitrochrysene |
| CYP1A2 | 2-acetylaminofluorene; aflatoxin B1; β-naphthylamine; 4-aminobiphenyl protein pyrolysis products [IQ; MeIQ; GluP-1; etc.] |
| CYP2A6 | NNK |
| CYP2A13 | NNK |
| CYP1B1 | 7,12-dimethylbenz[a]anthracene |
| CYP2E1 | benzene; chloroform; vinyl chloride; dimethylnitrosamine |
| CYP3A4 | aflatoxin B1; 6-aminochrysene; 1-nitropyrene |

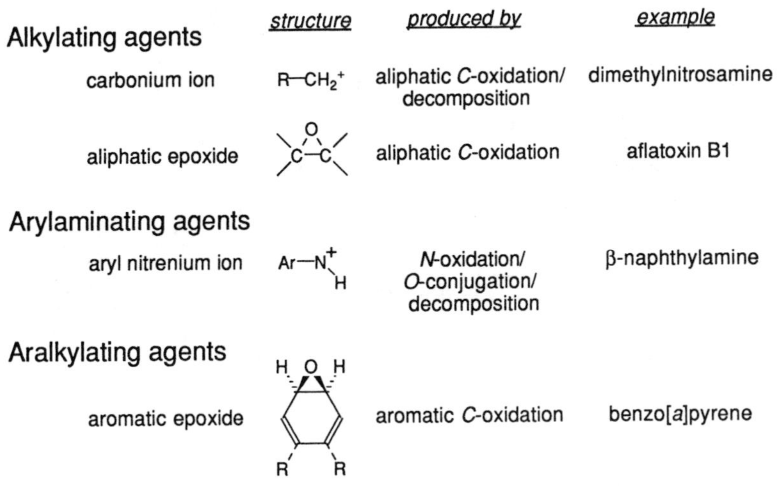

## Alkylating agents

|  | *structure* | *produced by* | *example* |
|---|---|---|---|
| carbonium ion | R—CH₂⁺ | aliphatic *C*-oxidation/ decomposition | dimethylnitrosamine |
| aliphatic epoxide | | aliphatic *C*-oxidation | aflatoxin B1 |

## Arylaminating agents

| aryl nitrenium ion | Ar—N⁺H | *N*-oxidation/ *O*-conjugation/ decomposition | β-naphthylamine |

## Aralkylating agents

| aromatic epoxide | | aromatic *C*-oxidation | benzo[*a*]pyrene |

**Figure 3.5.** Classes and structures of DNA-binding reactive electrophiles and the enzyme reactions that can produce them.

NH⁺). The latter are generated by cytochrome P450-mediated metabolism followed by conjugation with either acetate, sulfate, or glucuronic acid (Fig. 3.7). Competing metabolic pathways may be important in determining which DNA-reactive metabolites are formed in sufficient quantities to produce genotoxicity.

Polycyclic aromatic hydrocarbons and related compounds are capable of transferring an aralkyl (aromatic alkyl) group to DNA. Benzo[*a*]pyrene, for example, is converted in several steps involving the P450 enzymes CYP1A1 and CYP3A4 to the 7,8-diol-9,10-epoxide (BPDE), which is sufficiently electrophilic to attack bases of DNA (Fig. 3.8). Although exceptions exist, bioactivation of procarcinogens into their ultimate carcinogenic metabolites usually requires more than one enzyme-catalyzed step and it has been difficult to establish which enzyme pathways are the most relevant for carcinogenesis.

The contribution of specific activation pathways has been clarified in laboratory animals by deleting candidate enzymes through targeted deletion or mutation of genes (see Chap. 4, Sec. 4.3.11). For example, mice that are null for CYP1B1 are highly resistant to induction of lymphomas by dimethylbenz[*a*]anthracene (DMBA), indicating that CYP1B1 is essential for activation of DMBA in lymphoid tissues; however, CYP1B1 mice are not resistant to DMBA-induced lung tumors because alternative enzymes can activate DMBA in lung tissue (Gonzalez, 2001). Additional mouse models have provided new evidence that challenges the importance of

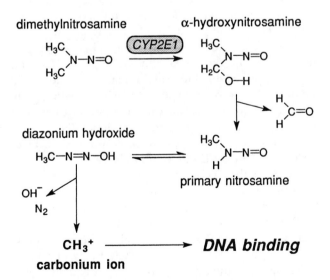

**Figure 3.6.** Metabolic activation pathway for dimethylnitrosamine.

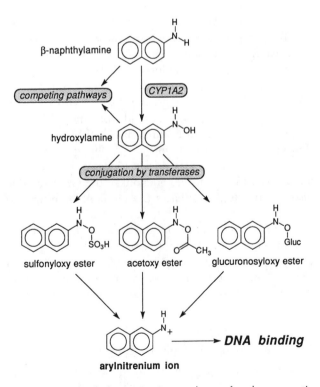

**Figure 3.7.** Metabolic activation pathway for the aromatic amine β-naphthylamine.

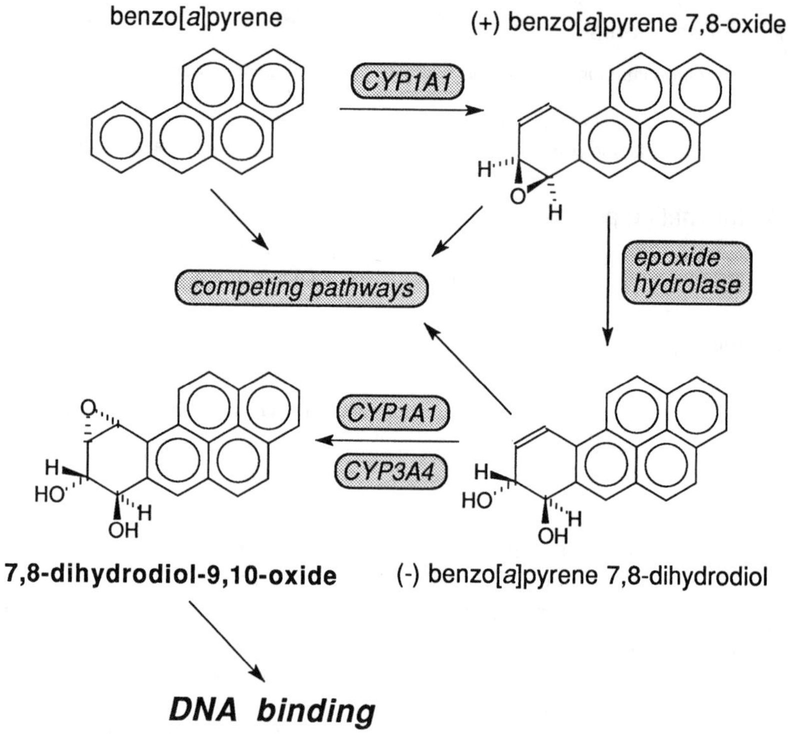

**Figure 3.8.** Metabolic activation pathway for the polycyclic aromatic hydrocarbon benzo[a]-pyrene.

CYP1A1 and CYP1A2 in the activation of aromatic hydrocarbons and aromatic amines, respectively. CYP1A1 levels are low in animals that are not exposed to aromatic hydrocarbons but can be induced to high levels via binding of the hydrocarbons to the aryl hydrocarbon receptor (AHR), a transcriptional regulator of CYP1A1 expression. Aryl-hydrocarbon-receptor–null mice are totally resistant to induction of skin tumors by BP, presumably due to failure of CYP1A1 induction in these animals (Shimizu et al., 2000). On the other hand, CYP1A1 null mice show greater toxicity and covalent BP-DNA adduct levels than wild-type mice following oral exposure to BP, indicating that CYP1A1-dependent detoxication of this chemical may be quantitatively more important than its role in bioactivation (Uno et al., 2004). Furthermore, knockout of the CYP1A2 gene also unexpectedly increases the covalent binding and toxicity of 4-aminobiphenyl, which had been thought to require bioactivation by this enzyme before DNA-binding can occur (Tsuneoka et al., 2003). Gene knockout experiments in mice will continue to be powerful tools to elucidate the roles of specific enzymes and receptors in chemical carcinogenesis (Nebert et al., 2004).

### 3.2.3 Genetic Polymorphisms of Carcinogen-Metabolizing Enzymes

In populations where all members are exposed to the same carcinogens, some individuals develop cancer and others do not. For example, many smokers develop lung cancer but some smokers do not. Reasons for this variation among individuals in susceptibility to chemical carcinogens are uncertain but there is considerable inter-individual variation, much of it genetically based, in several of the enzyme systems that activate and detoxify procarcinogens (Nebert et al., 1996). Epidemiologic studies have provided evidence that genetic traits that influence the activity of drug-metabolizing enzymes may be associated (albeit usually weakly) with altered susceptibility to chemical carcinogens. For example, the N-acetyltransferase (NAT1 and NAT2) enzymes are involved in activation and detoxification of aromatic and heterocyclic amine procarcinogens. There is an association between the "slow acetylator" phenotype, produced by allelic variants at the NAT2 gene locus and the incidence of bladder carcinoma, while the NAT2 rapid acetylator phenotype is associated with an increased risk for colorectal cancer. Allelic variation at the NAT1 gene locus (regulated independently from NAT2) may also play a role in predisposition to bladder cancer (reviewed in Grant et al., 1997).

CYP2A6 is the major enzyme in humans for metabolism of nicotine, and is also capable of bioactivating the tobacco smoke carcinogen, NNK (Fig. 3.1; Table 3.1). CYP2A6 is polymorphic in humans. Individuals with defective CYP2A6 alleles are less likely to become smokers and, if they smoke, will smoke fewer cigarettes than individuals with the normal CYP2A6 genotype (Tyndale and Sellers, 2001). Although risk for lung cancer has been reported to be reduced by 75 percent in subjects who are homozygous for a deletion-type mutation in CYP2A6 (Miyamoto et al., 1999), other studies have not shown such an association. More recent observations suggest that CYP2A13 may actually play a more important role than CYP2A6 in the bioactivation of NNK (Su et al., 2000), and that genetic variations in CYP2A13 function are linked to smoking-related risk for lung adenocarcinoma (Wang et al., 2003). In China, where high nitrosamine exposure is associated with a high incidence of esophageal cancer, a CYP2E1 polymorphism altered cancer risk approximately 5-fold (Lin et al., 1998).

More usually, epidemiologic studies of polymorphisms of drug-metabolizing enzymes indicate only small changes in relative risk. The effects of a carcinogen are influenced by multiple metabolic pathways as well as by DNA repair and cell cycle control, so that variation in a single biotransformation pathway would be expected to produce only modest associations with cancer incidence. Combining multiple risk factors could lead to stronger relative risks. For example, individuals with a combination of a null variant of the glutathione-S-transferase-mu gene and an allelic variant of the cytochrome P450 CYP1A1 gene have been shown to have a 9-fold increase in relative risk for lung cancer, which jumps to a 41-fold elevation when stratified by smoking history (Nakachi et al., 1993; Miller et al., 2001). Polymorphisms in CYP1A2 and NAT2 individually have little effect on risk of colorectal cancer; however, a "rapid" phenotype for CYP1A2 in combination with a "rapid" phenotype for NAT2 increases risk 3-fold (Kiyohara, 2000).

### 3.2.4 DNA Adducts and DNA Repair

As indicated in Figure 3.9, different types of DNA-reactive chemical agents tend to produce distinctive adducts on the individual DNA bases (Dipple, 1995). Highly charged alkylating agents tend to bind to the exocyclic oxygen atoms on the bases (e.g., $O^6$ deoxyguanosine), while less ionic species bind to ring nitrogen atoms such as N7 of deoxyguanosine. Arylaminating agents produce predominantly C8 deoxyguanosine adducts, although these may be formed by rearrangement subsequent to initial attack at the more nucleophilic N7 atom. Polycyclic aralkylating agents appear to bind preferentially to the exocyclic nitrogen atoms of adenine and guanine bases. The generation of adducts to bases in DNA affects the fidelity of DNA replication and can result in base substitutions. Several mechanisms have evolved that repair DNA and restore the original nucleotide sequence. These mechanisms are illustrated in Figure 3.10 and discussed in detail in Chapter 5, Section 5.4. Aspects of DNA repair that are particularly relevant to chemical carcinogenesis are summarized below.

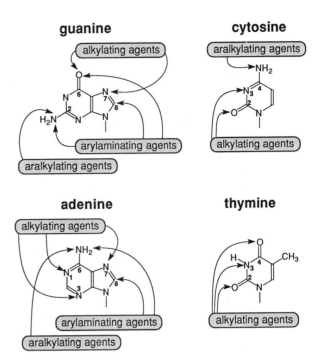

**Figure 3.9.** Sites of substitution on the four DNA bases by the three main chemical classes of genotoxic carcinogens. (Adapted from Dipple, 1995.)

In direct repair, the bond between the adduct and nucleotide is broken, there is direct removal of small alkyl substituents, and the normal DNA configuration is re-created. The most important lesion biologically is probably the $O^6$ methylated derivative of guanine, $O^6$-meG (Fig. 3.9), which can pair with thymine and result in a mutagenic transition of G:C to A:T when DNA is replicated. Such damage can be repaired by the enzyme

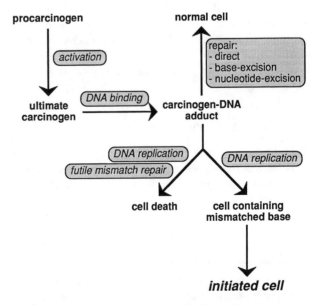

**Figure 3.10.** Possible outcomes following adduct formation.

$O^6$-alkylguanine DNA alkyltransferase (AGT), encoded by the gene $O^6$-methylguanine DNA methyl transferase (*MGMT*; Gerson, 2004). AGT selectively removes methyl groups from the $O^6$ position of guanine as well as adducts such as $O^6$-ethylG, $O^6$-butylG, and $O^4$-methylthymine (see Chap. 5, Sec. 5.4.1). In several types of cancer, oncogene activation results from a transition of G:C to A:T, consistent with failure to repair the alkylation of guanine. Targeted overexpression of AGT in the thymus protected transgenic mice against the development of thymic lymphomas induced by exposure to *N*-methyl-*N*-nitrosourea (MNU; Dumenco et al., 1993). Targeted expression of AGT in bone marrow also protected mice against the myelosuppressive effects of the chemotherapeutic agent chloroethylnitrosourea (Maze et al., 1996). Chemically damaged bases such as $O^6$-meG do not necessarily block DNA replication but may result in an $O^6$-meG-T mismatch, thereby activating DNA mismatch repair (see Chap. 5, Sec. 5.4.2). Mismatch repair removes the incorrect base specifically from the newly synthesized daughter strand of DNA. Since $O^6$-meG is in the parental strand during replication, DNA mismatch repair is inefficient in repairing this adduct; it removes the thymine from the daughter strand, but leaves $O^6$-meG in the parental strand. A deficiency in mismatch repair may therefore allow survival of genetically damaged cells and predispose to cancer.

Base excision repair (see Chap. 5, Sec. 5.4.3) removes nonbulky base adducts that do not distort the DNA helix. These adducts include 3-methyladenine, 7-methyladenine, $O^2$-hydroxymethylcytosine, or 8-hydroxyguanine residues produced by methylating agents such as MNU. These adducts and bulky DNA adducts such as BP-guanine, or guanine-cisplatin adducts, can also be removed by nucleotide excision repair (see Chap. 5, Sec. 5.4.4). Bulky adducts may inhibit DNA replication and/or result in DNA polymerase preferentially filling the noninstructive site with adenine. If this occurs opposite a guanine adduct, thymine will pair with the adenine during the next round of DNA replication, resulting in a G-to-T transversion.

### 3.2.5 Targets of Chemical Carcinogens

The relevant targets for mutagenesis by carcinogens include protooncogenes and tumor suppressor genes. When protooncogenes are activated by a mutational event, signals for cell growth are increased, but for tumor suppressor genes, which regulate cell growth negatively, relevant mutations result in a loss of function (see Chap. 7, Sec. 7.4). Commonly found mutations in chemically induced tumors in rodents are those which activate the *ras* family of oncogenes. For example, rat mammary tumors induced by a single dose of MNU con-

tain H-*ras* genes that have been activated by a single point mutation (G-to-A transition) at codon 12 of the gene (Zhang et al., 1991). In papillomas and carcinomas induced in mouse skin by 7,12-dimethylbenz[*a*]anthracene, there is an activating mutation in codon 61 (A-to-T transversion) of the H-*ras* gene (Quintanilla et al., 1986).

In humans, mutations in the tumor suppressor gene *p53* are present in more than 50 percent of tumors. The sites of mutation are not random but occur at discrete hot spots (see Chap. 4, Sec. 4.5.4 and Chap. 7, Sec. 7.4.2). Mutational hot spots probably occur for two different reasons: (1) the high efficiency of adduct formation or low efficiency of DNA repair at that site, and (2) specific mutations that predispose to oncogenesis are selectively retained in tumor cells during promotion and progression. The evidence linking particular chemical exposures to cancer has been greatly strengthened by the observation that chemicals leave molecular signatures in the form of characteristic patterns of mutation in *p53* and other genes. For example, lung tumors as well as nontumorous lung tissues from smokers with lung cancer carry a high mutational load at hotspot codons 157, 248, and 249 in the *p53* gene (Hussain et al., 2001) (see also Sec. 3.5.5). Most p53 mutations in lung cancer are G $\rightarrow$ T transversions, a type of mutation also observed in hepatocellular carcinoma (linked to aflatoxin and HBV exposure; see below and Chap. 6, Sec. 6.2.5), but rare in other tumors.

Transversions at these same codons can be produced in human bronchial epithelial cells in culture by exposing them to BPDE, the ultimate carcinogenic form of BP in laboratory animals (Fig. 3.8, Denissenko et al., 1996; Hussain et al., 2001). The correspondence between G $\rightarrow$ T mutational hot spots in the p53 gene in human cancers, and hot spots of adduct formation by PAHs from tobacco smoke in cell culture, provides a strong link between PAH exposure in smokers and the development of lung cancer (Yoon et al., 2001). Lung tumors that develop in nonsmokers contain a different spectrum of p53 mutations than the tumors from smokers and the total number of p53 mutations is greater in smokers and ex-smokers than in never-smokers (Hainaut and Pfeifer, 2001; Vähäkangas et al., 2001). Lung cancers from ex-smokers contain a p53 mutational spectrum similar to that in active smokers, indicating the persistence of molecular lesions that underlie the eventual manifestation of cancer.

More than half of the hepatocellular carcinomas (HCC) from aflatoxin-exposed populations in Africa and China have a G $\rightarrow$ T transversion at codon 249 of the p53 gene. This mutation is not present in HCC in patients with moderate or low aflatoxin exposure; thus the transversion at codon 249 is considered a molecular fingerprint linking aflatoxin exposure to the eventual development of HCC (Shen and Ong, 1996; Smela et al., 2001).

### 3.2.6 Nongenotoxic Carcinogens

A large fraction (~40 percent) of the chemicals that are carcinogenic in rodent bioassays (see Sec. 3.3.2) are not genotoxic, whereas most of the chemicals that are probable human carcinogens (IARC classification) are genotoxic (Lima and Van der Laan, 2000). Genotoxic carcinogens usually induce tumors in many animal species and at varied anatomic sites whereas nongenotoxic carcinogens tend to be much more restricted, producing tumors only in one or a few organs. This suggests that nongenotoxic carcinogens exert their tumorigenic effect by altering function in specific regulatory pathways. For example, dopamine antagonists induce mammary tumors in female rats by increasing secretion of prolactin from the pituitary which subsequently stimulates proliferation of mammary epithelium (Lima and Van der Laan, 2000). Nongenotoxic carcinogens, in general, share an important property with tumor promoters (see Sec. 3.2.1), namely, their ability to stimulate cell proliferation.

Chemicals known as peroxisome proliferators constitute an important class of nongenotoxic carcinogens in rodents (Michalik et al., 2004). These agents exert their biological effects by binding to peroxisome proliferator activated receptors (PPARs) which are nuclear receptors that modulate expression of growth regulatory genes and enzymes involved in oxidative stress (Corton et al., 2000). Several agents that activate PPARs (especially PPAR$\alpha$) are hepatocarcinogens in rodents. The mechanism seems to involve oxidative stress leading to DNA damage (even though the PPAR activators themselves are not direct genotoxins) in combination with stimulation of hepatocyte proliferation. Agents that activate PPARs include the hypolipidemic drugs, clofibrate and ciprofibrate, and antidiabetic drugs in the thiazolidinedione family. Phthalates, used in large quantities in industry as plasticizers, also can be potent PPAR activators. Because humans have been exposed to these PPAR activators, there is concern about potential cancer risk (Corton et al., 2000). However, there is no epidemiologic evidence that cancer risk is increased in people who have had prolonged exposure to PPAR activators. Proliferation of peroxisomes and hepatic cell proliferation are not observed in humans at exposure levels that produce these effects in rodents (Corton et al., 2000). The resistance of humans to liver carcinogenesis by PPAR activators (whereas rodents are highly susceptible) appears to lie at the level of the PPAR receptor. When the human PPAR gene is inserted into mice as a transgene, the human PPAR receptor supports induction of peroxisomal enzymes by peroxisome-proliferating chemicals, but does not stimulate the hepatocellular proliferation that is essential to carcinogenesis (Cheung et al., 2004). The disparity in cancer risk between rodents and humans exposed to PPAR activators highlights the difficulty of using rodents to screen for relevant human carcinogens.

## 3.3 IDENTIFICATION OF CARCINOGENS AND ASSESSMENT OF RISK

Establishing that a given chemical is a human carcinogen is a difficult and protracted process. Humans are exposed to many chemicals in foods, medicines and the environment, and there is a long latent period between exposure and tumor appearance. The most productive approach has involved astute clinical observation combined with carefully designed epidemiologic and laboratory studies in vitro and in vivo (Table 3.2).

### 3.3.1 In Vitro Assays for Carcinogens

In vivo bioassays are expensive, time consuming, and impractical as an initial screen of the thousands of chemicals that need to be assessed for carcinogenic potential. Thus in vitro assays of cell transformation have been developed. These assays were originally carried out with fibroblasts, which are relatively easy to grow in

**Table 3.2.** Assays for Carcinogens

Long-term Assays
  Clinical observation and epidemiology
  Bioassays in laboratory animals, principally rodents
Short-term Assays
  Detection of DNA damage
    Covalent adducts of the test compound with DNA after metabolic activation
    DNA strand breakage
  Detection of chromosomal damage
    Chromosomal abnormalities by cytogenetics
    Sister chromatid exchange
    Micronucleus frequency
    Sperm abnormalities
  Detection of mutational events
    Bacterial mutagenesis (Ames *Salmonella* assay, etc.)
    Sex-linked mutations and reciprocal translocations in *Drosophila*
    Mutational spectra in transgenic mice
  Unscheduled DNA synthesis in cells in culture
  Neoplastic transformation of mammalian cells in culture

culture, but they have also been applied to epithelial cells. Most studies of cell transformation in vitro have used immortalized cell lines that will grow indefinitely in culture, but which do not form tumors when reinjected into syngeneic (genetically identical) or immune-compromised mice. Such cell lines exhibit contact inhibition of growth, that is, they stop dividing when they come into close proximity with one another but remain viable. Occasionally in rodent cells (but very rarely in human cells) a spontaneous change occurs that causes the cells to lose contact inhibition, so that they continue to proliferate by spreading over adjacent cells and pile up to form a focus or colony of transformed cells. These foci can be identified by their dense, multilayer structure, basophilic staining, and the random orientation of the spindle-shaped cells. When cells from such foci are expanded and reinjected back into syngeneic or immune-compromised mice, they often form tumors. Transformed foci can be induced by treatment of the cells with many carcinogenic chemicals (as well as by radiation), or by oncogenic viruses and transfection of oncogenes (see Sec. 3.5.1 and Chap. 7, Sec. 7.2.6); thus focus-forming assays are quite suitable for screening putative carcinogens.

However, cell-transformation assays are time consuming and shorter-term tests have been developed that are based on the premise that carcinogens are mutagenic. Perhaps the most widely used short-term assay is the Ames assay (Ames et al., 1990; Fig. 3.11). This test uses mutant *Salmonella typhimurium* strains that are unable to synthesize the essential amino acid histidine and are therefore unable to grow if it is absent from the culture medium. Exposure of these bacteria to mutagens can result in reversion of the mutation back to histidine independence; consequently they regain the ability to grow in histidine-deficient medium. The number of revertant colonies that grow on agar plates after chemical exposure is thus a measure of the mutagenic potency of the test compound. Because chemicals often must be bioactivated in order to be mutagenic or carcinogenic, the assay is usually conducted in the presence of mammalian liver enzymes to bioactivate the procarcinogen.

Most of the chemical agents known to be important carcinogens in humans are mutagenic in bacteria and can also cause cytogenetic changes in rodent bone marrow. Many mutagens are also carcinogenic; however, most of the chemicals that are mutagenic in short-term assays have not been shown to be carcinogenic in humans. Assessment of the carcinogenic potential of nongenotoxic chemicals is particularly difficult because there is no apparent common mechanism on which to base large-scale routine in vitro screening assays for chemicals that are not mutagenic.

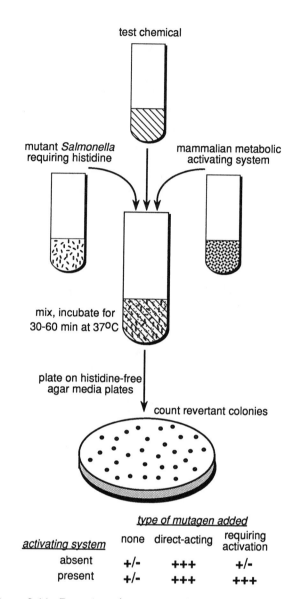

**Figure 3.11.** Detection of mutagenic chemicals in *Salmonella typhimurium* (Ames assay). (Adapted from Pitot and Dragan, 2001.)

### 3.3.2 Bioassays in Animals

Recently, transgenic animals (Chap. 4, Sec. 4.3.12) carrying readily retrievable mutational targets have been developed for in vivo mutational testing. After exposure of the animal to the potential chemical mutagen, it is possible to retrieve the mutational target (such as the *lac-I* gene in the commercial Big Blue® mouse) and determine mutational frequencies as well as the nature of the mutation(s). These animals provide valuable information regarding tissue and organ specificity. This approach is expensive and is used as a secondary assay after a chemical has been established as a mutagen through a primary screen in microorganisms.

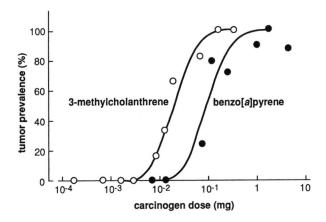

**Figure 3.12.** Dose-response curves for 3-methylcholanthrene and benzo[a]pyrene in male C3H mice. The carcinogens were injected subcutaneously and sarcomas arising at the site of a single injection were counted. (Adapted from Bryan and Shimkin, 1943.)

Direct carcinogenicity assays in rodents also serve as a useful surrogate to detect potential human carcinogens, although data from human epidemiologic studies (see Chap. 2) are required to establish human carcinogenicity. Studies in rodents are often criticized because they frequently employ doses of potential carcinogens in excess of the probable human exposure. At high doses, cytotoxic effects of the test chemical can confound the outcome by causing necrosis and regenerative proliferation in some tissues, especially liver. However, most chemicals that induce tumors at high dose will also induce some tumors at lower doses in studies using larger numbers of animals. High doses are used in animal studies for the practical reason of reducing the number of animals required. Most animal models can detect tumor incidences of about 5 percent, but not as low as 1 percent. In man an increase in total tumor incidence of even 1 percent would be unacceptable. Several genetically altered mouse strains have been generated to examine mechanisms of carcinogenesis and to provide more efficient models for testing suspect chemical carcinogens. These include mice bearing a mutated human H-*ras* gene as well as p53-deficient mice (Sills et al., 2001). A major advantage of these genetically altered mice is that tumors often appear much more rapidly than in wild-type mice, thereby reducing the duration and cost of assays for potential carcinogens.

The incidence of cancer in rodents caused by chemical agents generally increases with dose, but carcinogenic potency can differ between two closely related compounds (Fig. 3.12). Some generalizations concerning the quantitative relationship between exposure and responses to carcinogens are:

1. A single exposure to certain chemical carcinogens is sufficient to induce tumors in a high proportion of the animals. For example, a single dose of any one of several polycyclic aromatic hydrocarbons is capable of producing mammary carcinomas in over 90 percent of female rats if they are approaching sexual maturity.

2. Tumor production is often enhanced and the latency time to appearance of tumors reduced if chemical exposure is repeated; for example, induction of liver tumors in rodents treated with nitrosamines. Mechanistically, repeated exposure may enhance the likelihood that the required sequence of mutations will accumulate during the multistage process of carcinogenesis.

3. Tumor susceptibility varies widely among different animal species exposed to the same dose of the same chemical carcinogen. For example, rats are much more susceptible to liver tumors from feeding of aflatoxins than are mice. These variations in susceptibility may be due to differences in the activity of enzyme pathways that activate or detoxify chemical carcinogens. Genetically based diversity in metabolism and response to carcinogens also occurs across different strains within the same laboratory species and among different individuals in the human population.

4. Dose-response curves may vary in different tissues that are susceptible to a given carcinogen, even within the same animal. Figure 3.13 presents data from a large-scale dose-response study (about 24,000 mice) of the carcinogen 2-acetylaminofluorene (2-AAF). At lower doses liver tumors are induced, but the dose-response curve for induction of bladder cancer is much steeper than for liver, such that at higher doses of 2-AAF, bladder tumors are more common. The

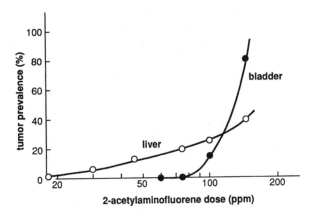

**Figure 3.13.** Dose-response curves for induction of liver and bladder tumors in female mice treated with 2-acetylaminofluorene; tumors were observed after treatment for 18 to 33 months. (Replotted from data in Cohen and Ellwein, 1991.)

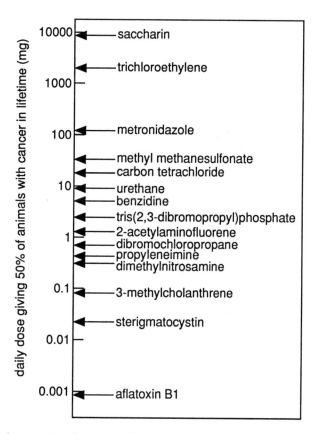

**Figure 3.14.** The range of carcinogenic potencies for various chemicals. The values shown on the y-axis indicate the amount of daily intake that is required to produce cancer in 50 percent of test animals over a lifetime of exposure. Note that the scale is logarithmic. (Adapted from data compiled by Ames, as cited in Maugh, 1978.)

difference in response between bladder and liver is not due to pharmacokinetic differences in carcinogen distribution or adduct formation, but to increased cell proliferation in bladder at the higher doses of 2-AAF (Cohen and Ellwein, 1991).

5. There is a very broad range of potencies among different chemical carcinogens. As shown in Figure 3.14, less than 1 μg/day of AFB1 is sufficient to produce tumors in 50 percent of rats after a lifetime of exposure, whereas compounds such as trichloroethylene or saccharin require more than 1 g/day to produce the same incidence of tumors.

### 3.3.3 Challenges in Identifying Human Carcinogens

Even after a particular chemical has been shown to be mutagenic by in vitro tests and to be carcinogenic in laboratory animals, the following problems make it difficult to determine whether or not that chemical causes cancer in humans:

1. The time interval between exposure to a potential carcinogen and the clinical detection of a tumor may

be 10 to 20 years in humans. This long latent period makes it difficult to link the disease to exposure to a particular agent.

2. It is often difficult to quantify the level of exposure, especially when it has occurred decades earlier. Most chemical residues and biomarkers of exposure have limited persistence (weeks to months) after exposure ends.

3. Humans are exposed to a multitude of chemicals and other potentially carcinogenic agents (viruses, ionizing radiation, etc.). These complex exposure patterns can confound attempts to attribute the disease to a particular agent.

4. People may differ widely from one another in their susceptibility to specific chemical carcinogens as a result of genetic variation at several loci, including those encoding genes involved in pathways of metabolic activation and detoxification of carcinogens (see Sec. 3.2.3).

5. The statistical power for detecting carcinogens in epidemiologic studies is low unless the population studied is very large or unless there is a dramatic increase in tumor incidence at a particular anatomic site (see Chap. 2, Sec. 2.2.3).

Reduction of risk first requires that the factors contributing to risk be identified. These factors may be external or they may be intrinsic to the population at risk. A systematic, stepwise approach is employed by regulatory agencies such as the Environmental Protection Agency (EPA) in the United States, which, in order to determine risk, attempts to integrate the multiple factors that interact in human carcinogenesis (Fig. 3.15). To predict and prevent human harm, the dose-response assessment may rely heavily upon data from laboratory animals despite the numerous caveats that apply in any attempt to extrapolate data from animals to carcinogenesis in humans.

### 3.3.4 Molecular Epidemiology

Molecular epidemiology makes use of molecular markers that may relate quantitatively to carcinogen exposure and/or to genetic markers that are associated with predisposition to cancer (Fig. 3.15 and Chap. 2, Sec. 2.3.3). In estimating risk, studies of cancer incidence can then be supplemented by surrogate molecular and biological end points rather than cancer outcomes per se. For example, the carcinogen dose received by individuals might be quantified through measurement of biomarkers of exposure such as adduct formation or mutational frequency in accessible cells. Figure 3.16 illustrates that the level of BP adducts in the DNA in lung tissue in smokers is highly correlated with the activity of CYP1A1. In other studies CYP1A1 induction has been correlated with the extent of smoke exposure. An in-

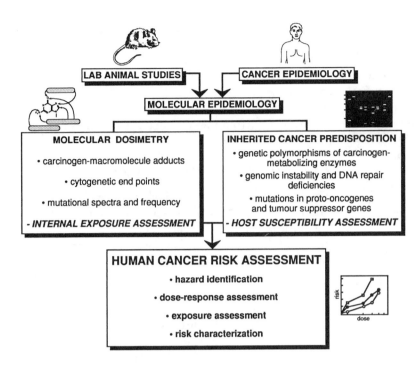

**Figure 3.15.** Strategy for using multiple approaches to assess chemical carcinogens for their risk of causing human cancer. (Adapted from Harris, 1991 and 1993.)

crease in lung CYP1A1 activity may therefore predict an increase in adduct formation and subsequent risk of lung cancer (see Sec. 3.2.3). Although this type of study is informative, it is limited by the requirement for lung biopsy to obtain tissue for analysis. In the prospective Physician's Health Study, white blood cells were used as a surrogate for lung tissue. It was found that smokers who displayed elevated levels of carcinogen DNA

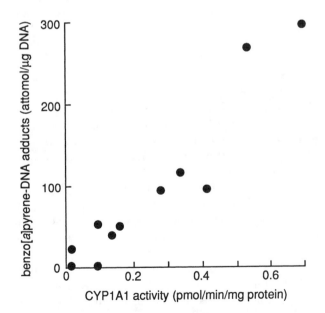

**Figure 3.16.** Correlation between cytochrome P4501A1 activity and formation of benzo[a]pyrene diol-epoxide adducts to DNA in lung samples from human lung cancer patients. (Adapted from Alexandrov et al., 1992.)

adducts in their white blood cells were more likely to be diagnosed with lung cancer one to thirteen years later than smokers who had lower concentrations of adducts (Tang et al., 2001). Higher adduct levels may arise from increased activation of carcinogens, decreased detoxification, decreased DNA repair, or a combination of these factors.

A major goal of molecular epidemiology is to identify individuals and populations who may have elevated cancer risk due to heritable predisposing factors so that preventive strategies can be implemented. Mutations in key genes such as *Rb* or *BRCA1* confer a very high cancer risk in individuals who harbor these mutations (see Chap. 2, Sec. 2.2 and Chap. 7, Sec. 7.4). However, such high penetrance mutations are relatively rare and do not constitute a major source of cancer risk for populations. Population risk may be attributable more to the relatively common genetic traits that alter the balance between activation and detoxication of carcinogens, for example, polymorphisms in cytochrome P450 enzymes and phase II conjugating enzymes (see also Chap. 2, Sec. 2.3.4). The individual risk from genetically based alterations in these enzymes usually is low; however, collectively, polymorphisms have a great impact on attributable cancer risk in populations (Perera and Weinstein, 2000). Particular combinations of polymorphisms can act additively or even synergistically to increase risk (see Sec. 3.2.3).

### 3.3.5 Management of Risk

Risk management applies risk assessment, along with identification of carcinogens and their sources, to the creation of regulations designed to eliminate or reduce exposure. Permissible exposure has been set by some regulatory agencies as the level that would result in less than one additional case of cancer for every million people exposed. The determination of this safe exposure level is very difficult. Experiments in various laboratory animals and studies in human populations have demonstrated that tumor incidence rises with increasing exposure to chemical carcinogens (Figs. 3.12 and 3.13). For example, the relative risk of lung cancer rises as the number of cigarettes smoked per day increases (Fig. 3.17). Of concern to regulatory agencies is chronic involuntary human exposure to low levels of cigarette smoke or to low levels of carcinogens in the workplace or environment. A practical challenge is therefore the prediction of risk at very low exposure levels. In practice, the risk from low-level exposure must be estimated by extrapolation downward from higher dose ranges where measurable responses (in animals or by molecular assays) can be observed.

There is usually uncertainty about the shapes of the response curves at low doses where infrequent tumor induction is superimposed upon a background of spontaneous tumors. When plotted against the logarithm of the dose, typical dose-response curves are sigmoidal (Fig 3.12), implying that there may be a threshold below which the increase in risk is insignificant. Several mathematical models have attempted to define the tu-

mor response at low exposure levels. The conservative position adopted by many regulatory agencies is that the carcinogenic dose-response curve is linear back to zero, that is, there is some finite cancer risk even at the lowest doses (albeit with very low probability). The debate about thresholds, no-effect levels, and the degree of cancer risk from low-level exposure applies to radiation and other carcinogens (Goldman, 1996).

## 3.4 CHEMOPREVENTION OF CANCER

There is great interest in blocking carcinogenesis by pharmacological means, that is, chemoprevention or chemoprophylaxis, especially in high-risk groups (Lippman and Hong, 2002a). Because the process of carcinogenesis is multistage, chemopreventive agents could act by many different mechanisms. Any chemical used prophylactically in an attempt to prevent cancer will require continuous administration and must pose very low risks to health. Candidates for chemopreventive agents fall into two principal categories: (1) the general population and (2) individuals who may be at high risk due to genetic predisposition or heightened levels of exposure. Epidemiologic studies show consistently that elevated intake of fruits and vegetables reduces cancer risk at many sites. Thus for the general population, the preferred chemopreventive strategy is simply to encourage diets rich in fruits and vegetables.

### 3.4.1 Agents That Decrease Bioactivation or Increase Detoxification of Carcinogens

As described in Section 3.2.2, most procarcinogens are activated to their carcinogenic forms by various enzymes of the cytochrome P450 family. Chemicals that inhibit P450 enzymes and/or induce phase II conjugating enzymes might, therefore, be effective anticarcinogens. For example, flavones and isothiocyanates found in cruciferous vegetables reduce metabolism and covalent binding of nitrosamines to DNA and subsequent tumorigenesis in laboratory animals. Flavonoids and coumarins also reduce tumor initiation by PAHs by inhibiting the P450 enzymes that activate PAHs (Hursting et al., 1999).

Indiscriminate inhibition of the full complement of P450 enzymes would not be safe as a chemopreventive strategy because P450 enzymes constitute the major pathway by which humans and other animals eliminate a wide range of potentially harmful chemicals. Rather, it is necessary (and challenging) to identify highly selective inhibitors that can prevent bioactivation of specific chemical agents under defined high-risk circumstances. Inhibitors of P450 enzymes protect against chemically induced cancers, but so do some P450 inducers. This paradox reflects competing roles of P450 enzymes. P450 enzymes bioactivate procarcinogens into

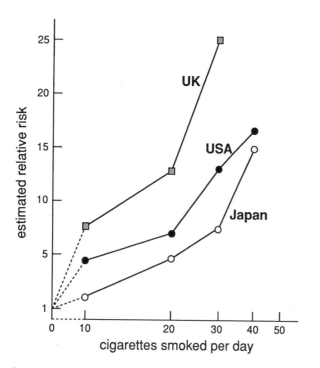

**Figure 3.17.** Dose-response relationship between the amount smoked and the risk of lung cancer in men from cohort studies from the United Kingdom, the United States, and Japan. (Replotted from data in Wynder and Hoffmann, 1994.)

reactive metabolites that bind to DNA but also enhance overall clearance of procarcinogens and carcinogens from the body. For example, induction of P450 enzymes in liver can protect animals exposed to procarcinogens by the oral route because the high P450 enzyme activity in liver accomplishes first-pass clearance of the carcinogen (see Chap. 16, Sec. 16), so that exposure of susceptible peripheral tissues is reduced (Okey, 1992; Nebert et al., 2004).

Phase II enzymes include glutathione-$S$-transferases that conjugate reactive metabolites with glutathione (see also Chap. 18, Sec. 18), and UDP-glucuronosyltransferases, which conjugate reactive metabolites with glucuronic acid. Genetic deficiencies in UDP-glucuronosyltransferases in rats lead to an increased sensitivity to genetic damage from the tobacco carcinogens NNK and BP (Kim and Wells, 1996). Some of these transferases can be induced by products of plant origin such as sulforaphane from broccoli and by antioxidants such as butylated hydroxyanisole (BHA). Induction of conjugating enzymes can be highly protective of animals against major chemical carcinogens. However, as described in Section 3.2.2, some conjugating enzymes can function as bioactivating systems that convert unreactive precursors into toxic or carcinogenic products, as in the bioactivation of methylene chloride by glutathione-$S$-transferases and of hydroxylated metabolites of aromatic amines by several enzyme systems. Thus, whether enzyme induction (or enzyme inhibition) is beneficial or harmful depends upon which chemical agent is the main threat. Unfortunately, manipulations that protect from one class of carcinogen might increase the risk from some other chemical class. Generally, however, a high level of phase II enzymes protects from chemical carcinogenesis in laboratory animals and probably also in people.

Until recently, agents that alter the balance between activation and detoxication of chemical carcinogens have not been used in man because they carry substantial risks of toxicity. However, oltipraz (a drug developed to treat schistosomiasis) has been found to inhibit the predominant AFB1-activating enzyme, CYP1A2, and induce a glutathione-$S$-transferase phase II enzyme that detoxifies reactive AFB1 metabolites by conjugation (Wang et al., 1999). This double action can substantially reduce covalent binding of AFB1 metabolites to DNA. This drug is undergoing clinical trials for prevention of hepatocellular carcinoma in regions of China where contamination of foodstuffs by aflatoxin is high and hepatocellular carcinoma is common.

Another cytochrome P450 modulator that has shown promise in preventing hormone-dependent tumors is indole-3-carbinole (I3C), which is found in broccoli, brussels sprouts, and other cruciferous vegetables. In animal studies, I3C protects from chemically induced mammary cancers and spontaneous endometrial carcinomas. Indole-3-carbinole induces CYP1A2, a form that hydroxylates estradiol-17$\beta$ and leads to lower circulating estrogen levels in both rodents and humans; it may thereby reduce the risk of estrogen-dependent tumors (Michnovicz and Bradlow, 1991). The protective effect of I3C may be due more to the removal of hormonal support later in the process of tumor progression than to a reduction in adduct formation in the earliest phases of carcinogenesis.

Some natural products of plant origin reduce adduct formation, not by altering enzyme activities but by scavenging reactive metabolites directly or acting as antioxidants. These agents include vitamin E ($\alpha$-tocopherol) and vitamin C (ascorbic acid), which inhibit chemical mutagenesis in cell culture and inhibit some chemically induced cancers in laboratory animals. However trials of these and other antioxidants, such as the food preservatives butylated hydroxytoluene (BHT) and butylated hydroxyanisole (BHA) have not been found to decrease the risk of cancer in high-risk populations.

### 3.4.2 Agents That Alter Promotion and Progression

As described in Section 3.2.1, promotion and progression involve processes of altered gene expression, inflammation, increased cell proliferation/decreased differentiation, deficient apoptosis of damaged cells, and cumulative genetic instability. Several of these processes provide potential sites for chemical intervention in the carcinogenic process.

Synthetic retinoids alter gene expression and stimulate apoptosis in damaged cells. Retinoids have demonstrated considerable efficacy as chemopreventive agents against several types of cancer in laboratory animals. Although results of initial clinical trials were disappointing, retinoids have shown some ability to delay appearance of secondary primary cancers of the head and neck (Lippman and Hong, 2002b). However, in two clinical intervention studies using $\beta$-carotene (natural retinoid) in smokers and in asbestos-exposed workers there was a paradoxical increase in lung cancer (Omenn et al., 1996; Vainio, 1999). Inflammation is known to be associated with increased cancer risk. Older-generation cyclooxygenase inhibitors such as aspirin and nonsteroidal anti-inflammatory agents (NSAIDS) reduce the risk of colorectal cancer in laboratory animals and in humans (Vainio, 1999) (see also Chap. 2, Secs. 2.3.2 and 2.3.4). Recently, anti-inflammatory targeting has been greatly improved by development of selective inhibitors of COX-2, an enzyme that predominantly generates inflammatory prostaglandins. Celecoxib, a selective COX-2 inhibitor, has shown particular promise for prevention of colon cancer in rodent models and now is in clinical trials in high-risk patients (Sporn and Suh, 2000; Lippman and Hong, 2002b).

Dramatic reductions in human cancer risk have been achieved with selective estrogen receptor modulators (SERMS), such as tamoxifen and raloxifene. These agents, which act as antagonists to the estrogen receptor in breast tissue, reduced breast cancer incidence by as much as 30 to 60% in multiple trials (reviewed in Cuzick et al., 2003 and in Serrano et al., 2004). SERMS exert some adverse effects in healthy women; thus aromatase inhibitors such as exemestane (which reduces estrogen biosynthesis) are entering clinical chemoprevention trials (Goss and Strassser-Weippl, 2004).

## 3.5 RADIATION CARCINOGENESIS

### 3.5.1 Cell Transformation by Radiation

The development of experimental models to evaluate the carcinogenic effects of ionizing radiation has been based on concepts similar to those for the study of chemical carcinogens, particularly the multistep carcinogenesis model. Assays of cell transformation similar to those described in Section 3.3.1 have provided the opportunity to examine mechanisms of radiation carcinogenesis. Irradiated cells are plated and allowed to grow to confluence. Transformed foci arise at a frequency that is dependent on radiation dose and the frequency of transformation can be increased by known tumor promoters such as croton oil or phorbol esters (see Sec. 3.2.1). Cell proliferation following the irradiation is important for the expression of a transformed phenotype. Surprisingly, for a given radiation dose, the yield of foci per dish is approximately the same over orders of magnitude in the number of cells plated (Little, 1994). This finding has been interpreted to indicate that at least two steps are involved in radiation transformation: (1) An initial radiation-induced event that occurs in a large fraction of the cells, and (2) a second rare event that occurs in only a few of the descendants of the irradiated cells (presumably during their proliferation). Studies have shown that this second event has the characteristics of a mutation. Similar findings have been reported for radiation transformation of rat mammary cells growing in vivo (Kamiya et al., 1995).

The frequency of spontaneous transformation in rodent fibroblasts is $10^{-4}$ to $10^{-5}$ per viable cell or lower. When such cells are irradiated with x- or $\gamma$-radiation, plated, and their survival and transformation frequencies measured, results as illustrated in Figure 3.18 are obtained. The number of transformants per irradiated cell increases with dose, over the range where little cell killing occurs (i.e., the shoulder of the survival curve, see Chap. 14, Sec. 14.3.1). At higher doses, as cell killing increases, the observed number of transformed foci decreases. Thus, there is an intermediate dose that gives maximal transformation (as has been seen for tumor

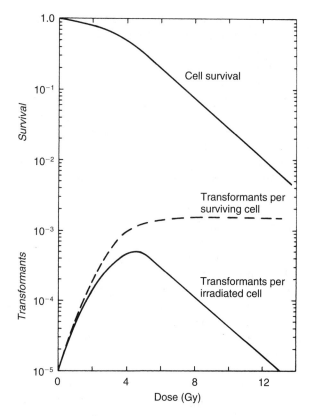

**Figure 3.18.** Typical results for cell survival, transformants per irradiated cell, and transformants per surviving cell for 10T1/2 cells exposed to low-LET ionizing radiation. When corrected for cell killing, the transformation frequency increases from a spontaneous level of $10^{-5}$ to a plateau value at 4 to 5 Gy of greater than $10^{-3}$. (Adapted from Little, 1977.)

induction in animals, see Sec. 3.5.3). Plotting transformants per surviving cell, as in Figure 3.18, indicates that the number of transformants increases for doses up to about 4 Gy and then plateaus, remaining constant up to about 12 Gy. When high linear energy transfer (LET) radiation is used (i.e., neutrons, $\alpha$ particles) more cells are killed by a given dose of radiation (see Chap. 14, Sec. 14.2.2) and more cells are transformed than by low LET radiation (x- or $\gamma$-rays); thus the effectiveness of high LET radiation for transformation is greater than that of x- or $\gamma$-rays and, as for cell survival (Chap. 14, Sec. 14.3.1), increases at low doses (Miller et al., 1995).

### 3.5.2 Mechanisms of Radiation Transformation

Carcinogenic chemicals appear to cause a low-probability initiation event which results in DNA damage that is then fixed in the genome (see Sec. 3.2.1). In contrast, data for radiation transformation point toward a high-frequency initial step followed by a rare second step (Little, 2000). The important initial effect of radiation appears to be the induction of genetic instability (Syluasen et al., 2001; Morgan et al., 2002), which then allows for a higher probability of rare mutations, which represent the second step(s) that lead, in turn, to malignant transformation. The observations that radiation tends to increase the incidence of the types of tumors which arise naturally in the population, and that the increased incidence of tumors is seen primarily at ages when spontaneously arising tumors of the same type would occur, are consistent with the idea that radiation acts to induce a mutator phenotype.

The mechanism(s) by which genetic instability is induced by radiation and maintained in the population are uncertain, but probably include: (1) mutations in genes involved in control of DNA synthesis or DNA repair, such as the mismatch repair system (see Chap. 5, Sec. 5.4.2), (2) the induction of chromosome instability, and (3) persisting aberrant production of oxygen radicals which can damage DNA (Little, 2000; Morgan et al., 2002). Irradiated cells maintain a higher incidence of mutations and chromosome instability for many generations after the irradiation both in vitro and in vivo (Morgan et al., 2002). These unstable cells acquire lesions such as point mutations, very different from the types of DNA damage induced directly by irradiation, and are more consistent with mutations that are observed in naturally arising cancers. This genetic instability appears to be dependent on species, strain, and tissue type; for example, there are differences in the susceptibility of mouse bone marrow cells to the induction of chromosome instability among different strains of mice. Differences in the susceptibility of different strains of mice to radiation-induced mammary cancer parallel differences in the sensitivity of their mammary epithelial cells to transformation (Ullrich et al., 1996). Mice resistant to transformation and mammary cancer development are also resistant to the development of genetic instability after irradiation (Ullrich and Ponnaiya, 1998).

The ultimate mechanism by which radiation induces malignant transformation is likely the activation of (proto)oncogenes or inactivation of tumor suppressor genes (see Chap. 7). Because DNA lesions associated directly with ionizing radiation are primarily deletion, translocation, or inversion of DNA sequences, inactivation of a tumor suppressor gene or inactivation of regulatory sequences would be a more likely effect of the initial radiation event (Cox, 1994). However, chromosome breakage followed by faulty repair and translocation or amplification of DNA segments are possible mechanisms by which activation of protooncogenes could occur (Chap. 7, Sec. 7.2).

### 3.5.3 Carcinogenesis by Ionizing Radiation in Animals

Single doses of x-rays or γ-rays in the range of 0.25 to 8 Gy given to the whole body can increase the frequency of malignant and benign tumors in irradiated animals. A variety of animals has been studied including dogs, monkeys, and rats, but the most intensive studies have been done with mice. Different tissues have different sensitivities for tumor induction and these vary for different animals or even strains of mice. Because tissues are not equally sensitive to radiation (but the initial damage is uniformly produced at the cell and tissue level), host factors presumably contribute to the overall process of cancer induction. Such factors may include levels of repair enzymes, rate of cell proliferation, endocrine function, and immune competence.

Specific genetic changes have been observed in some radiation-induced tumors. The *K-ras* oncogene was found to be activated through a single base change in mouse lymphomas that were induced by γ-radiation (Guerrero et al., 1984). Animal studies have also implicated mutations in the *Ret* gene in thyroid cancer and this has also been observed in humans (see Sec. 3.5.4). The induction of acute myeloid leukemia in mice has been shown to involve specific abnormalities on chromosome 2 (Bouffler et al., 1996). Some radiation-induced solid tumors have mutations in the p53 gene and both p53 knockout mice and mice carrying a mutant p53 transgene are highly susceptible to radiation-induced tumors (Lee and Bernstein, 1995). Radiation-induced genetic instability was found to be significantly greater in p53 knockout mice than in heterozygotes or wild-type animals (Liang at al., 2002), supporting the idea that absence or reduction of p53 expression enhances radiation-induced tumorigenesis by increasing genetic instability at various loci, such as those for tumor suppressor genes (see Chap. 7, Sec. 7.4).

The dose dependence for tumor induction by ionizing radiation differs for different tissues, but for single acute doses of x- or γ-rays given to the whole body, the relationship between tumor induction and dose appears to be sigmoidal (Fig. 3.19, curve A). At low doses there is little induction but as the dose increases there is a steep increase in the number of tumors followed by saturation or even a decrease at high doses. Factors which influence this dose-response curve are:

1. Many strains of mice have a spontaneous level of occurrence of the specific tumor under study (in this hypothetical example, 10 percent) even in the absence of radiation. Spontaneous tumors may complicate the assessment of tumor induction at low doses since radiation-induced tumors cannot be distinguished from them.

2. The induction curve for a specific tumor might have a low threshold dose so that the rate of tumor production could appear to be linear with dose.

3. As the dose of radiation increases, cell killing will increase, leading to a maximal rate of tumor induction and a possible decrease in incidence at higher doses.

4. There is a latent period between radiation treatment and tumor detection. Thus, an increase in the fre-

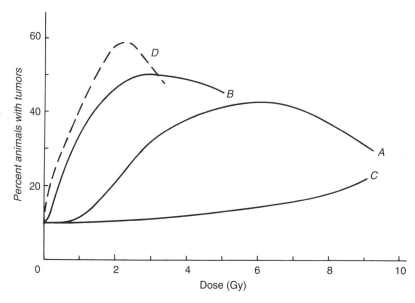

**Figure 3.19.** Schematic diagram of induction of a specific tumor type in mice exposed to various doses of ionizing radiation given to the whole body based on a review of a number of different in vivo results. (*Curve A*) Tumors induced by single acute doses of low-LET radiation. (*Curve B*) Tumors induced by single acute doses of high-LET radiation. (*Curve C*) Tumors induced by fractionated doses (e.g., 1 Gy/day) of low-LET radiation. (*Curve D*) Tumors induced by fractionated doses (e.g., 0.5 Gy/day) of high-LET radiation.

quency of tumors at a certain time after irradiation may represent an effect on the absolute level of tumor incidence or an earlier occurrence of tumors or both.

Tumor induction for a single dose of high LET radiation (such as neutrons or α-particles) given to the whole body occurs, in general, at lower doses than for low LET radiation (x- or γ-rays). This effect is illustrated for neutron irradiation in Figure 3.19 curve B, which indicates a small low-dose threshold portion so that tumor induction appears to be almost linear with dose. The curve continues to a maximum, which illustrates that a higher proportion of tumors occurs at a lower dose than for low LET radiation, and then may decrease. In Figure 3.19, a single dose of 3.3 Gy of low LET radiation gives 35 percent tumor induction, while a single dose of 1.1 Gy of neutrons gives the same effect. The effectiveness of neutrons (or other high LET radiations) relative to x- or γ-rays for tumor induction is highly dependent on dose and the biological effect being studied. This effect is accounted for in risk assessment by multiplying dose received from high LET sources by a quality factor to convert it to an equivalent dose of low LET radiation. This equivalent dose is expressed in Sieverts (Sv): 1 Sv is equivalent to 1 Gy of x- or γ-radiation.

Other than exposures due to accidents and nuclear explosions (which may expose individuals to high and/or low LET radiation), most radiation exposures of concern to man involve fractionated or low-dose rate low LET irradiation. Most studies of fractionated low-LET radiation in animals have resulted in a reduction of tumor incidence for a given total dose as illustrated by Figure 3.19, curve C, presumably because fractionation allows for extensive repair of damage and results in re-

duced carcinogenic effect. Continuous radiation at a low dose rate gives a curve similar to Figure 3.19, curve C. In contrast, fractionating high-LET radiation or exposure at low dose rates has little effect on tumor induction, giving the same results as for single acute doses (Fig. 3.19, curve B), or is more efficient in causing tumor induction (Fig. 3.19, curve D). Lack of repair of damage after high LET radiation means that fractionation or prolonging the time for radiation delivery is of little or no benefit in reducing the probability of tumor induction.

### 3.5.4 Human Data on Carcinogenesis by Ionizing Radiation

The carcinogenic risks of radiation exposure in people have been derived from many sources, including occupational exposures (e.g., radiologists and uranium miners), therapeutic exposures (e.g., unavoidable treatment of normal tissues in cancer therapy, or treatment of ankylosing spondylitis), and accidental exposures (see e.g., Bhatia and Sklar, 2002). A discussion of the data for therapeutic exposures in the context of recent in vitro studies is given in Hall (2004). However, most information is from studies of the atom-bomb survivors in Hiroshima and Nagasaki, who were exposed in 1945, and from studies of exposures during medical x-ray examinations, particularly of pregnant women, which resulted in fetal exposure to irradiation. These groups of people were exposed to acute doses of irradiation, thus extrapolation of the risks to low levels of continuous exposure has relied on more limited information from occupational exposures and on experimental studies and modeling. Radiation risk is defined as the increase in the number of cancer deaths over that expected for an unirradiated population. Excess absolute risk is expressed as the increased number of cancers per $10^4$ person-years after exposure to 1 Sievert. Excess relative risk is the increase in cancers above that expected in an unirradiated population expressed as a fraction of the level in the unirradiated population.

Information about the atom-bomb survivors is based on a leukemia registry established soon after the bombing and on a lifespan study of more than 120,000 individuals living in the two cities that was initiated in 1950. Of these individuals approximately 93,000 were atom-bomb survivors and 27,000 were not in the cities at the time of the bombing. Detailed dosimetry for about 87,000 of these individuals has been performed. The first evidence of a carcinogenic effect was an increase in the incidence of leukemias, due to the short latent period for this malignancy. The risk rose rapidly in the first five to ten years after exposure and then declined so that after twenty-five years there was little excess risk (Preston et al., 1994). An analysis of the incidence of hematologic malignancies (leukemia, lymphoma, and multiple myeloma) over the period 1950–1987 gave an estimated excess relative risk at 1 Sv for all leukemias of 3.9 (Preston et al., 1994). Lymphomas and multiple myeloma showed no significant increase. These numbers have not changed significantly in the subsequent ten years to 1997 (Preston et al., 2003). However, this analysis does not include leukemia cases that arose in the first five years after exposure because of the inadequacy of information for these early years. If these cases had been included, the estimated risk of leukemia would probably increase by 10 to 15 percent.

In a cohort of about 86,000 people in the atom-bomb lifespan study, a total of 9335 deaths from solid cancers occurred between 1950 and 1997, of which an estimated 440 (5 percent) were associated with radiation exposure (Preston et al., 2003). The excess relative risk for all solid cancers at age 70 for a person exposed to 1 Sv at age 30 was estimated to be 0.47 (90 percent confidence interval (CI), 0.41–0.53). This value varies with sex, age at exposure, and attained age. It is higher for females (0.63) than males (0.37), is higher for those exposed at younger ages, and is lower for those with greater attained age. Estimated values for excess relative risk and excess absolute risk for tumors of different organs are given in Preston et al. (2003). Females demonstrate a higher excess relative risk than males for a number of tumor sites but since these are largely the inverse of the natural incidence, the overall excess absolute risk is essentially the same for both sexes (12.6 cases per $10^4$ person-year-Sv for males vs. 13.5 for females). Estimates of lifetime risk of radiation-associated solid cancer deaths for persons exposed to 0.1 Sv at different ages are given in Table 3.3, together with estimated natural (background) risk.

**Table 3.3.** Estimated Lifetime Risk of Radiation-Associated Solid Cancers Deaths (RASC) After Exposure to 0.1 Sv

| Age at Exposure | Sex | Lifetime Risk of RASC (%) | Background Risk (%) |
|---|---|---|---|
| 10 | M | 2.1 | 30 |
| | F | 2.2 | 20 |
| 30 | M | 0.9 | 25 |
| | F | 1.1 | 19 |
| 50 | M | 0.3 | 20 |
| | F | 0.4 | 16 |

*Source*: Data from Preston et al. (2003).

There was no recorded carcinogenic effect of irradiation in utero in studies of atom-bomb survivors, but studies of children irradiated in utero with medical x-rays from about 1940 to 1975 have consistently demonstrated an increased risk of cancer induction, with an overall excess relative risk of about 1.5 for leukemias and solid tumors (Doll, 1995; Doll and Wakeford, 1997). The relative risk is related to the number of x-ray exposures (i.e., number of films taken), and hence to dose received by these children, and has declined with year of birth as the dose per film declined. For the period from about 1960 onwards, most of the doses would have been equal or less than 0.01 Sv and the relative risk is about 1.3. This leads to an excess risk of cancer of about 6 percent per 1 Sv, with 40 percent of this risk (2.5 percent per 1 Sv) being due to leukemia (Doll and Wakeford, 1997).

The exposure of large numbers of people to radioactive fallout from the accident at the nuclear power plant in Chernobyl in 1986 has provided information about risks associated with exposure to internally ingested isotopes. The only significant increase in tumor incidence to date is a high level of papillary thyroid tumors in exposed children, particularly young children (Williams, 2002). These tumors are associated with exposure to radioactive iodine, much of it probably ingested from contaminated milk. Iodine is concentrated in the thyroid gland giving much higher exposures to the gland (~1000-fold the average whole-body dose). The developing thyroid gland is much more sensitive than the mature gland in older children and adults. A majority of these tumors are associated with translocations of the *RET* (onco)gene similar to those observed in animal models. In contrast, mutations of the *RAS* gene or *p53* genes were not observed. Excess absolute risk per unit of thyroid dose was estimated as $2.1/10^4$ children-year-Sv. The relative risk for children one year old in Belarus (up to 1998) was estimated as 237 versus a relative risk of 6 for children ten years old. Experience with the atom-bomb survivors suggests that it will be many years before the full extent of the risks from this accident will be known.

Another important source of exposure to internal isotopes is radon in houses. Studies of uranium miners have shown that exposure to radon causes an increased risk of lung cancer (Darby et al., 1995; Lubin et al., 1995), which is roughly proportional to dose, but the analysis is confounded by a number of factors, particularly smoking. Lubin et al. (1995) have derived a formula for extrapolating these data to the general public and have estimated that the proportion of lung cancer deaths attributable to radon exposure in U.S. homes is 10 percent for men and 12 percent for women. It is less for smokers and greater for nonsmokers. For lung cancer risk it has been estimated that smoking one to nine cigarettes per day is equivalent to receiving a dose of 3.4 Sv or to living for thirty years in a home with a very high radon concentration (Boice and Lubin, 1996). These levels can be compared to average background levels of 2 to 3 mSv per year for radiation exposure.

Extrapolation from the available data to estimate carcinogenic risk of low doses of radiation presents similar problems to those described in Section 3.3.5 for exposure to chemicals (i.e., is there a threshold or should a linear extrapolation to zero dose be used?). The excess relative risk of solid cancer deaths from the recently published analysis of data from the atom-bomb survivors (Preston et al., 2003) is plotted against dose in Figure 3.20. The best-fit curve through these data has features similar to curve A in Figure 3.19, but it has a finite initial slope. Furthermore a linear extrapolation cannot be ruled out (Preston, 2003). For leukemia in the atom-bomb survivors a linear-quadratic fit was significantly better than a linear fit (Preston et al., 1994). A threshold or a linear-quadratic model (see Chap. 14, App. 14.1) are more consistent with data from animals, but the shape of the low-dose portion of the curve varies from one experimental system to another.

### 3.5.5 Carcinogenesis by Ultraviolet Radiation

There is a correlation between latitude (average sun exposure) and the incidence of malignant tumors of the skin with the tumors tending to occur on sun-exposed areas, such as the face. Genetic background is also a determining factor, especially low skin pigmentation (Celts, Scottish, Welsh), because this contributes to an increase in the effective dose delivered to the cells at risk in the basal layer of the epidermis. Chronic exposure to sunlight is required for carcinogenesis, suggesting the need for multiple interactions of UV radiation with the target cells.

Because of the limited penetration of UV radiation through tissue, studies of the carcinogenic effect of UV radiation in animals have been limited to induction of tumors in skin. Studies of UV carcinogenesis have focussed on exposures classed as UVC, UVB, and UVA, corresponding to wavelengths of 200 to 290 nm, 290 to 320 nm, and greater than 320 nm, respectively. Because of filtering of UV radiation by the ozone layer, wavelengths shorter than 290 nm (UVC) are believed to play little role in the exposure of the human population to solar radiation. Ultraviolet B is the most effective range of wavelengths for skin.

If low daily doses of UV radiation are given to the skin of mice over weeks to months then, as the daily dose and dose rate increase, the latency time for initial appearance of tumors (mostly fibrosarcomas and squamous cell carcinomas) decreases and the rate of tumor induction increases. A given total dose of UV radiation appears to be more effective as a carcinogen when administered at a lower exposure rate or as a fractionated course, in contrast to results with low-LET ionizing radiation. The relationship between tumor induction and wavelength in hairless mice has been found to peak at about 290 nm, similar to that observed for cell transformation in vitro and for the induction of skin erythema (sunburn) in humans. The relationship for induction of squamous cell carcinomas (SCC) in humans is similar and directly related to total sun exposure (De Gruijl and Forbes, 1995; De Gruijl et al., 2001). Basal cell carcinoma (BCC) and cutaneous melanoma (CM) in humans are more strongly associated with intermittent sun exposure and with a history of sunburn, particularly in childhood (De Gruijl et al., 2001).

In experiments in which multiple UV doses were given to mice there was a clear relationship between induction of pyrimidine dimers (i.e., cross-linked thymine

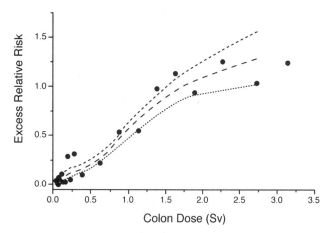

**Figure 3.20.** A plot of the excess relative risk at 1 Sv for solid cancer deaths in the atom-bomb survivors versus the estimated dose to the colon (as a representative internal organ). The data are averaged over sex for attained age of 70 after exposure at age 30. The dashed line is a smoothed estimate based on the points with upper and lower 1 standard error bounds. (Redrawn from Preston et al., 2003.)

or cytosine bases in DNA) in the target basal layer of the skin, and the subsequent incidence of tumors (Fry and Ley, 1983). In these experiments there was a lower dose range where no tumors were induced, followed by a significant increase with higher UV dose to the basal layer. Treatment of UV-irradiated animals with the tumor promoter 12-O-tetradecanoyl-phorbol-13-acetate (TPA) converted this curvilinear response to a linear no-threshold response. Tumors induced by UV radiation in mice tend to be strongly immunogenic. Repeated UV irradiation of mice induces not only tumors but also an immunological change that inhibits the ability to reject transplanted syngeneic tumors that were induced by UV radiation (Kripke, 1990). Ultraviolet radiation has a profound effect on cutaneous immunity, causing a reduction in the number of cutaneous antigen presenting (Langerhans) cells, and raised levels of suppressor T-lymphocytes, which act against a common UVB-induced antigen. Suppression of the immune response to UV-induced tumors can be transferred from one animal to another by these suppressor T-cells. Thus, the dose-response relationship for UV induction of tumors may be complex because the dose-response relationships for cancer induction and immune suppression may not be the same, and the appearance of tumors will be mediated by both effects. Transient immune effects have also been observed in humans following UV exposure (Streilein et al., 1996) and humans, who have a high average sun exposure and undergo immunosuppressive therapy for renal transplants have a higher frequency of squamous cell tumors of the skin than those in the general population (Hardie et al., 1980).

A high frequency of UV-induced tumors in mice demonstrate point mutations in the p53 gene and these mutations are primarily C-to-T transitions (Kress et al., 1992). More than 50 percent of skin cancers in humans (both SCC and BCC) also have characteristic *p53* mutations (Ziegler et al., 1993). Many of these mutations are CC-to-TT transitions that are characteristic of misrepair or lack of repair of pyrimidine dimers (Daya-Grosjean et al., 1995). Such dimers may be repaired by a number of processes including nucleotide excision repair (see Chap. 5, Sec. 5.4.4) and there is an increased risk of skin cancer in patients with xeroderma pigmentosum (XP), an inherited disease in which there is a deficiency in nucleotide excision repair (De Gruijl et al., 2001). The high incidence of *p53* mutations, which can be found in preneoplastic lesions, may cause genomic instability, which is consistent with the frequent loss of heterozygosity (LOH) seen in BCC (9q) and SCC (3p,9q,13p,17p,17q), although LOH has been observed in the absence of p53 mutations (see Chap. 7, Sec. 7.4.1).

The LOH at 9q appears to be associated with deletion or mutation of the patched (*PTC*) gene and 70 to 90 percent of BCC in XP patients have *PTC* mutations (Daya-Grosjean and Sarasin, 2000). The *PTC* gene is part of the Hedgehog (Hh) signaling pathway that can cause activation of the Gli transcription factors in human cells (Chap. 8, Sec. 8.4.3). One of the downstream targets of Gli is the *Bcl2* gene, which acts to inhibit apoptosis (see Chap. 10, Sec. 10.2.1). Activation of this pathway may also override the G1 arrest associated with the p21$^{WAF1}$ gene (see Chap. 5, Sec. 5.5). Transgenic mouse models with an activated Hedgehog pathway, or constitutive upregulation of Gli1 restricted to basal cells, show increased incidence of BCC. Activating *ras* mutations have also been reported in a minority of SCC and BCC (De Gruijl et al., 2001).

In familial cutaneous melanoma (CM) there are markers on 9p21 which map to the *INK4 a,b* locus, which codes for the cyclin-dependent kinase inhibitors p16 and p15. This locus also codes for the p14$^{ARF}$ protein, which can act to stabilize p53 by binding to the HDM2 gene and interfering with degradation of p53. Loss of *INK4a (p16)* appears to be the most important defect in familial CM and in sporadic CM point mutations typical of UV irradiation can be observed in this gene. Mutations in *N-RAS* have also been reported in CM from regularly sun-exposed sites, again occurring in the vicinity of dipyrimidine sites. Thus skin cancers are clearly associated with UV damage to DNA and genetic evidence links SCC to *p53* mutations and possibly RAS mutations, BCC to *PTC* and *p53* mutations and CM to mutations in *INK4a* and possibly *N-RAS* (De Gruijl et al., 2001; Cleaver and Crowley, 2002).

## 3.6 SUMMARY

Most chemical carcinogens form adducts with bases in DNA either directly or, more often, after metabolic activation. Cancers arise from multiple sequential unrepaired lesions at specific sites in oncogenes or tumor-suppressor genes. Genetic variation in the capacity to repair DNA alters cancer risk, as does variation in enzymes that activate or detoxify carcinogens. Methods to identify carcinogens rely on the premise that most carcinogens are genotoxic. Based on knowledge of the mechanisms by which carcinogens act, it may be possible to manipulate biochemical or cellular defense mechanisms to reduce cancer risk, and a number of clinical trials are in progress. However, the most effective method to reduce the human cancer burden is through reduction of exposure to known carcinogens, especially to such high-risk agents as tobacco smoke.

Ionizing and UV radiation can both give rise to tumors, but different DNA lesions probably initiate the process of carcinogenesis. For ionizing radiation, the critical damage probably leads to instability of the DNA, and this, in turn, leads to an increased probability of errors in DNA replication occurring in subsequent cell cycles. This may lead to changes in expression or activation of oncogenes or inactivation of tumor suppressor genes. Ionizing radiation induces tumors in different tissues with different efficiencies, implying the existence of modulating host factors. Carcinogenesis induced by UV light requires multiple exposures. Tumor induction increases with total dose and has a wavelength dependence similar to that for sunburn and for induction of pyrimidine dimers in DNA. Many skin tumors contain mutations in the *p53* gene that are a consequence of misrepair or lack of repair of pyrimidine dimers.

The risk of cancer in humans exposed to moderate doses of ionizing radiation (up to 4 Gy) has been estimated from studies of the Japanese atom-bomb survivors. Most tissues are affected, but the relative risk varies. Estimates of risk for low doses of radiation and for low exposures to chemical carcinogens spread over long periods of time are made by extrapolation of data relating to risk after larger (usually acute) doses. There is considerable uncertainty about these extrapolated estimates of risk.

## REFERENCES

Alexandrov K, Rojas M, Castegnaro M, et al: An improved fluorometric assay for dosimetry of benzo[*a*]pyrene diol epoxide-DNA adducts in smoker's lungs: comparisons with total bulky adducts and aryl hydrocarbon hydroxylase activity. *Cancer Res* 1992; 52:6248–6253.

Ames BN, Profet M, Gold L: Dietary pesticides (99.9% all natural). *Proc Natl Acad Sci USA* 1990; 87:7777–7781.

Ames BN, Gold LS: The causes and prevention of cancer: the role of environment. *Biotherapy* 1998; 11:205–220.

Bertram JS: The molecular biology of cancer. *Mol Aspects Med* 2001; 21:167–223.

Bhatia S, Sklar C: Second cancers in survivors of childhood cancer. *Nat Rev Cancer* 2002; 2:124–132.

Boice JD, Lubin JH: Lung cancer risks: comparing radiation with tobacco. *Radiat Res* 1996; 146:356–357.

Bouffler SD, Breckon G, Cox R. Chromosomal mechanisms in murine radiation acute myeloid leukemogenesis. *Carcinogenesis* 1996; 17:655–659.

Bryan WR, Shimkin MB: Quantitative analysis of dose-response data obtained with three carcinogenic hydrocarbons in strain C3H male mice. *J Natl Cancer Inst* 1943; 3:503–531.

Cheung C, Akiyama TE, Ward JM, Nicol CJ, Feigenbaum L, Vinson C, Gonzalez FJ: Diminished hepatocellular proliferation in mice humanized for the nuclear receptor peroxisome proliferator-activated receptor alpha. *Cancer Res* 2004; 64:3849–3854.

Cleaver JE, Crowley E: UV damage, DNA repair and skin carcinogenesis. *Front Biosci* 2002; 7:1024–1043.

Cohen SM, Ellwein LB: Genetic errors, cell proliferation, and carcinogenesis. *Cancer Res* 1991; 51:6493–6505.

Corton JC, Lapinskas PJ, Gonzalez FJ: Central role of PPARα in the mechanism of hepatocarcinogenic peroxisome proliferators. *Mutat Res* 2000; 448:139–151.

Cox R: Molecular mechanisms of radiation oncogenesis. *Int J Radiat Biol* 1994; 65:57–64.

Cuzick J, Powles T, Veronesi U, et al.: Overview of the main outcomes in breast-cancer prevention trials. *Lancet* 2003; 361:296–300.

Darby SC, Whitley E, Howe GR, et al: Radon and cancers other than lung cancer in underground miners: a collaborative analysis of 11 studies. *J Natl Cancer Inst* 1995; 87: 378–383.

Daya-Grosjean L, Dumaz N, Sarasin A: The specificity of p53 mutation spectra in sunlight induced human cancers. *J Photochem Photobiol B* 1995; 28:115–124.

Daya-Grosjean L, Sarasin A: UV-specific mutations of the human patched gene in basal cell carcinomas from normal individuals and xeroderma pigmentosum patients. *Mutat Res* 2000; 450:193–199.

De Gruijl FR, Forbes PD. UV-induced skin cancer in a hairless mouse model. *Bioessays* 1995; 17:651–660.

De Gruijl FR, van Kranen HJ, Mullenders LHF. UV-induced DNA damage, repair, mutations and oncogenic pathways in skin cancer. *J Photochem Photobiol B* 2001; 63:19–27.

Denissenko MF, Pao A, Tang M-S, Pfeifer GP: Preferential formation of benzo[*a*]pyrene adducts at lung cancer mutational hotspots in *P53*. *Science* 1996; 274:430–432.

Dipple A: DNA adducts of chemical carcinogens. *Carcinogenesis* 1995; 16:437–441.

Doll R. Hazards of ionizing radiation: 100 years of observations on man. *Br J Cancer* 1995; 72:1339–1349.

Doll R, Wakeford R. Risk of childhood cancer from fetal irradiation. *Br J Radiol* 1997; 70:130–139.

Dumenco L, Allay E, Norton K, Gerson S: The prevention of thymic lymphomas in transgenic mice by human O6-alkylguanine-DNA transferase. *Science* 1993; 259:219–222.

Fearon ER, Vogelstein B: A genetic model for coloroectal tumorigenesis. *Cell* 1992; 61:759–761.

Fry RJM, Ley RD: Ultraviolet radiation carcinogenesis. In Slaga TJ, ed: *Mechanisms of Tumor Promotion* Vol II. Boca Raton FL; CRC Press; 1983:73–96.

Gerson SL: MGMT: its role in cancer aetiology and cancer therapeutics. *Nat Rev Cancer* 2004; 4:296–306.

Goldman M: Cancer risk of low level exposure. *Science* 1996; 271:1821–1822.

Gonzalez FJ: The use of gene knockout mice to unravel the mechanisms of toxicity and chemical carcinogenesis. *Toxicol Lett* 2001; 120:199–208.

Goss PE, Strasser-Weippl K: Aromatase inhibitors for chemoprevention. *Best Practice Res Clin Endocrinol Metab* 2004; 18:113–130.

Grant DM, Hughes NC, Janezic SA, et al: Human acetyltransferase polymorphisms. *Mut Res* 1997; 376:61–70.

Guengerich FP: Metabolism of chemical carcinogens. *Carcinogenesis* 2000; 21:345–351.

Guerrero I, Villasante A, Corces V, Pellicer A: Activation of a c-K-ras oncogene by somatic mutation in mouse lymphoma induced by gamma radiation. *Science* 1984; 225:1159–1169.

Hainaut P, Pfeifer GP: Patterns of p53 G → T transversions in lung cancers reflect the primary mutagenic signature of DNA damage by tobacco smoke. *Carcinogenesis* 2001; 22: 367–374.

Hall EJ. The crooked shall be made straight; dose-response relationships for carcinogenesis. Henry S. Kaplan Distinguished Scientist Award Lecture 2003: *Int J Radiat Biol* 2004; 80:327–337.

Hardie IR, Strong RW, Hartley LCJ, et al: Skin cancer in Caucasian renal allograft recipients living in a sub-tropical climate. *Surgery* 1980; 87:177–180.

Harris CC: Chemical and physical carcinogenesis: advances and perspectives for the 1990s. *Cancer Res* 1991; 51:5023s–5044s.

Harris CC: p53 at the crossroads of molecular carcinogenesis and risk assessment. *Science* 1993; 262:1980–1981.

Hursting SD, Slaga TJ, Fischer SM, et al: Mechanism-based cancer presention approaches: targets, examples, and the use of transgenic mice. *J Natl Cancer Inst* 1999; 91:215–225.

Hussain SP, Amstad P, Raja K, et al: Mutability of p53 hotspot codons to benzo[a]pyrene diol epoxide (BPDE) and the frequency of p53 mutations in nontumorous human lung. *Cancer Res* 2001; 61:6350–6355.

Kamiya K, Yasukawa-Barnes J, Mitchen JM, et al: Evidence that carcinogenesis involves imbalance between epigenetic high frequency initiation and suppression of promotion. *Proc Natl Acad Sci USA* 1995; 92:1332–1336.

Kim PM, Wells PG: Genoprotection by UDP-glucuronosyltransferases in peroxidase dependent, reactive oxygen species-mediated micronucleus initiation by the carcinogens 4-(methylnitrosoamino)-1-(3-pyridyl)-1-butanone and benzo[a]pyrene. *Cancer Res* 1996; 56:1526–1532.

Kiyohara C: Genetic polymorphism of enzymes involved in xenobiotic metabolism and the risk of colorectal cancer. *J Epidemiol* 2000; 10:349–360.

Knudson AG: Two genetic hits (more or less) to cancer. *Nat Rev Cancer* 2001; 1:157–162.

Kress S, Sutter C, Strickland PT, et al: Carcinogen specific mutational pattern in the p53 gene in ultraviolet-B radiation induced squamous cell carcinomas of mouse skin. *Cancer Res* 1992; 52:6400–6403.

Kripke ML: Effects of UV radiation on tumor immunity. *J Natl Cancer Inst* 1990; 82:1392–1396.

Lee JM, Bernstein A: Apoptosis, cancer and the p53 tumour suppressor gene. *Cancer Metastasis Rev.* 1995; 14:149–161.

Liang L, Shao C, Deng L, et al: Radiation-induced genetic instability in vivo depends on p53 status. *Mut Res.* 2002; 502:69–80.

Lima BS, Van der Laan JW: Mechanisms of nongenotoxic carcinogenesis and assessment of human hazard. *Regul Toxicol Pharmacol* 2000; 32:135–143.

Lin DX, Tang YM, Peng Q, et al: Susceptibility to esophageal cancer and genetic polymorphisms in glutathione S-transferases T1, P1, and M1 and cytochrome P4502E1. *Cancer Epidemiol Biomarkers Prev* 1998; 7:1013–1018.

Lippman SM, Hong WK: Cancer prevention science and practice. *Cancer Res* 2002a; 62:5119–5125.

Lippman SM, Hong WK: Cancer prevention by delay. *Clin Cancer Res* 2002b; 8:305–313.

Little JB: Radiation carcinogenesis in vitro: implications for mechanisms. In Hiatt HH, Watson JD, Winston JA, eds. *Origins of Human Cancer*, Book B, *Mechanisms of Carcinogenesis.* Cold Spring Harbor, NY: Cold Spring Harbor Laboratory; 1977:923–939.

Little JB: Changing views of cellular radiosensitivity. *Radiat Res* 1994; 140:299–311.

Little JB: Radiation carcinogenesis. *Carcinogenesis.* 2000; 21:397–404.

Lubin JH, Boice JD, Edling C, et al: Lung-cancer in radon-exposed miners and estimates of risk from indoor exposure. *J Natl Cancer Inst* 1995; 87:817–827.

Maugh TH II: Chemical carcinogens: how dangerous are low doses? *Science* 1978; 202:37–41.

Maze R, Carney JP, Kelley MR, et al: Increasing DNA repair methyltransferase levels via bone marrow stem cell transduction rescues mice from the toxic effects of 1,3-bis(2-chloroethyl)-1-nitrosourea, a chemotherapeutic alkylating agent. *Proc Natl Acad Sci USA* 1996; 93:206–210.

Michalik L, Desvergne B, Wahli W: Peroxisome-proliferator-activated receptors and cancers: complex stories. *Nat Rev Cancer* 2004; 4:61–70.

Michnovicz JJ, Bradlow HL: Altered estrogen metabolism and excretion in humans following consumption of indole-3-carbinole. *Nutr Cancer* 1991; 16:59–66.

Miller MC III, Mohrenweiser HW, Bell DA: Genetic variability in susceptibility and response to toxicants. *Toxicol Lett* 2001; 120:269–280.

Miller RC, Marino SA, Brenner DJ, et al: The biological effectiveness of radon-progeny alpha particles. II Oncogenic transformation as a function of linear energy transfer. *Radiat Res* 1995; 142:54–60.

Miyamoto M, Umetsu Y, Dosaka-Akita H, et al: CYP2A6 gene deletion reduces susceptibility to lung cancer. *Biochem Biophys Res Commun* 1999; 261:658–660.

Morgan WF, Hartmann A, Limoli CL, et al: Bystander effects in radiation-induced genomic instability. *Mut Res* 2002; 504:91–100.

Nakachi K, Imai K, Hayashi S, Kawajiri K: Polymorphisms of the CYP1A1 and glutathione S-transferase genes associated with susceptibility to lung cancer in relation to cigarette dose in a Japanese population. *Cancer Res* 1993; 53:2994–2999.

Nebert DW, McKinnon RA, Puga A: Human drug-metabolizing enzyme polymorphisms: effects on risk of toxicity and cancer. *DNA Cell Biol* 1996; 15:273–280.

Nebert DW, Dalton TP, Okey AB, Gonzalez FJ: Role of aryl hydrocarbon receptor-mediated induction of the CYP1 enzymes in environmental toxicity and cancer. *J Biol Chem* 2004; 279:23847–23850.

Okey AB: Enzyme induction in the cytochrome P450 system. In: Kalow W, ed. *Pharmacogenetics of Drug Metabolism.* New York: Pergamon Press; 1992:549–608.

Omenn GS, Goodman GE, Thornquist MD, et al: Risk factors for lung cancer and for intervention effects in CARET, the beta-carotene and retinol efficacy trial. *J Natl Cancer Inst* 1996; 88:1550–1559.

Perera FP, Weinstein IB: Molecular epidemiology: recent advances and future directions. *Carcinogenesis* 2000; 21:517–524.

Pitot HC III, Dragan YP: Chemical carcinogenesis. In Klaaseen CD, ed. *Casarett & Doull's Toxicology: The Basic Science of Poisons*, 6th ed. New York: McGraw-Hill; 2001:241–319.

Preston DL, Kusumi S, Tomonaga S, et al: Cancer incidence in atomic bomb survivors. Part III: leukemia, lymphoma and multiple myeloma, 1950–1987. *Radiat Res* 1994; 137(Suppl):S68–S97.

Preston DL, Shimizu Y, Pierce DA, et al: Studies of mortality of atomic bomb survivors. Report 13: Solid cancer and non-cancer disease mortality: 1950–1997. *Radiat Res* 2003; 160: 381–407.

Quintanilla M, Brown K, Ramsden M, Balmain A: Carcinogen specific mutation and amplification of Ha-ras during mouse skin carcinogenesis. *Nature* 1986; 322:78–80.

Serrano D, Perego E, Costa A, Decensi A: Progress in chemoprevention of breast cancer. *Crit Rev Oncol/Hematol* 2004; 49:109–117.

Shen H-M, Ong C-N: Mutations of the p53 tumor suppressor gene and ras oncogenes in aflatoxin hepatocarcinogenesis. *Mut Res* 1996; 366:23–44.

Shimizu Y, Nakatsuru Y, Ichinose M, et al: Benzo[a]pyrene carcinogenicity is lost in mice lacking the aryl hydrocarbon receptor. *Proc Natl Acad Sci USA* 2000; 97:779–782.

Sills RC, French JE, Cunningham ML: New models for assessing carcinogenesis: an ongoing process. *Toxicol Lett* 2001; 120:187–198.

Smela ME, Currier SS, Bailey EA, Essigmann JM: The chemistry and biology of aflatoxin B1: from mutational spectrometry to carcinogenesis. *Carcinogenesis* 2001; 22:535–545.

Sporn MB, Suh N: Chemoprevention of cancer. *Carcinogenesis* 2000; 21:525–530.

Streilein JW, Taylor JR, Vincek V et al. Relationship between ultraviolet radiation-induced immunosuppression and carcinogenesis. *J Invest Dermatol* 1994; 103(Suppl 5):107S–111S.

Su T, Bao Z, Zhang QY, et al.: Human cytochrome P450 CYP2A13: predominant expression in the respiratory tract and its high efficiency metabolic activation of a tobacco-specific carcinogen, 4-(methylnitrosamino)-1-(3-pyridyl)-1-butanone. *Cancer Res* 2000; 60:5074–5079.

Syljuasen RG, Krolewski B, Little JB: Molecular events in radiation transformation. *Radiat Res* 2001; 155:215–221.

Tang D, Phillips DH, Stampfer M, et al: Association between carcinogen-DNA adducts in white blood cells and lung cancer risk in the Physicians Health Study. *Cancer Res* 2001; 61:6708–6712.

Tsuneoka Y, Dalton TP, Miller ML, et al.: 4-aminobiphenyl-induced liver and urinary bladder DNA adduct formation in Cyp1a2(−/−) and Cyp1a2(+/+) mice. *J Natl Cancer Inst* 2003; 95:1227–1237.

Tyndale R, Sellers EM: Variable CYP2A6-mediated nicotine metabolism alters smoking behavior and risk. *Drug Metab Dispos* 2001; 29:548–552.

Ullrich RL, Bowles ND, Satterfield LC, Davis CM. Strain-dependent susceptibility to radiation-induced mammary cancer is a result of a difference in epithelial cell sensitivity to transformation. *Radiat Res* 1996; 146: 353–355.

Ullrich RL, Ponnaiya B: Radiation-induced instability and its relation to radiation carcinogenesis. *Int J Radiat Biol.* 1998; 74:747–754.

Uno S, Dalton TP, Derkenne S et al.: Oral exposure to benzo[a]pyrene in the mouse: detoxication by inducible cytochrome P450 is more important than metabolic activation. *Mol Pharmacol* 2004; 65:1225–1237.

Vähäkangas KH, Bennett WP, Castrén K, et al: *p53* and K-*ras* mutations in lung cancers from former and never-smoking women. *Cancer Res* 2001; 61:4350–4356.

Vainio H: Chemoprevention of cancer: a controversial and instructive story. *Br Med Bull* 1999; 55:593–599.

Wang H, Tan W, Hao B, et al.: Substantial reduction in risk of lung adenocarcinoma associated with genetic polymorphism in CYP2A13, the most active cytochrome P450 for the metabolic activation of tobacco-specific carcinogen NNK. *Cancer Res* 2003; 63:8057–8061.

Wang JS, Shen X, He X, et al: Protective alterations in phase 1 and 2 metabolism of aflatoxin B1 by oltipraz in residents of Qidong, People's Republic of China. *J Natl Cancer Inst* 1999; 91:347–354.

Williams D: Cancer after nuclear fallout: lessons from the Chernobyl accident. *Nat Rev Cancer* 2002: 2:543–549.

Wynder EL, Hoffmann D: Smoking and lung cancer: scientific challenges and opportunities. *Cancer Res* 1994; 54: 5284–5295.

Yoon J-H, Smith LE, Feng Z, et al: Methylated CpG dinucleotides are the preferential targets for G-to-T transversion mutations induced by benzo[a]pyrene diol epoxide in mammalian cells: similarities with the p53 mutational spectrum in smoking-associated lung cancers. *Cancer Res* 2001; 61:7110–7117.

Yuspa SH: Overview of carcinogenesis: past, present and future. *Carcinogenesis* 2000; 21:341–344.

Zeigler A, et al: Mutation hotspots due to sunlight in the p53 gene of nonmelanoma skin cancers. *Proc Natl Acad Sci USA* 1993; 90:4216–4220.

Zhang R, Haag JD, Gould MN: Quantitating the frequency of initiation and cH-ras mutation in *in situ* N-methyl-N-nitrosourea-exposed rat mammary gland. *Cell Growth Differ* 1991; 2:1–6.

# 4

# Methods of Molecular Analysis

*Suzanne Kamel-Reid, Cheryl H. Arrowsmith, Patricia P. Reis, and Jeremy A. Squire*

## 4.1 INTRODUCTION

Advances in chromosomal and genetic analysis have occurred rapidly and have played a central role in the conceptual understanding of cancer. Initial genetic analysis of tumors was limited to gross chromosomal abnormalities, but impressive progress in molecular biology has yielded a diversity of molecular methods to understand alterations in cancer cells. This progress has resulted in the development of specific molecular tools to rapidly assay genetic changes in tumors. This chapter reviews the cytogenetic, molecular genetic, and proteomic methods used to study the molecular basis of cancer, and highlights methodologies that are likely to affect cancer management.

## 4.2 CHROMOSOMAL ANALYSIS OF CANCER CELLS

Cancer arises as a result of the accumulation of genetic changes that confer a selective advantage to the cells in which they occur. These changes consist of mutations in specific genes, as well as chromosomal aberrations. They usually occur in somatic cells, but some genetic changes are heritable and cause a predisposition to cancer. While molecular techniques can identify DNA mutations, cytogenetics provides an overall description of chromosome number, structure, and the extent and nature of chromosomal abnormalities.

Chromosomes are conventionally examined at the metaphase stage of mitosis, when they become condensed and have a defined, reproducible appearance under the microscope (Swansbury and Constant, 2003). DNA replication occurs before mitosis, so that each chromosome consists of two identical sister chromatids held together at the centromere. Exposure of the tumor cells to colcemid or a related agent arrests them in metaphase by disrupting the formation of the mitotic spindle fibers that normally separate the chromatids. The cells are then swollen in a hypotonic solution, fixed in methanol-acetic acid, and metaphase spreads are prepared by dropping the fixed cells onto glass microscope slides.

Chromosomes are recognized in preparations of metaphase cells by their size and shape and by the pattern of light and dark bands observed after staining using specific procedures. Methods for improving the yield of dividing cells and for high-resolution banding of elongated chromosomes, developed in the 1980s, allowed the precise definition of chromosomal aberrations in tumors as well as the identification of rearrangements. Using these techniques, most tumor cells can now be shown to have defects involving different chromosomes (reviewed in Swansbury and Constant, 2003). Chromosomes are identified by one of several staining techniques that produce a characteristic series of bands along the chromosomes. The most popular way of generating banded chromosomes is a brief proteolytic digestion with trypsin, followed by exposure to Giemsa stain. The number of detectable dark-stained G bands depends on the quality of the chromosome spread and the stage of the cell in mitosis. Cells spread at prophase can have over 800 identifiable bands. However, a typical metaphase spread prepared using conventional methods (Fig. 4.1) has approximately 550 bands (reviewed in Verma and Babu, 1995). Analysis of G-banded chromosome preparations is performed us-

ing bright-field microscopy and photography. Modern cytogenetics laboratories usually use electronic cameras and analyze metaphase chromosomes with the help of computers attached to the microscope. The end result of cytogenetic analyses is a karyotype, which, in written form, describes the chromosomal complement using the internationally accepted cytogenetic nomenclature summarized in Table 4.1. A more detailed description of the accepted international nomenclature for describing chromosomes can be found in Heim and Mitelman (1995). An example of a high quality G-banded karyotype from a leukemic cell is shown in Figure 4.1.

Many techniques are used to obtain dividing tumor cells for cytogenetic analysis. Leukemias and lymphomas are easily dispersed into single cells suitable for chromosomal analysis, and more data are available for these diseases than for solid tumors (Table 4.2). Cells from these tumors can be obtained from peripheral blood, bone marrow, or lymph node biopsies. Because malignant cells proliferate, it is usually not necessary to stimulate them to divide or to incubate them in tissue culture prior to analysis.

In contrast, cytogenetic analysis of solid tumors presents several difficulties. First, the cells are tightly bound

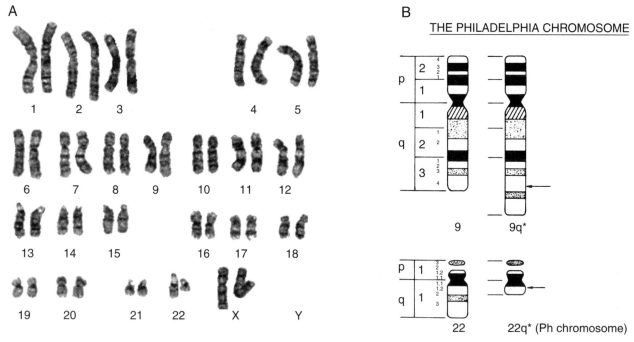

**Figure 4.1.** The photograph on the left (*A*) shows a typical karyotype from a patient with chronic myelogenous leukemia. By international agreement, the chromosomes are numbered according to their appearance following G-banding. Note the loss of material from the long arm of one copy of the chromosome 22 pair (*the chromosome on the right*) and its addition to the long arm of one copy of chromosome 9 (*also the chromosome on the right of the pair*). (*B*). A schematic illustration of the accepted band pattern for this rearrangement (p denotes the short arm and q the long arm of the chromosome). The arrows indicate the precise position of the break points that are involved. The karyotypic nomenclature for this particular chromosomal abnormality is t(9;22)(q34;q11). This description means that there is a reciprocal translocation between chromosomes 9 and 22 with break points at q34 on chromosome 9 and q11 on chromosome 22. The rearranged chromosome 22 is sometimes called the *Philadelphia chromosome* (or Ph chromosome), after the city of its discovery.

**Table 4.1.** Nomenclature for Chromosomes and Their Abnormalities

| Description | Meaning |
|---|---|
| −1 | Loss of one chromosome 1 |
| +7 | Gain of extra chromosome 7 |
| 2q- or del (2q) | Deletion of part of long arm of chromosome 2 |
| 4p + | Addition of material to short arm of chromosome 4 |
| t(9;22)(q34;q11) | Reciprocal translocation between chromosomes 9 and 22 with break points at q34 on chromosome 9 and q11 on chromosome 22 |
| iso(6p) | Isochromosome with both arms derived from the short arm of chromosome 6 |
| inv(16)(p13q22) | Part of chromosome 16 between p13 and q22 is inverted |

together and must be dispersed by mechanical means and/or by digestion with proteolytic enzymes (e.g., collagenase). These procedures can damage cells. Second, the mitotic index in solid tumors is often low, making it difficult to find enough metaphase cells to obtain good-quality cytogenetic preparations. Third, lymphoid and myeloid cells often infiltrate solid tumors and may be confused with the malignant cell population. Despite these difficulties, cytogenetic analyses of several types of solid tumors have identified a large number of chromosomal aberrations. Subsequent studies have allowed some of the oncogenes involved to be recognized and cloned (Tsang et al., 1999).

The study of solid tumors has been facilitated by new analytic approaches that combine elements of conventional cytogenetics with molecular methodologies. This new hybrid discipline is called *molecular cytogenetics*, and its application in tumor analysis usually involves the use of techniques based on *fluorescence in situ hybridization* or FISH (described in Sec. 4.4.1).

## 4.3 MOLECULAR ANALYSIS

Advances in technology have made it possible to identify and isolate specific genes, and it is often easier to isolate a gene than its protein product. The nucleotide sequence can be determined from an isolated gene, and the amino acid sequence of its product can be deduced. It is possible to synthesize small peptides corresponding to the proposed amino acid sequence of the product and to make antibodies against these sequences. Often the antibodies will react with the complete protein,

**Table 4.2.** Common Chromosomal Abnormalities in Lymphoid and Myeloid Malignancies

| Malignancy | Chromosomal Aberration[a] | Molecular Lesion |
|---|---|---|
| Acute myeloid leukemia (AML) | | |
| M1, M2 subtypes | t(8;21)(q22;q22) | *AML1-MTG8* fusion |
| M3 subtype | t(15;17)(q22;q11.2) | *PML-RARA* fusion |
| M4Eo subtype | inv(16)(p13;q22) or t(16;16)(p13;q22) | *MYH11-CBFB* fusion |
| M2 or M4 subtypes | t(6;9)(p23;q24) | *DEK-CAN* fusion |
| Therapy-related AML | ~5/del(5q), ~7/del(7q) | |
| Chronic myeloid leukemia (CML) | t(9;22)(q34;q11) (Ph[1] chromosome) | *BCR-ABL* fusion encoding p210 protein |
| CML blast crisis | t(9;22)(q34;q11), 8, +Ph[1], 19, or i(17q) | *BCR-ABL* fusion encoding p210 protein, *TP53* mutation |
| Acute lymphocytic leukemia (ALL) | t(9;22)(q34;q11) | *BCR-ABL* fusion encoding p190 protein |
| Pre-B ALL | t(1;19)(q23;p13.3) | *E2A-PBX1* fusion |
| Pre-B ALL | t(17;19)(q22;p13.3) | *E2A-HLF* fusion |
| B-ALL, Burkitt's lymphoma | t(8;14)(q24;q32) t(2;8)(p12;q24) t(8;22)(q24;q11) | Translocations between *myc* and *IgH, IgLκ* and *IgLλ* loci |
| B-Chronic lymphocytic leukemia | +12,t(14q32) | Translocations of *IgH* locus |

[a]For an interpretation of the nomenclature of chromosomal rearrangements, see Table 4.1.

*Source*: Adapted from Sheer and Squire (1996).

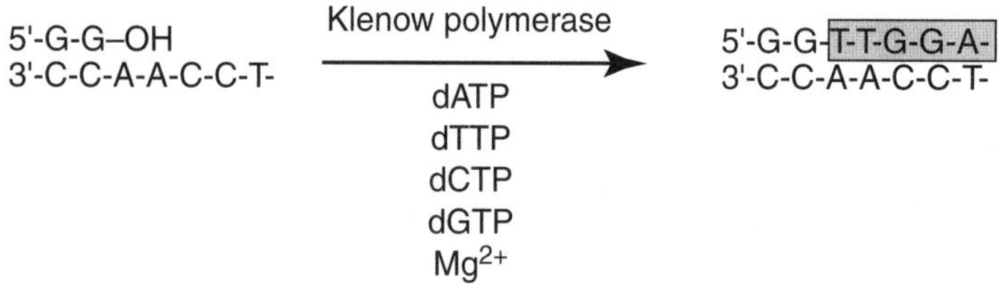

5'-G-G—OH                 Klenow polymerase            5'-G-G-T-T-G-G-A-
3'-C-C-A-A-C-C-T-     ⟶                                3'-C-C-A-A-C-C-T-
                              dATP
                              dTTP
                              dCTP
                              dGTP
                              Mg²⁺

**Figure 4.2.** Synthesis of a complementary strand of DNA (*stippled*) using the Klenow fragment of DNA polymerase I. The substrate is a 3'-hydroxyl end of a primer hybridized to a single-stranded template. The primer is usually a short, synthetic, single-stranded oligonucleotide. All four nucleotides and magnesium ions are also required for DNA polymerases.

allowing the subsequent isolation and purification of the gene product. The following sections describe those techniques commonly used for the genetic analysis of tumors. For additional information, the reader is referred to comprehensive reviews on molecular genetics (e.g., Ausubel et al., 2003).

### 4.3.1 Hybridization of Nucleic Acid Probes

The ability of single-stranded nucleic acids to hybridize, or renature, with their complementary sequence is fundamental to the majority of techniques used in molecular genetic analysis. The DNA of most organisms is double stranded; that is, it is composed of two complementary strands of specific sequences of the four nucleotide bases (A, C, G, or T). When double-stranded DNA is heated, the complementary strands separate (denature) to form single-stranded DNA. Given suitable conditions, the separated complementary regions of DNA can join together to re-form a double-stranded molecule. This renaturation process is called *hybridization*. DNA strands that are not highly complementary will not hybridize to one another or interfere with complementary strand hybridization. Duplexes can form between complementary single-stranded DNA molecules or between one DNA molecule and one RNA molecule.

The fidelity of base pairing in DNA replication is determined by DNA polymerase enzymes, which usually add only the correct base specified by the template strand in elongating a new strand. Commercial DNA polymerases have been isolated and purified from *Escherichia coli* bacteria. The most frequently used polymerase enzyme is the large fragment of DNA polymerase I, often referred to as the *Klenow fragment*. This enzyme adds nucleotides to the 3'-hydroxyl (3'-OH) end of an oligonucleotide hybridized to a template (Fig. 4.2), thus leading to synthesis of a complementary new strand of DNA. By including radionucleotides in the reaction mixture, the complementary copy of the template can be used as a highly sensitive radioactive probe in techniques that depend on DNA hybridization, such as southern blotting (see Sec. 4.3.4) or screening bacteria to isolate cloned DNA probes (see Sec. 4.3.3). The success of most of the molecular techniques described in the following sections results from the extraordinary sensitivity of the hybridization process and the fidelity of the polymerase.

### 4.3.2 Restriction Enzymes

Restriction enzymes are endonucleases that have the ability to cut DNA only at sites of specific nucleotide sequences and always cut the DNA at exactly the same place within the designated sequence. Restriction enzymes were first discovered in bacterial cells, where their functions include protection against infecting viruses and, perhaps, participation in DNA repair and recombination. Similar enzymes may exist in mammalian cells, but few have been characterized. Figure 4.3 illustrates some commonly used restriction enzymes together with

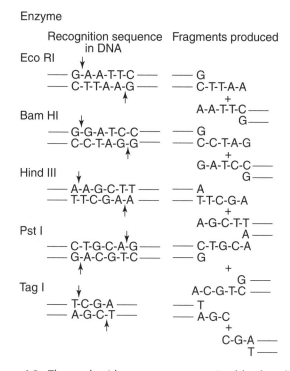

**Figure 4.3.** The nucleotide sequences recognized by five different restriction endonucleases are shown. On the left-hand side, the sequence recognized by the enzyme is shown; the sites where the enzymes cut the DNA are shown by the arrows. On the right side, the two fragments produced following digestion with that restriction enzyme are shown. Note that each recognition sequence is a palindrome; that is, the first two or three bases are complementary to the last two or three bases. For example, for Eco RI, GAA is complementary to TTC. Also note that following digestion, each fragment has a single-stranded tail of DNA. This tail is useful in allowing fragments cut with the same restriction enzyme to anneal with each other.

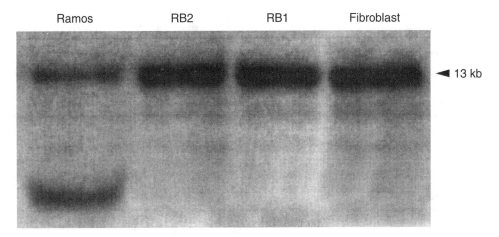

**Figure 4.4.** In the experiment shown, DNA was extracted from normal fibroblasts, from cells from two different retinoblastoma tumors (RB1, RB2), and from a Burkitt's lymphoma (Ramos). The DNA was digested with the restriction enzyme EcoR1 and probed with a DNA fragment specific for the c-*myc* oncogene. As shown in the figure, all of the samples have the usual germline-sized piece of DNA at 13 kb. However, in the Ramos tumor in which the t(8;14) translocation occurs in the middle of this oncogene, there is a new fragment of smaller size. Such an analysis illustrates the ease with which abnormalities in DNA can be detected by restriction endonuclease digestion and the southern blot technique.

the sequence of nucleotides that they recognize and the position at which they cut the sequence.

Restriction enzymes are important because they allow DNA to be cut into reproducible segments that can be analyzed precisely. For example, Figure 4.4 presents a study of the *MYC* gene using southern blotting of DNA (see Sec. 4.3.4) from a number of human cell lines. After DNA is cut with EcoR1, this gene is found on a DNA fragment of 13 kilobase (kb) pairs. In contrast, an identical analysis of the cell line Ramos yields a much smaller fragment, indicating either mutation or rearrangement near this gene.

An important feature of many restriction enzymes is that they create sticky ends. These ends occur because the DNA is cut in a different place on the two strands. When the DNA molecule separates, the cut end has a small single-stranded portion that can hybridize to other fragments having compatible sequences (i.e., fragments digested using the same restriction enzyme). The presence of sticky ends allows investigators to cut and paste pieces of DNA together, as described in Section 4.3.3.

### 4.3.3 Manipulation of Genes and Generation of a Cloned Probe or DNA Library

A gene contains DNA sequences that carry all of the information necessary to specify the amino acid sequence of the corresponding protein. In higher organisms, the gene consists of coding and noncoding regions. The coding regions, called *exons*, are usually interrupted by noncoding regions, called *introns*. After the mRNA is synthesized from the DNA template, the sequences complementary to the introns are removed (spliced out), so that the mRNA is complementary only to the coding sequence. A complementary DNA strand (cDNA) can be synthesized using mRNA as the template by a reverse transcriptase enzyme. The cDNA then contains only the exons of the gene from which the mRNA was transcribed.

Once a gene has been identified, the DNA segment of interest is usually inserted into a bacterial virus or plasmid to facilitate its manipulation and propagation. Figure 4.5 presents a schematic of how a restriction fragment of DNA containing the coding sequence of a gene can be inserted into a bacterial plasmid conferring resistance against the drug ampicillin to the host bacterium. The plasmid or virus is referred to as a *vector* carrying the passenger DNA sequence of the gene of interest. The vector DNA can be cut with the same restriction enzyme used to prepare the cloned gene, so that all the fragments will have compatible sticky ends and can be spliced back together. The spliced fragments can be sealed with the enzyme DNA ligase, and the reconstituted molecule can be introduced into bacterial cells. Because bacteria that take up the plasmid are resistant to the drug (e.g., ampicillin), they can be isolated and propagated to large numbers. In this way, large quantities of a gene can be obtained (i.e., cloned) and labeled with either radioactivity or biotin for use as a DNA probe for analysis in southern or northern blots (see Sec. 4.3.4). Cloned DNA can be used directly for nucleotide sequencing (see Sec. 4.3.8), or for transfer into other cells (see Sec. 4.3.10). Alternatively, the starting DNA may be a complex mixture of dif-

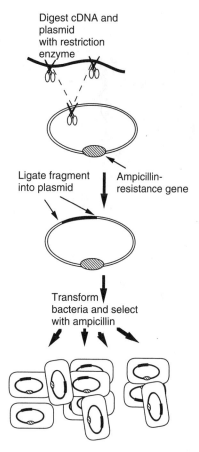

is outlined schematically in Figure 4.6B. The DNA to be analyzed is cut into defined lengths using a restriction enzyme, and the fragments are separated by electrophoresis through an agarose gel. Under these conditions the DNA fragments are separated based on size,

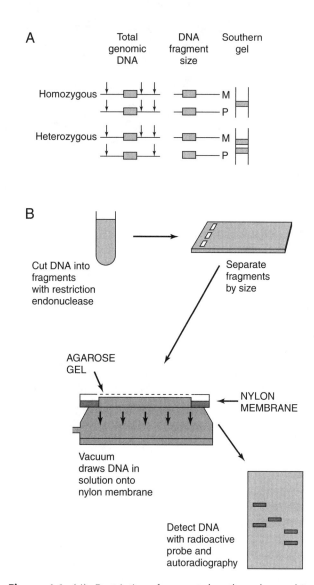

**Figure 4.5.** Insertion of a gene into a bacterial plasmid. The cDNA probe (*black line*) is digested with a restriction endonuclease (depicted by scissors) to generate a defined fragment of cDNA with sticky ends. The circular plasmid DNA is cut with the same restriction endonuclease to generate single-stranded ends that will hybridize and circularize with the cDNA fragment. The recombinant DNA plasmid can be selected for growth using antibiotics because the ampicillin resistance gene (*hatched*) is included in the construct. In this way large amounts of the human cDNA probe can be obtained.

ferent restriction fragments derived from human cells. Such a mixture could contain enough DNA so that the entire human genome is represented in the passenger DNA inserted into the vectors. When a large number of different DNA fragments have been inserted into a vector population and then introduced into bacteria, the result is a *DNA library*, which can be plated out and screened by hybridization with a specific probe. In this way an individual *recombinant DNA clone* can be isolated from the library and used for most of the other applications described in the following sections.

### 4.3.4 Blotting Techniques

Southern blotting is a widely used method for analyzing the structure of DNA that involves the blotting of DNA onto a supporting matrix. The southern blot technique

**Figure 4.6.** (*A*) Restriction fragment length polymorphism analysis of DNA. In a normal cell there are two copies of each piece of DNA, one derived from the maternal chromosome (M) and one from the paternal chromosome (P). The restriction sites for a specific restriction enzyme (*designated by the arrows*) are shown for each chromosome. Suppose that in an individual, the first restriction site to the right of a unique DNA sequence on the paternal chromosome has mutated and is missing. The result of this mutation is that the gene will be found on a smaller fragment of DNA from the maternal chromosome than from the paternal chromosome. Thus, a southern blot of DNA from the cells will show two bands, one identifying the maternal chromosome and one identifying the paternal chromosome. (*B*) Analysis of DNA by southern blotting. Schematic outline of the procedures involved in analyzing DNA fragments by the southern blotting technique. The method is described in more detail in Section 4.3.4.

with the smallest fragments migrating farthest in the gel and the largest remaining near the origin. Pieces of DNA of known size are electrophoresed at the same time and act as a molecular weight scale. A piece of nylon membrane is then laid on top of the gel and a vacuum pump is used to draw fluid through the gel into the membrane. This suction causes the DNA to migrate from the gel to the nylon membrane, where it is immobilized and cannot diffuse further. A common application of the southern technique is to determine the size of the fragment of DNA that carries a particular gene. For such an analysis, a cloned gene can be isolated and made radioactive. The nylon membrane containing all the fragments of DNA cut with a restriction enzyme is incubated in a solution containing the radioactively labeled gene (see Fig. 4.6). Under these conditions, the gene, usually called a probe, will anneal with homologous DNA sequences present on the membrane. Gentle washing will remove the single-stranded, unbound probe; hence the only DNA fragments remaining on the membrane that contain radioactively-labeled material will be those homologous sequences that hybridized with the labeled probe. To detect the region of the membrane containing the radioactive material, the nylon sheet is simply placed on top of a piece of x-ray film, enclosed in a dark container and placed at −70 °C for several hours to expose the film. The film is then developed and the places where the radioactive material is located show up as dark bands (see Fig. 4.4).

An almost identical procedure can be used to characterize messenger RNA. In this case, RNA is separated by electrophoresis, transferred to nylon membranes, and probed with a labeled, cloned fragment of DNA. The technique is called northern blotting and is used to evaluate the expression patterns of genes. An analogous procedure, called western blotting, has also been devised to characterize proteins. Following separation by denaturing gel electrophoresis, the proteins are immobilized by transfer to a charged synthetic membrane. To identify specific proteins, the membrane is incubated in a solution containing a specific primary antibody, then incubated with a secondary antibody that will bind to the primary antibody and is conjugated to horseradish peroxidase (HRP) or biotin. The antibody will bind only to the region of the membrane containing the protein of interest. The protein antibody conjugate can be detected by exposure to chemoluminescence detection reagents. The emitted fluorescent light is then identified by short exposure to photographic film, allowing the bands of interest to be identified.

## 4.3.5 The Polymerase Chain Reaction

A limitation of blotting techniques is that many cells are required to produce enough DNA or RNA for hybridization analysis, and signals are often so weak that visualization requires several days of autoradiography. The polymerase chain reaction (PCR) addresses this problem of sensitivity. A DNA polymerase enzyme called *Taq* polymerase (which is resistant to denaturation at high temperatures) and specific oligonucleotide primers are used to increase the amount of target DNA for analysis. Usually DNA of about 200 to 1000 base pairs is amplified. Analysis by PCR requires precise knowledge of the sequences flanking the region of interest. Two short oligonucleotides complementary to the flanking regions can then be synthesized or obtained commercially, and these are used as primers for *Taq* polymerase. To amplify DNA, all components of the reaction-target DNA, primers, deoxynucleotides, and *Taq* polymerase are placed in a small tube. The reaction sequence is accomplished by simply changing the temperature of the reaction mixture in a cyclical way (see Fig. 4.7A). A typical PCR reaction would involve:

1. Incubation at 94 °C to denature (separate) the DNA duplex and create single-stranded DNA.
2. Incubation at 53 °C to allow hybridization of new primers, which are in vast excess (this temperature may vary depending on the sequence of the primers).
3. Incubation at 72 °C to allow *Taq* polymerase to synthesize new DNA from the primers.

Repeating this cycle permits another round of amplification (Fig. 4.7B). Each cycle takes only a few minutes, the precise time depending on the nature of the primers and the length of DNA to be amplified. Generally, twenty-five to forty cycles can be completed in two to five hours. Twenty cycles can theoretically produce a million-fold amplification that can usually be visualized as a bright ethidium bromide-stained band after a short period of gel electrophoresis (Fig. 4.7C). Polymerase chain reaction products can then be sequenced or subjected to other methods of genetic analysis. Polymerase proteins with greater heat stability and copying fidelity have been recently developed, allowing for long-range amplification using primers separated by as much as 15 to 30 kilobases of intervening target DNA (Ausubel et al., 2003).

The polymerase chain reaction is exquisitely sensitive and its applications include the detection of minimal residual disease in hematopoietic malignancies and of circulating cancer cells from solid tumors. Experiments have shown that as low a ratio as one leukemic cell in $10^5$ to $10^6$ normal cells can be detected with the appropriate PCR conditions.

With a slight modification, PCR can also be used to study gene expression or screen for mutations in RNA. It is first necessary to use reverse transcriptase to make a complementary single-strand DNA copy (cDNA) of an mRNA prior to performing the PCR. The cDNA is used as a template for a PCR reaction as described above.

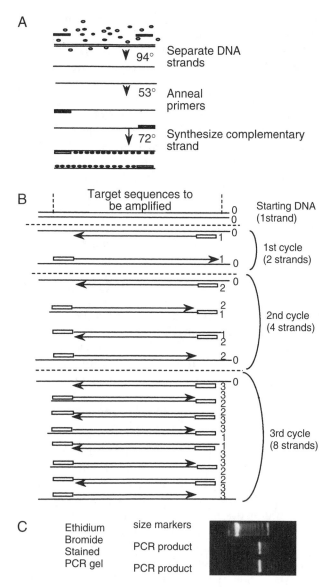

**Figure 4.7.** (*A*) Reaction sequence for one cycle of PCR. Each line represents one strand of DNA; the small rectangles are primers and the circles are nucleotides. (*B*) The first three cycles of PCR are shown schematically. (*C*) Ethidium-bromide–stained gel after 20 cycles of PCR. (See Sec. 4.3.5 for further explanation.)

This technique, which is usually called *reverse transcription PCR* (RT-PCR), allows amplification of cDNA corresponding to both abundant and rare RNA transcripts, thereby providing a convenient source of DNA that can be screened for mutations. The RT-PCR technique can also provide approximate quantitation of expression of a particular gene (Ausubel et al., 1996). It is ideal for the detection of tumors with reciprocal chromosome translocations because the fusion transcript generated by the rearrangement is present only in tumor cells and thus provides a unique substrate for RT-PCR. Polymerase chain reaction technology is used increasingly to detect gene rearrangements and molecular markers

for use in diagnosis and prognosis (Olavarria et al., 2001; Grimwade and Coco, 2002; reviewed in Ausubel, 2003).

### 4.3.6 Quantitative Real-Time Polymerase Chain Reaction

Although PCR has increased the ability to detect and manipulate low copy sequences, accurate quantification of these sequences has been problematic. The development of real-time quantitative PCR has eliminated the variability often associated with PCR, and has allowed the quantitation of low amounts of template. Similarly, quantitative reverse-transcription polymerase chain reaction has proven to be a sensitive method to detect low levels of mRNA (often obtained from small samples or microdissected tissues) and to quantify gene expression. Different chemistries are available for real-time detection of RNA and DNA. There is a very specific 5′ nuclease assay, which uses a fluorogenic probe for the detection of reaction products after amplification, and there is a less specific but much less expensive assay, which uses a fluorescent dye (SYBR Green I) for the detection of double-stranded DNA products. In both methods the fluorescence emission from each sample is collected by a charge-coupled device-camera and the data are automatically processed and analyzed by computer software.

Quantitative real-time PCR using fluorogenic probes can analyze multiple genes simultaneously within the same reaction and results in both amplification and analysis of samples with no need for post-PCR processing or gels. This methodology allows the simultaneous analysis of approximately 100 samples within two hours and is thus compatible with high-throughput sample analysis.

*SYBR Green I*    SYBR Green I fluorescent dye is a highly specific double-stranded DNA binding dye that allows the detection of product accumulation during each PCR cycle (Simpson et al., 2000). Unbound SYBR Green I dye exhibits little fluorescence. During primer annealing, a few molecules bind to the double-stranded primer-target sequence, resulting in light emission upon excitation. During the polymerization step, many molecules bind to the newly synthesized DNA, and there is an increase in fluorescence that is monitored in real time. At denaturation the SYBR Green molecules are released and the fluorescence signal decreases in intensity to background levels (Bustin, 2000). Figure 4.8 illustrates the SYBR Green I methodology. SYBR Green I dye is not sequence-specific and is thus able to bind and detect all double-stranded DNA, including nonspecific amplification products. Thus, a high quality reaction is necessary for accurate quantitative results.

*Fluorescent Probes and Molecular Beacons*    Real-time PCR generally uses separate PCR primers and probes, and the generation of a fluorescent signal depends on the molecular interactions between template, primers, and probe. Real-time PCR can also be performed using molecular beacons (see below). Both methods present comparable sensitivity and reproducibility (Hein et al., 2001). The use of the 5′ exonuclease activity of *Taq* polymerase in combination with a probe enables the detection of a specific PCR product as it accumulates during PCR and offers the advantage of a very sensitive quantification of small amounts of nucleic acid. In addition to the sense and antisense primers, a nonextendable oligonucleotide probe with a fluorescent reporter dye (e.g., FAM) attached to the 5′-end, and a quencher dye (e.g., TAMRA) at the 3′-end hybridizes downstream of the sense primer to the target sequence. In the molecular beacons, fluorophore and quencher may be separated by up to 40 bp and quenching is achieved by a process called *fluorescence resonance energy transfer*. The fluorophore is the donor molecule and transfers its energy to the quencher molecule that releases energy as a fluorescence emission. During the extension phase in the PCR reaction, *Taq* polymerase hydrolyzes the probe and leads to generation of a fluorescent signal that is directly proportional to the amount of PCR product (Fig. 4.9). This fluorescent signal is monitored in real time.

Real-time PCR has many potential clinical and research applications (Bustin and Dorudi, 1998), such as in the detection of aneuploidy (Wilke et al., 2000) and the detection of micrometastasis or minimal residual disease in a variety of tumors (Cheung and Cheung, 2001; Li et al., 2002), as well as in the molecular staging of tumors (D'Cunha et al., 2002). Molecular beacons have been used for the high-throughput screening of single nucleotide polymorphisms (SNPs) in real-time PCR assays (Mhlanga and Malmberg, 2001; see Sec. 4.3.7). When hybridizing to the target sequence, molecular beacons are forced to undergo a conformational change forming a probe-target hybrid that includes more base pairs and is thus more stable. This conformational change causes the fluorophore and the quencher molecule to move away from each other and fluorescence is thus emitted.

### 4.3.7 Single Nucleotide Polymorphisms (SNPs)

DNA sequences can differ at single nucleotide positions within the genome. These single nucleotide polymorphisms (SNPs) can occur as frequently as 1 out of every 1000 base pairs. Single nucleotide polymorphisms can occur in both introns and exons; in introns they generally have little effect, but in exons they can affect protein structure and function. For example, SNPs may be involved in altered drug metabolism due to their modifying effect on the cytochrome p450 metabolizing enzymes. They also contribute to disease (e.g., SNPs that

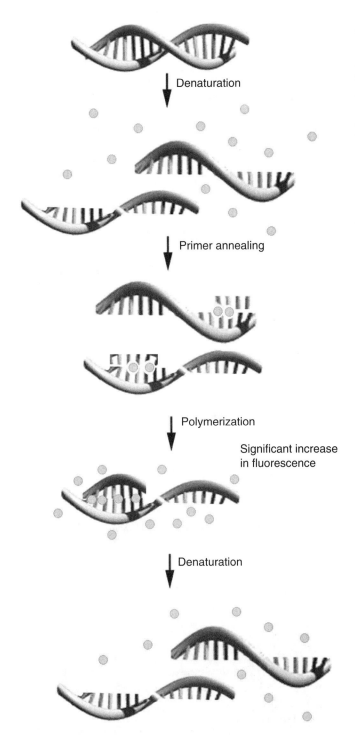

**Figure 4.8.** Real-time PCR using SYBR Green I dye. During denaturation, unbound SYBR Green I dye exhibits low fluorescence intensity. At the annealing temperature, a few dye molecules bind to the double-stranded DNA target, resulting in an increase in fluorescence emission. During the polymerization step, several molecules of the dye bind to the newly synthesized DNA and a significant increase in fluorescence is detected and can be monitored in real time.

Denaturation

Primer annealing

Polymerization

Significant increase in fluorescence

Denaturation

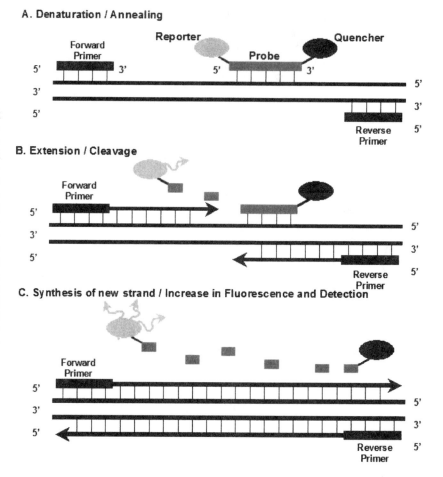

**Figure 4.9.** Real-time PCR using fluorescent probes and molecular beacons. During denaturation, both probe and primers are in solution and remain unbound from the DNA strand. During annealing, the probe specifically hybridizes to the target DNA between the primers (*A*). The 5' to 3'exonuclease activity of the DNA polymerase cleaves the probe, thus dissociating the quencher molecule from the reporter molecule, which results in fluorescence of the reporter, indicated by the arrow (*B*). The probe fragments are then displaced from the target DNA, polymerization continues, and an increase in fluorescence emission (*shown by arrows*) by the reporter can be detected (*C*). The amount of fluorescence detected is proportional to the amount of PCR product generated.

result in missense mutations) and disease predisposition (reviewed in Syvanen, 2001). There are many methods to characterize SNPs (reviewed in Syvanen, 2001), and they are being optimized for high-throughput applications. Most methods require PCR amplification of the sample to be genotyped prior to analysis (see Sec. 4.3.5), thus influencing the number of fragments that can be analyzed simultaneously. Denaturing high-performance liquid chromatography (DHPLC) allows the automated detection of single base substitutions, insertions, or deletions. It works under the same principle as single-strand conformation polymorphism (SSCP; see Sec. 4.3.9) analysis, such that under partially denaturing conditions, homoduplexes and heteroduplexes can be differentiated, thus identifying sequences with base pair mismatches. Suspected polymorphic/mutated sites must then be sequenced to verify the presence of such genetic variation (Wolford, 2000; Xiao and Oefner, 2001).

### 4.3.8 Sequencing of DNA

The primary method for characterizing genes and the proteins that they encode is to determine the sequence of the DNA. The most frequently used method is dideoxy-chain termination. The DNA to be sequenced is most often amplified by using PCR.

DNA sequencing is analogous to DNA replication in vitro, but it uses dideoxynucleotide triphosphates (ddNTPs) in the reaction. DNA sequencing is carried out in four separate reactions each containing one of the four ddNTPs (i.e., ddATP, ddCTP, ddGTP, or ddTTP) together with the other normal nucleotides. In each reaction the sequencing primers bind and start the extension of the chain at the same place. The extended primers, however, terminate at different sites when dideoxynucleotides are incorporated (see Fig. 4.10). This produces fragments of different size terminated at every nucleotide. Separation of the newly synthesized radioactive DNA on polyacrylamide gels allows visualization of each fragment produced in the sequencing reaction. The use of polyacrylamide gels allows fragments differing by a single base to be separated. Usually a sequence of 200 to 500 bases can be read from a single gel.

In automated fluorescent sequencing, fluorescent dye labels are incorporated into DNA extension products using 5'-dye labeled primers (dye primers) or 3'-dye labeled dideoxynucleotide triphosphates (dye terminators). Au-

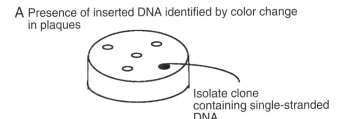

**A** Presence of inserted DNA identified by color change in plaques

Isolate clone containing single-stranded DNA

**B** Anneal the primer to DNA

DNA inserted into vector

Primer

dATP*
dTTP
dGTP
dCTP
dd CTP

+DNA polymerase
* = 32p

**C** Complementary Strand Extension

• = Dideoxy - ddCTP

GGG    G    GG G G

Primer

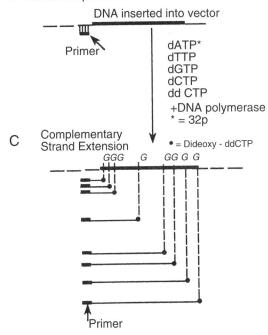

**D**                              Read Autoradiogram

G
G
G
T
T
T
A
T
T
A
C
G
T
C
A
T
A
A
G
G
G

G A T C

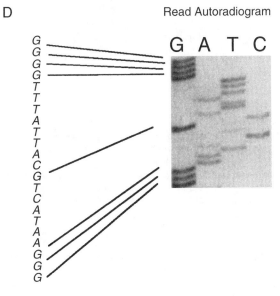

**Figure 4.10.** Colonies containing DNA cloned fragments can be identified and selected in bacterial culture (*A*). Amplification of DNA inserted into vector (*B*) is carried out in separate reactions each one containing one of the four ddNTPs (*C*). Dideoxy-chain termination sequencing, showing an extension reaction to read the position of the nucleotide guanidine (see Sec. 4.3.8 for details). (Part (*D*) Autoradiogram courtesy of Lilly Noble, University of Toronto, Canada).

tomated DNA sequencers can detect fluorescence from four different dyes that are used to identify A, C, G, or T extension reactions. Each dye emits light at a different wavelength when excited by an argon ion laser. All four colors and therefore all four bases are detectable and distinguished in the single lane of a gel. Automated fluorescent sequencing takes advantage of cycle sequencing in which successive rounds of denaturation, annealing, and extension result in linear amplification of extension products. The advantage to cycle sequencing is that it is robust and easy to perform, much less DNA template is required than single-temperature extension methods and high temperatures reduce the hybridization between primers and nonspecific annealing between primer and template.

The dye-labeled DNA fragments are injected and enter a small glass tube (capillary). Current is applied and the sample electrophoreses through the capillary. When the DNA fragments reach the detector window in the capillary, the laser excites the fluorescent dye labels. Emitted fluorescence from the dyes is collected by a cooled, charge-coupled device (CCD) camera at particular wavelength bands and stored as digital signals on a computer for processing. The sequencing analysis software interprets the results, identifying the bases from the fluorescent intensity at each data point (see Fig. 14.16*H*).

The sequence of a strand of DNA can be compared to data available on public databases such as www. ncbi.nlm.nih.gov to check for regions of sequence similarity. This method has permitted the classification of many genes or small functional parts of genes into families, such as the immunoglobulin supergene family. Genes within these families have homologies ranging from 65 to 100 percent similarity and likely evolved from a common ancestral gene. Such computer comparisons can identify homology to already known gene sequences and increase the speed and efficiency of the gene discovery process. Unique genomic sequence data can rapidly provide the precise chromosomal localization of the gene under study, so that it is then possible to determine whether there is an association between the gene location and the location of recurrent chromosome aberrations in tumors.

### 4.3.9 Identification of Mutations in Tumors

Molecular mutations of DNA may be as small as a single base-pair substitution or can involve deletion or rearrangement of thousands of base pairs of DNA. Smaller mutations present the biggest challenge because identification of a single nucleotide change among thousands of nucleotides may be required. Most methods depend on identifying mismatched bases when complementary strands of a mutant and its normal sequence are allowed to hybridize to form a heteroduplex (double-stranded DNA, where each strand originates from a different source).

*Single-Strand Conformation Polymorphism* Single-strand conformation polymorphism (SSCP) is a commonly used technique for screening for mutations (Ausubel et al., 2003). This technique is fast and easy to perform and detects regions with various types of DNA changes including single base substitutions. SSCP relies on the property of single-stranded DNA having a tendency to adopt complex conformational structures stabilized by weak intramolecular hydrogen bonds. When a mutation is present in the DNA, this will affect the conformation of that sequence and will result in a different electrophoretic mobility relative to the wild-type sequences when DNA in a gel is subjected to an electric field. In a typical SSCP experiment, PCR products are made in the presence of radiolabeled nucleotides using primers flanking the gene of interest. The PCR products are heat denatured to form single strands and subjected to electrophoresis; control samples are run on the same gels so that differences from the wild-type electrophoretic pattern can be detected. The fragments with potential mutations or polymorphisms are detected as shifts from the wild-type control fragments (Fig. 4.11). As SSCP does not provide information about the nature of the change found, DNA sequencing must be performed on that region of the gene.

*Protein Truncation Test*  The protein truncation test is an efficient method for detecting mutations that give rise to premature termination of protein synthesis from a gene. These mutations consist of small deletions or insertions, splice errors, and changes to nonsense codons. The protein truncation test is a PCR-based technique where DNA or cDNA can be used as a template. Polymerase chain reaction products derived from the DNA sequences, which are transcribed into proteins, are amplified using primers specific to the gene of interest. One of the primers is designed to introduce sequences for RNA and consequent protein synthesis into the PCR product. Using an in vitro transcription/translation system, PCR products are copied into mRNA and consequently into the corresponding size of protein molecules. If there is a truncation mutation within the PCR product, a shorter protein will be synthesized as compared to control samples. The synthesized protein products are electrophoresed on a polyacrylamide gel and those resulting from truncation mutations migrate faster and are detected as bands in the gel (Fig. 4.11).

*Heteroduplex Analysis*  Heteroduplex analysis identifies mismatched bases formed when complementary

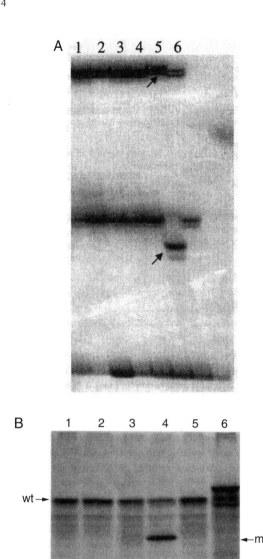

**Figure 4.11.** (*A*) Single-strand conformation polymorphism analysis. Example using the p53-tumor suppressor gene. Exon 9 of the p53 gene has been PCR amplified in a series of tumor DNA samples obtained from breast cancer patients. The PCR products are subjected to nondenaturing polyacrylamide gels and electrophoresed at low temperatures (10–20°C). The band shifts in lane 5 indicate alterations in the gene sequence in exon 9 of the p53 gene. DNA sequencing for band shifts detected by SSCP is always carried out to identify the nature of the sequence alteration. (*B*) The protein truncation test. Example using BRCA1 the hereditary breast and ovarian cancer gene. A region in exon 11 of BRCA1 gene has been analysed in a series of lymphocyte DNA samples from breast cancer patients. The wild-type protein products are indicated as *wt*. The faster running product indicated as *m* in lane 4 demonstrates the presence of a truncation mutation in this sample. (Courtesy of Dr. H. Ozcelik, University of Toronto, and Mount Sinai Hospital, Toronto.)

strands of a mutant and its normal sequence are allowed to hybridize to form a double-strand heteroduplex molecule. This PCR-based technique is sensitive enough to detect single base substitutions in fragments of DNA under 200 bp; however, due to its efficiency and simplicity, it has been used more often in the detection of nucleotide insertions and/or deletions in heterozygous individuals. Heteroduplex formation is carried out by subjecting PCR products to heat denaturation during which PCR molecules are separated into their single-stranded forms, followed by a cooling down step where single-stranded molecules re-anneal to form double-stranded molecules. Compared with homoduplex molecules where base pairing between the strands is complete, the mismatched heteroduplex molecules migrate much more slowly in polyacrylamide gels due to their shape, thus enabling the detection of mutations.

Denaturing high-pressure liquid chromatography is a powerful tool that allows high-throughput profiling of mutations by using temperature modulated heteroduplex analysis. Denaturing high-pressure liquid chromatography has proved effective for the detection of mutations that are difficult to identify using SSCP analysis, and minimizes the number of fragments that require sequencing to verify the presence of mutations. Fragments containing putative mutations can be eluted from the DHPLC column, amplified by PCR, and sequenced using automated sequencing. High sensitivity, accuracy of detection, ease of use, and low cost per sample, combined with automation, make this a powerful method for high-throughput mutational analysis.

*Microsatellite Instability* Short repetitive DNA sequences or microsatellites, consisting of mono-, di-, tri-, and tetranucleotide repeats are widely distributed throughout the genome (Ionov et al., 1993). These repeats are genetically unstable, undergoing alterations in length during DNA replication, either by expansion or contraction of the repeat sequences. Microsatellites form a great source of polymorphic genetic markers and have been used extensively in the construction of detailed linkage maps, whereby genes are associated with particular microsatellites, and in the identification and characterization of genes related to specific diseases. Microsatellite instability has been found to be associated with many sporadic and familial cancers, including hereditary non-polyposis colon cancer (Ionov et al., 1993; Liu et al., 1995), which can be caused by germline mutations in DNA mismatch repair genes (Chap. 2, Sec. 2.3.3). In the tumors of patients with hereditary non-polyposis colon cancer, microsatellite instability is widespread, introducing many somatic mutations into the genome, and probably thereby affecting the function of genes important in colon carcinogenesis. Tumors exhibiting such instability are termed *replication error positive*: they can be identified by analyzing a series of microsatellite repeat loci in the tumor and the normal tissue of the same individual. Oligonucleotide primers flanking the microsatellite loci are used for PCR amplification, with incorporation of a radioactive isotope or a fluorescent dye. Microsatellite instability, indicated by a change in the number of repeated units, can be observed by separating the PCR products according to their size on a polyacrylamide gel. The detection of a difference in the size of a repeat in the tumor tissue as compared to normal tissue indicates the presence of microsatellite instability.

### 4.3.10 Putting New Genes into Cells

The function of a gene can often be studied most effectively by placing it into a cell different from the one from which it was isolated. For example, one may wish to place a mutated oncogene, isolated from a tumor cell, into a normal cell to determine whether it causes malignant transformation. A number of transfection protocols have been developed for efficient introduction of foreign DNA into mammalian cells, including calcium phosphate or DEAE-dextran precipitation, spheroplast fusion, lipofection, electroporation, and transfer using viral vectors (Ausubel et al., 2003). For all methods, the efficiency of transfer must be high enough for easy detection, and it must be possible to recognize and select for cells containing the newly introduced gene.

The classic method for introducing DNA into cells for experimental manipulation is a technique in which calcium phosphate is used to precipitate DNA in large aggregates; for unknown reasons, some cells take up large quantities of such DNA. The mechanism by which *DEAE-dextran transfections* allow for introduction of foreign DNA into cells is similar: The positive charge of the DEAE-dextran polymer neutralizes the negative charge of the DNA polymer, forming a fine precipitate that can come into contact with the plasma membrane of the host cell. The DEAE-dextran/DNA complex is then internalized by pinocytosis.

Other delivery systems involve the use of *viral vectors*, because they can be targeted to a variety of cell types, they persist, and can infect nondividing cells. Retroviruses are very stable because their complementary DNA integrates into the host mammalian DNA, but only relatively small pieces of DNA (up to 10 kilobases) can be transferred. Adenovirus vectors take larger inserts (~36 kilobase) and have a very high efficiency of transfer. Nonviral vectors, such as liposomes, can be used for transient expression of introduced DNA. For *lipofection*, plasmid DNA is complexed with a liposome suspension in serum-free medium. This DNA/liposome complex is added directly to cells grown in tissue culture, and after a three- to five-hour incubation period, fresh medium containing serum is added. The cells are incubated to allow expression of the transfected gene. Electroporation, which entails administration of an electrical current to a cellular-DNA mixture, is also an efficient means of introducing DNA to many cell types.

Whichever method is used to introduce the DNA, it is usually necessary to select for retention of the transferred genes before assaying for expression. For this reason, a selectable gene, such as the gene encoding resistance to the antibiotic neomycin, can be introduced simultaneously by taking advantage of the fact that frequently cells that can take up one gene will also take up another.

### 4.3.11 Site-Directed Mutagenesis and Functional Inactivation of Genes

Following the sequencing of the human genome (and that of other species), a large number of genes are being cloned without any knowledge of their function. Important clues concerning the function of a new gene can be provided by the occurrence of regions of similarity in the amino-acid sequence that can lead to similarities in secondary protein structure. For example, many of the transcription-factor proteins have a characteristic sequence in which DNA-binding takes place

(e.g., leucine-zipper or zinc-finger domain; see Chap. 8, Sec. 8.2.8). One way of testing the putative function of such a sequence is to see whether a mutation within the critical site causes loss of function. In the example of transcription factors, a mutation might result in a protein that failed to bind DNA appropriately. Site-directed mutagenesis permits the introduction of mutations at a precise point in a cloned gene, resulting in specific changes in the amino-acid sequence and, hence, secondary structure of an encoded protein.

By site-directed mutagenesis, amino acids can be deleted, altered, or inserted, but for most experiments, the changes do not alter the reading frame or disrupt protein continuity. There are two main ways of introducing a mutation into a cloned gene (Ausubel et al., 2003). The first method relies on the chance occurrence of a restriction enzyme site in the region one wishes to alter. Typically, the gene is digested with the restriction endonuclease, and a few nucleotides may be inserted or deleted at this site by ligating a small oligonucleotide complementary to the sticky end of the restriction enzyme (see Fig. 4.12A). The second method is more versatile but requires more manipulation. The gene is first obtained in a single-stranded form by cloning into a vector such as M13 (see Sec. 4.3.3). A short oligonucleotide is synthesized containing the desired nucleotide change but otherwise complementary

**Figure 4.12.** Methods for site-directed mutagenesis. (*A*) Insertion of a new sequence at the site of action of a restriction enzyme by ligating a small oligonucleotide sequence within the reading frame of a gene. (*B*) Use of a primer sequence that is synthesized to contain a mismatch at the desired site of mutagenesis.

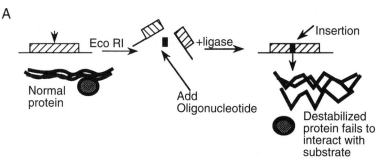

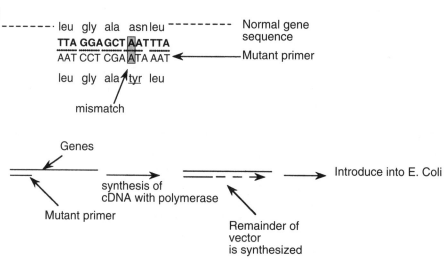

to the region to be mutated. The oligonucleotide will anneal to the single-stranded DNA but contains a mismatch at the site of mutation (see Fig. 4.12B). The hybridized oligonucleotide-DNA duplex is then exposed to DNA polymerase I (plus the four nucleotides and buffers), which will synthesize and extend a complementary strand with perfect homology at every nucleotide except at the site of mismatch in the primer used to initiate DNA synthesis. The double-stranded DNA is then introduced into bacteria, and because of the semi-conservative nature of DNA replication, 50 percent of the vector (M13 phage) produced will contain normal DNA and 50 percent will contain the DNA with the introduced mutation. Several methods allow easy identification of the mutant vector. Using these techniques, the effects of artificially generated mutations can be studied in cell culture or in transgenic mice (see Sec. 4.3.12).

Another approach to studying a gene by functional inactivation is to introduce a DNA or RNA sequence that will specifically inactivate the expression of a target gene. This can be achieved by introducing DNA or RNA molecules with a sequence that is homologous to that contained within a target gene but where the order of the bases is opposite to that of the usual complementary strand (i.e., 3':5' instead of 5':3'). Several investigators have demonstrated that antisense RNA or DNA molecules can combine in vitro specifically with their homologous sequences in mRNA and interfere with the expression of that gene (e.g., see Brantl, 2002). An extension of antisense technology is the recent observation that complementary RNA can directly interfere with gene expression (RNA interference: RNAi), leading to the specific disappearance of the selected gene products (Kittler and Buchholz, 2003; Yin et al., 2003). RNAi interferes with the stability of the mRNA transcript by initiating a degradation process of transcripts arising from the targeted gene. Specific gene inactivation in this way has the potential for therapy of tumors; for example, by inhibiting the expression of an oncogene. A limitation of all the above technologies is that once the nucleic acids enter a cell, they are vulnerable to a variety of cellular nucleases. To be biologically effective, a high concentration of molecules must be efficiently delivered to all cellular targets and must persist inside the cells for a prolonged period of time.

### 4.3.12 Transgenic and Knockout Mice

One way to investigate the effects of gene expression in specific cells on the function of the whole organism is to transfer genes directly into the germline and generate transgenic mice. For example, inappropriate expression of an oncogene in a particular tissue can provide clues about the possible role of that oncogene in normal development and in malignant transformation. Usually a cloned gene with the desired regulatory elements is mi-

croinjected into the male pronucleus of a single-cell embryo so that it can integrate into a host chromosome and become part of the genome of the growing organism. If the introduced gene is incorporated into the germline, the resulting mouse will become a founder for breeding a line of mice, all of which carry the newly introduced gene. Such mice are called *transgenic mice*, and the inserted foreign gene is called a *transgene*. Its expression can be studied in a variety of different cellular environments in a whole animal. Each transgene will have a unique integration site in a host chromosome and will be transmitted to offspring in the same way as a naturally occurring gene. However, the site of integration often influences the expression of a transgene, possibly because of the activity of genes in adjacent chromatin. Sometimes the integration event also alters the expression of endogenous genes (insertional mutation): this observation led to the development of gene-targeting approaches, so that specific genes could be inactivated or knocked out. The effect of the inserted or knocked out gene can then be studied for effects in the mice.

In vivo site-directed mutagenesis is the method by which a mutation is targeted to a specific endogenous gene. Instead of introducing a modified cloned gene at a random position as described above, a cloned gene fragment is targeted to a particular site in the genome by a procedure called *homologous recombination* (reviewed in Zimmer, 1992). This technique relies on the ability of a cloned mammalian gene or DNA fragment to preferentially undergo homologous recombination in a normal cell at its naturally occurring chromosomal position, thereby replacing the endogenous gene. The introduced mutation may result in the knocking out of gene expression, thus facilitating the study of gene function (Fig. 4.13). The same approach can be used to correct a disease mutation in the mouse and restore normal function, thereby allowing murine models for gene therapy to be developed.

In typical targeting experiments, the desired genetic modification is either generated in cloned DNA by techniques described in Section 4.3.3 or, more usually, the gene is disrupted by insertion of a drug resistance gene (e.g., *neo*) into the middle of an endogenous gene, making it impossible to produce the normal protein product. Initially the modified DNA is introduced into pluripotent stem cells derived from a mouse embryo called embryonic stem (ES) cells. The frequency of homologous recombination is low (less than one in a million cells) but is greatly influenced by a variety of factors such as the vector being used, the method of DNA introduction, the length of the regions of homology, and whether the targeted gene is expressed in ES cells.

Homologous recombination with cloned sequences creates predictable novel DNA junctions in the genome that can be conveniently detected by PCR. Oligonucleotide primers flanking the chosen site of recombination

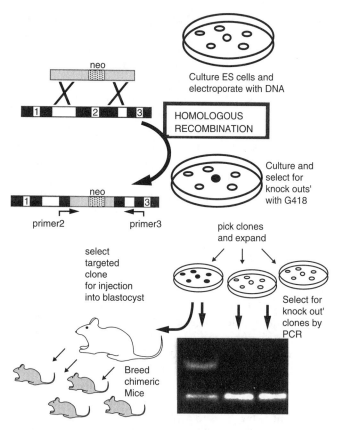

metes are derived from the ES cells, then a breeding line containing the modification of interest can be established. Recent technologic advances in gene targeting by homologous recombination in mammalian systems enable the production of mutants in any desired gene.

It is also possible to generate a *conditionally targeted mutation* within a mouse line using the *cre-loxP system*. This method takes advantage of the properties of the Cre recombinase enzyme first identified in P1 bacteriophage. Cre recognizes a 34 base pair DNA sequence (*loxP*). When two *loxP* sites are oriented in the same direction, the Cre recombinase will excise the sequence in between; when they are oriented in the reverse direction, Cre will induce the inversion of the intervening sequences. This system can be applied to the transgenic mouse in a number of ways (for review, see Babinet and Cohen-Tannoudji, 2001). For example, using the technique of homologous recombination, it is possible to replace a murine genomic sequence with the same sequence containing *loxP* sites, thus flanking a desired region by *loxP* sites. The resulting mice are normal, until the Cre recombinase is introduced. The manner of introduction of the recombinase may also be carefully chosen so that only a specific cell type may be affected, or only a particular phase of differentiation, or both, thus allowing for spatial and temporal control of gene mutation within the mouse genome. This system is particularly advantageous in examining the role of essential genes in the mouse. A mouse knocked out for the gene of interest may not be viable, while a conditional knockout mouse utilizing the *cre-loxP* system may allow one to study the effects of turning the gene on or off in a living animal. The *cre-loxP* system may also be used to generate chromosomal aberrations in a cell-type–specific manner, which can improve understanding of the biology of some human diseases, particularly leukemias.

**Figure 4.13.** Disruption of a gene by homologous recombination in embryonic stem (ES) cells. Exogenous DNA is introduced into the ES cells by electroporation or by one of the methods described in Section 4.3.10. The homologous region on the exogenous DNA is shown in *gray*, the selectable gene neomycin (neo) is *speckled*, and the target exons are *black*. The two recombination points are shown by X's and the exogenous DNA replaces some of the normal DNA of exon 2, thereby destroying its reading frame by inserting the small neo gene. Embryonic stem cells that have undergone a successful homologous recombination are selected as colonies in G418 because of the stable presence of the neo gene. PCR primers for exons 2 and 3 are used to identify colonies in which a homologous recombination event has taken place. ES cells from such positive cells (*dark colony*) are injected into blastocysts, which are implanted into foster mothers (*white*). If germline transmission has been achieved, chimeric mice are bred to generate homozygotes for the knocked out gene.

## 4.4 GENOMIC METHODS OF TUMOR ANALYSIS

The molecular analysis of tumors is a rapidly advancing field in which mechanisms of disease are being elucidated using new profiling methods that have been developed as part of the human genome project (Duggan et al., 1999). Until mapping and characterization of the entire human genome was initiated, the genetic assessment of diseased tissues and tumors relied heavily on single gene analyses or study of an individual protein. Such gene-by-gene methods were very time consuming and did not take into account the collective alterations of genes and proteins during oncogenesis. Global expression analysis using microarrays and the molecular cytogenetic methods described below now allow for the simultaneous analysis of thousands of genes at the DNA, RNA, or protein levels in a high-throughput fashion. These methodologies offer unprecedented opportunities to obtain molecular signatures of tumors.

will generate a diagnostic distinct PCR product only if the modified DNA fragment is present at the correct site of insertion. The ES cells that contain the modified gene are selected by growth in medium containing the drug G418, for which resistance is programmed by the 'neo' insert in the modified gene, and these cells are cloned and tested with PCR for homologous recombination. Once an ES cell line with the desired modification has been isolated and purified, ES cells are injected into a normal embryo, where they often contribute to all the differentiated tissues of the chimeric adult mouse. If ga-

Once a gene or gene function has been identified, it is necessary to map it to a specific chromosome. Mapping of genes provides clues about which genes are affected by chromosome breaks or other abnormalities. For example, the observation that the *abl* oncogene was located on chromosome 9 near the region of the breakpoint in the Ph chromosome stimulated investigators to examine the tumor cells for possible involvement of the *abl* oncogene in this rearrangement. As described below, fluorescence in situ hybridization (FISH) is a very versatile technique for both mapping genes and for characterizing genomic aberrations in tumors. However, both FISH and traditional linkage methods for gene mapping are gradually being superseded by other methods, such as computational analyses of human sequences, known as bioinformatics.

### 4.4.1 Fluorescence In Situ Hybridization

To perform FISH, DNA probes specific for a gene, chromosome segment, or whole chromosome are labeled, usually by incorporation of biotin and/or digoxigenin, and are then hybridized to metaphase chromosomes. The DNA probe will re-anneal to the denatured piece of DNA at its precise location on the chromosome (see Fig. 4.14). After washing off the unbound probe, the hybridized sequences are detected using avidin, which binds strongly to biotin, and/or antibodies to digoxigenin, coupled to fluorescein isothiocyanate, Texas Red, or another fluorochrome. The sites of hybridization are clearly visualized as fluorescent points of light where the probe is bound to chromatin. The chief advantage of FISH for gene mapping is that information is obtained directly about the positions of the probes in relation to chromosome bands or to other previously mapped reference probes.

Fluorescence in situ hybridization can be performed on interphase nuclei from tumor biopsies or cultured tumor cells, which enables cytogenetic aberrations to be visualized without the need for obtaining good quality metaphase preparations (see Fig. 4.14*G*). By using FISH with the N-*myc* probe against neuroblastoma cells, it is easy to detect massive copy number changes per cell (Fig. 4.14*C* through *E*). Chromosome aberrations can also be detected using specific centromere probes that give two signals from normal nuclei but one signal when there is only one copy of the chromosome (monosomy) or three signals when there is an extra copy (trisomy; Fig. 4.14*F*). Chromosome deletions can also be detected by using probes from the deleted region and counting the signals. If the probes used for FISH are close to specific translocation break points on different chromosomes, they will appear joined as a result of the translocation generating a color fusion signal (Fig. 4.14*G*). These procedures are particularly useful for rapid detection of aberrations such as the *bcr-abl* rearrangement in chronic myeloid leukemia (Chap. 7, Sec. 7.2.4).

Determination of the length of telomeres (Curran et al., 1998) was traditionally performed by southern blotting and densitometry, and provided an average value for a total cell population studied (see Chap. 5, Sec. 5.6.1). Telomere repeats can now be analyzed by using a fluorescein-labeled peptide nucleic acid (PNA) probe to calculate telomere length, a method called quantitative (Q)-FISH (Baerlocher et al., 2002). Quantitative fluorescence in situ hybridization can be performed on any cytogenetic preparation or on tissue sections of tumors (Vukovic et al., 2003). A flow cytometric approach (FLOW-FISH) can also be used for evaluation of the total telomere signal intensity among cells in a population based on in situ hybridization using the same PNA probe and DNA staining with propidium iodide (Baerlocher et al., 2002).

### 4.4.2 Comparative Genomic Hybridization

If the cytogenetic abnormalities are unknown, it is not possible to select a suitable probe for their detection by FISH. *Comparative genomic hybridization* (CGH) allows investigators to produce a detailed map of the differences between chromosomes in different cells. This method detects increases (amplifications) or decreases (deletions) of segments of DNA (Kallioniemi et al., 1992).

In typical CGH experiments, DNA from malignant and normal cells such as fibroblasts is labeled with two different fluorochromes and then hybridized simultaneously to normal chromosome metaphase spreads. Tumor DNA is labeled with biotin and detected with fluorescein (green fluorescence); the control DNA is labeled with digoxigenin and detected with rhodamine (red fluorescence). Regions of gain or loss of DNA sequences in the tumor, such as deletions, duplications, or amplifications, are seen as changes in the ratio of the intensities of the two fluorochromes along the target chromosomes (Fig. 4.15). An amplified sequence will generate increased green fluorescence, whereas a deletion will shift the red/green ratio toward red. For low-copy-number amplifications and hemizygous deletions, this change in fluorescence ratio is difficult to distinguish by eye and requires specialized image analysis software (see Fig. 4.16*D*). One disadvantage of CGH is that it can detect only large blocks (>5 Mb) of over- or underrepresented chromosomal DNA; balanced rearrangements such as inversions or translocations escape detection. Comparative genomic hybridization is now being applied to microarrays and the greatly improved resolution of microarray CGH has improved the potential of this technique enormously (see Sec. 4.4.4).

### 4.4.3 Spectral Karyotyping (SKY) and Multi-Fluor Fluorescence In Situ Hybridization (M-FISH)

Universal chromosome painting techniques have been developed in which it is possible to analyze all chromosomes simultaneously. Two essentially similar approaches

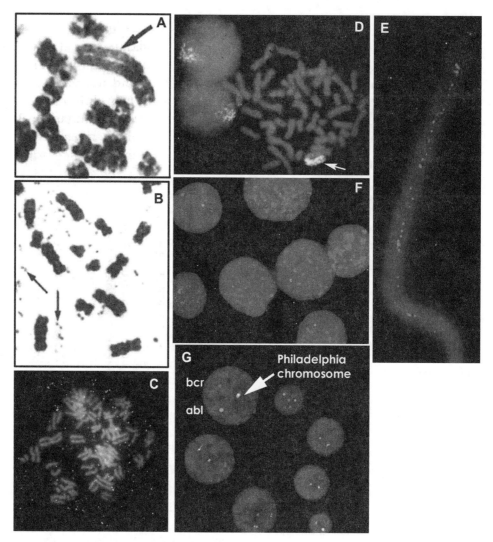

**Figure 4.14.** Analysis of oncogene rearrangements in tumors by conventional cytogenetics and FISH analysis. (*A*) An abnormally long chromosome (*arrow*). The extended region of this chromosome has no identifiable bands and is called a *homogeneously staining region* (HSR). (*B*) Multiple paired dots of chromatic material. These chromosomal abnormalities are called *double minutes* (DM). Both HSRs and DMs are associated with gene amplification. DMs are extrachromosomal circular DNA containing a few copies of the oncogene. HSRs are integrated multiple tandem repeats of the oncogene. (*C*) Metaphase preparation from a neuroblastoma that has N-*myc* amplification on DMs (green dots) detected by FISH. (*D*) A metaphase from another neuroblastoma that has N-*myc* amplification and an HSR. In this FISH preparation, the additional N-*myc* signals can be seen to decorate the HSR (*arrow*), the HSR is also apparent as clusters of yellow signal in the interphase nuclei. (*E*) A HSR in a neuroblastoma cell line with gene amplification of N-*myc*. In this preparation, the HSR has been stretched so that, in the extended form, multiple N-*myc* signals can be seen as a linear array. (Courtesy of Ajay Pandita, Pathology Department, University of Toronto.) (*F*) Interphase nuclei from a neuroblastoma with DMs. The bright pink dots within each nucleus are the FISH signals from the N-*myc* oncogene, which is known to be amplified to 50–100 copies per cell in this patient's tumor. In addition the single green dot indicates the loss of one copy of chromosome region 1p36. (*G*) Interphase cytogenetic analysis of a leukemia to identify the Philadelphia chromosome using FISH with the *bcr* and *abl* probes. The *abl* probe has been labeled with a red fluorochrome (*black dot*) and the *bcr* with a green fluorochrome (*shaded dot*). When the Philadelphia chromosome is present in a nucleus, both the red and green signals become superimposed, producing one strong yellow signal (*white dot*). If the nucleus does not have this abnormality, two red signals and two green signals will be present. (See color plate.)

have been developed: SKY (Veldman et al., 1997) and M-FISH (Speicher et al., 1996). Both techniques are based on the differential display of colored fluorescent chromosome-specific paints, which provide a complete analysis of the chromosomal complement in a given cell. Using combinations of 23 different colored paints as a cocktail probe, subtle differences in fluorochrome labeling of chromosomes after hybridization with this cocktail allows the computer to assign a unique color to each chromosome pair. Abnormal chromosomes can be identified by the pattern of color distribution along them and rearrangements between different chromosomes will

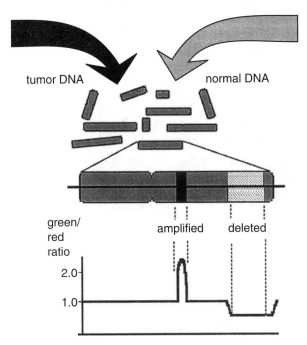

green/red ratio

2.0

1.0

amplified    deleted

**Figure 4.15.** Comparative genomic hybridization (CGH). Tumor DNA is labeled with a green fluorochrome (*black arrow*), normal reference DNA is labeled with a red fluorochrome (*shaded arrow*), and an equal mixture of each is hybridized to normal human metaphase chromosomes. Unlabeled repetitive human DNA is included to suppress binding of labeled DNA to repetitive elements. Regions of DNA gain are seen as an increased green fluorescence intensity on the target chromosomes (green to red ratio > 1.0); regions of DNA loss are seen as increased red fluorescence intensity (ratio < 1.0). Regions on the chromosome that are stained equally for both green and red indicate equal copy number for tumor and reference DNA. It can be seen that the DNA derived from the tumor being studied has both gene amplification (*black region*) and a deletion (*pale shading*) for this particular chromosome.

lead to a distinct transition from one color to another at the position of the breakpoint (Fig. 4.16). In contrast to comparative genomic hybridization, detection of such karyotype rearrangements using SKY and M-FISH is not dependent on change in copy number. This technology is particularly suited to solid tumors where the complexity of the karyotypes may often mask the presence of subtle chromosomal aberrations.

### 4.4.4 Microarray Analysis of Genes

Microarray analysis has been developed to assess expression of the increasing number of genes identified by the Human Genome Project (Brown and Botstein, 1999). The approach involves the production of DNA arrays or chips on solid supports for large-scale hybridization experiments. There are two variants of the chip: in one, DNA probe targets are immobilized to a solid inert surface such as glass and exposed to a set of fluorescently labeled sample DNAs; in the second, an

array of different oligonucleotide probes is synthesized in situ on the chip (Bowtell, 1999). The array is exposed to labeled DNA samples, and hybridized complementary sequences are determined by digital imaging. The resulting microarray, or DNA chip technology, allows large-scale gene discovery, expression, mapping, and sequencing studies as well as detection of mutations or polymorphisms. Microarrays of cDNAs have been used to study differential gene expression in bacteria, yeast, plant and human tissues, and cell lines. This approach allows for the simultaneous analysis of the differential expression of thousands of genes at once and is having a major impact on understanding the dynamics of gene expression in cancer cells. In this assay, mRNA from the sample of interest can serve as a template for producing complementary DNA (cDNA) in the presence of a reverse transcriptase enzyme. This cDNA is then fluorescently labeled and hybridized to the target gene sequences spotted on the cDNA microarray slide. The fluorescent intensity of each hybridized sequence in the array is read using a scanner. The scanner that records the intensity values is linked to custom digital image analysis software, which produces a color-coded image of the array, and a quantitative value is recorded for each target gene. Intensity of fluorescence correlates with expression of the gene for which the spot codes. Gene expression results can be clustered using different methods of data analysis (e.g., hierarchical clustering). This method is widely applied to databases of gene expression profiles, and it merges individual datapoints into a tree structure called a dendogram, based on their similarity (Fig. 4.17).

Recent advances have coupled CGH with the microarray technology. Instead of using metaphase chromosomes, CGH is applied to arrayed sequences of genomic DNA bound to glass slides and probed with genomes of interest. For example, tumor DNA can be compared to a normal reference DNA. The arrays are constructed typically using genomic clones that are evenly spaced along the whole genome and cover all chromosomal loci of interest (www.ncbi.nlm.nih.gov/). The greatly improved resolution of microarray CGH has permitted small genomic amplifications and deletions to be detected in tumors that may have gone unnoticed using older methods such as metaphase CGH or conventional cytogenetics.

### 4.4.5 Analysis of Tissue Sections and Single Cells

Tissue samples are usually fixed in formalin and then embedded in paraffin wax to preserve cell and tissue morphology for histopathological analysis. The ability to use FISH on paraffin-embedded archival specimens is dependent on the accessibility of the target DNA within the cell nucleus, and can be enhanced by pre-

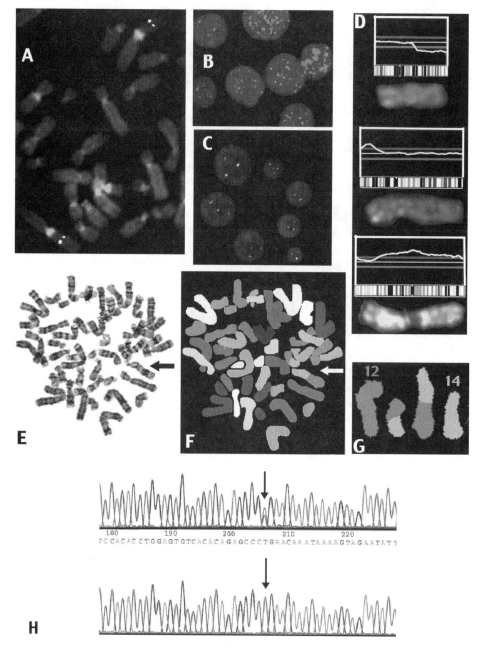

**Figure 4.16.** (*A*) Example of FISH mapping of a single copy genomic probe to chromosome 1. This is a DAPI (*blue counterstain*) banded normal metaphase preparation showing the location of positive signals (*yellow signals*) obtained with a cosmid probe containing an insert size of 40 kilobases of DNA from a gene on chromosome 1. A positive FISH signal is present on each chromatid of both pairs of chromosome 1 at band 1q25. (*B*) MYCN amplification in nuclei from neuroblastoma detected by FISH with a MYCN probe (*magenta speckling*) and a deletion of the short arm of chromosome 1. The signal (*pale blue/green*) from the remaining normal chromosome 1 is seen as a single spot in each nucleus. (*C*) Detection of a Philadelphia chromosome in interphase nuclei of leukemia cells. All nuclei contain one green signal (BCR gene), one pink signal (ABL gene), and an intermediate fusion yellow signal because of the 9;22 chromosome translocation. (*D*) The comparative genomic hybridization analysis profile from a neuroblastoma cell line. Chromosome 1 shows an overall gain of DNA indicated by an increase in the level of green signal (*bottom panel*). In this cell line most of chromosome 1 was trisomic. Chromosome 2 has a strong green signal at band 2p24 due to amplification (50 copies/cell) of MYCN in the cell line (*middle panel*). The long arm of chromosome 6 shows a loss (deletion) of DNA and a shift toward the red signal (*top panel*). (*E-G*) SKY analysis of blood lymphocytes from a patient with a translocation. (*E*) One of the aberrant chromosomes can be seen by classic G-banding (*arrow*); (*F*) the same metaphase spread has been subjected to SKY; and (*G*) the 12;14 reciprocal translocation is identified. (*H*) Automated sequencing of BRCA2, the hereditary breast cancer predisposition gene. Each colored peak represents a different nucleotide. The *lower panel* is a sequence of a wild-type DNA sample. The sequence of a mutation carrier in the upper panel contains a double peak (*indicated by an arrow*) in which the nucleotide T in intron 17 located at 2 bp downstream of the 5′ end of exon 18 is converted to a C. This mutation results in aberrant splicing of exon 18 of the BRCA2 gene. The presence of a T nucleotide, in addition to the mutant C, implies that only one copy of the two BRCA2 genes is mutated in this sample (see Sec. 4.3.9 for details). (See color plate.)

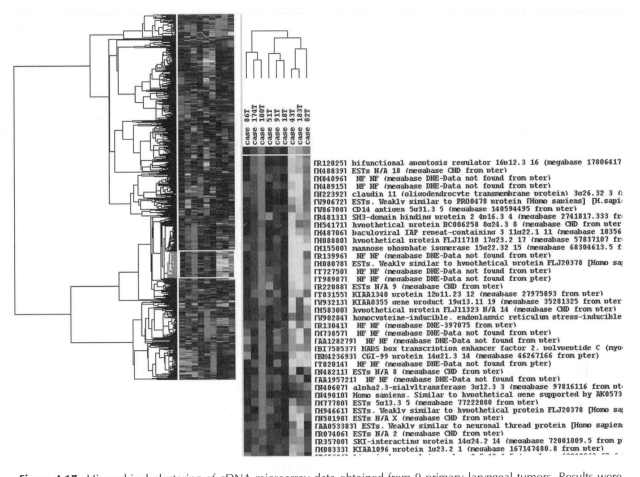

**Figure 4.17.** Hierarchical clustering of cDNA microarray data obtained from 9 primary laryngeal tumors. Results were visualized using Tree view software, and include the dendogram (clustering of samples) and the clustering of gene expression, based on genetic similarity. Tree view represents 946 genes that best distinguish these two groups of samples. Genes whose expression is higher in the tumor sample relative to the reference sample are shown in *red*; those whose expression is lower than the reference sample are shown in *green*; and no change in gene expression is shown in *black*. (Courtesy of Patricia Reis and Shilpi Arora, The Ontario Cancer Institute and Princess Margaret Hospital, Toronto.) (See color plate.)

treatment that increases the efficiency of hybridization. Analysis of tissue samples has been improved by development of tissue arrays, which contain multiple small circular pieces derived from punches of representative areas of paraffin sections from different tumors or normal tissues (Chen et al., 2003; Fig. 4.18). The arrays can contain pieces from hundreds of different tumors represented as 0.5 to 2 millimeter diameter discs of tissue containing several thousand cells, which retain the morphologic features of the original specimen from which the tissue punch was obtained. Tissue arrays are processed in much the same way as regular paraffin sections containing only one tissue sample.

Tissue in situ hybridization techniques rely on the hybridization of a specifically labeled nucleic acid probe to the cellular RNA in individual cells or tissue sections (Ausubel et al., 2003). Early studies described the localization of viral or abundant cellular messages in cul-

tured cells or tissue sections using radioactively labeled probes. Nonradioactive techniques for the detection of cellular mRNAs employ biotinylated probes, which are then detected by either a fluorescent or enzymatic system.

Successful in situ hybridization to cellular mRNA relies on several factors. Cytologic fixation should retain good cellular morphology but must not be so extensive that it inhibits probe access. Type of fixative and duration of fixation should be determined empirically for the tissue of interest. Limited proteolytic digestion with pepsin or proteinase K is commonly used to increase probe access to fixed tissues. The probe may be either DNA or RNA. DNA probes labeled by either nick translation or random primer labeling bind to the tissue specimen by hybridization, thus increasing the hybridization signal. Self-annealing of probe also occurs; however, this decreases the effective probe concentra-

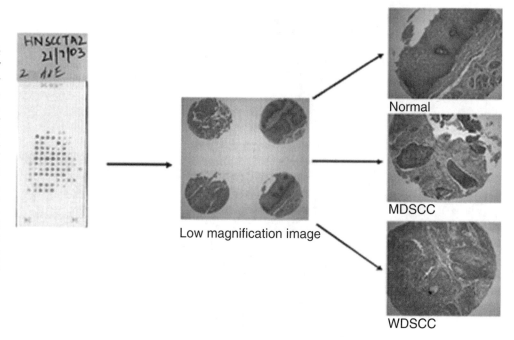

**Figure 4.18.** Hematoxylin & Eosin stained tissue array slide. This slide contains approximately 100 tissue spots, including control tissues, oral squamous cell carcinoma, and adjacent normal tissues. All samples are spotted in duplicate. MDSCC is moderately differentiated squamous cell carcinoma. WDSCC is well-differentiated squamous cell carcinoma. (Courtesy of Shilpi Arora, The Ontario Cancer Institute and Princess Margaret Hospital, Toronto.) (See color plate.)

Low magnification image

Normal

MDSCC

WDSCC

tion. Highly specific radioactive probes are easily synthesized in large quantities. RNA probes generally give lower backgrounds than equivalent DNA probes because nonspecifically bound probe is removed by subsequent ribonuclease treatment.

Another approach for molecular analysis using very small numbers of cells is random PCR. This technique allows for the global amplification of all DNA sequences present in microdissected cells, thereby increasing globally the amount of DNA for subsequent analysis. The method can also be adapted to generate representative amplification of the mRNA in a small number of cells. The technique has been useful in providing DNA for molecular genetic studies using microdissected DNA from paraffin blocks, cDNA from single-cell RT-PCR reactions, and chromosome band-specific probes derived for microdissected chromosomal DNA.

One problem associated with the molecular genetic analysis of small numbers of tumor cells is that substantial numbers of normal cells will often be present in tumors and can confound interpretation. This contamination is often scattered throughout a tumor section, and it is not possible to microdissect a pure population of tumor cells cleanly. This problem has recently been circumvented by the use of laser capture microdissection, in which tumor sections are coated with a clear ethylene vinyl acetate (EVA) polymer prior to microscopic examination (Emmert-Buck et al., 1996). Tumor cells can be captured for subsequent analysis by briefly pulsing the area of interest with an infrared laser. The EVA film becomes sticky and will selectively attach to the tumor cells directly in the laser path. When sufficient cells have been fused to the EVA film, it is placed

into nucleic acid extraction buffers and used for PCR or other molecular analyses.

## 4.5 PROTEIN-BASED METHODS: PROTEOMICS

Proteomics covers a spectrum of techniques for analysis of protein composition and function. Recent advances in computing power and analytical instrumentation such as mass spectrometry, nuclear magnetic resonance (NMR) spectroscopy, and x-ray diffraction, as well as increased knowledge of primary structure from the completion of the sequencing of the human genome, has stimulated this developing field. Mass spectrometry is used to analyze the mass and charge of proteins. Nuclear magnetic resonance and x-ray diffraction are the primary methods of structural biology, which are used to determine the three-dimensional structures (the relative positions of all atoms) of proteins and other biomolecules. These techniques have enhanced understanding of the molecular defects that occur in cancer and provided insight into how such defects may be treated. Knowledge of a protein's three-dimensional structure often illustrates the mechanism by which it recognizes other molecules, catalyzes enzymatic reactions, and how oncogenic mutations alter these functions. Furthermore, the structure also provides a basis for the design of therapeutic agents that could prevent oncogenic activity of mutant or overexpressed oncoproteins.

Mass spectrometry is able to identify individual proteins in complex biological samples and is becoming an important method for surveying the levels and combinations of proteins in normal and diseased tissues. X-ray crystallography, and NMR spectroscopy have matured to the point where researchers expect to determine systematically the structure of all proteins; this field of study is termed *structural proteomics* or *structural genomics* (Christendat et al., 2000). For each of these techniques, the preparation of the sample is the most critical area (Edwards et al., 2000); however, unlike MS methods, both NMR and x-ray diffraction techniques require large (milligram) quantities of pure protein. Here we review the essential aspects of each experimental technique and provide examples of the use of each in cancer research and the development of therapeutic agents.

### 4.5.1 Mass Spectrometry

One of the major challenges in proteomics is the separation of protein complexes within the cell. The small scale and high throughput of proteomic approaches makes conventional purification techniques cumbersome; rather, investigators have relied on techniques such as gel separation, and/or affinity purification of exogenously expressed proteins containing a protein tag that can be captured using an antibody or affinity resin. More recently, the advent of increasingly powerful mass spectrophotometers has allowed the analysis of complex protein mixtures (thousands of different proteins in a single sample) unaided by purification or gel separation (Ashman et al., 2001; Tyers and Mann, 2003). Others have developed a method of differentially labeling proteins with a normal and heavy isotope of a chemical affinity tag (ICAT, isotope coded affinity tag; Ranish et al., 2003). The subtle shift in peptide mass between the labeled and unlabeled samples allows for quantitative comparison of the two protein mixtures between the cell extracts. The advantage of the latter two techniques is that they do not rely on exogenously expressed protein, and multiple time points after a given stimulus allow a more accurate reflection of the dynamic nature of the cellular response.

The instrumentation used for mass spectrometry varies widely, both in configuration and in biological or clinical applications. Typically, a protein sample is first subjected to endoproteolytic digestion with trypsin, which generates peptides containing at least two positive charges: the free amino group and a carboxyterminal lysine or arginine residue. Such peptides bear double positive charge under the acidic conditions used for ionization, and hence tend to fragment efficiently at peptide bonds. The digested peptide mixture may then be separated by liquid chromatography (LC) on a low flow-rate capillary hydrophobic column. The emerging peptides are then ionized and separated according to their mass to charge (m/z) ratio by a series of electromagnetic quadrapole chambers, often in combination with an ion trap or time of flight (TOF) tube. Accurate determination of the m/z ratio (typically on the order of parts per million), in combination with knowledge of the charge state allows an accurate mass estimate of the

peptide fragment. Because peptides tend to fragment at the peptide bond, the ion series for a given peptide is related directly to primary sequence. Peptide fragments of increasing length from the amino terminus are referred to as the B series, and fragments of increasing length from the carboxy terminus are referred to as the Y series. Similar to reading a DNA sequencing ladder, the sequence composition of each polypeptide can be inferred from the differential masses of the B and Y series peptides and then matched to protein sequence by a database search. Alternatively for pure protein samples, the digestion mixture can be spotted on a solid phase substrate matrix and ionized by laser pulses, a configuration termed matrix-assisted laser desorption ionization (MALDI). This is followed by peptide mass determination by TOF analysis. While peptide sequence information can sometimes be extracted by MALDI-TOF, typically the lower ionization energy of this method yields only intact singly charged peptides that do not fragment well, but which are well suited for protein identification by matching the total peptide mass fingerprint to theoretical protein digests in database searches. These general principles have been elaborated to more sophisticated instrument platforms, such as Fourier transform ion cyclotron resonance (FT-ICR) mass spectrometers, which in theory have the dynamic range and resolution to systematically characterize many tens of thousands of peptides derived from very complex mixtures, such as crude cell extracts or biological fluids such as serum. It is anticipated that mass spectrometry-based approaches may ultimately allow the routine and rapid diagnosis of distant site diseases such as cancer by virtue of representation of minute quantities of specific disease-associated antigens in the blood.

The full potential of MS for the analysis of cellular proteins is just beginning to be explored. Even changes in protein phosphorylation within a cell are being mapped at a genome-wide level (Mann et al., 2001; Zhou et al., 2002). In addition, protein-based arrays are being developed that reflect the abundance of particular proteins via capture with affinity tags or via antibody recognition. Proteomic footprints of particular disease states, or those occurring in response to certain treatments, can be assessed, and compared against mRNA expression analyses to provide a more complex and accurate picture for diagnosis, treatment customization, and prognosis (Verma et al., 2001; Zhou et al., 2001).

### 4.5.2 X-ray Crystallography

*X-ray crystallography* is a technique in which a high intensity x-ray beam is directed through a highly ordered crystalline phase of a pure protein or biomolecular complex. The regular array of electron density within the crystalline protein molecules diffracts the x-rays so that the diffracted x-rays interfere constructively, giving rise to a unique diffraction pattern. From the diffraction pattern the distribution of electrons in the molecule (an electron density map) is calculated and a molecular model of the protein is then progressively built into the electron density map.

Protein crystallization is a trial-and-error procedure in which a variety of solvent conditions are tested in multiwell plates. Highly pure protein (usually from recombinant sources) is divided into a series of small drops of aqueous buffers often containing one or more cosolvents or precipitants. The drop is left to slowly evaporate or equilibrate with a reservoir solution (in the same well), and if conditions are favorable, the protein slowly comes out of solution in a crystalline form. This represents the limiting step in crystallography because the conditions may vary greatly from one protein to another, and it is impossible to know *a priori* under which conditions, if any, a given protein will crystallize. Not every protein will crystallize, and often researchers try individual domains or multiple domains within a given protein or homologous proteins from other species in order to find a combination of protein and conditions that will yield a crystal that diffracts well.

An additional complication for protein crystallography is the requirement for introduction of either metal ions or selenium (incorporated into the protein as seleno-methionine) to aid in interpretation of the x-ray diffraction pattern. These heavy atoms diffract x-rays anomalously and therefore can be used to calculate the phases of the diffracted x-rays and subsequently the electron density map. The final step of fitting the atoms of the protein into the electron density map requires the use of interactive computer graphics programs, or semi-automated programs if the data are of sufficient quality and resolution. Initially the electron density map contains many errors, but it can be improved through a process called refinement, in which the atomic model is adjusted to improve the agreement with the measured diffraction data. The quality of an atomic model is normally judged through the standard crystallographic R factor, which is a measure of how well the atomic model fits the experimental data.

The fine details revealed by high-resolution x-ray structures are useful for understanding the principles of molecular recognition in protein-ligand complexes. The structure of imatinib (Gleevec; STI571) bound to the c-Abl kinase domain is a remarkable example of the application of this approach. This therapeutic agent is a rationally-developed, potent, and selective inhibitor for Abl tyrosine kinases, including the chronic-myelocytic-leukemia–related translocation product of *bcr-abl*, making it an effective therapy for chronic myelocytic leukemia. Scientists at Ciba-Geigy (now Novartis) used high-throughput screening of compound libraries to identify the 2-phenylaminopyrimidine class of kinase inhibitors. The pharmaceutical properties of these compounds were then optimized through successive rounds of medicinal chemistry and evaluation of structure-activity relationships. The structural mechanism of the inhibition of bcr-abl by imatinib has been shown by x-ray crystallography to involve both binding by the inhibitor to the nucleotide binding pocket of the active site of the catalytic domain of the kinase, as well as stabilization of an inactive conformation of the enzyme (Fig. 4.19) (Schindler et al., 2000). The latter effect is specific to the c-Abl kinase and two closely related kinases (PDGR receptor and c-kit) and explains the high specificity of this inhibitor.

### 4.5.3 Nuclear Magnetic Resonance Spectroscopy

Nuclear magnetic resonance (NMR) spectroscopy takes advantage of a fundamental property of the nuclei of atoms called the nuclear spin (Cavanagh et al., 1996).

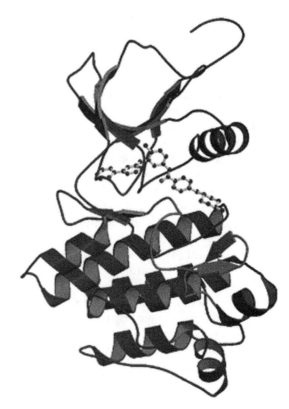

**Figure 4.19.** X-ray crystallography reveals the mechanism of inhibition by the therapeutic drug, imatinib. The three-dimensional structure of the catalytic domain of c-Abl, which is overexpressed in CML due to the BCR-ABL translocation, is shown bound to imatinib. The polypeptide backbone of the protein is represented as ribbons and coils showing how the protein chain folds up into a specific three-dimensional shape. The domain can be roughly divided into two regions, an N-terminal lobe and a C-terminal lobe, with the interface forming the active site of the enzyme. Imatinib (represented with ball and sticks for atoms and bonds, respectively) binds in a crevice, or pocket, in the active site and locks the protein into an inactive conformation by preventing the activation loop from assuming the active conformation.

When placed in a static magnetic field, nuclei with non-zero spin will align their magnetic dipoles with (low-energy state) or against (high-energy state) the magnetic field. Under normal circumstances there is a small difference in the population distribution between the two energy states, thereby creating a net magnetization that is manipulated using electromagnetic pulses. Each nucleus absorbs the energy from these pulses at a characteristic frequency that is dependent on its chemical properties and the surrounding environment, including the conformation of the molecule and its nearest neighbor nuclei. Structures of noncrystalline proteins in aqueous solution are derived from a series of NMR experiments that reveal interactions of nuclei close together in three-dimensional space, even though they are distant within the primary sequence of the protein. These data allow calculation of an ensemble of protein conformations that satisfy a large number (hundreds to thousands) of experimental restraints. This necessitates extensive data collection (often more than ten experiments lasting hours to days) and computer-assisted analysis of the spectra in order to calculate a structure.

The main nucleus observed by NMR is that of hydrogen, ($^1$H). However, proteins have hundreds to thousands of $^1$H signals, many with the same resonance frequency. This problem is solved by the use of multidimensional NMR, in which protein samples are labeled with the NMR-active stable isotopes, $^{15}$N and $^{13}$C. The incorporation of stable isotopes is required to resolve the large number of signals in two, three, or four dimensions, each dimension corresponding to $^1$H, $^{15}$N, and/or $^{13}$C resonance frequencies. Due to the poor signal-to-noise ratio of the NMR signals in large proteins, the size of proteins amenable to high resolution NMR structural studies is currently limited to ~30 kiloDaltons or less. Recent developments in methodology have made it possible to study larger molecules, but this requires the use of partial or full deuteration (i.e., incorporation of heavy hydrogen) in combination with special NMR techniques, resulting in lower-resolution structural information. Overexpression of proteins in *E. coli* with affinity tags (a specifc protein sequence that is efficiently bound by a specific antibody or metal ion) has facilitated incorporation of the appropriate isotopes and convenient one-step purification by affinity chromatography. Samples typically need to be concentrated; this requirement makes it difficult to study proteins with low solubility or those that are prone to aggregation or precipitation. Therefore much time is required for optimizing the stability and solubility of a protein prior to study by NMR spectroscopy.

### 4.5.4 Structural Analysis of the p53 protein

Structural studies of the tumor suppressor protein p53 (Chap. 7, Sec. 7.4.2) provide a good example of the use of both NMR and X-ray crystallography in cancer research, revealing information on cancer-related mutations, p53 domains, and their interaction with other molecules. p53 is a phosphoprotein which functions as a tumor suppressor, mainly as a DNA-binding transcriptional regulator of genes involved in apoptosis and cell-cycle progression (Bargonetti and Manfredi, 2002). The p53 protein is composed functionally and structurally of five domains (Fig. 4.20). The acidic, N-terminal transactivation domain (residues 1 to 70) has been shown by NMR to be largely unstructured in the absence of binding partners, but small regions adopt helical or other more rigid conformations when bound to a number of regulatory molecules, such as the oncoprotein Mdm2. A proline-rich domain (residues 60 to 97) interacts with signaling modules such as SH3 domains (see Chap. 8, Sec. 8.2.4). The central region of p53 (residues 100 to 300) contains its squence-specific DNA binding domain. A tiny sequence of thirty residues comprises the oligomerization (Tet) domain (320 to 360); tetramerization of p53 is required for efficient binding to the four-fold pseudo repeats found in p53 responsive elements. Finally, the negatively charged C-terminal regulatory domain (360 to 393) has also been shown by NMR to be largely disordered when not bound to other proteins or DNA. This modular architecture of p53, originally suggested by increased protease susceptibility of the N- and C-termini and the linker between the DNA-binding and tetramerization domains, has recently been confirmed by NMR studies of oligomeric forms of the protein. This modular and flexible domain structure is also likely responsible for the failure of tetrameric forms of the protein to crystallize either on their own or complexed with DNA.

The crystal structure of a monomeric DNA binding domain bound to a portion of the p53 responsive element revealed important details of how this protein recognizes DNA and the effects of cancer-related mutations (Cho et al., 2002). The majority of cancer-causing mutations involve residues that are in direct contact with DNA. Hot-spot mutations include Arg248, the most frequently mutated residue in human cancer, and Arg273; these are both intimately involved in interactions with DNA. Other mutations, which are not directly involved in DNA binding, are at residues important in the structural integrity of the DNA binding domain. For example, mutation of Val143 to alanine in the hydrophobic core of this domain results in a destabilization of the domain, which explains why this mutant is temperature sensitive.

Nuclear magnetic resonance and x-ray studies of the tetramerization domain have shown how mutations at the interface between subunits (e.g., found in patients with the Li-Fraumeni syndrome) can lead to a predisposition to cancer due to impaired p53 function (Davison et al., 1998). They also explain how overexpression

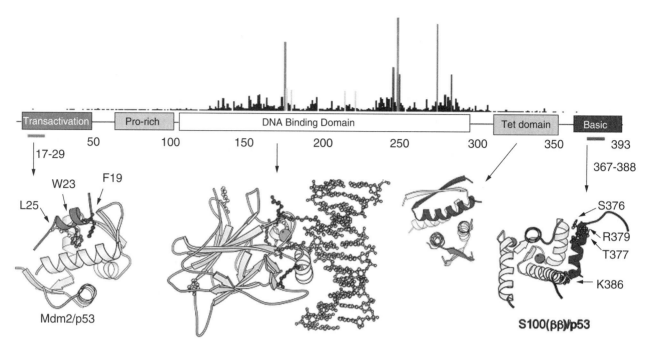

**Figure 4.20.** Linear schematic of p53 outlining the different functional and structural domains. The primary sequence of p53 is represented as a horizontal line with domains shown as *colored rectangles* with residue numbers underneath. The frequency of cancer-associated mutations at each amino acid residue is indicated as a histogram above the primary sequence. Hotspot mutations are colored in *red* (R248, R273, R175), in *blue* (G245, R282, R249), and in *yellow* (C176, H179, Y220, and F212). The corresponding residues are colored in the same manner and drawn in *ball-and-stick* representation in the x-ray crystal structure of the DNA binding domain bound to DNA and zinc ion (*blue sphere*) shown in the lower central panel. Most of these hotspot mutations result in disruption of amino acid side chains either directly involved in DNA binding, or in supporting either the helix or loops that interact with DNA. Those more distal from the DNA interface have an overall destabilizing effect on the domain. The *lower left panel* shows the x-ray structure of Mdm2 (*cyan*) bound to a p53-derived peptide (*red*) from the transactivation domain. The three hydrophobic residues (F19, W23, and L25) on one face of the p53 helix responsible for the interaction with Mdm2 are shown in *ball-and-stick* representation. The NMR-derived structure of the tetramerisation domain revealed a dimer of dimers (*yellow/blue and yellow/pink*). The NMR-derived structure of the complex between S100(ββ) and a peptide derived from the basic regulatory domain of p53 (*dark blue*) revealed the manner in which posttranslational phosphorylation by protein kinase C (at residues S376 and T377) and acetylation by p300 (at residues R379 and K386) are blocked by the interaction. Calcium ions in S100(ββ) are represented by the *red spheres*. (See color plate.)

of a single allele of mutant p53 can act in a dominant negative manner by bringing together mutant and wild-type DNA binding domains in one tetrameric molecule, thereby resulting in reduced DNA-binding activity.

p53 also interacts with a variety of proteins that modulate its activity and post-translational modifications. For example, Mdm2 and S100B are two oncogenes that negatively regulate p53 by binding to the solvent accessible and unstructured N- and C-terminal regions, respectively. The crystal structure of a domain of Mdm2 bound to an N-terminal peptide of p53 showed that hdm2 induces a helical conformation in this region of p53 and physically masks the transactivation domain from interaction with other proteins in the transcription apparatus (Kussie et al., 1996). Similarly, the NMR structure of an S100(B) complex with the C-terminal domain (Rustandi et al., 2000) contributed to the understanding of the mechanism of inactivation of p53 in cancers involving the amplification of this protein; the

interaction sterically blocks four posttranslational modification sites at the C-terminal domain of p53, preventing the activation of p53. The structures of the Mdm2-p53 and S100(B)-p53 complexes can be used as the basis for rational drug design to disrupt the interactions in cancers where the increased levels of these proteins is the primary mechanism of uncontrolled growth.

## 4.6 SUMMARY

Advances in techniques of chromosomal and genetic analysis have occurred rapidly, and have played a central role in the conceptual understanding of cancer. These advances have allowed a dramatic increase in the understanding of all aspects of tumor cell biology. Techniques such as FISH, SKY, CGH, northern blotting, real-time PCR, and SNP analysis, among others, are being used routinely in the analysis of clinical samples and the diagnosis and prognosis of disease, while other techniques such as microarray technology promise to revolutionize the manner in which diseases are diagnosed and treated.

Chromosomal abnormalities are identified by cytogenetic, and, more recently, molecular cytogenetic approaches. While these methods have been applied more extensively to leukemias and lymphomas than to solid tumors, they yield useful information about genes potentially associated with malignancy. Advances in technology and analysis have made it possible to identify and isolate specific genes, and to determine the sequences and putative functions of their protein products. Techniques of molecular analysis have allowed for rapidly increased understanding of the correlation between alterations in gene expression and the development of tumors. Microarray technology, SKY, CGH and tissue in situ hybridization analysis and recently developed proteomic approaches, allow the identification and better understanding of genes and proteins whose structure and/or function are modified in disease, ultimately providing more opportunities for the understanding of the mechanisms of disease, and the identification of unique targets in human tumors for therapeutic intervention.

## ACKNOWLEDGMENTS

The authors wish to thank Ayeda Ayed, Antonio Pineda-Lucena, Mike Tyers, and Brett Larsen, for their editorial contributions to this chapter.

## REFERENCES

Ashman K, Moran MF, Sicheri F, et al: Cell signalling—the proteomics of it all. *Sci STKE* 2001; 103:PE33.

Ausubel LJ, Kwan CK, Sette A, et al: Complementary mutations in an antigenic peptide allow for crossreactivity of autoreactive T-cell clones. *Proc Natl Acad Sci USA* 1996; 93:15317–15322.

Ausubel FA, Brent R, Kingston RE, et al, eds: *Current Protocols in Molecular Biology*. New York: Wiley; 2003.

Babinet C, Cohen-Tannoudji M: Genome engineering via homologous recombination in mouse embryonic stem (ES) cells: an amazing versatile tool for the mammalian biology. *An Acad Bras Cienc* 2001; 73:365–383.

Baerlocher GM, Mak J, Tien T, Lansdorp P: Telomere length measurement by fluorescence in situ hybridization and flow cytometry: tips and pitfalls. *Cytometry* 2002;47:89–99.

Bargonetti J, Manfredi JJ: Multiple roles of the tumor suppressor p53. *Curr Opin Oncol.* 2002; 14:86–91.

Bowtell DD: Options available—from start to finish—for obtaining expression data by microarray. *Nat Genet* 1999; 21(Suppl 1):25–32.

Brantl S: Antisense-RNA regulation and RNA interference. *Biochim Biophys Acta* 2002; 1575:15–25.

Brown PO, Botstein D: Exploring the new world of the genome with DNA microarrays. *Nat Genet* 1999; 21:33–37.

Bustin SA: Absolute quantification of mRNA using real-time reverse transcription polymerase chain reaction assays. *J Mol Endocrinol* 2000; 25:169–193.

Bustin SA, Dorudi S: Molecular assessment of tumour stage and disease recurrence using PCR-based assays. *Mol Med Today* 1998; 4:389–396.

Cavanagh J, Fairbrother WJ, Palmer AG, and Skelton NJ: *Protein NMR Spectroscopy, Principles and Practice*. San Diego: Academic Press, 1996.

Chen B, Van Den Brekel MW, Buschers W, et al: Validation of tissue array technology in head and neck squamous cell carcinoma. *Head Neck* 2003; 25:922–930.

Cheung IY, Cheung NK: Quantitation of marrow disease in neuroblastoma by real-time reverse transcription-PCR. *Clin Cancer Res* 2001; 7:1698–1705.

Cho Y, Gorina S, Jeffrey PD, Pavletich NP: Crystal structure of a p53 tumor suppressor-DNA complex: understanding tumorigenic mutations. *Science* 1994; 265:346–355.

Christendat D, Yee A, Dharamsi A, et al: Structural proteomics of an archaeon. *Nat Struct Biol* 2000; 7:903–909.

Curran AJ, St Denis K, Irish J, et al: Telomerase activity in oral squamous cell carcinoma. *Arch Otolaryngol Head Neck Surg* 1998; 124:784–788.

Davison TS, Yin P, Nie E, et al: Characterization of the oligomerization defects of two p53 mutants found in families with Li-Fraumeni and Li-Fraumeni-like syndrome. *Oncogene* 1998; 17:651–656.

D'Cunha J, Corfits AL, Herndon JE 2nd, et al: Molecular staging of lung cancer: real-time polymerase chain reaction estimation of lymph node micrometastatic tumor cell burden in stage I non-small cell lung cancer—preliminary results of Cancer and Leukemia Group B Trial 9761. *J Thorac Cardiovasc Surg* 2002; 123:484–491.

Duggan DJ, Bittner M, Chen Y, et al: Expression profiling using cDNA microarrays. *Nat Genet* 1999; 21:10–14.

Edwards AM, Arrowsmith CH, Christendat D, et al. Protein production: feeding the crystallographers and NMR spectroscopists. *Nat Struct Biol* 2000;(Suppl):970–972.

Emmert-Buck MR, Bonner RF, Smith PD, et al: Laser capture microdissection. *Science* 1996; 274:998–1001.

Grimwade D, Lo Coco F: Acute promyelocytic leukemia: a model for the role of molecular diagnosis and residual disease monitoring in directing treatment approach in acute myeloid leukemia. *Leukemia* 2002; 16:1959–1973.

Heim S, Mitelman F: *Cancer Cytogenetics*. New York: Wiley; 1995.

Hein I, Lehner A, Rieck P, et al: Comparison of different approaches to quantify Staphylococcus aureus cells by real-time quantitative PCR and application of this technique for examination of cheese. *Appl Environ Microbiol* 2001; 67:3122–3126.

Hughes S, Lim G, Beheshti B, et al: Use of whole genome amplification and comparative genomic hybridization to detect chromosomal copy number alterations in cell line material and tumour tissue. *Cytogenet Genome Res* 2004;105: 18–24.

Ionov Y, Peinado MA, Malkhosyan S, et al: Ubiquitous somatic mutations in simple repeated sequences reveal a new mechanism for colonic carcinogenesis. *Nature* 1993; 363: 558–561.

Ishikawa, F: FISH goes with the flow. *Nat Biotechnol* 1998; 16:723–724.

Kallioniemi A, Kallioniemi OP, Sudar D, et al: Comparative genomic hybridization for molecular cytogenetic analysis of solid tumors. *Science* 1992; 258:818–821.

Kittler R, Buchholz F: RNA interference: gene silencing in the fast lane. *Semin Cancer Biol* 2003; 13:259–265.

Kussie PH, Gorina S, Marechal V, et al.: Structure of the MDM2 oncoprotein bound to the p53 tumor suppressor transactivation domain. *Science* 1996;274:948–953.

Li A, Forestier E, Rosenquist R, Roos G: Minimal residual disease quantification in childhood acute lymphoblastic leukemia by real-time polymerase chain reaction using the SYBR green dye. *Exp Hematol* 2002; 30:1170–1177

Liu J, Fujiwara TM, Buu NT, et al: Identification of polymorphisms and sequence variants in the human homologue of the mouse natural resistance-associated macrophage protein gene. *Am J Hum Genet* 1995; 56:845–853.

Mann M, Ong SE, Gronborg M, et al: Analysis of protein phosphorylation using mass spectrometry: deciphering the phosphoproteome. *Trends Biotechnol* 2002; 20:261–268.

Mhlanga MM, Malmberg L: Using molecular beacons to detect single-nucleotide polymorphisms with real-time PCR. *Methods* 2001; 25:463–471.

Mitelman F, et al: *An International System for Human Cytogenetic Nomenclature* (ISCN). 1995.

Olavarria E, Kanfer E, Szydlo R, et al: Early detection of BCR-ABL transcripts by quantitative reverse transcriptase-polymerase chain reaction predicts outcome after allogeneic stem cell transplantation for chronic myeloid leukemia. *Blood* 2001; 97:1560–1565.

Ranish JA, Yi EC, Leslie DM, et al: The study of macromolecular complexes by quantitative proteomics. *Nat Genet* 2003; 33:349–355.

Rustandi RR, Baldisseri DM, Weber DJ: Structure of the negative regulatory domain of p53 bound to S100B ($\beta\beta$). *Nat Struct Biol* 2000;7:570–574.

Schindler T, Bornmann W, Pellicena P, et al: Structural mechanism for STI-571 inhibition of abelson tyrosine kinase. *Science* 2000; 289:1938–1942.

Sheer D, Squire J: Clinical applications of genetic rearrangements in cancer. *Semin Cancer Biol* 1996; 7:25–32.

Simpson DA, Feeney S, Boyle C, et al: Retinal VEGF mRNA measured by SYBR green I fluorescence: a versatile approach to quantitative PCR. *Mol Vis* 2000; 6:178–183.

Speicher MR, Gwyn Ballard S, Ward DC: Karyotyping human chromosomes by combinatorial multi-fluor FISH. *Nat Genet* 1996; 12:368–375.

Swansbury J: Introduction to the analysis of the human G-banded karyotype. *Methods Mol Biol* 2003; 220:259–269.

Syvanen AC: Accessing genetic variation: genotyping single nucleotide polymorphisms. *Nat Rev Genet* 2001; 10:2961–2972.

Tsang P, Pan L, Cesarman E, et al: A distinctive composite lymphoma consisting of clonally related mantle cell lymphoma and follicle center cell lymphoma. *Hum Pathol* 1999; 30:988–992.

Tyers M, Mann M: From genomics to proteomics. *Nature* 2003; 422:193–197.

Veldman T, Vignon C, Schrock E, et al: Hidden chromosome abnormalities in haematological malignancies detected by multicolour spectral karyotyping. *Nat Genet* 1997; 15:406–410.

Verma M, Wright GL Jr, Hanash SM, et al: Proteomic approaches within the NCI early detection research network for the discovery and identification of cancer biomarkers. *Ann NY Acad Sci* 2001; 945:103–115.

Verma RS, Babu A: *Human Chromosomes*. New York: McGraw-Hill; 1995.

Vukovic B, Park PC, Al-Maghrabi J, et al: Evidence of multifocality of telomere erosion in high-grade prostatic intraepithelial neoplasia (HPIN) and concurrent carcinoma. *Oncogene* 2003; 22:1978–1987.

Wilke K, Duman B, Horst J: Diagnosis of haploidy and triploidy based on measurement of gene copy number by real-time PCR. *Hum Mutat* 2000; 16:431–436.

Wolford JK, Blunt D, Ballecer C, Prochazka M: High-throughput SNP detection by using DNA pooling and denaturing high performance liquid chromatography (DHPLC). *Hum Genet* 2000; 107(5):483–487.

Xiao W, Oefner PJ: Denaturing high-performance liquid chromatography. A review. *Hum Mutat* 2001; 17:439–474.

Yin JQ, Gao J, Shao R, et al: si-RNA agents inhibit oncogene expression and attenuate human tumor cell growth. *J Exp Ther Oncol* 2003; 3:194–204.

Yurkanis-Bruice, P: *Organic Chemistry*, third ed. Upper Saddle River, NJ: Prentice Hall; 2001.

Zimmer A: Manipulating the genome by homologous recombination in embryonic stem cells. *Ann Rev Neurosci.* 1992; 15:115–137.

Zhou H, Watts JD, Aebersold R: A systematic approach to the analysis of protein phosphorylation. *Nat Biotechnol* 2001; 19:375–378.

# 5

# Genomic Stability and DNA Repair

*Robert G. Bristow and Lea Harrington*

## 5.1 INTRODUCTION

There is overwhelming evidence that mutations can cause cancer. Major evidence for the genetic origin of cancer includes: (1) the observation of Ames (Ames et al., 1981) that many carcinogens are also mutagens (Chap. 3, Sec. 3.3.1) and (2) the finding that genetically determined traits associated with a deficiency in the enzymes necessary to repair lesions in DNA are associated with an increased risk of cancer (see Sec. 5.3). Mutations may occur in the germline of an individual and be represented in every cell in the body, or they may occur in a single somatic cell and be identified in a tumor following clonal proliferation. As described in Chapter 7, all species have numerous genes called *cellular oncogenes* (or *protooncogenes*), that are homologous to the transforming oncogenes carried by specific RNA retroviruses. Some human tumors have mutations in these oncogenes that may have led to their activation. However, there is no evidence for germline mutations in cellular oncogenes, perhaps because such mutations

in the germline are lethal even in the heterozygous state. In contrast, there is good evidence for germline mutations affecting *tumor suppressor genes*, which can lead to familial clustering of cancer or transmission of predisposition to tumors. In such cases, the loss-of-function of a tumor suppressor gene is inherited in a Mendelian manner.

DNA mutations that result in the instability of the genome can lead to an increased risk for cancer, presumably because the initial germline mutation increases the likelihood of somatic mutations occurring in direct-acting genes. In this chapter, genetic and epigenetic factors that control genomic stability are discussed in Section 5.2. The biochemical pathways that act to repair specific DNA lesions, and enact cell cycle checkpoints following DNA damage, are described in Section 5.4. Finally, the importance of the appropriate maintenance of chromosomal length and telomerase activity is highlighted in Section 5.5 in relation to cell immortalization and transformation. Throughout the chapter, examples are given of the importance of each of these areas in human cancer carcinogenesis, diagnosis, and treatment.

## 5.2 GENETIC INSTABILITY AS THE BASIS FOR MALIGNANT TRANSFORMATION

### 5.2.1 Causes of Genetic Instability

Cellular carcinogenesis is known to require sequential mutations in DNA (Chap. 2, Sec. 2.3.3 and Chap. 11, Sec. 11.1.2). This damage can be the result of endogenous processes such as errors in the replication of DNA and the intrinsic chemical instability of certain DNA bases during the process of oxidative cellular metabolism. DNA damage can also result from exogenous ionizing or ultraviolet (UV) radiation and chemical carcinogens (see Chap. 3). These agents create DNA base damage or base-pair mismatching, DNA crosslinks, DNA single-strand breaks (DNA ssb) or DNA double-strand breaks (DNA dsb), leading to chromosomal fragmentation, translocation, and deletion. Unless the cell can protect and maintain the integrity of the genome, these genetic alterations may cause cancer by activating protooncogenes and/or inactivating tumor suppressor genes. Some inactivating mutations occur in genes responsible for maintaining genomic integrity or DNA repair facilitating the development of a *mutator* cellular phenotype (Fig. 5.1; Loeb, 1991). It has been estimated that premalignant and normal tissues derived from certain heritable DNA repair syndromes already contain

approximately 10,000 genomic alterations per cell (Stoler et al., 1999). These data support a model in which DNA instability is a cause, rather than a consequence, of cancer progression. The successful maintenance of genomic stability is therefore an important defense against the process of neoplastic transformation.

In addition to mutation, there are other mechanisms that lead to genetic instability, including *gene amplification*, and the epigenetic modification of chromatin-associated, transcriptional states through *gene methylation* and *gene acetylation*. In cells that display gene amplification, gene expression is aberrantly and constitutively enhanced above the level of physiologically normal levels. Gene-amplified cells can display discrete cytogenetic changes (see Chap. 4, Sec. 4.4.2 and Fig. 18.8), such as *double-minute (DM) chromosomes* or *homogeneously staining regions (HSRs)*. Additionally, some cells acquire drug-resistance via gene amplification. The rate at which drug-resistant variants arise in a cell population is therefore an indirect measure of genetic instability. Using specific markers of drug resistance such as the *DHFR* or *MDR* genes (see Chap. 18, Sec. 18.2), it has been observed that gene amplification occurs at a high frequency in transformed cells ($10^{-3}$–$10^{-5}$), yet is almost undetectable in normal diploid fibroblasts (a frequency of less than $10^{-9}$).

If the amplified gene is an oncogene or a regulator of DNA replication or cell cycle progression, gene overexpression may result in increased cellular proliferative advantage leading to clonal selection and malignant transformation. Some amplified oncogenes, such as *HER2* (*NEU/ERB-B2*) in breast cancer and the *N-MYC* gene in neuroblastoma, are predictors of poor prognosis in those patients who harbor these tumors. For example, the amplification of the *HER2* gene can occur in up to 25 percent of human breast cancers and is associated with a greater risk of distant metastasis. However, it may also provide a therapeutic target as described in Chapter 17, Section 17.6.2.

The structure and activity of chromatin can be altered by posttranslational modifications (e.g., acetylation, phosphorylation, methylation, and ubiquitylation). *Methylation* of DNA is the main epigenetic modification in humans and has been observed in over half of the tumor suppressor genes that cause familial cancers. Usually, there is an associated gain of methylation in normally unmethylated CpG islands within the DNA. Methylation-induced transcriptional silencing begins early during the process of genetic instability and can affect many genes that are important in tumor progression. These genes include those involved in cell cycle control (e.g., $p16^{INK4a}$), transcription, hormone biology (e.g., estrogen and progesterone receptor genes), intracellular signal transduction [e.g., the Von Hippel-Lindau (*VHL*) gene], apoptosis, DNA repair, and tumor suppressor genes (e.g., *pRB*). Furthermore, given that methyl-

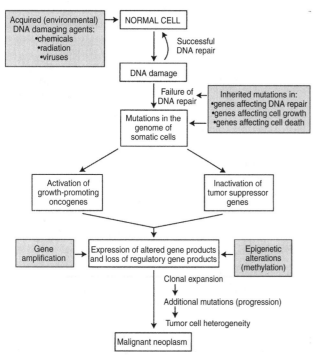

**Figure 5.1.** Genetic and epigenetic mechanisms of genetic instability.

ation is a potentially reversible state, this creates a target for novel cancer therapeutic strategies involving gene re-activation. For example, both retinoic acid and 5'-aza-deoxycytidine can reverse DNA methylation and re-activate expression of normal regulatory genes, thereby leading to the regression of some human leukemias.

Histones are the core proteins of nucleosomes and their acetylation status regulates, in part, gene expression by altering chromatin coiling. Two groups of enzymes, the histone deacetylases (HDACs) and the acetyl transferases, determine the level of histone acetylation. Deacetylated histones are generally associated with silencing of gene expression; in contrast, the acetylation of histones is generally associated with gene expression. Histone deacetylase inhibitors promote acetylation, leading to the uncoiling of chromatin and are emerging as an exciting new class of potential anticancer agents for the treatment of solid and hematological malignancies. Examples of these agents include short-chain fatty acids (e.g., sodium butyrate, valproic acid), hydroxyaminic acids (e.g., SAHA, TSA), synthetic benzamide derivatives, and cyclic tetrapeptides. Depending on the cell type, inhibition of HDACs in cancer cells can lead to transcriptional activation of about 2 percent of human genes, including tumor suppressor genes. Treating cells with HDAC inhibitors can increase cell cycle arrest, induction of apoptosis, and differentiation in cancer cells. Several HDAC inhibitors have shown impressive antitumor activity in vivo at nanomolar concentrations and are currently in phase I and phase II clinical trials alone, or in combination with demethylating agents (Fig. 5.2; Momparler, 2003).

Normal tissues may have different inherent abilities to maintain their genetic integrity when faced with exogenous or endogenous damaging stimuli. For example, genetic stability is maintained in stem cells when compared to somatic cells, in part due to altered DNA repair pathways (see Sec. 5.3). Evidence from primary stromal versus primary epithelial cell cultures suggests that normal epithelial cells may be predisposed to genetic instability. Stromal cells (e.g., fibroblasts) eventually lose the ability to proliferate in culture [termed *cellular senescence* as a result of loss of chromosomal telomere DNA (see Sec. 5.5.2)]. However other cell types, such as human mammary epithelial cultures, exhibit genetic alterations due to sequential loss of DNA repair and checkpoint control during cell proliferation that enable an increased number of population doublings. During this process rare cells can escape cellular senescence and become immortalized (Tlsty, 1990). Differences between stromal and epithelial cultures also exist for the relative ability to initiate cell cycle checkpoints following DNA damage. These and other observations may account for the increased incidence of epithelial-based tumors compared to stromal-based tumors in humans (Fig. 5.3).

Clinical studies are underway that attempt to document specific tissue biomarkers of genetic instability in premalignant human tissues. This information can be used to ascertain whether a specific individual at risk for cancer will benefit from treatment with chemopreventive agents based on their susceptibility and the carcinogenic insult. Tissue biomarkers can be related to DNA repair, cell cycle checkpoint control, altered oncogenes or tumor suppressor genes, or chromosomal aberrations. For example, as part of several chemoprevention trials (see Chap. 3, Sec. 3.4), biopsies have been obtained from tissues in high-risk patients (e.g., bronchial biopsies from chronic smokers; oral or laryngeal biopsies from individuals with premalignancy) and examined for chromosome instability using in situ hybridization (see Chap. 4, Sec. 4.4; Hittelman, 2001). Many biopsy specimens show evidence of chromosome instability within the carcinogen-exposed tissue and

**Figure 5.2.** Action of histone deacetylase inhibitors (HDAC inhibitors). With inhibition of histone deacetylases (HDACs), histones are acetylated, and the DNA that is tightly wrapped around deacetylated histone cores relaxes. Accumulation of acetylated histones in nucleosomes leads to increased transcription of a subset of genes (for example, *p21^WAF*) which, in turn, leads to downstream effects that result in cell-growth arrest, differentiation, and/or apoptotic cell death and as a consequence, inhibition of tumor growth. Ac, acetyl group; HAT, histone acetyltransferase, TFC-transcription factor complex. (Reproduced with permission from Marks et al., 2001.) (See color plate.)

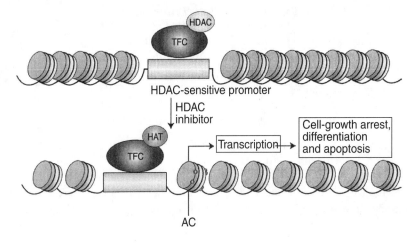

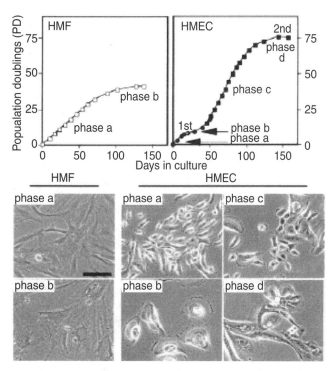

**Figure 5.3.** Genetic instability in epithelial tissues compared to stromal tissues. Data from Romanov et al. (2001) showing that human mammary fibroblasts (HMFs; left upper panel) undergo a limited number of cell divisions (*phase a*) before entering an irreversible arrest, called senescence (*phase b*). In contrast, human mammary epithelial cells (HMECs; *upper right panel*) exhibit an initial growth phase (*phase a*) that is followed by a transient growth plateau (termed selection or *phase b*) from which proliferative cells emerge to undergo further population doublings (*phase c;* approximately 20–70 doublings) before entering a second growth plateau (*phase d*). Seen in the panels below are representative cell images from each phase for each cell type. Rare HMECs can emerge from senescence, exhibit eroding telomeric sequences and ultimately generate the types of chromosomal abnormalities seen in the earliest lesions of breast cancer. (Reproduced with permission from Romanov et al., 2001.)

multifocal clonal outgrowths can persist for many years. The latter may account for continued lung cancer risk following smoking cessation. Future work in this area will involve the discovery of new compounds that can reverse genetic instability in a given tissue of interest, with the potential for preventing cancer.

### 5.2.2 Human DNA Repair Disorders and Cancer Risk

Repair of DNA plays an important role in determining cancer predisposition, thus providing further evidence that genetic change is a primary event in malignant transformation. Functional analyses of DNA repair proteins in vivo have recently benefited from molecular recom-

binant technologies, whereby a specific DNA repair gene is either aberrantly expressed or rendered null (i.e., gene knockout) in murine embryonic stem cells (see Chap. 4, Sec. 4.3.12). These studies suggest that some, but not all, DNA repair proteins are required for mammalian development as a number of the knocked-out genes were embryonic lethal (e.g., mice null for *RAD51* and *RAD50*). Furthermore, these repair-deficient mice were also prone to chromosomal instability and to the early onset of specific cancers.

A number of human disease syndromes are associated with pronounced cellular sensitivity to DNA-damaging agents due to hereditary deficiencies in DNA repair or to deficiencies in signaling pathways that are activated by DNA damage (Table 5.1). Patients with several of these syndromes show marked chromosomal instability and predisposition to malignancy and are therefore *cancer prone*. For example, the disorders, xeroderma pigmentosum (XP), ataxia telangiectasia (AT), Bloom's syndrome (BS), and Fanconi's anemia (FA) are all autosomal recessive, cancer-prone diseases that are associated with defective DNA repair. Patients suffering from XP are sun-sensitive and have an extreme predisposition to skin cancer—an increase in incidence of perhaps 1000-fold. Patients with AT have a very high incidence of lymphomas, often before the age of 20. The incidence of lymphomas is also increased markedly in FA and BS patients. Human hereditary non-polyposis colon cancer (HNPCC) is caused by a deficiency in DNA mismatch repair (see Chap. 2, Sec. 2.3.3). Finally, there are at least two diseases, Cockayne's syndrome (CS) and trichothiodystrophy (TTD), that involve deficiencies in DNA repair and do not exhibit an increase in malignancy, but instead exhibit signs of early aging.

### 5.3 BIOCHEMISTRY OF DNA REPAIR PATHWAYS

An improved understanding of the mechanisms of DNA repair came from the isolation of repair-deficient rodent cells [e.g., Chinese hamster ovary (CHO) mutants] with unusual sensitivity to different classes of DNA damaging agents. Some mutants exhibited extreme sensitivity to ultraviolet light and crosslinking agents such as mitomycin C, but little or no sensitivity to x-rays. Other cells exhibited sensitivity to x-rays and chemical agents known to cause DNA breakage, but little or no sensitivity to UV light or crosslinking agents. These various phenotypes, which are similar to those characterized previously in bacteria and yeast, indicate the involvement of several distinct DNA repair pathways and associated gene products. Some of these repair pathways are so highly conserved from yeast to humans that yeast proteins can substitute for human proteins and vice versa; this has been helpful in the cloning and func-

**Table 5.1.** Cancer Prone Human Syndromes With Defective DNA Repair

| Syndrome | Affected Repair Pathway | Defective Protein | Main Type of Genomic Defect | Major Cancer Predisposition |
| --- | --- | --- | --- | --- |
| Xeroderma pigmentosum (XP) | Nucleotide excision repair | XP CS | Point mutations | UV-induced skin cancer |
| Ataxia telangiectasia (AT) | DNA dsb response | ATM | Chromosome aberrations | Lymphomas |
| AT-like disorder (ATLD) | DNA dsb response | MRE11 | Chromosome aberrations | Lymphomas |
| Nijmegen breakage syndrome (NBS) | DNA dsb response | NBS1 | Chromosome aberrations | Lymphomas |
| BRCA1/BRCA2 | Homologous recombination | BRCA1 BRCA2 | Chromosome aberrations | Breast (ovarian) cancer |
| Werner syndrome | Homologous recombination | WRN helicase | Chromosome aberrations | Various cancers |
| Bloom syndrome | Homologous recombination | BLM helicase | Chromosome aberrations— sister-chromatid exchange | Leukemia, lymphoma, others |
| Hereditary non-polyposis colorectal cancer (HNPCC) | Mismatch repair | MLH1 MSH2 | Microsatellite instability | Colorectal cancer |
| Fanconi's anemia | DNA crosslink repair | FANC-D2 | Chromosome aberrations | Leukemia, others |

tional characterization of the human homologs of yeast DNA repair genes.

An important property in DNA repair is the fidelity of the repair pathway leading to the concepts of error-prone, and error-free, DNA repair. Many DNA lesions can block transcription of RNA, thereby inactivating the gene which contains damaged DNA. Persistent blockage of RNA synthesis can lead to cell death but these lesions are often repaired through the *transcription-coupled repair* pathway (TCR; see Sec. 5.3.4 below). Transcription-coupled repair is designed to displace the stalled RNA polymerase and drive a high-priority repair mechanism. For lesions that block DNA replication, several error-prone DNA polymerases have been described which have increased flexibility and low fidelity to allow for replicative bypass (i.e., translesion DNA synthesis) of the damage contained within DNA. These polymerases can temporarily be used by the cell following DNA damage and can then be substituted by more accurate DNA polymerases. One model suggests that the increased use of these lower-fidelity *translesion DNA polymerases* contributes to high error-rates during DNA replication and may lead to malignant transformation (Fig. 5.4).

In the following sections, discrete biochemical pathways of DNA repair are described. These pathways can

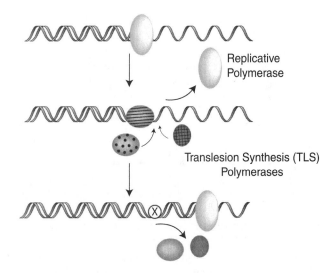

**Figure 5.4.** Translesion DNA synthesis (TLS). The 'DNA polymerase switch model' for TLS and mutagenesis (Cordonnier and Fuchs, 1999). This figure shows the replicative DNA polymerase locked at a lesion contained within the DNA template. Cells contain several different DNA polymerases that have varying polymerase fidelity and these can transiently replace the replicative DNA polymerase, which results in replication errors. After a short patch of "translesion" synthesis in the vicinity of the lesion, these "faulty" polymerases are replaced again by the high-fidelity replicative DNA polymerase that resumes processive DNA synthesis.

be divided into different classes depending on the specific DNA lesion they are designed to repair, and include: (1) direct damage reversal, (2) mismatch repair, (3) base excision repair, (4) nucleotide excision repair, and (5) homologous and nonhomologous repair of DNA double-strand breaks.

### 5.3.1 Direct Reversal Repair of O(6)-Methylguanine: Alkylating Agents and RAS Activation

DNA-reactive carcinogens and anticancer drugs induce many structurally-distinct mutagenic and cytotoxic DNA lesions. Alkylating agents react with nucleophilic sites in the bases and phosphotriester bonds of DNA. Upon exposure to $N$-nitroso compounds [such as $N$-methyl-$N$-nitrosourea (MeNU) or $N$-ethyl-$N$-nitrosourea (EtNU)], about a dozen different alkylation products are formed in cellular DNA including O(6)-methylguanine [$O^6$-meG; see Chap. 3, Sec. 3.2.4]. When unrepaired, these lesions cause G:C $\rightarrow$ A:T mutations by anomalous base pairing during the process of DNA replication. O6–alkylguanine DNA alkyltransferase is therefore a key enzyme involved in the prevention of malignant transformation by removing $O^6$-meG adducts. It acts on double-stranded DNA by flipping the O(6)-guanine adduct out of the DNA helix and into a binding pocket to mediate DNA repair.

Studies in transgenic mice in which alkyltransferase expression levels are increased or decreased confirm the importance of this repair pathway in protecting against mutations. Furthermore, intertissue variations in the levels of alkyltransferase enzymes may account for the differential organ-specific susceptibility to these types of carcinogens (see Chap. 3, Sec. 3.2.4). For example, lesions formed in DNA upon exposure to MNU or EtNU can induce rat mammary adenocarcinomas at high yield in which G:C $\rightarrow$ A:T transitions at the second position of codon 12 (GGA) of the $H$-ras oncogene and represents a frequent carcinogenic signature (see Chap. 3, Sec. 3.2.5).

Some human tumor cells do not express alkyltransferase despite having an intact gene, due to methylation of CpG-rich islands in its promoter region. In other tumor cells, high alkyltransferase activity is observed and is associated with increased resistance to chemotherapeutic agents such as temozolomide or BCNU. This resistance can be abolished by the drug, O(6)-benzylguanine, which degrades alkyltransferases using the ubiquitin-proteosomal system (see Chap. 9, Fig. 9.4). This drug is in clinical trials as a potential chemosensitizer when used with alkylating agents. Other clinical trials are in progress to determine whether the toxicity of alkylating agents can be reversed by increasing the repair capacity of bone marrow cells through gene therapy.

### 5.3.2 Mismatch Repair and Hereditary Non-Polyposis Colorectal Cancer

*Hereditary non-polyposis colorectal cancer* (HNPCC) is the most common form of hereditary colorectal cancer accounting for 2 to 5 percent of all colorectal cancers (see Chap. 2, Sec. 2.3.3). In addition to colorectal cancer, HNPCC patients also have an excess of endometrial, small-bowel, and renal cancer. This familial cancer syndrome occurs secondary to genetic instability acquired through deficient DNA *mismatch repair* (MMR; Harfe et al., 2000). The MMR system recognizes and restores mismatched nucleotides that can arise by erroneous DNA replication or within DNA insertion-deletion loops (ranging from one to ten bases). These loops can result from errors in DNA polymerase function during DNA replication. Insertion-deletion loops affect repetitive DNA sequences, and cells from HNPCC exhibit

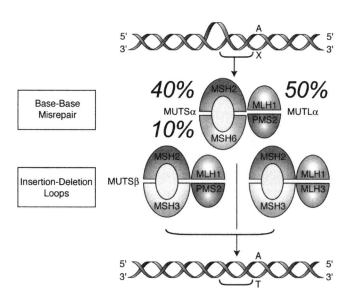

**Figure 5.5.** Mismatch repair (MMR) pathway. At least six different MMR proteins, in the form of MUTSα or MUTSβ heterodimers, are required for the repair of DNA base mismatches or insertion-deletion loops introduced during DNA replication. For the initial recognition of DNA replication errors, the MSH2 protein forms a heterodimer with either MSH6 or MSH3 depending on the type of lesion to be repaired (e.g., MSH6 is required for the correction of single-DNA base mispairs, whereas both MSH3 and MSH6 may contribute to the correction of DNA insertion-deletion loops). The majority of human MMR mutations associated with hereditary non-polyposis colorectal cancer (HNPCC) occur in the MSH2 and MLH1 proteins (40% and 50% as shown), whereas the remaining 10% of the mutations are associated with the MSH6 protein. (Adapted from Friedberg, 2001.)

gains or losses of short DNA repeat units within microsatellite regions, giving rise to *microsatellite instability* (MSI; Kolodner et al., 1999). These represent runs of approximately four to forty repeated mononucleotides or dinucleotides such as TTTT or CACACA and occur at multiple sites within the genome. Microsatellite instability can be detected using DNA gel electrophoresis and is an important clinical marker for MMR deficiency.

Mutations in six human MMR genes have been associated with HNPCC and MSI (Fig. 5.5). The protein products of MMR genes form heterodimer complexes, and different protein pairs recognize specific mismatched nucleotides in DNA. For example, the MSH2 protein forms a heterodimer with two additional MMR proteins, MSH6 or MSH3, and the resulting complexes are called hMutS-$\alpha$ or hMutS-$\beta$ respectively. MSH6 is required for the recognition of DNA base-base misrepair, whereas MSH3 and MSH6 have partially redundant functions for the recognition of DNA insertion-deletion loops. A second heterodimer of the MMR gene products MLH1 and PMS2 (i.e., hMutL-$\alpha$) coordinates the interplay between the initial mismatch recognition complex and subsequent protein interactions required to complete MMR. The latter proteins include PCNA (see Chap. 7, Sec. 7.4.2), DNA polymerases $\delta$ and $\varepsilon$, ssDNA-binding protein, and possibly DNA helicases (Hoeijmakers, 2001).

More than 300 different MMR mutations have been documented in human cancers, mainly affecting MLH1 (approximately 50 percent), MSH2 (approximately 40 percent) and MSH6 (approximately 10 percent). Genetically predisposed individuals with HNPCC carry a defective copy of an MMR gene in every cell. Somatic inactivation of the remaining wild-type copy in a target tissue, typically colon, gives rise to a profound repair defect and increased rates of mutation in cells (i.e., a mutator phenotype) with progressive accumulation of mutations in adenomatous polyposis coli *(APC)*, *p53* or other genes (Loeb, 1991; Jiricny et al., 2000; Peltomaki, 2001).

Knowing the status of MMR and MSI in sporadic colon cancers may be useful information for understanding prognosis following surgery or in choosing appropriate chemotherapy. For example, MMR-deficient cells may be more sensitive to topoisomerase inhibitors (e.g., camptothecin and etoposide) but more resistant to cisplatin. Resistance to cisplatin and its resulting DNA adducts is thought to be due to increased ability for adduct-bypass secondary to faulty mismatch recognition and repair. Furthermore, the absence of MSI appears to be a predictive marker for colon cancer sensitivity to adjuvant chemotherapy (i.e., 5-fluorouracil and leucovorin) following primary surgery (Ribic et al., 2003).

### 5.3.3 Oxidative Damage and Base Excision Repair

Spontaneous oxidative damage is known to occur in cells, producing $10^4$ to $10^5$ oxidative residues, (e.g., 8-oxo-guanine) per cell per day among the $3 \times 10^9$ bases in the genome. If a cell cannot repair this continual onslaught of base damage, malignant transformation may occur. DNA base damage, occurring as a result of endogenous oxidative processes or exogenous DNA damage (e.g., ionizing radiation) is repaired by the *base excision repair* (BER) pathway. Base excision repair involves the enzymatic removal of the damaged DNA base by DNA glycosylases. This initial removal step leaves an apurinic or apyrimidinic (AP) site (Fig. 5.6). The major BER pathway is *short-patch BER* and involves the replacement of a single nucleotide following DNA backbone cleavage at the AP site. A minor BER pathway is the *long-patch BER pathway*, which exists for the repair

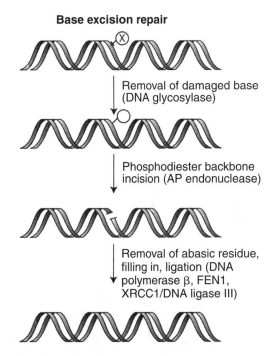

**Base excision repair**

Removal of damaged base
(DNA glycosylase)

Phosphodiester backbone
incision (AP endonuclease)

Removal of abasic residue,
filling in, ligation (DNA
polymerase $\beta$, FEN1,
XRCC1/DNA ligase III)

**Figure 5.6.** Base excision repair (BER) of oxidative damage. Oxidative damage creates DNA base damage which is repaired by the BER pathway. The major pathway is *short-patch BER* and involves the replacement of a single nucleotide following the DNA backbone cleavage at the apurinic or apyrimidinic (AP) site. Where the lesions in DNA are methylated or deaminated bases, the abasic site in the DNA is first nicked by APE1, an AP endonuclease. The AP site is prepared for the concerted actions of DNA polymerase-$\beta$, FEN1 and the XRCC1-DNA ligase III complex. These proteins remove the 5'-terminal baseless sugar residue and subsequently seal the DNA nick by DNA synthesis using the opposite strand as a template. A second *long-patch BER* pathway, exists for the repair of 2-13 damaged nucleotides. (Adapted from Friedberg, 2001.)

of two to thirteen damaged nucleotides. Although all DNA glycosylases cleave glycosylic bonds, they differ in their base substrate specificity and in their reaction mechanisms. For example, the OGG1 protein is an 8-oxo-guanine DNA glycosylase and therefore can remove spontaneous or ionizing radiation-induced lesions to prevent cellular mutations. The gene locus of OGG1 on chromosome 3p25–26 is frequently lost in lung cancers, consistent with a role for the protein in preventing carcinogenesis.

No human disorders have been related directly to inherited BER deficiencies and knockout mice engineered to lack core BER proteins die in embryo, attesting to the important role of BER in development. In contrast, mouse knockout models for a variety of glycosylase genes have shown only mild increases in the incidence of genetic mutations. This may be due to partial redundancy in the glycosylases or due to overlap with the transcription-coupled repair processes described below. However, BER may also be defective in cells that have mutations in tumor suppressor proteins. For example, the p53 protein can stimulate BER by in-

teracting directly with APE1 and DNA-polymerase-$\beta$. In cells that express mutant p53 proteins, this interaction is lost and as a result these cells have an increased number of unrepaired oxidative lesions and increased mutagenesis (Offer et al., 2001).

### 5.3.4 Nucleotide Excision Repair and Xeroderma Pigmentosum (XP)

Nucleotide excision repair (NER) is a complex DNA repair pathway involving more than thirty genes designed to repair ultraviolet-induced photoproducts or cyclobutane pyridimine dimers (CPD). Many of the NER genes were originally cloned from complementation analyses of cells from patients and are referred to as XPA-XPG (i.e., xeroderma pigmentosum A, B, C, D, E, G proteins) or CSA or CSB (i.e., Cockayne syndrome A and B proteins). As some of the NER proteins (e.g., TFIIH) are also involved in the control of RNA transcription, some of the syndromes resulting from their deficiency are also referred to as *transcription factor disorders* (Fig. 5.7; Berneburg et al., 2001).

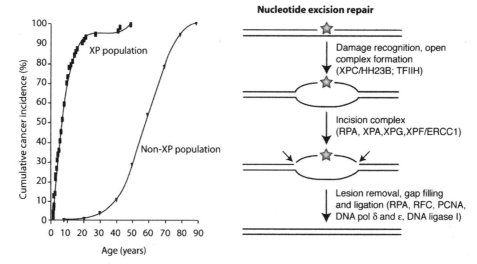

**Figure 5.7.** Nucleotide excision repair (NER) and skin cancer risk. *Left:* Incidence of skin cancer in xeroderma pigmentosum (XP) compared to normal population with similar exposure to the sun. The 1000-fold excess risk of UV-induced skin cancer is secondary to defective NER of UV-induced DNA lesions in XP patients. *Right:* One of the first steps in global NER (GG-NER) is the recognition of UV-induced photoproducts or cyclobutane pyridimine dimer (CPD) lesions (indicated by the star) in the DNA that are recognized as disrupted DNA base pairing by the XPC-HH23B protein complex. If a UV-induced lesion is contained within a DNA strand undergoing transcription, the RNA polymerase is displaced by the Cockayne Syndrome CSB and CSA proteins to facilitate transcription-coupled NER (TCR-NER; not shown). Thereafter, in either GG-NER and TCR-NER, the XPB and XPD helicases of the multi-subunit TFIIH transcription factor open 30 base pairs of DNA around the damaged template. XPA and RPA proteins then probe and stabilize the open template followed by action of the XPG and ERCC1-XPF proteins which cleave the 3′ and 5′ borders of the opened DNA region on the damaged strand to generate a 24–34 base oligonucleotide containing the damaged DNA. DNA synthesis then ensues using the intact nondamaged DNA template to code for the required base pairs. The entire process of NER takes several minutes to complete. (Adapted from Friedberg, 2001.)

The process of NER is highly conserved in eukaryotic cells and consists of the following four steps: (1) recognition of the damaged DNA; (2) excision of an oligonucleotide of twenty-four to thirty-two residues containing the damaged DNA by dual incision of the damaged strand on each side of the lesion; (3) filling in of the resulting gap by DNA polymerase; and (4) ligation of the nick (Balajee and Bohr, 2000). In human cells, NER requires at least six core proteins for damage recognition and incision (i.e., XPA, XPC-hHR23B, RPA, TFIIH, XPG, and XPF–ERCC1) and other factors for DNA synthesis and ligation (e.g., PCNA, RFC, DNA polymerase $\delta$ or $\epsilon$ and DNA ligase I; de Laat et al., 1999).

Nucleotide excision repair consists of two subpathways termed *global genome repair* (GG-NER) that is transcription-independent and removes lesions from the entire genome, and *transcription-coupled repair* (TCR-NER). The GG-NER pathway surveys the entire genome for lesions which distort the DNA. These lesions are removed rapidly. In contrast, CPDs are repaired very slowly by GG-NER and are removed more efficiently from the transcribed strand of expressed genes by TCR-NER. TCR-NER focuses on DNA lesions that block the activity of RNA polymerases and overall transcriptional activity. The elongating transcriptional machinery is thought to facilitate the recognition of DNA lesions on the transcribed strand in TCR-NER. (Hoeijmakers, 2001).

The human XP, CS, and TTD disorders exhibit cellular ultraviolet sensitivity (Hoeijmakers, 2001). However, only XP patients are cancer-prone with a dramatic 1000-fold increase in the incidence of UV-induced skin cancer (Fig. 5.7). This is due to mutations in one of seven XP genes (i.e., *XPA-XPG*) in their cells. Furthermore, secondary genetic events, such as mutations in the *p53* gene, are common in the skin tumors in XP patients consistent with ongoing genomic instability. Cockayne syndrome is characterized by a TCR-related defect secondary to mutations in *CSB* and *CSA* genes. Cockayne syndrome patients exhibit neurodegeneration and premature aging relating to inappropriate apoptosis in target tissues. Trichothiodystrophy patients share many features of CS patients, but also have brittle hair, nails, and scaly skin, secondary to reduced expression of epidermal matrix proteins. Similar to their human counterparts, XP-related gene knockout mice exhibit decreased NER and increased UV-induced carcinogenesis.

### 5.3.5 DNA Double-Strand Break Repair: Homologous Recombination RAD51 and BRCA2

Double-strand breaks (dsb) in DNA result from exogenous agents such as ionizing radiation (IR) and certain chemotherapeutic drugs, from endogenously gener-

ated reactive oxygen species, and from mechanical stress on the chromosomes (Zhou et al., 1998). They can also be produced when DNA replication forks encounter DNA single-strand breaks or following defective replication of chromosome ends (i.e., telomeres; see Sec. 5.5). In addition, DNA dsbs are generated to initiate recombination between homologous chromosomes during meiosis or occur as intermediates during developmentally regulated rearrangements, such as V(D)J recombination and immunoglobulin class-switch recombination (see Chap. 20, Sec. 20.2.4). The programmed rearrangements are initiated by specific enzymes that generate DNA dsbs in the target locus [i.e., the RAG1 and RAG2 proteins in V(D)J recombination] but the recombination intermediates seem to be resolved by the same pathways that are used to repair DNA dsbs induced by ionizing radiation (Jeggo, 1997; van Gent et al., 2001).

In human cells, recombinational repair of DNA dsbs occurs either by *homologous recombination* (HR; Fig. 5.8) or *nonhomologous end joining* (NHEJ; Fig. 5.9). Although it was originally thought that NHEJ was the dominant mode of DNA dsb in mammalian tissues, it appears that one pathway may be preferentially used depending on tissue type, the extent of DNA damage, the cell cycle phase in which the cell is damaged, and the relative need for repair fidelity. There may also be cooperation between the two pathways (Richardson and Jasin, 2000). In homologous recombination, extensive homology is required between the region of the DNA dsb and the sister chromatid or homologous chromosome from which repair is directed. This pathway is thought to predominate in repair of DNA dsbs in germline tissues and during S and G2 phases of the cell cycle. The HR pathway results in error-free repair of DNA dsbs because the intact undamaged template is used to pair new DNA bases between the damaged and undamaged strands during DNA synthesis.

Nonhomologous end joining does not require homology and the NHEJ proteins simply link the ends of DNA breaks together; this usually results in the loss or gain of a few nucleotides. Nonhomologous end joining is error-prone and operates predominantly to repair damage in somatic cells during the G1 phase of the cell cycle. There is evidence to suggest that RAD52 (a HR-related protein), and KU, a DNA end-binding protein that functions in NHEJ, compete for binding to dsbs and channel the repair of dsbs into HR or NHEJ respectively, depending on the cellular context (van Gent et al., 2001). There is a separate, but related, DNA dsb repair pathway that ligates DNA dsbs using small sections of microhomologous DNA and involves the MRE11 and BRCA2 proteins (Fig. 5.10).

Biochemical and genetic studies in yeast have been fundamental in the ability to clone human homologs

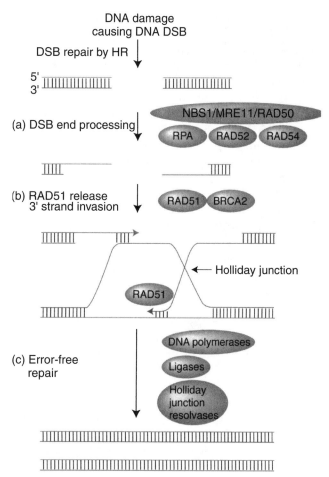

of proteins involved in HR. In the yeast, *Saccharomyces cerevesiae*, the *RAD52* epistaxis group of genes are involved in HR including *RAD50*, *RAD51*, *RAD52*, *RAD54*, *RAD55*, *RAD57*, *RAD59*, *MRE11*, and *XRS2* (the latter re-termed *p95* or *NBS1-nibrin* in mammalian cells). $RAD51^{-/-}$ mice are embryonic lethal, attesting to the importance of this critical HR protein in meiosis and development. Careful observations during the initial stages of embryogenesis in $RAD51^{-/-}$ mice have shown that lethality is preceded by chromosomal rearrangements and deletions. It is thought that DNA replication errors and replication-associated DNA

**Figure 5.8.** Homologous recombination (HR) repair of DNA double strand breaks (DSB). The initiating step for homologous recombination is thought to be the processing of the 3′ end of the DNA break by the NBS1/MRE11/RAD50 protein complex. Following binding of the RAD52 and RAD54 proteins, Replication Protein A (RPA) facilitates the assembly of the Rad51-BRCA2 complex on the single-strand 3′ DNA overhang to form a RAD51-nucleoprotein filament. The formation of the complex and invasion of the RAD51 filament is facilitated by the RAD51 accessory proteins XRCC2, XRCC3, RAD51B, RAD51C and RAD51D (not shown). The RAD51 nucleofilament DNA is then able to pair with a homologous region in duplex DNA forming a Holliday junction after alignment of sister chromatids. Complex chromatin alterations and configurations are required to unwind the DNA and allow for DNA strand exchange. After identification of the identical sister chromatid sequences, the intact double-stranded copy is then used as a template to repair the DNA break by subsequent DNA synthesis using DNA polymerases, ligases and Holliday junction resolvases. Homologous recombination results in error-free (i.e., high-fidelity) repair of DNA double-strand breaks and predominates in the S and G2 phases of the cell cycle.

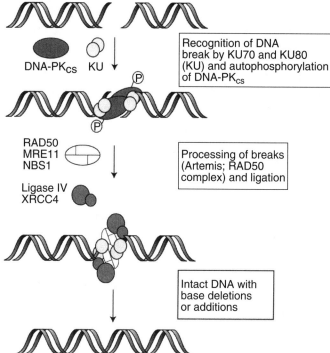

**Figure 5.9.** Non-homologous end-joining (NHEJ) repair of DNA double-strand breaks. DNA-PKcs, KU70, KU80, DNA-ligase IV, and XRCC4 are all critical components of the NHEJ repair pathway. DNA-PK is composed of a heterodimeric DNA-binding component, named KU70/KU80 which binds to either blunt or staggered DNA ends at the double-strand break and recruits the large catalytic subunit kinase, DNA-PKcs to the break. DNA-PKcs undergoes autophosphorylation after binding to the DNA break and may recruit additional proteins to the damaged site as potential phosphorylation substrates. The NBS1-MRE11-RAD50 protein complex and the Artemis protein may be involved in processing of DNA ends during the initial binding and activation of DNA-PK kinase activity. The XRCC4-ligase IV heterodimer finally ligates the breaks to create intact DNA strands. Non-homologous recombination can result in error-prone (i.e., low-fidelity) repair of DNA double-strand breaks and predominates in the G1 phase of the cell cycle. (Adapted from van Gent et al., 2001.)

A

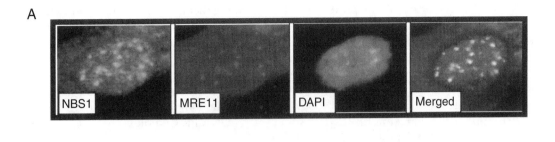

B

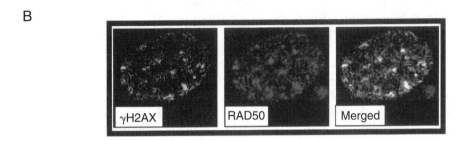

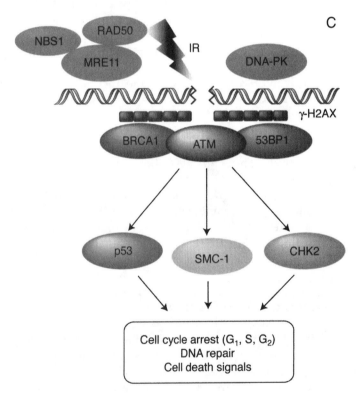

**Figure 5.10.** (*A* and *B*). Immunofluorescence micrographs showing focal recruitment of DNA repair proteins to sites of DNA damage. In *panel A,* a human fibroblast is immunostained for NBS1 (*green*) and MRE11 (*red*) proteins at 8 hours following exposure to 12 Gy of ionizing radiation. The nuclear volume is stained in blue with DAPI stain. The 1:1 merging of the MRE11 and NBS1 fluorescent signals (*seen as yellow foci in far right panel*) is consistent with colocalization of the two proteins within an NBS1/MRE11/RAD50 complex at sites of DNA damage. Reproduced with permission of Maser et al. (1997). In *panel B,* modified histone molecules (γ-H2AX), produced in response to DNA damage colocalize, with the DNA repair protein RAD50 (unpublished data from Al Rashid and Bristow; 2003). (*C*) DNA double-strand breaks activate the γ-H2AX response leading to the recruitment of the NBS1/MRE11/RAD50 complex and of the DNA-PK$_{CS}$, ATM, BRCA1 and 53BP1 proteins involved in signaling of DNA damage. In particular, the recruitment of the ATM kinase can lead to the subsequent phosphorylation of the p53, CHK2, and SMC-1 (structural maintenance of chromosome-1) which control the cell cycle checkpoints in the G1, S, and G2 phases of the cell cycle, leading to DNA repair and/or activation of cell death. (Adapted after Abraham, 2001.) (See color plate.)

strand breaks are converted into DNA dsbs in HR-defective cells (Lim and Hasty, 1996). In cells derived from *RAD54$^{-/-}$* mice (which are developmentally normal), there is also decreased homologous recombination and increased sensitivity to DNA crosslinking agents such as mitomycin-C. Interestingly, *RAD54$^{-/-}$* embryonic cells are sensitive to ionizing radiation, yet somatic fibroblasts are not, supporting a greater role for HR in DNA dsb repair and genomic stability within germline tissues (Essers et al., 1997). Although in *S. cerevesiae RAD52* is essential for DNA dsb repair, *RAD52$^{-/-}$* mice are viable and fertile and do not show a DNA dsb repair deficiency. Homologous recombination therefore appears to be more complex in mammalian cells than in yeast, possibly due to functional redundancy in many of the proteins.

The BRCA2 breast cancer susceptibility protein (see also Chap. 7, Sec. 7.4.5) may also play a role in the homologous repair of DNA dsbs. Both BRCA1 and BRCA2 proteins form discrete nuclear foci during S-phase at the sites of DNA damage following exposure to DNA damaging agents. Although RAD51 colocalizes at subnuclear sites with BRCA1, their interaction is thought to be indirect, with only 1 to 5 percent of BRCA1 in somatic cells associating with RAD51 (Marmorstein et al., 1998). In contrast, the BRCA2 protein contains eight repeats, each with 30 to 40 residues, which are the major sites for the direct binding to RAD51 by a significant fraction of the total intracellular pool of BRCA2 (Davies et al., 2001). As such, BRCA2-deficient cells have ten-fold lower levels of homologous recombination when compared to BRCA2-proficient cells (Moynahan et al., 2001). One model suggests that a BRCA2-RAD51 complex promotes the accurate assembly of DNA repair proteins required to offset DNA breaks that accumulate during DNA replication; these could otherwise lead to gross chromosomal rearrangements, loss of heterozygosity at tumor suppressor gene loci, and carcinogenesis.

Aberrant HR is also observed in the cancer-prone Bloom's (BS) and Werner's (WS) syndromes with increased spontaneous level of sister chromatid exchange (SCE), chromosomal deletions, and translocations. BS and WS have mutations in the BLM and WRN proteins, respectively. These are RecQ helicase proteins, which normally act at multiple steps in DNA replication including the stabilization of replication forks and removal of DNA recombination intermediates, in order to maintain genome integrity. Fanconi's anemia is a rare autosomal recessive disease characterized by bone marrow failure, developmental anomalies, a high incidence of leukemia, and cellular hypersensitivity to crosslinking agents such as Mitomycin C. Five of the seven known Fanconi's anemia proteins bind together in a complex and influence the function of a sixth, FANC-D2, which colocalizes with BRCA1 and NBS1 in nuclear foci after genotoxic stress (Nakanishi et al., 2002; De la Torre et al., 2003).

A number of human cancers, including ovarian, breast, prostate, and pancreatic cancer, have mutations or altered expression and function of the *MRE*11, *RAD51/RAD52/RAD54*, and *BRCA1/2* genes. This suggest that tumorigenesis is associated with altered homologous recombination in sporadic tumors. Increased levels of RAD51 expression in certain cancer cell lines have also been associated with altered phosphorylation, ubiquitination, and transcription of the RAD51 protein due to abnormal c-ABL- and STAT5-mediated tyrosine kinase signaling pathways in cancer cell lines (Chap. 8, Sec. 8.5.1). This can lead to acquired radioresistance and chemoresistance. New preclinical strategies have therefore been designed to reverse the RAD51-mediated resistant phenotype including the use of antisense to *RAD51* or by using the tyrosine kinase inhibitor, imatinib (Daboussi et al., 2002).

### 5.3.6 DNA Double-Strand Break Repair: Nonhomologous End Joining and the DNA-PK Complex

Major protein complexes implicated in the NHEJ pathway are the DNA-PK protein kinase and XRCC4/Ligase IV complexes (Fig. 5.9). Human DNA-PK consists of a ~460 kDa DNA-PK catalytic subunit (DNA-PK$_{CS}$), and a DNA end-binding KU heterodimer (consisting of 70 kD and 80 kD protein subunits). The catalytic subunit shows homology to the PI-3K kinase superfamily (Chap. 8, Sec. 8.2.7) at its C-terminus, which contains the protein kinase domain required for phosphorylating DNA-PK-associated proteins during repair. Mutations in either *DNA-PK$_{CS}$* or in one of the *KU* genes results in sensitivity to ionizing radiation and reduced ability to repair radiation-induced DNA dsbs. XRCC4 forms a stable complex with DNA ligase IV, and probably links the initial lesion detection by KU 70/80 and DNA-PK$_{CS}$, scaffolding to the actual ligation reaction carried out by DNA ligase IV (Fig. 5.9; Pang et al., 1997). An extensive list of DNA-PK phosphorylation targets has been described, including DNA-PK$_{CS}$ leading to autophosphorylation. Some of the cellular phenotypes displayed by mammalian DNA-PK mutant cells can be attributed to the failure to interact with phosphorylation substrates that do not directly participate in the end-joining process. These substrates are involved in apoptosis, intracellular signaling, and cell cycle regulation (Khanna and Jackson, 2001).

Much information regarding the cellular activity of the DNA-PK complex stems from research utilizing the SCID (severe combined immunodeficiency) mouse which is immunodeficient due to lack of mature T and B cells and radiosensitive due to defective proteins involved in V(D)J recombination (Chap. 20, Sec. 20.2.4). This is secondary to an inability to process the broken DNA molecules produced by the RAG1 and RAG2 proteins at the immunoglobulin or T-cell receptor loci. The DNA-PK$_{CS}$ protein in the SCID mouse is mutant and unstable due to a loss of the last eighty-three amino acids prior to the C-terminus kinase domain. DNA-PK activity is therefore severely reduced in tissues derived from this animal. More recently, mice have been generated in which the *DNA-PK$_{CS}$* gene has been completely disrupted. Fibroblasts derived from *DNA-PK$_{CS}$*-, *KU70*-, or *KU80*-deficient animals have defects in the kinetics and overall amount of DNA dsb rejoining following ionizing radiation. These animals also show chromosomal instability in their normal cells and are susceptibile to lymphoma, suggesting that these genes act as tumor suppressor genes (Khanna and Jackson, 2001).

The NBS1/MRE11/RAD50 protein complex acts in both HR and NHEJ pathways and also in maintenance of telomeres (see Sec. 5.5). Mutations in the NBS1 gene result in *Nijmegen Breakage Syndrome* (NBS), a recessive disorder with some phenotypic similarities to ataxia telangiectasia (AT) including chromosomal instability, radiosensitivity, and an increased incidence of lymphoid tumors (Little, 1994; Featherstone and Jackson, 1998). Mutations in human MRE11 have been linked to the *ataxia telangiectasia-like disorder* (ATLD). Cells from NBS, AT, and ATLD patients are hypersensitive to DNA dsb-inducing agents and show radioresistant DNA synthesis after exposure to ionizing radiation (Girard et al., 2000). Disruption of the mammalian *Rad51* or *Mre11* genes results in nonviable cells, attesting to their importance in development. Biochemical studies of the yeast and human protein complexes have shown that MRE11 has a $3'$ to $5'$ $Mn^{2+}$-dependent exonuclease activity on DNA substrates with blunt or $5'$ protruding ends and endonuclease activity on hairpin and single-stranded ssDNA substrates. This suggests that MRE11 might be a nuclease that stimulates the use of microhomology during NHEJ (see Fig. 5.9).

Although impaired DNA dsb repair and increased radiosensitivity have been reported for a DNA-PK$_{CS}$-deficient human glioblastoma tumor cell line, there are no human cancer syndromes attributed to defects in DNA-PK protein function. The relative levels of DNA-PK$_{CS}$ protein are generally lower in rodent than in human tissues, and DNA-PK$_{CS}$ and KU80 protein expression varies widely among different tissue types. However, there is no evidence that tumor cell radiosensitivity is simply correlated to the relative expression level of DNA-PK$_{CS}$ protein expression (Chan et al., 1998).

### 5.3.7 Nuclear Foci of DNA Repair Proteins

Using innovative microscopic and fluorescent technologies, researchers can specifically generate and visualize discrete DNA dsbs. These studies have shown that the MRE11 and RAD50 proteins co-aggregate in a dose-dependent manner as discrete ionizing-radiation induced nuclear complexes (i.e., foci) within irradiated human fibroblasts (Fig. 5.10; Maser et al., 1997). This complex requires the NBS1 protein to chaperone the complex from the cytoplasm to the nuclear sites of damage as these foci were not visualized in irradiated fibroblasts that lacked functional NBS1 protein (Carney et al., 1998; Nelms et al., 1998). Similar observations have been made for nuclear foci containing RAD51, RAD54, RAD52, BRCA1, and BRCA2 proteins following irradiation and during DNA replication (Paull et al.,

2000). Observations of DNA-damage sensing and other DNA repair proteins (e.g., RAD50/MRE11/NBS1, MMR-related proteins, BS helicase, 53BP1, BRCA1/2) have led to the concept of a super-complex of BRCA1-associated proteins (i.e., *the BASC complex*) acting as a surveillance "repairosome" within the nucleus following DNA damage (Wang et al., 2000; Rappold et al., 2001). Mammalian cells respond to DNA dsbs by phosphorylating serine 139 in the unique and evolutionary conserved carboxy-terminus of H2AX, one of the histone proteins in higher order chromatin structure (Rogakou et al., 1999). This alternate H2AX phosphoform ($\gamma$-H2AX) can be detected by specific antibodies. Kinetic experiments suggest that $\gamma$-H2AX is formed in thousands of copies as an immediate DNA damage response per double-strand break (Modesti and Kanaar, 2001). $\gamma$-H2AX also colocalizes with BRCA1, 53BP1, RAD50, and RAD51 over a period of six to eight hours following irradiation, and is phosphorylated by ATM and DNA-PK$_{CS}$ (see Sec. 5.4). Histone modification in mammalian cells may therefore assist repair of DNA damage by recruiting repair factors to damaged sites, but it remains to be seen whether these changes can be used in cancer diagnosis or treatment.

## 5.4 DNA DAMAGE CHECKPOINTS AND DNA REPAIR

Mammalian cells have evolved complex interrelated responses to DNA damage including cell cycle checkpoints, DNA repair, and apoptosis. Cell cycle checkpoints are sites of cell cycle arrest in the G1, S, and G2 phases that ensure successful and accurate DNA replication and repair prior to mitosis. Two general types of cell cycle checkpoints exist (Hoeijmakers, 2001; Kao et al., 2001). The mitotic spindle assembly checkpoint is responsible for ensuring that the mitotic spindle is correctly formed prior to division. Additionally, there are DNA integrity checkpoints that delay the cell cycle in response to DNA damage or to defects in DNA replication (i.e., G1 to S, intra-S, and G2 to M checkpoints; Nelson and Kastan, 1994).

Characterization of cells derived from people with the syndrome, ataxia telangiectasia (AT), illustrate cellular and clinical endpoints of aberrant DNA repair and checkpoint control due to mutations in one gene, *ATM*. The *ATM* (AT mutated) gene encodes a large protein that possesses a highly conserved C-terminal kinase domain related to phosphatidylinositol 3-kinase (PI-3K; Chap. 8, Sec. 8.2.7; Durocher and Jackson, 2001). Other members of this kinase family, such as DNA-PKcs and ATR (AT mutated and rad3-related), also function in DNA repair and cell cycle checkpoint control following DNA damage. An initial step in the response to DNA damage requires the activity of these PI-3K-related serine/threonine kinases to recognize the damaged DNA template or altered chromatin conformation: ATM protein detects ionizing radiation-induced DNA damage and ATR detects UV-induced DNA damage. Both ATM and ATR are thought to localize initially to sites of DNA damage and subsequently phosphorylate the CHK2 and CHK1 kinase proteins. The CHK2 and CHK1 kinases coordinate the G1 and G2 cell cycle checkpoints in response to ionizing or ultraviolet irradiation by interacting with the CDC25A, CDC25C and p53 proteins (see Fig. 5.10C and 5.11).

Most mutations in ATM result in truncation and destabilization of the protein, but certain missense and splicing errors have been shown to produce a less severe phenotype. Cerebellar degeneration, immunodeficiency, chromosomal instability, and cellular and clinical sensitivity to ionizing radiation all characterize the AT syndrome (Rotman and Shiloh, 1998; Weissberg et al., 1998). The pleiotropic clinical symptoms associated with AT may be explained partly by modification of cellular metabolism. For example, the loss of ATM function is associated with increased oxidative damage, particularly in cerebellar Purkinje cells, implicating a role for ATM in the response to reactive oxygen species and possibly explaining the cerebellar degeneration observed in AT-affected individuals (Fig. 5.11; Rotman and Shiloh, 1998).

The association between mutation of the *ATM* gene and a high incidence of lymphoid malignancy in patients with AT, together with the development of lymphoma in *atm* deficient mice, indicates that inactivation of the *atm* gene may be of importance in the pathogenesis of sporadic lymphoid malignancy. Loss of heterozygosity at 11q22-23 (the location of the *atm* gene) is a common event in lymphoid malignancy. Frequent inactivating mutations of the *atm* gene have been reported in patients with Hodgkin's and non-Hodgkin's lymphoma, rare sporadic T-cell prolymphocytic leukemia (T-PLL), B cell chronic lymphocytic leukemia (B-CLL), and most recently, mantle cell lymphoma (MCL). Furthermore, AT heterozygotes may have a slightly increased risk of breast cancer when compared to the normal population. These data strongly suggest that *atm* functions as a tumor suppressor gene (see Chap. 7, Sec. 7.4; Rotman and Shiloh, 1998).

Many data have been derived from studying cells derived from AT patients and *atm* $^{-/-}$ mice in culture. These cells display hypersensitivity to ionizing but not ultraviolet radiation, exhibit chromosomal instability, and a mild DNA dsb rejoining defect. ATM-deficient cells also have radioresistant DNA synthesis (persistent DNA synthesis after irradiation that is not observed in normal cells) and further defects in the G1-S, S, and

G2-M phase DNA damage checkpoints. One model suggests that ATM or ATR kinase activity requires colocalization with its substrate (i.e., p53 or other proteins) at sites of DNA damage to initiate DNA repair and the cell cycle checkpoints. ATM is held inactive as a dimer until DNA damage leads to autophosphorylation of ATM monomers activating its kinase activity (Bakkenist and Kastan, 2003). ATM initiates a G1-to-S cell cycle checkpoint by a posttranslational stabilization of the p53 protein via direct phosphorylation of serine 15 on p53 (Canman et al., 1998). ATM also phosphorylates threonine residue 68 on the CHK2 protein which then phosphorylates p53 at serine 20 (see Chap. 7, Sec. 7.4.2).

Additional evidence for a functional relationship between CHK2 and p53 is provided by the demonstration of *CHK2* mutations in people with Li-Fraumeni–like syndromes that do not carry mutations in *p53* (classic Li-Fraumeni syndrome is an inherited human cancer predisposition condition generally caused by germline heterozygous mutations in the *p53* gene). These phosphorylations lead to p53 subnuclear stabilization by interfering with a nuclear export site contained within the amino terminus of the p53 protein and by preventing degradation of p53 by MDM-2 (see Chap. 7, Sec. 7.4.2; Liang and Clarke, 2001). Because p53 acts primarily as a transcription factor, current models regard its stabilization, following DNA damage, as a mechanism to activate the cyclin D/E-kinase complex inhibitor, p21$^{WAF}$. This results in continual hypo-phosphorylation of the retinoblastoma (pRB) protein and results in a G1 cell cycle arrest. A second rapid G1 checkpoint pathway is also activated which targets the CDC25A phosphatase which is essential for G1/S transition(Chap. 9, Sec. 9.2.1; Falck et al., 2001).

Further important targets of ATM-mediated phosphorylation are the BRCA1, NBS1, and SMC-1 proteins that initiate both DNA repair and an S-phase DNA damage checkpoint (Fig. 5.11; Cortez et al., 1999; Gatei et al., 2000; Lim et al., 2000).

Following their activation by ATM and ATR, CHK1 and CHK2 phosphorylate a conserved site (Ser-216) on protein phosphatase CDC25C, which results in it being bound and inactivated by the 14-3-3-$\sigma$ protein (see Chap. 9, Sec. 9.2.1). The inactive CDC25C is then incapable of removing an inhibitory phosphate group on Tyr-15 of CDC2, preventing entry into mitosis. In addition, a p53-dependent transcriptional repression of the *CDC2* and *cyclin B* promoters may also contribute to the maintenance of the G2/M checkpoint in mammalian cells. It is hypothesized that this may allow for last-minute repair of chromosomal or chromatid damage prior to cellular division. Taken together, the crosstalk between ATM and ATR and factors involved in DNA repair, DNA damage signaling, and cell cycle control acts

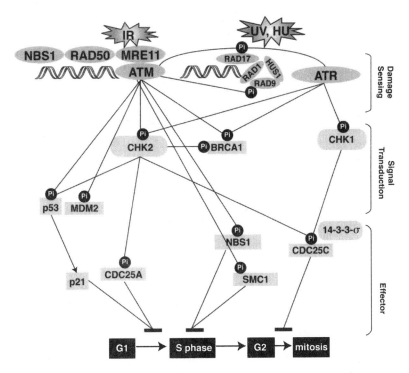

**Figure 5.11.** The response to DNA damage includes a series of protein–protein interactions, which alter protein phosphorylation (denoted as Pi). The ATM and ATR proteins are PI-3K kinases that initial sense damage induced by ionizing radiation (IR) or by ultraviolet (UV) radiation or Hydroxyurea (HU; which mimics the damage produced by stalled DNA replication forks). Initial sensing can also be mediated by the NBS1-MRE11-RAD50 complex and by RAD17-RAD1-HUS1-RAD9 at the site of DNA breaks. This is followed by signal transduction of the type and extent of the damage to proteins by phosphorylating CHK2, p53, MDM2, BRCA1, and CHK1, which mediate cell cycle checkpoint responses using downstream effector proteins to arrest the cells until the DNA damage can be repaired. The phosphorylation of the p53 and CHK2 proteins leads to altered activity of the cdk-inhibitor p21$^{WAF}$ and the CDC25A protein, which prevents the G1 to S transition. The phosphorylation of NBS1 and SMC1 arrest the cells in S-phase. Altered phosphorylation or cytoplasmic sequestration (by 14-3-3-$\sigma$) of the CDC25C protein prevents cells from undergoing mitosis following DNA damage (the relative activity of cyclin-cdk complexes in response to these phosphorylations is further detailed in Chap. 9, Sec. 9.2). (Adapted from Qin, 2003.)

to maintain genomic stability and inhibit carcinogenesis (Fig. 5.11).

Chromosome segregation is crucial for cells to maintain the integrity of their genome (Jasin, 2000). Mitotic exit occurs after ubiquitination and proteolytic degradation of cyclin B by the anaphase-promoting complex (APC), which inactivates cyclin-dependent kinase 1 (Chap. 9, Sec. 9.2.1). The *mitotic spindle checkpoint* monitors the interaction between chromosomes and microtubules at highly specialized chrosomomal regions called *kinetochores* (Musacchio and Hardwick, 2002). This checkpoint delays chromosome segregation during anaphase to correct any defects in the mitotic spindle apparatus; if defects persist, the cell undergoes cell death. The kine-

tochore-associated MAD2, BUBR1, BUB1, and BUB3 proteins are critical constituents of the spindle-checkpoint pathway: MAD2 and BUBR1 regulate mitotic progression by direct interaction and inhibition of the APC machinery and BUB1 and BUB3 also mediate mitotic arrest after disruption of microtubules. Cells that lack either BUB1 or BUB3 do not undergo mitotic arrest when treated with spindle-disrupting agents, such as the chemotherapy drugs docetaxel or vinblastine (Fig. 5.12).

Genetic defects in the spindle checkpoint can lead to chromosome loss during mitosis and meiosis with links to the pathogenesis of several human tumors. For example, in human colon and breast carcinoma cells, BUB1 mutations have been identified that facilitate the

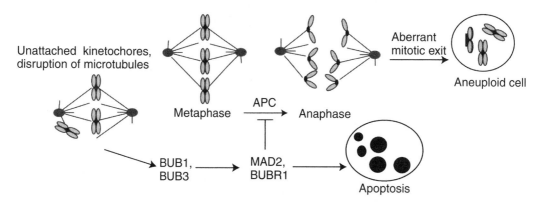

**Figure 5.12.** Mitotic spindle checkpoint. Improper chromosome alignment on the mitotic spindle due to unattached kinetochores or disruption of microtubules by DNA damage or spindle poisons can activate the mitotic spindle checkpoint. An intact spindle-checkpoint induces metaphase arrest through inhibition of the anaphase-promoting complex (APC) by the BUB1, BUB3, BUBR1 and MAD2 proteins. Defective spindle-checkpoint function results from either loss of BUB1- and BUB3-dependent signaling or abrogation of MAD2, BUBR1-mediated inhibition of the APC. This can lead to aberrant mitotic exit generating aneuploid cells or cell death. (Adapted from Stewart, 2003.)

transformation of cells that lack the breast cancer susceptibility gene, *BRCA2*. In other studies, *MAD2* haploinsufficiency significantly elevated the rate of lung tumor development in *mad2*$^{+/-}$ mice compared with age-matched controls (Stewart et al., 2003).

## 5.5 TELOMERE LENGTH REGULATION AND CANCER

Human cells have evolved a complex network of proteins that bind to chromosomal ends, or *telomeres*, and protect them from being inappropriately recognized as DNA damage. Increasing evidence suggests that disruption of this nucleoprotein complex, either through loss of telomere DNA sequences or direct disruption of protein function at the telomere, may signal a DNA damage response leading to cessation of cell division or cell death. Cells that continually proliferate, such as cancer cells, must thus find a mechanism to maintain telomeres. Most often, cancer cells achieve this protection through the activation of an enzyme that adds new telomere DNA onto chromosome ends, called *telomerase*. Together, telomerase and the nucleoprotein complex that protects telomeres ensure the maintenance of the telomere structure in dividing mammalian cells.

### 5.5.1 Telomeres Protect Chromosomal Ends from Degradation

Pioneering genetic experiments in the fruit fly and maize laid the foundation for our appreciation of the importance of telomeres in genome stability (reviewed in Greider, 1996). These initial experiments determined that DNA damage could result in the loss of the terminal knob of linear chromosomes, called the telomere. Loss of DNA sequences can lead to chromosome loss and a cycle of chromosome breakage, chromosome fusion, and chromosome bridges during subsequent cell division. Most linear chromosomes terminate in a long, noncoding repetitive tract of G-rich telomeric-DNA (Greider, 1996), which varies in sequence and length from organism to organism. In humans, telomeres are composed of 4 to 15 kilobase pairs (kbp) of the hexanucleotide sequence 5′-TTAGGG-3′ followed by 100 to 150 nucleotides of a single-stranded TTAGGG 3′ overhang (McElligott and Wellinger, 1997; Wright et al., 1997). The 3′ single-stranded overhang is looped back on itself in a structure termed the t-loop (Griffith et al., 1999; Murti and Prescott, 1999; Munoz-Jordan et al., 2001). Internal to the telomeric tract resides several kilobases of degenerate telomeric sequence, called subtelomeric DNA. The subtelomeric and telomeric regions exist in a nucleoprotein complex containing several telomere-binding proteins and chromatin associated proteins. This nucleoprotein complex possesses a distinct nucleosomal structure that is thought to protect the chromosome ends from being perceived as damaged DNA, or as a DNA double-strand break (reviewed in Greider, 1996; McEachern et al., 2000; Fig. 5.13).

Because DNA polymerases fail to extend to the 5′ ends of linear DNA, a special cellular mechanism must compensate for the gradual erosion elicited by incomplete replication of the chromosomal termini. This mechanism requires the addition of new G-rich single-stranded telomere DNA to chromosome ends by telomerase, which carries its own telomere-complementary RNA template called the telomerase RNA (Greider and Blackburn, 1985; Fig. 5.13). New telomeric sequences added by telomerase therefore compensate for the gradual erosion of chromosome ends, thus maintain-

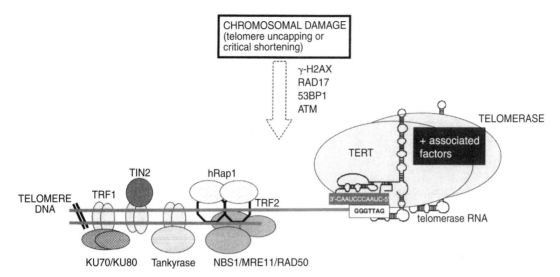

**Figure 5.13.** Protein-protein interactions at the chromosomal telomere. A schematic representation of telomerase at the telomere, showing the two critical components for catalysis: the telomerase RNA (drawn according to its predicted secondary structure), and the telomerase reverse transcriptase (TERT). It is presumed that the t-loop (see text) must dissociate to allow access of telomerase to the 3' overhang. The RNA template of telomerase (*grey box*) allows extension of the telomere DNA (*white box*), one nucleotide at a time. Important proteins also found at the telomere include the TIN2, TRF1, KU70/KU80, Tankyrase, NBS1, MRE11, RAD50, TRF2, and hRAP1 proteins as discussed in the text. Chromosomal damage, in the form of severe telomere shortening or telomere uncapping, elicits a DNA damage response with phosphorylation of the histone H2AX (γ-H2AX) at the site of damage and recruitment of 53BP1, RAD17, or ATM involved in the sensing of repair of DNA damage (see Sec. 5.3.7).

ing telomere length and chromosome stability. This highly conserved complex exists as a large, multisubunit enzyme (Nugent and Lundblad, 1998). Telomerase contains an essential protein subunit that resembles a reverse transcriptase, called *telomerase reverse transcriptase* (TERT) (Nugent and Lundblad, 1998). The telomerase RNA and TERT appear to comprise the catalytic core of the enzyme complex (Weinrich et al., 1997; Beattie et al., 1998). Certain telomerase-associated proteins carry out a number of roles in enzyme assembly and recruitment to the telomere, whereas others appear to play ancillary or redundant roles in telomerase function (Nugent and Lundblad, 1998).

### 5.5.2 Telomere Control in Normal Cell Proliferation and Senescence

Both genetic and biochemical data support the theory that maintenance of telomere length is crucial for the long-term survival of mammalian cells in culture (McEachern et al., 2000). In humans, normal somatic cells lack telomerase activity due to transcriptional repression of the TERT catalytic protein subunit of telomerase, and therefore show telomere shortening with each subsequent cell doubling (Greider, 1998). Human somatic cells do not replicate indefinitely in culture.

The eventual loss of replicative potential is termed *cellular senescence* or the *Hayflick limit*, a phenotype which correlates with the loss of telomere DNA (Greider, 1998). In the absence of the tumor suppressor genes *p53* or *pRB*, human somatic cells can undergo additional population doublings before eventually reaching a proliferative block, called crisis. At crisis, cells exhibit extensive genome instability and most will die. Only a small fraction of cells (about 1 in $10^7$) survive by either activating expression of the endogenous hTERT gene, or via other telomerase-independent mechanisms collectively referred to as ALT (for *alternate telomere length maintenance*; see Sec. 5.5.3; Reddel et al., 2001).

The hypothesis that cellular senescence is causally linked to critically short telomeres is supported by the finding that reintroduction of TERT into human somatic cells renders them capable of indefinite proliferation; this is the only single gene known to indefinitely prolong the life span of human cells in culture (Bodnar et al., 1998; Vaziri and Benchimol, 1998). Despite being immortal in a culture dish, TERT reconstituted human somatic cells appear to preserve their normal morphology, response to external stress, and chromosomal karyotype (Fig. 5.14; Vaziri et al., 1999).

In mice, the disruption of the gene encoding the RNA subunit of telomerase leads to telomere shorten-

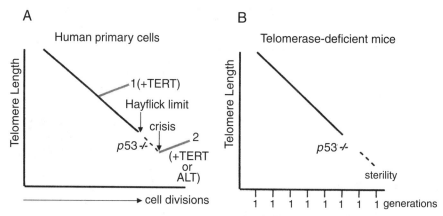

**Figure 5.14.** Long-term viability of primary cells that lack telomerase activity. As seen in (*A*), reintroduction of TERT indefinitely extends the cells' lifespan and telomeres stabilize at varying lengths (see *1*); however, other cells can survive "crisis" spontaneously when TERT or ALT (i.e., mechanisms that maintain telomeres in a telomerase-independent manner) is activated (see *2*), leading to transformation. This occurs at an increased rate in p53$^{-/-}$ cells as discussed in the text. Cells from telomerase-deficient mice (*B*) acquire critically short telomeres leading to telomere-teleomere fusion, which activates a p53-dependent apoptotic response. This apoptotic response is particularly evident in germline tissues resulting in sterility of these mice.

ing in all tissues (Blasco et al., 1997). Following six generations of breeding, visible defects are observed in several organs that contain proliferating cells in telomerase-deficient mice (Lee et al., 1998). Critically short telomeres lead to telomere-telomere fusions, which in turn appear to activate a p53-dependent apoptotic response (see Chap. 7, Sec. 7.4.2; Lee et al., 1998; Chin et al., 1999). This programmed cell death is particularly evident in germline tissues resulting in sterility of these mice (Lee et al., 1998). Crossing telomerase-deficient mice with p53-deficient mice can extend the number of fertile generations (Chin et al., 1999), but, eventually, the germline cells from telomerase/p53 deficient mice also undergo apoptosis. This observation suggests that p53-independent mechanisms are also involved in monitoring telomere integrity and genome instability in dividing cells (Chin et al., 1999).

Many human tissues express little or no detectable telomerase activity and loss of telomere DNA has been correlated with increasing tissue age (Autexier and Greider, 1996; Greider, 1996). While it is a critical factor in cellular senescence in vitro, there is as yet no direct evidence that shortened telomeres are physiologically relevant to normal aging in any human tissues. In some diseased states, such as HIV infection, liver disease, and in some DNA repair deficiencies, certain individuals may show shortened telomeres in the cells derived from target organs, but this may be an indirect effect of increased proliferation at these sites (Greider, 1998). Interestingly, mutations in the human telomerase RNA have been linked recently with human diseases, such as dykeratosis congenita and aplastic ane-

mia, and the early bone marrow failure and myeloid proliferative disorders that mark these disease are thought to arise as a consequence of shortened telomeres (Mason and Bessler, 2004). In keeping with the finding that mice with short telomeres are more resistant to skin papillomas, overexpression of TERT in the murine skin leads to increased papilloma formation when compared to normal, nontransgenic skin (Gonzalez-Suarez et al., 2000; Gonzalez-Suarez et al., 2001). These results have led to the speculation that telomerase may play other roles in cell proliferation besides maintenance of telomere length. However, overexpression of telomerase activity may also lead to subtle changes in the dynamics of telomere length equilibrium, which in turn may protect highly proliferating cells from genomic instability and apoptosis.

### 5.5.3 Telomere-Bound Proteins and DNA Repair

Several proteins that bind to double-stranded and single-stranded telomeres play key roles in ensuring the stability of the telomere in eukaryotic cells. In yeast, single-stranded and double-stranded telomere binding proteins have been extensively characterized, and play an important role in telomere protection, sensing of telomere length, and recruitment of telomerase to the telomere. Human homologs of the yeast double-stranded telomere-binding protein, RAP1, have now been characterized: TRF1, TRF2, and RAP1. TRF1 appears to negatively regulate telomerase access to the telomere, and its DNA binding activity is in turn influenced by poly-ADP ribosylation via a protein that possesses poly ADP ribosylation (PARP) activity, called tankyrase (Smith, 2001).

Analysis of TRF2 in humans has uncovered additional intriguing parallels to the DNA damage pathway (see Table 5.2). TRF2 forms a complex with several proteins previously characterized for their role in nonhomologous end joining described in Sec. 5.3, including KU70/KU80, NBS1, MRE11, and RAD50 (Song et al., 2000; Zhu et al., 2000). While the precise role of this complex is not yet known, KU70 deficient cells show an increased rate of telomere-telomere fusions (Samper et al., 2000), and as stated previously, patients with NBS (Nijmegen Breakage Syndrome) show sensitivity to DNA damage and an increased incidence of certain types of cancer (Petrini, 2000). These repair proteins therefore appear to play a somewhat paradoxical role in protecting chromosome ends from inappropriate recombination. TRF2 itself is also important for telomere

integrity. In human cell lines, overexpression of TRF2 variants that are unable to bind DNA results in telomere-telomere fusions and cell cycle arrest in a manner that is dependent on p53 and ATM (Karlseder et al., 1999). These data suggest that loss of function of the TRF2 complex results in an immediate DNA damage response that is p53 and ATM dependent. Removal of TRF2 from telomeres, either through telomere uncapping or critical telomere shortening, leads to the immediate activation of a DNA damage checkpoint, and critically shortened or damaged telomeres recruit similar DNA-repair proteins as observed elsewhere in the genome at DNA breaks (Takai et al., 2004, d'Adda di Fagagna et al., 2004). Recent evidence suggests that TRF2 acts directly to suppress ATM activation; thus, the loss of TRF2 at the telomere may provide the trigger for a DNA damage response (Karlseder et al., 2004).

**Table 5.2.** DNA Repair Proteins That May Also Play a Role at the Telomere

| Name | Function in DNA Repair | Function at the Telomere |
| --- | --- | --- |
| p53 | Transcription factor and essential in a wide variety of responses to DNA damage | Important for triggering apoptosis upon loss of TRF2 function or when telomeres become critically shortened |
| ATM | PI-3K related, important for signal transduction in response to DNA damage | In humans, ATM is important for apoptosis upon loss of TRF2 function; ATM and ATR colocalize with telomere DNA in ALT cell lines |
| PARP | Important for recruiting DNA repair machinery to sites of DNA damage; poly-ADP ribosylates p53 and DNA-PK | Human PARP-deficient cells have shorter telomeres and an increase in telomere-telomere fusions, especially in absence of p53 |
| KU70/80 | Important for DSB repair, including NHEJ, homologous recombination, and VDJ recombination | Murine KU-deficient cells possess increased telomere-telomere fusions. |
| DNA-PK | Important for DSB repair during non-homologous recombination. PI-3K related | DNA-PKcs-deficient cells show increased telomere-telomere fusions |
| MRE11 | MRE11 forms complex with NBS1 and RAD50 following DNA damage | MRE11/RAD50/NBS1 form a complex with TRF2 at t-loops |
| RAD51 | Important for DSB repair during homologous recombination | Promotes viability in absence of telomerase in yeast; in humans, RAD51 colocalizes with a fraction of telomeres in PML bodies in ALT cell lines |
| RAD52 | Essential for strand invasion in DSB repair and breakage-induced replication (BIR) | Essential for survival in absence of telomerase activity in yeast |
| WRN | Has 3'-5' exonuclease activity and is a RecQ-helicase | Colocalizes with telomere DNA in PML bodies within ALT cell lines; WRN deficient cell lines show accelerated telomere shortening in culture. |
| BLM | Cells from Bloom's patients are sensitive to DNA damage | BLM colocalizes to a fraction of telomeres in PML bodies within ALT cell lines |
| BRCA1 | Tumor suppressor protein; BRCA1-deficient mice arrest early in development with elevated levels of $p21^{WAF}$ and this phenotype is partially rescued by deletion of p53 | BRCA1 colocalizes to PML bodies; BRCA1/p53-deficient murine cells show increase in telomere-telomere fusions |

In cells that maintain telomeres in a telomerase-independent manner (i.e., via ALT), a fraction of telomeres are found in a novel promyelocytic body (the PML body) that also contains several DNA repair proteins (see Table 5.2; Yeager et al., 1999; Grobelny et al., 2000; Lombard and Guarente, 2000; Wu et al., 2000). The functional significance of these PML bodies is not understood, although they may represent a site for telomere-telomere recombination and repair. A similar DNA damage-sensing pathway also appears to play an important role in homeostasis of telomere length in yeast. Mec1 and Tel1, two homologs of the PI-3K family, appear to be important for signaling cell cycle arrest when telomere integrity is compromised. In the absence of both proteins, cell division is limited (Ritchie et al., 1999). These data suggest that the PI-3K signaling pathway is probably activated by an unknown trigger in response to altered telomere structure.

### 5.5.4 Aberrant Telomere Control and Malignant Transformation

In contrast to normal cells, most human tumors and many transformed human cell lines contain telomerase activity and do not exhibit telomere shortening with increasing cell division (Shay and Wright, 2001). In cancerous cells, it is thought that telomerase activity confers a proliferative advantage through maintenance of telomere length and increased genome stability. Support for this hypothesis is found in several studies that examined the effect of telomerase inhibition on the replicative potential of human tumor cell lines. Inhibition of telomerase elicits telomere shortening in most human cancer cells, and eventually these cells succumb to cell death when telomeres reach an ill-defined critically short length (Hahn et al., 1999; Herbert et al., 1999; Zhang et al., 1999). In addition, misincorporation of mutant telomere repeats induces rapid cell death regardless of initial telomere length (Kim et al., 2001). In contrast to normal human cells, most human tumor cell lines lack functional p53 proteins. Like mouse cells that are deficient in both p53 and telomerase, these cells possess an ability to undergo cell death in response to critically short telomeres that is not dependent on p53.

The rare cancer cells that are able to survive in the absence of telomerase are thought to maintain telomeres via homologous recombination between chromosome ends (Reddel et al., 2001). In ALT cell lines, telomeres that are marked with a reporter construct can jump to new telomere locations, an observation that is consistent with telomere-telomere recombination (Dunham et al., 2000). Because ALT cells do not express telomerase activity, inhibition of telomerase function has no effect on the continued growth of these cell types (Hahn et al., 1999).

Our understanding of telomere biology will no doubt lead to the development of potent and selective inhibitors of telomerase that require testing in clinical trials. New telomere/telomerase targeting compounds includes antisense oligonucleotides, G-quadruplex stabilizing substances, small molecule inhibitors of telomerase, telomerase expression-related strategies such as telomerase promoter-driven suicide gene therapy, and telomerase immunotherapy. However, assaying the efficacy of telomerase inhibitors may be difficult as telomere erosion will be slow and antiproliferative effects may not be elicited immediately. Nevertheless, these novel treatment strategies may be relatively tumor specific, given the disparity in telomerase activity between normal and cancerous cells (see Chap. 17, Sec. 17.6.2).

### 5.6 SUMMARY

Genetic stability is crucial to the prevention of carcinogenesis. Many proteins involved in cell cycle checkpoint control, chromosomal stability, DNA repair, and telomerase activity act in concert during cell proliferation to maintain the integrity of the genome. Determining the tissue-specificity of the proteins involved in these responses will be important to understand the relative susceptibility of different tissues to endogenous and exogenous carcinogenic insult. Human DNA repair-deficient, and DNA damage checkpoint-deficient, syndromes and murine genetic knockout models provide important cellular and biochemical clues as to the temporal activity of many proteins within DNA damage signaling cascades.

Our understanding of these pathways is leading to the development of molecular cancer diagnostics and therapies specific to certain proteins that normally act as gatekeepers of genomic stability. Examples include gene therapy or pharmacological means designed to re-institute normal p53 tumor suppressor gene function or DNA repair and telomere-specific therapies. Further improvements will no doubt stem from careful genomic and proteomic approaches in a variety of tissues to derive tissue-specific information relating to models of carcinogenesis and chemoprevention.

### REFERENCES

Abraham RT: Cell cycle checkpoint signaling through the ATM and ATR kinases. *Genes Dev* 2001; 15:2177–2196.

Ames BN, Cathcart R, Schwiers E, Hochstein P: Uric acid provides an antioxidant defense in humans against oxidant- and radical-caused aging and cancer: a hypothesis. *Proc Natl Acad Sci USA* 1981; 78:6858–6862.

Autexier C, Greider CW: Telomerase and cancer: revisiting the telomere hypothesis. *Trends Biochem Sci* 1996; 21:387–391.

Bakkenist CJ, Kastan MB: DNA damage activates ATM through intermolecular autophosphorylation and dimer dissociation. *Nature* 2003; 421:499–506.

Balajee AS, Bohr VA: Genomic heterogeneity of nucleotide excision repair. *Gene* 2000; 250:15–30.

Beattie TL, Zhou W, Robinson MO, Harrington L: Reconstitution of human telomerase activity in vitro. *Curr Biol* 1998; 8:177–180.

Berneburg M, Lehmann AR: Xeroderma pigmentosum and related disorders: defects in DNA repair and transcription. *Adv Genet* 2001; 43:71–102.

Blasco MA, Lee HW, Hande MP, et al: Telomere shortening and tumor formation by mouse cells lacking telomerase RNA. *Cell* 1997; 91:25–34.

Bodnar AG, Ouellette M, Frolkis M, et al: Extension of life-span by introduction of telomerase into normal human cells. *Science* 1998; 279:349–352.

Canman CE, Lim DS, Cimprich KA, et al: Activation of the ATM kinase by ionizing radiation and phosphorylation of p53. *Science* 1998; 281:1677–1679.

Carney JP, Maser RS, Olivares H, et al: The hMre11/hRad50 protein complex and Nijmegen breakage syndrome: linkage of double-strand break repair to the cellular DNA damage response. *Cell* 1998; 93:477–486.

Chan DW, Gately DP, Urban S, et al: Lack of correlation between ATM protein expression and tumour cell radiosensitivity. *Int J Radiat Biol* 1998; 74:217–224.

Chin L, Artandi SE, Shen Q, et al: p53 deficiency rescues the adverse effects of telomere loss and cooperates with telomere dysfunction to accelerate carcinogenesis. *Cell* 1999; 97:527–538.

Cortez D, Wang Y, Qin J, Elledge SJ: Requirement of ATM-dependent phosphorylation of BRCA1 in the DNA damage response to double-strand breaks. *Science* 1999; 286:1162–1166.

Daboussi F, Dumay A, Delacote F, Lopez BS: DNA double-strand break repair signalling: the case of RAD51 post-translational regulation. *Cell Signal* 2002; 14:969–975.

d'Adda di Fagagna F, Reaper PM, et al: A DNA damage checkpoint response in telomere-initiated senescence. *Nature.* 2003; 426:194–198.

Davies AA, Masson JY, McIlwraith MJ, et al: Role of BRCA2 in control of the RAD51 recombination and DNA repair protein. *Mol Cell* 2001; 7:273–282.

De la Torre C, Pincheira J, Lopez-Saez JF: Human syndromes with genomic instability and multiprotein machines that repair DNA double-strand breaks. *Histol Histopathol* 2003; 18:225–243.

de Laat WL, Jaspers NG, Hoeijmakers JH: Molecular mechanism of nucleotide excision repair. *Genes Dev* 1999; 13:768–785.

Dunham MA, Neumann AA, Fasching CL, Reddel RR: Telomere maintenance by recombination in human cells. *Nat Genet* 2000; 26:447–450.

Durocher D, Jackson SP: DNA-PK, ATM and ATR as sensors of DNA damage: variations on a theme? *Curr Opin Cell Biol* 2001; 13:225–231.

Essers J, Hendriks RW, Swagemakers SM, et al: Disruption of mouse RAD54 reduces ionizing radiation resistance and homologous recombination. *Cell* 1997; 89:195–204.

Falck J, Lukas C, Protopopova M, et al: Functional impact of concomitant versus alternative defects in the Chk2-p53 tumour suppressor pathway. *Oncogene* 2001; 20:5503–5510.

Featherstone C, Jackson SP: DNA repair: the Nijmegen breakage syndrome protein. *Curr Biol* 1998; 8:R622–R625.

Friedberg EC: How nucleotide excision repair protects against cancer. *Nat Rev Cancer* 2001; 1:22–33.

Gatei M, Young D, Cerosaletti KM, et al: ATM-dependent phosphorylation of nibrin in response to radiation exposure. *Nat Genet* 2000; 25:115–119.

Girard PM, Foray N, Stumm M, et al: Radiosensitivity in Nijmegen Breakage Syndrome cells is attributable to a repair defect and not cell cycle checkpoint defects. *Cancer Res* 2000; 60:4881–4888.

Gonzalez-Suarez E, Samper E, Flores JM, Blasco MA: Telomerase-deficient mice with short telomeres are resistant to skin tumorigenesis. *Nat Genet* 2000; 26:114–117.

Gonzalez-Suarez E, Samper E, Ramirez A, et al: Increased epidermal tumors and increased skin wound healing in transgenic mice overexpressing the catalytic subunit of telomerase, mTERT, in basal keratinocytes. *EMBO J* 2001; 20:2619–2630.

Greider CW: Telomere length regulation. *Annu Rev Biochem* 1996; 65:337–365.

Greider CW: Telomeres and senescence: the history, the experiment, the future. *Curr Biol* 1998; 8:R178–R181.

Greider CW, Blackburn EH: Identification of a specific telomere terminal transferase activity in Tetrahymena extracts. *Cell* 1985; 43:405–413.

Griffith JD, Comeau L, Rosenfield S, et al: Mammalian telomeres end in a large duplex loop. *Cell* 1999; 97:503–514.

Grobelny JV, Godwin AK, Broccoli D: ALT-associated PML bodies are present in viable cells and are enriched in cells in the G(2)/M phase of the cell cycle. *J Cell Sci* 2000; 113 24:4577–4585.

Hahn WC, Stewart SA, Brooks MW, et al: Inhibition of telomerase limits the growth of human cancer cells. *Nat Med* 1999; 5:1164–1170.

Harfe BD, Jinks-Robertson S: DNA mismatch repair and genetic instability. *Annu Rev Genet* 2000; 34:359–399.

Herbert B, Pitts AE, Baker SI, et al: Inhibition of human telomerase in immortal human cells leads to progressive telomere shortening and cell death. *Proc Natl Acad Sci USA* 1999; 96:14276–14281.

Hittelman WN: Genetic instability in epithelial tissues at risk for cancer. *Ann NY Acad Sci* 2001; 952:1–12.

Hoeijmakers JH: Genome maintenance mechanisms for preventing cancer. *Nature* 2001; 411:366–374.

Jasin M: Chromosome breaks and genomic instability. *Cancer Invest* 2000; 18:78–86.

Jeggo PA: DNA-PK: at the cross-roads of biochemistry and genetics. *Mutat Res* 1997; 384:1–14.

Jiricny J, Nystrom-Lahti M: Mismatch repair defects in cancer. *Curr Opin Genet Dev* 2000; 10:157–161.

Kao GD, McKenna WG, Yen TJ: Detection of repair activity during the DNA damage-induced G2 delay in human cancer cells. *Oncogene* 2001; 20:3486–3496.

Karlseder J, Broccoli D, Dai Y, et al: p53- and ATM-dependent apoptosis induced by telomeres lacking TRF2. *Science* 1999; 283:1321–1325.

Karlseder J, Hoke K, Mirzoeva OK, et al: The telomeric protein TRF2 binds the ATM kinase and can inhibit the ATM-dependent DNA damage reponse. *PLoS Biol.* 2004; 2(8):E240.

Khanna KK, Jackson SP: DNA double-strand breaks: signaling, repair and the cancer connection. *Nat Genet* 2001; 27:247–254.

Kim MM, Rivera MA, Botchkina IL, et al: A low threshold level of expression of mutant-template telomerase RNA inhibits human tumor cell proliferation. *Proc Natl Acad Sci USA* 2001; 98:7982–7987.

Kolodner RD, Marsischky GT: Eukaryotic DNA mismatch repair. *Curr Opin Genet Dev* 1999; 9:89–96.

Lee HW, Blasco MA, Gottlieb GJ, et al: Essential role of mouse telomerase in highly proliferative organs. *Nature* 1998; 392:569–574.

Liang SH, Clarke MF: Regulation of p53 localization. *Eur J Biochem* 2001; 268:2779–2783.

Lim DS, Hasty P: A mutation in mouse rad51 results in an early embryonic lethal that is suppressed by a mutation in p53. *Mol Cell Biol* 1996; 16:7133–7143.

Lim DS, Kim ST, Xu B, et al: ATM phosphorylates p95/nbs1 in an S-phase checkpoint pathway. *Nature* 2000; 404:613–617.

Little JB: Failla Memorial Lecture. Changing views of cellular radiosensitivity. *Radiat Res* 1994; 140:299–311.

Loeb LA: Mutator phenotype may be required for multistage carcinogenesis. *Cancer Res* 1991; 51:3075–3079.

Lombard DB, Guarente L: Nijmegen breakage syndrome disease protein and MRE11 at PML nuclear bodies and meiotic telomeres. *Cancer Res* 2000; 60:2331–2334.

Marks P, Rifkind RA, Richon VM, et al: Histone deacetylases and cancer: causes and therapies. *Nat Rev Cancer* 2001; 1:194–202.

Marmorstein LY, Ouchi T, Aaronson SA: The BRCA2 gene product functionally interacts with p53 and RAD51. *Proc Natl Acad Sci USA* 1998; 95:13869–13874.

Maser RS, Monsen KJ, Nelms BE, Petrini JH: hMre11 and hRad50 nuclear foci are induced during the normal cellular response to DNA double-strand breaks. *Mol Cell Biol* 1997; 17:6087–6096.

Mason PJ, Bessler M: Heterozygous telomerase deficiency in mouse and man: when less is definitely not more. *Cell Cycle* 2004; 3:1127–1129.

McEachern MJ, Krauskopf A, Blackburn EH: Telomeres and their control. *Annu Rev Genet* 2000; 34:331–358.

McElligott R, Wellinger RJ: The terminal DNA structure of mammalian chromosomes. *EMBO J* 1997; 16:3705–3714.

Modesti M, Kanaar R: DNA repair: spot(light)s on chromatin. *Curr Biol* 2001; 11:R229–R232.

Momparler RL. Cancer epigenetics. *Oncogene* 2003; 22:6479–6483.

Moynahan ME, Pierce AJ, Jasin M: BRCA2 is required for homology-directed repair of chromosomal breaks. *Mol Cell* 2001; 7:263–272.

Munoz-Jordan JL, Cross GA, de Lange T, Griffith JD: t-loops at trypanosome telomeres. *EMBO J* 2001; 20:579–588.

Murti KG, Prescott DM: Telomeres of polytene chromosomes in a ciliated protozoan terminate in duplex DNA loops. *Proc Natl Acad Sci USA* 1999; 96:14436–14439.

Musacchio A, Hardwick KG: The spindle checkpoint: structural insights into dynamic signalling. *Nat Rev Mol Cell Biol* 2002; 3:731–741.

Nakanishi K, Taniguchi T, Ranganathan V, et al: Interaction of FANCD2 and NBS1 in the DNA damage response. *Nat Cell Biol* 2002; 4:913–920.

Nelms BE, Maser RS, MacKay JF, et al: In situ visualization of DNA double-strand break repair in human fibroblasts. *Science* 1998; 280:590–592.

Nelson WG, Kastan MB: DNA strand breaks: the DNA template alterations that trigger p53-dependent DNA damage response pathways. *Mol Cell Biol* 1994; 14:1815–1823.

Nugent CI, Lundblad V: The telomerase reverse transcriptase: components and regulation. *Genes Dev* 1998; 12:1073–1085.

Offer H, Milyavsky M, Erez N, et al: Structural and functional involvement of p53 in BER in vitro and in vivo. *Oncogene* 2001; 20:581–589.

Pang D, Yoo S, Dynan WS, et al: Ku proteins join DNA fragments as shown by atomic force microscopy. *Cancer Res* 1997; 57:1412–1415.

Paull TT, Rogakou EP, Yamazaki V, et al: A critical role for histone H2AX in recruitment of repair factors to nuclear foci after DNA damage. *Curr Biol* 2000; 10:886–895.

Peltomaki P: Deficient DNA mismatch repair: a common etiologic factor for colon cancer. *Hum Mol Genet* 2001; 10:735–740.

Petrini JH: The Mre11 complex and ATM: collaborating to navigate S phase. *Curr Opin Cell Biol* 2000; 12:293–296.

Qin J, Li L: Molecular anatomy of the DNA damage and replication checkpoints. *Radiat Res* 2003; 159:139–148.

Rappold I, Iwabuchi K, Date T, Chen J: Tumor suppressor p53 binding protein 1 (53BP1) is involved in DNA damage-signaling pathways. *J Cell Biol* 2001; 153:613–620.

Reddel RR, Bryan TM, Colgin LM, et al: Alternative lengthening of telomeres in human cells. *Radiat Res* 2001; 155:194–200.

Ribic CM, Sargent DJ, Moore MJ, et al: Tumor microsatellite-instability status as a predictor of benefit from fluorouracil-based adjuvant chemotherapy for colon cancer. *N Engl J Med* 2003; 349:247–257.

Richardson C, Jasin M: Coupled homologous and nonhomologous repair of a double-strand break preserves genomic integrity in mammalian cells. *Mol Cell Biol* 2000; 20:9068–9075.

Ritchie KB, Mallory JC, Petes TD: Interactions of TLC1 (which encodes the RNA subunit of telomerase), TEL1, and MEC1 in regulating telomere length in the yeast Saccharomyces cerevisiae. *Mol Cell Biol* 1999; 19:6065–6075.

Rogakou EP, Boon C, Redon C, Bonner WM: Megabase chromatin domains involved in DNA double-strand breaks in vivo. *J Cell Biol* 1999; 146:905–916.

Romanov SR, Kozakiewicz BK, Holst CR, et al: Normal human mammary epithelial cells spontaneously escape senescence and acquire genomic changes. *Nature* 2001; 409:633–637.

Rotman G, Shiloh Y: ATM: from gene to function. *Hum Mol Genet* 1998; 7:1555–1563.

Samper E, Goytisolo FA, Slijepcevic P, et al: Mammalian Ku86 protein prevents telomeric fusions independently of the length of TTAGGG repeats and the G-strand overhang. *EMBO Rep* 2000; 1:244–252.

Shay JW, Wright WE: Telomeres and telomerase: implications for cancer and aging. *Radiat Res* 2001; 155:188–193.

Smith S: The world according to PARP. *Trends Biochem Sci* 2001; 26:174–179.

Song K, Jung D, Jung Y, et al: Interaction of human Ku70 with TRF2. *FEBS Lett* 2000; 481:81–85.

Stewart ZA, Westfall MD, Pietenpol JA: Cell-cycle dysregulation and anticancer therapy. *Trends Pharmacol Sci* 2003; 24:139–145.

Stoler DL, Chen N, Basik M, et al: The onset and extent of genomic instability in sporadic colorectal tumor progression. *Proc Natl Acad Sci USA* 1999; 96:15121–15126.

Takai H, Smogorzewska A, de Lange T: DNA damage foci at dysfunctional telomeres. *Curr Biol.* 2003; 13:1549–1556.

Tlsty TD: Normal diploid human and rodent cells lack a detectable frequency of gene amplification. *Proc Natl Acad Sci USA* 1990; 87:3132–3136.

van Gent DC, Hoeijmakers JH, Kanaar R: Chromosomal stability and the DNA double-stranded break connection. *Nat Rev Genet* 2001; 2:196–206.

Vaziri H, Benchimol S: Reconstitution of telomerase activity in normal human cells leads to elongation of telomeres and extended replicative life span. *Curr Biol* 1998; 8: 279–282.

Vaziri H, Squire JA, Pandita TK, et al: Analysis of genomic integrity and p53-dependent G1 checkpoint in telomerase-induced extended-life-span human fibroblasts. *Mol Cell Biol* 1999; 19:2373–2379.

Wang Y, Cortez D, Yazdi P, et al: BASC, a super complex of BRCA1-associated proteins involved in the recognition and repair of aberrant DNA structures. *Genes Dev* 2000; 14: 927–939.

Weinrich SL, Pruzan R, Ma L, et al: Reconstitution of human telomerase with the template RNA component hTR and the catalytic protein subunit hTRT. *Nat Genet* 1997; 17:498–502.

Weissberg JB, Huang DD, Swift M: Radiosensitivity of normal tissues in ataxia-telangiectasia heterozygotes. *Int J Radiat Oncol Biol Phys* 1998; 42:1133–1136.

Wright WE, Tesmer VM, Huffman KE: Normal human chromosomes have long G-rich telomeric overhangs at one end. *Genes Dev* 1997; 11:2801–2809.

Wu G, Lee WH, Chen PL: NBS1 and TRF1 colocalize at promyelocytic leukemia bodies during late S/G2 phases in immortalized telomerase-negative cells. Implication of NBS1 in alternative lengthening of telomeres. *J Biol Chem* 2000; 275:30618–30622.

Yeager TR, Neumann AA, Englezou A, et al: Telomerase-negative immortalized human cells contain a novel type of promyelocytic leukemia (PML) body. *Cancer Res* 1999; 59:4175–4179.

Zhang X, Mar V, Zhou W, et al: Telomere shortening and apoptosis in telomerase-inhibited human tumor cells. *Genes Dev* 1999; 13:2388–2399.

Zhou PK, Sproston AR, Marples B, et al: The radiosensitivity of human fibroblast cell lines correlates with residual levels of DNA double-strand breaks. *Radiother Oncol* 1998; 47:271–276.

Zhu XD, Kuster B, Mann M, et al: Cell-cycle-regulated association of RAD50/MRE11/NBS1 with TRF2 and human telomeres. *Nat Genet* 2000; 25:347–352.

# 6

# Viruses and Cancer

*Christopher D. Richardson*

## 6.1 INTRODUCTION

Viruses are implicated in approximately 15 percent of all cancers. They can cause malignancies that include nasopharyngeal carcinoma, Burkitt's lymphoma, cervical carcinoma, T-cell leukemias, hepatocellular carcinoma, and Kaposi's sarcoma. Oncogenes and tumor suppressor proteins were first identified through the study of cancer-causing viruses. For example, research with simian virus 40 led to the discovery of the tumor suppressor gene *p53* and *retinoblastoma* (*Rb*) (see Chap. 7, Sec. 7.4). Oncogenic viruses fall into two groups: the DNA tumor viruses that contain either linear or circular double-stranded DNA and the RNA-containing tumor viruses (also called *retroviruses*). DNA tumor viruses usually cause malignant transformation by inhibiting the normal function (growth control) of tumor suppressor genes, whereas retroviruses usually deregulate signal transduction pathways (see Chap. 8).

Stehelin et al. (1976) demonstrated that Rous sarcoma virus (a retrovirus that causes sarcomas in chickens) contained nucleotide sequences that were not found in similar nontransforming retroviruses. These novel retroviral sequences, however, were closely related to nucleotide sequences present in the DNA of normal chickens. This important discovery indicated that a viral transforming gene (in this case v-*src*) was derived from a normal cellular gene. Many other retroviruses have been shown to contain different oncogenes derived from and closely related to their cellular counterparts. The normal cellular genes from which the retroviral oncogenes (v-*onc*) are derived are referred to as *protooncogenes* (or c-*onc*). The process by which protooncogenes become integrated into the viral genome and are converted to viral oncogenes with overt transforming activity is complex; it involves recombination between the retroviral and cellular genomes following integration of a retrovirus adjacent to a cellular protooncogene. This process, known as *transduction*, is accompanied by alterations in the structure and regulation of oncogene sequences. Many of the oncogenes found in transforming retroviruses have also been identified independently in spontaneously arising tumors of nonviral origin, where they appear to be activated by other mechanisms, including point mutation, gene amplification, and chromosomal translocation (see Chap. 7, Sec. 7.2).

Protooncogenes encode a wide range of protein products involved in the control of cell proliferation and differentiation, including growth factors, growth factor receptors, components of signal transduction pathways, and transcription factors that regulate the synthesis of mRNA (see Chap. 7, Sec. 7.3 and Chap. 8, Sec. 8.2). Tumor suppressor genes, in contrast, represent genes that are likely to play a role in negatively regulating cell growth (Chap. 7, Sec. 7.4). In this chapter, the mechanisms of cellular transformation by oncogenic viruses are described. These mechanisms provide clues to more general mechanisms of transformation due to increases in dominantly acting oncogenes or inactivation of tumor suppressor genes.

## 6.2 DNA TUMOR VIRUSES

### 6.2.1 Simian Virus 40 and Polyomavirus

The papovaviruses, including Simian virus 40 (SV40), JC virus, BK virus, and polyomavirus, have yielded valuable information about the process of cellular transformation by DNA viruses. These viruses may cause tumors in rodents but have not been associated directly with human cancer. Polyomavirus was found to cause tumors in the salivary glands of mice and subsequently in many other organs, leading to the name by which it is known. The SV40 virus was identified as a contaminant in poliomyelitis virus vaccines prepared in rhesus monkey cells and caused widespread concern after it was discovered that the virus yielded tumors in newborn hamsters. The virus was injected unwittingly into millions of people. Epidemiologic studies of people who received the vaccine gave no evidence that it can cause cancer in humans. However, the fact that *SV40* gene sequences were recently identified in a small number of human tumors, including ependymomas, mesotheliomas, and osteosarcomas renewed fears that the virus might contribute to human carcinogenesis, and the presence of SV40 DNA sequences and T antigens in these tumors is being scrutinized (reviewed by Pennisi, 1997; Jasani et al., 2001). The JC and BK viruses have been associated with progressive multifocal leukoencephalopathy. Sporadic reports have also described their presence in some primary brain tumors, osteosarcomas, lymphomas, and colon cancers.

The papovaviruses interact with susceptible cells in two different ways. In permissive cells that support productive infection, the lytic cycle proceeds in two phases: an early phase in which nonstructural, regulatory proteins are synthesized and a late phase during which viral DNA is replicated, coat protein is made, and progeny virions are assembled. Viral DNA is not integrated in the cellular genome during the lytic cycle. Release of mature virus particles results in lysis and cell death. Monkey cells are permissive for SV40 infection, whereas mouse cells are permissive for polyoma infection. A second type of interaction leads to a small proportion of surviving transformed cells that contain viral DNA integrated randomly into host chromosomes. Transformation occurs more commonly in cells that are unable to efficiently support viral replication. In contrast to normal cells, virus-transformed cells show little or no contact inhibition and therefore grow to high cell density in culture; they give rise to multilayered and disorganized cell colonies, show anchorage-independent growth in a semisolid medium containing agar or methylcellulose, and exhibit a decreased requirement for serum. Moreover, the cells transformed in culture after infection give rise to tumors when inoculated into susceptible animals.

Papovaviruses are small, nonenveloped icosahedral viruses that contain circular, double-stranded DNA genomes of about 5 kilobases in length (Fig. 6.1). Early gene products are transcribed immediately after the virus enters the cell and the genome is transported to the nucleus of the host cell. Late genes are transcribed after viral DNA replication begins, and produce viral structural proteins (VP1, VP2, VP3) and agnoprotein, in the case of SV40. The major capsid protein, VP1 interacts with the host cell receptor, which is believed to be the major histocompatability complex class I protein (MHC I) in the case of SV40, and sialic acid for polyomavirus. Agnoprotein appears to facilitate the localization of VP1 to the nucleus, is involved in virus assembly, and helps in the release of virus from the host cell. Viral DNA replication, transcription, and virion assembly occur in the nucleus. The early genes of SV40 include *large-T* and *small-t antigens* (Fig. 6.1) and the early genes of polyomavirus are *large-T, middle-T,* and *small-t antigens*. These gene products possess transforming properties.

The large-T antigens of the papovaviruses are complex multifunctional proteins and the functional domains of SV40 T antigen are summarized in Figure 6.1*B* (Ali and DeCaprio, 2001; Pipas and Levine, 2001). The domains are more or less similar for the closely related polyoma large-T antigen. More than 95 percent of large-T antigen is associated with the nucleus but a small portion is found linked to the plasma membrane. The protein is phosphorylated, O-glycosylated, ADP-ribosylated, is associated with $Zn^{++}$, binds adenosine triphosphate (ATP), and possesses a nuclear localization signal (NLS). The large-T antigen binds to the viral DNA origin of replication and functions as the switch between early and late transcription. This protein has DNA helicase activity (i.e., unwinds double-stranded DNA), and hydrolyzes ATP in the process. Large-T antigen contains three domains involved in the transformation and immortalization of rodent cells (Conzen and Cole, 1995). The J domain, favors transcription of both viral and cellular promoters. Through the J domain, the T antigen interacts with the Rb tumor suppressor protein (p105)

A

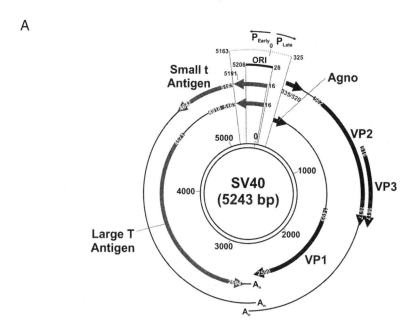

B

## SV40 Large T Antigen

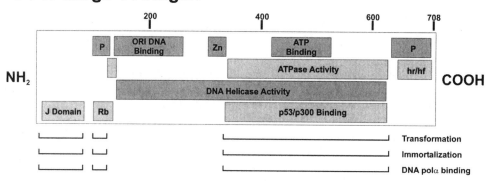

**Figure 6.1.** Simian virus 40 (SV40) genome and domains of large-T antigen. (*A*) The SV40 genome consists of a circular duplex DNA molecule. Two primary sets of transcripts are expressed from opposite strands of the genome that are further processed to produce early and late viral mRNAs. Early gene products are shown in gray while late gene products are presented in black. One of the two early mRNAs encodes large-T antigen, and the other includes sequences that encode the small-t antigen. The amino-terminal 82 residues of these proteins are identical. The large black boxes denote protein coding regions; the lines indicate noncoding regions; the intron sequences that are removed by splicing are indicated by thin lines. The late mRNA encodes the structural proteins (VP1, VP2, VP3) as indicated. Agno is a small late-protein that facilitates virus assembly and release. (*B*) Schematic representation of the functional domains of large-T antigen. Both p53 and pRb, the products of two cellular tumor suppressor genes, interact with large T antigen. The Rb protein binds to both the J and Rb domains. The p53 and CBP/p300 proteins bind to a similar region. T antigen has DNA helicase and ATPase activity for its replication function with cellular DNA polymerase and DNA binding proteins. This protein is the switch between early and late transcription, and T antigen binds to the origin of replication through the ORI DNA binding domain. The protein is phosphorylated, binds $Zn^{++}$, and has a host range or species specific domain (hr/hf). The LXCXE sequence motif for binding to pRb, p107, and p130 lies in the Rb domain.

as well as the related proteins p107 and p130 (see Chap. 7, Sec. 7.4.4). It contains a characteristic LXCXE (leucine-cysteine-glutamine) motif that is found in proteins that interact with molecules in the Rb family (see

also Fig. 6.3). The Rb protein and related proteins p107 and p130 function in part by binding to and inactivating the transcription factor designated E2F. The binding of large-T antigen to pRb and related proteins disrupts the pRb-E2F interaction, resulting in the release of E2F and the activation of E2F-responsive genes, which are associated with cell cycle progression (see Chap. 9, Sec. 9.2.1). Another transformation domain found in the T antigen of SV40, but not that of polyomavirus, forms complexes with p53 and led to the discovery of this tumor suppressor gene. T antigen binding to p53 inhibits apoptosis and favors cell cycle progression. Transfection of the gene encoding *large-T antigen* may alone cause the malignant transformation of normal rodent cells, although the presence of the small-t antigen contributes to the full expression of an SV40-transformed phenotype. Transgenic mice that contain the *SV40 large-T antigen* gene develop a high incidence of tumors in organs in which the gene is expressed (Furth, 1998).

The small-t antigens of SV40 and polyomavirus also function in transformation (Rundell and Parakati, 2001). Small-t antigen is dispensable for lytic growth of the virus but it does favor cell cycle progression (G1-S) through activation of growth factor signal transduction pathways, via interaction with the catalytic and structural subunits of protein phosphatase 2A (PP2A). By displacing the structural subunit, small-t antigen inhibits phosphatase activity and upregulates kinase activity in the mitogen-activated kinase (MAPK), stress kinase (SAPK), protein kinase C (PKC), phosphatidylinositol-3 kinase (PI-3 kinase), protein kinase B (PKB/AKT), and NF-kB pathways (Pallas et al., 1990; Yang et al., 1991; Sontag et al., 1997) (see Chap. 8, Sec. 8.2). The middle-T antigen of polyomavirus localizes to the plasma membrane and interacts with components of signal transduction pathways including c-src and PI-3 kinase to upregulate MAPK and PKB/AKT activity (Auger et al., 1992; Chap. 8, Sec. 8.2). Because middle-T antigen also contains most of the sequence of small-t antigen, it can also complex with, and inhibit the effects of, PP2A (Pallas et al., 1990). The interactions of all three T antigens with specific cellular components favor cell cycle progression, cell division, activation of growth factor pathways, and inhibition of apoptosis. These three proteins account for all of the oncogenic properties of the papovaviruses.

## 6.2.2 Human Adenoviruses

Adenoviruses are common and can cause acute infections of the upper respiratory tract, infantile gastroenteritis, pharyngitis, juvenile hepatitis, and conjunctivitis. Most people have antibodies directed against one or more of these viruses. Human adenovirus type 12 is known to cause tumors in newborn hamsters but adenoviruses have never been associated with human tumors during epidemiological studies or searches for viral DNA in tumor tissue. Human cells infected with adenovirus undergo lytic infection, while rodent cells are less permissive for growth of the virus and readily survive infection to undergo transformation. The ability of human adenoviruses to induce tumors in rodents and transform cells in culture have made them an important tool with which to study the process of malignant transformation.

Adenoviruses are icosahedral particles with antennae-like fibers emanating from the vertices of the icosahedron. They are composed of eleven structural proteins (Fig. 6.2*A*). The 35-kilobase linear, double-stranded DNA genome is organized into early and late transcription units (Fig. 6.2*B*). It contains five early transcription units (E1A, E1B, E2, E3, and E4), two delayed early units, and one major late unit that is spliced to generate five families of late mRNAs (L1 to L5) which code for the structural viral proteins. Cells transformed with adenoviruses contain an incomplete viral genome that always includes the viral *E1A* (early region 1A) and *E1B* genes integrated into host DNA. This minimal region of adenovirus DNA was shown to be capable of transforming rat embryo cells following DNA-mediated gene transfer.

Two mRNA species, 12S and 13S, are produced by differential splicing from the *E1A* gene and encode similar proteins of 243 and 289 amino acids, respectively, that function as transcription activators. These two proteins differ internally by an additional 46 amino acids that are unique to the 13S product. Multiple transcripts also originate from the *E1B* gene, giving rise to two major proteins of 19 kDa and 55 kDa, which function to block apoptosis. E2 encodes three proteins (E2A, E2B, and E2C) that function in DNA replication. E3 proteins are also multiply spliced gene products that are designated by their molecular masses and function to interfere with the immune response. E4 proteins are a diverse family of proteins that mediate transcription, mRNA transport, modulate DNA replication, and inhibit apoptosis.

In gene-transfer experiments, both *E1A* gene products immortalize primary rodent cells and complement an activated *Ras* gene to transform these cells. *E1B* can replace *Ras* in this type of assay to promote transformation. Additional functions attributed to E1A protein include its ability to either activate or repress transcription from cellular and viral genes dependent on enhancer sequences. Comparison of the E1A amino acid sequence among several adenovirus serotypes shows the presence of three conserved regions (CR1, CR2, and CR3). Mutational analysis of the E1A region has revealed that CR1 (amino acids 40 to 80) and CR2 (amino acids 121 to 139) are necessary for transformation, whereas CR3 (amino acids 140 to 188) is dispensable (Moran and Mathews, 1987). The E1A regions required for control of cell growth, blockade of differentiation, and transformation comprise the nonconserved amino terminus together with CR1 and CR2. The

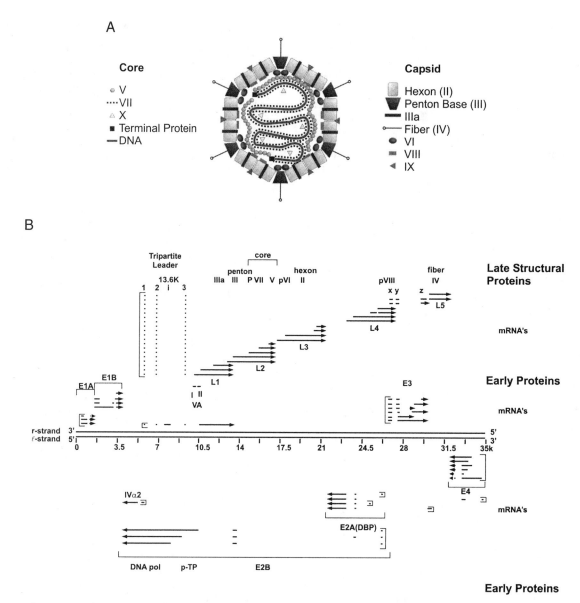

**Figure 6.2.** The structure of human adenovirus and a representation of RNA transcripts and proteins made from the adenovirus genome. (*A*) The virus consists of capsid and core proteins. Capsid proteins include hexon, penton base, IIIa, fiber, VI, VIII, and IX proteins. The core contains the double-stranded DNA genome, major core proteins (V, VII), terminal proteins, and minor core protein (X). (*B*) The genome is a template for early gene transcripts (E1A, E1B, E2, E3, E4) and late gene transcripts (L1, L2, L3, L4, L5). Early gene products cause transformation, inhibit apoptosis, regulate DNA replication, and block the immune response. Late gene products code for structural proteins (penton, core, hexon, pVIII, and fiber) and mRNA is transcribed from the major late promoter and contains the small exons of the tripartite leader.

CR2 region contains the LXCXE motif that binds to pRb (see Fig. 6.3) and is also present in SV40 large-T antigen and in the E7 protein of human papillomaviruses. E1A can activate transcription by E2F by promoting its dissociation from pRb through binding (Whyte et al., 1988) and promotes cell cycle progression, moving the infected cell into S phase. E1A also blocks acetylation of histones and inhibits the transcription of certain genes. Both of these processes are thought to play a role in E1A-mediated transformation.

The E1B55K protein has been shown to bind to p53 and to inhibit its transactivation function as well as p53-dependent apoptosis (Harada and Berk, 1999). Unlike E1A, expression of E1B55K alone is not sufficient to stimulate resting cells to enter S phase. The E1B19K protein has many activities, all of which tend to block apoptosis and favor cell survival. It is a member of the anti-apoptotic Bcl-2 family and has been shown to block both Fas- and TNF-mediated apoptosis by interacting with Bax (Han et al., 1996). In addition, E1B19K can upregulate the SAPK pathway (Chap. 8, Sec. 8.2.6) to increase transcription and expression of c-jun which serves as a survival pathway in many cell types (See and Shi, 1998).

Adenoviruses have also been shown to antagonize the immune system. The E1A protein and virus-associated RNAs inhibit the protective effects of interferons $\alpha$ and $\beta$. E3 proteins block induction of apoptosis by CTLs and macrophages, and interfere with the processing and presentation of peptide antigens. Gene products of the E3 region can be deleted without affecting infections in culture, but these mutations dramatically reduce infections in vivo.

Adenoviruses have been considered as potential vaccination and gene therapy delivery systems (Chap. 21, Sec. 21.2.2). Foreign genes have been introduced into the E1, E3, or E4 regions and virus has been propagated in cell lines that contain the complementary deleted region. An efficient immune response directed against the coat proteins of the virus limits multiple use of these reagents. Although most patients appear to tolerate high doses of these reagents, one unfortunate incident produced a fatal outcome in an individual 4 days into the gene therapy trial (Marshall, 1999). This death probably resulted from a severe immune reaction directed against the adenovirus proteins in the liver. In another very novel approach, an adenovirus was engineered to be selectively toxic in malignant cells containing a defective p53 gene. The virus, called Onyx-015 (or dl-1520), was defective in synthesis of the E1B55K protein and was postulated to grow in and kill only cells lacking a functional *p53* gene, providing potential selectivity against a variety of human tumors (Bischoff et al., 1996; Ries et al., 2000) (Chap. 21, Sec. 21.2). The agent has been used in trials for treatment of head and neck tumors and hepatocellullar carcinomas, with limited success (Heise et al., 1997).

### 6.2.3 Human Papillomaviruses

Human papillomaviruses (HPV) are nonenveloped DNA viruses that infect epithelial cells to cause warts in the skin, condylomas in mucous membranes, cancer of the cervix, and other tumors of the urogenital tract. Papillomaviruses contain a single molecule of circular double-stranded DNA that is about 8 kilobases in length and encodes eight early genes (*E1* to *E8*) and two late genes (*L1* and *L2*). In addition there is a noncoding regulatory region called the long control region (LCR; Fig. 6.3*A*). The functions of the various proteins are as follows: L1 is the major capsid protein while L2 is a minor capsid protein that associates with genomic DNA. E1 directs initiation of DNA replication and E2 is a transcription activator that has an auxilliary role in replication. The function of E3 is not known while E4 disrupts

cytokeratins and is important for viral release. E5 is a membrane protein with transforming properties that interacts with growth factor receptors. E6 is a transforming protein that targets p53 for degradation by the ubiquitin pathway (see Chap. 9, Sec. 9.2.1). E7 is a transforming protein that binds to Rb. The function of E8 is not known.

Papillomaviruses have been difficult to study and propagate in culture because they replicate in stratified squamous epithelium, a property that cannot be duplicated in monolayer cell cultures. The virus reaches the basal layers of the epithelium where it can replicate through a process of mechanical stress and damage to the keratinized epithelium. Virus is taken into the host cell through receptor mediated endocytosis and is transported to the nucleus. Early gene transcription and translation of early proteins and limited replication of the viral genome occur in the basal squamous epithelial cell. The transcription and production of late capsid proteins (L1, L2), high levels of DNA replication, and virus assembly occur in the keratinized epithelium. Virus is released as the stratum corneum is sloughed from the surface of the skin or mucosa.

More than one hundred different types of HPV have been identified. These viruses infect only epithelial cells and are associated mostly with benign mucosal and cutaneous lesions, such as warts in the skin and anogenital regions. Low-risk anogenital warts can be caused by several HPV types—including HPV6, 10, and 11—that infect the genital tract and are associated also with low grades of cervical intraepithelial neoplasia that regress spontaneously; they are rarely found in malignant tumors. Anogenital warts are prevalent among young sexually active adults and their incidence increased six-fold between 1966 and 1981.

Cervical cancer is the third most common cancer in women worldwide and is a sexually transmitted disease that is associated with high-risk HPV types—including HPV16, 18, 31, 33, and 45—that are found in about 90 percent of all cervical cancers (zur Hausen, 2000). However, these HPV types have also been detected in nonmalignant cervical tissue, and only a small proportion of women with clinically apparent high-risk HPV infection eventually develop cervical carcinoma, possibly because many of these infections may be transient. Human papillomavirus infection is not sufficient for tumor development and other cofactors—such as smoking, use of oral contraceptives, recurrent infection, early pregnancy, and immunologic and hormonal status—may play a role in progression to malignancy. Human papillomavirus has also been associated with non-melanoma skin cancers, anal cancer, vulvar cancer, penile cancer, and respiratory malignant papillomas. Immunosuppressed individuals, transplant recipients, and AIDS patients are at higher risk for HPV-related malignancies.

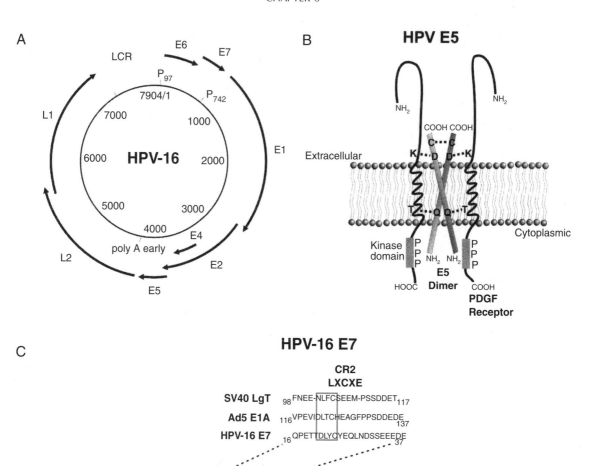

**Figure 6.3.** (*A*) Organization of the HPV-16 genome. The papillomavirus genome is double-stranded circular DNA, but the genes are expressed from only one strand in a unidirectional manner. The coding regions for viral proteins in all three possible translation phases are indicated by the solid heavy lines and are based on the complete DNA sequence. E and L stand for early and late proteins, respectively. There are 9 genes which code for early proteins (E1, E2, E4, E5, E6, E7, and E8) and the late structural proteins (L1, L2). P97 and P742 are the promoters used in transcription. (*B*) E5 protein of papillomavirus dimerizes through an intermolecular disulfide bond linkage and interacts with platelet derived growth factor receptor (PDGFR). Aggregation of the receptor occurs through ionic (lysine-aspartic acid, K-D) or hydrogen bond (threonine-glutamine, T-Q) interactions to activate the receptor associated tyrosine kinase. (*C*) E7 protein binds pRB through an LXCXE (Leu-amino acid-Cys-amino acid-Glu) motif in a CR2 region along with residues in the CR1 domain. It targets the pRB protein for degradation. A CR3 domain contains metal binding and dimerization motifs which can transactivate some genes recognized by E2F. In many respects the E7 protein is very similar in structure and function to the SV40 large-T antigen and adenovirus E1A proteins.

The HPV genome is maintained in benign warts as an episome (a nonintegrated, circular form). In malignant cells, HPV DNA is integrated randomly into various chromosomes, resulting in substantial deletions or disruption of the viral genome, particularly the *E2* gene, which has a negative regulatory effect on the expression of the HPV proteins E6 and E7. These latter two proteins are always retained and consistently expressed in cervical tumor tissue and cervical tumor cell lines, suggesting that one or both of these proteins is required for transformation by HPV. A comparison of high-risk HPVs, such as HPV16 and HPV18, with low-risk viruses such as HPV2, HPV4, HPV6, and HPV11 has allowed the mapping of transformation properties to the *E5*, *E6*, and *E7* genes. The E5 protein can dimerize and interact with growth factor receptors, such as those for the epidermal growth factor (EGFR) and platelet-derived growth factor (PDGFR), leading to activation of the MAPK pathway (Chap. 8, Sec. 8.2.6) and cell proliferation (Fig. 6.3*B*). Gene transfer experiments (see Chap. 4, Sec. 4.3.10) with primary human fibroblasts or keratinocytes demonstrate that either the *E6* or *E7* genes from the high-risk HPV types but not from the low-risk HPV types extend the life span of these cells in culture (Hawley-Nelson et al., 1989; Munger et al., 1989). These cells, however, enter a crisis period in culture and will not form tumors when injected into nude mice. Human papillomavirus E6 proteins interact with and inactivate the p53 tumor suppressor protein. E6 may also have additional functions that operate in the transformation process because it can still promote hyperplasia in a p53 null background. Human papillomavirus E7 proteins contain domains similar to the adenovirus E1A protein and large T antigen of SV40; the transforming ability of E7 proteins depends on their binding to pRb tumor suppressor proteins (Dyson et al., 1989) through a domain that contains the LXCXE motif (Fig. 6.3*C*). Binding of E7 to pRb favors the degradation of the tumor suppressor and results in the release of the bound E2F transcription factor from pRb to induce cellular DNA synthesis and progression into the S phase of the cell cycle. The E7 protein from low-risk HPV types binds to pRb with at least a ten-fold lower efficiency than the E7 protein of HPV16 and HPV18. The E7 protein can also interact with cyclin-dependent kinase inhibitors such as p27 and p21 (Chap. 9, Sec. 9.2), which may promote the replication of papillomavirus DNA in differentiating squamous epithelial cells. Thus, related mechanisms of transformation seem to be evident for papovaviruses, adenoviruses, and papillomaviruses (Fig. 6.3*D*). Prophylactic and therapeutic vaccines directed against the more lethal types of papillomaviruses are being explored.

### 6.2.4 Epstein-Barr Virus

An aggressive lymphoma that affects African children was first described by Dennis Burkitt and is known as *Burkitt's lymphoma.* Cultured cells from these lymphomas were found by Epstein and Barr to release a herpesvirus that subsequently became known as *Epstein-Barr virus* (EBV). Epstein-Barr virus is transmitted horizontally, usually via contaminated saliva, infecting more than 90 percent of the human population by the age of 20, often without any manifestation of disease. Epstein-Barr virus strains can be classified into two main types, type 1 and type 2, based on polymorphisms (Chap. 4, Sec. 4.3.7) (genetic differences) within certain viral genes.

Type 1 strains are more common in western countries, whereas both type 1 and type 2 strains are prevalent in central Africa and New Guinea. Strong epidemiologic and clinical data have associated EBV infection with three lymphoproliferative diseases of B-cell origin—infectious mononucleosis, Burkitt's lymphoma, and lymphoma of the immunocompromised host (e.g. in the setting of organ transplantation and HIV infection). There is also a very strong association between EBV infection and undifferentiated nasopharyngeal carcinoma (NPC), and it is implicated in the pathogenesis of Hodgkin's disease (Weinreb et al., 1996). EBV may also be associated with some gastric carcinomas (Takada, 1999). Geographic and ethnic variation have been recognized in the incidence of these EBV-associated malignancies, indicating involvement of other genetic and environmental factors.

Epstein-Barr virus contains a double-stranded DNA genome that codes for immediate-early, early, and late gene products. The B-lymphocyte is the preferential target cell of EBV. The complement regulatory protein CD21, which normally protects a cell from self-destruction, is the cell receptor for this virus. Two forms of infection can occur in the B-cell using two different sets of gene products and promoters: (1) latent infection that is accompanied by B-cell proliferation, and (2) lytic infection that is characterized by synthesis of structural proteins, generation of linear viral genomes, packaging, and the generation of mature virions.

Upon entry into the host cell, the viral genome travels to the nucleus and circularizes to form an episome or plasmid, thereby establishing a latent infection (Fig. 6.4*A*). Latency is characterized by the synthesis of six EBV nuclear antigens (EBNA-LP, EBNA-1, EBNA-2, EBNA-3A, EBNA-3B, and EBNA-3C). Three latent membrane proteins (LMP1, LMP2A, LMP2B) are also synthesized during latency. EBNA-1 protein is required for DNA replication of the extrachromosomal viral plasmids in EBV-infected cells. It binds to the viral origin of replication and is essential for maintenance of multiple viral genomes in an episomal form. EBNA-1 also binds to chromosomes to enable the EBV episome to partition to progeny cells. EBNA-LP and EBNA-2 activate transcription from viral and cellular genes. EBNA-2 protein transactivates expression of cellular and viral genes through interaction with at least two sequence-specific DNA-binding proteins. LMP1 has transforming effects in rodent fibroblast cell lines; it permits them to grow under low serum conditions, generate colonies in soft agar, and causes them to form tumors in nude mice (Wang et al., 1985; Fig. 6.4*B*). In B-lymphocytes it causes cell clumping, increased villous projections, upregulates vimentin and other proteins, and protects cells from apoptosis through induction of BCL-2 protein

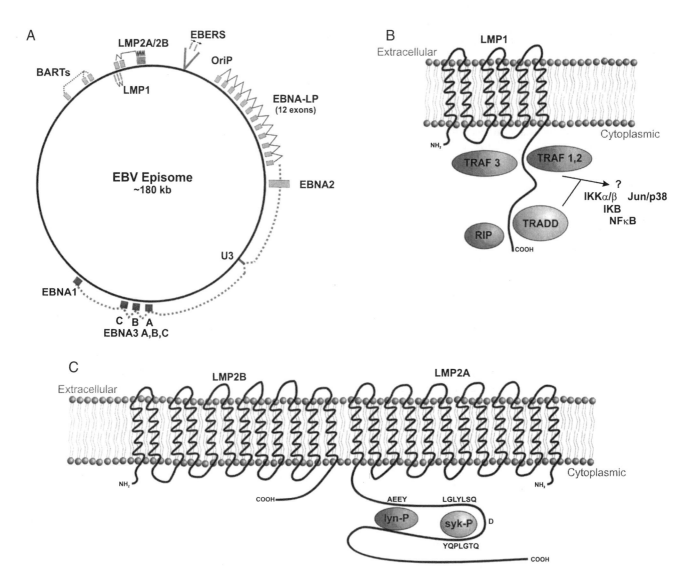

**Figure 6.4.** (*A*) Latency-associated genes of the genome from Epstein-Barr virus (EBV). When EBV infects a cell, the genome becomes circularized and forms an episome or plasmid. The gene products associated with latency are called: Epstein-Barr nuclear antigens (EBNA) leader protein, 1, 2, 3A, 3B; 3C, latent membrane proteins (LMP) 1, 2A, 2B; Epstein-Barr early RNAs (EBERS), BamHI RNA transcripts (BARTs). The transcribed gene products are multiply spliced and the exons are represented as gray rectangular boxes. The latency-associated origin of replication is OriP. (*B*) LMP1 is a transforming protein that activates transcription and stimulates cell growth through interaction with TNF receptor associated proteins (TRA's, TRADD, RIP). It stimulates cell survival pathways by activating NFκB through phosphorylation of inhibitor of NFκB (IKB) and activation of c-jun through upregulation of the SAPK pathway. (*C*) LMP2A is a receptor-like protein that contains tyrosine phosphorylation domains that sequester src-like tyrosine kinases (lyn and syk) and prevent reactivation of the infected B cell from its latent state.

(Chap. 10, Sec. 10.2.1). LMP-1 can also cause hyperplasia and lymphomas when expressed as a transgene in mice. LMP2 proteins span the membrane of the host cell 12 times (Fig. 6.4C). LMP2A protein is a substrate for and associates with src family tyrosine kinases. LMP2B lacks the amino terminus, which is involved in this interaction. The function of LMP2A is to block activation of lytic EBV infection by sequestering the protein kinases that would mediate reactivation following crosslinking of the surface immunoglobulin that serves as the B-cell receptor (Longnecker, 2000; Dykstra et al.,

2001). This association targets the kinases for ubiquitin-mediated degradation (see Chap. 9, Sec. 9.2.1). LMP2A can also activate PI-3 kinase and PKB/AKT (Chap. 8, Sec. 8.2) to enhance survival of the latently-infected B-cell.

Viral latency is designed to promote the survival of the EBV episome in the face of an efficient attack by cytotoxic T-lymphocytes on the infected cell. Latency attempts to minimize the number of viral proteins and antigenic epitopes being expressed and yet retain the genetic material of EBV within the infected cell. Initially the circularized viral genome expresses all the proteins and RNA transcripts associated with latency. This promotes a state of lymphoproliferation and replication of the viral episome. This state, referred to as latency III, is present in the rapidly proliferating B-lymphocytes found in infectious mononucleosis or posttransfusion lymphoma. In latency states I and II, fewer viral proteins are expressed (they include EBNA1 and EBERS); this is the characteristic state of nasopharyngeal carcinoma cells, T-cell lymphomas, and gastric carcinomas. In vitro this state can be mimicked by fusing EBV infected lymphoblastic cell lines with EBV-negative epithelial, fibroblast, or hemopoietic cells. Latency II alone is characteristic of cells in Hodgkin's disease.

Reactivation of EBV from the latent state to produce structural proteins and virions can occur through a number of stimuli. These include crosslinking of B-cell receptors with antibodies or treatment with phorbol esters, which mimic phosphatidyl inositol/diacylglycerol, and activate MAPK and PKC, leading to transcription of a number of genes that are generally involved in DNA replication (see Chap. 8, Secs. 8.2.4 and 8.2.7). Late genes are subsequently transcribed and specify the structural proteins of EBV. In addition, an interleukin 10 analogs (BCRF1), is transcribed in the late phase of infections. It has B-cell growth properties, downregulates natural killer (NK) cells, blocks cytotoxic T-cell activity, and inhibits interferon $\gamma$ production to favor a Th2 immune response (Chap. 20; Hsu et al., 1990). Cooperation between the latent and lytic states of EBV infection is an efficient mechanism by which to propagate the viral genome and minimize the exposure of viral proteins to immune surveillance.

*Infectious mononucleosis* is a benign disease where symptoms range from mild transient fever to several weeks of pharyngitis, lymphadenopathy, swollen spleen and lymph nodes, and general malaise. Infectious mononucleosis is characterized by the proliferation of latently infected EBV-infected B-cells coupled with the effects of reactive T-cells, which eventually clear the pathogen. Epstein-Barr virus is released from the oropharynx in localized lytic infections that appear to occur when latently infected B-cells are in contact with mucosal surfaces. Linear EBV DNA, characteristic of lytic infection, is detectable in only a fraction of tonsillar lymphocytes. Epithelial cells in these local regions may become permissive to EBV infection. At the peak of an acute infection, 0.1 to 1 percent of the circulating B-cells are positive for Epstein-Barr early RNAs (EBERS) and the latency antigens. Expanding B-cell populations carry somatically rearranged Ig genes that are characteristic of antigen primed polyclonal memory B-cells and are capable of producing antibodies. Upon resolution of infectious mononucleosis through the action of cytotoxic T-lymphocytes directed against both lytic and latent antigen epitopes, an asymptomatic carrier state is established.

*Burkitt's lymphoma* is the most common childhood cancer in equatorial Africa and is also found in coastal New Guinea. Climatic factors, the high incidence of *Plasmodium falciparum* malaria, as well as EBV infection, predispose children in these areas to the disease. Both type 1 and type 2 isolates of EBV have been found to be associated with Burkitt's lymphoma. Tumors present at extranodal sites, most frequently in the jaw during molar tooth development, but also in the orbit of the eye, the central nervous system, and in the abdomen. It affects three times as many boys as girls. The tumors are monoclonal, are composed of germinal center B-cells, and contain chromosome translocations between c-*myc* and the IgG heavy chain locus (8:14) or c-*myc* and the IgG light chain loci (8:2 or 8:22; Chap. 7, Sec. 7.2.4). These translocations are believed to result in deregulation of c-*myc* expression as a result of proximity to the Ig enhancer sequences, thus preventing the normal downregulation of c-*myc* expression in maturing B-lymphocytes. Malaria or AIDS together with EBV may supply lymphoproliferative signals that favor translocations. High c-myc expression in the EBV-transformed B-cell can substitute for the growth promoting effects of the EBV latency genes. Burkitt's lymphoma is endemic in Africa, but it can also occur fifty to a hundred times less frequently in Europe and North America. A third form of the disease now affects patients infected with HIV and is called AIDS-related Burkitt's lymphoma. The lymphomas are immunologically silent and avoid surveillance by cytotoxic T-lymphocytes through inhibition of proteosome-dependent antigen presentation, downregulation of MHC I, and low levels of co-stimulatory and cell adhesion molecules on the cell surface (Chap. 20, Secs. 20.4 and 20.5). Normally only EBNA1 and EBERS are expressed in Burkitt's lymphoma, accounting for a lack of immunogenicity against the tumors. In 30 percent of tumors, the p53 gene is also mutated.

*Nasopharyngeal carcinoma* (NPC) is a relatively rare disease in Europe and North America but is much more common among Southeast Asian populations, particularly those of Southern China. The link between NPC and EBV was first suggested by the presence of elevated antiviral antibodies in the sera of patients. DNA hybridization studies and polymerase chain reaction (PCR) amplification (see Chap. 4, Secs. 4.3.4 and 4.3.5) have subsequently confirmed that EBV is present in most tumor samples. Real-time quantitative PCR can be used to measure the EBV DNA load in the plasma and can be correlated with tumor burden and recurrence following treatment. The role of EBV in NPC is poorly understood, although racial, genetic, and environmental cofactors appear to be important (Liebowitz, 1994). MHC I haplotype, dietary factors (nitrosamines in dried fish), x-rays, chemical carcinogens, cytochrome P450 mutations, and physical irritants (dust and smoke) have all been implicated as risk factors for NPC. Four EBV proteins, in addition to EBERS, have been detected in NPC cells, namely, the nuclear antigen EBNA-1, LMP1, LMP2A, and LMP2B. The profound growth-stimulating effect of LMP1 on keratinocyte cultures suggests that LMP1 expression may exert similar effects in the nasopharyngeal epithelium. It has been suggested that EBV infection of nasopharyngeal epithelial cells could provide an expanded pool of target cells susceptible to further genetic changes in oncogenes and tumor suppressor genes necessary for malignant transformation of these cells and development of NPC.

*Hodgkin's disease* is a lymphoma characterized by a malignant population of mononuclear B-cells and multinuclear Reed-Sternberg cells set within a background of reactive nonmalignant lymphocytes. Reed-Sternberg cells carry the genotype of a cell that has inappropriately escaped apoptotic death and have the properties of monoclonal postgerminal center (memory) B-cells. They do not express conventional B- or T-cell markers but do express a range of cytokines that have the capacity to divert cytotoxic lymphocytes(CTL) recognition away from them. An association between EBV and Hodgkin's disease is now supported by a variety of circumstantial evidence. Epstein-Barr virus DNA sequences and transcripts have been detected in malignant Reed-Sternberg cells and their mononuclear variants by in situ hybridization and PCR–based assays (Weiss et al., 1989). LMP1 protein has also been detected by immunohistochemical staining of lymph nodes from patients with Hodgkin's disease (Herbst et al., 1991). The association of EBV with this disease varies greatly from country to country, and Hodgkin's disease in developing countries differs from that in western countries in terms of epidemiologic, pathologic, and clinical characteristics. Thus, 100 percent of Kenyan children with Hodgkin's disease were found to be positive for EBV particles (53 of 53 cases), while only 51 percent of children from the United States and the United Kingdom (46 of 90 cases) showed evidence of EBV in their malignant cells (Weinreb et al., 1996). Differences may be explained by geographic variation of EBV isolates.

### 6.2.5 Hepatitis B Virus

Most individuals infected with the hepatitis B virus (HBV) develop either an acute transient illness or an asymptomatic infection that leaves them immune. However, severe liver failure associated with fulminant hepatitis can occur in about 1 percent of those infected with HBV and usually results in death. About 10 percent of infected individuals develop chronic hepatitis, which can progress to more severe conditions such as cirrhosis and liver cancer. There are estimated to be 500 million chronic carriers of HBV worldwide and 2 billion seropositive individuals have been exposed to the virus. There is strong epidemiological evidence indicating the importance of chronic HBV infection in the development of human hepatocellular carcinoma. More than 80 percent of individuals with liver cancer have been chronically infected by HBV. Hepatitis B is widespread throughout Asia, Africa, and regions of South America and in some regions hepatocellular carcinoma is the leading cause of cancer death. Transmission of HBV is primarily through blood and sexual contact. Introduction of the recombinant vaccine derived from the membrane protein of HBV (Recombivax HB®) which is administered as a three-dose regimen promises to limit the incidence of this virus in North America. However, the high prevalence of this virus throughout the world, together with 15 to 20 percent frequency of vaccine failure, makes it unlikely that this virus will be totally eradicated.

Hepatitis B virus is an enveloped DNA-containing virus. The envelope contains three related forms of surface-exposed glycoproteins (L, M, S) that act as the major surface antigenic determinants (HBsAg; Fig. 6.5A). The larger surface antigen (L) interacts with an unidentified HBV receptor on the plasma membranes of hepatocytes. Viral membranes surround an icosahedral nucleocapsid composed of core protein (C). This nucleocapsid contains at least one HBV polymerase protein (P) as well as the HBV genome. Viral DNA found in viral particles is composed of one 3.2-kilobase strand (minus strand) base-paired with a shorter plus strand of variable length. Small fragments of remnant RNA pregenome can also be found in the virus as a consequence of replication. Because the $5'$ ends of both strands invariably overlap by about 300 bases, the DNA retains a circular configuration, although neither strand is itself a closed circle. The genome of HBV is organized very efficiently and its coding capacity consists of four overlapping reading frames which specify core protein (C), envelope surface proteins (L, M, S), polymerase (P), and the viral oncogene (X; Fig. 6.5B). Different HBV proteins are generated by the transcription and translation of mRNAs from several start sites and in-frame initiation codons.

Hepatitis B virus cannot be propagated in cultured cells, and many of the steps of viral replication, such as attachment, host cell entry, and virion assembly are poorly understood. However, several cell lines are capable of supporting HBV DNA synthesis, following transfection with viral DNA. Genome replication is complex and occurs after viral DNA is transported into the nucleus where the gap is repaired to produce covalently closed-circular DNA by using host cell enzymes (Fig. 6.5C). Integration of HBV DNA into host chromosomes

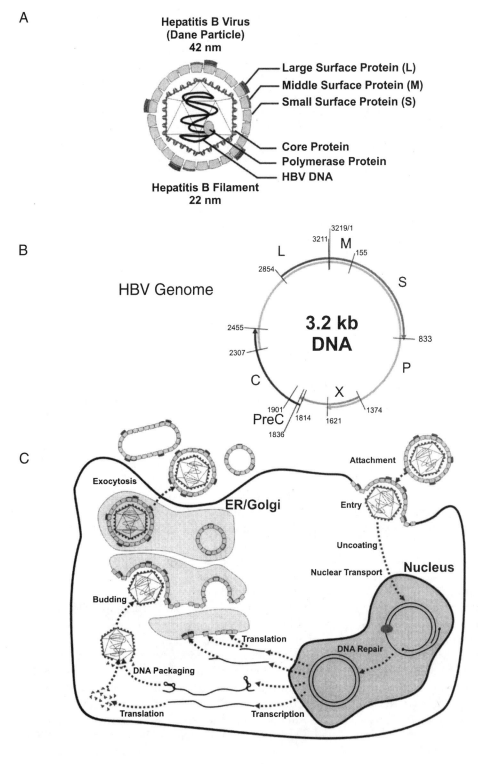

**A**

**Hepatitis B Virus
(Dane Particle)
42 nm**

Large Surface Protein (L)
Middle Surface Protein (M)
Small Surface Protein (S)

Core Protein
Polymerase Protein
HBV DNA

**Hepatitis B Filament
22 nm**

**B**

HBV Genome

3219/1
3211
M
155
L
S
2854
2455
833
2307
P
C
X
1901
1374
PreC
1814
1621
1836

**3.2 kb
DNA**

**C**

Exocytosis
ER/Golgi
Attachment
Entry
Uncoating
Nuclear Transport
Nucleus
Budding
Translation
DNA Repair
DNA Packaging
Translation
Transcription

**Figure 6.5.** (*A*) Essential features of the structure of hepatitis B virus. The envelope contains surface-exposed glycoproteins (L, M, S), and surrounds an icosahedral nucleocapsid composed of core protein. The nucleocapsid contains at least one HBV polymerase protein as well as the HBV genome. Viral DNA in the virion is composed of one 3.2-kilobase strand (minus strand) base-paired with a shorter plus strand of variable length. (*B*) The genome of HBV is compact and consists of four overlapping reading frames that specify core protein (C), envelope surface proteins (L,M,S), polymerase (P), and the viral oncogene (X or HBx). Different HBV proteins are generated by transcription and translation of mRNAs from several promoter start sites and in-frame initiation codons. A larger form of core protein (pre-C) possesses a signal peptide, which causes it to associate with the endoplasmic reticulum (ER), and allows the core antigen (HB$_e$Ag) to be secreted from the cell. The shorter form of core protein remains in the infected cell and functions as the major nucleocapsid protein. The X protein is a multifunctional polypeptide that acts as a weak oncogene in HBV infections. (*C*) HBV initiates infection by binding to an unknown receptor on the hepatocyte and the membranes of the virus fuse with those of the host cell. The nucleocapsid core enters the cytoplasm and is transported to the nucleus where the viral DNA (single-stranded DNA gap) is repaired by host enzymes to form a double-stranded circle. Enhancers and promoters within the HBV DNA are recognized by host cell RNA polymerase to produce RNA transcripts required for vital protein synthesis (C, S, P, X). Host RNA polymerase also directs the synthesis of an RNA pregenome that also serves as a template for the vital DNA genome.

is not required for replication. Once recircularized, enhancers and promoters within the HBV DNA direct the synthesis of RNA transcripts required for viral protein synthesis (C, S, P, X) and the formation of an RNA pregenome that serves as a template for viral DNA replication. The viral polymerase (P) is actually a reverse transcriptase that first directs the synthesis of minus strand DNA from the RNA pregenome. An RNAse activity associated with the polymerase subsequently degrades the RNA pregenome, and the viral polymerase uses the RNA fragments to prime synthesis of the positive sense DNA strand. Complete replication of this positive strand DNA never occurs and the virus is secreted from the host cell by a process of exocytosis, following virus assembly.

Integrated HBV DNA is found frequently in the cellular DNA of hepatocellular carcinomas. The implications of viral DNA integration are controversial. In an animal model for studying transformation by HBV, woodchuck hepatitis viral DNA is commonly integrated adjacent to oncogenes such as c-*myc* and N-*myc* to yield insertional activation of these genes (see Chap. 7, Sec. 7.2). However, HBV is not believed to act as an insertional mutagen of *C-MYC* and *N-MYC* genes in humans. Hepatitis B virus integration in human cells frequently induces deletions and translocations in a seemingly random way. Insertion of HBV DNA, and the subsequent disruption of cellular genes encoding the α-retinoic acid receptor and cyclin A have been reported. However, the importance of these events in the development of liver cancer is not known.

Only two viral genes, *HBx* and *M* (*preS2/S*), are usually retained intact after viral DNA integration. Products of both these genes can upregulate signal transduction pathways and stimulate transcription of genes characteristic of growth and survival (e.g., c-jun, c-fos; Hildt et al., 1996; Feitelson, 1999). HBx is a multifunctional protein whose role in HBV infections and carcinogenesis has remained elusive. It was originally called the promiscuous transactivator because HBx increases the synthesis of many viral and cellular gene products. However, most HBx resides in the cytoplasm and a nuclear function for this protein seems unlikely. HBx has been implicated in the development of hepatocellular carcinoma because transgenic mice that synthesize HBx are predisposed to liver tumors within a year of their birth. HBx may be a survival factor that upregulates several signal transduction pathways including c-src kinase, ras/raf/MAPK, SAPK/JNK, protein kinase C, JAK/STAT, PI-3 kinase, protein kinase B (see Chap. 8, Sec. 8.2; reviewed in Diao et al., 2001). HBx can interact with and sequester the tumor suppressor, p53, within the cytoplasm, which again would support a role in oncogenesis (Wang et al., 1994; Truant et al., 1995). In addition, HBx can bind and sequester Damaged DNA Binding Protein 1 (DDB1), interfering with DNA repair (Becker et al., 1998). This process could contribute to the generation of mutations during hepatocarcinogenesis.

### 6.2.6 Kaposi's Sarcoma-Associated Herpesvirus

Kaposi's sarcoma-associated herpesvirus (KSHV) or human herpesvirus 8 (HHV-8) was identified as the pathogen responsible for a number of malignancies including Kaposi's sarcoma (KS), body cavity-based or primary effusion lymphoma, and multicentric Castleman's disease. Kaposi's sarcoma is a vascular tumor of endothelial cells that affects elderly men in Mediterranean and African populations (endemic KS). However, with the onset of AIDS, a more aggressive and often lethal form of KS appeared. The virus infects the spindle cells of the skin, which are probably derived from lymphatic endothelial cells, and causes a proliferation of small red blotches over the entire body through a process of angiogenesis (Fig. 6.6). Body cavity-based or primary effusion lymphoma is a B-cell lymphoma, which occurs as malignant effusions in visceral cavities. These lymphomas are often co-infected with EBV, and in the setting of AIDS the tumors are extremely aggressive. Multicentric Castleman's disease is a reactive lymphadenopathy characterized by expanded germinal centers and proliferation of endothelial vessels within involved lymph nodes. Although classified as a hyperplasia and considered nonneoplastic, it often precedes the development of non-Hodgkins lymphoma; it appears to be caused by viral secretion of IL-6. The KSHV tumors are usually found in immunosuppressed individuals and the virus is endemic in many populations without causing disease. Kaposi's sarcoma-associated herpesvirus has also been associated with other diseases including multiple myeloma, sarcoidosis, and posttransplantation skin tumors, but a causative role has not been established.

Kaposi's sarcoma-associated herpesvirus is a large, enveloped double-stranded DNA in the same family as the Epstein-Barr virus (Moore and Chang, 2001). The virus can now be propagated in culture using immortalized dermal microvascular endothelial cells (Moses et al., 1999). The genome of KSHV encodes 87 gene products that include latency factors, viral structural proteins, replicative enzymes, and host genes acquired through a process of molecular piracy that help the virus to evade immune surveillance and inhibits apoptosis (Fig. 6.6*A*). Many of the genes share homology with those of the Epstein-Barr virus, and KSHV also encode latency and lytic gene products.

The KSHV episome is maintained in the cell through use of latency-associated factors including latency associated nuclear antigen (LANA), which binds to viral DNA and also both inhibits p53-dependent transcription and binds to the retinoblastoma protein pRb. It has similar properties to EBNA1 of EBV and large-T antigen of SV40. Viral chemokines secreted by KSHV serve to inhibit the cell mediated $T_H1$ immune response and shift it to the humoral $T_H2$ arm of the immune system (Chap. 20, Sec. 20.2.3). They bind to chemokine receptors which signal attraction of the $T_H2$ lymphocytes. These viral chemokines are also highly angiogenic and contribute to vascularization of the tumors (Stine et al., 2000). A functional receptor with sequence similarity to the IL-8 receptor (vIL-8R) can induce cellular transformation and secretion of vascular endothelial

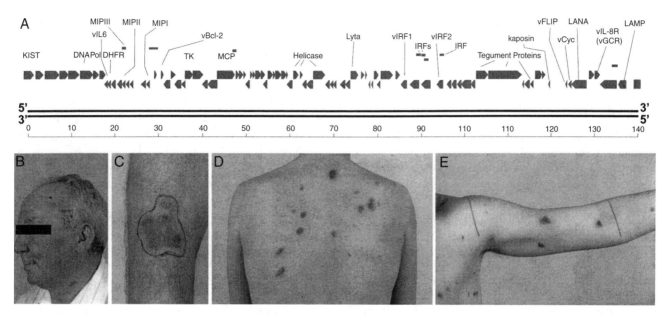

**Figure 6.6.** (*A*) Double-stranded DNA genome of the Kaposi's sarcoma virus. The genome contains 87 open reading frames (ORFs) coding for latency proteins, reactivation proteins, and structural proteins. Host genes that help the virus evade immune surveillance and inhibit apoptosis have been acquired from chromosomes through a process of molecular piracy. These genes include vFLIP, vBcl-2, v-cyclin, interferon response factors (IRFs), and membrane cofactor protein (MCP), KIST, vIL6, MIP chemokines, LANA, vIL-8R (vGCR), and LAMP. (*B-E*) Skin lesions associated with Kaposi sarcoma. Lesions present as red blotches on the skin due to the infection of spindle cells. Angiogenesis occurs in the surrounding tissue. *Panels B and C* are examples of endemic or Mediterranean Kaposi's sarcoma, while panels D and E illustrate epidemic or AIDS-related Kaposi sarcoma. (Photographs courtesy of Dr. Fei-Fei Liu, Ontario Cancer Institute.) (See color plate.)

growth factor, VEGF (Chap. 12, Sec. 12.2.1). Activation of this receptor results in calcium influx into infected cells and activation of the MAPK pathway. The expression of this receptor in transgenic mice results in an angioproliferative disorder similar to KS (Yang et al., 2000). The secreted viral IL-6 (vIL-6) cytokine has 62 percent sequence similarity to its host cellular homologue. It binds to host cell receptors and stimulates cell growth, VEGF production, and transformation of spindle cells and B-cells. Kaposi's sarcoma-associated herpesvirus can also lead to upregulation of a homolog of D-type cyclin, vCYC, which can interact with a cellular cyclin dependent kinase (CDK6) to phosphorylate the retinoblastoma protein pRb and favor the G1 to S phase transition in the cell cycle (Chap. 9, Sec. 9.2; Chang et al., 1996; Godden-Kent et al., 1997). The vCYC-CDK6 complex is resistant to the CDK inhibitors p16, p21, and p27 and phosphorylates the p27 inhibitor to trigger its degradation (Swanton et al., 1997). Thus, vCYC has properties of a transforming protein, and overexpression of cellular D-type cyclins have previously been observed in some B-cell lymphomas and parathyroid tumors.

During latent infections, KSHV expresses two membrane proteins, KSHV immunoreceptor tyrosine activa-tion motif-based signal transducer (KIST) and latency-associated membrane protein (LAMP). KIST appears to have an analogous function to the LMP1 protein of EBV. Like LMP1, the KIST protein has transformation properties in Rat-1 fibroblasts. Latency-associated membrane protein has similarities to both the LMP1 and LMP2A protein of EBV (see Fig. 6.4) and possesses up to twelve membrane spanning domains; the cytoplasmic C terminus contains an src protein kinase-binding motif. Overexpression of LAMP seems to block the function of KIST, and prevents intracellular calcium mobilization. This protein may block reactivation of lytic infection from the latent state. However, this protein may also have transformation properties. As is the case with EBV, lytic replication, characterized by virus particle formation, can be triggered by chemical agents including butyrate and phorbol esters (TPA and PMA) that inhibit histone deacetylases and activate MAPK signaling, respectively. The virus also specifies interferon response factors (vIRF1 and vIRF2) that antagonize their cellular homologues and block the antiviral effects of interferon. In addition, KSHV encodes vBCL-2 and vFLIP that act like their cellular homologs to inhibit apoptosis (see Chap. 10, Sec. 10.2). Viral infections appear to respond to nucleotide analogues such as acyclovir. Kaposi sarcoma may also be treated with topical liquid nitrogen, intralesional vinblastine, vincristine, doxorubicin, bleomycin, paclitaxel, or the angiogenesis inhibitor, thalidomide.

## 6.3 RETROVIRUSES

### 6.3.1 Life Cycle

Retroviruses are enveloped viruses of about 120 nm in diameter (Fig. 6.7A). The outer envelope is a lipid bilayer that is derived from the plasma membrane of the host cell through a budding process. It contains a viral glycoprotein that is encoded by the viral *env* gene. This glycoprotein is usually cleaved during the assembly process to yield two subunits, SU and TM, which remain tightly associated with each other. The envelope surrounds a nucleocapsid core composed of capsid proteins derived from the viral *gag* gene. The core includes two identical single strands of viral RNA that are linked together in a dimer structure through their 5′ termini and code for the capsid proteins, protease, integrase, viral polymerase, and envelope proteins (gag-pro-pol-env; Fig 6.8A). In addition, some classes of retroviruses (e.g., HIV and HTLV) contain accessory genes that encode proteins, which help in the processes of mRNA synthesis and viral assembly, while others may contain an oncogene that contributes to cellular transformation. Bound to the RNA are several copies of the enzyme reverse transcriptase (RT) encoded by the viral *pol* gene.

The life cycle of a retrovirus occurs through a sequence of discrete steps, illustrated in Figure 6.7B. Adsorption of the virus to a cell is mediated by an interaction between the envelope proteins of the virus and specific receptor molecules on the cell surface, and leads to membrane fusion between the viral envelope and host cell plasma membrane. A fusion peptide found on the envelope protein mediates this event. Specificity at the level of virus adsorption accounts in large part for the restricted host and cell range of many types of retroviruses. Human immunodeficiency virus, for example, attaches to and enters a cell through the CD4 cell surface antigen: as a result, only CD4-positive cells are susceptible to infection by HIV. Host coreceptor molecules, such as the chemokine receptors CXCR4 and CCR5, can add further specificity at the level of membrane fusion and entry (Berger et al., 1999). Other receptors for retroviruses include the low-density lipoprotein receptor, the tv-b locus (TNF family receptor), multispanning membrane amino acid transporter proteins, or the sodium-dependent phosphate symporter. Retroviruses infect mice, birds, reptiles, mink, cats, cows, monkeys, and to a lesser extent humans, to cause tumorigenesis. Compared to other viruses, these agents are fragile; overcrowding, close contact, and intimate behavior facilitates their transfer from one host to another. Retroviruses cause few cancers in humans and

much of what is known about these viruses has been derived from isolates from mice and chickens. The protooncogenes targeted by these viruses have been instrumental in the elucidation and understanding of signal transduction pathways.

Once the virus is inside the cell, loss of the viral envelope produces a core particle that is permeable to entry by deoxyribonucleotides. The RNA is converted to double-stranded DNA through the activity of the virus-encoded RT that occurs in a large cytoplasmic complex consisting of nucleocapsid, RT, integrase, and viral RNA. The +ve sense RNA genome serves as a template in this process and a large pool of deoxyribonucleotides may trigger this process. Reverse transcription is primed by cellular tRNA. Initially, a small nucleotide repeat sequence at both ends of the viral RNA is extended to form long terminal repeats (LTR) that are incorporated into the double-stranded DNA (see Fig. 6.8). These linear DNA molecules then cross the nuclear membrane. Simple retroviruses require the breakdown of the nuclear membrane during the normal process of cellular mitosis, whereas linear DNA of HIV-related viruses can cross the nuclear membrane of a nondividing cell. One or a few molecules of viral DNA integrate randomly into the host chromosomes in association with the viral integrase molecule. The integrated form of the virus is called the *provirus*.

Once integrated, the proviral DNA acts as a template for transcription. Although both LTRs are identical and contain promoter and enhancer sequences necessary for synthesis of viral RNA, the upstream LTR acts to promote transcription whereas the downstream LTR specifies termination. Between the LTRs are coding sequences for the *gag*, *pro*, *pol*, and *env* genes (Fig. 6.8A). In a simple retrovirus, two transcripts are synthesized from the proviral DNA. A full-length genomic transcript serves as the mRNA for the synthesis of both gag and gag-pro-pol fusion proteins. This transcript can also be packaged into virus particles and therefore acts as the genome of the virus. Gag, gag-pro-pol, and genomic RNA assemble beneath the env protein at the plasma membrane of the infected cell and the complete virion buds from the cell. Maturation of the viral particle occurs during the budding process as the viral protease (pro) cleaves the gag-pro-pol precursor into matrix (MA), capsid (CA), nucleocapsid (NC), protease (Pro), reverse transcriptase (RT), and integrase (IN) polypeptides. This maturation is crucial to produce a fully infectious virion, and protease is the target of inhibitors (indinavir or squinavir) currently used to treat AIDS. Retroviral infections are surprisingly benign and do not have immediate cytopathic effects on the infected host cell. However, over the long term, disease can become apparent due to the acquisition of host genes or insertional mutagenesis into the host chromosome by these viruses.

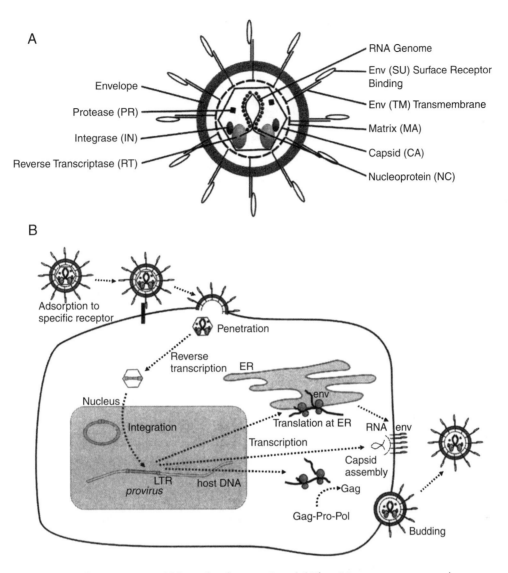

**Figure 6.7.** The structure and life cycle of a retrovirus. (*A*) The virion possesses a membrane that contains an envelope protein that is cleaved into 2 subunits—surface receptor (SU) and transmembrane (TM) components. Beneath the envelope is a matrix protein (MA) that holds the membrane and the nucleocapsid together. The nucleocapsid consists of a capsid protein (CA), nucleoprotein (NC), reverse transcriptase (RT), integrase (IN), and protease (PR). The genome consists of two identical RNA strands. (*B*) The retrovirus attaches to a specific receptor on the host cell. Its membrane subsequently fuses with that of the cell and the nucleocapsid is released into the cytoplasm. The single-stranded viral RNA genome is reverse-transcribed to a double-stranded DNA form, which has at its ends long terminal repeats (LTR). The viral DNA migrates to the nucleus and integrates into the chromosomal DNA. The single viral transcript can form the genome for progeny viruses or can be processed and translated to generate viral structural proteins, gag or gag-pro-pol, and env. The gag and pol proteins are processed by the virus-associated protease to yield capsid (CA), matrix (MA), polymerase (pol), and integrase (IN) proteins. The envelope protein mRNA is translated at the rough endoplasmic reticulum and the protein precursor is cleaved to surface receptor (SU) and transmembrane (TM) subunits in the Golgi. Viral assembly occurs beneath the membrane of the host cell and the mature virus buds from the plasma membrane.

### 6.3.2 Acute Transforming Viruses

Transforming retroviruses can be separated into two major groups based on their different mechanisms of transformation. Some viruses contain a viral oncogene, and these have been termed *acute* or *rapidly transforming viruses* (see also Chap. 7, Sec. 7.2.1). More than twenty viral oncogenes have been identified; each of these has been found to have a counterpart in normal cells. Other viruses do not contain an oncogene and are

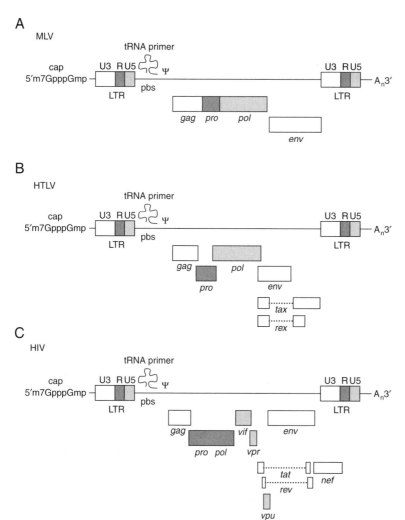

**Figure 6.8.** Genomic organization of oncogenic retroviruses. (*A*) Single-stranded RNA genome of Moloney leukemia virus (MLV) showing long terminal repeats (LTRs) and coding regions for gag, pro, pol, and envelope proteins. The RNA genome is capped and possesses a poly A sequence at its 3′ terminus. $\psi$ represents the packaging signal with which capsid protein associates. (*B*) In addition to the long-terminal repeats (LTRs) and the typical *gag*, *pol*, and *env* genes found in other replication-competent retroviruses, a novel region exists at the 3′ end of the HTLV (human T cell leukemia virus) genome encoding two regulatory proteins, Tax (transactivator) and Rex (regulator of expression). Three different mRNA species have been identified for HTLV-1. The full-length genomic mRNA encodes the gag and pol proteins and is also packaged into virions. A singly spliced mRNA encodes the env protein and the doubly spliced mRNA encodes Tax and Rex. (*C*) The genome of HIV (human immunodeficiency virus) also codes for structural proteins, regulatory proteins (Tat and Rev), and accessory proteins (vpr, vpu, and nef).

referred to as *chronic* or *slowly transforming viruses*. They elicit their transforming properties by insertion of the viral genome into the host chromosomal DNA. Again, these cancer viruses affect mice and birds, and as yet have not been implicated in human tumorigenesis.

Acute transforming viruses are almost always replication-defective due to replacement of viral sequences required for replication with host-derived oncogene sequences. For example, MC29 is a defective virus containing v-myc and is missing all of the *pol* gene and parts of *gag* and *env*. As a result, these transforming viruses require the presence of replication-competent helper viruses that assist in viral replication and assembly by supplying the necessary viral gene products. Because viral oncogenes come under the control of the efficient retroviral promoter present on the LTRs and are no longer tightly regulated by cellular mechanisms that normally act on the natural promoter, these genes can be expressed at inappropriately high levels. The viral oncogenes are frequently mutated because of the poor fidelity of retroviral replication, and often contain point mutations, deletions, substitutions, and insertions when compared with the protooncogenes from which they are derived. In addition, viral oncogenes differ from protooncogenes in that they do not contain intron (i.e., noncoding) sequences. Retroviruses containing oncogenes can transform cells in culture after several days and can induce leukemias and sarcomas in infected animals relatively quickly. Expression of the v-*onc* gene transforms every infected cell. Consequently, polyclonal tumors develop from many different infected progenitor cells. Examples of oncogenes and their cellular counterparts that have been transduced by acute transforming viruses are summarized in Table 6.1. They include growth factors (v-Sis), growth factor receptors (v-erbB), intracellular tyrosine kinases (v-src, v-fps, v-fes, v-abl), serine/threonine kinases (v-Akt, v-Raf), members of the G protein family (H-ras, K-ras), transcription factors (v-myc, v-erbA, v-fos, v-jun), and many others.

### 6.3.3 Chronic Tumor Viruses

The replication-competent chronic tumor viruses do not contain viral oncogenes but transform infected cells

**Table 6.1.** Oncogenes Recovered in Transducing Retroviruses

| Oncogene | Retrovirus | Function of Cellular Homolog |
| --- | --- | --- |
| Sis | Simian sarcoma virus | Platelet derived growth factor |
| ErbB1 | Avian erythroblastosis virus (ES4) | Epidermal growth factor receptor |
| Fms | Feline sarcoma virus (McDonough) | CSF-1 receptor |
| Sea | Avian erythroblastosis virus (S13) | Growth factor receptor |
| Kit | Feline sarcoma virus (HZ4) | Stem cell growth factor receptor |
| ErbA | Avian erythroblastosis virus (R) | Thyroid hormone receptor |
| H-ras | Murine sarcoma virus (Harvey) | G protein, GTPase, signaling |
| K-ras | Murine sarcoma virus (Kirsten) | G protein, GTPase, signaling |
| Crk | Avian sarcoma virus (1, CT10) | Adaptor protein, signaling, T cell |
| Cbl | Casitas mouse lymphoma virus | Adaptor protein, lymphocytes, signaling |
| Src | Rous sarcoma virus (RSV) | Non-receptor tyrosine kinase, signaling |
| Abl | Abelson murine leukemia virus | Non-receptor tyrosine kinase, signaling |
| Fps | Fujinami avian sarcoma virus | Non-receptor tyrosine kinase, signaling |
| Fes | Feline sarcoma virus (S-T) | Non-receptor tyrosine kinase, signaling |
| Fgr | Feline sarcoma virus (G-R) | Non-receptor tyrosine kinase, signaling |
| Yes | Avian sarcoma virus (Y73, Esh) | Non-receptor tyrosine kinase, signaling |
| Mos | Moloney mouse sarcoma virus | Serine-threonine kinase, germ cell |
| Raf | Mouse sarcoma virus (3611) | Serine-threonine kinase, MAPK pathway |
| Mil | Avian myelocytoma virus (MH2) | Serine-threonine kinase, Raf homolog |
| Akt | Avian sarcoma virus (AK-8) | Serine-threonine kinase, PKB |
| Jun | Avian sarcoma virus (17) | Transcription factor (AP-1 complex) |
| Fos | Mouse sarcoma virus (F-B-J) | Transcription factor (AP-1 complex) |
| Myc | Avian myelocytoma virus (MC29, MH2) | Transcription factor |
| Myb | Avian myeloblastosis virus (BAI/A) | Transcription factor |
| Ets | Avian myeloblastosis virus (E26) | Transcription factor, GATA-1 |
| Rel | Avian reticuloendotheliosis virus | Transcription factor, NFκB family |
| Ski | Avian retrovirus (Sloan-Kettering) | Transcription factor, muscle, MyoD |
| Qin | Avian retrovirus (ASV31) | Transcription factor, forkhead family |

through a mechanism known as *insertional mutagenesis,* in which proviral integration leads to the aberrant activation or sometimes inactivation of adjacent cellular genes (see also Chap. 7, Sec. 7.2.2). Protooncogenes may be activated by LTR promoter insertion, LTR enhancer insertion, viral poly-A site insertion that stabilizes mRNA, or viral leader insertion that increases and stabilizes mRNA. In other instances a cellular gene may be activated or inactivated by insertion of the retrovirus in the middle of a cellular gene depending upon the arrangement of exons. Several of the protooncogenes identified initially as progenitors to transducing retroviral oncogenes (c-*erb*B1, c-*mos*, c-*myb*, c-*myc*, c-H-*ras*, c-K-*ras*, c-*fms*, c-*fli1*) have also been identified through insertional mutagenesis. Cytokines regulating cell growth (*IL-2, IL-3, IL-10*) have also been found to be activated by retroviral integration in several animal species. Usu-

ally more than one insertional mutation event is required to produce tumors in animals.

Avian leukemia virus (ALV) is a typical slow-acting retrovirus. In ALV-induced B-cell lymphomas, malignant clones transformed by these viruses contain proviruses integrated in the vicinity of the c-*myc* gene (Neel et al., 1981). In many tumors, the provirus is integrated upstream of c-*myc* and in the same transcriptional orientation. In such cases the 3′ LTR, which normally acts to terminate viral transcription, promotes transcription of c-*myc* sequences. The resulting hybrid RNA transcripts contain both viral and c-*myc* sequences and are present at levels 30- to 100-fold higher than that of c-*myc* RNA in normal tissues. Such c-*myc* transcripts appear to encode a normal c-myc protein. This mechanism is called *promoter insertion.* In other tumors, the provirus is integrated upstream of c-*myc* but oriented in the transcriptional direction opposite to that of the gene, or it is integrated downstream of the gene. The strong enhancer properties of the LTRs are then believed to be responsible for activation of c-*myc* transcription, and this mechanism of transformation is known as *enhancer insertion*. The majority of B-cell lymphomas induced by ALV contain proviral sequences adjacent to c-*myc*, but the *myc* oncogene requires the cooperative function of a second oncogene. Because integration adjacent to c-*myc* is a random, rare event and secondary genetic events are required for tumor progression, ALV-induced leukemia may arise slowly and is clonal in origin.

Other examples of transformation by chronic tumor viruses include insertion of the mouse mammary tumor virus (MMTV) next to the *wnt-1/int-1* or *hst/int-2* genes leading to mammary tumors in mice. The hst/int-2 protein belongs to the fibroblast growth factor family and can be upregulated in Kaposi's sarcoma, stomach cancer, and teratocarcinomas, as well as in mouse mammary tumors. The *Lck* gene, normally found in T cells, NK cells, and some B cells, was found to be upregulated in lymphoma cell lines derived from thymomas of murine leukemia virus-infected mice. Other oncogenes, which have been found to be activated through proviral insertion include *Ahi-1, Evi-1, Evi-2, Fli-1, Mlvi-1, Mlvi-3,* and *Pvt-1*.

Proviral insertion may disrupt or alter the protein-coding sequence of resident cellular genes. For example, in ALV-induced erythroblastosis, proviral insertions commonly map to a small region in the middle of the epidermal growth factor receptor (EGFR) gene (c-*erb*B1). The resulting transcripts contain viral *gag* and *env* sequences fused to c-*erb*B1 sequences. The amino acid sequence predicted from these hybrid transcripts contain amino acids encoded by *gag* and *env* fused to carboxy-terminal amino acid sequences encoded by c-*erb*B1. Thus, expression of an altered, truncated EGFR molecule appears necessary for the development of ALV-induced erythroblastosis.

### 6.3.4 Human T-Cell Leukemia Viruses

HTLV-1 and HTLV-2 are the only retroviruses that are known to lead directly to cancers in humans. The related HIV viruses are associated with tumorigenesis through immune suppression and subsequent reactivation of many of the DNA-containing viruses discussed in the preceding sections. However, HTLV-1 by itself can cause adult T-cell leukemia (ATL), a rare but virulent cancer that is endemic in Southern Japan, the Caribbean, northern South America, parts of Africa, and the southeastern United States. Transmission of this disease may occur through blood transfusion, breast feeding, and sexual intercourse. Nucleotide sequence determination of the viral genomes has shown that the Japanese and American isolates were closely related strains of a single retrovirus now called human T-cell leukemia virus (HTLV-1; Wong-Staal and Gallo, 1985; Yoshida, 1987).

There are four molecular subtypes of HTLV-1 (A-D) which reflect the geographical locations from which the virus is isolated. The virus exhibits little genetic variation and there is about 98 percent homology between different HTLV-1 strains. In some chronically infected patients the virus can also cause a neurodegenerative disease called tropical spastic paraparesis (TSP). HTLV-2 is much less common than HTLV-1 and a convincing role for this virus in human disease has yet to be demonstrated, although a few patients have exhibited neurological disease.

Unlike the common oncogenic retroviruses of animals, HTLV-1 does not carry a host-derived oncogene and does not activate cellular protooncogenes by insertional mutation. Rather HTLV-1 is believed to initiate a multistep process leading to ATL. These steps include an asymptomatic carrier state, preleukemic state, chronic/smoldering ATL, lymphoma type, and acute ATL. Both HTLV-1 and HTLV-2 can immortalize human peripheral blood T-cells in vitro, as well as T-cells from monkeys, rabbits, cats, and rats but the cellular receptor for the virus is not known. The virus can infect either CD4$^+$ or CD8$^+$ T-cells, but transformed cells from ATL patients are usually CD4$^+$ and only occasionally CD8$^+$. Following infection of T-lymphocytes by HTLV-1, all the cells upregulate IL-2 receptors on their surface, and the provirus is found randomly integrated into the cellular genome. The infected cell population undergoes a transient polyclonal expansion followed by a latency period that is variable in duration; it can be as short as a few years if infection occurs in adulthood or as long as 40 years if infection occurs in infancy. The latent state may be maintained by immunologic clearance of the infected cells and an infected individual has about a 1 percent chance of developing ATL over a lifetime. If the disease progresses to pre-ATL, 50 percent of patients still have the chance of undergoing spontaneous regression. When ATL is clinically evident, however, all the leukemic cells in the patient have a common proviral integration site in the host DNA, but no two patients have the same integration site. These observations suggest that ATL is derived from a single infected progenitor cell but that subsequent genetic events are required. Patients exhibit severe skin lesions, lymphocytes with multilobed nuclei, and are extremely susceptible to secondary infections by other viruses, bacteria, or fungi. The mean survival time for a patient with acute ATL is about 6 months despite intensive therapy.

The genome of HTLV-1 is illustrated in Figure 6.8*B*. In addition to *gag, pol,* and *env* genes, HTLV encodes two other proteins, Tax and Rex. The Tax protein has been shown to be the transforming component of HTLV-1; it is critical for viral replication and functions as a transcriptional coactivator of viral and cellular gene expression (Yoshida et al., 1995). Tax protein does not bind directly to promoter sequences, and its mode of action is through the modification of host transcription factors, including CREB and NFκB (Chap. 8, Sec. 8.2.8). Mutations in Tax have shown that both CREB and NFκB activities are required for efficient transformation. Cellular genes that are responsive to transcriptional activation by Tax include *IL-2α*, the α subunit of the interleukin-2 (IL-2) receptor, granulocyte-macrophage colony-stimulating factor, and the protooncogenes *c-sis* and *c-fos*. Tumor cells from ATL patients as well as T-lymphocytes transformed in culture with HTLV-1 display an activated T-cell phenotype characterized by expression of IL-2 cell surface receptors and cell adhesion molecules such as ICAM-1. Expression of the HTLV-1 *tax* gene in transgenic mice leads to various abnormalities, including the development of fibroblastic tumors and leukemia (Nerenberg et al., 1987). Targeting transgenic Tax expression to T-cells of mice produced large granular lymphocytic leukemia (Grossman et al., 1995). Thus, expression of the *tax* gene has the potential to perturb normal cellular functions leading to malignancy.

The other HTLV-1 accessory protein, Rex, is essential for viral replication and acts posttranscriptionally to upregulate the levels of virion structural proteins to assure the production of infectious virus. It is analogous to Rev of HIV and stimulates the transport of unspliced mRNA to the cytoplasm of the infected cell.

## 6.3.5 Human Immunodeficiency Virus

Human immunodeficiency virus is a member of the retrovirus family and has been classified as a lentivirus. The RNA genome of HIV encodes core (*gag*), polymerase (*pol*), and envelope (*env*) gene products in addition to accessory proteins (Tat, Rev, Nef, Vif, Vpr, and Vpu) that play key roles in the pathogenesis of the viral infection (Fig. 6.8C). Tat is a transactivating protein of the LTR promoter and Rev interacts with and directs the export of unspliced viral mRNAs to the cytoplasm and favors synthesis of viral structural proteins. Vif increases viral infectivity of certain cell types and Vpr promotes nuclear localization of proteins from the cytoplasm. Vpu enhances the release of virus from the cell. Nef is critical in maintaining high virus loads, increases circulating virions, and downregulates surface expression of CD4 and MHC I (Chap. 20, Sec. 20.2). The virus initiates infection by binding to the CD4 receptor on T-cells and macrophages, and penetrates into the host cell through use of chemokine coreceptors and a process of membrane fusion. Viral replication occurs as described in Figure 6.7B and HIV

causes immune suppression through destruction of lymphoid tissue and depletion of CD4$^+$ T-cells. Combinations of antiretroviral nucleotide analogs and viral protease inhibitors are now used to suppress plasma viral loads for prolonged periods. This treatment is known as highly active antiretroviral therapy (HAART).

Although HIV does not cause cancer directly, it is an immune suppressive virus that can lead to the appearance of several types of malignancies during late-stage infections (Scadden, 2003). These AIDS-related malignancies are the result of reactivation of infections with human papillomaviruses, EBV, and human herpesvirus-8 (KHSV) (Sec. 6.2.6). The cancers include smooth muscle sarcomas (leiomyosarcoma), Hodgkin's disease, nasopharyngeal carcinoma, AIDS-related lymphomas (non-Hodgkin's lymphoma), cervical cancer, anal carcinomas, squamous-cell neoplasia, primary effusion lymphoma, and Kaposi's sarcoma. Highly active antiretroviral therapy can be effective in treating less aggressive cancers, but tumor-specific therapy may be indicated.

## 6.4 HEPATITIS C VIRUS

Hepatitis C virus (HCV) is a member of the family of viruses that includes yellow fever virus, West Nile virus, and dengue fever virus (reviewed in Tellinghuisen and Rice, 2003). Following the discovery of hepatitis B virus in 1965, and the characterization of hepatitis A virus in 1973, it became apparent that other agents responsible for blood-borne hepatitis also existed and caused non-A, non-B hepatitis (NANBH). This led to the discovery of the hepatitis C virus. The HCV virion is low in abundance and has only been observed in a few studies. It is about 50 nanometers in diameter and consists of an envelope that contains the two viral glycoproteins, E1 and E2. Surrounding the positive sense, single-stranded RNA genome is the core or nucleocapsid protein. There are six known genotypes of this virus that reflect their geographical distribution. Hepatitis replication is slow and inefficient and the virus establishes persistent viral infections that are not cytotoxic. Two major barriers have hampered research in the HCV field: the virus cannot be propagated in cultured cells and the lack of a small animal in which to grow and to study the immunology of this pathogen, and to evaluate antiviral agents. Chimpanzees are the only primates besides humans that support the replication of HCV. A recent breakthrough in the form of a severe combined immunodeficient, urokinase-transgenic mouse into which human liver cells have been introduced promises to offer a useful tool with which to study antiviral agents and production of the virus in vivo (Mercer et al., 2001).

Hepatitis C virus is blood borne and is spread through transfusions, intravenous drug use, and multiple use of needles for inoculations. The acute phase of hepatitis C is often mild and undiagnosed in both adults and children. Malaise, nausea, right upper quadrant pain, and dark urine may appear in about one third of patients. Liver transaminase (ALT) levels in the blood may increase and jaundice is only occasionally evident. However, HCV proceeds to establish persistent viral infections and chronic disease in 60 to 80 percent of these patients leading to cirrhosis and hepatocellular carcinoma. Damage to the hepatocytes in the liver occurs through the effects of cytotoxic T-cells and the action of Fas ligand and perforin on these target cells. The virus undergoes genetic variation in the face of a mounting humoral response and a region that encodes the E2 protein, called the hypervariable 2 (HVP2) region, is particularly prone to mutagenesis (Farci et al., 2001). Low-grade persistent viral infections appear to survive in the face of a vigorous immune response against the virus: the virus may survive immune surveillance through the generation of mutants that escape T-cell cytotoxicity (Cooper et al., 1999; Wong et al., 2001).

The genome of HCV is not transcribed to DNA and does not integrate into the host chromosome. In vitro studies have shown that the core protein of HCV can enter the nucleus and protect the cell from Fas- and TNF $\alpha$-mediated apoptosis through activation of the transcription factor NF$\kappa$B (Marusawa et al., 1999). Transgenic mice expressing core protein develop HCV primary liver carcinomas after about 16 months (Moriya et al., 1998). Other proteins also influence host cells but whether the gene products of HCV contribute to liver cancer remains unknown (Koike et al., 2002). The virus has also developed means to evade the interferon antiviral system (He and Katze, 2002; Foy et al., 2003).

## 6.5 SUMMARY

Viruses have proven to be important agents in promoting a diverse set of cancers. DNA viruses such as SV40, adenoviruses, and papillomaviruses generally downregulate the activity of tumor suppressors such as p53 and Rb proteins, and were instrumental in the discovery and characterization of these cellular products. Histone acetylation is also modulated by these three viruses and favors the transcription of other genes involved in transformation. Transducing retroviruses can pirate cellular genes coding for growth factors, receptors, tyrosine kinases, G-proteins, adaptors, and transcription factors while chronic retroviral tumor viruses can activate similar genes through insertional mutagenesis. Many viruses contain genes that block apoptosis or inhibit immune recognition of the infected host cell, which favors cell survival. Each virus discussed in this chapter is unique in the manner in which it deregulates cell growth. However, transformation of the host cell is always achieved through viral manipulation of the cell cycle, apoptotic, and signal transduction pathways to favor growth and survival. Details may differ, but similar basic principles underlie the process of cellular transformation by these agents.

## REFERENCES

Ali SH, DeCaprio JA: Cellular transformation by SV40 large T antigen: interaction with host proteins. *Semin Cancer Biol* 2001; 11:15–23.

Auger KR, Carpenter CL, Shoelson SE, et al: Polyoma virus middle T antigen-pp60c-src complex associates with purified phosphatidylinositol 3–kinase in vitro. *J Biol Chem* 1992; 267:5408–5415.

Becker SA, Lee TH, Butel JS, Slagle BL: Hepatitis B virus X protein interferes with cellular DNA repair. *J Virol* 1998; 72:266–272.

Berger EA, Murphy PM, Farber JM: Chemokine receptors as HIV-1 coreceptors: roles in viral entry, tropism, and disease. *Annu Rev Immunol* 1999; 17:657–700.

Bischoff JR, Kirn DH, Williams A, et al: An adenovirus mutant that replicates selectively in p53-deficient human tumor cells. *Science* 1996; 274:373–376.

Chang Y, Cesarman E, Pessin MS, et al: Identification of herpesvirus-like DNA sequences in AIDS-associated Kaposi's sarcoma. *Science* 1994; 266:1865–1869.

Chang Y, Moore PS, Talbot SJ, et al: Cyclin encoded by KS herpesvirus. *Nature* 1996; 382:410.

Conzen SD, Cole CN: The three transforming regions of SV40 T antigen are required for immortalization of primary mouse embryo fibroblasts. *Oncogene* 1995; 11:2295–2302.

Cooper S, Erickson AL, Adams EJ, et al: Analysis of a successful immune response against hepatitis C virus. *Immunity* 1999; 10:439–449.

Diao J, Garces R, Richardson CD: X protein of hepatitis B virus modulates cytokine and growth factor related signal transduction pathways during the course of viral infections and hepatocarcinogenesis. *Cytokine Growth Factor Rev* 2001; 12:189–205.

Dykstra ML, Longnecker R, Pierce SK: Epstein-Barr virus coopts lipid rafts to block the signaling and antigen transport functions of the BCR. *Immunity* 2001; 14:57–67.

Dyson N, Howley PM, Munger K, et al: The human papilloma virus-16 E7 oncoprotein is able to bind to the retinoblastoma gene product. *Science* 1989; 243:934–937.

Fanning E, Knippers R: Structure and function of simian virus 40 large tumor antigen. *Annu Rev Biochem* 1992; 61:55–85.

Farci P, Shimoda A, Coiana A, et al: The outcome of acute hepatitis C predicted by the evolution of the viral quasispecies. *Science* 2000; 288:339–344.

Feitelson MA: Hepatitis B virus in hepatocarcinogenesis. *J Cell Physiol* 1999; 181:188–202.

Foy E, Li K, Wang C, et al: Regulation of interferon regulatory factor-3 by the hepatitis C virus serine protease. *Science* 2003; 300:1145–1148.

Furth PA: SV40 rodent tumour models as paradigms of human disease: transgenic mouse models. *Dev Biol Stand* 1998; 94:281–287.

Godden-Kent D, Talbot SJ, Boshoff C, et al: The cyclin encoded by Kaposi's sarcoma-associated herpesvirus stimulates cdk6 to phosphorylate the retinoblastoma protein and histone H1. *J Virol* 1997; 71:4193–4198.

Grossman WJ, Kimata JT, Wong FH, et al: Development of leukemia in mice transgenic for the tax gene of human T-cell leukemia virus type I. *Proc Natl Acad Sci USA* 1995; 92:1057–1061.

Han J, Sabbatini P, Perez D, et al: The E1B 19K protein blocks apoptosis by interacting with and inhibiting the p53-inducible and death-promoting Bax protein. *Genes Dev* 1996; 10:461–477.

Harada JN, Berk AJ: p53-independent and -dependent requirements for E1B-55K in adenovirus type 5 replication. *J Virol* 1999; 73:5333–5344.

Hawley-Nelson P, Vousden KH, Hubbert NL, et al: HPV16 E6 and E7 proteins cooperate to immortalize human foreskin keratinocytes. *EMBO J* 1989; 8:3905–3910.

He Y, Katze MG: To interfere and to anti-interfere: the interplay between hepatitis C virus and interferon. *Viral Immunol* 2002; 15:95–119.

Heise C, Sampson-Johannes A, Williams A, et al: ONYX-015, an E1B gene-attenuated adenovirus, causes tumor-specific cytolysis and antitumoral efficacy that can be augmented by standard chemotherapeutic agents. *Nat Med* 1997; 3:639–645.

Herbst H, Dallenbach F, Hummel M, et al: Epstein-Barr virus latent membrane protein expression in Hodgkin and Reed-Sternberg cells. *Proc Natl Acad Sci USA* 1991; 88: 4766–4770.

Hildt E, Saher G, Bruss V, et al: The hepatitis B virus large surface protein (LHBs) is a transcriptional activator. *Virology* 1996; 225:235–239.

Hsu DH, de Waal Malefyt R, Fiorentino DF, et al: Expression of interleukin-10 activity by Epstein-Barr virus protein BCRF1. *Science* 1990; 250:830–832.

Jasani B, Cristaudo A, Emri SA, et al: Association of SV40 with human tumours. *Semin Cancer Biol* 2001; 11:49–61.

Koike K, Tsutsumi T, Fujie H, et al: Molecular mechanism of viral hepatocarcinogenesis. *Oncology* 2002; 62(Suppl 1):29–37.

Liebowitz D: Nasopharyngeal carcinoma: the Epstein-Barr virus association. *Semin Oncol* 1994; 21:376–381.

Longnecker R: Epstein-Barr virus latency: LMP2, a regulator or means for Epstein-Barr virus persistence? *Adv Cancer Res* 2000; 79:175–200.

Marshall E: Gene therapy death prompts review of adenovirus vector. *Science* 1999; 286:2244–2245.

Marusawa H, Hijikata M, Chiba T, et al: Hepatitis C virus core protein inhibits Fas- and tumor necrosis factor alpha-mediated apoptosis via NF-kappaB activation. *J Virol* 1999; 73:4713–4720.

Mercer DF, Schiller DE, Elliott JF, et al: Hepatitis C virus replication in mice with chimeric human livers. *Nat Med* 2001; 7:927–933.

Moore PS, Chang Y: Molecular virology of Kaposi's sarcoma-associated herpesvirus. *Philos Trans R Soc Lond B Biol Sci* 2001; 356:499–516.

Moran E, Mathews MB: Multiple functional domains in the adenovirus E1A gene. *Cell* 1987; 48:177–178.

Moriya K, Fujie H, Shintani Y, et al: The core protein of hepatitis C virus induces hepatocellular carcinoma in transgenic mice. *Nat Med* 1998; 4:1065–1067.

Moses AV, Fish KN, Ruhl R, et al: Long-term infection and transformation of dermal microvascular endothelial cells by human herpesvirus 8. *J Virol* 1999; 73:6892–6902.

Munger K, Phelps WC, Bubb V, et al: The E6 and E7 genes of the human papillomavirus type 16 together are necessary and sufficient for transformation of primary human keratinocytes. *J Virol* 1989; 63:4417–4421.

Neel BG, Hayward WS, Robinson HL, et al: Avian leukosis virus-induced tumors have common proviral integration sites and synthesize discrete new RNAs: oncogenesis by promoter insertion. *Cell* 1981; 23:323–334.

Nerenberg M, Hinrichs SH, Reynolds RK, et al: The tat gene of human T-lymphotropic virus type 1 induces mesenchymal tumors in transgenic mice. *Science* 1987; 237:1324–1329.

Pallas DC, Shahrik LK, Martin BL, et al: Polyoma small and middle T antigens and SV40 small t antigen form stable complexes with protein phosphatase 2A. *Cell* 1990; 60:167–176.

Pennisi E: Monkey virus DNA found in rare human cancers. *Science* 1997; 275:748–749.

Pipas JM, Levine AJ: Role of T antigen interactions with p53 in tumorigenesis. *Semin Cancer Biol* 2001; 11:23–30.

Ries SJ, Brandts CH, Chung AS, et al: Loss of p14ARF in tumor cells facilitates replication of the adenovirus mutant dl1520 (ONYX-015). *Nat Med* 2000; 6:1128–1133.

Rundell K, Parakati R: The role of the SV40 ST antigen in cell growth promotion and transformation. *Semin Cancer Biol* 2001; 11:5–13.

Scadden DT: AIDS-related malignancies. *Annu Rev Med* 2003; 54:285–303.

See RH, Shi Y: Adenovirus E1B 19,000-molecular-weight protein activates c-Jun N-terminal kinase and c-Jun-mediated transcription. *Mol Cell Biol* 1998; 18:4012–4022.

Sontag E, Sontag JM, Garcia A: Protein phosphatase 2A is a critical regulator of protein kinase C zeta signaling targeted by SV40 small t to promote cell growth and NF-kappaB activation. *EMBO J* 1997; 16:5662–5671.

Stehelin D, Varmus HE, Bishop JM, Vogt PK: DNA related to the transforming gene(s) of avian sarcoma viruses is present in normal avian DNA. *Nature* 1976; 260:170–173.

Stine JT, Wood C, Hill M, et al: KSHV-encoded CC chemokine vMIP-III is a CCR4 agonist, stimulates angiogenesis, and selectively chemoattracts TH2 cells. *Blood* 2000; 95:1151–1157.

Swanton C, Mann DJ, Fleckenstein B, et al: Herpes viral cyclin/Cdk6 complexes evade inhibition by CDK inhibitor proteins. *Nature* 1997; 390:184–187.

Takada, K. Epstein-Barr virus and gastric carcinoma. *Mol Pathol* 2000; 53:255–261.

Tellinghuisen TL, Rice CM: Interaction between hepatitis C virus proteins and host cell factors. *Curr Opin Microbiol* 2002; 5:419–427.

Truant R, Antunovic J, Greenblatt J, et al: Direct interaction of the hepatitis B virus HBx protein with p53 leads to inhibition by HBx of p53 response element-directed transactivation. *J Virol* 1995; 69:1851–1859.

Wang D, Liebowitz D, Kieff E: An EBV membrane protein expressed in immortalized lymphocytes transforms established rodent cells. *Cell* 1985; 43:831–840.

Wang XW, Forrester K, Yeh H, et al: Hepatitis B virus X protein inhibits p53 sequence-specific DNA binding, transcriptional activity, and association with transcription factor ERCC3. *Proc Natl Acad Sci USA* 1994; 91:2230–2234.

Weinreb M, Day PJ, Niggli F, et al: The consistent association between Epstein-Barr virus and Hodgkin's disease in children in Kenya. *Blood* 1996; 87:3828–3836.

Weiss LM, Movahed LA, Warnke RA, et al: Detection of Epstein-Barr viral genomes in Reed-Sternberg cells of Hodgkin's disease. *N Engl J Med* 1989; 320:502–506.

Whyte P, Buchkovich KJ, Horowitz JM, et al: Association between an oncogene and an anti-oncogene: the adenovirus E1A proteins bind to the retinoblastoma gene product. *Nature* 1988; 334:124–129.

Wong DK, Dudley DD, Dohrenwend PB, et al: Detection of diverse hepatitis C virus (HCV)-specific cytotoxic T lymphocytes in peripheral blood of infected persons by screening for responses to all translated proteins of HCV. *J Virol* 2001; 75:1229–1235.

Wong-Staal F, Gallo RC: The family of human T-lymphotropic leukemia viruses: HTLV-I as the cause of adult T cell leukemia and HTLV-III as the cause of acquired immunodeficiency syndrome. *Blood* 1985; 65:253–263.

Yang SI, Lickteig RL, Estes R, et al: Control of protein phosphatase 2A by simian virus 40 small-t antigen. *Mol Cell Biol* 1991; 11:1988–1995.

Yang TY, Chen SC, Leach MW, et al: Transgenic expression of the chemokine receptor encoded by human herpesvirus 8 induces an angioproliferative disease resembling Kaposi's sarcoma. *J Exp Med* 2000; 191:445–454.

Yoshida M: Expression of the HTLV-1 genome and its association with a unique T-cell malignancy. *Biochim Biophys Acta* 1987; 907:145–161.

Yoshida M, Suzuki T, Fujisawa J, et al: HTLV-1 oncoprotein tax and cellular transcription factors. *Curr Top Microbiol Immunol* 1995; 193:79–89.

zur Hausen H: Papillomaviruses causing cancer: evasion from host-cell control in early events in carcinogenesis. *J Natl Cancer Inst* 2000; 92:690–698.

# 7

# Oncogenes and Tumor Suppressor Genes

*Sara Oster, Linda Penn, and Vuk Stambolic*

## 7.1 INTRODUCTION

These are revolutionary times in cancer research. For years scientists have been seeking the answers to such complex questions as, "What is the difference between normal and tumor cells?", "Why are normal cells under strict growth control and tumor cells able to grow in an uncontrolled manner?", "How can the tumor cells be eradicated in the absence of collateral damage to neighboring normal cells?". With oncogenes and tumor suppressor genes now established as holding a key role in cancer etiology, these questions can be addressed.

There is substantial evidence that multiple genes must be mutated or deregulated in a single cell to cause malignant transformation and cancer growth. Thankfully this is a rare event. Most cells that harbor even a single mutation are either targeted for repair or are cleared from the organism by protective mechanisms including immune surveillance or activation of cellular suicide programs. Not all mutations contribute to tumor development: the genetic material in each of our cells is estimated to encode approximately 30,000 genes, and mutations in less than 10 percent of these genes contribute to the carcinogenic process.

Genes that may contribute to tumorigenesis play key roles in regulating critical cellular processes such as cell division, life span, differentiation, angiogenesis, invasion, and death. They can be divided into two categories: oncogenes and tumor suppressor genes. Two copies or alleles of each gene exist in every cell. Specific mutation of one allele converts the normal "protooncogene" to the activated, transforming oncogene that can contribute to the carcinogenic process. The oncogene is dominant over the protooncogene and generally results in a protein product that is deregulated and/or constitutively active (Fig. 7.1). Oncogenic conversion is a gain-of-function mutation. By contrast, tumor suppressor genes are recessive and mutations leading to loss or inactivation of both alleles are required for transformation. Tumor suppressors are also known as recessive oncogenes or anti-oncogenes and their inactivation represents a loss-of-function mutation (Fig.

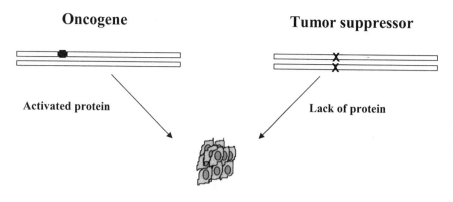

**Oncogene**

**Tumor suppressor**

**Activated protein**

**Lack of protein**

**Cancer**

**Figure 7.1.** Oncogenes and tumor suppressors. An *oncogene* is a gene whose activation represents a gain of function mutation. A *tumor suppressor* is a gene whose activation represents a loss of function mutation. A combination of both classes of mutations is often found in human cancers.

7.1). Both oncogene activation and tumor suppressor inactivation collaborate in the stepwise progression to tumorigenesis. In this chapter we will focus on these cancer genes and outline how they have been identified, the genetic abnormalities associated with deregulation, the nature of the specific gene products, their mechanisms of action, and recent advances to counteract these tumor-promoting lesions with novel anticancer therapeutics.

## 7.2 ONCOGENES

An oncogene is a gene whose protein product contributes to the development and/or progression of cancer. The first oncogenes were discovered over twenty-five years ago as transforming agents of viruses that caused tumors in chickens and rodents. Cellular counterparts were then identified that play critical roles within the cell. The expression and/or activities of these cellular protooncogenes are usually tightly regulated in a normal cell and deregulation of these molecules can lead to cancer. There are many ways in which cellular protooncogenes can be activated to become cancer-causing oncogenes as depicted in Figure 7.2 with respect to the c-myc oncogene. Both genetic and functional methods have been employed to identify novel oncogenes. Genetic approaches include identifying transforming sequences in cancer causing retroviruses, determining DNA sequences affected by retroviral insertion, and characterizing amplified genes or genes commonly involved in chromosomal translocations. Functional approaches to identify oncogenes are based on properties that they impart to the cell and can be identified by expression cloning. Mechanisms of oncogene activation and the genetic and functional approaches to identify them are discussed in more detail below.

### 7.2.1 Acute Transforming Retroviruses

In the early and mid-1900s it was established that certain types of cancer in rodents, birds, and cats were

transmissible by retroviruses (see Chap. 6, Sec. 6.3.2). The genetic material of these acute transforming retroviruses was subsequently cloned and sequenced. This analysis revealed that tumor-producing retroviruses had incorporated genetic material derived from the normal host cell into the viral genome. Moreover, genetic analysis of acute transforming retroviruses from tumors in animals of different species showed that a restricted set of host genetic material was transduced into a variety of retroviruses (Butel, 2000). These discoveries suggest that a limited subset of cellular oncogenes could contribute to the transformation process. The nomenclature for the oncogene derived from the retrovirus was prefaced with the v- (virus) designation while the cellular counterpart was distinguished by the c- (cell) specification. Approximately fifty oncogenes have been identified by this approach (Table 7.1).

At the time of their initial identification as oncogenes, neither the mechanism of activation nor the functional role of the proteins encoded by these genes in the normal or tumor cell was understood. Subsequent experiments compared properties of viral oncogenes with the cellular protooncogenes of the host. Each oncogene was activated in a unique manner, which resulted in deregulated activity of the protein product. For example, comparison of the tyrosine protein kinase c-Src with v-Src at the level of amino acid sequence showed that the latter harbored several point mutations as well as a deletion of eleven amino acids at the carboxyl end (Fig. 7.3). Introduction of each of these mutations into the c-src proto-oncogene showed that the C-terminal deletion was the key transforming event that activated c-Src (Bjorge et al., 2000). Further analysis of this region revealed that deletion of a negative regulatory tyrosine residue of the c-Src protein specifically deregulated both the protein kinase and transforming activities of c-Src (Fig. 7.3). Activation by mutation of negative regulatory domains occurs in other oncogenes including the tyrosine kinase v-abl and the transcription factor v-myb, although the activating

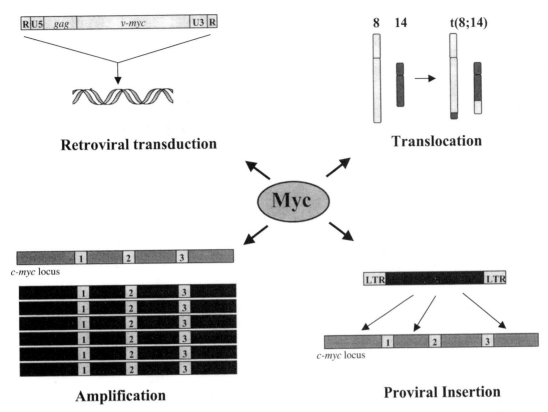

**Figure 7.2.** Mechanisms of oncogene activation. The oncogene c-myc is used as an example to illustrate some of the potential mechanisms of oncogene activation. Retroviral transduction occurs when a retrovirus containing the viral form of the oncogene inserts into the host DNA and the gene is aberrantly expressed from the viral transcription machinery. Translocation can result in activation of an oncogene when the protooncogene is translocated to a region of DNA which leads to constitutive expression of the oncogene. A common translocation observed in Burkitt's lymphoma patients is the fusion of a portion of chromosome 8 with chromosome 14, which results in the myc gene being constitutively transcribed by the active immunoglobulin regulatory region. Amplification of the genomic locus containing the protooncogene can lead to activation as the gene is highly expressed in cells with multiple copies. Proviral insertion into any one of a number of regulatory regions of the *c-myc* locus can cause aberrant expression of the protooncogene and lead to oncogene activation. Oncogene activation leads to deregulated expression of the oncoprotein product.

mutations are distinct for each oncogene. Oncogene deregulation can also be achieved in the absence of mutation in the coding region of the gene. Comparison of the c-Myc and v-Myc transcription factors showed that overexpression of the normal protein product by the strong retroviral transcriptional promoter and enhancers was sufficient to activate Myc and drive transformation.

### 7.2.2 Proviral Insertion

A second class of animal retroviruses was shown to cause transformation but tumors arose only after prolonged latency periods (see also Chap. 6, Sec. 6.3.3). These retroviruses do not transduce host genetic material; instead, their mechanism of action is a consequence of their point of integration into the host genome. Retroviruses that integrate near the locus of a cellular pro-

tooncogene can confer a selective growth advantage to the cell. The strong transcriptional promoters and/or enhancers of the retrovirus are able to drive deregulated expression of the neighboring protooncogene; this activates the oncogene and in turn contributes to neoplastic transformation.

Several oncogenes have been identified by characterizing the cellular genes juxtaposed to sites of retroviral integration in the host genome of tumor cells. In avian leukosis virus-induced bursal lymphomas transcription of the c-myc gene is significantly elevated in response to provirus insertion near the *c-myc* locus (Fig. 7.2). Integration can occur upstream or downstream of the gene and in the same or opposite orientation. Similarly, analyses of genes near the integration site of the mouse mammary tumor virus (MMTV) in mouse mammary carcinomas, revealed a series of novel oncogenes known as *int-1* and *int-2*. It is uncertain whether retro-

**Table 7.1.** Examples of Oncogenes and Their Protein
Products

| Oncogene/ Protein Product | Function |
|---|---|
| **Growth Factors** | |
| v-sis | Platelet derived growth factor |
| int-1 | Matrix protein |
| int-2 | Fibroblast growth factor-related protein |
| KS3 | Fibroblast growth factor-related protein |
| **Growth Factor Receptors** | |
| FGFR3 | Fibroblast derived growth factor receptor |
| PDGFR | Platelet derived growth factor receptor |
| IGF-1R | Insulin growth factor receptor |
| VEGFR | Vascular endothelial growth factor receptor |
| EGFR | Epidermal growth factor receptor |
| v-kit | Stem cell growth factor receptor |
| v-fms | CSF-1 receptor |
| Her2/NEU | Heregulin receptor |
| met | Hepatic growth factor receptor |
| flt3 | FLT3 ligand receptor |
| trk | Nerve growth factor receptor |
| **Ras oncogenes** | |
| H-ras | GTPase |
| K-ras | GTPase |
| N-ras | GTPase |
| **Cytoplasmic kinases** | |
| BCR-ABL | Protein tyrosine kinase |
| src | Protein tyrosine kinase |
| v-fes | Protein tyrosine kinase |
| v-fps | Protein tyrosine kinase |
| v-fgr | Protein tyrosine kinase |
| hck | Protein tyrosine kinase |
| pim | Protein serine/threonine kinase |
| v-raf | Protein serine/threonine kinase |
| v-mos | Protein serine/threonine kinase |
| **Transcription factors** | |
| c-myc | Transcription factor |
| N-myc | Transcription factor |
| L-myc | Transcription factor |
| v-fos | Transcription factor |
| v-jun | Transcription factor |
| v-rel | Transcription factor |
| v-ets | Transcription factor |
| **Anti-apoptotic proteins** | |
| bcl-2 | Anti-apoptotic protein |
| twist | Anti-apoptotic protein |

Modified from BSO 3rd Ed. and Genetic Basis of Human Cancer.

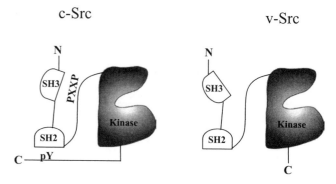

**Figure 7.3.** Activating and inhibiting mutations of *src*. The protein encoded by the *src* protooncogene is inhibited by an intramolecular interaction of the phosphotyrosine in the C-terminus with the SH2 domain. In v-src, the C-terminal region containing this tyrosine is deleted, leading to constitutive activation.

viral insertion plays a direct role in the etiology of human cancer. However, the analysis of proviral insertions in animal tumor cells has identified oncogenes that play a role in both animal and human neoplasia.

### 7.2.3 Gene Amplification

Deregulated expression of cellular protooncogenes can occur by amplification of the intact locus (Fig. 7.2). For example, genomic analysis of cells derived from neuroblastoma has revealed frequent amplification of the c-myc family member, N-myc. Similar analysis of small cell lung carcinoma showed amplification of all three transforming members of the myc gene family; *C-MYC*, *N-MYC*, and *L-MYC* (Oster et al., 2002). Examples of amplification of other oncogenes include the epidermal growth factor receptor (*EGFR*) in glioblastomas, *HER-2/NEU* and *CYCLIN D1* in breast cancer, and *C-ABL* in chronic myeloid leukemia. Amplification can manifest as either homogenously staining regions within a chromosome or double-minute particles that are not associated with intact chromosomes (see Chap. 4, Fig. 4.14). Oncogene amplification is often associated with poor prognosis and late stage disease.

### 7.2.4 Reciprocal Translocation

Comparisons of chromosomes derived from normal and tumor cells from the same patient by standard Giemsa stain or G-banding have revealed gross genetic abnormalities in tumor DNA (see Chap. 4, Sec. 4.2). Specific translocations have been associated with specific types of cancer. Thus, in chronic myelogenous leukemia (CML) a reciprocal translocation of a small portion of the long arms of chromosome 9 and 22 is consistently evident, and the modified chromosome is referred to as the Philadelphia (Ph) chromosome. Several reciprocal translocations were subsequently identified from other malignancies. The genes at or near these breakpoints have been cloned and characterized and have led to the identification of several oncogenes involved in human cancers.

At a molecular level, reciprocal translocations can result in two types of structural alterations that lead to oncogene activation. The first mechanism is typified by the Ph chromosome and leads to the generation of a chimeric gene that encodes a novel fusion protein (Fig. 7.4). The translocation t(9;22)(q34;q11) results in the C-ABL protooncogene on chromosome 9 being juxtaposed to the BCR (breakpoint cluster region) gene on chromosome 22. This translocation leads to the formation of the novel BCR-ABL fusion protein, which encodes a protein with more potent tyrosine protein kinase activity compared to the wild-type C-ABL protein (Fig. 7.4). Reciprocal translocation leads to the formation of several other fusion proteins including the transcription factor FLI1-EWS in Ewing's sarcoma and the homeobox protein PAX7-FKHR in rhabdomyosarcoma.

The second mechanism of oncogenic activation resulting from reciprocal translocation leads to the overexpression and deregulation of an intact cellular protooncogene. This type of reciprocal translocation occurs in Burkitt's lymphoma (BL) (see Chap. 6, Sec. 6.2.4) where 100 percent of BL tumors harbor a translocation in which the C-MYC protooncogene is juxtaposed to an immunoglobulin (IG) locus (Fig. 7.2). The strong transcriptional activity of the IG locus in antibody producing B-cells, is reprogrammed in BL to drive the tran-

scription of the C-MYC gene. This leads to the deregulated overexpression and activation of C-MYC, which directly contributes to disease. Indeed, the IG locus is a hotspot for translocation in other B-cell neoplasms. For example, in B-cell follicular lymphoma the IG locus is juxtaposed to the BCL-2 gene, which contributes to tumor development by functioning as a strong inhibitor of cell death or apoptosis (see Chap. 10, Sec. 10.21). Similarly the T-cell receptor (TCR) loci are hot spots for reciprocal translocation that contribute to the development of acute T-cell leukemia. For example, translocations involving the TCR loci have been documented with genes such as those encoding the transcription factors C-MYC, LYL-1, TAL-1 (also known as SCL1 or TCL-5), as well as HOX-11.

### 7.2.5 Novel Genetic Abnormalities That Activate Oncogenes

Recent technological advances have increased both the sensitivity and specificity of detection of chromosomal abnormalities (see Chap. 4, Sec. 4.4). This improvement in detection promises to lead to additional hotspots of genetic abnormality that are associated with disease and with novel oncogenes. In addition, oncogenes like C-MYC are often overexpressed in cells of human cancers yet this deregulated expression is not always associated with an abnormality of the locus, such as amplification or translocation. This suggests that C-MYC

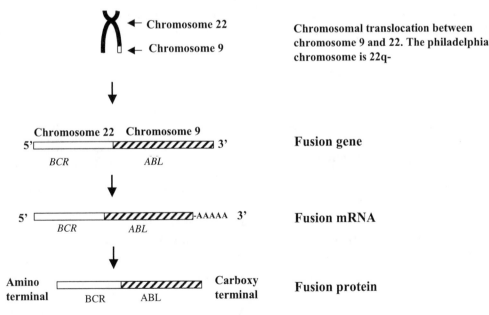

**Figure 7.4.** Reciprocal translocation leads to a chimeric gene which encodes a novel protein. Translocation of the genetic material of chromosome 9 and chromosome 22 leads to the formation of an oncogenic fusion protein. The aberrant 22q- is referred to as the Philadelphia chromosome. This translocation leads to a fusion of the genes BCR and ABL, resulting in an mRNA molecule which encodes the fusion oncoprotein BCR-ABL.

activation may occur by novel mechanisms. Expression of *C-MYC* is highly regulated in normal, nontransformed cells at several levels including gene transcription, posttranscriptional regulation, translational and posttranslational regulation. Changes at any of these levels of regulation might deregulate *C-MYC* expression. For example, point mutations that result in stabilization of *MYC* mRNA or enhanced transcription through the internal ribosomal entry site would lead to increased expression. In addition, *MYC* may be indirectly activated by mutations in upstream signaling pathways (Oster et al., 2002). These new analyses will further contribute to understanding cancer development and the oncogenes involved.

### 7.2.6 Expression Cloning

Oncogenes from tumor cells can be identified by their ability to functionally transform nonmalignant cells. The first examples of functional cloning involved experiments in which DNA from tumor cells was transfected into immortal, nontransformed NIH 3T3 fibroblasts (see Chap. 4, Sec. 4.3.10; Fig. 7.5). Nontransformed cells are inhibited by cell-cell contact and require a substratum for proliferation. Cells that have been transformed with certain oncogenes grow to form foci independent of cellular contact or adhesion to a substratum. In this functional assay, cells that formed foci contained DNA that was capable of transforming the NIH 3T3 cells and thus contained a potential oncogene. Isolation and sequencing of the transfected DNA led to the identity of members of the RAS family of oncogenes. Other genes have also been identified by this method, including the receptor tyrosine kinases,

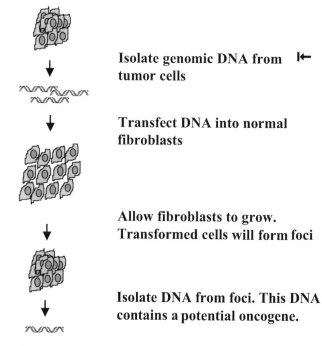

**Isolate genomic DNA from tumor cells**

**Transfect DNA into normal fibroblasts**

**Allow fibroblasts to grow. Transformed cells will form foci**

**Isolate DNA from foci. This DNA contains a potential oncogene.**

**Figure 7.5.** Transfection of DNA from tumor cells into nontransformed cells can lead to the identification of oncogenes. By this method, DNA is isolated from tumor cells and used to transfect normal fibroblasts. These cells are then grown to confluence and those cells that form foci may contain oncogenes.

*neu, met, trk, erbB-2/her-2,* and the growth factors *hst* and *ks3.*

Expression of only a subset of oncogenes can lead cells to form foci in vitro and additional methods to identify novel oncogenes have been developed. For example, *bcl-2* is an oncogene that encodes a protein that confers cell

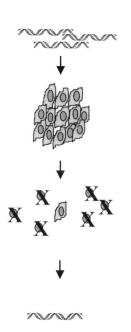

**Isolate genomic DNA from tumor cells**

**Transfer DNA into cells**

**Culture cells in medium containing agonists that trigger cells to undergo apoptosis or in medium depleted for key survival cytokines. Most cells will undergo apoptosis under these conditions.**

**Expand those cells that survive and identify the tumor DNA that conferred apoptosis resistance to the cell. These are potential oncogenes.**

**Figure 7.6.** Expression cloning. Expression cloning can be used to identify anti-apoptotic oncogenes. By this approach cells infected with retrovirus carrying a cDNA library are subsequently subjected to apoptotic conditions. The surviving clones are expanded and the library-derived cDNA isolated. The latter may represent a novel oncogene, like *bcl-2*, that can block apoptosis in the stepwise progression to tumorigenesis. Oncogenes that encode proteins that possess additional types of transforming activity can be cloned using an expression cloning strategy coupled with an appropriate assay for the activity under investigation.

survival by preventing apoptosis (see Chap. 10, Sec. 10.2.1; Reed, 1998). Bcl-2 does not contribute to focus formation in in vitro transforming assays, but it can contribute to cancer progression in vivo. This oncogenic activity can be detected using expression cloning combined with a unique cell based assay (Fig. 7.6). By this approach cells are infected with retroviruses carrying a cDNA library and subjected to conditions that induce apoptosis. Surviving clones are expanded and the cDNA representing a potential oncogene is isolated. Indeed, this assay has been used to clone novel anti-apoptotic genes that can cooperate in transformation with the *myc* oncogene. Fibroblast cells overexpressing *c-myc* were infected with a cDNA library carried in retroviral vectors and subsequently subjected to conditions that would normally induce cell death. DNA was rescued from those cells that did not die under these conditions and sequenced. The genes isolated in this study, *twist* and *dermo,* were subsequently shown to antagonize cell death and contribute to transformation (Maestro et al., 1999). Functional screens to identify genes that contribute to various processes in oncogenesis will be useful to identify oncogenes that do not display the prototypic function of inducing cellular growth. By using these types of functional screens in conjunction with novel high-throughput assays to assess biological activities, it will be possible to isolate genes that characterize a wide array of functional classes, such as anti-apoptotic, pro-invasion, or pro-angiogenesis proteins.

## 7.3 FUNCTION OF ONCOGENIC PROTEINS

Oncogenic proteins have often been categorized by their subcellular localization and by their biochemical activity. Most oncoproteins participate in signaling pathways through which the cell receives and executes instructions from the extracellular milieu that leads to a wide variety of biological activities, including mitogenesis, differentiation, lineage determination, cell migration, extracellular matrix production, and apoptosis. Oncogene products can be classified as (1) growth factors; (2) growth factor receptors; (3) Ras oncoproteins; (4) cytoplasmic protein kinases; (4) transcription factors; (5) anti-apoptotic proteins; or (6) other oncoproteins (Fig. 7.7). Examples of oncogenes whose protein products fall into these classes are listed in Table 7.1. Proteins within a single category, based on subcellular localization, do not necessarily affect a similar biological outcome. The specific regulatory roles of oncoproteins in signal transduction are described in Chapter 8.

The protein products of cellular oncogenes can affect numerous, diverse biological processes. A commonly accepted multihit hypothesis indicates that cooperation between multiple oncogenes and/or loss of tumor suppressors from different functional classes is necessary for transformation to proceed (Hanahan and Weinberg, 2000). Before a cell becomes cancerous a number of biological changes must take place: these include the ability to (1) proliferate independently of growth signals; (2) circumvent programmed cell death; (3) replicate indefinitely; (4) induce vascular formation; and (5) invade tissues. These processes are reviewed in detail in Chapters 9 through 12. The majority of the oncogenes listed in Table 7.1 induce cellular proliferation independently of growth signals. This disproportionate distribution is likely a consequence of the historical effort in cancer research to understand the molecular mechanisms of cellular proliferation. With researchers embarking on expression cloning strategies to identify novel oncogenes, additional oncogenes that

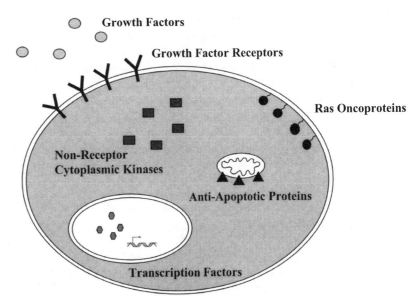

**Figure 7.7.** Oncogenes are involved in cytoplasmic signaling pathways and nuclear gene regulation. They include growth factors and growth factor receptors, *ras* oncogenes, nonreceptor cytoplasmic kinases, anti-apoptotic proteins, and nuclear transcription factors.

fall into other functional categories will undoubtedly be discovered, such as pro-angiogenesis, pro-invasion, and anti-apoptotic proteins. Some oncogenes can lead to multiple biological outcomes and fit into multiple categories. For example, the *myc* oncogene can induce cellular proliferation, immortalization, angiogenesis, and tissue invasion (Pelengaris et al., 2002).

An important goal of research focused on oncogenes is to identify critical inducers of oncogenesis that are potential drug targets for the treatment of the disease. Recent experiments have shown that inhibition of the function of a single oncogene can reverse the tumor phenotype despite the fact that cancer is generally thought to involve a stepwise progression with multiple genetic mutations. Thus, in transgenic animals expressing the inducible oncogenes *myc* or *ras*, tumors were formed when these genes were activated. However, when these genes were turned off tumors regressed (Pelengaris et al., 2002). While this indicates that a cancerous phenotype may be reversed by the inhibition of a single oncogene, it is more likely that a combination or cocktail of anti-cancer agents will best target the tumor cells for destruction. Indeed, molecular inhibitors to specific oncoproteins have recently been developed and many are undergoing evaluation in clinical trials.

We will describe the categories of oncogenes itemized in Table 7.1, highlighting specific examples, and discuss some of the therapeutic inhibitors that have been generated to oncoproteins of each class.

### 7.3.1 Growth Factors and Their Receptors

The control of cell proliferation is highly regulated by extracellular signals known as growth factors. Growth factors are high affinity ligands for transmembrane receptors belonging to the family of receptor tyrosine kinases (RTKs; Reilly, 2003). Signal transduction by RTKs is a multistep process which includes ligand binding and receptor dimerization, intermolecular phosphorylation of the intracellular domain on tyrosine residues, recruitment and then activation of cytoplasmic signaling molecules that transmit signals to the nucleus (see also Chap. 8, Sec. 8.2). Receptor tyrosine kinase mediated signaling is highly regulated in nontransformed cells, but is constitutively activated in cancers. Activation can occur by ligand overexpression, mutations within the RTK protein itself that deregulate receptor signaling, or overexpression of the receptor due to mechanisms such as translocation and gene amplification. Overexpression by any means can activate RTKs by increasing the concentration of the protein at the plasma membrane leading to ligand independent dimerization.

Activation of growth factors or their receptors is evident in a wide range of human cancers. The ERBB family of receptors includes EGFR, ERBB2/HER2/NEU,

ERBB3, and ERBB4 that can in some instances be bound and activated by ligands. Activation can contribute to a variety of cancers including breast, ovarian, brain, glioblastoma, colorectal, and small cell lung cancer (Blume-Jensen and Hunter, 2001). Activation of the *KIT* receptor is evident in mastocytomas and gastrointestinal tumors while activating mutations of the *MET* receptor have been described in kidney and hepatocellular carcinomas. *FGFR3* is activated in multiple myeloma and *FLT3* activation is evident in acute myelogenous leukemia. VEGF/VEGFR contribute to a potent angiogenic response in a variety of tumors (see Chap. 12, Sec. 12.2; Ferrara et al., 2003).

Receptor tyrosine kinases are popular drug targets because of their cell surface localization which is relatively accessible to targeting. Successful drugs that specifically target oncoproteins of this class include trastuzumab, a monoclonal antibody that binds to and inhibits the HER-2/NEU oncoprotein, as well as erlotinib and gefitinib that inhibit EGFR. Several agents have been developed to target VEGF/VEGFR using a diverse set of strategies and many are under investigation in clinical trials (Ferrara et al., 2003; Sridhar and Shepherd, 2003).

### 7.3.2 *Ras* Oncogenes

The *ras* family of oncogenes includes three common transforming members, *N-ras, K-ras, H-ras*. Each of these genes encodes a 21 kilodalton membrane associated G-coupled protein whose primary function within the cell is to phosphorylate effector molecules in response to signaling cues (see also Chap. 8, Sec. 8.2.5). *Ras* oncogenes were first identified by transfection studies in NIH 3T3 cells, as described in Section 7.2.6 (Boettner and Van Aelst, 2002). In nontransformed cells, Ras activity is highly regulated and Ras resides primarily in its inactive state bound to GDP. Ras is activated by upstream signaling cascades and stimulated to release GDP by guanine nucleotide exchange factors (GEFs) and to exchange it with GTP. This leads to an allosteric change that allows binding of Ras effector molecules and transduction of signaling cascades. Inhibitory GTPase activating proteins (GAPs) stimulate the GTPase activity of Ras leading to hydrolysis of GTP bound to Ras. By phosphorylation of effector molecules Ras leads to multiple signaling pathways, including activation of Raf, Ral-GEF and PI-3K pathways (see Chap. 8, Sec. 8.2.5). *Ras* can be activated by a single point mutation, which leads to constitutive activation of growth promoting pathways.

RAS proteins are mutated or overexpressed in up to 30 percent of human cancers (Bos, 1989; Boettner and Van Aelst, 2002). These include, but are not limited to, acute myelogenous leukemia, pancreatic carcinoma, and colorectal cancer. Because RAS activation holds such a key role in the etiology of human cancers, RAS was one of the first oncoproteins to be targeted for anti-cancer therapy. RAS activation and localization to cellular membranes is essential for function and is dependent upon a particular posttranslational modification called prenylation. Farnesyltransferase (FTase) was identified as the enzyme that catalyzes the addition of a farnesyl lipid moiety to the CAAX motif at the carboxyl-end of H-RAS. This spawned the development of FTase inhibitors (FTIs) as RAS antagonists. However, it has recently been shown that K-RAS is the RAS family member that is primarily activated in human cancers, yet K-RAS is prenylated by another mechanism involving geranylgeranylation. Thus, the FTIs target many farnesylated cellular proteins, but not activated K-RAS. FTase inhibitors remain in early phase clinical trials; however, the molecular target(s) remain unknown (Caponigro et al., 2003). Geranylgeranyltransferase inhibitors (GGTIs) are in development (Sebti and Hamilton, 2001; Sun et al., 2003). Both prenylation pathways can be inhibited by targeting the upstream enzyme of the mevalonate pathway, HMG-CoA reductase, which has been shown to trigger tumor-specific apoptosis in vitro. The statin family of drugs target HMG-CoA reductase and are used in the treatment of hypercholesterolemia (Corsini et al., 1995). Due to their immediate availability and tumor-specific action, statins are also in early phase clinical trials as novel anti-cancer agents (Wong et al., 2002). Anti-sense molecules have also been developed to target *RAS* expression directly (Stahel and Zangemeister-Wittge, 2003). However, targeting proteins downstream of RAS has shown promise and may be the direction of choice for future drug targeting of RAS activated pathways.

### 7.3.3 Cytoplasmic Kinases

Cytoplasmic kinases play an essential role in transmitting the activated signal from the cell surface receptor through the cytoplasm to the nucleus. This cascade of kinase events enables several unique and overlapping signal transduction pathways to be regulated according to the signal transmitted (Chap. 8, Sec. 8.2). The kinases are required for several cellular outcomes, including proliferation, differentiation, and death. The kinase cascades that are well established as holding a key role in regulating cell growth and survival are those that lie downstream of activated Ras. For example, Ras phosphorylates Raf-1 kinase which, in turn, phosphorylates and activates MEK1 that then catalyzes the phosphorylation of ERK1 and ERK2 on specific tyrosine and threonine residues (Chap. 8, Sec. 8.2.5). Because a large subset of the many tumors harboring activated *RAS* would be sensitive to inhibitors of downstream components of this pathway, the RAF and MEK kinase have

been targeted. Two types of inhibitors have been developed to RAF; an anti-sense compound that degrades RAF mRNA (ISIS 5132) and a small-molecule inhibitor that blocks Raf kinase activity (BAY 43-9006) (Hilger et al., 2002; Stahel and Zangemeister-Wittge, 2003). Both agents are undergoing evaluation in clinical trials. Investigation of a small-molecular weight inhibitor of MEK kinase (PD 184352 or CI-1040) has shown that the compound is well tolerated (Allen et al., 2003). These and other studies have established the RAF-MEK-ERK signaling cascade as a potential target for therapeutic approaches (Sebolt-Leopold et al., 1999; Lee and McCubrey, 2002).

Another cytoplasmic kinase that holds a key role in tumorigenesis and has been successfully targeted by novel therapeutics is BCR-ABL. The BCR-ABL fusion oncoprotein is evident in the leukemic blast cells of 95 percent of chronic myelogenous leukemia (CML) and in some acute lymphoblastic leukemias. This fusion protein is created by the translocation between the long arms of chromosomes 9 and 22, t(9;22)(q34;q11), also known as the Philadelphia chromosome (Fig. 7.4). Depending on the precise region of the translocation two major fusion proteins can be formed and are named according to their molecular weight, P210 and P190. The Ph chromosome is evident in some normal subjects that do not present with leukemia, indicating that the translocation in itself is insufficient to induce cancer. The fusion of BCR and ABL leads to constitutive tyrosine kinase activity of the ABL portion of the protein. ABL was identified as an oncogene when it was discovered that this gene represented the transforming sequences in Abelson leukemia viruses. ABL is a non-receptor protein tyrosine kinase that contains SH2 and SH3 interaction domains, nuclear localization signals, a DNA-binding domain, and actin binding domains in its N terminal sequences, as well as SH3 binding sites in its C-terminal sequences (see Chap. 8, Secs. 8.2.3 and 8.2.4 for discussion of SH2 and SH3 proteins). The ABL kinase is activated in response to a variety of DNA damaging agents and plays a role in the p53 dependent response to DNA damage. BCR is a signaling protein that contains many binding sites for adaptor molecules along its length. The P210 BCR-ABL fusion protein can also bind to numerous adapter signaling molecules which can lead to activation of signaling pathways for cellular proliferation such as the Ras/MAP kinase pathway and the PI-3 kinase pathway (see Chap. 8, Sec. 8.2.7). The kinase activity of ABL is absolutely required for the oncogenic activity of BCR-ABL, and sequences encoded by BCR appear to potentiate this activity.

One of the most successful applications of targeted therapy is the use of an anti-BCR-ABL agent in the treatment of CML (Deininger, 2004; Shah and Sawyers, 2003). Imatinib mesylate targets the ATP-binding region of the BCR-ABL tyrosine kinase and has shown remarkable efficacy with limited side effects even when used as a single agent against CML. The most durable responses are evident in earlier stage patients. BCR-ABL activity is restored in the majority of cases of acquired resistance due to point mutations that preclude drug interaction. A phase III trial compared interferon-$\alpha$ and cytarabine, previously the most effective therapy for CML, with imatinib in newly diagnosed patients. This study recruited >1000 patients in nearly 200 centers worldwide. Imatinib proved to be the agent of choice in terms of hematological response, cytogenetic response, and progression-free survival (O'Brien et al., 2003). Other tyrosine kinases are also sensitive to imatinib, including C-KIT (stem cell factor) and platelet-derived growth factor receptor (PDGFR). These observations have enabled imatinib to be used in the treatment of additional cancers, including gastrointestinal stromal tumors (Griffin, 2001; Capdeville and Silbermann, 2003).

### 7.3.4 Transcription Factors

Aberrant gene regulation is a hallmark of cancer cells and is a consequence of direct and indirect activation of transcription factor activity in the nucleus. The products of several genes are localized in the nucleus and play a key role in the carcinogenic process. These include steroid receptors in breast and prostate cancers, several transcriptional factors downstream of serine kinase cascades including Jun, Myc and Ets, and latent transcription factors such as STATs (signal transducers and activators of transcription; see Chap. 8, Sec. 8.3.1). In nontransformed cells these transcriptional regulators are tightly controlled but are deregulated in cells of malignant origin. Despite their role in oncogenesis, transcription factors have not been popular targets for drug development due to their less accessible subcellular localization (Darnell, 2002). Nonetheless, agents that block transcription factor function have begun to emerge and they fall into two classes. One targets general transcriptional processes such as histone deacetylation (HDAC) and the other targets specific oncogenic transcription factors including MYC.

HDACs remove acetyl groups from core nucleosomal histones to repress gene transcription and blocking this activity can specifically target transformed cells both in vitro and in vivo (Penn, 2001). Inhibitors of HDAC show little toxicity to normal cells. Mechanistically HDAC inhibitors alter only about 2 percent of gene expression with specific induction of certain target genes. Many have been developed and several have advanced to phase I trials.

Targeting of specific transcription factors is under investigation and one of the potential nuclear targets is MYC (Oster et al., 2002; Hermeking, 2003). MYC is an attractive therapeutic target as blocking MYC can lead to dramatic tumor regression in animal models (Pelengaris et al., 2002). Moreover, blocking MYC expression leads to a rapid growth inhibitory response due to the short half-life of both MYC mRNA and MYC protein, and even small decreases in Myc expression can affect cell transformation (Oster et al., 2002). Much effort is focused on the use of antisense molecules (Biroccio et al., 2003; Stahel and Zangemeister-Wittke, 2003). Peptide and small-molecule inhibitors directed to the MYC carboxyl end are also under investigation (Boffa et al., 2000; Pescarolo et al., 2001). Another approach is to introduce ectopic MAD family members to antagonize MYC activity (Oster et al., 2002). Novel approaches to target MYC expression, MYC activity, and MYC/protein or MYC/DNA interactions hold promise for inhibiting tumor cell proliferation or triggering apoptosis of tumor cells.

### 7.3.5 Anti-apoptotic Proteins

Novel strategies in anti-cancer drug development are directed toward stimulation of apoptosis (Chap. 10, Sec. 10.4). Apoptosis is highly controlled by a regulatory network of signaling pathways. Ultimately the release of cytochrome c from the inner mitochondrial membrane space to the cytoplasm triggers apoptosis and results in the activation of caspases that then destroy the cell. A key regulator of apoptosis at the level of cytochrome c release is an oncogene (bcl-2), which is often overexpressed in tumor cells. B-cell lymphoma gene-2 (bcl-2), is a pro-survival molecule that encodes the prototypic members of a family of proteins, which includes other pro-survival proteins like Bcl-$X_L$ and Mcl-1, and pro-apoptotic molecules like Bax and Bid (see Chap. 10, Sec. 10.2.1). BCL-2 was first identified as a translocation in human follicular lymphomas that juxtaposed the BCL-2 gene to the immunoglobulin heavy chain gene leading to overexpression of BCL-2. Overexpression of BCL-2 protein has also been observed in other leukemias, such as B-cell chronic lymphocytic leukemia, acute myeloid leukemia, multiple myeloma, and solid tumors of the breast, bowel, lung, and skin. Indeed, constitutive overexpression of bcl-2 in transgenic mice results in prolonged cell survival and malignancy. Bcl-2 is predominantly localized to the outer membranes of mitochondria as well as those of the nucleus and endoplasmic reticulum and its subcellular localization may play an important role in its function. Bcl-2 family members share conserved regions termed BH domains. It is through these domains that Bcl-2 family members can form heterodimers and homodimers, to modulate protein function. It appears as though the ratio of anti-apoptotic to pro-apoptotic members of the Bcl-2 family may dictate the fate of the cell in response to growth or anti-growth signals.

Because BCL-2 and related anti-apoptotic proteins are expressed at high levels in many types of cancer, they are suitable targets for pharmaceutical intervention. The first generation inhibitors were antisense molecules (augmerosen, G3139) that targeted the first six codons of the BCL-2 coding sequence. G3139 has only a moderate effect when administered alone but shows improved efficacy when used in combination with chemotherapy. These compounds provide proof-of-principle that regulating apoptosis can sensitize tumor cells to die in response to low-dose chemotherapy (Biroccio et al., 2003; Shangary and Johnson, 2003). Other inhibitors of apoptosis are under development (Letai, 2003).

## 7.4 TUMOR SUPPRESSOR GENES

Approximately 1 percent of all human cancers arise in individuals with a hereditary cancer syndrome. Even though such conditions are relatively rare, investigations of the affected individuals and of mutations of genes associated with their disease have proven invaluable in understanding the genetics and etiology of cancer. Most inherited cancer syndromes are a consequence of germline transmission of inactivating, loss-of-function mutations in tumor suppressor genes. Unlike oncogenes, whose mutations are associated with sporadic tumors and act in a dominant manner, mutations of tumor suppressor genes are recessive at the somatic level, and the remaining wild-type allele is inactivated during cancer development. Phenotypic and clinical manifestations of numerous inherited cancer predisposition syndromes, together with the known genetic events associated with them, are catalogued in an expanding Online Mendelian Inheritance in Man (OMIM) database (www.ncbi.nlm.nih.gov/omim).

The existence of genes with an ability to inhibit tumor growth was first proposed when it was demonstrated that growth of mouse tumor cells in syngenic animals could be suppressed by their fusion to nonmalignant cells. However, prolonged propagation of these hybrid cells in culture resulted in their reversion to a tumorigenic phenotype and chromosomal aberrations (Harris et al., 1969). Subsequent studies revealed that loss of specific chromosomes or parts of chromosomes coincided with the appearance of tumorigenic revertants (Stanbridge et al., 1982). Moreover, cellular transfer of particular individual chromosomes impaired the tumorigenicity of several cancer cell lines, further supporting the notion that genes, or groups of genes, are capable of tumor suppressor function (Saxon et al., 1986; Weissman et al., 1987). Parallel with cellular studies, Knudson investigated the epidemiology of familial retinoblastoma, an autosomal dominant hereditary form of retinal cancer (Knudson, 1971). In contrast to sporadic cases of retinoblastoma, patients with familial disease were likely to develop a more severe, bilateral or multifocal disease at an earlier age of onset. Based on these observations, Knudson proposed that two mutations, or two hits, were required for retinoblastoma to appear in both sporadic and familial cases. In familial retinoblastoma, the first mutation is transmitted through the germline and is present in all cells, whereas the second mutation needs to occur somatically. In other words, a second hit in only one retinal cell is sufficient for the tumor to arise, in agreement with the dominant inheritance of familial retinoblastoma. In sporadic (noninherited) retinoblastoma, both mutations, or hits, have to occur within the same somatic cell, statistically a far less likely event. Knudson's two-hit hypothesis highlighted the importance of recessive mutations in tumorigenesis and offered evidence for the cooperation of inherited and somatic genetic alterations in human cancer.

### 7.4.1 Genetic Deletions and Loss of Heterozygosity

Genetic defects of tumor suppressor genes also occur frequently in sporadic cancer, both during tumor initiation and progression. Cytogenetic studies of peripheral blood lymphocytes of patients with familial cancers offered important information about the location of tumor suppressor genes. For instance, 5 percent of retinoblastoma patients had interstitial deletions on chromosome 13q14, whereas Wilms tumor patients frequently had deletions on chromosome 11p13, pointing to the chromosomal position of tumor suppressor genes associated with these diseases (Francke, 1976; Francke et al., 1979). More recent studies indicate that large deletions account for only a limited number of inherited mutations, whereas small deletions and point mutations are more commonly found in tumors. Information relating to genetic alterations in cancer can be accessed through an interactive Mitelman Database of Chromosome Aberrations in Cancer (http://cgap.nci.nih.gov/Chromosomes/Mitelman).

Genetic material in all somatic cells is comprised of equal contributions of maternal and paternal chromosomal material. Small DNA sequence differences (polymorphisms) between parental chromosomes, termed *heterozygosity*, are present at most genetic loci (see Chap. 4, Sec. 4.3.7). While subtly altering gene function, polymorphisms are not associated with genetic diseases, but are responsible for phenotypic traits, such as skin, eye and hair color, and baldness. However, in tumors, the wild-type allele of a tumor suppressor gene is commonly replaced by a mutated one through the processes of mitotic recombination, chromosomal nondysjunction, or gene conversion, resulting in the absence of DNA polymorphism, termed *loss of heterozygosity* or LOH (Fig. 7.8). Loss

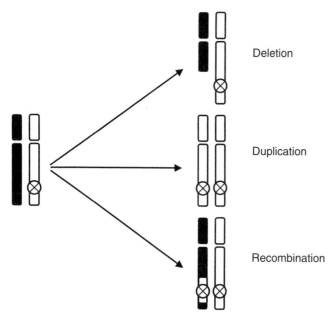

**Figure 7.8.** Loss of heterozygosity (LOH). A mutated gene (represented by the circled x) is present on one chromosome. Loss of heterozygosity occurs when the second allele and the surrounding polymorphic markers are lost via large deletion (*top*), chromosome nondysjunction and duplication of the remaining copy (*middle*), or mitotic recombination (*bottom*).

of heterozygosity can also arise from a complete absence of the wild-type allele, as in the case of large deletions or partial or complete chromosomal loss. Frequent LOH of a specific polymorphic chromosomal marker in a particular tumor type implies that the chromosomal area in the vicinity of that marker contains a candidate tumor suppressor gene. Thus, DNA sequence polymorphisms and identification of regions of LOH provided a means to search for allele loss in tumors (Knudson, 1993).

Cytogenetic studies and linkage analysis which serve to establish cosegregation of particular genetic markers with appearance of cancer in large multigenerational families, as well as LOH analysis, facilitated the search for tumor suppressor genes associated with a specific type of cancer. However, cloning of the individual tumor suppressor genes requires more precise analyses of the chromosomal region containing the candidate gene. Experimental strategies for isolation of tumor suppressor genes include DNA database homology searches, subtractive hybridization approaches aimed at identifying differences between normal and tumor cells, such as representational difference analysis (RDA), and finally positional cloning of the candidate gene (see Chap. 4, Secs. 4.3.8, 4.3.9, and 4.4.1). Once the candidate tumor suppressor gene is cloned, mutation rates associated with both the familial and sporadic cases of a particular type of cancer need to be reevaluated and confirmed to consider a gene a tumor sup-

pressor. In addition to direct mutations, loss-of-function of a tumor suppressor gene can also be a result of epigenetic changes, such as altered DNA methylation, transcription, or mRNA stability. Furthermore, the function of certain tumor suppressor genes can be counteracted by the action of activated oncogenes and genes carried by oncogenic viruses. Loss of tumor suppressor genes in the later stages of tumorigenesis can be associated with selective growth properties once the tumor is confronted with apoptotic, growth suppressing, or hypoxia-induced signals. Further, mutations of certain tumor suppressor genes can occur at the point of transition from the premalignant to invasive tumor lesions and directly contribute to the metastatic potential of affected cells (see Chap. 11, Sec. 11.7).

More than twenty tumor suppressor genes have been identified thus far and their cellular and biochemical function examined (Table 7.2). Individual tumor suppressors lack significant amino acid sequence homology and display varied molecular means of action, but can be broadly divided into gatekeepers and caretakers, as proposed by Kinzler and Vogelstein (1997). Gatekeepers directly affect tumor growth by counteracting cellular proliferation or promoting cell death. Mutations of gatekeepers are rate limiting for tumor growth and are frequently found in both hereditary and sporadic tumors. In contrast, mutations of caretakers lead to genomic instability, increasing the mutation rate and promoting activation of oncogenes and inactivation of gatekeeping tumor suppressor genes.

Mutations of caretakers are not commonly found as initiating events in sporadic tumors, presumably because additional mutations are needed for a tumor to arise. However, genetic defects in caretakers are associated with inherited diseases characterized by increased sensitivity to DNA damage, such as xeroderma pigmentosum, ataxia telangiectasia, Fanconi anemia, and Bloom and Werner syndromes (see Chap. 5, Sec. 5.2.3). Some tumor suppressors display characteristics of both gatekeepers and caretakers. The following sections will describe the function and inheritance of some frequently mutated tumor suppressor genes.

### 7.4.2 The *p53* Gene

The *p53* tumor suppressor gene is mutated in more than 50 percent of all human cancers, which results in a selective growth advantage for cells harboring its mutations (Greenblatt et al., 1994). Genetic studies in mice have demonstrated that *p53* is not essential for normal growth and development. However, mice carrying *p53* mutations are highly susceptible to tumor development, particularly of lymphoid origin, confirming the role of *p53* as a tumor suppressor (Donehower et al., 1992). Human carriers of a heterozygous *p53* mutation suffer

**Table 7.2.** A Partial List of Some of the Best-characterized Caretaker and Gatekeeper Tumor Suppressor Genes/Proteins

| Tumor Suppressor | Biological Function | Mechanism of Action | Tumor Type |
|---|---|---|---|
| **Caretakers** | | | |
| XP-A to G, CS-A, B | Nuclear excision repair | Various, implicated in several aspects of DNA repair | Xeroderma pigmentosa, Cockayne syndrome, trichothiodystrophy |
| TTD-A | | | |
| ATM | Radiosensitivity | Protein kinase | Ataxia-telangiectasia |
| BLM | Genomic stability | DNA and RNA helicase | Bloom syndrome |
| FANC | Sensitivity to chromosome breakage | unknown | Fanconi anemia |
| hMSH2, hMLH1, hPMS2, hPMS1 | DNA mismatch repair | Recognition of mismatched DNA | Hereditary non-polyposis colorectal cancer |
| WRN-H | Genomic stability | Unknown | Werner syndrome |
| **Gatekeepers** | | | |
| RB | Cell cycle regulation | Association with several cell cycle regulators | Retinoblastoma |
| p53 | Cell cycle regulation, apoptosis | Transcription factor | Li-Fraumeni syndrome numerous cancers |
| PTEN | Apoptosis, proliferation | Phosphatidylinositol 3' phosphatase | Cowden's syndrome, numerous cancers |
| BRCA1, BRCA2 | Double-strand DNA repair, transcription | Direct binding to double-strand DNA breaks, transcription activation | Breast, ovarian and other types of cancer |
| WT | Unknown transcriptional targets | Transcription factor | Wilms tumors |
| NF1 | Cell growth and differentiation | GTPase activating protein | Neurofibromatosis type 1 |
| APC | proliferation | Regulates stability of several proteins | Adenomatous polyposis coli, sporadic colorectal tumors |

from Li-Fraumeni syndrome (OMIM #151623), a rare autosomal dominant disorder characterized by early onset mesenchymal and epithelial malignancies at multiple sites (Malkin et al., 1990). Tumors in Li-Fraumeni patients display LOH and absence of the wild-type *P53* allele in tumor cells.

The human *P53* gene is located on human chromosome 17p13 and encodes a 393 amino acid phosphoprotein. In response to cellular stresses induced by DNA damage, hypoxia, or oncogene activation, intracellular levels of p53 increase. p53 structural features suggest a function in regulation of gene expression. The N-terminus of p53 contains an acidic transactivation domain (a domain often found in proteins that directly regulate gene expression), whereas the central portion of the protein includes a DNA-binding domain. Furthermore, C-terminus of p53 carries a strong nuclear localization signal. Indeed, p53 mutants with impaired regulation of transcription fail to suppress growth of p53-deficient cells, indicating that this function of p53 is essential for its role as a tumor suppressor. Numerous genes that contain DNA

elements specifically targeted by p53 within their promoters have been discovered, indicating that p53 might have multiple functions in tumor suppression.

Following cellular DNA damage, activation of p53 induces an arrest of cells in G1 phase of the cell cycle. It is believed that a transient p53-induced G1 arrest allows DNA repair to occur before replication, thus preventing cells with damaged DNA from entering S phase (Chap. 5, Sec. 5.4). Some of the most prominent transcriptional targets of p53 are p21[waf1] (el-Deiry et al., 1993), a 21 kDa inhibitor of cyclin-dependent kinases important for proper G1-S cell cycle transition (see Chap. 9, Sec. 9.2.2) and GADD45 (Kastan et al., 1992), an inhibitor of cell proliferation (Fig. 7.9). Both p21[waf1] and GADD45 can bind to the proliferating cell nuclear antigen (PCNA), a component of cyclin-dependent kinase complexes and a protein involved in DNA replication and DNA repair. Thus, p53-mediated induction of p21[waf1] and GADD45 results in simultaneous inhibition of cyclin-dependent kinases and prevention of S-phase entry, and interference with DNA replication by

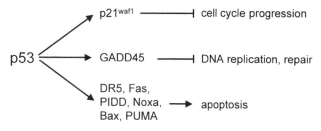

**Figure 7.9.** Mechanism of p53 action. Transcriptional targets of p53 include molecules involved in regulation of cell cycle, DNA replication, and repair and apoptosis.

virtue of PCNA binding. In addition, p53 has been implicated in DNA repair via direct interaction with DNA helicases encoded by the xeroderma pigmentosa genes XPB and XPD, which are part of the cellular nucleotide excision repair machinery (see Chap. 5, Sec. 5.3.4; Wang et al., 1996). In support of the importance of p53 in regulation of cell cycle arrest following DNA damage and DNA repair, cells lacking p53 have an increased incidence of genetic instability and gene amplification (Kastan et al., 1991).

p53 also has a function in programmed cell death or apoptosis (see Chap. 10, Sec. 10.2.4). In response to exposure to radiation or various chemotherapeutic drugs that induce double strand DNA breaks, p53 initiates an apoptotic program in a number of cell types. A growing number of p53 targets with an active role in promoting apoptosis have been identified, including DR5, Fas, PIDD, Noxa, Bax, PUMA, and others (reviewed in Vousden, 2000). In cells mutant for p53, failure to induce apoptosis after DNA damage can result in propagation of cells containing multiple mutations, directly contributing to tumorigenesis.

Regulation of p53 is complex (reviewed in Vousden, 2002). Under normal conditions, p53 protein interacts with Mdm-2, which antagonizes p53 transcriptional activity, promotes its nuclear export and targets p53 for ubiquitin-mediated degradation (see Chap. 9; Fig. 9.4). Subsequent to cellular exposure to DNA-damaging agents, p53 protein becomes multiply phosphorylated at various serine and threonine residues, preventing its association with Mdm-2 and resulting in p53 stabilization and activation. Interestingly, p53 directly activates transcription of Mdm-2, effectively initiating an inhibitory loop that terminates p53 responses. Mdm-2 is also subject to tight regulation by phosphorylation, as well as interaction with the Arf tumor suppressor gene product. Arf sequesters Mdm-2 to the nucleolus where it cannot access p53 and directly inhibits Mdm-2 ubiquitin ligase activity. p53 protein is also a common target of DNA tumor virus proteins, including SV40 large tumor antigen, the adenoviral E1B protein, and the pa-

pillomavirus E6 protein, as well as certain cellular oncogenes. The transforming potential of these molecules is often directly dependent on their ability to interact with p53 and impair its function. Thus, molecules involved in the regulation of p53 form an elaborate oncogene-tumor suppressor gene network. The existence of such networks has been demonstrated for the majority of known tumor suppressor genes. Any malfunction within these networks due to inherited or sporadic mutations could result in neoplastic transformation.

### 7.4.3 Phosphatase and Tensin Homolog Deleted on Chromosome 10 (*PTEN*)

*PTEN* was discovered as a candidate tumor suppressor gene deleted at human chromosome 10q23 in a number of advanced tumors (Li et al., 1997; Steck et al., 1997). Systematic search for *PTEN* alterations in human cancer demonstrated a high rate of *PTEN* mutations in glioblastomas, prostate, thyroid, breast and skin tumors and in cell lines (reviewed in Stambolic et al., 1999). In contrast to other tumors where *PTEN* mutations are found in the advanced phases of the disease, *PTEN* mutations also occur at all stages of endometrial cancer, suggesting *PTEN* involvement in the process of tumor initiation in this organ.

In addition to mutations in sporadic tumors, germline mutations of *PTEN* cause Cowden syndrome (OMIM #158350), an autosomal dominant hamartoma syndrome. The affected individuals have high incidence of benign hamartomatous tumors throughout the body early in life, as well as increased occurrence of cancers of the breast, thyroid, brain, and endometrium (Eng, 2003). Mice heterozygous for *PTEN* are also highly susceptible to tumors (Podsypanina et al., 1999; Stambolic et al., 2000). Young $PTEN^{+/-}$ mice fail to exhibit characteristics of patients with Cowden syndrome but develop lymphoid malignancies with 15 to 20 percent penetrance. However, past six months of age, a majority of $PTEN^{+/-}$ female mice develop endometrial and breast neoplasia, whereas a proportion of males develop prostate cancer. Importantly, tumors that develop in $PTEN^{+/-}$ animals are associated with LOH at the *PTEN* locus.

The human *PTEN* gene encodes a 403 amino acid polypeptide with a high degree of homology to protein phosphatases. The importance of an intact PTEN phosphatase domain for its tumor suppressor function is highlighted by the discovery that the majority of tumor-associated *PTEN* mutations map to the region encoding the phosphatase domain (Rasheed et al., 1997; Marsh et al., 1998). Moreover, unlike wild-type PTEN, catalytically-inactive PTEN is not able to suppress growth and tumorigenicity of PTEN-deficient glioblastoma cells (Furnari et al., 1997). Despite homology to

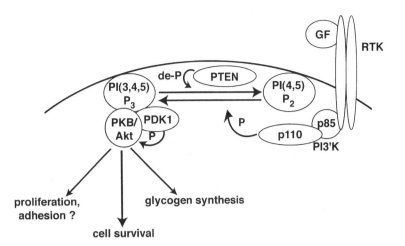

**Figure 7.10.** Phosphatidylinositol 3′ signaling. Following interaction of growth factors (GF) with receptor tyrosine kinases (RTK), the regulatory subunit of PI-3K (p85) is recruited to the receptor, resulting in activation of the catalytic subunit (p110) and an increase in intracellular levels of phosphatidylinositol (3,4,5) trisphosphate [PI(3,4,5)$P_3$]. Proteins containing pleckstrin homology domains, including phosphatidylinositol-dependent kinase 1 (PDK1) and protein kinase B (PKB/Akt), specifically interact with PI(3,4,5)$P_3$, resulting in activation of PKB/Akt and affecting numerous cellular processes. PTEN acts as a negative regulator of these pathways, as shown.

protein phosphatases, PTEN functions by dephosphorylating a lipid second messenger, phosphatidylinositol (3,4,5) trisphosphate [PI(3,4,5)$P_3$], the primary product of phosphatidylinositol 3′ kinase activity (PI-3K) and antagonizing PI-3K function (Fig. 7.10; Chap. 8, Sec. 8.2.7; Cantley and Neel, 1999; Stambolic et al., 1999). PI-3K is a component of multiple cellular signaling pathways implicated in regulation of cell proliferation, survival, and adhesion, organization of the cytoskeleton, and glucose metabolism (Di Cristofano and Pandolfi, 2000). A role for PI-3K in tumorigenesis is underscored by the identification of activating mutations in both upstream and downstream components of PI-3K signaling pathways in human cancer. For example, amplification of genes encoding the receptor tyrosine kinases that activate PI-3K, such as platelet-derived growth factor receptor (PDGFR) and epidermal growth factor receptor (EGFR), have been reported in glioblastoma patients (see Chap. 8, Sec. 8.2.2). Moreover, overexpression of PKB/Akt, a major target and effector of PI-3K-mediated cellular survival signaling has been shown in certain ovarian, pancreatic and breast cancers (Stambolic et al., 1999).

Consistent with the role for PTEN as a negative regulator of phosphatidylinositol signaling, loss of PTEN in mammalian cells results in increased PI(3,4,5)$P_3$ levels and PKB/Akt activation. Cells mutant for PTEN exhibit significantly lower sensitivity to cytotoxic stresses that normally induce apoptosis, such as osmotic shock, ultraviolet irradiation, heat treatment, or stimulation with tumor necrosis factor-$\alpha$ (Stambolic et al., 1998). Sensitivity to apoptotic stimuli and activity of PKB/Akt in PTEN-deficient cells could be restored to wild-type levels by expression of exogenous PTEN. Expression of PTEN was also shown to inhibit cell proliferation, migration, integrin-mediated cell spreading, and formation of focal adhesions (Di Cristofano and Pandolfi, 2000). The balance between PI-3K, PI(3,4,5)$P_3$, PKB/Akt, and their downstream targets on one side, and PTEN on the other, functions as a molecular indicator that governs the survival and/or proliferation potential of individual cells. Any alterations of this balance due to either amplification of positive regulators of survival and proliferation, or inactivating mutations of the negative ones, can lead to tumorigenesis.

### 7.4.4 The Retinoblastoma Gene (*Rb*)

The retinoblastoma gene (*RB*) was the first human tumor suppressor to be identified as a result of its frequent mutations in familial retinoblastoma, a rare pediatric eye tumor (OMIM #180200). In addition to retinoblastoma, mutations of *RB* can be found in other human malignancies, including osteosarcoma, small-cell lung carcinoma, prostate, and breast cancer (Weinberg, 1995; Sherr, 1996).

The human *RB* gene is located on chromosome 13q14 and encodes a 928 amino acid phosphoprotein. The Rb protein has a key function in regulation of cell cycle progression, as expression of Rb arrests cells in G1 phase of the cell cycle (see Chap. 9, Sec. 9.2.1). Protein phosphorylation is critical for Rb function. The kinases that phosphorylate Rb belong to a family of serine/threonine kinases named cyclin-dependent kinases (CDKs), which are tightly regulated by their cyclin partners. Phosphorylation of 16 potential CDK target sites on Rb oscillates during the cell cycle. While the hyperphosphorylated (inactive) form of Rb is most prevalent in proliferating cells, hypophosphorylated (active) Rb can be found in quiescent or differentiating cells. At least three cyclin-CDK complexes target Rb during cell cycle progression. Cyclin D/cdk4/6 phosphorylates Rb during early G1, cyclin E-cdk2 is responsible for late G1 Rb phosphorylation, whereas cyclin A-cdk2 maintains hyperphosphorylation of Rb during S phase (Sherr, 1996). Hyperphosphorylation of Rb results in its inactivation and allows the cell cycle to proceed (see Chap. 9, Sec. 9.2.1).

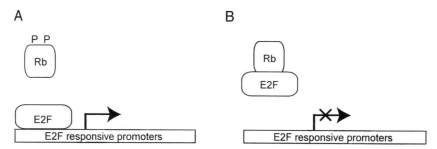

**Figure 7.11.** Rb achieves its function through interaction with the E2F transcription factor. (*A*) During the G1/S and G2/M phases of the cell cycle, Rb protein is mutiply phosphorylated preventing its association with E2F, resulting in full expression of E2F target genes. (*B*) At the beginning of G1 phase of the cell cycle, via the action of specific phosphatases, Rb protein is dephosphorylated, allowing its association with E2F and repression of E2f target genes.

Many of the cell cycle regulatory functions of Rb can be explained by its interaction with the E2F family of transcription factors (Dyson, 1998; Nevins, 2001; Fig. 7.11). Rb binding inhibits E2F activity and transcription of numerous E2F target genes and also actively represses transcription of certain E2F targets. Genes regulated by E2F include virtually the entire group of initiation factors that participate in DNA replication, as well as DNA polymerase $\alpha$, the proliferating cell nuclear antigen (PCNA), and proteins involved in nucleotide biosynthesis. In addition, E2F also promotes synthesis of both cyclin E and cdk2 that form the complex responsible for Rb inhibition and activation of DNA replication (Nevins, 2001). Considering the known spectrum of E2F target genes, Rb function is essential for some of the most critical steps in cell division and any genetic alterations that affect Rb regulation could contribute to tumorigenesis. This view is strongly supported by frequent mutations of another tumor suppressor, p16[INK4a], an inhibitor of cyclin D/cdk4 activity (see Chap. 9, Sec. 9.2.2). In the absence of p16[INK4a], cyclin D/cdk4 activity is elevated leading to inhibition of Rb, E2F accumulation, and transactivation of its target genes (Sherr, 2001). Thus, loss of p16[INK4a] is functionally equivalent to loss of function of Rb. Moreover, amplification of both *CYCLIN D1* and *CDK4* has been reported in several types of cancer. Similarly to p53, Rb is also inhibited by interaction with oncoproteins expressed by the DNA tumor viruses, such as E1A, SV40 large T antigen, and human papillomavirus E7 (see Chap. 6, Sec. 6.2; DeCaprio et al., 1988; Whyte et al., 1988; Dyson et al., 1989). In addition to regulation of the cell cycle, Rb controls apoptosis in several cell types furthering its potential function in tumor suppression (Harbou and Dean, 2000).

### 7.4.5 *BRCA1* and *BRCA2*

Breast cancer is the most prevalent cancer in women, and increased incidence of breast cancer in certain families has been documented since the nineteenth century. However, the first breast cancer susceptibility genes have only been identified recently. Mutations of *BRCA1*, located on human chromosome 17q21, and *BRCA2*, located on 13q12-13, account for a majority of familial breast cancer cases. The inheritance of *BRCA1* and *BRCA2* mutations is autosomal dominant, suggesting that these genes act as tumor suppressors. Besides breast cancers, mutations of *BRCA1* have been found in familial ovarian cancer and prostate cancer, whereas *BRCA2* mutations can be found in male breast, ovarian, prostate, pancreatic, gall bladder, bile duct, and stomach cancer (Welcsh and King, 2001).

Considering the partially overlapping tumor spectra in carriers of *BRCA1* and *BRCA2* mutations, it has been postulated that the two gene products might have a complementary function in cells. The 1,863 amino acid *BRCA1* and the 3,418 amino acid *BRCA2* proteins do not display significant similarity to any known protein or to each other. Nevertheless, human and mouse cells that lack functional BRCA1 or BRCA2 accumulate chromosomal breaks, aneuploidy, and centrosome amplification (Scully et al., 2000), suggesting a common function for these molecules in maintenance of chromosomal stability. Both proteins are predominantly nuclear and ubiquitously expressed. Following DNA damage, BRCA1 is rapidly recruited to DNA break sites and directly binds single-stranded and double-stranded DNA breaks (Scully and Livingston, 2000). It is believed that BRCA1 binds DNA breaks as part of a large molecular complex that also includes BRCA2, Rad51, and Rad50, essential components of cellular DNA break repair machinery (Fig. 7.12; see Chap. 5, Secs. 5.3.5 and 5.3.6; Scully and Livingston, 2000). The physiological significance of these interactions is strengthened by the impairment of RAD51 function in cells lacking BRCA1 and BRCA2. Moreover, these cells exhibit hypersensitivity to ionizing radiation, a genotoxic stress that induces double-stranded DNA breaks.

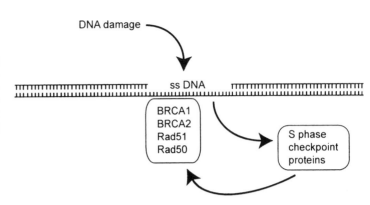

**Figure 7.12.** BRCA1 and BRCA2 are recruited to sites of DNA breaks. Appearance of single- or double-stranded DNA breaks activates S phase checkpoint proteins, which signal to recruit a large macromolecular complex containing BRCA1, BRCA2, Rad51, and Rad50 to the site of the DNA break. Such complex serves as an organizing center for the cellular DNA break repair machinery.

In view of the fundamental function of BRCA1 and BRCA2 in the maintenance of genetic integrity, it is surprising that their mutations are implicated in a relatively limited group of human cancers. Investigations of mice with targeted deletions of BRCA1 and BRCA2, respectively, provided insight into their relationship and tumorigenesis. Mouse embryos nullizygous for BRCA1 or BRCA2 die during embryogenesis displaying defects in proliferation and induction of a p53 target gene *p21^{waf1}*, a potent cell cycle inhibitor (see Chap. 9, Sec. 9.2.2) Based on these findings, it has been proposed that genomic instability caused by BRCA dysfunction results in activation of a DNA-damage-induced, p53-dependent cell cycle arrest, leading to catastrophic death of the embryo. In support of this scenario, deletion of p53 or *p21^{waf1}* delays the death of both BRCA1- and BRCA2-mutant embryos. Similarly, in adult cells, deletion of BRCA1 or BRCA2 would be expected to result in cell cycle arrest and subsequent death of the mutant cell. However, if the BRCA1 or BRCA2 mutation occurs in a cell that already has a defect in one of the cell cycle checkpoint genes, such a cell might continue to proliferate, accumulating further genetic aberrations and leading to neoplasia (Chap. 5., Sec. 5.4). Alternatively, genomic instability caused by BRCA dysfunction could be closely followed by genetic inactivation of one of more cell cycle checkpoint genes resulting in a similar outcome.

Breast development results from a proliferative burst during puberty under the influence of estrogenic hormones. Unlike the other rapidly proliferating epithelia, such as the endometrium or the intestinal epithelium, breast tissue is clonal. In other words, the progeny of the first proliferative burst is retained throughout life. Hypothetically, any cancer-predisposing mutation that occurs within the breast epithelial precursor cells would be maintained in a significant proportion of the adult breast tissue. Considering that BRCA mutations are almost exclusively associated with familial breast cancer, it is possible that loss of one of the BRCA alleles (haploinsufficiency) leads to increased genomic instability and elevated frequency of tumorigenic mutations during breast development. The timing of genetic events during breast tumor progression is still poorly understood.

Cellular functions of BRCA genes described thus far firmly establish their role as caretaker tumor suppressor genes. However, both BRCA genes contain strong transcriptional activation domains. Moreover, they interact with various transcription factors, including p53 and c-myc (Scully and Livingston, 2000). A search for transcriptional targets of BRCA1 has identified the previously described *p21^{waf1}* and the estrogen receptor as potential downstream effectors of BRCA1 function. BRCA1 also appears to be a component of the human SWI/SNF chromatin remodeling complex, which could affect expression of many genes in a more general manner (Bochar et al., 2000). Taken together, these findings imply additional gatekeeper functions for BRCA genes in tumor suppression mediated by regulation of specific transcriptional targets.

## 7.5 SUMMARY

Despite relatively good understanding of oncogene and tumor suppressor gene mutations associated with certain types of human cancer and the biochemical pathways affected by them, the in vivo circumstances under which tumors develop are probably far more complex. Investigations of genes whose mutations are involved in tumorigenesis revealed the existence of cellular oncogene/tumor suppressor gene networks. Mutations targeting different components of these networks could have similar outcomes with respect to tumor development. Further, immediate cellular environment, including metabolic, mitogenic, and positional clues, activity of various modifier genes within individual cells, as well as selective pressure for tumor growth, play key roles in cancer initiation, progression, and metastasis. Genetic screening of patients for oncogene and tumor suppressor mutations might serve as a foundation for devising customized clinical regimens aimed at treating cancer.

## REFERENCES

Allen LF, Sebolt-Leopold J, Meyer MB. CI-1040 (PD184352), a targeted signal transduction inhibitor of MEK (MAPKK). *Semin Oncology* 2003; 30:105–116.

Berg T, Cohen SB, Dsharnais J, et al: Small-molecule antagonists of Myc/Max dimerization inhibit Myc-induced transformation of chicken embryo fibroblasts. *Proc Natl Acad Sci USA* 2002; 99:3830–3835.

Birroccio A, Leonetti C, Zupi G: The future of antisense therapy: combination with anticancer treatments. *Oncogene* 2003; 22:6579–6588.

Bjorge JD, Jakymiw A, Fujita DJ: Selected glimpses into the activation and function of Src kinase. *Oncogene* 2000; 19:5620–5635.

Blume-Jensen P, Hunter T: Oncogenic kinase signalling. *Nature* 2001: 411:355–365.

Bochar DA, Wang L, Beniya H, et al: BRCA1 is associated with a human SWI/SNF-related complex: linking chromatin remodeling to breast cancer. *Cell* 2000; 102:257–265.

Boettner, B, Van Aelst L: The RASputin effect. *Genes Dev* 2002; 16:2033–2038.

Boffa LC, Scarfi S, Mariani MR, et al: Dihydrotestosterone as a selective cellular/nuclear localization vector for antigene peptide nucleic acid in prostatic carcinoma cells. *Cancer Res* 2000; 60:2258–2262.

Bos JL: Ras oncogenes in human cancer: a review. *Cancer Res* 1989; 49:4682–4689.

Butel JS: Viral carcinogenesis: revelation of molecular mechanisms and etiology of human disease. *Carcinogenesis* 2000; 21:405–426.

Cantley LC, Neel BG: New insights into tumor suppression: PTEN suppresses tumor formation by restraining the phosphoinositide 3–kinase/AKT pathway. *Proc Natl Acad Sci U S A* 1999; 96:4240–4245.

Capdeville R, Silbermann S: Imatinib: A targeted clinical drug development. *Semin Hematol* 2003; 40:15–20.

Caponigro F, Casale M, Bryce J: Farnesyl transferase inhibitors in clinical development. *Expert Opin Investig Drugs* 2003; 12:943–954.

Corsini A, Maggi FM, Catapano AL: Pharmacology of competitive inhibitors of HMG-CoA reductase. *Pharmacol Res* 1995; 31:9–27.

Darnell JE: Transcription factors as targets for cancer therapy. *Nat Rev Cancer* 2002; 2:740–749.

DeCaprio JA, Ludlow JW, Figge J, et al: SV40 large tumor antigen forms a specific complex with the product of the retinoblastoma susceptibility gene. *Cell* 1988; 54:275–283.

Deininger MW: Basic science going clinical: molecularly targeted therapy of chronic myelogenous leukemia. *J Can Res Clin Oncol.* 2004; 130:59–72.

Di Cristofano A, Pandolfi PP: The multiple roles of PTEN in tumor suppression. *Cell* 2000; 100:387–390.

Donehower LA, Harvey M, Slagle BL, et al: Mice deficient for p53 are developmentally normal but susceptible to spontaneous tumours. *Nature* 1992; 356:215–221.

Dyson N: The regulation of E2F by pRB-family proteins. *Genes Dev* 1998; 12:2245–2262.

Dyson N, Howley PM, Munger K, Harlow E: The human papilloma virus-16 E7 oncoprotein is able to bind to the retinoblastoma gene product. *Science* 1989; 243:934–937.

el-Deiry WS, Tokino T, Velculescu, VE, et al: WAF1, a potential mediator of p53 tumor suppression. *Cell* 1993; 75:817–825.

Eng C: PTEN: one gene, many syndromes. *Hum Mutat* 2003; 22:183–198.

Ferrara N, Gerber H-P, LeCouter J: The biology of VEGF and its receptors. *Nat Med* 2003; 9:669–676.

Francke U: Retinoblastoma and chromosome 13. *Cytogenet Cell Genet* 1976; 16:131–134.

Francke U, Holmes LB, Atkins L, Riccardi VM: Aniridia-Wilms' tumor association: evidence for specific deletion of 11p13. *Cytogenet Cell Genet* 1979; 24:185–192.

Furnari FB, Lin H, Huang HS, Cavenee WK: Growth suppression of glioma cells by PTEN requires a functional phosphatase catalytic domain. *Proc Natl Acad Sci USA* 1997; 94:12479–12484.

Greenblatt MS, Bennett WP, Hollstein M, Harris CC: Mutations in the p53 tumor suppressor gene: clues to cancer etiology and molecular pathogenesis. *Cancer Res* 1994; 54:4855–4878.

Griffin J: The biology of signal transduction inhibition: basic science to novel therapies. *Semin Oncol* 2001; 28:3–8.

Hanahan D, Weinberg RA: The hallmarks of cancer. *Cell* 2000; 100:57–70.

Harbou JW, Dean DC: The Rb/E2F pathway: expanding roles and emerging paradigms. *Genes Dev* 2000; 14:2393–2409.

Harris H, Miller OJ, Klein G, et al: Suppression of malignancy by cell fusion. *Nature* 1969; 223:363–368.

Hermeking H: The MYC Oncogene as a cancer drug target. *Curr Cancer Drug Targets* 2003; 3:163–175.

Hilger RA, Scheulen ME, Strumberg D: The Ras-Raf-MEK-ERK pathway in the treatment of cancer. *Onkologie* 2002; 25:511–518.

Kastan MB, Onyekwere O, Sidransky D, et al: Participation of p53 protein in the cellular response to DNA damage. *Cancer Res* 1991; 51:6304–6311.

Kastan MB, Zhan Q, el-Deiry WS, et al: A mammalian cell cycle checkpoint pathway utilizing p53 and GADD45 is defective in ataxia-telangiectasia. *Cell* 1992; 71:587–597.

Kinzler KW, Vogelstein B: Cancer-susceptibility genes. Gatekeepers and caretakers. *Nature* 1997; 386: 761–763.

Knudson AG: Antioncogenes and human cancer. *Proc Natl Acad Sci USA* 1993; 90:10914–10921.

Knudson AG Jr: Mutation and cancer: statistical study of retinoblastoma. *Proc Natl Acad Sci USA* 1971; 68:820–823.

Lee JT Jr, McCubrey JA: The Raf/MEK/ERK signal transduction cascade as a target for chemotherapeutic intervention in leukemia. *Leukemia* 2002; 16:486–507.

Letai A: BH3 domains as BCL-2 inhibitors: prototype cancer therapeutics. *Expert Opin Biol Ther* 2003; 3:293–304.

Li J, Yen C, Liaw D, et al: PTEN, a putative protein tyrosine phosphatase gene mutated in human brain, breast, and prostate cancer. *Science* 1997; 275:1943–1947.

Maestro R, Tos AP, Hamamori Y, et al: Twist is a potential oncogene that inhibits apoptosis. *Genes Dev* 1999; 13:2207–2217.

Malkin D, Li FP, Strong LC, et al: Germ line p53 mutations in a familial syndrome of breast cancer, sarcomas, and other neoplasms. *Science* 1990; 250:1233–1238.

Marsh DJ, Coulon V, Lunetta KL, et al: Mutation spectrum and genotype-phenotype analyses in Cowden disease and Bannayan-Zonana syndrome, two hamartoma syndromes with germline PTEN mutation. *Hum Mol Genet* 1998; 7:507–515.

Nevins JR: The Rb/E2F pathway and cancer. *Hum Mol Genet* 2001; 10:699–703.

O'Brien SG, Guilhot F, Larson RA, et al: Imatinib compared with interferon and low-dose cytarabine for newly diagnosed chronic-phase chronic myeloid leukemia. *N Engl J Med* 2003; 348:994–1004.

Oster SK, Ho CS, Soucie EL, Penn LZ: The myc oncogene: MarvelouslY Complex. *Adv Cancer Res* 2002; 84:81–154.

Pelengaris S, Khan M, Evan G: c-MYC: more than just a matter of life and death. *Nat Rev Cancer* 2002; 2:764–776.

Penn LZ: Apoptosis modulators as cancer therapeutics. *Curr Opin Investig Drugs* 2001; 2:684–692.

Pescarolo MP, Bagnasco L, Malacarne D, et al: A retro-inverso peptide homologous to helix 1 of c-Myc is a potent and specific inhibitor of proliferation in different cellular systems. *FASEB J* 2001; 15:31–33.

Podsypanina K, Ellenson LH, Nemes A, et al: Mutation of Pten/Mmac1 in mice causes neoplasia in multiple organ systems. *Proc Natl Acad Sci USA* 1999; 96:1563–1568.

Rasheed BK, Stenze, TT, McLendon RE, et al: PTEN gene mutations are seen in high-grade but not in low-grade gliomas. *Cancer Res* 1997; 57:4187–4190.

Reed JC: Bcl-2 family proteins. *Oncogene* 1998; 17:3225–3236.

Reilly JT: Receptor tyrosine kinases in normal and malignant haematopoiesis. *Blood Rev* 2003; 17;241–248.

Saxon PJ, Srivatsan ES, Stanbridge EJ: Introduction of human chromosome 11 via microcell transfer controls tumorigenic expression of HeLa cells. *EMBO J* 1986; 5:3461–3466.

Scully R, Livingston DM: In search of the tumour-suppressor functions of BRCA1 and BRCA2. *Nature* 2000; 408: 429–432.

Scully R, Puget N, Vlasakova K: DNA polymerase stalling, sister chromatid recombination and the BRCA genes. *Oncogene* 2000; 19:6176–6183.

Sebolt-Leopold JS, Dudley DT, Herrera R, et al: Blockade of the MAP kinase pathway suppresses growth of colon tumors in vivo. *Nat Med* 1999; 5:810–816.

Sebti SM, Hamilton AD: Farnesyltransferase and geranylgeranyltransferase I inhibitors as novel agents for cancer and cardiovascular disease. In: Sebti SM, Hamilton AD, eds. *Farnesyltransferase Inhibitors in Cancer Therapy*. Totowa, NJ: Humana Press Inc; 2001: 197–219.

Shah NP, Sawyers CL: Mechanisms of resistance to STI571 in Philadelphia chromosome-associated leukemias. *Oncogene* 2003; 22:7389–7395.

Shangary S, Johnson DE: Recent advances in the development of anticancer agents targeting cell death inhibitors in the Bcl-2 protein family. *Leukemia* 2003; 17:1470–1481.

Sherr CJ: Cancer cell cycles. *Science* 1996; 274:1672–1677.

Sherr CJ: The INK4a/ARF network in tumour suppression. *Nat Rev Mol Cell Biol* 2001; 2:731–737.

Sridhar SS, Shepherd FA: Targeting angiogenesis: a review of angiogenesis inhibitors in the treatment of lung cancer. *Lung Cancer* 2003; 42:S81–S91.

Stahel RA, Zangemeister-Wittke U: Antisense oligonucleotides for cancer therapy—an overview. *Lung Cancer* 2003; 41:S81–S88.

Stambolic V, Mak TW, Woodgett JR: Modulation of cellular apoptotic potential: contributions to oncogenesis. *Oncogene* 1999; 18:6094–6103.

Stambolic V, Suzuk A, de la Pompa JL, et al: Negative regulation of PKB/Akt-dependent cell survival by the tumor suppressor PTEN. *Cell* 1998; 95:29–39.

Stambolic V, Tsao MS, Macpherson D, et al: High incidence of breast and endometrial neoplasia resembling human Cowden syndrome in pten+/− mice. *Cancer Res* 2000; 60:3605–3611.

Stanbridge EJ, Der CJ, Doersen CJ, et al: Human cell hybrids: analysis of transformation and tumorigenicity. *Science* 1982; 215:252–259.

Steck PA, Pershouse MA, Jasser SA, et al: Identification of a candidate tumour suppressor gene, MMAC1, at chromosome 10q23.3 that is mutated in multiple advanced cancers. *Nat Genet* 1997; 15:356–362.

Sun J, Ohkanda J, Coppola D, et al: Geranylgeranyltransferase I inhibitor GGTI-2154 induces breast carcinoma apoptosis and tumor regression in H-Ras transgenic mice. *Cancer Res.* 2003; 634:8922–8929.

Vogelstein B, Kinzler KW: The Genetic Basis of Human Cancer. New York: McGraw-Hill Professional, 2002.

Vousden KH: p53: death star. *Cell* 2000; 103:691–694.

Vousden KH: Activation of the p53 tumor suppressor protein. *Biochim Biophys Acta* 2002; 1602:47–59.

Wang XW, Vermeulen W, Coursen JD, et al: The XPB and XPD DNA helicases are components of the p53–mediated apoptosis pathway. *Genes Dev* 1996; 10:1219–1232.

Weinberg RA: The retinoblastoma protein and cell cycle control. *Cell* 1995; 81:323–330.

Weissman BE, Saxon PJ, Pasquale SR, et al: Introduction of a normal human chromosome 11 into a Wilms' tumor cell line controls its tumorigenic expression. *Science* 1987; 236:175–180.

Welsch PL, King MC: BRCA1 and BRCA2 and the genetics of breast and ovarian cancer. *Hum Mol Genet* 2001; 10:705–713.

Whyte P, Buchkovich KJ, Horowitz JM, et al: Association between an oncogene and an anti-oncogene: the adenovirus E1A proteins bind to the retinoblastoma gene product. *Nature* 1988; 334:124–129.

Wong WW-L, Dimitroulakos J, Minden MD, Penn LZ: HMG-CoA reductase inhibitors and the malignant cell: the statin family of drugs as triggers of tumor-specific apoptosis. *Leukemia* 2002; 16:508–519.

# 8

# Cellular Signaling

*Melanie A. McGill and C. Jane McGlade*

## 8.1 INTRODUCTION

The ability of cells to receive and respond to extracellular signals is a critical process in the embryonic development of multicellular organisms as well as for the maintenance and survival of mature tissues in the adult. Changes in the physical or chemical environment of the cell can result in modifications of cell metabolism, structure, movement, or growth. Cellular responses are brought about by elaborate networks of intracellular signals transmitted by changes in protein phosphorylation and enzymatic activity, localization, and the formation of protein-protein complexes. Cellular responses are triggered by the recognition of extracellular signals at the cell surface, resulting in the activation of linked cytoplasmic and nuclear biochemical cascades. These signal transduction pathways control cellular processes from the generalized control of cell proliferation and survival to specialized functions such as the immune response and angiogenesis. When dysregulated, signaling pathways involved in normal growth, adhesion, and development contribute to malignant transformation in human cells. With this knowledge has come the development of new cancer therapeutics that specifically target aberrant signal transduction pathways. This chapter will explore how selected signal transduction pathways are organized and regulated with a particular focus on pathways that control cellular properties relevant to the malignant phenotype.

## 8.2 SIGNALING PATHWAYS TRIGGERED BY GROWTH FACTORS

### 8.2.1 Extracellular Growth Factors

In multicellular organisms, cell regulation is controlled by secreted polypeptide molecules called *growth factors* or *cytokines*, by antigen stimulation of immune cells, or by cell contact with neighboring cells and surrounding extracellular matrix. Our most detailed understanding of signal transduction pathways comes from studies of soluble growth factors and their interaction with complementary growth factor receptors expressed on responsive cells. Interaction of growth factors with receptors on the cell surface leads to the modification of intracellular biochemical signaling pathways that control cellular responses, especially cell proliferation. Cellular regulation also occurs through direct cell-to-cell contact or cell contact with its surrounding extracellular matrix (as discussed in Sec. 8.3.3).

Growth factors were first identified in cell culture medium required to sustain mammalian cell survival and proliferation. One of the characteristics of malignant transformation was found to be relative independence from the action of external growth factors. A large number of polypeptide growth factors have been identified with diverse functions in normal embryonic development and tissue homeostasis, but only a few have been associated with the process of malignant transformation. Polypeptide growth factors influence cellular processes such as growth, proliferation, differentiation, survival, and metabolism via their interaction with specific transmembrane receptor protein tyrosine kinases (RPTKs; van der Geer et al., 1994). Most growth factors, secreted by one cell type, bind to specific receptor proteins on a different cell. These receptor molecules span the plasma membrane and thus connect the receipt of an extracellular signal to the intracellu-

lar environment (Fig. 8.1). Most growth factors are small monomeric (i.e., single chain) polypeptides, such as epidermal growth factor (EGF) and members of the fibroblast growth factor (FGF) family. There are also dimeric polypeptide growth factors (i.e., those containing two chains of amino acids), such as platelet-derived growth factor (PDGF). In addition to being freely diffusible, growth factors can also reside in spatially restricted domains within an organism, either through binding to components in the extracellular matrix, or because they are produced as membrane-anchored molecules that reside on the surface of the producing cells. The properties of selected growth factors and their receptors are summarized in Table 8.1.

### 8.2.2 Growth Factor Receptor Tyrosine Kinases

Receptors for growth factors are membrane-spanning cell surface molecules that share the ability to phosphorylate themselves and other cytoplasmic proteins on

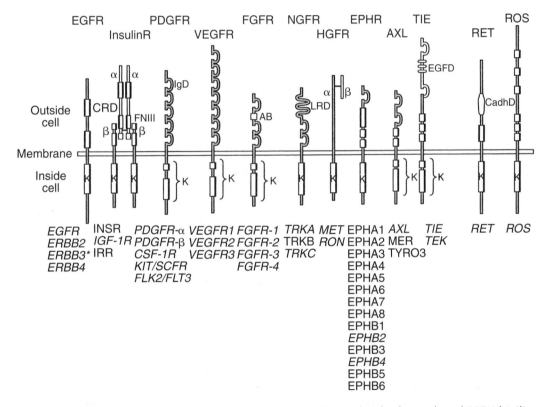

**Figure 8.1.** The receptor protein tyrosine kinases. Representative molecules from selected RPTK families are shown and additional family members are listed underneath: EGFR, epidermal growth factor receptor; PDGFR, platelet-derived growth factor receptor; VEGFR, vascular endothelial growth factor receptor; FGFR, fibroblast growth factor receptor; NGFR, nerve growth factor receptor; HGFR, hepatocyte growth factor receptor; EPHR, ephrin receptor; AXL, a tyro3 RPTK; TIE, tyrosine kinase receptor in endothelial cells. All members have a conserved intracellular kinase domain (k). Some of the common structural elements found in the extracellular ligand binding domain include the CRD (cysteine-rich domain), FNIII (fibronectin type III repeats), IgD (immunoglobulin-like domain), AB (acid-rich box), LRD (leucine-rich domain); EGFD (epidermal growth factor-like domain); and CadhD (cadherin-like domain). Italic type indicates RPTK members that are implicated in human malignancies. Asterisk indicates the RPTK has no intrinsic kinase activity.

**Table 8.1.** Properties of Selected Polypeptide Growth Factors

| Growth Factor | Description | Receptors |
|---|---|---|
| Platelet-derived growth factor, PDGF<br>PDGFA, PDGFB, PDGFC, PDGFD | Secreted disulfide-linked homodimers; PDGFA and PDGFB also form heterodimers | Homo- or heterodimers of transmembrane tyrosine kinases PDGFRα and PDGFRβ |
| Epidermal growth factors | Mature peptides derived from proteolytic cleavage of transmembrane precursors | Transmembrane tyrosine kinases |
|    Epidermal growth factor (EGF) | | EGFR/Her1/ErbB-1 |
|    Transforming growth factor-α (TGF-α) | | EGFR/Her1/ErbB-1 |
|    Amphiregulin | | EGFR/Her1/ErbB-1 |
|    Epigen | | EGFR/Her1/ErbB-1 |
|    Heparin-binding(HB)-EGF | | EGFR/Her1/ErbB1; Her4/ErbB4 |
|    Betacellulin | | EGFR/Her1/ErbB1; Her4/ErbB4 |
|    Epiregulin | | EGFR/Her1/ErbB1; Her4/ErbB4 |
| No natural ligand identified | | EGFR2/Her2/Erb2; EGFR3/Her3/Erb-3 |
| Fibroblast growth factors | Small secreted polypeptides that require heparin sulfate for activation | Transmembrane tyrosine kinases |
|    FGF1, 2 | Acidic and basic FGF, respectively | FGFR-1, 2, 3, 4 |
|    FGF3 | | FGFR-1, 2 |
|    FGF4, 6 | | FGFR-1, 2, 4, &3 (FGF4) |
|    FGF5 | | FGFR-1,2 |
|    FGF7, 10 | | FGFR-2, 1 (FGF10) |
|    FGF8 | | FGFR-1, 2, 3, 4 |
|    FGF9 | | FGFR-2, 3, 4 |
|    FGF11, 12, 13, 14 | FGF homology factors remain intracellular | ? |
|    FGF15 | | ? |
|    FGF16, 17, 18, 19 | | FGF17 binds FGFR-1, 2 |
|    FGF20 | | |
| Transforming growth factor-β family (TGF-β) | Biologically active as dimer; synthesized as an inactive proform that is cleaved and secreted | Complex of one of 7 Type I and one of 5 Type II receptors which possess ser/thr kinase activity |
|    TGF-β1-5<br>   Bone morphogenetic protein (BMP)<br>   Nodals<br>   Activins | | |
| Insulin-like growth factor | Mature peptide consists of B and A domains linked by a C and D domain | Dimer of transmembrane tyrosine kinases |
|    IGF-1 | | IGF-1R |
|    IGF-2 | | IGF-1R, IGF-2R |
| Neurotrophins | Secreted as mature noncovalently linked homodimeric proteins generated from pre-pro-precursors | Specific receptor tyrosine kinases and common receptor p75$^{NTR}$ |
|    Nerve growth factor (NGF) | | Trk A, p75$^{NTR}$ |
|    Brain-derived neurotrophic factor (BDNF) | | Trk B, p75$^{NTR}$ |
|    Neurotrophin-3 (NT-3) | | Trk C, p75$^{NTR}$ |
|    Neurotrophin-4/5 (NT-4/5) | | p75$^{NTR}$ |
| Hepatocyte growth factor (HGF) | Glycosylated heterodimer | Tyrosine kinase, c-Met |
| Ephrins | Membrane tethered ligands | Transmembrane tyrosine kinases |
|    A-class<br>     EphrinA1-ephrinA5 | Glycosylphosphatidylinositol (GPI) anchored ligands | EphA1-A8 |
|    B-class<br>     EphrinB1-ephrinB3 | Transmembrane ligands with intrinsic signaling properties | EphB1-EphB4, EphB6<br>EphA4 also binds ephrinB2, and B3 |

tyrosine residues, thereby activating a signaling cascade (van der Geer et al., 1994; Blume-Jensen and Hunter, 2001). This large family of molecules (over 60 have been identified) are referred to as receptor protein tyrosine kinases (RPTKs), and are subdivided into twenty different families based on distinct structural components (van der Geer et al., 1994). Figure 8.1 shows a schematic representation of the major RPTK families. The main distinguishing feature among RPTK subgroups resides in the extracellular growth-factor-binding domain at the amino terminus. Usually several hundred amino acids in length, these extracellular domains can be grouped by sequence homology, by the position of conserved cysteine amino acids, or by the presence of sequence motifs also found in other functionally unrelated molecules such EGF repeats, immunoglobulin repeats, or fibronectin type III repeats. The extracellular domains of RPTKs are also commonly modified posttranslationally by glycosylation.

The extracellular domain is connected to the intracellular (cytoplasmic) domain by a single short hydrophobic helix transmembrane component (Fig. 8.1). The cytoplasmic domain is comprised of regulatory sequences and a conserved kinase domain, which catalyzes the transfer of a phosphate group from adenosine triphosphate (ATP) onto a protein substrate. Most growth factor receptors are protein tyrosine kinases that specifically phosphorylate the amino acid tyrosine in protein substrates. The core catalytic domain is typically about 260 amino acids in length and is as much as 90 percent identical between members of this protein kinase family (Hanks and Quinn, 1991; Robinson et al., 2000).The amino acids flanking the kinase domain and

adjacent to the plasma membrane (juxtamembrane region) of growth factor receptors frequently contain sites of tyrosine phosphorylation and these regions often have important roles in both signal transmission and in regulation of catalytic activity. Such regulatory sequences can also reside within the catalytic domain of receptor kinases. Members of the PDGFR and VEGFR families of receptors are distinguished by possessing a split kinase domain in which important autophosphorylation sites are present on a kinase insert within the catalytic domain (van der Geer et al., 1994).

Binding of the growth factor or ligand induces conformational changes in the extracellular domain of the receptor that facilitates dimerization (i.e., joining together) or clustering of receptor tyrosine kinases (Fig. 8.2). Some ligands, such as PDGF, are themselves dimeric forms of a single subunit and naturally induce a symmetric ligand/receptor dimer. Structural studies have revealed how other ligands that exist as monomers, such as EGF, can induce receptor dimerization (Schlessinger, 2002). These studies revealed that binding of EGF to EGFR (ErbB1 or Her1) induces a conformational change that exposes a dimerization loop that mediates association of neighboring ligand-occupied receptors. Similar dimerization loops are found in the other members of the EGFR family (ErbB2, ErbB3, and ErbB4), allowing the formation of heterodimers between different members of the ErbB family. Dimerization of receptors also leads to conformational switches within the cytoplasmic domain required for full catalytic activity. Some RPTKs, such as the insulin receptor, exist as inactive dimers that undergo a conformational change following ligand binding, which re-

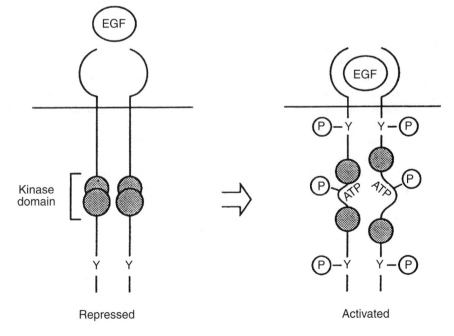

**Figure 8.2.** Growth factor receptor dimerization and activation. In the absence of ligand (EGF) binding the intracellular kinase domain is inactive, held in a repressed conformation by intramolecular interactions. Ligand binding induces receptor dimerization, relief of inhibitory constraints, and autophosphorylation of the intracellular domains on tyrosine residues. These autophosphorylation sites function to both enhance the catalytic activity and serve as docking sites for intracellular signaling molecules that bind to phosphotyrosine. P, phosphate; Y, tyrosine.

sults in the close juxtaposition of the catalytic domains (Yip and Ottensmeyer, 2003). The juxtamembrane region of receptors from the Eph and PDGFR families represses the activity of the kinase domain and this repression is relieved by ligand binding (Hubbard, 2001).

Ligand binding, receptor dimerization, and the consequent conformational changes in the growth factor receptor bring together two catalytic domains, resulting in intermolecular autophosphorylation (transphosphorylation) of tyrosine residues within the catalytic domain and in the noncatalytic regulatory regions of the cytoplasmic domain. Phosphorylation of key residues within the kinase activation loop induces the opening of the catalytic site and allows access to ATP and protein substrates, while phosphorylated residues in noncatalytic regions create docking sites for downstream signaling molecules that are essential for signal propagation (Fig. 8.2; Pawson, 2002).

Abnormal RPTKs involved in cancer are deregulated by loss of one or more of the autoinhibitory mechanisms described above, making their catalytic activity ligand independent. For example, the *ErbB2/neu* oncogene encodes an RPTK that is frequently amplified in human breast and other tumors. Increased expression is thought to increase the concentration of active dimers generating continuous and inappropriate cellular signaling. Similarly, mutations in the juxtamembrane regulatory region of the Kit receptor are associated with gastrointestinal stromal tumors (Blume-Jensen and Hunter, 2001).

### 8.2.3 Cytoplasmic Signaling Molecules

Signaling pathways downstream of activated RPTKs are constructed through interactions of specific proteins that create networks of signaling molecules. These signaling networks consist of both preformed and rapidly associating protein complexes that transmit information throughout the cell. A unifying feature of cytoplasmic signaling proteins is the presence of one or more conserved noncatalytic domains that mediate sequence specific protein-protein interactions. The modular nature of these domains allows them to be used in diverse groups of cytoplasmic signaling molecules (Pawson and Scott, 1997). Many of these domains bind specifically to short (typically less than 10 amino acids) contiguous regions of their target protein. In some cases the binding of specific domains to their target requires phosphorylation of amino acids within the sequence-specific binding motif. Proteins that contain either SH2 (Src Homology 2) or PTB (phosphotyrosine binding domains), which recognize tyrosine phosphorylated sequence motifs, are central to the formation of signaling complexes following activation of growth factor receptor tyrosine kinases (Fig. 8.3; Schlessinger and Lemmon, 2003).

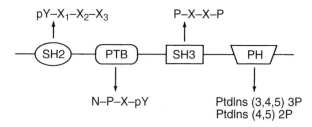

**Figure 8.3.** Examples of modular interaction domains. Representation of the protein modules most commonly found in intracellular signaling proteins that are linked to growth factor receptor signaling cascades. Each is shown with its consensus peptide or phospholipid (PtdIns) binding target. For each example shown there are notable exceptions. For example, the SH2 domain of SLAM associated protein (SAP) can bind ligands in the absence of tyrosine phosphorylation; several PTB domains including those of the X11 and Numb proteins binds to NPXY motifs in the absence of phosphorylation, and the SH3 domain of Gads, binds to an R-X-X-K motif. The domains are represented as if linked together on a single polypeptide to illustrate how the presence of multiple domains within signaling molecules would facilitate the assembly of larger signaling complexes. N, asparagine; P, proline; Y, tyrosine; X, any amino acid; R, arginine; K, lysine.

The SH2 domain was identified as a conserved region containing approximately 100 amino acids found outside the catalytic domain of Src family cytoplasmic tyrosine kinases (Pawson and Gish, 1992). The specificity of SH2 domain recognition is determined both by the requirement for phosphotyrosine, common to almost all SH2 domains, and by three to four amino acids (often termed the +1, +2, and +3 residues relative to the phosphotyrosine) on the carboxy-terminal side of the tyrosine residue. Individual SH2 domains bind selectively to distinct phosphopeptide motifs, and the preferred consensus binding sequences for many SH2 domains have been defined (Songyang et al., 1993). A distantly related SH2 domain, also called a TKB domain, is found in the cytoplasmic protein c-Cbl. Although TKB and SH2 domains have no primary amino acid sequence similarity, three-dimensional structural analysis has shown that the phosphotyrosine recognition properties of these domains are similar (Meng et al., 1999).

In 1994 a second, structurally unrelated protein module that specifically binds phosphotyrosine-containing peptides was identified. In contrast to SH2 domains, PTB (Phospho-Tyrosine Binding) domains recognize phosphotyrosine in a specific sequence motif where amino acids on the amino terminal side of the tyrosine are critical for binding specificity (van der Geer and Pawson, 1995; Forman-Kay and Pawson, 1999). Some PTB domains recognize specific nonphosphorylated sequences, suggesting that at least two distinct subfamilies of PTB domains exist.

Activation of growth factor receptors results in the autophosphorylation of the receptor at multiple tyrosine residues, and results in the creation of a number of docking sites for cytoplasmic proteins which contain SH2 or PTB domains (Schlessinger and Lemmon, 2003). Several other strategies for creating these docking sites are employed by, for example, the insulin receptor (IR) where the major substrate IRS-1 becomes phosphorylated at multiple sites following stimulation, and the T-cell receptor (see Sec. 8.3.2), where activation of associated cytoplasmic tyrosine kinases, such as Lck, results in the phosphorylation of the membrane-associated protein LAT. Tyrosine phosphorylation of IRS-1 and LAT creates multiple docking sites for SH2-domain-containing proteins (Myers et al., 1994; Samelson, 2002). SH2 and PTB domains therefore play crucial roles in linking an external signal received by a membrane receptor to cytoplasmic signaling pathways.

### 8.2.4 Formation of Multiprotein Complexes and Signal Transmission

Since the original description of the SH2 domain, dozens of additional protein modules have been identified, and, for most, their three-dimensional structures have been described and distinct target specificities have been defined (Pawson and Nash, 2003). All of these interaction modules are independently folding domains such that their amino and carboxy termini are in close proximity and the ligand binding surfaces are available when they are incorporated into a larger polypeptide. In addition to tyrosine phosphorylated peptides described above, the specific binding partners for protein modules include phosphoserine- or phosphothreonine-containing peptides, proline-rich peptides, and carboxy terminal motifs. Some families of interaction domains bind to phospholipids in membranes, while others form homo- or heterotypic interactions with similar domains. Many cytoplasmic signaling molecules possess multiple interaction domains either as multiple copies of one domain or in combinations of different domains.

Two additional protein interaction domains often found in signaling molecules downstream of growth factor receptors are the SH3 (Src homology 3) and PH (Pleckstrin homology) domain (Fig. 8.3). SH3 domains are approximately sixty amino acids in length and can bind to proline rich motifs in target proteins. The interaction is not dependent on changes induced by phosphorylation. SH3 domains are known to function in the assembly of multiprotein complexes, and as regulatory domains in intramolecular interactions. Several additional domains that bind proline rich motifs include the WW domain and the EVH1 domain that are found in important signaling proteins (Zarrinpar et al., 2003).

Pleckstrin homology domains are protein modules of approximately 120 amino acids in length that interact specifically with membrane phosphoinositides (phosphorylated forms of phosphatidylinositol; PtdIns). Phosphoinositides are found at low levels within the cell and can be rapidly modified by phosphorylation in response to signaling. Importantly, PH domains recognize specific phosphoinositides such as $PtdIns(3,4,5)P3$ that are transiently produced following growth factor receptor activation. An important function of PH domains, therefore, is the recruitment of PH domain containing proteins to the membrane in the vicinity of an activated growth factor receptor. Additional phosphoinositide binding modules such as the PX (phox homology) and FYVE domains, which preferentially bind to distinct phosphoinositides, also function to recruit signaling molecules to discrete membrane locations (Lemmon, 2003).

Most cytoplasmic signaling molecules that are targets of tyrosine kinases contain one or more SH2 domains. Subsets of these also contain one or more SH3 domains. Some signaling proteins have no catalytic function (e.g., nck, crk, and grb2) and are composed entirely of SH2 and SH3 domains. This type of molecule has been termed an *adaptor protein* because it functions by interacting with signaling enzymes which do not contain SH2 domains (or other phosphotyrosine containing modules such as PTB or TKB domains), thereby coupling them to a tyrosine kinase signaling complex (Pawson and Scott, 1997). The structure of these adaptor molecules is such that each has a different capacity to form protein complexes due to the binding specificity of its SH2 and SH3 domains, and the result is an organized network of protein-protein interactions essential to coordinate an appropriate cellular response.

Figure 8.4 illustrates three examples of protein module function in the activation of growth factor receptor signal transduction. The phospholipase enzyme PLCγ contains two SH2 domains that mediate its recruitment to activated growth factor receptors. PLCγ is then tyrosine phosphorylated by the activated RPTK, which stimulates its phospholipase activity. Hydrolysis of the membrane phosphoinositide $PtdIns(4,5)P2$ by phospholipases plays an important role in signal transduction by generating the second messengers DAG (diacylglycerol) and IP3 (inositol 1,4,5 triphosphate). Diacylglycerol is an activator of downstream protein kinases (e.g., PKC), while IP3 mobilizes $Ca^{2+}$ from intracellular stores affecting $Ca^{2+}$ dependent processes in the cell.

The SH2 and SH3 domain-containing adaptor protein, grb-2 (growth factor receptor bound-2) plays a critical role in the activation of the small GTPase protein, Ras, a central transducer of growth factor receptor signals. As described in Section 8.2.5, Ras proteins are membrane-associated molecules that actively signal when bound to the guanine nucleotide GTP. The

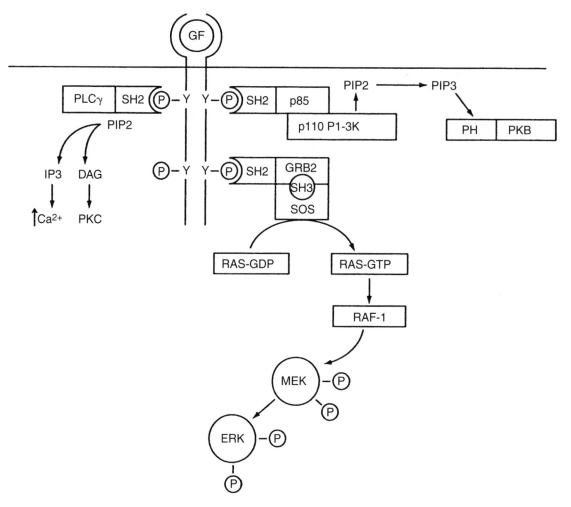

**Figure 8.4.** Recruitment of cytoplasmic signaling molecules by receptor protein tyrosine kinases. Binding of a receptor to a growth factor leads to phosphorylation of the intracellular domain on tyrosine residues; this allows the SH2 domain-mediated association of enzymes such as phospholipase C which hydrolyzes phosphatidyl inositol (PIP2) into inositol triphosphate (IP3) and diacylglycerol (DAG). Adaptor molecules such as GRB2 (growth factor receptor bound 2) and p85 also bind to activated receptors via their SH2 domains. GRB2 is associated with the guanine nucleotide exchange factor SOS (Son-of-Sevenless). SOS is recruited to activated receptor complexes then catalyzes the exchange of GDP for GTP on RAS. The heterodimeric phosphoinositide kinase, PI-3 kinase, comprises a catalytic subunit, p110, and an adaptor or regulatory subunit, called p85, that contains two SH2 domains. Binding of the p85/p110 complex to activated growth factor receptors via the p85 SH2 domain activates catalytic activity of p110, which phosphorylates phosphoinositides. The products of this reaction, PIP2 and PIP3, serve as membrane anchoring sites for PH domain containing proteins such as PKB. See text for additional details.

SH2 domain of grb-2 associates with activated growth factor receptors while its SH3 domains are bound to proline based motifs in SOS (Son-of-Sevenless), a guanine nucleotide exchange protein that activates Ras. Therefore, receptor activation leads to the recruitment of the grb2-SOS complex close to its target, Ras, leading to its activation and downstream signaling.

Activation of growth factor receptors also results in the activation of phosphoinositide kinases called PI-3 kinases that phosphorylate the 3′ hydroxyl group of the inositol ring. PI-3 kinase is made up of a catalytic subunit, p110, and an adaptor or regulatory subunit, called p85, that contains two SH2 domains. Following receptor activation, the PI-3 kinase heterodimer is recruited to the activated receptor by the p85 SH2 domains, where binding to specific phosphotyrosine interaction motifs leads to allosteric activation of the p110 catalytic subunit causing phosphorylation of phosphoinositides to produce PIP2 and PIP3.

### 8.2.5 Ras Proteins

Ras proteins control signaling pathways that regulate normal cell growth and malignant transformation.

Three distinct Ras protein isoforms—H-ras, K-ras, and N-ras—have been identified in mammals and are part of a large family of small (low molecular weight) guanine nucleotide triphosphate (GTP) binding proteins. The three Ras proteins have a molecular weight of 21 kilodaltons (hence the designation p21$^{Ras}$) and share 85 percent sequence homology. Despite interacting with a common set of activators and effectors, genetic studies in mice indicate that Ras proteins have subtly different functions during development (Downward, 1990; Downward, 2003). The Ras proteins are GTPases that cycle between an active GTP-bound "on" and an inactive GDP-bound "off" configuration in response to extracellular signals, essentially functioning as a molecular binary switch (Fig. 8.5). Ras is activated by the effects of guanine nucleotide exchange factors (GEFs) such as SOS, described above, that release Ras-bound GDP and allow GTP binding. Termination of Ras activity occurs through the hydrolysis of GTP, converting it to GDP by action of GTPase-activating proteins (GAPs) which promote the intrinsic GTPase activity of the Ras proteins themselves. Therefore, a balance of the activities of GEFs and GAPs determines the activity of normal Ras proteins. Both the GEFs and a number of the GAP family members, which are often represented by p120$^{GAP}$, are themselves regulated by receptor tyrosine kinase signaling cascades (Sprang, 1997). Several oncogenic mutations of *Ras* have been identified that inhibit its intrinsic GTPase activity, trapping it in the activated GTP-bound state. Deregulated and constitutively active mutations of *Ras* lead to cell transformation.

In the active GTP-bound form, Ras proteins bind to a number of distinct effector proteins that in turn, activate downstream signaling cascades. One of the best characterized is its interaction with the protein kinase Raf-1. Ras-GTP binding to Raf-1 activates its kinase activity, and consequently the downstream cascade of protein kinases, including MEK and ERK (see Sec. 8.2.6). Additional Ras-GTP effectors include RAL GDS (RAL guanine nucleotide dissociation stimulator), a GEF for another small GTPase, RAL, and the p110 catalytic subunit of PI-3K (Fig. 8.5). Through these diverse effectors, Ras proteins regulate cell cycle progression, cell survival, and cytoskeletal organization.

The normal function of Ras proteins requires them to be posttranslationally modified. Newly synthesized Ras proteins are processed by a protein farnesyl transferase that adds an isoprenoid chain group to a cysteine residue in the carboxy terminus of Ras proteins. This covalently-linked farnesyl group is required for Ras association with intracellular membranes. Both H-ras and N-ras are also subsequently modified by the addition of two palmitoyl long-chain fatty acids that are important for the correct localization of these proteins to specific membrane locations. Recent evidence suggests that Ras proteins are activated and propagate signals from specific microdomains within the plasma membrane, as well as from distinct subcellular compartments such as the Golgi and endosomes (Hancock, 2003).

Abnormalities in Ras protein activity have been identified in many human malignancies, due to either mutations which render it active and locked in a GTP-bound state, or to deregulated signaling from upstream pathways. As such, Ras proteins are promising targets for anti-cancer therapeutics, as described in Chapter 7, Section 7.3.2 (Downward, 2003).

Members of a related family of small GTPases, which includes Rho, Rac, and Cdc42 are important regulators of cell morphology, motility, and the actin cytoskeleton. Similar to the Ras proteins, Rho proteins also cycle between GTP and GDP bound states and are regulated by Rho specific GEFs and GAPs. In addition, the activity of Rho proteins is regulated by GDP dissociation inhibitors (GDIs), which bind and sequester Rho proteins in the GDP bound "off" state. Growth factor receptor, integrin (Sec. 8.3.3) and Wnt (Sec. 8.4.1) signaling can

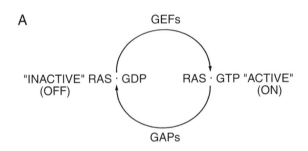

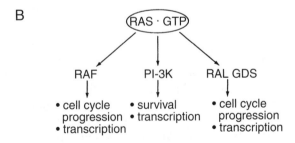

**Figure 8.5.** Ras protein activation and downstream signaling. (*A*) The small GTPase Ras cycles between an inactive GDP bound state and the active GTP bound state. Ras activation is regulated by guanine nucleotide exchange factors (GEFs) that promote exchange of GDP for GTP. GTP hydrolysis requires GTPase activating proteins (GAPs) which enhance the weak intrinsic GTPase activity of RAS proteins. (*B*) Once in its active GTP bound form, RAS interacts with different families of effector proteins including RAF protein kinases, phosphoinositide 3–kinases (PI-3K), and RAL GDS, a GEF for the RAS related protein RAL. Activation of these downstream pathways leads to cellular responses including gene transcription, cell cycle progression, and survival.

activate Rho proteins, and GTP bound Rho interacts with effector proteins that regulate a range of cellular behaviors, such as actin polymerization, cell polarity, and activation of MAPK signaling cascades. Rho proteins are required for cellular transformation by oncogenic Ras proteins, and their activation promotes tumor metastasis (see Chap. 11, Sec. 11.5.2). Although mutant, activated forms of Rho are not found in human tumors, elevated expression of Rho proteins in breast and colon cancer, for example, is correlated with tumor progression (Sahai and Marshall, 2002). The critical effector pathways that mediate the tumorigenic effects of Rho proteins are an area of ongoing investigation.

In addition to Rho and Ras family members, another distinct class of heterotrimeric guanine nucleotide-binding proteins (G proteins) function in the transmission of signals from membrane-spanning receptors for hormones, neurotransmitters, and chemokines. Space constraints prevent a thorough discussion of G protein coupled receptors and their function in relation to cancer, and the reader is referred to Hamm, 1998 and Neves and coworkers, 2002 (and references therein) for a more detailed discussion of G protein signaling networks.

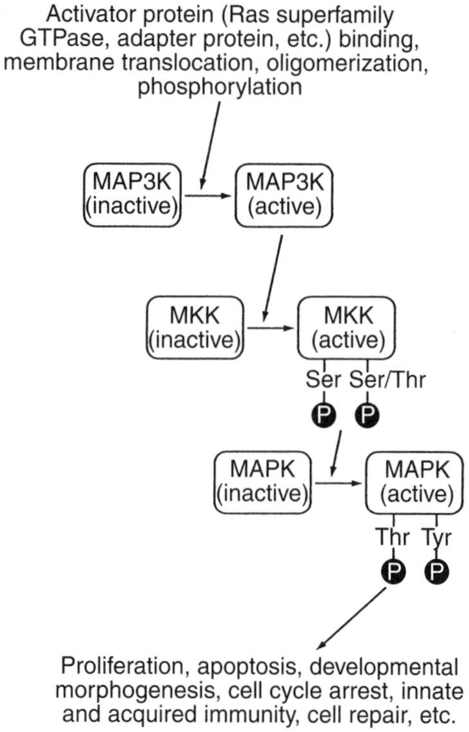

### 8.2.6 Mitogen Activated Protein Kinase Signaling Pathways

The mitogen activated protein kinases (MAPK) regulate highly conserved signaling pathways in all eukaryotic cells. Mammalian cells contain multiple distinct MAPK pathways that respond to divergent signals, including growth factors and environmental stresses such as osmotic stress and ionizing radiation (Chang and Karin, 2001; Kyriakis and Avruch, 2001). All MAPK pathways include a core three-tiered signaling unit, in which MAPKs are activated by the sequential activation of linked serine/threonine kinases (Fig. 8.6). The MAPKs are activated by phosphorylation of threonine (Thr) and tyrosine (Tyr) residues in a T-X-Y motif in the kinase activation loop. This phosphorylation is achieved by a family of dual specificity kinases, referred to as MEKs or MKKs (MAPK-kinase). MEK activity is regulated by serine and threonine phosphorylation catalyzed by kinases called MAP3Ks (MAPK-kinase-kinase). A number of distinct families of MAP3Ks are activated by diverse upstream stimuli that link the activation of the MAPK signaling unit to extracellular signals. These structurally related pathways are controlled by stimuli having very different physiologic consequences (i.e., mitogenesis or the stress response) and have become functionally distinct (Fig. 8.6). Pathway integrity is maintained by scaffold molecules that bind and physically link specific core pathway components. Similarly, although all MAPKs

**Figure 8.6.** The MAPK core signaling module. MAPK pathways include a core three-tiered signaling unit, in which MAPKs are activated by the sequential activation of linked serine/threonine kinases. The MKKs are unique dual specificity kinases that phosporylate both tyrosine (Tyr) and threonine (Thr) residues within an activation motif found in the MAPKs. P, phosphate; Ser, Serine.

phosphorylate very similar consensus motifs in their target substrates, specificity of protein substrate selection is ensured by docking domains that mediate binding of kinases to their substrates (Sharrocks et al., 2000).

Three distinct MAPK pathways in mammalian cells have been extensively characterized, the extracellular signal regulated kinase 1 and 2 (ERK1/2), the c-Jun N-terminal kinase or stress activated protein kinase (JNK/SAPK), and the p38 pathways (Fig. 8.7). As described in Section 8.2.5 and Figure 8.4, activation of Ras proteins causes the activation of Raf-1, a MAP3K upstream of ERK1/2. ERK kinase activation is part of a final common pathway used by growth factor receptors such as those for EGF, PGDF, FGF, and by more diverse stimuli from cytokine receptors and antigen receptors. Raf-1 directly activates MEK-1/2 by phosphorylating it on serine residues, which enhances the availability of the catalytic site to potential substrates. Activated MEK-1/2 is a dual specificity kinase that phosphorylates the ERK kinases. MEK-induced phosphorylation of ERK occurs on threonine and tyrosine at the TEY [single-letter amino acid abbreviation for threonine (T), glutamic acid (E), tyrosine (Y)] motif, which induces both catalytic activation of ERK and its translocation to the nucleus. Nuclear ERK interacts with specific transcription factors, such as ELK-1, that contain an ERK docking site, leading to their phosphorylation and activation of specific transcriptional targets.

The SAPK and p38 pathways mediate responses to cellular stresses such as extremes of heat, exposure to ultraviolet and ionizing radiation, anticancer drugs, and exposure to potentially damaging biologic agents such as the cytokines IL-1 and tumor necrosis factor (TNF). The core components of the SAPK and p38 parallel those of the ERK pathway, although the upstream activation steps are less well defined (Fig. 8.7). Stress activated protein kinase is phosphorylated by the dual specificity kinases SEK1 and MKK7, and p38 is activated by MKK3 and MKK6. As in the ERK pathway, both the SAPK and p38 kinase pathways are triggered by MAP3K, serine/threonine kinases. In keeping with the heterogeneity of cellular stimuli that activate the SAPK and p38 pathways, three families of MAPK3s are known to act upstream of these pathways; the MEK kinases (MEKKs), the mixed lineage kinases (MLKs), and the thousand and one kinases (TAOs). The large and diverse family of MEKKs includes members such as MEKK1, which is selective for activation of the SAPK pathway, and others such as MEKK4, which activates both SAPK and p38 pathways. Members of the MLK family are selective for the activation of SAPK, and TAOs appear to be specific for p38 activation. Activation of SAPK and p38 pathway MAP3Ks is, in some cases, regulated by the small GTP-binding proteins Rac and Cdc42, which may act in a similar way to the Ras proteins described above. However, the precise mechanisms by which these proteins respond to stress are still under active investigation.

Activation of MAPK pathways brings about changes in gene expression that drive the cellular responses to external stimuli. Cell proliferation, differentiation, and sur-

vival can all be regulated through MAPK signaling. Nuclear transcription factors are key MAPK targets that directly affect gene transcription (Sec. 8.2.8). For example, ERKs phosphorylate and activate the ELK-1 transcription factor, while SAPK activates c-Jun, p38 phosphorylates MEF2A, and most MAPKs activate the Ets family of transcription factors. However, activated MAPKs can also act on cytoplasmic targets such as the effector kinases, MAP-KAP-2, and MNK1, which regulate protein translation.

Given the broad biological outcomes of MAPK signaling, it is not surprising that dysregulation of these pathways has been implicated in malignant transformation. Increased levels of activated ERKs are found frequently in human tumors, and often are attributable to the presence of mutations in Ras or other upstream components in the growth factor signaling cascades. Recently, the Raf-1 related kinase BRAF was identified as a human oncogene (Davies et al., 2002). Mutations in BRAF that result in kinase activation are found in greater than 60 percent of human melanomas and at lower frequency in a wide range of other human tumors. This discovery indicates that mutated forms of core MAPK components may be important targets for cancer therapy.

### 8.2.7 Phosphoinositide Signaling Pathways

Phosphoinositides are phospholipids of cell membranes that are dynamically regulated in response to growth factor signaling (Katso et al., 2001). They contribute to signal propagation by two main mechanisms introduced in Section 8.2.4: by serving as precursors of the second messengers IP3 and DAG, or by binding to signaling proteins that contain specific phosphoinositide binding modules. Figure 8.8 illustrates some of the important phospholipid products that function in growth factor signal transduction pathways. In response to growth factor signaling phosphoinositides can be phosphorylated or dephosphorylated by lipid kinases and phosphatases at distinct positions on the inositol ring. Activation of phosphoinositide 3-kinase, PI-3K, which specifically phosphorylates the 3' position, leads to the rapid production of phosphatidylinositol-3,4,5-triphosphate, PtdIns(3,4,5)P3. Some of the PtdIns(3,4,5)P3 is immediately converted to PtdIns(3,4)P2 by the action of 5' inositol phosphatases such as the SH2 domain containing protein SHIP. Signaling proteins containing PH domains bind to both PtdIns(3,4,5)P3 and PtdIns(3,4)P2 (Cantley, 2002).

The PH-domain-containing protein serine/threonine kinases PDK1 and Akt/PKB are recruited in the vicinity of activated receptors. There, PKB is activated by conformational changes evoked by phospholipid binding and its subsequent phosphorylation by the constitutively active PDK1. A number of important sub-

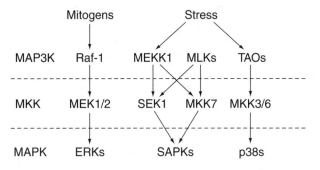

**Figure 8.7.** Mammalian MAPK signaling pathways. Parallel MAPK signaling pathways include MAP3Ks that respond to distinct stimuli, and activate the dual specificity MKKs, which in turn activate the MAPKs. The activated ERKs, SAPKs, and p38 family members induce distinct cellular responses as described in the text.

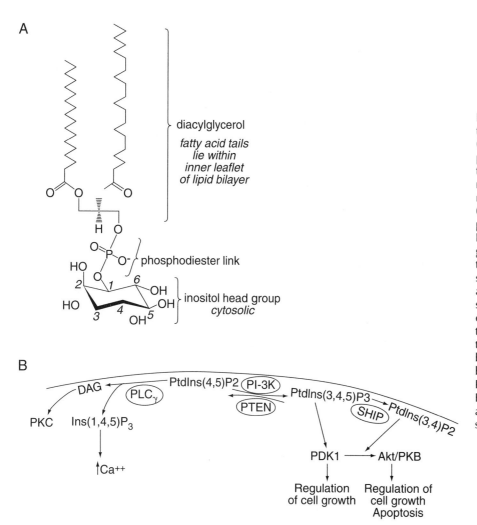

**Figure 8.8.** Phosphoinositide metabolism in growth factor signaling. (*A*) The chemical structure of phosphatidyl inositol (PtdIns). The positions in the inositol ring that are modified by phosphorylation are numbered. (*B*) PtdIns, hydrolases (PLC), kinases (PI-3K), and phosphatases (PTEN, SHIP) involved in PtdIns signaling downstream of growth factor receptors are illustrated. PLC activation produces the second messengers Ins(1,4,5)P3(IP$_3$) and DAG that activate downstream signaling via release of intracellular calcium stores and activation of protein kinase C (PKC). PH domain containing kinases PDK1 and Akt/PKB bind to 3′ phospholipids generated by PI-3K, leading to their activation. PDK1 phosphorylates and activates PKB, leading to the phosphorylation and inactivation of downstream substrates.

strates for activated PKB have been identified that fall into two main classes as regulators of apoptosis, or regulators of cell growth (see Chap. 9, Secs. 9.2 and 9.3 and Chap. 10, Sec. 10.2). PDK1 phosphorylates protein targets in addition to PKB. One of its substrates is ribosomal p70 S6-kinase, a key regulator of cell growth through control of the protein translation machinery.

The importance of phosphoinositides in human cancers was clearly revealed by the discovery that numerous human malignancies are associated with inactivating mutations in the PTEN gene (see Chap. 7, Sec. 7.4.3). PTEN is a 3′-phosphoinositide phosphatase that dephosphorylates the 3′ position of PtdIns(3,4,5)P3 and PtdIns(3,4)P2, and therefore functions as a major negative regulator of PI-3K signaling. Loss of PTEN leads to accumulation of 3′-phosphoinositides, causing deregulated PKB activity and malignant transformation (Jiang and Zhang, 2002).

### 8.2.8 Transcriptional Response to Signaling

Activation of signaling pathways leads to transcription of new genes that coordinate cell growth, cellular dif-ferentiation, cell death, and other biological effects. Transcription of genes is catalyzed by the enzyme RNA polymerase II and regulated by supporting molecules collectively termed *transcription factors* (Woychik and Hampsey, 2002). Transcription factors can activate or repress gene expression by binding to specific DNA recognition sequences, typically six to eight base pairs in length, found in the promoter regions at the start of genes. The formation of RNA transcripts is influenced by the interaction of these gene-specific factors with elements of a common core of molecules regulating the activity of RNA polymerase II (Woychik and Hampsey, 2002). The activity of transcription factors can be modified, most often by phosphorylation, through the activity of many of the signaling pathways described above, but most notably by the MAPKs. Transcription factor activity may also be enhanced through interaction with small molecules (e.g., steroid hormones; see Chap. 19, Sec. 19.2) or by signal-induced release from inhibitory interactions such as for NFκB (normally bound by the inhibitor IκB, that is released upon phosphorylation). Transcription factors are modular, consisting of a DNA binding region that binds to specific DNA sequences, as described below, and an activation or repression domain, which interacts with other proteins to stimulate or repress transcription from a nearby promoter (Brivanlou and Darnell, 2002).

Based on the structure of their DNA binding domains, transcription factors can be placed into four groups: homeodomain (sometimes called helix-turn-helix), zinc-finger, leucine-zipper, and helix-loop-helix (HLH) (Fig. 8.9). A common principle underlying specific protein-DNA interactions is the interaction of an α-helix, sometimes referred to as the recognition helix of the transcription factor, with the major groove of the DNA (Muller, 2001).

The homeodomain factors contain a sixty amino acid DNA binding domain called a homeobox that is simi-

lar to the helix-turn-helix domain first described in bacterial repressors. The name derives from homeobox genes in *Drosophila* that determine identity of body structure. In vertebrates, homeodomain proteins have similar properties and function as master regulators during development. The homeodomain contains three helical regions. The third helical region, as well as amino acids at the amino terminal end of the homeodomain, directly contact the DNA.

Zinc-finger transcription factors contain a sequence of twenty to thirty amino acids having two paired cysteine or histidine residues that are coordinated by a zinc ion. Binding of the zinc ion folds these polypeptide sequences into compact domains with α-helices that insert into the DNA. Members of this group of transcription factors mediate differentiation and growth signals,

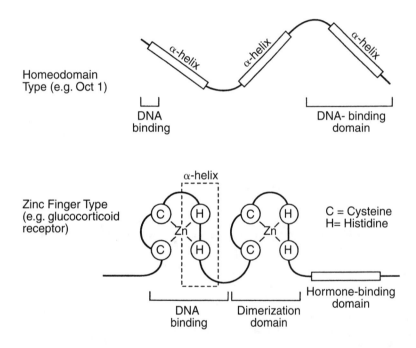

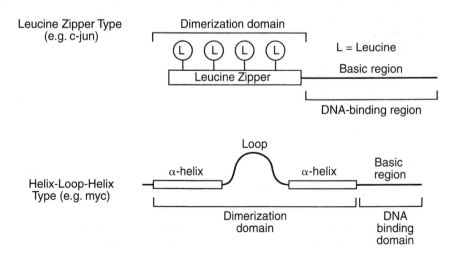

**Figure 8.9.** Classes of transcription factor DNA binding domains. The general structure of the four major classes of DNA binding domains found in modular transcription factors is illustrated.

including those due to binding of steroid hormones to receptors; they have been implicated in malignancy (Chap. 19).

Leucine-zipper transcription factors contain helical regions with leucine residues occurring at every seventh amino acid, which protrude from the same side of the α-helix. These leucines form a hydrophobic interaction surface with leucine zippers of similar proteins. Additional members of this family contain other hydrophobic amino acids in the α-helices that make up the dimerization domain. The DNA binding regions of the α-helices contain basic amino acids that interact with the DNA backbone. These factors, also referred to as *basic zipper proteins* bind to DNA as homo- or heterodimers, and include the fos/jun pair (called the AP1 transcription factor), which becomes activated by cellular stress. Members of this group also tend to become activated by proliferative and developmental stimuli.

Basic helix-loop-helix factors are similar to the basic zipper factors described above, but include a loop region separating the two α-helical regions that form the dimerization domain. DNA binding by homo- or heterodimers requires basic amino acids adjacent to the helix-loop-helix motif.

Activation and repression domains are structurally diverse regions, ranging from the random coil conformation of acidic activation domains to the highly structured ligand binding domains of hormone receptors. Both transcription activators and repressors exert their effects by binding to multisubunit co-activators or co-repressors that act to modify chromatin structure and assembly of RNA polymerase complexes. Enzymes that regulate histone acetylation and phosphorylation are key components of transcriptional activator and repressor complexes. Histone acetylation near the promoter regions of genes facilitates the interaction of the DNA with transcription factors while deacetylation results in more condensed chromatin structures that inhibit assembly of the transcription machinery at the promoter (Berger, 2002; e.g., Myc, see Chap. 7, Sec. 7.3.4).

Mutation of transcription factors, which can cause dysregulated activation and expression of genes or lead to inappropriate repression of others, can lead to transformation and has been implicated in human cancers (see Chap. 7, Sec. 7.3.4). While we understand how mutation or overexpression of these factors alters their activity, we do not yet fully understand how these changes affect the gene expression or repression patterns that bring about the oncogenic state.

### 8.2.9 Biological Outcomes

Growth factor signaling results in changes in expression of large numbers of genes that program physiologic responses such as cell cycle progression, cellular differentiation, cell growth, survival, or apoptosis. Changes in gene expression proceed in two stages following activation of signaling pathways. The expression of immediate early genes, which often encode transcription factors, and whose expression does not require new protein synthesis, is followed by a secondary phase of gene expression (sometimes called the delayed response genes) that are often targets of the immediate early genes (Hill and Treisman, 1999).

Normal cells in the G1 phase of the cell cycle respond to external stimuli by either withdrawing from the cell cycle (G0) or advancing through the restriction point toward cell division. Progression from G1 and entry into S phase normally requires stimulation by mitogens, such as growth factors. For example, the D type cyclins are expressed as part of the delayed early response to stimulation of growth factor signaling cascades. These D type cyclins assemble with cyclin dependent kinases, and the active complex phosphorylates and inactivates the Rb protein, releasing the E2F transcription factor family that in turn activates the transcription of genes required for S phase entry (see Chap. 9, Sec. 9.2). One of the most common properties of cancer cells is the ability to undergo G1 phase progression in the absence of external mitogenic stimuli. Activating mutations in any of the growth factor signaling components upstream of the G1 checkpoint control can lead to cyclin D accumulation, which drives continuous cell cycling (see Chap. 9, Sec. 9.3; Sherr, 1996; Evan and Vousden, 2001).

A second important consequence of growth factor signaling is cell survival. Normal cells require continuous exposure to survival factors, such as soluble growth factors, or cell matrix interactions, to suppress apoptosis. Tissue homeostasis is maintained through the limited supply or spatial restriction of these factors that limit cell expansion. Evasion of this control mechanism is another common feature of tumor cells. Activating mutations in survival pathways, such as activating mutations in PKB or loss of function mutations in PTEN, can confer resistance to apoptotic signals which would normally limit deregulated cell proliferation (see Chap. 7, Sec. 7.4.3; Evan and Vousden, 2001).

### 8.2.10 Downregulation of Growth Factor Signaling

The activity of receptor and cytoplasmic tyrosine kinases is tightly regulated. Many of the proteins that antagonize tyrosine kinase signaling are also recruited to active receptor complexes through SH2, PTB, or TKB domain-mediated interactions. For example, the opposing action of protein tyrosine phosphatases can eliminate docking sites for proteins containing SH2 domains, or inhibit tyrosine kinase activity by dephosphorylation of regulatory phosphorylation sites in the kinase activation loop (Chernoff, 1999).

Regulation of receptor levels at the cell membrane is another mechanism used to regulate activity. The rapid removal of receptors from the cell surface by endocytosis allows a cell to return to an unstimulated, basal state after receiving and responding to a specific signal. Internalized receptors can either be permanently inactivated through transport to the lysosome where they are degraded, or be recycled back to the plasma membrane where they are available for receiving other signals. This process of internalization and degradation is tightly linked to ubiquitin modification of both the receptor itself, and accessory molecules (Fig. 8.10). Ubiquitin is a 76 amino acid peptide that is attached to target proteins through a multistep process. Free ubiquitin is first attached to an ubiquitin-activating enzyme (E1) and subsequently transferred to an ubiquitin-conjugating enzyme (E2), which in partner with an ubiquitin ligase (E3) transfers ubiquitin to the specific protein substrate (Hershko and Ciechanover, 1998). The specificity of this process is determined by the E3 ligase component that selectively binds substrates (Tyers and Willems, 1999; see also Chap. 9, Sec. 9.2.1). Iterative ubiquitination then serves as a signal to target the attached protein for degradation by the proteasome. For cell surface proteins, ubiquitination signals entry into

the endocytic pathway and trafficking to multivesicular bodies (MVB) and to lysosomes for degradation (Fig. 8.10; Hicke, 1999; Rotin et al., 2000). For example, the protooncogene c-Cbl is a TKB containing E3 ligase that promotes the ubiquitination of several RPTKs such as EGFR, as well as the cytosolic tyrosine kinases that regulate antigen receptor signaling (see Sec. 8.3.2). Following response to EGF, ubiquitin is attached to the EGFR leading to its incorporation into internal vesicles of the MVB which leads to its degradation in lysosomes. Mutant forms of Cbl that lack ubiquitin ligase activity result in the recycling of the activated EGFR back to the plasma membrane and prolong EGFR signaling.

## 8.3 RECEPTORS LINKED TO CYTOPLASMIC TYROSINE KINASES

The activation of tyrosine kinases also plays a central role in transmission of signals from a number of cell surface receptors that do not possess intrinsic tyrosine kinase activity. In the examples that follow, cytoplasmic tyrosine kinases are recruited to cell surface molecules soon after receptor activation. Many of the intracellular events that occur resemble those evoked by receptor tyrosine kinases as described in Section 8.2. Figure 8.11 shows schematic diagrams of a selection of cytoplasmic tyrosine kinases. A common feature of these cytoplasmic TKs is the presence of conserved protein modules, such as SH2 and SH3 domains. These protein modules function to regulate kinase activity and also to couple these molecules to extracellular receptors. The unique features of receptor signaling pathways, which utilize cytoplasmic tyrosine kinases, are described below.

### 8.3.1 Cytokine Receptor Signaling

Cytokines regulate the growth and differentiation of multiple lineages through interaction with structurally and functionally related receptors of the cytokine receptor superfamily. These receptors do not contain intrinsic tyrosine kinase activity, but rather transmit intracellular signals through their association with the Janus kinase (JAK) family of tyrosine kinases. Many cytokines are pleiotropic in nature and exhibit distinct biological responses in different cell types. However, there are multiple cytokines that exhibit functional redundancy and elicit similar biological responses in a single type of cell. This redundancy can be explained in part by the fact that different cytokines often share identical receptor subunits.

Cytokine receptors contain unique extracellular ligand binding regions, a single transmembrane domain, and a cytoplasmic domain (Fig. 8.12). With the exception of the receptors for G-CSF and erythropoietin that are single chains, most cytokine receptors exist as a multisubunit complex. These complexes are composed of

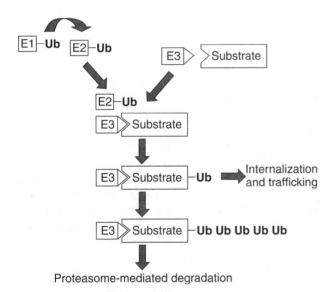

**Figure 8.10.** Ubiquitination pathway. Proteins are ubiquitinated in a multistep process involving at least three enzymes. Free ubiquitin is first attached to an E1 ubiquitin-activating enzyme and then subsequently transferred to an E2 ubiquitin-conjugating enzyme. The E2 in partner with an E3 ubiquitin ligase, transfers the ubiquitin moiety to the specific protein substrate. Addition of an ubiquitin chain or polyubiquitination of a substrate targets it for degradation by the proteasome, whereas a single ubiquitin moiety or mono-ubiquitination of a substrate, such as cell surface receptors, can serve as a signal for receptor internalization and trafficking to multivesicular bodies and lysosomes.

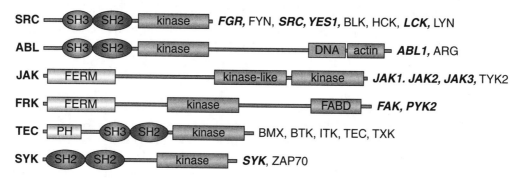

**Figure 8.11.** Cytoplasmic protein tyrosine kinases. The general structure of several cytoplasmic protein tyrosine kinase families is illustrated. Members of each family are listed beside each diagram. Those in bold and italic type are duplicated in human malignancies.

four distinct signaling chains; the gp130 subunit [interleukin (IL)-6Rβc, where "c" denotes that the chain is common to other cytokine receptors], IL-3Rβc, IL-2Rβc, and IL-2Rγc chains (Fig. 8.12A). Receptors

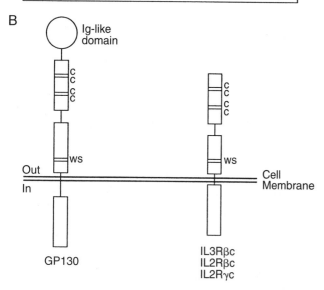

**Figure 8.12.** Cytokine receptors. (A) Common cytokine receptor subunits. Cytokine receptors share four subunits that function as connectors to cytoplasmic signaling cascades. CNTF, ciliary neurotropic factor; LIF, leukemia inhibitory factor; OM, oncostatin M; GM-CSF, granulocyte-macrophage colony-stimulating factor. (B) Cytokine receptors are composed of a unique extracellular domain that binds ligands, a transmembrane domain, and a cytoplasmic region. Ig-like, immunoglobulin-like; c, cysteine; WS motif, WSXWS where W is tryptophan, S is serine, and X is any amino acid.

containing the gp130 subunit can transmit signals from many different ligands including IL-6, ciliary neurotrophic factor (CNTF), leukemia inhibitory factor (LIF), oncostatin M (OM) and IL-11. These cytokines have diverse functions such as modulating inflammatory and immune responses, and embryonic development. Similarly, the response to IL-3, IL-5, and granulocyte-macrophage colony stimulating factor (GM-CSF) overlaps in various hematopoietic cells due to the common use of the IL-3Rβc subunits in receptors for these cytokines. The IL-2 receptor is composed of three subunits: the α, β, and γ chains. The β subunit is used by the IL-15 receptor, while the γ subunit is used as part of the receptors for IL-4, IL-7, IL-9, and IL-13.

Similar to RPTK signaling, cytokine binding induces receptor dimerization and subsequent initiation of downstream signaling events (Fig. 8.13A). As the cytoplasmic domain of the common receptor subunits do not possess intrinsic tyrosine kinase activity, the noncovalent association with the JAK family of cytoplasmic tyrosine kinases is required for signal transmission (Ihle and Kerr, 1995; O'Shea et al., 2002). The JAKs contain a FERM domain, which is a potential SH2 domain, a kinase-like domain, and a functional tyrosine kinase domain (Fig. 8.11). They bind to the juxtamembrane region of the cytokine receptor subunits. Receptors such as the erythropoietin receptor bind only one member of the JAK family, however, others, such as the gp130 receptor, bind to at least three distinct JAK proteins. Upon receptor dimerization, JAKs become activated, leading to phosphorylation of specific tyrosine residues on the receptor. This generates docking sites for SH2 domain containing proteins such as the STAT (signal transducers and activators of transcription) family of transcription factors (Fig. 8.13A). STATs are then phosphorylated inducing homo- or heterodimerization and subsequent transport to the nucleus where they regulate gene expression. STATs contain a conserved amino terminal DNA binding domain that is specific to the STAT family of proteins, a conserved SH2 domain, and

A

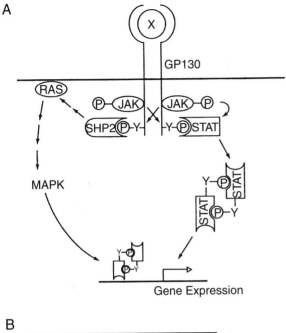

MAPK

Gene Expression

B

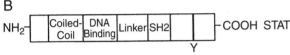

C

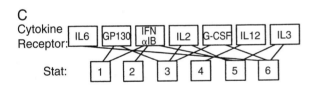

**Figure 8.13.** Cytokine receptor signaling. (*A*) Cytokine binding induces receptor dimerization resulting in JAK activation and receptor phosphorylation. STATs then bind the phosphorylated receptor, and are subsequently phosphorylated inducing dimerization and transport to the nucleus where they activate downstream target genes. (*B*) Structure of the STATs. STATs contain a DNA binding domain, an SH2 domain, and a conserved tyrosine residue in the carboxy terminus. (*C*) Cytokine receptors utilize multiple STAT molecules to elicit cellular responses.

a carboxy-terminal tyrosine residue that mediates dimerization (Fig. 8.13*B*). Stimulation of various cytokine receptors results in an overlapping pattern of STAT activation (Fig. 8.13*C*).

Although the JAK/STAT pathway is the primary downstream signaling pathway of cytokine receptors, other pathways such as the MAPK cascade may be activated upon stimulation of the cytokine receptor. For example, the binding of IL-6 to gp130 subunit induces phosphorylation of JAK and subsequent phosphorylation of Shp2 and activation of grb2/SOS/Ras/MAPK pathway (see Sec. 8.2.5; Heinrich et al., 2003). Furthermore, tyrosine kinases, such as members of the Src

family, also associate with and are activated by receptors composed of the IL-2βc or the gp130 subunits. A number of cytokines also induce the activation of the p85 subunit of phosphatidylinositol-3 kinase, thus linking cytokine and lipid-kinase signaling pathways (Ihle and Kerr, 1995).

### 8.3.2 Antigen Receptor Signaling

The antigen receptors on B- and T-lymphocytes are multichain receptors that couple to both Src and Syk family cytoplasmic tyrosine kinases (Fig. 8.11). These receptors are activated by recognition of foreign antigens, and although a number of lymphocyte specific proteins play key roles in the membrane proximal signaling events, the pathways activated downstream of the receptors, for example, Ras and PLCγ, are similar to those described for growth factor receptor signaling (Weiss and Littman, 1994).

The T-cell receptor (TCR) expressed on the surface of lymphocytes recognizes antigens when presented by the major histocompatibility complex (MHC) on antigen presenting cells (Fig. 8.14; see Chap. 20, Sec. 20.2). Stimulation of the TCR gives rise to diverse cellular responses that drive thymocyte development, T-cell activation, apoptosis, and homeostasis (Chen et al., 1996). The TCR is a heterodimer consisting of covalently linked α and β polypeptide chains that contain a variable ligand-binding domain at the amino-terminal end and a constant region proximal to the membrane that belongs to the immunoglobulin (Ig) superfamily. The TCR is associated with the multisubunit CD3 complex, which is present as two separate heterodimers of CD3γ-CD3ε, CD3ε-CD3δ, and a TCR-ζ homodimer (Fig. 8.14). The cytoplasmic domains of the CD3 chains contain immunoreceptor tyrosine-based activation sequence motifs (ITAM), and these serve as the signal-transducing unit for the TCR. *Immunoreceptor tyrosine-based activation sequence motif* is the term given to sites of tyrosine phosphorylation that conform to consensus binding motifs for SH2 containing proteins. The engagement of TCR-CD3 complex activates Src family tyrosine kinases Lck and Fyn. CD45 dephosphorylates Lck tethered to the CD4 coreceptor leading to activation of Lck that rapidly phosphorylates the ITAM sequences. Tyrosine phosphorylation of the ζ chain ITAMs establishes a binding site for the tandem SH2 domain containing protein kinase, ZAP-70 (Weiss and Littman, 1994). Activated SRC family and ZAP-70 tyrosine kinases phosphorylate downstream substrates such as enzymes and adaptor proteins. Hematopoietic-specific adaptor proteins play an important role in transmitting signals downstream of the TCR (Fig. 8.14; Jordan et al., 2003). Two central adaptor proteins, LAT and SLP-76, are rapidly phosphorylated on tyrosine residues in response to TCR engage-

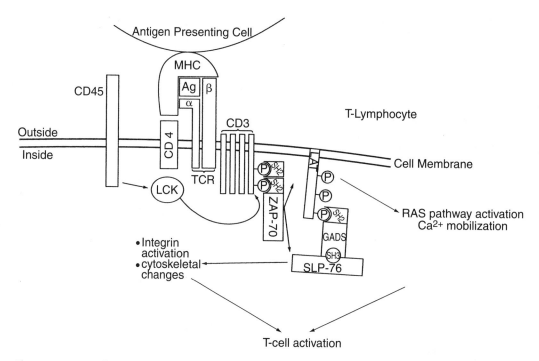

**Figure 8.14.** T-cell receptor signaling. Engagement of the TCR receptor leads to rapid activation of the Src family kinase Lck, which phosphorylates the intracellular domains of the associated CD3 complex. The SH2 domain-containing tyrosine kinase ZAP-70 binds to phosphorylated CD3 chains and in turn is activated and phosphorylates two critical adaptor molecules, the membrane anchored LAT protein and the cytoplasmic SLP-76 protein. Phosphorylated LAT and SLP-76 function as docking sites for the recruitment of multiple SH2 domain containing signaling molecules and activate multiple downstream signaling events, including gene transcription culminating in T-cell activation, and cytokine production.

ment. Tyrosine phosphorylated LAT and SLP-76 in turn recruit SH2 domain containing proteins. These multiprotein complexes are connected by the adapter protein GADS and collectively coordinate the activation of the Ras and ERK pathways, the mobilization of $Ca^{2+}$, integrin activation, and the rearrangement of the cytoskeleton, leading to alterations in gene transcription that are essential for T-cell activation (Fig. 8.14).

T-cell responses are normally limited by activation induced cell death, and this process is essential to maintain T-cell homeostasis. Loss of this regulatory process leads to excessive lymphoid proliferation and can lead to autoimmunity and lymphoma (see Chap. 20, Sec. 20.3).

### 8.3.3 Integrin Activated Signaling Pathways

Mammalian cells express on their surface a variety of cell adhesion molecules that mediate their attachment to the extracellular matrix (ECM) and/or their interaction with the same or different cell types. Most adhesion molecules are transmembrane proteins, but some are anchored in the plasma membrane by an L-terminal glycophosphatidylinositol moiety. Interactions between cells and the ECM are essential for cell survival and cell proliferation, and can regulate differ-

entiation. Loss of interactions between the cell and ECM results in induction of apoptosis in both epithelial and endothelial cells. However, a common property of malignant cells is that they continue to survive and proliferate in the absence of interactions with the ECM.

Integrins are transmembrane cell surface receptors expressed in all cell types that serve as the primary physical link between the ECM and actin cytoskeleton enabling direct communication across the plasma membrane (Calderwood et al., 2000; Brakebusch and Fassler, 2003). They recognize and bind to specific ECM ligands and transduce signals leading to the activation of intracellular signaling pathways that regulate cell migration, cell polarity, cell proliferation, and survival. Integrins are comprised of membrane spanning $\alpha$ and $\beta$ subunits that associate noncovalently to form a heterodimer on the cell surface. Receptor diversity and versatility in ligand binding is determined by the extracellular domains, and through the specific pairing of eight $\beta$ subunits and eighteen $\alpha$ subunits. The cytoplasmic domains of both $\alpha$ and $\beta$ integrin subunits are conserved among vertebrate species and *Drosophila*, and serve as a platform for both actin binding proteins such as $\alpha$-actinin and talin, and intracellular signaling components such as protein kinases.

The binding of integrins to ECM ligands induces integrin clustering and subsequent recruitment of actin filaments and signaling proteins to the integrin cytoplasmic domain. These large transmembrane adhesion complexes composed of the ECM and intracellular signaling components are called *focal adhesion plaques* (FAPs) (see Chap. 11, Sec. 11.5.1). The formation of FAPs assures cell adhesion to the ECM in addition to the targeted localization of actin filaments and signaling components necessary for the establishment of cell polarity, directed cell migration, and maintenance of cell proliferation and survival. The integrin-actin cytoskeleton connection is highly dynamic and subject to many regulatory processes. It is differentially regulated in different locations of the cell, such as at the leading and trailing edge. In addition to providing a physical link between the ECM and the cytoskeleton, binding of integrins to their ligands elicits a variety of intracellular signaling events (Liu et al., 2000; Hynes, 2002; Martin et al., 2002). For example, integrin signaling regulates the formation of filopodia, lamellipodia, and stress fibers through the Rho family of small GTPases Cdc42, Rac, and Rho. It can also stimulate tyrosine phosphorylation and subsequent activation of a number of cellular proteins including focal adhesion kinase (FAK) and Src protein kinases that regulate remodeling of FAPs. Furthermore, activation of the Ras family of GTPases by integrins is important for activation of serine-threonine kinases such as ERK, PAK, and JNK that regulate gene expression and cell cycle progression (see Sec. 8.2).

Up- or downregulation of integrins has been regularly observed in tumor progression. For example, increased expression of $\alpha v \beta 3$-integrin is associated with metastasis (see Chap. 11, Sec. 11.5.1; Nip and Brodt, 1995), and is observed in tumor induced migration of vascular endothelial cells (see Chap. 12, Sec. 12.3). The changes observed in integrin expression seem to be tumor and integrin specific. Carcinomas such as those of breast, prostate, and colon appear to lose expression of $\alpha 3 \beta 1$, $\alpha 2 \beta 1$, and $\alpha 5 \beta 1$ while expression of $\alpha 6 \beta 1$ remains unchanged. $\alpha 6 \beta 1$ has also been implicated in tumor invasion. An activating mutation in the $\beta 1$-integrin subunit may be involved in the formation of squamous cell carcinoma of the tongue (Evans et al., 2003). This tumor is characterized by the absence of spontaneous differentiation as a result of sustained activation the MAPK signaling pathway by the activated $\beta 1$-integrin mutant.

## 8.4 DEVELOPMENTAL SIGNALING PATHWAYS

Signaling events that influence cellular biology may also be initiated through transmembrane receptors that are not linked to or dependent on tyrosine kinase activity. These pathways have profound effects on normal cellular physiology and embryonic development, and have important implications for both cancer induction and therapeutics. Only a few signaling pathways are required to generate the cellular and morphological diversity of cell types and patterns found in the animal kingdom. Often these same signaling pathways are used within different cellular contexts to produce a large number of different cellular signals. During embryonic development, most cell-cell interactions involve Wnt, Hedgehog, transforming growth factor-$\beta$, Notch, JAK/STAT, and nuclear hormone pathways. All these pathways activate specific target genes by regulation of downstream transcription factors. Many of these signaling pathways that are essential for the development of an organism are deregulated in disease states such as cancer.

### 8.4.1 Wnt Signaling

The Wnt proteins comprise one of the major families of signaling molecules necessary for development of a multicellular organism. They constitute a large family of secreted glycoproteins that are highly conserved throughout evolution. The receptors for Wnt proteins are seven transmembrane receptors of the Frizzled family (Fig. 8.15). Together with the co-receptors LRP5 and LRP6, ligand bound Frizzled receptors initiate signaling to downstream intracellular targets. The strength of receptor affinity for the Wnt ligand results in activation of at least four alternate intracellular pathways; the canonical Wnt pathway which leads to regulation of gene expression through $\beta$-catenin; the planar cell polarity pathway which activates cytoskeleton reorganization through Rho and JNK; the Wnt/Ca pathway which involves the activation of PLC and PKC; and a less well-defined pathway that regulates spindle orientation and asymmetric cell division (Cadigan and Nusse, 1997; Huelsken and Birchmeier, 2001; Huelsken and Behrens, 2002).

The canonical Wnt pathway regulates the ability of $\beta$-catenin to activate specific target genes in the nucleus (Akiyama, 2000; Moon et al., 2002). $\beta$-catenin is the key mediator of the Wnt signal functioning as a cotranscriptional activator. Here Wnt activation prevents proteasomal degradation and leads to stabilization of $\beta$-catenin in the cytoplasm (Fig. 8.15). In the absence of Wnt, $\beta$-catenin levels are kept low through association with the so-called destruction complex, which includes the tumor suppressor protein APC and GSK3$\beta$. $\beta$-catenin is phosphorylated by GSK3$\beta$, leading to its ubiquitination and subsequent degradation by the proteasome. Upon Wnt activation, the Frizzled receptors inactivate GSK3$\beta$, resulting in reduced phosphorylation and subsequent stabilization of $\beta$-catenin. Stabilized $\beta$-catenin accumulates in the cytoplasm and then shut-

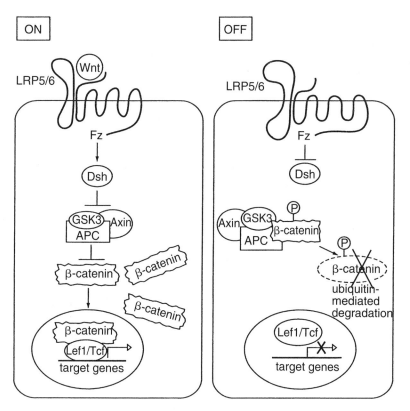

**Figure 8.15.** Wnt signaling. In the canonical Wnt signaling pathway, Wnt binding to the Frizzled (Fz)/LRP5/6 complex inactivates the kinase GSK3 in a process involving Dsh, thereby stabilizing β-catenin. β-catenin accumulates in the cytoplasm and shuttles to the nucleus where it functions as a cotranscriptional activator with Lef1/Tcf to regulate transcription of target genes. In the absence of Wnt, β-catenin is phosphorylated by GSK3 and targeted for ubiquitin-dependent proteasomal degradation. Dsh, dishevelled; APC, adenomatous polyposis coli.

tles to the nucleus where it interacts with the Lef1/TCF family of transcription factors to regulate transcription of specific target genes. These transcription factors bind directly to DNA but are incapable of activating gene transcription independently of β-catenin. Known target genes include c-myc, cyclin D1, and metalloproteinase7.

The first Wnt gene discovered, mouse Wnt-1, was identified by its ability to form mouse mammary tumors when ectopically expressed upon retroviral insertion. Constitutive activation of the canonical Wnt pathway has been observed in a number of human cancers, but amplification, rearrangement, or mutation of the Wnt gene has not been identified. Aberrant Wnt signaling that leads to cancer development most likely results from inappropriate gene activation mediated by β-catenin (Polakis, 2000; Kikuchi, 2003). APC is a tumor suppressor that was identified as a gene responsible for the onset of familial adenomatous polyposis, an autosomal dominantly inherited disease that predisposes patients to multiple colorectal polyps and cancers. In *Drosophila* genetic ablation of APC results in upregulation of β-catenin signaling, revealing its strong regulation of β-catenin. Mutant forms of APC that are unable to stimulate degradation of β-catenin are incapable of blocking target gene expression, and may therefore activate a transcriptional complex contributing to tumor growth. The spectrum of APC mutations found in human cancers typically result in truncation of the protein suggesting it is the regulation of β-catenin levels and not the binding of APC

and β-catenin that is important. Although APC mutations are common in colorectal cancer, including the majority of sporadic colorectal tumors, their frequency in other cancers is quite low.

Mutations in β-catenin have been observed in a variety of human cancers including pediatric kidney cancer, hepatocarcinoma, medulloblastoma, melanoma, gastric, pancreatic, ovarian, and prostate cancer. Mutations occur frequently in the regulatory region of β-catenin preventing phosphorylation of the β-catenin protein. Phosphorylation of β-catenin is necessary for its degradation and thus loss of phosphorylation and degradation leads to upregulation of downstream target genes. Finally, hepatocellular carcinomas (HCC) often contain mutations in the Wnt signaling pathway. Downstream targets of β-catenin, c-myc, and cyclin D genes are amplified in a subset of HCCs (de La Coste et al., 1998; Huang et al., 1999). Furthermore, there is an association of nuclear accumulation of β-catenin with the invasive and intravascular compartments of the tumors. Accumulation of β-catenin is associated with poor prognosis.

## 8.4.2 Notch Receptor Signaling

Notch signaling influences cellular differentiation, proliferation, and apoptotic events at all stages of development; it functions as an essential communication mechanism to direct the fate of neighboring cells. Genetic abnormalities in the Notch pathway have been implicated in cancers and neurogenerative disorders.

Notch is a ligand-activated cell surface receptor initially identified in *Drosophila*, but subsequently identified in the roundworm *Caenorhabditis elegans* and vertebrates (Jarriault et al., 1995; Artavanis-Tsakonas et al., 1999; Kopan, 2002). Although the central components of the Notch signaling pathway are conserved, the consequences of the Notch signal depend largely on the cellular context. In mammals, four Notch receptor homologs with similar structural features, Notch1–4, are expressed in both overlapping and distinct patterns throughout mammalian tissues. The Notch receptor is a large single-pass transmembrane protein that contains a number of conserved protein-protein interaction motifs within its three domains (Fig. 8.16*A*). The large extracellular domain contains a number of EGF-like repeats involved in ligand binding, and three cysteine-rich Lin12/Notch repeat (LNR) regions thought to play an inhibitory role in receptor activation. This LNR region is followed by a single transmembrane domain, and an intracellular domain composed of a RAM23 site that interacts with proteins from the CSL [CBF1/Su(H)/Lag1] family of transcription factors, six tandem ankyrin repeats involved in mediating protein-protein interactions with regulators of the receptor, and a proline, glutamine, serine, and threonine rich (PEST) sequence associated with high rates of protein turnover.

The current model of Notch signaling proposes a number of complex cleavage events that occur during receptor maturation and transmission of the Notch signal. During its maturation, Notch is first processed into two distinct fragments that interact to form a heterodimer on the cell surface (Fig. 8.16*B*). In this heterodimeric form, Notch is able to bind transmembrane ligands of the DSL (Delta/Serrate/Lag2) family presented on neighboring cells. Upon ligand binding, a second cleavage event occurs releasing the Notch extracellular domain. This event then triggers a third cleavage, and release of the active intracellular fragment of Notch that can translocate to the nucleus where it interacts with transcription factors to regulate downstream target genes. It is this nuclear translocation event that is important for transmission of the Notch signal.

Notch has been reported to act as both an oncogene and tumor suppressor, depending on the cellular context, dose, and timing (Joutel and Tournier-Lasserve, 1998; Nam et al., 2002; Radtke and Raj, 2003). Changes in the Notch signal either through a gain or loss of Notch function have been observed in different cancers suggesting that perturbations in the Notch signal can lead to disease (Maillard and Pear, 2003). Constitutive activation of the Notch receptor has been strongly linked to malignant transformation. The first connection between aberrant Notch signaling and tumor formation was recog-

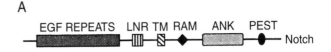

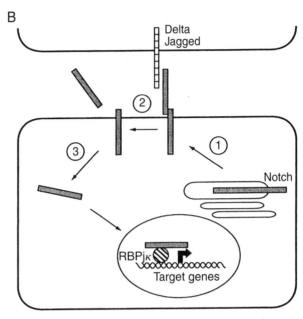

**Figure 8.16.** Notch receptor signaling. (*A*) Schematic representation of the Notch receptor. EGF, epidermal growth factor-like repeats; LNR, Lin12/Notch repeat region; TM, transmembrane domain; ANK, ankyrin repeats; PEST, proline, glutamate, serine, threonine rich region. (*B*) Model of Notch pathway. Notch is first processed in the trans-Golgi network into a heterodimer, which is found on the cell surface (1). In this heterodimeric form, Notch binds transmembrane ligands such as Delta and Jagged presented on neighboring cells. Ligand binding causes a second cleavage event that releases the extracellular domain of Notch (2). This then triggers a final cleavage event that releases the active intracellular domain of Notch that translocates to the nucleus where it functions as a co-transactivator with the CSL family of transcription factors (such as the example shown, RBPjκ) to regulate target genes.

nized when a recurrent t(7;9)(q34;q34.3) chromosomal translocation was identified in a subset of human T-cell acute lymphoblastic leukemias (Ellisen et al., 1991). This balanced translocation involving the human *NOTCH1* gene and the *TCRβ* locus created a truncated constitutively activated form of the Notch1 receptor which functions as a potent oncogene. Aberrant Notch signaling appears to be involved in a wide variety of human neoplasms, including pancreatic cancer. Notch is also highly expressed in human cervical and renal cancer cells. In mice, viral insertion of MMTV into the *Notch4* locus contributes to the generation of mammary carcinomas. It has also been shown that Notch may act as a suppressor of skin carcinogenesis where it interacts with other developmental signaling pathways such as the Wnt and Hedgehog pathways (Kopan and Turner, 1996; Nicolas et al., 2003). Thus, it is the dysregulation of Notch signaling that contributes to disease states and not its specific up- or downregulation.

### 8.4.3 Hedgehog Signaling

Hedgehog (Hh) proteins are secreted 19 kilodalton glycoproteins that act as key mediators of fundamental processes in embryonic development. They are essential to the growth, patterning, and morphogenesis of many different tissues and organs including the skin, brain, gut, lung, and bone, and more recently are thought to play a role in hematopoiesis (Ingham and McMahon, 2001; Nybakken and Perrimon, 2002; Cohen, 2003). The Hh signaling pathway is highly conserved throughout evolution, and much of what is known about signaling in vertebrates has been inferred from studies in *Drosophila*. In humans there are three homologs of the *Drosophila* hedgehog gene; sonic hedgehog (*SHH*), desert hedgehog (*DHH*), and Indian hedgehog (*IHH*). Of the three human hedgehog proteins, SHH is the most widely expressed, and apparently the most potent.

The hedgehog proteins signal through a membrane-receptor complex that includes the Patched (Ptc) and Smoothened (Smo) transmembrane receptors (Fig. 8.17). Ptc is the ligand binding component of the receptor complex, and Smo, a protein with homology to a G protein coupled receptor, is responsible for transducing the hedgehog signal. In the absence of Hh ligands, Ptc silences the Hh pathway by maintaining Smo in an inactive state, thereby inhibiting downstream signaling events. In the presence of Hh ligand, Hh binding to Ptc releases the inhibition of Smo and this in turn activates the transcription factors Gli1, Gli2, and Gli3 in vertebrates and cubitus interruptus (Ci) in *Drosophila*, leading to the regulation of downstream target genes. How Smo activation is coupled to the cytoplasmic proteins involved in Hh signaling is poorly understood. A large cytoplasmic complex composed of the serine/threonine protein kinase Fused (Fu), Suppressor of fused [Su(Fu)], the kinesin-like protein Costal-2 (Cos2), and the transcription factor Ci/Gli is anchored to microtubules in the absence of Hh. Upon Hh stimulation this complex dissociates, releasing Ci/Gli, which translocates to the nucleus and transmits the necessary signals. Recently Cos2 and Fu have been shown to phys-

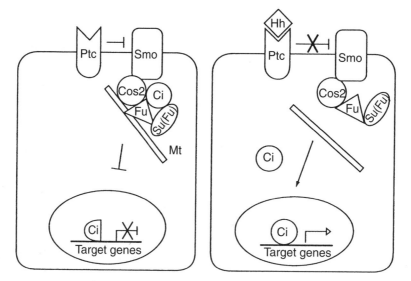

**Figure 8.17.** Hedgehog signaling. Binding of Hedgehog (Hh) to the receptor complex Patched (Ptc) and Smoothened (Smo) releases the inhibition of Smo by Ptc. Activated Smo then signals through an ill-defined mechanism that results in nuclear translocation of Ci (Gli in vertebrates) that then regulates target gene expression. Ci/Gli is found in a complex with Fused (Fu), Suppressor of Fused [Su(Fu)] and Costal2 (Cos2) bound to microtubules (MT). Upon activation of Smo this complex is disassembled, releasing Ci/Gli and allowing nuclear translocation and upregulation of downstream target genes including Wingless (Wnt in vertebrates), Decapentaplegic (bone morphogenetic protein BMP in vertebrates), and Patched itself. In *Drosophila*, Ci is a bifunctional transcriptional regulator. In the absence of Hh, a truncated form of Ci functions as a transcriptional repressor binding to target genes and blocking transcription. In the presence of Hh, full-length Ci binds target genes and upregulates transcription.

ically interact with the cytoplasmic tail of Smo, and this interaction is necessary for Smo signal transduction ( Jia et al., 2003; Lum et al., 2003; Ruel et al., 2003). Various inhibitors that function at different levels of the pathway have also been identified and ensure tight regulation of the pathway. Because Ptc and other inhibitors function to silence the Hh pathway in the absence of active Hh ligands, it is believed that the Hh-Gli pathway is kept in an "off" state and is only active at the times and locations at which the Hh signals act.

Abnormal activation of the Hedgehog signaling pathway has been implicated in the development of sporadic cancers such as basal-cell carcinomas, medulloblastomas, some gliomas, digestive tract tumors, and pancreatic cancers (Taipale and Beachy, 2001; Mullor et al., 2002; Ruiz i Altaba et al., 2002). Furthermore, inactivating mutations in the patched gene have been identified in familial tumors and result in the overexpression of activated GLI1 function and are responsible for the basal-cell nevus syndrome (Gorlin's syndrome). This hereditary syndrome is associated with a predisposition to basal-cell carcinomas (BCC), medulloblastomas, and rhabdomyosarcomas. Mutations in another regulatory component of the Shh pathway, Su(Fu) have been identified in patients with medulloblastomas (Taylor et al., 2002). Additional evidence implicating the Shh-Gli pathway comes from animal models. For example, overexpression of Gli1 or Gli2 in mice can induce skin tumors that strongly resemble human BCC, and mice with a single functional Ptc allele develop medullablastomas. The Hedgehog pathway likely plays a role in the initiation and/or maintenance of other sporadic tumors that are derived from tissues or cell groups that use this pathway for proliferation during development. Indeed Gli expression is constitutive in both lung and prostate cancer.

### 8.4.4 Signal Transduction by the TGF-β Superfamily

Members of the transforming growth factor-β (TGF-β) superfamily regulate a number of developmental and homeostatic processes such as cell proliferation, differentiation, apoptosis, cell adhesion, and migration. They constitute a highly conserved family of proteins with at least thirty vertebrate members and over a dozen structurally and functionally related proteins found in invertebrates such as *C. elegans* and *Drosophila*. There are two general branches of this superfamily, the TGF-β/activin/Nodal branch and bone morphogenic protein (BMP)/GDP branch, whose members have diverse but often complementary effects. Some members are widely expressed during embryogenesis and in adult tissues whereas others are expressed in only a few cell types and for limited periods of time during development.

Transforming growth factor-β (1–3), the prototypic members of this superfamily, are secreted growth fac-

tors synthesized as inactive precursors and proteolytically processed into a mature secreted ligands. Upon dimerization, TGF-β becomes biologically active and binds to a cell surface receptor complex consisting of two distinct single-pass transmembrane proteins known as the type I and type II receptors, both of which contain an intracellular serine-threonine kinase domain (Fig. 8.18; Moustakas et al., 2001; Attisano and Wrana, 2002; Dennler et al., 2002). Ligand binding induces association of the type I and type II receptors into a tetrameric complex. This leads to unidirectional phosphorylation and subsequent activation of the kinase domain of the type I receptor by the type II receptor. The activated type I receptor then signals to the SMAD (for

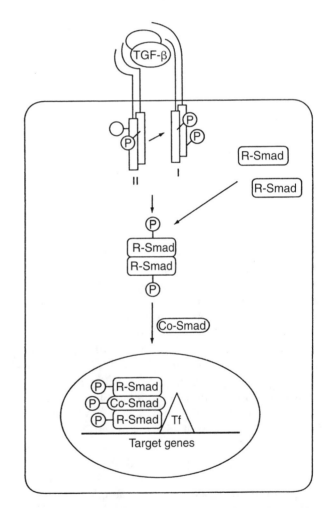

**Figure 8.18.** TGF-β signaling. TGF-β ligand binding induces the association of type II and type I receptor heterodimers into a tetrameric complex. This results in phosphorylation and subsequent activation of the type I receptor that then phosphorylates a member of the R-Smad class of proteins (Smads 1, 2, 3, 5, or 8). Phosphorylated R-Smads interacts with the Co-Smad, Smad4 and this complex then accumulates in the nucleus. In the nucleus the activated Smad complex associates with DNA binding cofactors, coactivators and corepressors that regulate transcription of target genes. Tf, transcription factors.

Sma and Mad proteins from *C. elegans* and *Drosophila*, respectively) family of intracellular mediators, which function to carry the signal from the cell surface directly to the nucleus. There are three distinct classes of SMADs: receptor-regulated or R-SMADs, common mediator or Co-SMADs, and inhibitory SMADs. The activated type I receptor directly phosphorylates and activates the R-SMADs leading to interaction with Co-SMADs, such as SMAD4. This heterodimeric complex then translocates to the nucleus to regulate gene expression. The inhibitory SMADs conteract the effects of R-SMADs and antagonize TGF-$\beta$ signaling.

The biological response to TGF-$\beta$ signaling appears to be almost entirely determined by the type I receptor. In vertebrates there are seven distinct type I receptors that interact with one of five type II receptors. The signal from the type I receptor is funneled through one of two groups of SMAD proteins. Specific R-SMADs recognize different DNA binding proteins and regulate distinct target genes and thereby generate diverse biological responses. For example, phosphorylation and activation of the R-SMADs, SMAD2, and SMAD3, transduce a TGF-$\beta$-like signal, whereas activation of the R-SMADs, SMAD1, SMAD5, and SMAD8, transduce signals initiated by BMPs. There is also some evidence that TGF-$\beta$ can signal through SMAD independent processes via the activation of RhoA, Ras, and TGF-$\beta$ activated kinase 1, Tak1 (Massague et al., 2000).

Mutations in the TGF-$\beta$ family of ligands are responsible for a variety of human diseases including human cancer, hereditary chondrodysplasias, and pulmonary hypertension (de Caestecker et al., 2000; Massague et al., 2000). Transforming growth factor-$\beta$ itself plays an important role in cancer progression by functioning as both an anti-proliferative factor and as a tumor promoter. If TGF-$\beta$ signaling is blocked, there is an increase in cell growth leading to tumor formation. In addition, numerous components of the TGF-$\beta$ pathway are tumor suppressors that are mutated in cancer. Point mutations in the receptors have been identified in human colon and gastric cancers. Mutations in SMAD2 have been identified in colorectal and lung cancers, and SMAD4 mutations are found in a large number of colorectal, pancreatic, and lung cancers. These point mutations in the SMAD proteins leads to loss of phosphorylation of SMAD2, for example, and subsequent loss of association with SMAD4.

## 8.5 SUMMARY

It has been estimated that upwards of 6400 genes in the human genome (approximately 20 percent of human coding genes as estimated by the Human Genome Project) encode proteins involved in signal transduction. This multitude of extracellular signals, cell surface receptors, and intracellular signaling proteins is highly organized into regulatory circuits. However, a diverse array of extracellular signals activate common core signaling pathways and can in turn lead to very different cellular responses. As well, seemingly small changes within individual components of a growth factor pathway can have catastrophic effects on cellular function. Although researchers have made significant advances in understanding the molecular details of many signaling pathways, our understanding of how these changes bring about the phenotypic changes associated with malignancy is limited.

Some of the most promising recent developments in cancer therapies are based upon our understanding of growth factor signaling and the identification of aberrantly activated signaling components. The development of powerful new genomic techniques that facilitate genome wide screens for cancer genes, proteomics and advances in mass spectral analysis that can define the global changes in protein modifications within specific tumor types, and microarray analysis to reveal complex gene expression patterns that define specific cancers will all contribute to our knowledge of both normal and cancer cell signal transduction mechanisms. Together these approaches will also lead to the identification of new cancer causing genes and new drug targets, and the therapeutics developed in response to them will have the potential to be tumor specific. In addition, the establishment of mouse models of human cancer will allow the rapid validation of new therapeutic targets and development of small molecule inhibitors that can specifically antagonize the activity of an aberrantly activated signal transduction pathway, or potentially augment a defective tumor suppressor pathway.

## REFERENCES

Akiyama T: Wnt/beta-catenin signaling. *Cytokine Growth Factor Rev* 2000; 11:273–282.

Artavanis-Tsakonas S, Rand MD, Lake RJ: Notch signaling: cell fate control and signal integration in development. *Science* 1999; 284:770–776.

Attisano L, Wrana JL: Signal transduction by the TGF-beta superfamily. *Science* 2002; 296:1646–1647.

Berger SL: Histone modifications in transcriptional regulation. *Curr Opin Genet Dev* 2002; 12:142–148.

Blume-Jensen P, Hunter T: Oncogenic kinase signalling. *Nature* 2001; 411:355–365.

Brakebusch C, Fassler R: The integrin-actin connection, an eternal love affair. *EMBO J* 2003; 22:2324–2333.

Brivanlou AH, Darnell JE Jr: Signal transduction and the control of gene expression. *Science* 2002; 295:813–818.

Cadigan KM, Nusse R: Wnt signaling: a common theme in animal development. *Genes Dev* 1997; 11:3286–3305.

Calderwood DA, Shattil SJ, Ginsberg MH: Integrins and actin filaments: reciprocal regulation of cell adhesion and signaling. *J Biol Chem* 2000; 275:22607–22610.

Cantley LC: The phosphoinositide 3–kinase pathway. *Science* 2002; 296:1655–1657.

Chang L, Karin M: Mammalian MAP kinase signalling cascades. *Nature* 2001; 410:37–40.

Chen CH, Six A, Kubota T, et al: T cell receptors and T cell development. *Curr Top Microbiol Immunol* 1996; 212:37–53.

Chernoff J: Protein tyrosine phosphatases as negative regulators of mitogenic signaling. *J Cell Physiol* 1999; 180:173–181.

Cohen MM Jr: The hedgehog signaling network. *Am J Med Genet* 2003; 123A:5–28.

Davies H, Bignell GR, Cox C, et al: Mutations of the BRAF gene in human cancer. *Nature* 2002; 417:949–954.

de Caestecker MP, Piek E, Roberts AB: Role of transforming growth factor-beta signaling in cancer. *J Natl Cancer Inst* 2000; 92:1388–1402.

de La Coste A, Romagnolo B, Billuart P, et al: Somatic mutations of the beta-catenin gene are frequent in mouse and human hepatocellular carcinomas. *Proc Natl Acad Sci USA* 1998; 95:8847–8851.

Dennler S, Goumans MJ, ten Dijke P: Transforming growth factor beta signal transduction. *J Leukoc Biol* 2002; 71:731–740.

Downward J: The ras superfamily of small GTP-binding proteins. *Trends Biochem Sci.* 1990; 15:469–472.

Downward J: Targeting RAS signalling pathways in cancer therapy. *Nat Rev Cancer* 2003; 3:11–22.

Ellisen LW, Bird J, West DC, et al: TAN-1, the human homolog of the Drosophila notch gene, is broken by chromosomal translocations in T lymphoblastic neoplasms. *Cell* 1991; 66:649–661.

Evan GI, Vousden KH: Proliferation, cell cycle and apoptosis in cancer. *Nature* 2001; 411:342–348.

Evans RD, Perkins VC, Henry A, et al: A tumor-associated beta 1 integrin mutation that abrogates epithelial differentiation control. *J Cell Biol* 2003; 160:589–596.

Forman-Kay JD, Pawson T: Diversity in protein recognition by PTB domains. *Curr Opin Struct Biol* 1999; 9:690–695.

Hamm H: The many faces of G protein signaling. *J Biol Chem* 1998; 273:669–672.

Hancock JF: Ras proteins: different signals from different locations. *Nat Rev Mol Cell Biol* 2003; 4:373–384.

Hanks SK, Quinn AM: Protein kinase catalytic domain sequence database: identification of conserved features of primary structure and classification of family members. *Methods Enzymol* 1991; 200:38–62.

Heinrich PC, Behrmann I, Haan S, et al: Principles of interleukin (IL)-6–type cytokine signalling and its regulation. *Biochem J* 2003; 374:1–20.

Hershko A, Ciechanover A: The ubiquitin system. *Annu Rev Biochem* 1998; 67:425–479.

Hicke L: Gettin' down with ubiquitin: turning off cell-surface receptors, transporters and channels. *Trends Cell Biol* 1999; 9:107–112.

Hill CS, Treisman R: Growth factors and gene expression: fresh insights from arrays. *Sci STKE.* 1999:PE1.

Huang H, Fujii H, Sankila A, et al: Beta-catenin mutations are frequent in human hepatocellular carcinomas associated with hepatitis C virus infection. *Am J Pathol* 1999; 155:1795–1801.

Hubbard SR: Theme and variations: juxtamembrane regulation of receptor protein kinases. *Mol Cell* 2001; 8:481–482.

Huelsken J, Behrens J: The Wnt signalling pathway. *J Cell Sci* 2002; 115:3977–3978.

Huelsken J, Birchmeier W: New aspects of Wnt signaling pathways in higher vertebrates. *Curr Opin Genet Dev* 2001; 11:547–553.

Hynes RO: Integrins: bidirectional, allosteric signaling machines. *Cell* 2002; 110:673–687.

Ihle JN, Kerr IM: Jaks and Stats in signaling by the cytokine receptor superfamily. *Trends Genet* 1995; 11:69–74.

Ingham PW, McMahon AP: Hedgehog signaling in animal development: paradigms and principles. *Genes Dev* 2001; 15:3059–3087.

Jarriault S, Brou C, Logeat F, et al: Signalling downstream of activated mammalian Notch. *Nature* 1995; 377:355–358.

Jia J, Tong C, Jiang J: Smoothened transduces Hedgehog signal by physically interacting with Costal2/Fused complex through its C-terminal tail. *Genes Dev* 2003; 17:2709–2720.

Jiang G, Zhang BB: PI 3-kinase and its up- and down-stream modulators as potential targets for the treatment of type II diabetes. *Front Biosci* 2002; 7:d903–d907.

Jordan MS, Singer AL, Koretzky GA: Adaptors as central mediators of signal transduction in immune cells. *Nat Immunol* 2003; 4:110–116.

Joutel A, Tournier-Lasserve E: Notch signalling pathway and human diseases. *Semin Cell Dev Biol.* 1998; 9:619–25.

Katso R, Okkenhaug K, et al: Cellular function of phosphoinositide 3-kinases: implications for development, homeostasis, and cancer. *Annu Rev Cell Dev Biol* 2001; 17:615–675.

Kikuchi A: Tumor formation by genetic mutations in the components of the Wnt signaling pathway. *Cancer Sci* 2003; 94:225–229.

Kopan R: Notch: a membrane-bound transcription factor. *J Cell Sci* 2002; 115:1095–1097.

Kopan R, Turner DL: The Notch pathway: democracy and aristocracy in the selection of cell fate. *Curr Opin Neurobiol* 1996; 6:594–601.

Kyriakis JM, Avruch J: Mammalian mitogen-activated protein kinase signal transduction pathways activated by stress and inflammation. *Physiol Rev* 2001; 81:807–869.

Lemmon MA: Phosphoinositide recognition domains. *Traffic* 2003; 4:201–213.

Liu S, Calderwood DA, Ginsberg MH: Integrin cytoplasmic domain-binding proteins. *J Cell Sci.* 2000; 113:3563–3571.

Lum L, Zhang C, Oh S, et al: Hedgehog signal transduction via smoothened association with a cytoplasmic complex scaffolded by the atypical kinesin, Costal-2. *Mol Cell* 2003; 12:1261–1274.

Maillard I, Pear WS: Notch and cancer: best to avoid the ups and downs. *Cancer Cell* 2003; 3:203–205.

Martin KH, Slack JK, Boerner SA, et al: Integrin connections map: to infinity and beyond. *Science* 2002; 296:1652–1653.

Massague J, Blain SW, Lo RS: TGFbeta signaling in growth control, cancer, and heritable disorders. *Cell* 2000; 103: 295–309.

Meng W, Sawasdikosol S, Burakoff SJ, Eck MJ: Structure of the amino-terminal domain of Cbl complexed to its binding site on ZAP-70 kinase. *Nature* 1999; 398:84–90.

Moon RT, Bowerman B, Boutros M, Perrimon N: The promise and perils of Wnt signaling through beta-catenin. *Science* 2002; 296:1644–1646.

Moustakas A, Souchelnytskyi S, Heldin CH: Smad regulation in TGF-beta signal transduction. *J Cell Sci* 2001; 114:4359–4369.

Muller CW: Transcription factors: global and detailed views. *Curr Opin Struct Biol* 2001; 11:26–32.

Mullor JL, Sanchez P, Altaba AR: Pathways and consequences: hedgehog signaling in human disease. *Trends Cell Biol* 2002; 12:562–569.

Myers MG Jr, Sun XJ, White MF: The IRS-1 signaling system. *Trends Biochem Sci* 1994; 19:289–293.

Nam Y, Aster JC, Blacklow SC: Notch signaling as a therapeutic target. *Curr Opin Chem Biol* 2002; 6:501–509.

Neves SR, Ram PT, Iyengar R: G protein pathways. *Science* 2002; 296:1636–1639.

Nicolas M, Wolfer A, Raj K, et al: Notch1 functions as a tumor suppressor in mouse skin. *Nat Genet* 2003; 33:416–421.

Nip J, Brodt P: The role of the integrin vitronectin receptor, alpha v beta 3 in melanoma metastasis. *Cancer Metastasis Rev* 1995; 14:241–252.

Nybakken K, Perrimon N: Hedgehog signal transduction: recent findings. *Curr Opin Genet Dev* 2002; 12:503–511.

O'Shea JJ, Gadina M, Schreiber RD: Cytokine signaling in 2002: new surprises in the Jak/Stat pathway. *Cell* 2002; 109(Suppl):S121–S131.

Pawson T: Regulation and targets of receptor tyrosine kinases. *Eur J Cancer.* 2002; 38(Suppl 5): S3–S10.

Pawson T, Gish GD: SH2 and SH3 domains: from structure to function. *Cell* 1992; 71:359–362.

Pawson T, Nash P: Assembly of cell regulatory systems through protein interaction domains. *Science* 2003; 300:445–452.

Pawson T, Scott JD: Signaling through scaffold, anchoring, and adaptor proteins. *Science* 1997; 278:2075–2080.

Polakis P: Wnt signaling and cancer. *Genes Dev* 2000; 14:1837–1851.

Radtke F, Raj K: The role of Notch in tumorigenesis: oncogene or tumour suppressor? *Nat Rev Cancer* 2003; 3:756–767.

Robinson DR, Wu YM, Lin SF: The protein tyrosine kinase family of the human genome. *Oncogene* 2000; 19:5548–5557.

Rotin D, Staub O, Haguenauer-Tsapis R: Ubiquitination and endocytosis of plasma membrane proteins: role of Nedd4/Rsp5p family of ubiquitin-protein ligases. *J Membr Biol* 2000; 176:1–17.

Ruel L, Rodriguez R, Gallet A, et al: Stability and association of Smoothened, Costal2 and Fused with Cubitus interruptus are regulated by Hedgehog. *Nat Cell Biol* 2003; 5:907–913.

Ruiz i Altaba A, Sanchez P, Dahmane N: Gli and hedgehog in cancer: tumours, embryos and stem cells. *Nat Rev Cancer* 2002; 2:361–372.

Sahai E, Marshall CJ: RHO-GTPases and cancer. *Nat Rev Cancer* 2002; 2:133–142.

Samelson LE: Signal transduction mediated by the T cell antigen receptor: the role of adapter proteins. *Annu Rev Immunol* 2002; 20:371–394.

Schlessinger J: Ligand-induced, receptor-mediated dimerization and activation of EGF receptor. *Cell* 2002; 110:669–672.

Schlessinger J, Lemmon MA: SH2 and PTB domains in tyrosine kinase signaling. *Sci STKE.* 2003:RE12.

Sharrocks AD, Yang SH, Galanis A: Docking domains and substrate-specificity determination for MAP kinases. *Trends Biochem Sci* 2000; 25:448–453.

Sherr CJ: Cancer cell cycles. *Science* 1996; 274:1672–1677.

Songyang Z, Shoelson SE, Chaudhuri M, et al: SH2 domains recognize specific phosphopeptide sequences. *Cell* 1993; 72:767–778.

Sprang SR: G protein mechanisms: insights from structural analysis. *Annu Rev Biochem* 1997; 66:639–678.

Taipale J, Beachy PA: The Hedgehog and Wnt signalling pathways in cancer. *Nature* 2001; 411:349–354.

Taylor MD, Liu L, Raffel C, et al: Mutations in SUFU predispose to medulloblastoma. *Nat Genet* 2002; 31:306–310.

Tyers M, Willems AR: One ring to rule a superfamily of E3 ubiquitin ligases. *Science* 1999; 284: 603–604.

van der Geer P, Hunter T, Lindberg RA: Receptor protein-tyrosine kinases and their signal transduction pathways. *Annu Rev Cell Biol* 1994;10:251–337.

van der Geer P, Pawson T: The PTB domain: a new protein module implicated in signal transduction. *Trends Biochem Sci* 1995; 20:277–280.

Villavicencio EH, Walterhouse DO, Iannaccone PM: The sonic hedgehog-patched-gli pathway in human development and disease. *Am J Hum Genet* 2000; 67:1047–1054.

Weiss A, Littman DR: Signal transduction by lymphocyte antigen receptors. *Cell* 1994; 76:263–274.

Wicking C, McGlinn E: The role of hedgehog signalling in tumorigenesis. *Cancer Lett* 2001 173:1–7.

Woychik NA, Hampsey M: The RNA polymerase II machinery: structure illuminates function. *Cell* 2002; 108:453–463.

Yip CC, Ottensmeyer P: Three-dimensional structural interactions of insulin and its receptor. *J Biol Chem* 2003; 278:27329–27332.

Zarrinpar A, Bhattacharyya, Lim WA: The structure and function of proline recognition domains. *Sci STKE* 2003:RE8.

# 9

# Cell Proliferation and Tumor Growth

*Jeff C.H. Donovan, Joyce Slingerland, and Ian F. Tannock*

## 9.1 OVERVIEW OF THE CELL CYCLE

Progression through the cell cycle is coordinated by a tightly regulated series of events. Cells can be recognized by morphological criteria in mitosis (M), and radiolabeled precursors of DNA have demonstrated that DNA synthesis takes place only in a specific period in the cell cycle termed the *synthesis* or S phase. The *gaps* (G) between M and S phase and between S phase and M are called, respectively, the G1 and G2 phases (Fig. 9.1). Following M, cells may also enter a quiescent G0 phase in the absence of stimuli triggering further cell division cycles. Most cells in normal adult tissues are in a quiescent G0 state. In the presence of a sustained mitogenic stimulus, cells in G0 or G1 progress to a *restriction point* (R), beyond which a cell is committed to enter S phase. After the R point, growth factors present in the environment are no longer required for progression into S phase and completion of G2 and M phases. In cancer cells, deregulation of multiple control mechanisms results in cells with different degrees of autonomy from extracellular growth-stimulatory or growth-inhibitory signals, making them more likely to meet the requirements for transition through the R point.

Progression through the cell cycle is regulated by the synthesis, assembly, and activation of key cell cycle regulatory complexes comprised of cyclins and cyclin-dependent kinases (Cdks, Fig. 9.1), followed by their subsequent inactivation disassociation and degradation. Multiple mechanisms regulate the timing of these processes, including transcriptional and translational controls, posttranslational control via ubiquitin-mediated proteolysis, as well as regulation of the subcellular localization of proteins. These processes are described in Section 9.2, and the dysregulation that may occur in cancer is described in Section 9.3.

Knowledge of the rate of tumor growth and the cell cycle distribution of constituent cells (and their rate of cell death) comes from studies of cell population kinetics. These properties influence the responsiveness of cells to anticancer treatment. Estimation of the distribution of a cell population among the phases of the cell cycle, and of phase duration, has depended on recognizing cells that are marked with a specific precursor of DNA synthesis, or on fluorescent stains that bind to

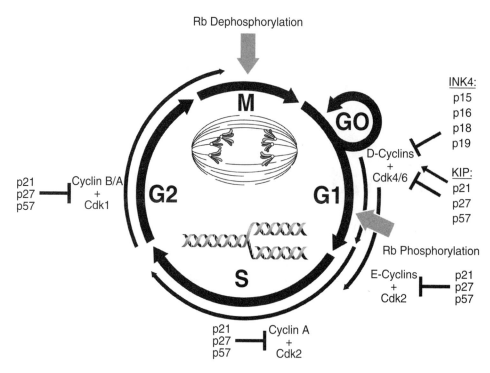

**Figure 9.1.** Overview of the cell cycle. The cell cycle is classically divided into the G1 (G, gap), S (DNA synthesis), G2 and M (mitotic) phases. The majority of cells in living organisms are in a quiescent G0 phase. Transition between these phases is governed by positive effectors (cyclins and cyclin-dependent kinases) and negative (INK4 and KIP family) regulators (Cdk inhibitors). Phosphorylation of the retinoblastoma protein (Rb) removes its restraining effect on the G1-to-S phase transition. p21 and p27 play both activating and inhibitory roles for D-type cyclin-Cdk (see text). The figure shows only cyclin/Cdks and Cdk inhibitors whose relevance to cancer is best understood.

DNA and indicate cellular DNA content. These methods are described in Section 9.4, together with a review of the cell kinetics of selected normal tissues and of human tumors, and their implications for cancer therapy.

An understanding of the molecular events that regulate the cell cycle, and the mechanisms whereby malignant cells escape from cell cycle controls and the proliferation arrest imposed by a finite life span, are key to understanding how cancerous cells differ from normal cells. These concepts are not only of biological interest; they are important for understanding how anticancer drugs and radiation affect normal tissues and tumors.

## 9.2 REGULATION OF THE CELL CYCLE

### 9.2.1 Cycle-Dependent Kinases and Cyclins

Mammalian Cdks comprise a family of ten serine-threonine protein kinases (Cdk 1–10) that catalyze different cell cycle transitions (some of these Cdks are shown in Fig. 9.1). A Cdk molecule binds to an activator molecule known as a cyclin, and this binding is an absolute requirement for Cdk activation (Sherr, 1994). In addition, Cdks are regulated by site-specific phosphorylation and by the binding of Cdk inhibitors (Sherr, 2000).

*Regulation of Cdks by Phosphorylation* Activation of Cdks requires the phosphorylation of a conserved threonine residue, located in the activation loop of the kinase (e.g., Thr 161 for Cdk1, Thr 160 for Cdk2), and this is catalyzed by the Cdk-activating kinase (CAK; Fig. 9.2). Phosphorylation of Thr within the activation loop elicits a conformational change, which together with cyclin binding, is required for kinase activity. Cdk-activating kinase is active throughout all phases of the cell cycle, but its access to the Cdk substrate is cell cycle regulated (Solomon and Kaldis, 1998). Inhibition of CAK action on, or access to the Cdks, prevents phosphorylation and activation of Cdks and leads to cell cycle arrest. Phosphorylation at conserved inhibitory sites (threonine 14 and tyrosine 15 on Cdks) leads to inhibition of Cdks and this is catalyzed by the Wee-1 and Myt-1 kinases (Fig. 9.2).

The cell division cycle (Cdc) phosphatases Cdc25A, Cdc25B, and Cdc25C remove the inhibitory phosphates from the threonine 14 and tyrosine 15 sites on Cdks and, like CAK, are also required for full Cdk activation. The expression and activity of these phosphatases is periodic across the cell cycle. Cdc25A expression and activity is maximal in late G1 and contributes to the acti-

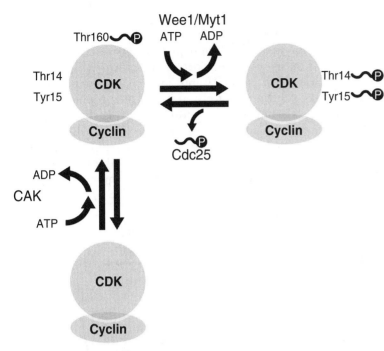

**CDK Active**   **CDK Inactive**

**CDK Inactive**

**Figure 9.2.** The cyclin-dependent kinases are essential mediators of transit throughout the cell cycle. Cdks require a cyclin binding partner for activation and are regulated by phosphorylation. Activating phosphorylation of Threonine (Thr160) by CAK and dephosphorylation of inhibitory Thr14/Tyr15 residues by Cdc25 family members is essential for Cdk activation. The Wee1/Myt1 kinases oppose Cdk activation by the Cdc25 phosphatases.

vation of Cdk2; active Cdk2 in turn potentiates Cdc25A activation creating a positive feedback loop. Overexpression of Cdc25A reduces the time required for G1-to-S phase transit, indicating that this phosphatase controls a rate-limiting step required for S-phase entry.

Cdc25B and Cdc25C are involved in the regulation of the G2/M transition and act in the nucleus on the cyclin-B–associated Cdk1 (see Draetta and Eckstein, 1997 for review). Binding of proteins of the 14-3-3 family to Cdc25B and Cdc25C leads to cytoplasmic sequestration of these proteins away from their nuclear targets (Fig. 9.3). This mechanism impairs Cdc25C action following DNA damage (see Chap. 5, Sec. 5.4). Cdc25C is predominantly cytoplasmic during interphase but nuclear during mitosis. During interphase, Cdc25C is phosphorylated on serine 216, a site that facilitates binding of proteins of the 14-3-3 family. 14-3-3 binding to Cdc25C contributes to retention of Cdc25C in the cytoplasm during S and G2 phases because access of the nuclear import machinery to the Cdc25C nuclear localization signal is blocked. Entry into mitosis is associated with a progressive decrease in Cdc25C phosphorylation at serine 216, a decrease in 14-3-3 binding, and nuclear accumulation of Cdc25C. This transition is accompanied by accelerated cyclin B nuclear import. Cdc25A and Cdc25B, but not Cdc25C, have been shown

to have oncogenic potential when overexpressed in mammalian cells (Yoneda, 2000).

*Activation of Cdks by Binding to Cyclins*   The family of mammalian cyclins include cyclins A to H and all share a conserved sequence of about 100 amino acids, referred to as the *cyclin box*. Different cyclins bind and activate different Cdks, and activated cyclin-Cdk complexes, in turn, phosphorylate various target proteins to ultimately mediate progression through the different cell cycle phases (Fig. 9.1). Cyclin levels change significantly during cell cycle progression, allowing for precise timing of Cdk activation and ensuring that these kinases are catalytically active only at specific times during the cell cycle. This is regulated by both the specific subcellular localization and the timed expression and degradation of various cyclins and Cdk inhibitors throughout the cell cycle. In general, the peak nuclear expression of a specific cyclin occurs at or just prior to the peak activity of the partner kinase, and following activation, the respective cyclins are degraded rapidly by the ubiquitin-mediated proteosomal pathway.

Protein degradation by the ubiquitin pathway occurs via the covalent attachment of multiple ubiquitin molecules containing 76 amino acids to a protein followed by recognition and degradation of the polyubiquiti-

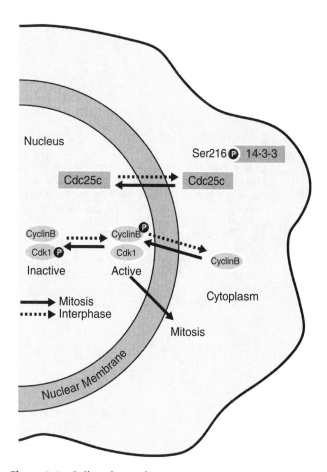

**Figure 9.3.** Cell cycle regulation at mitosis. Cyclin B/Cdk1 activation is essential for the entrance into and progression through mitosis. Cdc25c, which is retained in the cytoplasm by 14-3-3 proteins until the onset of mitosis, contributes to Cdk1 activation. Cyclin B1, like Cdc25c, is also predominantly cytoplasmic during interphase. Cyclin B1 phosphorylation facilitates its accumulation in the nucleus.

nated protein by the 26 S proteosome (Fig. 9.4; for review see Shah et al., 2001). The enzymes that mediate attachment of ubiquitin to the substrate are the E, ubiquitin activating enzyme, the E2 ubiquitin conjugating enzymes and the E3 ubiquitin ligases. E3 ubiquitin ligases of the SCF-type are involved in the proteolytic degradation of many different cell cycle regulators. Their name is derived from the multiple proteins which comprise the enzyme: Skp1, Cullin, Roc1/Rbx1, and an F-box protein. While the Skp1, Cullin, and Rbx-1 components are constant subunits of the SCF enzyme, the specific F-box protein recruited to the E3 complex determines the specific protein targeted for degradation. The F-box components for many mammalian cell cycle regulators have recently been identified (see discussion below; Craig and Tyers, 1999).

Progression through G1 and into S phase is regulated by the activities of the cyclin-D–, cyclin-E–, and cyclin-A–associated kinases (Morgan, 1995). One of the important substrates of these kinases is the retinoblastoma protein, Rb (Fig. 9.5). In early G1 phase, Rb is hypophosphorylated and bound to a member of the E2F/DP-1 family of transcription factors. The Rb/E2F or Rb/DP-1 complexes recruit additional molecules such as histone deacetylases (HDACs) to repress the transcription of genes whose products are required for DNA synthesis such as dihydrofolate reductase. However, activation of cyclin D and later cyclin-E–dependent kinases during progression from G1 to S phase leads to the accumulation of pRb in a hyperphosphorylated state. This not only relieves the Rb-HDAC–mediated transcriptional repression but allows E2F family members to dissociate from the hyperphosphorylated Rb, and activate transcription of genes required for S phase

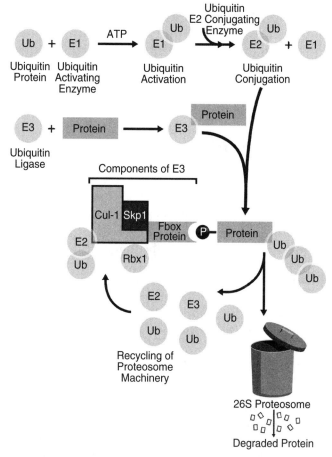

**Figure 9.4.** Protein degradation by the 26 S proteosome. Many proteins are marked for degradation by the 26 S proteosome following the attachment of multiple ubiquitin molecules. The ubiquitin-activating enzyme, E1, transfers ubiquitin moieties to one of several ubiquitin-conjugating enzymes, or E2s. The E2 catalyzes the attachment of ubiquitin to the substrate protein, generally with the assistance of an additional enzyme complex known as the ubiquitin ligase or E3. The ubiquitin proteolytic pathway is made up of multiple E2s and E3s with differing specificities. This ensures the discrimination between a large number of proteins targeted for degradation under different conditions.

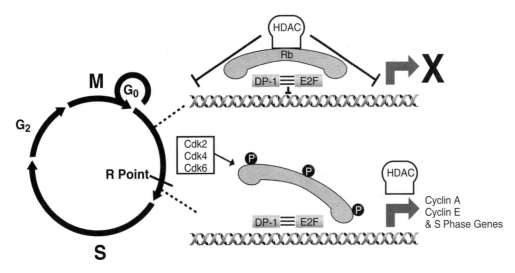

**Figure 9.5.** Regulation of the retinoblastoma (Rb) protein. In early G1, the E2F-Rb-HDAC and DP-1-Rb-HDAC complexes (HDAC, histone deacetylase) act as transcriptional repressors, thus inhibiting the transcription of genes required for entrance into and progression through S phase, such as cyclin E and cyclin A. Activation of cyclin D-Cdk4 and cyclin D-Cdk6 in early G1 and cyclin E-Cdk2 in late G1 leads to the phosphorylation of Rb. Because the hyperphosphorylated form of Rb has reduced affinity for binding of E2F and DP-1, they are liberated to activate transcription.

entrance, such as cyclin E and cyclin A, as well as enzymes needed for DNA synthesis. The phosphorylation of the retinoblastoma protein is one indicator of cell cycle progression through the restriction point.

In most cells, cyclin D-Cdk complexes are activated by mitogenic stimuli early in G1 followed by activation of cyclin E-Cdk2 in mid-G1 phase (Fig. 9.1). The D- and E-type cyclins promote movement through the G1/S transition: microinjection of antibodies to cyclin D1, cyclin E1, or cyclin E2 can prevent G1 to S phase progression (Sherr and Roberts, 1999; Sherr, 2000). Overexpression of both the D-type cyclins and cyclin E1 can shorten the time needed to progress from G1 into S phase. Moreover, concurrent overexpression of both cyclins further shortens the G1-to-S phase interval, suggesting that cyclin D1 and cyclin E complexes may regulate independent pathways.

Cyclin A-Cdk2 activation in late G1 phase follows cyclin E-Cdk2 activation and is essential for initiation of and progression through S phase and for the onset of mitosis (Fig. 9.1; Sherr, 1994). Antibodies to cyclin A block S phase entry and overexpression accelerates S phase entry. Cyclin A-Cdk2 also plays a key role in the duplication of centrosomes, the structures that are critical for proper chromosome segregation during mitosis (Meraldi et al., 1999).

In mammalian cells, two B-type cyclins (cyclin B1 and cyclin B2) associate with Cdk1 (also known as cdc2) to regulate entry into and exit from mitosis (Fig. 9.3; reviewed in Takizawa and Morgan, 2000). The subcellular localization of the B-type cyclins, like many proteins,

is determined by the equilibrium achieved between nuclear import and nuclear export. Prior to mitosis (during the S and G2 phase), cyclin B1 shuttles between the nucleus and cytoplasm, but the vast majority of cyclin B1 is retained in the cytoplasm due to impairment of nuclear import and activation of rapid nuclear export (Fig. 9.3; reviewed in Yoneda, 2000).

At the G2/M transition, cyclin B1 becomes phosphorylated, which prevents its association with an export mediator protein, resulting in a reduction in nuclear export and thus accumulation in the nucleus. Accelerated nuclear import may also facilitate cyclin B1 nuclear accumulation (Fig. 9.3). The ubiquitin-mediated degradation of cyclin B1 is activated in late G2/M phase and promotes exit from mitosis. As described earlier in this section, the Cdc25C phosphatase plays an important role at the G2/M transition by regulating cyclin B-Cdk1 activation and hence entry into mitosis (Takizawa and Morgan, 2000). The retinoblastoma protein is dephosphorylated in mitosis, prior to the G1 phase of the next cell cycle.

### 9.2.2 Inhibitors of Cyclin-Dependent Kinases

In addition to phosphorylation and binding to cyclins, Cdks are subject to regulation by the binding of Cdk inhibitory (CKI) proteins (Fig. 9.6). There are two families of CKIs: the *Ki*nase *I*nhibitory *P*rotein (KIP) family and the *I*nhibitor of Cd*k4* (INK4) family (Sherr and Roberts, 1999; Sherr, 2000). Overexpression of either KIP or INK proteins leads to G1 arrest.

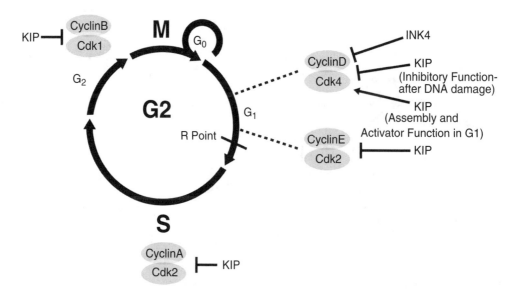

**Figure 9.6.** The Cdk inhibitors. A schematic diagram showing mechanisms of regulation of Cdks by the KIP and INK4 families of Cdk inhibitors. The KIP molecules inhibit cyclin-Cdk complexes including cyclin E-Cdk2 and cyclin A-CdK2. They facilitate assembly and activation of D-type cyclin-Cdks. The INK4 family of inhibitors act to destabilize cyclin-Cdk association and prevent reassociation of the displaced cyclin.

*The KIP Family of Cdk Inhibitors* The KIP family members, which include p21[Cip1], also known as p21[Waf1], p27[Kip1], and p57[Kip2] (referred to simply as p21, p27, and p57) share homology at their N-terminal Cdk inhibitory domain, and in vitro they can inhibit all cyclin-Cdk complexes (Fig. 9.6). The KIP proteins have binding sites for both the cyclins and Cdks, and only a single KIP molecule is required for cyclin-Cdk inhibition. In vivo, KIP expression and activity is tightly regulated.

p21 was identified both as a novel protein bound to Cdk2 and as a protein whose gene expression is upregulated by p53 following cellular stress or DNA damage (see Chap. 5, Sec. 5.4). p21 binds tightly to both the cyclin and Cdk subunits. p27 was identified in cells arrested in the G1 phase by contact inhibition, and by exposure of cells to transforming growth factor beta (TGF-β; reviewed in Slingerland and Pagano, 2000). Accumulation of p27 in cyclin E-Cdk2 complexes induces and/or maintains G1 arrest in response to several antiproliferative signals. p27 plays an essential role in maintaining G1 arrest in serum starved fibroblasts as well as in antiestrogen treated breast cancer cells (Coats et al., 1996; Cariou et al., 2000). The observation that p27 knockout mice are larger than p27 wild-type mice, and have hyperplasia of multiple organs, supports an important anti-proliferative role for this KIP member (Blain et al., 2003). Unlike p21, which appears to be regulated at the transcriptional level, p27 is largely regulated by translational controls and by control of its ubiquitin-mediated proteolysis.

In early G1 phase, p27 translation falls abruptly and its proteolysis is stimulated in a mitogen-dependent, cyclin E/Cdk2-independent manner (Connor et al., 2003). Later in G1, cyclin E-cdk2 activity increases and cyclin E/Cdk2 phosphorylates p27 at Thr 187, allowing for recognition of p27 by the F-box protein Skp2 leading ultimately to the ubiquitin-mediated proteolysis of p27 (see Fig. 9.4). Thus, p27 acts as an inhibitor of cyclin E-Cdk2 in early G1 phase, but as a Cdk2 substrate in late G1 phase (Sherr, 1994; Slingerland and Pagano, 2000). Skp2 levels are low in quiescent cells (where p27 levels are high) and growth factor stimulation leads to induction of Skp2.

The *p57* gene was cloned following a search for genes homologous to *p27* and *p21*; p57 can bind and inhibit cyclin-Cdks. The *p57* gene is located on chromosome 11 at 11p15.5, a locus that frequently undergoes loss of heterozygosity in several cancers, including Wilms' tumor, and tumors associated with the Beckwith-Wiedemann syndrome, a childhood multiorgan overgrowth syndrome.

In addition to their role as inhibitors of Cdk activity, KIP family members have an essential role in the assembly, activation, and nuclear localization of the D-type cyclin-Cdk complexes (LaBaer et al., 1997; Cheng et al., 1999). The importance of KIPs in regulating cyclin D-Cdk complexes has been demonstrated in vivo. Mouse embryo fibroblasts lacking p21 and p27 fail to assemble cyclin D and Cdk4 complexes, express lower cyclin D1 levels, and are unable to accumulate cyclin

D1 in the nucleus (Cheng et al., 1999). The ability of KIP proteins to act as assembly factors for D-type cyclins and Cdk4 and Cdk6 is regulated independently of their ability to function as inhibitors of Cdk2 and Cdk1 complexes. Thus, KIP proteins can carry out two separate functions: the binding and inhibition of cyclin E-Cdk2 complexes and the assembly and activation of cyclin D-Cdk complexes.

*The INK4 Family of Cdk Inhibitors* Unlike the KIP family, members of the INK4 family act in G1 phase to inhibit primarily Cdk4 and Cdk6 (Fig. 9.6). The four members, p15$^{INK4B}$, p16$^{INK4A}$, p18$^{INK4C}$, and p19$^{INK4D}$ are structurally related. INK4 proteins act to destabilize the association of the D-type cyclins with Cdk4 or Cdk6 leading to an inactive INK4-bound Cdk that lacks an activating cyclin (Sherr and Roberts, 1999; Sherr, 2000).

The product of the *p16* gene was identified as a Cdk4-associated protein and also as the *MST1* gene on chromosome 9p13 that is frequently deleted in many human cancers. p16 plays an important role in the proliferative arrest of cells at senescence (see Sec. 9.2.6). Study of p16 knockout mice has indicated that this protein plays a tumor suppressor role (Sharpless et al., 2001); such mice are prone to tumor development and cell lines derived from p16-null mice undergo spontaneous immortalization with high frequency.

The *p15* gene was cloned following demonstration that it was induced in response to exposure of cells to the antiproliferative cytokine, TGF-$\beta$ (Hannon and Beach, 1994; see also Chap. 8, Sec. 8.4.4). Arrest in G1 phase by TGF-$\beta$ occurs via pathways involving induction of the *p15* gene, stabilization of the p15 protein, and accumulation of p15 in Cdk4 and Cdk6 complexes (reviewed in Donovan and Slingerland, 2000). The *p18*

gene, the third member of the INK family, may mediate inhibition of Cdk4 and Cdk6 during differentiation. p18 knockout mice develop gigantism and widespread organomegaly similar to p27 knockouts, suggesting an important role for p18 in growth control. The observation that p27−/− p18−/− double null mice are larger than either single null mice alone suggests that p27 and p18 may regulate different pathways (Franklin et al., 1998). The most recently discovered INK4 member, p19, is thought to inhibit Cdk4 and Cdk6 activity during cell cycle progression in late G1 and early S phase. Unlike the other INK4 proteins, p19 has not been implicated in tumor development.

### 9.2.3 The Role of Myc in Cell Cycle Control

The product of the *myc* gene is a transcription factor that, together with its dimerization partner, Max, plays a key role in cell proliferation. The expression of Myc is strictly dependent on mitogenic signals and is suppressed by growth inhibitory or differentiation signals. Constitutive Myc expression leads to cell cycle entry in the absence of growth factors. Microinjection of anti-Myc antibodies inhibits G1-to-S phase progression and c-Myc null cells proliferate slowly and have reduced cyclin D-Cdk4/6 and cyclin E-Cdk2 activity (Mateyak et al., 1999). The transcriptional targets of Myc include many important positive regulators of the cell cycle, including cyclins D1 and D2, Cdk4, E2F-2, Cdc25A, Cdc25B, along with the catalytic subunit of telomerase, hTERT (see also Chap. 5, Sec. 5.5.2). The p15 and p27 proteins are also regulated by Myc (Fig. 9.7).

The Myc protein contributes to p27 regulation in several ways in the G1 phase. First, Myc may antagonize p27 inhibitory function. Overexpression of p27 in Rat1

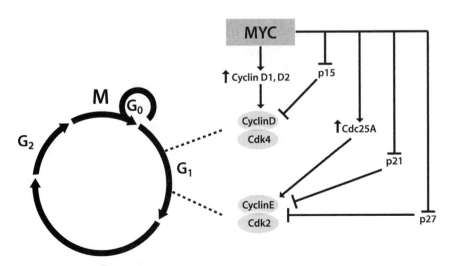

**Figure 9.7.** Regulation of the G1 phase by Myc. Myc activates transcription of cyclin D1, cyclin D2, and Cdc25A, and represses transcription of p15, p21, and p27. These Myc-dependent events lead ultimately to the activation of cyclin D/Cdk4 and cyclin E/Cdk2 and progression from G1 into S phase.

fibroblasts leads to G1 arrest, but the simultaneous over-expression of p27 and Myc prevents cell cycle arrest due to the sequestration and inactivation of p27 by Myc-induced protein(s) that prevent p27 from binding and inhibiting cyclin E-Cdk2 (Vlach et al., 1996). This suppression may occur through Myc-dependent induction of cyclin D1, cyclin D2, or other proteins that ultimately sequester p27 away from cyclin E-Cdk2, thereby preventing the inhibition of Cdk2 kinase activity. Second, in addition to antagonizing KIP function, Myc may also directly repress p27 and p21 transcription through the formation of Myc-Mad heterodimers (Luscher, 2001). Finally, Myc has been shown to directly activate the expression of Cul-1, an essential component of the SCF complex that promotes p27 degradation. Myc enhancement of Cul-1 expression leads to a reduction in p27 protein (O'Hagan et al., 2000). The Myc protein may also prevent cell cycle arrest in response to TGF-$\beta$ via its effects on p15 (Warner et al., 1999). Exposure of susceptible cells to TGF-$\beta$ normally leads to induction of p15 gene expression and this contributes to the G1 arrest. Myc overexpression can antagonize the induction of p15 following exposure to TGF-$\beta$ (Staller et al., 2001). Given the many ways in which overexpression of *myc* can deregulate the cell cycle, it is not surprising that Myc can cooperate with Ras to transform primary rat embryo fibroblasts into malignant cells. Activation of Myc is quite common in human tumors, including leukemias, lymphomas, and lung cancer (see Chap. 7, Secs. 7.2.5 and 7.3.4).

### 9.2.4 The Role of Ras in Cell Cycle Control

Our understanding of the multiple pathways that connect extracellular signals to the cell cycle machinery has expanded considerably since the discovery nearly two decades ago that Ras activity is required for cell cycle progression. Overexpression of Ras in serum-starved NIH 3T3 cells triggered them to enter S phase; conversely, microinjection of anti-ras antibodies in the presence of complete serum prevented S-phase entry. Ras activity plays a role not only in the transition from G0 to G1 phases, but in all transitions in the cell cycle. A critical effect of Ras in late G1 phase is the activation of pathways that contribute to phosphorylation of the retinoblastoma protein. Although Ras activation in cancer cells promotes proliferation, sustained activation of Ras triggers senescence in normal cells (see Sec. 9.2.6). Thus, most studies examining the effects of Ras on the cell cycle have been carried out using immortal or tumor-derived cell lines.

Mitogens that stimulate quiescent cells to progress from G0 into S phase lead to Ras activation. Activation of Ras rapidly triggers the Ras-Raf-mitogen-activated

protein kinase (MAPK) pathway, and also activates the Ras-phosphoinositol-3-kinase (PI-3K)-protein kinase B (PKB) pathway (see Chap. 8, Secs. 8.2.6 and 8.2.7). Both of these pathways play important roles in the regulation of the cell cycle (Kerkhoff and Rapp, 1998).

Multiple Ras effector pathways regulate cyclin-D1 levels (Fig. 9.8). Ras-Raf-MAPK activation induces transcription of the cyclin D1 gene and may regulate the assembly and activation of cyclin D1-Cdk4 complexes (Cheng et al., 1998). In addition, the PI-3K-PKB pathway activates translation of cyclin D1 (Muise-Helmericks et al., 1998), and leads to stabilization of the cyclin D1 protein (Diehl et al., 1998).

Multiple Ras effector pathways also regulate p27 (Fig. 9.8). Constitutive Ras-MEK-MAPK signaling has been shown to accelerate p27 proteolysis in some cell types, and inhibition of the pathway by pharmacological MEK inhibitors increased p27 levels and prevented S-phase

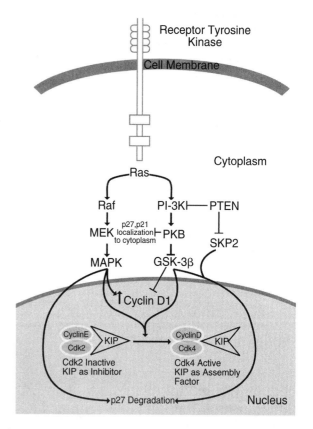

**Figure 9.8.** Cell cycle regulation by Ras signaling. The MAPK and PI-3K Ras effector pathways are two of the best characterized signaling pathways involved in cell cycle regulation. The PI-3K-PKB pathway mediates increased cyclin D1 translation, the stabilization of cyclin D1 (via GSK-3$\beta$ inhibition), the cytoplasmic mislocalization of p21 and p27, the conversion of KIP proteins to cyclin D-Cdk4 and Cdk6 assembly factors, and also activates degradation of p27. PTEN is frequently deleted in human cancers. SKP2 expression is increased in PTEN deleted cells and may contribute to loss of p27.

entry. In other cell types, including NIH 3T3 cells, MEK activation did not reduce p27 protein levels, but rather facilitated p27 sequestration by cyclin D1-Cdk4 complexes (Cheng et al., 1998). Activation of MEK/MAPK in breast cancer cells can also change the phosphorylation status of p27 leading to loss of its cyclin E-Cdk2 inhibitory activity and loss of responsiveness to the therapeutic effects of tamoxifen (Donovan et al., 2001).

Protein kinase B can phosphorylate and inhibit the forkhead transcription factors that themselves activate *p27* gene transcription. Thus, in some cell types, PKB activation decreases *p27* gene expression (Medema et al., 2000). *PTEN*, a tumor suppressor gene that encodes a lipid phosphatase that opposes the action of PI-3K (Fig. 9.8; see also Chap. 7, Sec. 7.4.3), has been shown to increase p27 stability by reducing the levels of the p27 F-box protein Skp2 (Mamillapalli et al., 2001). The observation that *p27* antisense oligonucleotides abolished the PTEN-induced arrest and that p27 levels are reduced in cells from PTEN null mice, lends further support to the notion that PTEN may act through p27 to cause cell cycle arrest.

The PI-3K pathway has been shown to play a role in regulating p21 and p27 localization and inhibitory function. Phosphorylation of p21 by PKB at threonine 145 leads to multiple effects including a reduction in the ability of p21 to bind and inhibit Cdk2 (Rossig et al., 2001), and cytoplasmic sequestration of p21 away from nuclear cyclin/Cdk2 targets (Zhou et al., 2001). Phosphorylation of p27 by PKB at threonine 157 leads to mislocalization of this Cdk inhibitor in the cytoplasm by impairing its nuclear import (Liang et al., 2002). In cells with constitutive PKB activation, the ability of p27 to arrest the cell cycle is impaired. Mislocalization of p27 to the cytoplasm is seen in up to 40 percent of human breast cancers and is associated with PKB activation, poor tumor differentiation, and poor prognosis.

### 9.2.5 Cell Cycle Regulation During Differentiation

In mammalian cells, cell cycle arrest accompanies terminal differentiation, and levels of Cdk inhibitors increase in most tissues during this process. Precise regulation of differentiation is required to ensure the proper number of differentiated cells at the appropriate time. Signals that induce differentiation also mediate G1 arrest.

p21 is localized in nonproliferating differentiated cells and its expression is prominent in skeletal muscle. p21 is regulated in differentiating cells by both p53-dependent and p53-independent pathways and is implicated in retinoic acid and vitamin-D3–induced differentiation of HL-60 leukemia cells. p27 is also induced during differentiation of HL-60 cells by vitamin D3 (Sherr and Roberts, 1999).

Targeted inactivation of Cdk inhibitor genes in mice has proven to be a useful approach to assess the role of the Cdk inhibitors in differentiation (reviewed in Blain et al, 2003). Many of the Cdk inhibitors have redundant functions during embryogenesis, and combined loss of two Cdk inhibitors is often required to disrupt cell cycle control. For example, normal differentiation is observed in the lens fiber of the eye in $p27^{-/-}$ or $p57^{-/-}$ single null mice, and only with the combined loss of both Cdk inhibitors in the $p27^{-/-}$ $p57^{-/-}$ double null mice is differentiation altered (Zhang et al., 1998a). Other Cdk inhibitors, however, do not compensate some functions. p27 knockout mice, for example, have multiorgan hyperplasia indicating an important anti-proliferative role for this protein that is not compensated by other Cdk inhibitors (reviewed in Sherr and Roberts, 1999).

In most cases, proliferation and differentiation are inversely coupled: mechanisms leading to cell cycle arrest facilitate differentiation, and mechanisms that prevent cell cycle arrest inhibit differentiation. Tumor cells, in general, have developed a block to normal differentiation and many have gained unlimited proliferative capacity (see Sec. 9.4.4). Limiting the proliferative capacity of some tumor cells by imposing cell cycle arrest causes them to resume normal differentiation. For example, enforced expression of p21 or the combination of p16 overexpression with the pharmacologic Cdk2 inhibitor roscovitine caused erythroleukemia cells to undergo G1 arrest and commit to terminal erythroid differentiation (Matushansky et al., 2000). In many cell types, however, cell cycle arrest is necessary but not sufficient for differentiation.

### 9.2.6 Cell Cycle Regulation at Senescence

Normal cells do not proliferate indefinitely when grown in culture. Rather, their proliferative potential is constrained to a finite number of population doublings leading to terminal growth arrest or senescence. The Cdk inhibitors mediate the G1 arrest that occurs when normal cultured cells undergo senescence following telomere shortening (see Chap. 5, Sec. 5.5.2). Senescence may function as a mechanism of tumor suppression since this form of proliferative arrest limits the accumulation of genetic errors in the progeny of a single cell. Abrogation of cellular senescence is required for continued tumor growth and metastatic progression. Investigation of effectors of cell cycle arrest at senescence has identified a number of molecular targets whose deregulation is required for immortalization and cancer progression.

The p21 and p16 proteins increase in senescent fibroblasts and contribute to the G1 arrest (Fig. 9.9). p16-

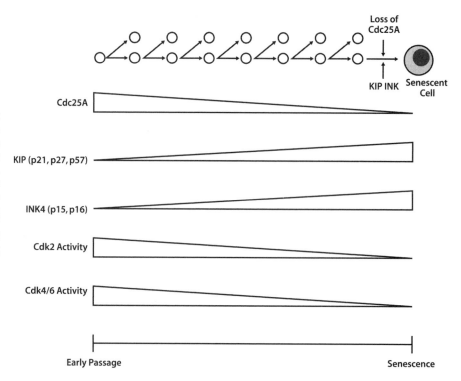

**Figure 9.9.** Cell cycle regulation at senescence. Senescence is a mechanism of tumor suppression that limits the number of population doublings and thus proliferative potential of cells. Although different cell types appear to invoke slightly different senescence mechanisms, all lead to Cdk inhibition and cell cycle arrest in G1. Loss of Cdc25A, increased INK4 proteins, and increased p21 and KIP-Cdk binding contribute to inhibition of the G1 Cdks.

null mouse embryonic fibroblasts showed an increased rate of immortalization compared to the wild-type cells, indicating a role for this Cdk inhibitor in senescence. In human keratinocytes, loss of p16 is required to escape senescence (Dickson et al., 2000). In contrast, BALB/c murine fibroblasts with a specific p16/INK4A deletion can still undergo senescence (Zhang et al., 1998b). These apparent discrepancies may be due to differences in the mechanisms that regulate senescence between fibroblasts and epithelial cells and between human and mouse cells. Human fibroblasts and epithelial cells seem to be dependent on p16 for their proliferative arrest at senescence, while mouse cells rely on other mechanisms, including the p19$^{ARF}$ protein (reviewed in Sherr, 2000).

p21 was discovered as a gene induced in senescent fibroblasts (Noda et al., 1994). p21 levels rise as fibroblasts and keratinocytes approach senescence. Elimination of p21 through homologous recombination extends the life span of human diploid fibroblasts in culture (Brown et al., 1997). In contrast, elevation of p21 or p27 is not observed as human prostatic or mammary epithelial cells approach senescence. In senescent human mammary epithelial cells, both an elevation in p15 and a reduction in CDC25A contribute to inhibition of the G1 Cdks (Sandhu et al., 2000a), whereas p16 plays an important role at senescence in human prostatic epithelial cells (Sandhu et al., 2000b). p27 may play a role in senescence in some cell types, including human fibroblasts, due to the increased activity of the

PTEN tumor suppressor. p57 may also have a role at senescence in some cell types, including human urothelial cells (Schwarze et al., 2001).

Cell cycle arrest also occurs in response to DNA damage including that caused by therapeutic agents. This process prevents the replication of damaged DNA during S-phase and is described in Chapter 5, Section 5.4.

## 9.3 DEREGULATION OF THE CELL CYCLE IN CANCER

In the past decade, the comparison of cell cycle regulators in normal cells with finite life span and in tumor-derived cells has demonstrated that the cell cycle is consistently deregulated during tumor development. Deregulation of cell cycle proteins often has significant prognostic implications for patient outcome. The development and progression of cancer involves processes that abort differentiation, prevent cellular senescence (thereby allowing immortalization), and abrogate sensitivity to growth inhibitory stimuli. Loss of sensitivity to growth inhibitory stimuli can result from elevated expression of the positive regulators, the cyclins and the Cdc25 phosphatase family, or from the deletion, mutation, or reduction of the levels of the Cdk inhibitors. In addition, malignant cells have developed the ability to bypass the restriction on S-phase entrance normally imposed by DNA damage checkpoints. This leads to an accumulation of genetic changes that promote the selective outgrowth of cells with a proliferative advantage.

**Table 9.1.** Mechanisms of Cell Cycle Deregulation in Human Cancer

| Cell Cycle Gene/Protein | Alteration (Genetic, Protein) |
|---|---|
| CYCLIN D1 | Amplification, translocation, increased protein |
| CYCLIN E | Amplification, translocation, increased protein |
| CYCLIN A | Viral integration, amplification |
| CDK4 | Amplification, point mutation, translocation |
| p27/p21 | Deletion, rare mutation, decreased protein, cytoplasmic mislocalization |
| p15/p16 | Deletion, point mutation, hypermethylation, decreased protein |

### 9.3.1 Upregulation of the Positive Effectors

*Overexpression of Cyclins* Increased cyclin expression is seen in many tumors and may result from translocation, gene amplification, or mutation (Table 9.1). Elevated cyclin expression in G1 phase may func-

tion not only to shorten the G1-to-S phase interval, but also to make cells less responsive to growth inhibitory stimuli. CYCLIN E1 is often overexpressed in breast, stomach, colon, and endometrial cancers, and particularly in breast cancer, this is predictive of aggressive behavior and patient mortality (Table 9.2; Keyomarsi et al., 2002). Of all the positive cell cycle effectors that are known to be deregulated in human cancers, CYCLIN E1 may have the greatest value as a prognostic factor.

Genetic changes leading to overexpression of *CYCLIN D* genes—including rearrangement, translocation, and amplification—are common in human malignancies, including lymphomas, squamous-cell carcinomas of the head and neck, lung and esophagus, as well as breast and bladder carcinoma (Tables 9.1 and 9.2). In transgenic mice overexpression of *CYCLIN D1*, under the control of the mouse mammary tumor virus (MMTV) promoter, resulted in mammary hyperplasia and mammary adenocarcinoma (Wang et al., 1994). Despite the oncogenic potential of cyclin D1 in tissue culture and mice, and the observation that CYCLIN D1 is overexpressed in 45 percent of breast cancers, there is no con-

**Table 9.2.** Prognostic Significance (for poor outcome) of Altered Positive Regulators in Cancer

| Cell Cycle Protein | Type of Cancer | Alteration | Univariate[a] | Multivariate[a] |
|---|---|---|---|---|
| CYCLIN D1 | Pancreatic | ↑ 62–70% | X | |
| | Lung | ↑ 20% | X | |
| | Esophageal | ↑ 26% | | X |
| CYCLIN D2 | Gastric | ↑ 23% | | X |
| CYCLIN D3 | Non-Hodgkin's lymphoma | ↑ 21% | | X |
| | Superficial melanoma | ↑ 20% | | X |
| CYCLIN E1 | Breast | ↑ 25–30% | | X |
| | Non-small cell lung | ↑ 53% | X | |
| | Gastric | ↑ 40–53% | X | |
| | Large cell lymphoma | ↑ 30% | X | |
| | Liver | ↑ 36% | X | |
| | Ovarian | ↑ 50% | | X |
| CYCLIN A | Breast | ↑ 30–43% | | X |
| CYCLIN B | Non-small cell lung | ↑ 20% | | X |
| | Breast | ↑ 40–70% | | X |
| | Breast (high grade) | ↑ 32% | X | |
| | Esophageal | ↑ 20% | | X |
| | Colorectal | ↑ 43% | | X |
| CDC25A | Breast | ↑ 47% | X | |
| | Esophageal | ↑ 46% | | X |
| | Ovarian | ↑ 30–50% | | X |
| CDC25B | Colorectal | ↑ 43% | | X |
| | Breast | ↑ 32% | | |
| CDK4 | Laryngeal | ↑ 47% | | X |
| | Esophageal | ↑ 43% | | X |
| CDK2 | Oral | ↑ 20–40% | X | |
| | Laryngeal | ↑ 63.7% | X | |

[a]See Chapter 22, Section 22.3.2 for discussion of univariate and multivariate analyses.

sistent association between poor prognosis in breast cancer and elevated CYCLIN D1 levels (reviewed in Barnes, 1997). CYCLIN D1 overexpression is generally seen in the context of estrogen receptor (ER) positivity (Chap. 19, Sec. 19.3.1), and indeed is associated with a good prognosis in a number of studies. Overexpression of the other D-type cyclins may have prognostic significance in other types of tumor, as summarized in Table 9.2.

CYCLIN A is overexpressed in several tumors, including those of the liver and breast, and its expression in these tumors is an independent predictor of earlier relapse and poor prognosis (Table 9.2). CYCLIN B1 overexpression also predicts for poor prognosis in many cancers, including breast and esophageal squamous carcinoma (Tsihlias et al., 1999).

*Overexpression of CDC25 Phosphatases*   Another group of positive regulators of the cell cycle, the CDC25 phosphatase family members, are overexpressed in many cancers. CDC25A overexpression is an independent predictor of decreased survival in patients with ovarian cancer and squamous cell carcinoma of the esophagus (Table 9.2; Broggini et al., 2000; Nishioka et al., 2001). CDC25A overexpression in breast cancer may also identify a group of patients with poor prognosis. In a study of 144 breast cancer patients with tumors less than 1 cm in size, CDC25A overexpression, detected in nearly 50 percent of breast carcinomas, was associated with elevated CYCLIN E-CDK2 kinase activity (Cangi et al., 2000). In addition, the combination of high CDC25A and low p27 protein levels was the strongest predictor of poor survival by univariate analysis. CDC25B overexpression is seen in up to 32 percent of high-grade breast tumors and associated with reduced disease-free survival in patients who did not receive adjuvant chemotherapy (Cangi et al., 2000). CDC25B overexpression was also seen in 77 of 181 (43%) colorectal carcinomas and predicted for poor outcome by multivariate analysis (Table 9.2; Takemasa et al., 2000).

Translocation and amplification of genes that increase the expression of the Cdks have been reported (Table 9.1). CDK4 overexpression was reported in laryngeal squamous cell carcinomas (Dong et al., 2001) and esophageal squamous cell carcinomas (Matsumoto et al., 1999) and predicted for poor survival (Table 9.2). In breast cancers, CDK4 amplification is also found and CDK4 mutations that prevent the binding of p16 have been reported in melanomas.

While these relatively small studies showing increased CYCLIN, CDC 25 phosphatase or CDK expression demonstrate cell cycle deregulation in many human cancers, their putative prognostic value will need to be confirmed in larger studies.

### 9.3.2 Inactivation of Cdk Inhibitors

As negative regulators of the cell cycle, the KIP and INK4 families of Cdk inhibitors are frequently targets for inactivation in cancer (Tables 9.1 and 9.3; reviewed in Tsihlias et al., 1999; Viglietto and Fusco, 2002).

Mutations of the genes encoding the KIP family members *p21* and *p27* are infrequent in human tumors, but alterations at the level of gene expression and protein stability are common. One consequence of *p53* mutation is the disruption of the p53/p21 response that coordinates DNA repair with cell cycle arrest, leading to the accumulation of genetically altered cells (see also Chap. 5, Sec. 5.4). The prognostic value of p21 protein levels is controversial in human cancer. In breast cancer, for example, a few relatively small studies have demonstrated an association between low p21 levels and poor prognosis, whereas other studies have indicated poorer prognosis with high p21 levels. These studies provided mostly univariate analyses and thus the independent predictive value of p21 is not known (see Tsihlias et al., 1999). Loss of p21 may predict for poor prognosis in other cancers. In patients with colorectal cancer, reduced p21 protein was shown to be an independent prognostic factor by multivariate analysis (Zirbes et al., 2000). Hypermethylation of the p21 gene promoter, which causes decreased p21 expression, was observed in the bone marrow cells of patients with acute lymphoblastic leukemia, and a multivariate analysis demonstrated that this was an independent prognostic factor in predicting reduced disease-free survival (Roman-Gomez et al., 2002).

Of the Cdk inhibitors examined to date, p27 may be the most clinically relevant prognostic factor (Table 9.3; for review see Alkarain et al., 2004). Immunohistochemical analysis of p27 protein levels is inexpensive, readily automated, and relatively easy for pathologists to score. Reduction in p27 protein levels has been observed in primary cancers of the breast, colon, lung, prostate, stomach, and esophagus, and its loss is associated independently with increased tumor grade and poor patient prognosis (Slingerland and Pagano, 2000; Viglietto and Fusco, 2002). The reduced p27 levels in human tumors results from increased degradation of the protein via the ubiquitin-proteosome pathway (Slingerland and Pagano, 1998). Extracts from several cancers with low p27 protein levels have demonstrated an elevated capacity to degrade recombinant p27. In some, but not all, cases, the F-box protein SKP2 may contribute to the increased p27 degradation (see Fig. 9.8). In human lymphomas, oral cancers, and colorectal cancers, increased SKP2 expression has been found to correlate positively with the grade of malignancy and inversely with p27 levels.

**Table 9.3.** Prognostic Significance (for poor outcome) of Altered Negative Regulators in Cancer

| Cell Cycle Gene/Protein | Type of Cancer | Frequency | Univariate | Multivariate |
|---|---|---|---|---|
| P21 decreased protein | Colorectal | 33% | | X |
| p21 hypermethylation | Acute lymphoblastic leukemia | 41% | | X |
| p27 decreased protein | Breast | 50–90% | | X |
| | Colon | 60% | | X |
| | Gastric | 44% | X | |
| | Prostate | 65–90% | | X |
| | Ovarian | 33–53% | | X |
| | Non-small cell lung | 85% | | X |
| | Oral | 75% | | X |
| | Esophageal | 50% | | X |
| | Non-Hodgkin's lymphoma | 50–82% | | X |
| p16 hypermethylation | Non-small cell lung | 31% | | X |
| | Multiple myeloma | 42% | X | |
| | Colorectal | 37% | X | |
| p16 decreased protein | Melanoma | 45% | X | |
| p16 deletion | Ewing sarcoma | 30% | X | |
| p15 hypermethylation | Acute promyelocytic leukemia | 73% | | X |
| p15 deletion | Adult T-cell leukemia | 25% | | X |

In addition to reduction in KIP levels, mislocalization of p27 from the nucleus to the cytoplasm has been associated with poor prognosis. Protein kinase B can phosphorylate p27 leading to its mislocalization in the cytoplasm, and almost half of primary breast cancers demonstrate both nuclear and cytoplasmic p27. Normal breast epithelial cells show only nuclear p27. In general there is a strong association between cytoplasmic p27 and elevated PKB activity in primary breast cancers. Amplification of the oncogene encoding the HER-2 receptor tyrosine kinase is observed in up to 30 percent of breast cancers (Chap. 7, Sec. 7.3.1). HER-2 activation is associated with poor prognosis and has been implicated in the enhanced ubiquitin-mediated degradation of p27 and its cytoplasmic relocation through activation of the MAPK and PI-3K pathways, respectively (Fig. 9.8; Viglietto and Fusco, 2002). Thus, the inactivation of proliferative restraints imposed by p27 may arise through accelerated p27 proteolysis and through its cytoplasmic mislocalization; both may contribute to poor prognosis in breast cancer (Liang et al., 2002).

In contrast to members of the KIP family, genes of the INK4 family, such as *p15* and *p16*, are commonly mutated or inactivated in human tumor cell lines and in about one third of primary tumors (Tables 9.1 and 9.3; Ruas and Peters, 1998). Mutational inactivation of *p15* or *p16* allows CYCLIN D1-CDK4 activation, which

in turn impairs RB function. The proteins in the p16/CYCLIN D1/CDK4/RB axis are frequently disrupted in human cancer. Moreover, there appears to be a lack of selective pressure for mutational inactivation of more than one protein in the p16/CYCLIN D1/CDK4/RB axis. Thus, it is not surprising that p16 and RB exhibit a reciprocal pattern of expression in most tumors: those tumors that have lost p16 retain RB, and those tumors that have mutated RB retain p16. Tumors that retain both RB and p16 function often show increased expression of CYCLIN D1 or CDK4. These data further support the notion that p16 and RB belong to a common tumor suppressive pathway.

p16 knockout mice are prone to tumor development and cell lines derived from such mice undergo spontaneous immortalization with high frequency (see Sec. 9.2.6). The prognostic role for *p16* in several types of cancers has been reviewed (Drexler, 1998; Tsihlias et al., 1999). Germline point mutations in the *p16* gene confer susceptibility to melanoma and pancreatic adenocarcinoma (Lynch et al., 2002). Mutant *p16* alleles that encode defective inhibitor proteins have been identified. Homozygous *p16* deletions have been observed in many cancers, including primary bladder carcinoma, glioma, mesothelioma, T-cell acute lymphoblastic leukemia, melanoma, prostatic adenocarcinoma, ovarian adenocarcinoma, and renal cell carcinoma (reviewed in Rocco and Sidransky, 2001). Inactivation of *p16* by methylation has also been observed in a number of cancers, including those of the head and neck, breast, prostate, brain, lung, colon, esophagus, and bladder, and is thought to be a major mechanism of gene inactivation in many different tumor types. The carcinogens in tobacco smoke have been implicated as exogenous agents that promote DNA methylation. In one study, methylation of *p16* was significantly associated with pack-years smoked and predicted for survival after surgery in a multivariate analysis of fifty-eight patients with stage I adenocarcinoma of the lung (Kim et al., 2001).

Deletions of *p15* often accompany loss of *p16* due to the close proximity of these genes on chromosome 9p and deletions of both are relatively common in acute lymphoblastic leukemia. Silencing of the *p15* promoter by methylation may play an important role in several types of malignancies, especially lymphomas, and may predict for reduced survival (Wong et al., 2000). A limited number of small studies of p18 and p19 in human cancers have infrequently identified these Cdk inhibitors to be the targets of deletions or mutations in cancer. Mice deficient in p18 are highly susceptible to pituitary as well as other types of tumors (Latres et al., 2000) but no malignant phenotype has been associated with *p19*-deficient mice.

### 9.3.3 Development of Drugs to Target the Cell Cycle

An understanding of normal cell cycle regulation and the mechanisms by which it becomes deregulated in human disease may lead ultimately to improved therapeutic strategies, or to a greater ability to identify different prognostic subsets of patients. Like many protein kinases, the Cdks are targets for drug development. Remarkably, it took only a decade from the time the first human Cdk homolog, Cdk1 (cdc2), was identified to the first clinical trials of various Cdk inhibitors. The list of potential inhibitors is expanding, but several, including flavopiridol and UCN-01, are in early clinical trials, either alone or in combination with other conventional therapies. Flavopiridol is a potent inhibitor of Cdks 1, 2 and 4, while UCN-01 is an inhibitor of both protein kinase C and Cdk activity. Small molecular inhibitors of the Cdc25 family are also being designed. Inhibition of the proteosome has been proposed as a mechanism to promote cell cycle arrest and apoptosis in cancer cells by interfering with the deregulated degradation of cell cycle regulatory molecules. Pharmacological inhibitors of receptor tyrosine kinases and specific inhibitors of MAPK and PI-3K signaling, both of which are required for cell cycle progression, are also being explored for clinical use. Many of the presently used chemotherapeutic agents, which promote cell cycle arrest or apoptosis in a nonspecific manner (see Chap. 17) may eventually be replaced by more tumor-specific and rationally-designed agents.

## 9.4 TUMOR GROWTH AND CELL KINETICS

Mechanisms that control the cycling of cells have been described in previous sections. In normal tissues that undergo cell renewal, these mechanisms contribute to a balance between cell proliferation, growth arrest and differentiation, and loss of mature cells by programmed cell death or apoptosis (Chap. 10). Tumors grow because the homeostatic mechanisms that maintain the appropriate number of cells in normal tissues are defective, leading to imbalance between cell proliferation and cell death, so that there is expansion of the cell population. The use of autoradiography with tritiated thymidine in the 1950s and 1960s, and the subsequent application of flow cytometry, have allowed a detailed analysis of tumor growth in terms of the kinetics of proliferation of their constituent cells. The proliferative rate of tumor cells varies widely between tumors; nonproliferating cells are common, and there is often a high rate of cell death. The rate of cell proliferation in tumors may be an important factor in determining prognosis or response to radiation or chemotherapy. Several normal tissues, including bone marrow and intestine, contain cells with high rates of proliferation, and damage to these cells is often dose-limiting for chemotherapy.

### 9.4.1 Growth of Human Tumors

Tumor growth can be determined by estimating tumor volume as a function of time. Exponential growth of tumors will occur if the rates of cell production and of cell loss or death are proportional to the number of cells present in the population. Exponential growth implies that the time taken for a tumor to double its volume is constant and often leads to the false impression that the rate of tumor growth is accelerating with time (Fig. 9.10). Increase in the diameter of a human tumor from 0.5 to 1.0 cm may escape detection, whereas increase in the diameter of a tumor from 5 to 10 cm is more dramatic and is likely to cause new clinical symptoms. Both require three volume doublings; during exponential growth they will occur over the same period of time.

Estimates of the growth rates of untreated human tumors have been limited by the following constraints: (1) Only tumors that are unresponsive to therapy can ethically be followed without treatment; limited data are available from older studies, mostly for metastases, but almost all patients now receive treatment. There have been few measurements of the growth of primary tumors. (2) Accurate measurements can be made only on tumors from selected sites. The majority of studies have

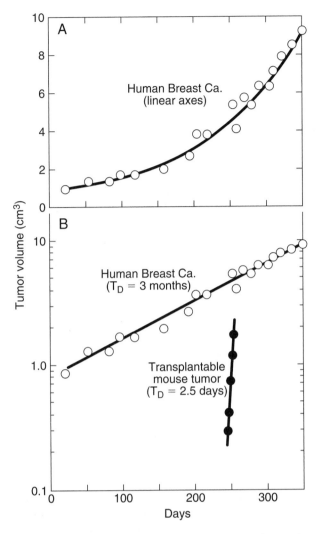

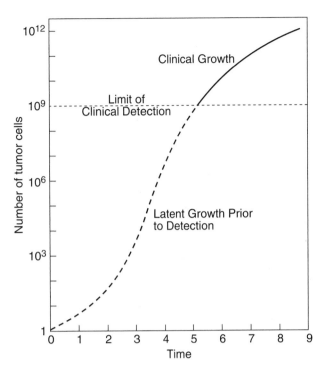

**Figure 9.11.** Hypothetical growth curve for a human tumor, showing the long latent period prior to detection. Tumors may show an early lag phase and progressive slowing of growth at large size.

rized in Table 9.4. A few general conclusions may be stated:

1. There is wide variation in growth rate, even among tumors of the same histologic type and site of origin.
2. Representative mean doubling times for lung metastases of common tumors in humans are in the range of 2 to 3 months.

**Figure 9.10.** Growth curves for a lung metastasis from a human breast cancer. *A.* Plotted on linear axes. *B.* Same data plotted using a logarithmic scale for tumor volume. (Data of RP Hill and RS Bush, unpublished. Included with permission.) A growth curve for a rapidly growing transplantable tumor in the mouse is included in *B* for comparison. $T_D$, volume doubling time.

examined lung metastases using serial x-rays, although computed tomographic and magnetic resonance imaging scans (see Chap. 13, Secs. 13.2.1 and 13.2.4) now allow accurate estimates of tumor volume in most organs of the body. (3) The limited observation period between the time of tumor detection and either death of the host or the initiation of some form of therapy represents only a small fraction of the history of the tumor's growth (Figs. 9.11 and 9.12).

Despite these limitations, there are many published estimates of the growth rate of human tumors. Steel (1977) reviewed published measurements of the rate of growth of 780 human tumors, and estimates of volume doubling time for several types of tumor are summa-

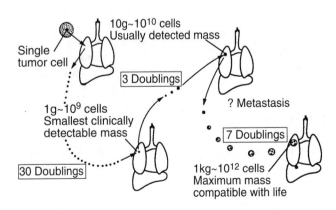

**Figure 9.12.** A human solid tumor must undergo about thirty to thirty-three doublings in volume from a single cell before it achieves a detectable size at a weight of 1 to 10 grams. Metastases may have been established prior to detection of the primary tumor. Only a few further doublings of volume lead to a tumor whose size is incompatible with life. (Adapted from Tannock, 1983.)

**Table 9.4.** Volume Doubling Time ($T_D$) for Representative Human Tumors

| Tumor Type | Number of Tumors | Volume Doubling Time,[a] Weeks |
|---|---|---|
| Primary lung cancer | | |
| Adenocarcinoma | 64 | 21 |
| Squamous cell carcinoma | 85 | 12 |
| Anaplastic carcinoma | 55 | 11 |
| Breast cancer | | |
| Primary | 17 | 14 |
| Lung metastases | 44 | 11 |
| Soft tissues metastases | 66 | 3 |
| Colon/rectum | | |
| Primary | 19 | 90 |
| Lung metastases | 56 | 14 |
| Lymphoma | | |
| Lymph node lesions | 27 | 4 |
| Lung metastases of | | |
| Carcinoma of testis | 80 | 4 |
| Childhood tumors | 47 | 4 |
| Adult sarcomas | 58 | 7 |

[a]Geometric mean values.

*Source*: Adapted from Steel (1977).

3. There is a tendency for childhood tumors and adult tumors that are known to be responsive to chemotherapy (e.g., lymphoma, cancer of the testis) to grow more rapidly than less responsive tumors (e.g., cancer of the colon).
4. Metastases tend to grow more rapidly than the primary tumor in the same patient.

Tumors are unlikely to be detected until they grow to about 1 gram, and tumors of this size will contain about one billion ($10^9$) cells. There is indirect evidence that many tumors arise from a single cell (see Sec. 9.4.4), and a tumor containing about $10^9$ cells will have undergone about thirty doublings in volume prior to clinical detection (because of cell loss, this will involve more than thirty consecutive divisions of the initial cell). After ten further doublings in volume, the tumor would weigh about 1 kilogram ($10^{12}$ cells), a size that may be lethal to the host. Thus, the range of size over which the growth of a tumor may be studied represents a rather short and late part of its total growth history (Figs. 9.11 and 9.12). There is evidence (e.g., for breast cancer) that the probability of metastatic spread increases with the size of the primary tumor, but the long preclinical history of the tumor may allow cells to metastasize prior to detection. Thus, early clinical detection may be expected to reduce but not to prevent the subsequent appearance of metastases.

The growth rate of a tumor in its preclinical phase can only be estimated indirectly. In patients, one may study the time to appearance of recurrent tumors after treatment that is curative in only some of the patients, so that growth in others may be assumed to derive from a small number of residual cells. These studies support the concept that growth is more rapid in the preclinical phase of a disease such as breast cancer, but there is little evidence for deceleration of growth during the clinical phase of rapidly progressive malignancies such as Wilms' tumor or Burkitt's lymphoma.

Deceleration of growth of large tumors is probably due to increasing cell death and decreasing cell proliferation as tumor nutrition deteriorates (see Sec. 9.4.5). Also, tumors often contain a high proportion of nonmalignant cells such as macrophages, lymphocytes, and fibroblasts, and the proliferation and migration of these cells will influence changes in tumor volume. Tumor growth may also be slow at very early stages of development (Fig. 9.11). Tumor cells may have to overcome immunologic and other host defense mechanisms, and they cannot expand to a large size until they have induced proliferation of blood vessels (*angiogenesis*) to support them (see Chap. 12).

### 9.4.2 Cell Population Kinetics

*Thymidine Autoradiography*   Much of the available information about cell population kinetics was derived by using autoradiography to detect the selective uptake of radioactive thymidine into cellular DNA, although these methods have been supplanted by automated techniques based on flow cytometry. The proportion of thymidine-labeled cells at a short interval after administration of tritiated ($^3$H) thymidine (the *labeling index*) is a measure of the proportion of cells in S phase. In the *percent-labeled-mitoses* (PLM) method, serial biopsies (or serial specimens from identical animals) are taken at intervals after a single injection of $^3$H-thymidine, and the proportion of mitotic cells that are labeled is estimated from autoradiographs prepared from these biopsies (see Steel, 1977, for details). While this method is labor intensive, it has provided most of the available estimates of the duration of different cell cycle phases in human tumors and normal tissues.

In most normal tissues of the adult, only a small proportion of the cells is actively proliferating. The remaining cells have either lost their capacity for proliferation through differentiation, or are G0 cells that can proliferate in response to an appropriate stimulus. Examples of the latter include stem cells in the bone marrow (see Sec. 9.4.3) and cells in skin that participate in wound healing. Most tumors also contain nonproliferating cells, and the term *growth fraction* describes the proportion of cells in the tumor population that is proliferating. Growth fraction can be determined by thymidine labeling and autoradiography, but preferred methods are based on distinguishing proliferating and nonproliferating cells by the presence or absence of specific enzymes or antigens, using flow or static cytometry (see below). Although approximate, the estimate of growth fraction is useful because most anticancer drugs are more toxic to proliferating cells (Chap. 17, Sec. 17.2.4) and growth fraction therefore indicates the proportion of tumor cells that might be sensitive to cycle-dependent chemotherapy.

The frequent occurrence of extensive necrosis and of apoptotic cells in tumors (see Chap. 10) and the ability of tumor cells to metastasize from a primary tumor indicate that there is considerable cell death or loss from many tumors. The rate of cell loss from tumors can be estimated by comparing the rate of cell production (from assessment of the labeling index or fraction of S phase cells by flow cytometry) with the rate of tumor growth. The overall rate of cell production may be characterized by the potential doubling time of the tumor ($T_{pot}$), which is the expected doubling time of

the tumor in the absence of cell loss. The value of $T_{pot}$ is usually much shorter than the measured volume doubling time because of extensive cell loss in human tumors (Steel, 1977).

*Flow Cytometry*   Flow cytometry is a method that allows the separation and sorting of cells based on cellular fluorescence. A schematic illustration of a flow cytometer is shown in Figure 9.13. Cells can be tagged with fluorescent markers to a wide range of molecules, including cell surface receptors, molecules involved in signaling pathways, and proteins that are expressed specifically in different phases of the cell cycle. Cells are then directed in single file through a laser beam to excite the fluorescent marker, and the fluorescence emission is collected and displayed as a fluorescence distribution. Cells can also be sorted on the basis of their fluorescence intensity.

Cells can be stained with a fluorescent dye whose binding (to DNA) is proportional to DNA content, and flow cytometry then allows enumeration of cells containing different amounts of DNA (Fig. 9.14). Several fluorescent dyes are available which stain DNA, includ-

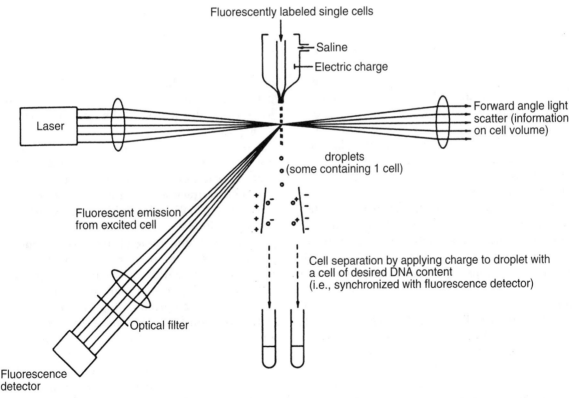

**Figure 9.13.** The principle of flow cytometry and cell sorting. Single cells stained with a fluorescent marker are directed through a laser beam. Fluorescence measurements allow quantitation of the marker, and forward angle light scatter gives information about cell volume. Charge may be applied to droplets containing cells with different levels of fluorescence, so that they may be deflected in an electrostatic field and sorted.

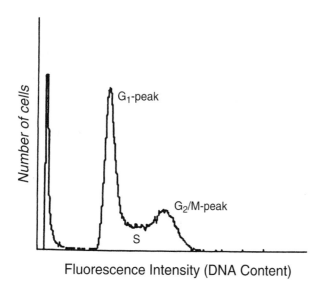

**Figure 9.14.** DNA distribution for a human bladder cancer cell line produced by flow cytometry. Cells were stained with acridine orange such that fluorescence is proportional to DNA content. The peak at the origin represents cellular debris.

ing ethidium bromide, propidium iodide, acridine orange, and Hoechst 33342. Most dyes require fixation of the cells to allow access of dye to the DNA, although selected DNA specific dyes (e.g., Hoechst 33342) can enter viable cells; the Hoechst dye allows isolation of viable cells according to DNA content. Often, fluorescent reagents are applied concurrently or sequentially to allow for analysis or separation of cells on the basis of two or more criteria (such as the expression of a specific protein and DNA content). Information about cell size may be obtained from analysis of scattered light. Multiparameter analyses are particularly useful in the study of heterogeneous tissue samples and in the classification of acute leukemias.

Computer analysis of a fluorescent DNA distribution (Fig. 9.14) provides estimates of the proportion of cells with 2N DNA content (i.e., G1 and most nonproliferating cells), with 4N DNA content (G2 and mitotic cells), and with intermediate DNA content (S phase cells). In tumors, the presence of aneuploidy (i.e., a G1-phase DNA content different from that of normal cells) and of variable DNA content among G1 cells complicates analysis of DNA distributions and the estimation of cell cycle parameters. The proportion of S phase cells obtained from a DNA distribution is analogous to the thymidine labeling index and gives a broad indication of the proliferative rate.

Flow cytometry can be used to estimate cell cycle phase distribution, growth fraction, and kinetic properties of cell populations. Minimally toxic nonradioactive precursors, such as 5-bromodeoxyuridine (BrdUrd), are incorporated into newly synthesized DNA (like tritiated thymidine) and can be recognized by flow

cytometry using commercially available fluorescently tagged monoclonal antibodies. Analysis by flow cytometry at different times later with application of a DNA stain can allow one to follow the tagged cells as they move through the cell cycle in a method that is analogous to the percent-labeled-mitosis method. The method may be used to estimate cell cycle phase durations of an unperturbed cell population, or to identify a population of cells that has been arrested in a given phase of the cell cycle following treatment with radiation or drugs.

Several methods allow proliferating and nonproliferating cells to be distinguished by flow cytometry. A variety of cellular antigens [e.g., those recognized by the monoclonal antibody, Ki-67 and proliferating cell nuclear antigen (PCNA)] appear to be expressed uniquely in cycling cells and can be recognized by fluorescence-labeled antibodies. The Ki-67 antigen has been used most often as a marker for proliferating cells although its function remains poorly understood (Brown and Gatter, 2002). Fluorescently tagged monoclonal antibodies that recognize cyclins and other molecules involved in cell cycle regulation can be used to determine their expression at different times during the mitotic cycle (see Sec. 9.2.1). Expression of these cell cycle dependent molecules in human tumor cells can also be related to prognosis (see Sec. 9.3 and Table 9.2).

A technique for dissolving the paraffin, followed by dispersion and staining of the cells, has allowed flow cytometry to be applied to the study of fixed tissue that is stored in paraffin blocks. Provided that attention is paid to quality control, this technique can provide a useful retrospective analysis of the relationship between kinetic parameters of human tumors and the subsequent outcome of the patients (Hedley et al., 1993). For several types of tumor, both DNA index (i.e., the DNA content of G1 tumor cells relative to that of normal cells) and S-phase fraction (or other index of cell proliferation such as Ki-67 index) give prognostic information that is additional to the traditional prognostic factors of tumor stage and grade (Table 9.5). In general, aneuploid tumors have a poorer prognosis than diploid tumors, and tumors with a more rapid rate of cell proliferation have a poorer prognosis than tumors with a slower rate of cell proliferation (Table 9.5).

The relationship between proliferative parameters and response to treatment with chemotherapy is complex. There may be a higher chance of response to chemotherapy in malignancies with a rapid rate of cell proliferation, although intrinsic drug sensitivity of the cells is likely to be the major determinant of response. In contrast, malignancies with a rapid rate of cell proliferation grow more rapidly both in the absence of effective treatment and in recovery after partially effective therapy. A further confounding factor arises be-

**Table 9.5.** Prognostic Significance of Cellular DNA Content and Measures of Cell Proliferation (S Phase Fraction or Ki-67 Index) Determined by Flow Cytometry for Selected Tumors

| Tumor Type | Properties of | |
| | Aneuploid Tumors | Tumors with a High Rate of Cell Proliferation |
| --- | --- | --- |
| Bladder cancer | Correlates with higher grade (and poorer outcome) for superficial tumors<br>Less useful for muscle-invasive tumors | Equivocal studies |
| Breast cancer | Equivocal studies | Increased risk of recurrence and death for node-negative and node-positive patients (independent risk factor) |
| Colorectal cancer | Weak prognostic factor for poor survival (Problem of quality control in studies) | Prognostic factor for poor survival |
| Prostate cancer | Prognostic factor for poor survival (Independent risk factor in some studies) | Prognostic factor for poor survival |
| Non-Hodgkin's lymphoma | No proven utility | Strong prognostic factor for poor survival |
| Multiple myeloma | Prognostic factor for poor survival | No data |
| Acute leukemia | Conflicting data | Not prognostic |

*Source*: Adapted from Hedley et al. (1993).

cause analysis of DNA distributions does not provide information about the proliferative status of *clonogenic cells*, such as stem cells, in normal tissues or tumors (Secs. 9.4.3 and 9.4.4). However, cells can be sorted on the basis of their DNA content after staining with nontoxic fluorescent drugs, thus allowing subsequent study of their clonogenic capacity and other properties. This method can be used after treatment with radiation or anticancer drugs to provide information about the cell cycle distribution of clonogenic cells that survive such treatment.

### 9.4.3 Cell Proliferation in Normal Tissues

Thymidine labeling and flow cytometry have been used to compare the overall rate of cell proliferation in a variety of normal tissues (Table 9.6). The side effects of chemotherapy that are common to many drugs (e.g., myelosuppression, mucositis, hair loss, and sterility) are observed in rapidly proliferating tissues, reflecting the greater activity of most anticancer drugs against proliferating cells (Chap. 17, Sec. 17.2.4). Acute effects of radiation injury are also observed in these tissues, because radiation-damaged cells often die when they attempt mitosis (Chap. 15, Sec. 15.5.2). The pattern of proliferation and differentiation of hemopoietic cells in the bone marrow and epithelial cells in the intestine are described below as examples of renewal tissues in which the pattern of cell proliferation is an important determinant of anticancer therapy.

*Bone Marrow* Morphologically recognizable cells in bone marrow and blood have an orderly progression of differentiation from myeloblasts to polymorphonuclear granulocytes, from pronormoblasts to red blood cells, and from megakaryocytes to platelets (Fig. 9.15). The earlier bone-marrow precursor cells cannot be recognized morphologically, but can be enriched by flow cytometry using fluorescent markers to antigens that are expressed selectively on their surface. For example, stem cells may be recognized by the expression of the CD34 antigen and the tyrosine kinase receptors known as c-kit and Flk-2/Flk-3. The pluripotential stem cell may undergo self-renewal or may produce progeny that are early precursor cells for lymphocytes or for cells which under appropriate conditions in culture will form colonies containing cells of the granulocyte (G), erythroid (E), megakaryocyte (Meg), and monocyte (M) series. Further proliferation and differentiation produces precursor cells whose progeny are bone-marrow cells of a specific lineage (Fig. 9.15).

**Table 9.6.** Proliferative Rates of Selected Normal Tissues in Adults

| Rapid | Slow | None |
| --- | --- | --- |
| Bone marrow | Lung | Muscle |
| GI mucosa | Liver | Bone |
| Ovary | Kidney | Cartilage |
| Testis | Endocrine glands | Nerve |
| Hair follicles | Vascular endothelium | |

*Note*: Acute side effects of chemotherapy occur commonly in rapidly proliferating tissue.

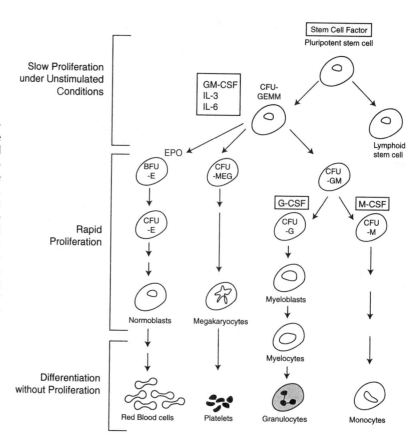

**Figure 9.15.** Schematic diagram of the differentiation of hematopoietic precursor cells in the bone marrow, leading to the production of red blood cells, platelets, granulocytes, and monocytes. Various cells are stimulated to proliferate and/or differentiate by the growth factors IL-3, IL-6, GM-CSF, G-CSF, M-CSF, erythropoietin (EPO), stem cell factor, and others (see Table 9.7); only their main target cells are indicated here. Under normal conditions, the early precursor cells proliferate slowly, intermediate precursors proliferate rapidly (in the megakaryocytic series there is nuclear replication without cell division) to expand the population, and later precursors of the functional cells differentiate without further cell division.

The growth factors that stimulate hematopoietic precursor cells to proliferate and differentiate into lineage-specific cells have been characterized (Table 9.7). Several of these growth factors act in concert to stimulate stem cells to proliferate, including stem-cell factor (also known as Kit-ligand), Interleukin-1 (IL-1), IL-3, and IL-6 (Moore, 1995). Considerable clinical experience has been obtained with the recombinant growth factors, granulocyte-macrophage colony-stimulating factor (GM-CSF), granulocyte colony-stimulating factor (G-CSF), and erythropoietin. Granulocyte-macrophage colony-stimulating factor and G-CSF have been shown to decrease the duration and extent of myelosuppression after chemotherapy, and G-CSF is used widely to lower the incidence of infection and hospitalization. Erythropoietin is used to treat anemia and accompanying fatigue, including anemia associated with cancer, and to decrease the need for blood transfusion. These growth factors may influence stem cell proliferation, but they exert greater activity to stimulate committed precursor cells, as indicated in Table 9.7.

Older thymidine-labeling studies demonstrated a very high rate of cell proliferation of recognizable precursors of granulocytes and red cells; these are among the most rapidly proliferating cells in the human body, with a mean duration of S phase ($T_s$) and mean cell cycle time ($T_c$) of about 12 and 24 hours. The more mature cells in each series undergo differentiation without pro-

liferation (Fig. 9.15). Stem cells and other early precursor cells proliferate quite slowly under resting conditions (Messner, 1995), and their more rapidly proliferating progeny provide replacement for the normal loss of mature cells, as shown in Figure 9.15. However, stem cells may proliferate rapidly to restore the bone-

**Table 9.7.** Selected Hematopoietic Growth Factors and the Target Cell Population That Is Stimulated[a]

| Growth Factor | Target Cell Population |
|---|---|
| Stem-cell factor (Kit ligand) | Bone marrow stem cells |
| Interleukin 1 (IL-1) | Stimulates stromal cells to produce other factors (IL-6, GM-CSF, G-CSF) |
| Interleukin 3 (IL-3) Interleukin 6 (IL-6) Granulocyte macrophage colony-stimulating factor (GM-CSF) | Early multipotential cells (CFU-GEMM and others) |
| Granulocyte colony-stimulating factor (G-CSF) | Early cells in granulocytic series (CFU-G) |
| Erythropoietin (Epo) | Early red cell precursors (BFU-E, CFU-E) |

[a]The interaction of growth factors to stimulate different types of cells is complex, and several growth factors have auxiliary effects to stimulate other types of precursor cells.

marrow population following depletion of more mature functional cells (e.g., by cancer chemotherapy) or after bone-marrow ablation and transplantation.

The pattern of proliferation and differentiation in the bone marrow provides an explanation for the decrease in mature granulocytes at 10 to 14 days after cycle-active chemotherapy and their recovery by 21 to 28 days (Chap. 17, Sec. 17.4.1). The rapidly proliferating intermediate precursor cells (Fig. 9.15) are most likely to be killed by chemotherapy. Effects on cells in the peripheral blood are not seen immediately because the later maturing cells are nonproliferating and tend to be spared by chemotherapy. Recovery of the bone marrow occurs when earlier precursors are stimulated to proliferate, following release of growth factors that follows loss of the mature functional cells. Treatment with agents that are selectively toxic to proliferating cells (as is true for most types of chemotherapy) during this recovery phase is to be avoided to prevent killing of cycling bone-marrow stem cells.

*Intestine* The functional part of the small intestine consists of numerous villi that project into the lumen and provide a large absorptive surface (Fig. 9.16). The villi are lined by a single layer of differentiated epithelial cells that do not proliferate, and apoptotic cell death

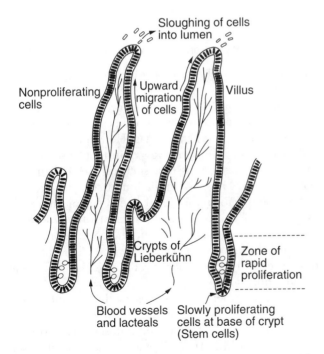

**Figure 9.16.** Model for cell proliferation and migration in the small intestine. Slowly proliferating cells in the bases of the crypts probably act as stem cells for the entire cell population. Other cells in the lower two-thirds of the crypts proliferate rapidly, with nuclei of mitotic cells visible in the lumens of the crypts. Cells migrate up the villi to replace those sloughed into the lumen.

and shedding of cells into the lumen occur at the top of the villi. These cells are replaced by upward migration of cells lining the crypts, which lie between and at the base of the villi. There is a high rate of cell proliferation in the crypts of the intestine, but cell proliferation occurs more slowly at the bases of the crypts (Fig. 9.16). Slowly proliferating cells in this region are analogous to bone-marrow stem cells in that they act as precursors for the entire crypt and surrounding villi. Control of cell proliferation in the intestine is complex and proliferation of stem cells in the crypts is influenced by a number of growth factors including EGF, TGF-$\beta$3, keratinocyte growth factor (FGF-7), and IL-11 (Berlanga-Accosta et al., 2001; Booth and Potten, 2001). Some cycle dependent drugs (e.g., cytosine arabinoside, CPT-11; Chap. 16, Secs. 16.4.4 and 16.5.1) and radiation may cause severe mucosal irritation of the intestine and diarrhea, although toxicity to this organ is less often dose limiting for anticancer drugs than that to the bone marrow.

### 9.4.4 Tumors as Clonal Populations

Renewal tissues such as bone marrow and intestinal mucosa represent a hierarchy of cells produced by cell division and differentiation from a small number of stem cells. Most tumors arise in renewal tissues, and there is substantial evidence that many tumors contain a limited population of stem cells with the capacity to regenerate the tumor after treatment. Other cells in the tumor population may have lost the capacity for cell proliferation (e.g., through differentiation) or have only limited potential for cell proliferation (analogous to morphologically recognizable precursor cells in bone marrow, such as myelocytes). The following evidence supports the validity of a stem-cell model for human tumors:

1. There is evidence (described below) that cells within many different types of tumor are derived clonally from a single cell.
2. Tissue-specific differentiation occurs in tumors, and an inverse relationship has been observed between indices of cell proliferation and differentiation. There is evidence that differentiated cells (which cannot generate a tumor on transplantation) are derived from undifferentiated cells that can generate tumors when transplanted into new hosts (Pierce and Speers, 1988). This relationship is similar to that observed in normal renewing tissues.
3. Cells from human tumors may generate colonies in a semisolid medium such as dilute agar provided that an adequate nutrient environment (including essential growth factors) is provided (Hamburger and Salmon, 1977; Courtenay et al., 1978). The proportion of cells that generate colonies is low (typically

< 1 percent) suggesting a low proportion of tumor stem cells. This low colony-forming efficiency might be due, however, to the imperfect microenvironment provided by the tissue culture medium.

4. Experience with radiation therapy suggests that in many human tumors only a small proportion of the cells has the ability to repopulate the tumor. Successful achievement of local control with moderate doses of radiation therapy would be expected only if a small fraction of the tumor cells were stem cells that must be killed by the radiation (Moore et al., 1983).

5. Recent experiments have determined that there is a population of cells in some human tumors that express distinct markers on their cell surface and have the properties of stem cells, including self-renewal and suppression of senescence (reviewed in Pardal et al., 2003). Thus in human leukemia, such cells express the gene *Bmi-1* (Lessard and Sauvageau, 2003; Park et al., 2004), while in human breast cancer a small subpopulation with the phenotype CD44(+)CD24(−/low) lineage markers(−) appear to be responsible for tumor development (Al-Hajj et al., 2003).

Evidence for the monoclonal origin of human tumors is provided by the observation that a unique identifying feature (a clonal marker) may be found in all of the constituent cells. Initial evidence accrued from analysis of X-linked genes or gene products in cells from tumors in women who are heterozygous at these genetic loci. One of the X chromosomes becomes inactivated at random in all cells of females during early life. The normal tissues of heterozygous females are therefore mosaics that contain approximately an equal number of cells in which one or the other (but not both) of the two alleles of a gene on the X chromosomes are expressed. However, cells in tumors arising in such individuals usually express only one allele of such genes—for example, they express only one form (isoenzyme) of the X-linked glucose-6-phosphate dehydrogenase (e.g., Fialkow, 1974). Other clonal markers include chromosomal rearrangements such as the Philadelphia chromosome in chronic myelogenous leukemia; uniquely rearranged immunoglobulins or T-cell receptors expressed by B-cell lymphomas or multiple myelomas and T-cell lymphomas (Chap. 20, Sec. 20.2.4); and molecular markers whose detection has been facilitated by the availability of gene sequencing.

The above techniques have demonstrated clonality in at least 95 percent of the wide range of tumors that have been examined (e.g., Fialkow, 1974; Vogelstein et al., 1987). Fearon and colleagues (1987) demonstrated clonal origin of thirty colonic adenomas (premalignant tumors) and twenty colonic carcinomas using analysis of X-linked genes; they also found a second clonal marker, loss of chromosome 17p sequences in most of the carcinomas but not in the adenomas. This observation suggests that sequential selection of clonal populations occurs during progression from benign to premalignant to malignant tumors. The continued accrual of genetic changes in subpopulations contributes to the heterogeneity observed among the cells of most tumors (Chap. 11, Sec. 11.1.2). Although cells in most tumors share a common antecedent cell, this could occur either because of transformation of a single cell, or because tumors arose from multiple transformed cells but one of their progeny developed a sufficient growth advantage that its descendants became dominant in the tumor.

The stem-cell model has major implications for the treatment of human tumors. When the aim of treatment is cure or long-term control, then therapy must aim to eradicate stem cells, because only these cells maintain the potential to regenerate the tumor population. If stem cells represent a small subpopulation within some tumors, as suggested by the results of treatment with radiotherapy, then short-term changes in tumor volume may not reflect the effects of treatment on stem cells. Rather, stem cell effects must be evaluated by placing the cells in an environment where they may express their potential to generate a large number of progeny—that is, by performing a colony-forming assay (see Chap. 14, Sec. 14.3.1 and Chap. 17, Sec. 17.2.3).

### 9.4.5 Cell Proliferation in Tumors

Typical values for the proportion of cells in S phase are in the range of 3 to 15 percent for many types of human solid tumors. Higher rates of cell proliferation are evident in faster-growing malignancies, including acute leukemia and some lymphomas. However, the rate of cell proliferation is usually less than that of some cells in normal renewing tissues, such as the intestine or bone marrow. Thus, accumulation of cells in tumors is not due simply to an increased rate of cell proliferation as compared to the normal tissue of origin. Rather, there is defective maturation and the population of malignant cells increases because the rate of cell production exceeds the rate of cell death or removal from the population.

A large number of estimates of the duration of S phase ($T_s$) and of the potential doubling time ($T_{pot}$) have been derived from labeled mitoses (PLM) studies or BrdUrd (or IdUrd) labeling and flow cytometry (see Sec. 9.4.2). Representative data from these studies are shown in Table 9.8. Mean values for $T_s$ tend to be in the range of 12 to 24 hours. Typical values of mean cell cycle time are in the range of 2 to 3 days, but this estimate is subject to uncertainty because the distribution

**Table 9.8.** Estimates of Mean Duration of S Phase ($T_S$), Cell Cycle Time ($T_C$), and Potential Doubling Time ($T_{pot}$) for Selected Human Tumors[a]

| Tumor Type | Number of Estimates | Mean Values of | | | Range | Method |
|---|---|---|---|---|---|---|
| | | $T_S$, hours | $T_C$, days | $T_{pot}$, days | | |
| Breast | 6 | 21 | 2.5 | 20 | | PLM |
| Lung | 6 | 20 | 4.5 | — | | PLM |
| | 3 | 24 | — | 6 | 3–11 | BrdUrd |
| Head/neck | 4 | 20 | 2.5 | | | |
| | 47 | 11 | — | 4.5 | 2–15 | IdUrd |
| Stomach | 21 | 14 | — | 8 | | BrdUrd |
| Colon/rectum | 10 | 17 | 3.0 | 5 | | PLM |
| | 4 | 24 | — | 6.5 | 5–10 | BrdUrd |
| Brain | 15 | 15 | — | 12 | 6–27 | BrdUrd |
| Melanoma | 6 | 21 | 2.5 | — | | PLM |
| | 2 | 9 | — | 5 | 3.5–7 | BrdUrd |
| Lymphoma | 7 | 12 | 2.0 | — | | PLM |
| Acute leukemia | 17 | 22 | 2.5 | 9 | 6–18 | PLM |
| | 44 | 13 | — | 9 | 3–7 | BrdUrd |

[a]$T_{pot}$ was calculated from $T_S$ and concurrent LI using BrdUrd, IdUrd, or $^3$H-thymidine incorporation.

*Source*: Data obtained using the PLM method were reviewed in Steel (1977) and Tannock (1978). Data obtained by the BrdUrd/IdUrd method are from Wilson et al. (1988), Riccardi et al. (1989), and Begg et al. (1990).

of cell cycle times is broad, and both the PLM and BrdUrd techniques tend to give information about the faster proliferating cells in the population. Estimates of $T_{pot}$ (range of 4.5 to 20 days), which reflects the proliferative capacity of cells, are much longer than estimates of mean cycle time $T_c$, implying that many human tumors have a low growth fraction. If some of the slowly proliferating or nonproliferating cells in human tumors retain the properties of a tumor stem cell (i.e., they can repopulate the tumor if stimulated to divide), the low growth fraction may be a factor that contributes to the relative resistance of human tumors to cycle-active chemotherapy. Estimates of mean values of $T_{pot}$ are in turn much lower than estimates of volume doubling time for common human tumors (typically 2 to 3 months, Table 9.4). It follows that the rate of cell loss in many human tumors is in the range of 75 to 90 percent of the rate of cell production.

Studies of human and animal tumors have demonstrated considerable heterogeneity in labeling and mitotic indices within different parts of the same tumor or its metastases. One of the factors that contributes to heterogeneity of cell proliferation is a variable degree of differentiation that may occur within the tumor: in general, there is an inverse relationship between differentiation and proliferative rate. A second factor is the generation of variant clonal subpopulations (see Sec. 9.4.4) with different proliferative capacities. A third and perhaps dominant factor is variability in the availability of oxygen and other nutrients in the microenvironment. Necrosis occurs commonly in solid tumors, and both in human and experimental tumors an orderly relationship can sometimes be observed with the edge of a necrotic region being parallel to a tumor blood vessel and separated from it by a distance that in humans is commonly about 100 to 200 micrometers (Thomlinson and Gray, 1955). In some tumors, this relationship may lead to the formation of either cylindrical cords of viable tissue with a central blood vessel and surrounding necrosis or to tumor nodules with a surrounding vascular network and central necrosis (Chap. 15, Sec. 15.4.2). These structures suggest that necrosis may occur when the concentration of essential nutrients that diffuse from tumor blood vessels has fallen to a critically low value, and/or when toxic breakdown products of cells have reached a critically high level. Intermittent blood flow in tumor capillaries may also lead to hypoxic regions of tumors. Apoptosis may be triggered by ischemia, although apoptotic cells are often distributed widely among the viable tumor cell population.

The presence of tumor cords or nodules has allowed study of cell proliferation in relation to the blood supply. Not surprisingly, well-nourished cells close to blood vessels have a more rapid rate of cell proliferation than poorly nourished cells close to a region of necrosis (e.g., Tannock, 1970). A similar gradient of cell proliferation is seen when tumor cells are grown as spheroids, which are multicellular aggregates grown in vitro that resemble tumor nodules, and which have a decreasing gradient of nutrient metabolites from their surface

(Sutherland, 1988). The presence of slowly proliferating cells at a distance from functional blood vessels has implications for tumor therapy: such cells may be resistant to radiation because of hypoxia (Chap. 15, Sec. 15.4.1) and to cytotoxic chemotherapeutic drugs because of their low proliferative rate (Chap. 17, Sec. 17.2.4) and limited drug access (Chap. 18, Sec. 18.3.3). Exposure to hypoxia (or other nutrient deprivation) may also promote rapid progression of the tumor cells to a more malignant phenotype (Chap. 11, Sec. 11.1.2).

Cell proliferation and cell death in tumors depend on tumor vasculature. Thus, the rate of tumor growth is likely to depend on the rate of expansion of functional tumor blood vessels by angiogenesis. In experimental animals, the proliferation rate of capillary endothelial cells appears to be slower than that of surrounding tumor cells (Denekamp and Hobson, 1982), which may lead to decreasing tumor vasculature and slowing of growth in larger tumors (Chap. 12, Sec. 12.3).

## 9.5 SUMMARY

The entry of resting cells into cycle, and the orderly progression of cells to synthesize DNA and subsequently to divide at mitosis is tightly regulated by the synthesis, activation, and subsequent degradation of a number of cell cycle regulatory proteins. Different cyclin-dependent kinases (Cdks) are activated by phosphorylation after binding to corresponding cyclins, and allow progression through the cell cycle. The KIP (including the p21, p27, and p57 proteins) and the INK families of proteins inhibit Cdks, so that both positive and negative effectors contribute to regulation of cell cycle progression. Expression of molecules that regulate the cell cycle may become disturbed in malignant cells with a resulting loss of control of cell proliferation. Increased expression of cyclins and Cdks, and/or reduced levels of Cdk inhibitors have been associated with poor prognosis in several types of human cancer.

The growth of tumors is dependent on the rate of proliferation and death of the cells within them. In many human tumors the rate of cell production is only slightly higher than the rate of cell death and many cells may not be actively cycling, so that the median doubling time of tumors (typically about 2 months for common human solid tumors) is much longer than the cell cycle time of the proliferating tumor cells (typically about 3 days). Factors that influence the rates of proliferation and cell death in tumors include nutrient molecules in the microenvironment, which in turn depend on angiogenesis and the expansion of the vascular network of the tumor, and the molecular signals that are influenced by endogenous and exogenous factors. The rate of cell proliferation is a major determinant of the response of tumors to cycle-active chemotherapy. Improved understanding of the molecular controls of cell proliferation is leading to the development of new agents that target specific effector molecules or pathways.

## REFERENCES

Al-Hajj M, Wicha MS, Benito-Hernandez A, et al: Prospective identification of tumorigenic breast cancer cells. *Proc Natl Acad Sci USA* 2003; 100:3983–3988.

Alkarain A, Jordan R, Slingerland J: p27 deregulation in breast cancer: prognostic significance and implications for therapy. *J Mammary Gland Biol Neoplasia* 2004; 9:67–80.

Barnard JA, Beauchamp RD, Coffey RJ, et al: Regulation of intestinal epithelial cell growth by transforming growth factor type β. *Proc Natl Acad Sci USA* 1989; 86:1578–1582.

Barnes DM: Cyclin D1 in mammary carcinoma. *J Pathol* 1997; 181:267–269.

Begg AC, Hofland I, Moonen L, et al: The predictive value of cell kinetic measurements in a European trial of accelerated fractionation in advanced head and neck tumours: an interim report. *Int J Radiat Oncol Biol Phys* 1990; 19:1449–1453.

Berlanga-Acosta J, Playford RJ, Mandir N, Goodland RA: Gastrointestinal cell proliferaton and crypt fission are separate but complementary means of increasing tissue mass following infusion of epidermal growth factor in rats. *Gut* 2001; 48:803–807.

Blain SW, Scher HI, Cordon-Cardo C, Koff A: p27 as a target for cancer therapeutics. *Cancer Cell* 2003; 3:111–115.

Blomberg I, Hoffmann I: Ectopic expression of Cdc25A accelerates the G(1)/S transition and leads to premature activation of cyclin E- and cyclin A-dependent kinases. *Mol Cell Biol* 1999; 19:6183–6194.

Booth D, Potten CS: Protection against mucosal injury by growth factors and cytokines. *J Natl Cancer Inst Monogr* 2001; 29:16–20.

Broggini M, Buraggi G, Brenna A, et al: Cell cycle-related phosphatases CDC25A and B expression correlates with survival in ovarian cancer patients. *Anticancer Res* 2000; 20:4835–4840.

Brown DC, Gatter KC: Ki67 protein: the immaculate deception? *Histopathology* 2002; 40:2–11.

Brown JP, Wei W, Sedivy JM: Bypass of senescence after disruption of p21[CIP1/WAF1] gene in normal diploid human fibroblasts. *Science* 1997; 277:831–834.

Cangi MG, Cukor B, Soung P, et al: Role of Cdc25A phosphatase in human breast cancer. *J Clin Invest* 2000; 106:753–761.

Camou S, Donovan JC, Flanagan WM et al: Downregulation of p21WAF1/CIP1 or p27 Kip1 abrogates antiestrogen-mediated cell cycle arrest in human breast cancer cells. *Proc Natl Acad Sci USA* 2000; 97:9042–9046.

Carrano AC, Eytan E, Hershko A, Pagano M: SKP2 is required for ubiquitin-mediated degradation of the CDK inhibitor p27. *Nature Cell Biol* 1999;1:193–199.

Cheng M, Olivier P, Diehl JA, et al: The p21(Cip1) and p27(Kip1) CDK 'inhibitors' are essential activators of cyclin D-dependent kinases in murine fibroblasts. *EMBO J* 1999; 18:1571–1583.

Cheng M, Sexl V, Sherr CJ, Roussel MF: Assembly of cyclin D-dependent kinase and titration of p27Kip1 regulated by mitogen-activated protein kinase kinase (MEK1). *Proc Natl Acad Sci USA* 1998; 95:1091–1096.

Coats S, Flanagan M, Nourse J, Roberts JM: Requirement of p27Kip1 for restriction point control of the fibroblast cell cycle. *Science* 1996; 272:877–880.

Connor MK, Kotchetkov R, Cariou S, et al: CRM1/Ran-mediated nuclear export of p27(Kip1) involves a nuclear export signal and links p27 export and proteolysis. *Mol Biol Cell* 2003; 14:201–213.

Courtenay VD, Selby PJ, Smith IE, et al: Growth of human tumour cell colonies from biopsies using two soft-agar techniques. *Br J Cancer* 1978; 38:77–81.

Craig KL, Tyers M: The F-box: a new motif for ubiquitin dependent proteolysis in cell cycle regulation and signal transduction. *Prog Biophys Mol Biol* 1999; 72: 299–328.

Denekamp J, Hobson B: Endothelial-cell proliferation in experimental tumours. *Br J Cancer* 1982; 46:711–720.

Dickson MA, Hahn WC, Ino Y, et al: Human keratinocytes that express h-TERT and also bypass a p16(INK4a)-enforced mechanism that limits life span become immortal yet retain normal growth and differentiation characteristics. *Mol Cell Biol* 2000; 20:1436–1447.

Diehl JA, Cheng M, Roussel MF, Sherr CJ: Glycogen synthase kinase-3beta regulates cyclin D1 proteolysis and subcellular localization. *Genes Dev* 1998; 12:3499–3511.

Dong Y, Sui L, Sugimoto K, et al: Cyclin D1–CDK4 complex, a possible critical factor for cell proliferation and prognosis in laryngeal squamous cell carcinomas. *Int J Cancer* 2001; 95:209–215.

Donovan J, Slingerland J: Transforming growth factor-beta and breast cancer: cell cycle arrest by transforming growth factor-beta and its disruption in cancer. *Breast Cancer Res* 2000; 2:116–124.

Donovan JC, Milic A, Slingerland JM: Constitutive MEK/MAPK activation leads to p27Kip1 deregulation and anti-estrogen resistance in human breast cancer cells. *J Biol Chem* 2001; 276: 40888–40895.

Draetta G, Eckstein J: Cdc25 protein phosphatases in cell proliferation. *Biochim Biophys Acta* 1997; 1332:M53–M63.

Drexler HG: Review of alterations of the cyclin-dependent kinase inhibitor INK4 family genes p15, p16, p18 and p19 in human leukemia-lymphoma cells. *Leukemia* 1998; 12:845–859.

Fearon ER, Hamilton SR, Vogelstein B: Clonal analysis of human colorectal tumors. *Science* 1987; 238:193–197.

Fialkow PJ: The origin and development of human tumors studied with cell markers. *N Engl J Med* 1974; 291:26–35.

Franklin DS, Godfrey VL, Lee H, et al: CDK inhibitors p18(INK4c) and p27(Kip1) mediate two separate pathways to collaboratively suppress pituitary tumorigenesis. *Genes Dev* 1998; 12:2899–2911.

Gille H, Downward J. Multiple ras effector pathways contribute to G(1) cell cycle progression. *J Biol Chem* 1999; 274:22033–22040.

Girard F, Strausfeld U, Fernandez A, Lamb N: Cyclin A is required for the onset of DNA replication in mammalian fibroblasts. *Cell* 1991; 67:1169–1179.

Hamburger AW, Salmon SE: Primary bioassay of human tumor stem cells. *Science* 1977; 197:461–463.

Hannon GJ, Beach D: p15 INK4B is a potential effector of TGF-β-induced cell cycle arrest. *Nature* 1994; 371:257–261.

Hedley DW, Shankey VT, Wheeless LL. DNA cytometry consensus conference. *Cytometry* 1993; 14:471–500.

Hengst L, Gopfert U, Lashuel HA, Reed SI: Complete inhibition of Cdk/cyclin by one molecule of p21(Cip1). *Genes Dev* 1998; 12:3882–3888.

Kaldis P, Solomon MJ: Analysis of CAK activities from human cells. *Eur J Biochem* 2000; 267:4213–4221.

Kerkhoff E, Rapp UR: Cell cycle targets of Ras/Raf signalling. *Oncogene* 1998; 17:1457–1462.

Keyomarsi K, Tucker SL, Buchholz TA, et al: Cyclin E and survival in patients with breast cancer. *N Engl J Med* 2002; 347:1566–1575.

Kim DH, Nelson HH, Wiencke JK, et al: P16(INK4a) and histology-specific methylation of CpG islands by exposure to tobacco smoke in non-small cell lung cancer. *Cancer Res* 2001; 61:3419–3424.

LaBaer J, Garrett M, Stevenson L, et al: New functional activities for the p21 family of CDK inhibitors. *Genes Dev* 1997; 11:847–862.

Latres E, Malumbres M, Sotillo R, et al: Limited overlapping roles of P15(INK4b) and P18(INK4c) cell cycle inhibitors in proliferation and tumorigenesis. *EMBO J* 2000; 19:3496–3506.

Lessard J, Sauvageau G: Bmi-1 determines the proliferative capacity of normal and leukaemic stem cells. *Nature* 2003; 423:255–260.

Liang J, Zubovitz J, Petrocelli T, et al: PKB/Akt phosphorylates p27, impairs nuclear import of p27 and opposes p27–mediated G1 arrest. *Nature Med* 2002; 8:1153–1160.

Luscher B: Function and regulation of the transcription factors of the Myc/Max/Mad network. *Gene* 2001; 277: 1–14.

Lynch HT, Brand RE, Hogg D, et al.: Phenotypic variation in eight extended CDKN2A germline mutation familial atypical multiple mole melanoma-pancreatic carcinoma-prone families: the familial atypical mole melanoma-pancreatic carcinoma syndrome. *Cancer* 2002; 94:84–96.

Mamillapalli R, Gavrilova N, Mihaylova VT, et al: PTEN regulates the ubiquitin-dependent degradation of the CDK inhibitor p27(KIP1) through the ubiquitin E3 ligase SCF(SKP2). *Curr Biol* 2001; 11:263–267.

Mateyak MK, Obaya AJ, Sedivy JM: C-Myc regulates cyclin D-Cdk4 and -Cdk6 activity but affects cell cycle progression at multiple independent points. *Mol Cell Biol* 1999; 19:4672–4683.

Matsumoto M, Furihata M, Ishikawa T, et al: Comparison of deregulated expression of cyclin D1 and cyclin E with that of cyclin-dependent kinase 4 (CDK4) and CDK2 in human oesophageal squamous cell carcinoma. *Br J Cancer* 1999; 80:256–261.

Matushansky I, Radparvar F, Skoultchi AI: Reprogramming leukemic cells to terminal differentiation by inhibiting specific cyclin-dependent kinases in G1. *Proc Natl Acad Sci USA* 2000; 97:14317–14322.

Medema RH, Kops GJ, Bos JL, Burgering BM: AFX-like Forkhead transcription factors mediate cell-cycle regulation by Ras and PKB through p27kip1. *Nature* 2000; 404:782–787.

Meraldi P, Lukas J, Fry AM, et al: Centrosome duplication in mammalian somatic cells requires E2F and Cdk2–cyclin A. *Nat Cell Biol* 1999; 1: 88–93.

Messner HA: Assessment and characterization of hemopoietic stem cells. *Stem Cells* 1995; 13(Suppl 3):13–18.

Moore JV, Hendry JH, Hunter RD: Dose-incidence curves for tumour control and normal tissue injury, in relation to the response of clonogenic cells. *Radiother Oncol* 1983; 1:143–147.

Moore MAS: Hematopoietic reconstruction: new approaches. *Clin Cancer Res* 1995; 1:3–9.

Morgan DO: Principles of Cdk regulation. *Nature* 1995; 374:131–134.

Muise-Helmericks RC, Grimes HL, Bellacosa A, et al: Cyclin D expression is controlled post-transcriptionally via a phosphatidylinositol 3–kinase/Akt-dependent pathway. *J Biol Chem* 1998; 273:29864–29872.

Nishioka K, Doki Y, Shiozaki H, et al: Clinical significance of CDC25A and CDC25B expression in squamous cell carcinomas of the oesophagus. *Br J Cancer* 2001; 85:412–421.

Noda A, Ning Y, Venable SF, et al: Cloning of senescent cell-derived inhibitors of DNA synthesis using an expression screen. *Exp Cell Res* 1994; 211:90–98.

O'Hagan RC, Ohh M, David G, et al: Myc-enhanced expression of Cul1 promotes ubiquitin-dependent proteolysis and cell cycle progression. *Genes Dev* 2000; 14:2185–2191.

Pardal R, Clarke MF, Morrison SJ: Applying the principles of stem-cell biology to cancer. *Nat Rev Cancer* 2003; 3:895–902.

Park IK, Morrison SJ, Clarke MF: Bmi1, stem cells, and senescence regulation. *J Clin Invest* 2004; 113:175–179.

Pierce GB, Speers WC: Tumors as caricatures of the process of tissue renewal: prospects for therapy by directing differentiation. *Cancer Res* 1988; 48:1996–2004.

Pines J: Cyclins, CDKs and cancer. *Semin Cancer Biol* 1995; 6:63–72.

Resnitsky D, Hengst L, Reed SI: Cyclin A-associated kinase activity is rate limiting for entrance into S phase and is negatively regulated in G1 by p27Kip1. *Mol Cell Biol* 1995; 15:4347–4352.

Reynisdottir I, Massague J: The subcellular locations of p15(Ink4b) and p27(Kip1) coordinate their inhibitory interactions with cdk4 and cdk2. *Genes Dev* 1997; 11:492–503.

Riccardi A, Danova M, Dionigi P, et al: Cell kinetics in leukemia and solid tumours studied with in vivo bromodeoxyuridine and flow cytometry. *Br J Cancer* 1989; 59:898–903.

Rocco JW, Sidransky D: P16(MTS-1/CDKN2/INK4a) in cancer progression. *Exp Cell Res* 2001; 264:42–55.

Roman-Gomez J, Castillejo JA, Jimenez A, et al: 5′ CpG island hypermethylation is associated with transcriptional silencing of the p21(CIP1/WAF1/SDI1) gene and confers poor prognosis in acute lymphoblastic leukemia. *Blood* 2002; 99:2291–2296.

Rossig L, Jadidi AS, Urbich C, et al: Akt-dependent phosphorylation of p21(Cip1) regulates PCNA binding and proliferation of endothelial cells. *Mol Cell Biol* 2001; 21:5644–5657.

Ruas M, Peters G: The p16ink4a/CDKN2A tumor suppressor and its relatives. *Biochim Biophys Acta* 1998; 1378:F115–F177.

Sandhu C, Donovan J, Bhattacharya N, et al: Reduction of Cdc25A contributes to cyclin E1–Cdk2 inhibition at senescence in human mammary epithelial cells. *Oncogene* 2000a; 19:5314–5323.

Sandhu C, Peehl DM, Slingerland J: P16 INK4A mediates cyclin-dependent kinase 4 and 6 inhibition in senescent prostatic epithelial cells. *Cancer Res* 2000b; 60:2616–2622.

Schwarze SR, Shi Y, Fu VX, et al: Role of cyclin-dependent kinase inhibitors in the growth arrest at senescence in human prostate epithelial and uroepithelial cells. *Oncogene* 2001; 20:8184–8192.

Shah SA, Potter MW, Callery MP: Ubiquitin proteasome pathway: implications and advances in cancer therapy. *Surg Oncol* 2001; 10:43–52.

Sharpless NE, Bardeesy N, Lee KH, et al: Loss of p16Ink4a with retention of p19Arf predisposes mice to tumorigenesis. *Nature* 2001; 413:86–91.

Sherr CJ: G1 phase progression: cycling on cue. *Cell* 1994; 79:551–555.

Sherr CJ: The Pezcoller lecture: cancer cell cycles revisited. *Cancer Res* 2000; 60:3689–3695.

Sherr CJ, Roberts JM: CDK inhibitors: positive and negative regulators of G1-phase progression. *Genes Dev* 1999; 13:1501–1512.

Slingerland J, Pagano M: Regulation of the cell cycle by the ubiquitin pathway. *Results Probl Cell Differ* 1998; 22:133–147.

Slingerland J, Pagano M: Regulation of the cdk inhibitor p27 and its deregulation in cancer. *J Cell Physiol* 2000; 183:10–17.

Solomon MJ, Kaldis P: Regulation of cdks by phosphorylation. *Results Probl Cell Differ* 1998; 22;79–109.

Staller P, Peukert K, Kiermaier A, et al: Repression of p15ink4b expression by Myc through association with Miz-1. *Nat Cell Biol* 2001; 3: 392–399.

Steel GG: *Growth Kinetics of Tumours: Cell Population Kinetics in Relation to the Growth and Treatment of Cancer.* Oxford, UK: Clarendon Press, 1977.

Sutherland RM: Cell and environment interactions in tumour microregions: The multicell spheroid model. *Science* 1988; 240:177–184.

Sutterluty H, Chatelain E, Marti A, et al: p45SKP2 promotes p27Kip1 degradation and induces S phase in quiescent cells. *Nat Cell Biol* 1999; 1:207–214.

Takemasa I, Yamamoto H, Sekimoto M, et al: Overexpression of CDC25B phosphatase as a novel marker of poor prognosis of human colorectal carcinoma. *Cancer Res* 2000; 60:3043–3050.

Takizawa CG, Morgan DO: Control of mitosis by changes in the subcellular location of cyclin-B1–Cdk1 and Cdc25C. *Curr Opin Cell Biol* 2000; 12:658–665.

Tannock IF: Population kinetics of carcinoma cells, capillary endothelial cells, and fibroblasts in a transplanted mouse mammary tumor. *Cancer Res* 1970; 30:2470–2476.

Tannock IF: Cell kinetics and chemotherapy: a critical review. *Cancer Treat Rev* 1978; 62:1117–1133.

Tannock IF: Biology of tumor growth. *Hosp Pract* 1983; 18:81–93.

Thomlinson RH, Gray LH: The histological structure of some human lung cancers and the possible implications for radiotherapy. *Br J Cancer* 1955; 9:539–549.

Tsihlias J, Kapusta L, Slingerland J: The prognostic significance of altered cyclin-dependent kinase inhibitors in human cancer. *Annu Rev Med* 1999; 50:401–423.

Viglietto G, Fusco A: Understanding p27(kip1) deregulation in cancer: down-regulation or mislocalization? *Cell Cycle* 2002; 1:394–400.

Vlach J, Hennecke S, Alevizopoulos K, et al: Growth arrest by the cyclin-dependent kinase inhibitor p27Kip1 is abrogated by c-Myc. *EMBO J* 1996; 15:6595–6604.

Vogelstein B, Fearon ER, Hamilton SR, et al: Clonal analysis using recombinant DNA probes from the X-chromosome. *Cancer Res* 1987; 46:4806–4813.

Wang TC, Cardiff RD, Zukerberg L, et al: Mammary hyperplasia and carcinoma in MMTV-cyclin D1 transgenic mice. *Nature* 1994; 369:669–671.

Warner BJ, Blain SW, Seoane J, Massague J: Myc downregulation by transforming growth factor beta required for activation of the p15(Ink4b) G(1) arrest pathway. *Mol Cell Biol* 1999; 19:5913–5922.

Wilson GD, McNally NJ, Dische S, et al: Measurement of cell kinetics in human tumours in vivo using bromodeoxyuridine incorporation and flow cytometry. *Br J Cancer* 1988; 58:423–431.

Wong IH, Ng MH, Huang DP, Lee JC: Aberrant p15 promoter methylation in adult and childhood acute leukemias of nearly all morphologic subtypes: potential prognostic implications. *Blood* 2000; 95:1942–1949.

Yoneda Y: Nucleocytoplasmic protein traffic and its significance to cell function. *Genes Cells* 2000; 5:777–787.

Zhang P, Wong C, Depinho RA, et al: Cooperation between the Cdk inhibitors p27(KIP1) and p57(KIP2) in the control of tissue growth and development. *Genes Dev* 1998a; 12:3162–3167.

Zhang S, Ramsay ES, Mock BA: Cdkn2a, the cyclin-dependent kinase inhibitor encoding p16ink4a and p19arf, is a candidate for the plasmacytoma susceptibility locus, Pctr1. *Proc Natl Acad Sci USA* 1998b; 95:2429–2434.

Zhou BP, Liao Y, Xia W, et al: Cytoplasmic localization of p21Cip1/WAF1 by Akt-induced phosphorylation in HER-2/neu-overexpressing cells. *Nat Cell Biol* 2001; 3:245–252.

Zirbes TK, Baldus SE, Moenig SP, et al: Prognostic impact of p21/waf1/cip1 in colorectal cancer. *Int J Cancer* 2000; 89:14–18.

# 10

# Cell Death

*Razqallah Hakem and Lea Harrington*

## 10.1 INTRODUCTION: APOPTOSIS VERSUS NECROSIS

Cell death is a fundamental process in normal development and tissue homeostasis of multicellular organisms. In mammals, tight regulation of both cell proliferation and cell death is required during development as well as during postnatal life. It is estimated that in a typical adult human 10 billion cells die daily.

Cell death results from at least two different processes: apoptosis (or programmed cell death) and necrosis (Table 10.1; Leist and Jaattela, 2001; Van Cruchten and Van Den Broeck, 2002). Necrosis serves to remove damaged cells from an organism and is essentially a passive process. In contrast, apoptosis is a process in which cells actively participate in their own death. Originally apoptosis and necrosis were distinguished by the different sequence of morphological changes associated with these modes of cell death. Changes associated with apoptosis include membrane blebbing, cytoplasm shrinkage, alteration of asymmetrical distribution of membrane components, and condensation of the nucleus (Fig. 10.1). Cells at late stages of apoptosis become fragmented into apoptotic bodies that are eliminated by phagocytic cells without triggering an inflammatory reaction. In contrast, necrosis-associated cellular changes are manifested by swelling of the cell and mitochondria followed by focal rupture of membranes. More advanced stages of necrosis are associated with disintegration of all cellular components and inflammation.

Although programmed cell death was reported by various developmental biologists and cytologists during the past two centuries, it was only in the early 1970s that it was named *apoptosis* (from the Greek word for "leaves falling from a tree"). The discovery that apoptosis is genetically regulated, and that its dysregulation is associated with various types of human disease including cancer and autoimmune disorders, has stimulated intense interest among biologists to understand the mechanisms leading to apoptosis.

The first evidence that apoptosis is a genetically regulated process arose from studies of *Caenorhabditis elegans* (Metzstein et al., 1998). During the development of this nematode, 131 of the 1090 somatic cells die by apoptosis. Genetic screens for mutants deficient for this

**Table 10.1.** Different Characteristics of the Two Major Cell Death Processes: Apoptosis and Necrosis

| Apoptosis | Necrosis |
| --- | --- |
| Membrane blebbing, no loss of integrity | Loss of membrane integrity |
| Shrinking of cytoplasm | Swelling of cytoplasm and mitochondria |
| Alteration of membrane asymmetry | Membrane asymmetry preserved |
| Condensation of nucleus | |
| Mono- and oligonucleosomal length fragmentation of nuclear DNA | Random digestion of DNA (smear of DNA after agarose gel electrophoresis) |
| Ends with fragmentation of cell into smaller bodies | Ends with total cell lysis |
| Energy (ATP)-dependent | Energy independent |
| Activation of caspases | |
| Involves at least two different pathways | |
| No inflammatory response | Inflammatory response |

programmed cell death have identified several specific genes required for normal apoptosis. Thus, loss-of-function mutations of *egl-1*, *ced-3*, or *ced-4* or gain-of-function mutations of *ced-9* result in survival of the 131 cells programmed to die.

Studies in *C. elegans* have shown that the pro-apoptotic molecule CED4 binds to CED3 and CED9. Further genetic studies in this species indicated that CED4 functions downstream of CED9 but upstream of CED3, giving rise to the pathway illustrated in Figure 10.2. The genetic studies of apoptosis in *C. elegans* largely facilitated our understanding of the general mechanisms of apoptosis. Robert Horvitz and John Sulston were awarded the Nobel Prize in Physiology or Medicine (2002) for their genetic studies of programmed cell death in the model system nematode *C. elegans*.

A

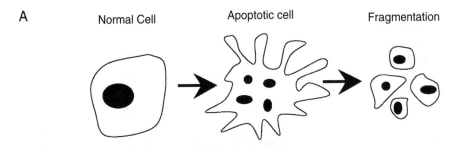

B

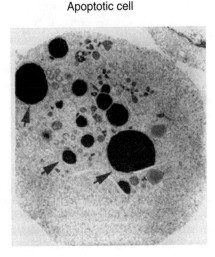

**Figure 10.1.** (*A*) Illustration of morphological features of apoptosis. In response to apoptotic stimuli, normal cells exhibit different morphological changes that are a hallmark for apoptosis. These changes include membrane blebbing and nuclear fragmentation followed by separation of the apoptotic cell into apoptotic bodies. (*B*) Electron microscopy showing an apoptotic embryonic stem cell 24 hours post-UV-irradiation (80 mJ/cm$^2$). Arrows indicate fragmented and condensed nuclear chromatin.

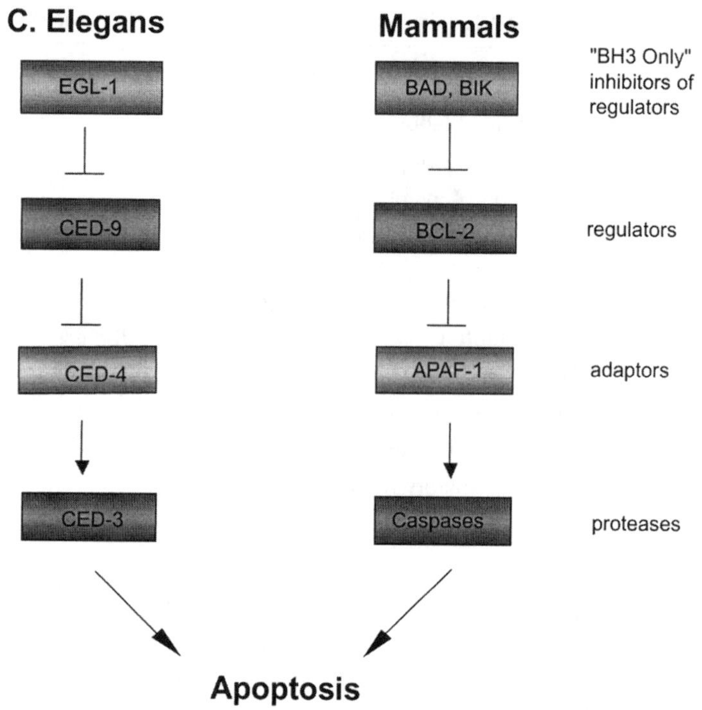

## C. Elegans            Mammals

**Figure 10.2.** Schematic representation of the apoptotic pathway and its components EGL-1, CED-9, CED-4, and CED-3 in *C. elegans* (*left*). Mammalian cells have evolved several orthologs to *C. elegans* proteins involved in the regulation of apoptosis (*right*; see text).

## 10.2 APOPTOSIS IN MAMMALS

In mammalian cells apoptosis can be triggered in response to endogenous stimuli (such as growth factor deprivation) as well as to exogenous stimuli [such as ultraviolet (UV) and γ-irradiation or other DNA damaging agents such as chemotherapeutic drugs]. Apoptosis can also be induced in response to inadequate cell-matrix interactions and this specific type of apoptosis is known as *anoikis* (Frisch and Screaton, 2001).

The direct involvement of various human tumor suppressor genes (such as *P53*, *PTEN*) and oncogenes (such as *AKT*, *BCL-2*) in the control of apoptosis is a strong demonstration of the requirement for a tight regulation of this cellular process.

The regulation of apoptosis in mammalian cells is complex and involves a variety of molecules, including both anti-apoptotic proteins, such as Bcl-2 and Bcl-X$_L$, and pro-apoptotic proteins, such as Apaf-1 and caspases (Fig. 10.3; Gross et al., 1999; Hengartner, 2000). Mitochondria have also been shown to play a major role in the early steps of apoptosis by releasing factors such as cytochrome *c* and apoptosis-inducing factor (AIF) that activate apoptotic pathways. In contrast to cytochrome *c*, the mechanism of action of AIF during apoptosis is poorly understood. In mammalian cells there are multiple homologs of the nematode *C. elegans* apoptotic proteins CED9, CED4, and CED3, which form two major pathways (see Figs. 10.2 and 10.3).

Biochemical studies have been instrumental in identifying the components of the apoptotic machinery in

mammals. In addition, mice with disruptions or alterations in specific apoptotic genes have been generated using gene targeting technology (see Chap. 4, Sec. 4.3.12) and have served as crucial tools in gaining a better understanding of the mammalian apoptotic pathways.

### 10.2.1 Bcl-2 Family Members and Apoptosis

The mammalian anti-apoptotic *BCL-2* gene was the first identified homologue of the *C. elegans ced-9* gene (Gross et al., 1999; Cory and Adams, 2002). *BCL-2* was identified in studies of human follicular B-cell lymphoma with the translocation t(14; 18). This chromosomal translocation results in overexpression of *BCL-2* and the inhibition of apoptosis within these cells (Chap. 7, Sec. 7.2.4). Expression of BCL-2 has been detected frequently in human cancers. In mammalian cells, Bcl-2 overexpression has been shown to prolong cell survival and to protect cells from a variety of apoptotic signals, including glucocorticoids, γ-irradiation, phorbol esters, ionomycin, and anti-CD3 monoclonal antibodies (mAbs). Various studies have implicated Bcl-2 as an inhibitor of cytochrome *c* release from mitochondria.

Bcl-2 is the prototypical member of a growing family of homologous proteins that includes anti-apoptotic proteins such as Bcl-2, Bcl-X$_L$, Bcl-w, A1, and Mcl-1 and pro-apoptotic proteins such as Bax, Bcl-X$_s$, Bak, Bad, Bik, Bim, and Bid (Gross et al., 1999; Cory and Adams, 2002). Members of the Bcl-2 family share several conserved domains called the Bcl-2 homology (BH) re-

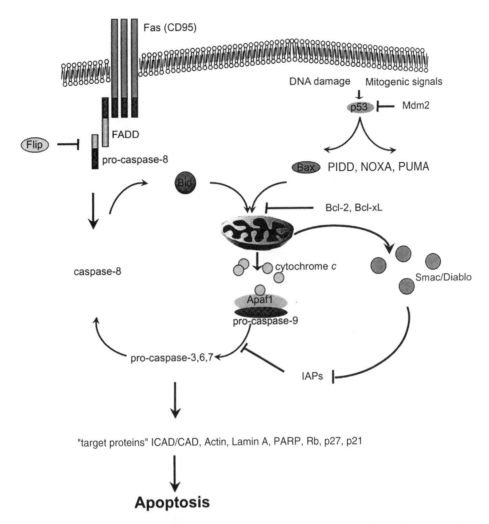

**Figure 10.3.** Schematic representation of the two major apoptotic pathways in mammalian cells: Death receptor and mitochondrial apoptotic pathways. The death receptor pathway is exemplified by the events that occur following engagement of Fas (CD95) by its ligand FasL (CD95L). Fas/FasL interaction leads to the trimerization of the Fas receptor and the recruitment of the adaptor protein FADD to the cytoplasmic tail of Fas. The interaction Fas/FADD is mediated by their respective death domains. Fas/FADD interaction allows the recruitment of the death-effector-domain–containing initiator caspase-8 (and caspase-10). The recruitment of these caspases to this complex results in their activation and subsequent processing of the downstream effectors caspase-3, -6, and -7. Effector caspases cleave various cellular proteins leading to commitment of the cell to apoptosis. The mitochondrial apoptotic pathway is triggered in response to various stimuli, including mitogenic signals and DNA damage. Activation of the tumor suppressor and transcriptional factor p53 in response to cellular stress signals leads to the transcriptional activation of several pro-apoptotic genes including Bax. Bax cooperates with activated Bid, a target for caspase 8 processing, to form openings in the outer mitochondrial membrane leading to the release of cytochrome *c* and Smac/Diablo to the cytoplasm. Cytochrome *c* clustering with Apaf-1 and caspase-9 results in the activation of caspase-9, whereas Smac/Diablo inactivates inhibitors of apoptosis (IAPs). Active caspase-9 cleaves downstream caspases that lead to apoptosis. The cleavage of caspase-8 by activated downstream caspases and caspase-8–mediated activation of Bid links the two apoptotic pathways.

gions. The BH1, BH2, BH3 and BH4 domains allow the formation of homo- and heterodimers between Bcl-2 family members and are thought to be vital for the function of these proteins (Fig. 10.4).

The in vivo functions of some Bcl-2 family members have been investigated in transgenic and mutant mice generated by gene targeting (Ranger et al., 2001). Mice overexpressing Bcl-2 in B-cells develop follicular hy-

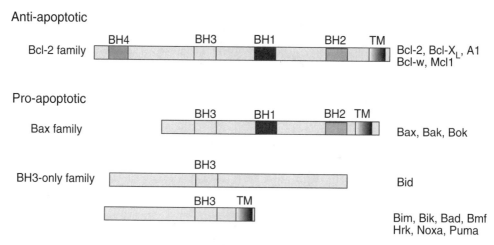

**Figure 10.4.** The members of the Bcl-2 family of anti-apoptotic and pro-apoptotic proteins are classified into three functional groups. The first group contains four Bcl-2 homology domains (BH1–BH4), a transmembrane domain (TM), and a short C-terminal hydrophobic tail that localizes these proteins to the outer surface of the mitochondria and the endoplasmic reticulum. This group I of anti-apoptotic proteins includes Bcl-2, Bcl-X$_L$, A1, Bcl-w, and Mcl1. Group II and group III consist of pro-apoptotic proteins. Members of the second group in the Bcl-2 family have the same domains as group I but lack the N-terminal BH4 domain. Members of this group include Bax, Bak, and Bok. The third group in the Bcl-2 family shares only BH3 as a common domain. This group includes various pro-apoptotic proteins such as Bid, Bim, Bik, Bad, Noxa, and Puma.

perplasia, with some mice acquiring aggressive monoclonal lymphomas. Similarly, overexpression of *Bcl-2* in T-cells leads to the development of peripheral T lymphomas in one third of transgenic mice. These results suggest that the normal function of Bcl-2 is to protect these cell types from apoptosis under certain physiological conditions.

Mice deficient for *Bcl-2* or *Bax* appear normal at birth but then develop different phenotypes (Ranger et al., 2001). Mutation of *Bcl-2* leads to impaired kidney development and loss of mature B- and T-cells as a consequence of increased apoptosis. However, mice deficient for Bax display lymphoid hyperplasia, impaired spermatogenesis, and testicular atrophy, and are infertile. Deletion of another anti-apoptotic Bcl-2 family member, *Bcl-X$_L$*, resulted in embryonic lethality at about embryonic day 13 (Ranger et al., 2001). Studies of these mutant mice have indicated an important role for Bcl-X$_L$ in programmed cell death during the development of the embryonic nervous system and lymphoid organs. These studies point to potential tissue-specific roles for distinct pro-apoptotic and anti-apoptotic proteins.

### 10.2.2  Apaf-1 and Apoptosis

Apoptosis protease activating factor-1 (Apaf-1), the first identified mammalian homolog of CED4, is critical for apoptosis (Zou et al., 1997). Apaf-1 is a 130 kilodalton protein composed of three functional domains: a short N-terminal caspase recruitment domain (CARD), a cen-

tral CED4 homology domain, and a long C-terminal "WD-40" repeat domain. In the presence of cytochrome *c* and 2′-deoxyadenosine 5′-triphosphate, Apaf-1 can interact with pro-caspase-9 through their mutual CARDs. Apaf-1 has also been shown to form oligomers. Oligomerization of Apaf-1 triggers autocatalysis of pro-caspase-9 leading to its processing and activation. In vitro studies have indicated that caspase-9, Apaf-1, cytochrome *c*, and dATP are all required for the activation of the effector caspases 3, 6, and 7 (Fig. 10.3).

Bcl-X$_L$ is able to interact with Apaf-1 and caspase-9 and form a ternary complex. Through this interaction, Bcl-X$_L$ mediates a negative control on the activation of caspase-9. In addition, the expression of *Apaf-1* was found to be transcriptionally induced by p53, further demonstrating the important role that p53 plays in controlling apoptosis (Moroni et al., 2001; Robles et al., 2001).

In vivo evidence for the essential role in apoptosis of *cytochrome c* and *Apaf-1* came from studies of mice with targeted disruption of these genes. Murine embryos deficient for *cytochrome c* die in utero by mid-gestation, but cell lines established from early *cytochrome c* null embryos are viable under conditions that compensate for defective oxidative phosphorylation (Li et al., 2000). As compared to cell lines established from wild-type embryos, cells lacking *cytochrome c* are resistant to apoptotic stimuli such as UV-irradiation and serum withdrawal, but have increased sensitivity to other apoptotic stimuli such as tumor necrosis factor (TNF). The mechanism leading to increased sensitivity in the absence of *cytochrome c* remain unknown. Deletion of *Apaf-1* in mice resulted in perinatal lethality (Yoshida et al., 1998). *Apaf-1* mutant embryos displayed decreased apoptosis of neuronal cells in the developing brain. When compared to wild-type controls, Apaf-1 deficient cells are less sensitive to a variety of apoptotic stimuli, including γ-irradiation, dexamethasone, and chemotherapeutic agents, but not to anti-Fas (CD95) antibody treatment.

Other putative mammalian homologs of CED4 have been described but their role in apoptosis remains to be confirmed.

### 10.2.3 Caspases and Apoptosis

The first mammalian caspase (ICE or caspase-1) was identified in 1993 on the basis of its similarity to the *C. elegans* protein CED3. More than fourteen mammalian caspases have been cloned (Hengartner, 2000). Caspases are cysteine proteases present in the cytosol in inactive forms. In order to become active, the pro-caspases must be proteolytically cleaved at specific aspartate residues. Active caspases are heterotetrameric complexes composed of two large subunits (~ 20 kilodalton) and two small subunits (~ 10 kilodalton; Fig. 10.5). All caspases contain an active site pentapeptide (QACXG; X is R, Q, or G).

While caspases are known primarily for their involvement in apoptosis, some caspases such as caspase-1 and caspase-11 also play crucial roles in inflammation. In fact caspase-1 was originally known as interleukin-1β-converting enzyme (ICE).

Caspases have a wide range of expression throughout mammalian tissues and often are coexpressed in the same cell or tissue types. The finding that caspases are able to sequentially process and activate other caspases, together with the structural studies of these proteins, has allowed the classification of caspases into initiators (e.g., caspase-8, caspase-9, and caspase-10) or executioners of apoptosis (such as caspase-3, caspase-6,

and caspase-7). Initiator pro-caspases contain large pro-domains, whereas executioner pro-caspases contain small pro-domains.

Various caspase substrates have been identified including cytoskeleton proteins (such as actin and gelsolin), nuclear proteins (such as lamin A and B) proteins involved in DNA repair (such as PARP, RAD51, and DNA-PKCs; see also Chap. 5, Sec. 5.2), cell cycle proteins (such as p21, p27, CDC27, and Rb; see also Chap. 9, Sec. 9.2) and apoptotic proteins (caspases, Bcl-2, Bcl-X$_L$, Bid, Bax, and ICAD). The caspase activated DNase (CAD) is inactive when associated with its inhibitor ICAD (also known as DNA fragmentation factor DFF). In response to apoptotic stimuli, ICAD is cleaved by caspases allowing the release of the active endonuclease CAD that produces the characteristic internucleosomal DNA cleavage (Earnshaw et al., 1999; Sec. 10.3.4).

The existence of multiple mammalian caspases suggests the possibility that each may have a specific role in apoptosis induced by a particular cell death signal or in a given tissue. Mice deficient for specific caspases have been generated (Zheng et al., 1999). *Caspase-3*$^{-/-}$ and *caspase-9*$^{-/-}$ mice show a similar brain defect characterized by ectopic masses of supernumerary cells that escape apoptosis during brain development (Hakem et al., 1998). Most of these mice die in utero or just after birth. *Caspase-2* mutation leads to defective cytolysis of B lymphoblasts mediated by perforin and granzyme B, and female mice with this mutation contain excess ovarian germ cells, with oocytes showing resistance to chemotherapy-induced apoptosis. *Caspase-12*$^{-/-}$ mice resist apoptosis induced by stimuli causing stress to the endoplasmic reticulum but undergo apoptosis in response to other stimuli. Other mice, such as those deficient for caspase-7 or caspase-8, show various developmental defects and die prenatally. In contrast, the absence of a dramatic phenotype in certain caspase mutant mice such as *caspase-6* mutants raises the possibility of functional redundancy among caspases.

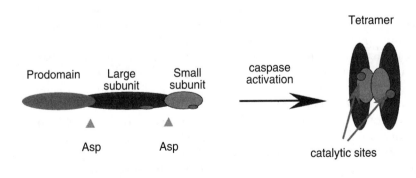

Tetramer

Prodomain    Large subunit    Small subunit

caspase activation

Asp    Asp

catalytic sites

Pro-caspase (inactive)

Active caspase

**Figure 10.5.** Schematic representation of caspases. Caspases exist in an inactive form (pro-caspases) that require proteolytic cleavage by upstream caspases. In the case of initiator caspases such as caspase-8, their aggregation leads to cross-activation. Cleavage of pro-caspases at specific Aspartate (Asp) residues leads to a large and a small subunit that form a heterodimer with two catalytic sites in the active caspase form.

Taken together, these studies reveal that caspases, like their anti-apoptotic counterparts, are regulated by both tissue-specific and tissue-overlapping mechanisms.

### 10.2.4 P53 and Apoptosis

P53, a transcription factor that is the most commonly mutated tumor suppressor gene in human cancers, controls several cellular pathways including apoptosis (Fig. 10.3) and the cell cycle (Hanahan and Weinberg, 2000; see also Chap. 9, Sec. 9.2.1). Inherited mutations of the *p53* gene are associated with Li-Fraumeni syndrome, a disease characterized by an increased risk for breast and lung carcinomas, soft tissue sarcomas, brain tumors, osteosarcoma, and leukemia. In some cervical cancers, viral proteins such as human papillomavirus (HPV) E6 can functionally inactivate p53 (Chap. 6, Sec. 6.2, Sec. 6.2.3).

p53 can be activated by two major pathways: the first triggered by mitogenic signals and the second triggered in response to DNA damage. Several p53 transcriptional targets have been identified, including genes involved in cell cycle regulation (see Chap. 9, Sec. 9.2) and an increasing number of genes that control apoptosis. Activated p53 leads to the transcriptional activation of pro-apoptotic genes including *apaf-1*, *caspase-1*, *bax*, *bid*, puma, *PIDD*, *DR5*, *noxa*, and *fas* (*CD95*). Conversely, p53 activation can repress the expression of the anti-apoptotic gene *bcl-2*. p53 also influences the expression of *PTEN*, another tumor suppressor gene involved in the control of the Akt protein kinase B (Akt/PKB) survival pathway (see Chap. 7, Sec. 7.4.3; Chap. 8, Sec. 8.2.7).

p53, though important, is not absolutely required for apoptosis. For example, p53-independent apoptosis takes place in *p53* null thymocytes in response to dexamethasone. Furthermore, p53-independent apoptosis contributes to cell death triggered upon loss of telomere integrity in both human and murine cells deficient for p53 and telomerase elongation activity (see Chap. 5, Sec. 5.5).

### 10.2.5 The Mitochondrial Apoptotic Pathway

Two principal mammalian apoptotic pathways have been identified: the mitochondrial pathway and the death receptor (DR) pathway (Fig. 10.3; Ashkenazi, 2002). Mitochondria play central roles in apoptosis through their sequestration of cytochrome c. Death stimuli can signal release of cytochrome c from the mitochondrial intermembrane space into the cytosol, a process that is inhibited by Bcl-2 or Bcl-$X_L$ and promoted by Bid and Bax. Cytosolic cytochrome c complexes with Apaf-1, which recruits and activates pro-caspase-9 in the presence of dATP or adenosine triphos-

phate (ATP; Hengartner, 2000). Caspase-9 activation in turn leads to activation of other caspases, including caspase-3, -6, and -7, which catalyze the cleavage of various cellular substrates leading to cell death. Caspase activity can be modulated by various members of the family of inhibitor of apoptosis proteins (IAPs). Inhibitor of apoptosis proteins were discovered originally in baculoviruses and shown to suppress the host cell death response to viral infection (Deveraux and Reed, 1999). Subsequently, IAPs were identified in various species including human. Several IAPs including XIAP, c-IAP1, and c-IAP2 have been shown to directely bind and inhibit caspases such as caspase-3, -7, and -9. Inhibitor of apoptosis proteins are inhibited by Smac/DIABLO, a protein that is released with the cytochrome c from mitochondria and binds to IAPs to relieve their inhibition of caspases (Fig. 10.3).

### 10.2.6 The Death Receptor Apoptotic Pathway

The mammalian death receptor (DR) apoptotic pathway is triggered by ligands which bind to the death receptor members of the TNF receptor family: Fas (CD95), TNF receptor type 1 (TNFR-1), Trail (TNF-related apoptosis-inducing ligand) receptors DR4, DR5, DR3 and DR6 (Nagata, 1999). For example, stimulation of Fas by FasL or TNFR-1 by TNF has been implicated in the elimination of unwanted lymphocytes and transformed cells.

Death receptors share the presence of a death domain in their cytoplasmic tails (Ashkenazi, 2002). Death receptor signaling is exemplified by the events that occur following engagement of Fas by its ligand FasL on the cell surface (Fig. 10.3). Following Fas/FasL interaction, the Fas receptor proteins aggregate to form a trimer and recruit the adaptor protein FADD (Fas-associated death domain protein) that contains two protein interaction domains, a death domain (DD) and a death effector domain (DED). Fas/FADD interaction allows the recruitment of DED-containing initiator caspases such as caspase-8 and caspase-10 to the complex, resulting in their activation. Activated caspase-8 and caspase-10 in turn process downstream caspases such as caspase-3, thereby finalizing the commitment to apoptosis.

The DR and mitochondrial pathways are linked by caspase-8 cleavage of BID (a pro-apoptotic member of the Bcl-2 family) that generates a proteolytic fragment that cooperates with Bax and forms supramolecular openings in the outer mitochondrial membrane leading to release of mitochondrial cytochrome c. Hence, BID may serve to amplify death signals initiated by engagement of the DR, as BID deficiency does not affect caspase-8 activation, but drastically diminishes caspase-3 processing.

Mice mutant for components of the death receptor pathway have illustrated the importance of this pathway in apoptosis. Defective apoptosis has been observed in mice and cells deficient for Fas, FasL, caspase-8, or FADD (Ranger et al., 2001).

## 10.3 ASSESSMENT OF APOPTOSIS

A number of assays have been developed to study apoptosis, and they are based on detection of: (1) alteration of the membrane structure, (2) release of cytochrome c to the cytosol, (3) activation of caspases, and (4) fragmentation of nuclear DNA.

### 10.3.1 Alteration of the Membrane Structure

Apoptosis is associated with alterations of the structure of the plasma membrane in cells (Earnshaw et al., 1999). In normal cells the distribution of phospholipids in the membrane bilayer is asymmetric with the inner layer containing anionic phospholipids such as phosphatidylserine and the outer membrane almost exclusively containing neutral phospholipids. In apoptotic cells the asymmetric distribution of phospholipids is perturbed and phosphatidylserines become exposed on the outer surface of the plasma membrane. This membrane alteration associated with apoptosis can be detected using Annexin-V, a calcium-dependent phospholipid-binding protein with high affinity for phosphatidylserines (Fig. 10.6A).

After staining cells with fluorescent-conjugated Annexin-V, nonapoptotic cells will not exhibit staining while apoptotic cells should stain positively. The stained samples can be analyzed using a flow cytometer (Chap. 9, Sec. 9.4.2) or under a fluorescence microscope. Propidium iodide (PI) is often included with Annexin-V in these apoptotic assays because cells with a compromised cell membrane will allow PI to diffuse into the cell and bind the cellular DNA. Apoptotic cells can therefore be detected and sorted in two parameter flow cytometric plots as Annexin-V positive/PI negative (early apoptosis) or Annexin-V positive/PI positive (late apoptosis), as shown in Figure 10.6B.

### 10.3.2 Release of Cytochrome c to the Cytosol

In response to apoptotic stimuli, cytochrome c is released from the mitochondria to the cytosol where it binds to Apaf-1 and pro-caspase-9, forming the apoptosome and triggering apoptosis (Zimmermann et al., 2001). This release of cytochrome c can be detected by immunohistochemistry using a monoclonal antibody that recognizes cytochrome c. In this assay, live cells stained with anti-cytochrome c show punctate staining corresponding to the localization of cytochrome c in mitochondria. In contrast, cells in the process of apoptosis show diffuse staining corresponding to the release of cytochrome c from mitochondria to the cytosol. An alternative approach is to use a western blot assay

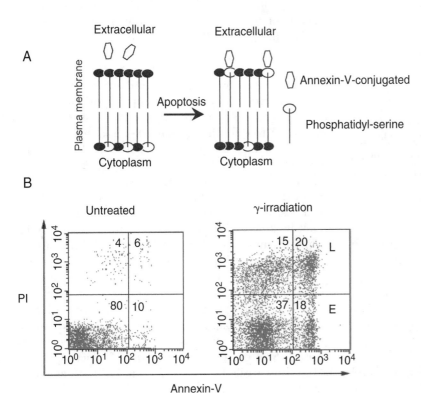

**Figure 10.6.** (A) Phosphatidylserines (phospholipids) localize exclusively to the inner cytoplasmic face of the plasma membrane. Following an apoptotic stimulus, the distribution of the membrane phosphatidylserines changes and they became present at the outer cell membrane of apoptotic cells. This redistribution of phosphatidylserines makes them accessible to Annexin-V, a calcium-dependent phospholipid binding protein. Apoptosis can be monitored by assessing the binding of conjugated Annexin-V such as Annexin-V FITC to cells, apoptotic cells (Annexin-V positive) and viable cells (Annexin-V negative) can be identified. (B) Fluorescence dot blots of Annexin V- FITC and propidium iodide (PI)-stained thymocytes either untreated or 24-hour post-γ-irradiation (600 rads). The percentages of cells in each quadrant are indicated.

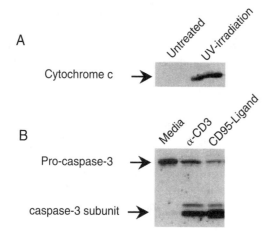

**Figure 10.7.** (*A*) Cytochrome c translocation to the cytoplasm in response to UV radiation mediated apoptosis. Embryonic stem cells were either untreated or treated with UV-radiation (80 mJ/cm2) and cultured for an additional 6 hours. Cytosolic fractions were prepared from these cells and western blots performed using anti-cytochrome c monoclonal antibody. (*B*) Processing of pro-caspase 3 in naive T-cells (media) or activated T-cells treated for 24 hours with anti-CD3 MAbs or with CD95–Ligand. Western blots were performed with an anti-Caspase 3 MAb that recognizes the pro-caspase 3 and the processed subunit.

using an antibody that recognizes cytochrome c. Cellular cytosolic fractions can be prepared by ultracentrifugation of lysed cells and cytochrome c should be detected in the cytosolic fraction from cells treated with apoptotic stimuli but not that from untreated cells, as shown in Figure 10.7*A*.

### 10.3.3 Processing of Caspases and Their Substrates

To become active, the pro-caspases (inactive caspases) must be proteolytically cleaved at specific aspartate residues (Earnshaw et al., 1999). The processing of pro-caspases can be analyzed by western blotting using specific anti-caspase antibodies (see Fig. 10.7*B*). Alternatively, activation of caspases can be indirectly assessed by western blot analysis of the processing of caspase substrates, such as PARP and Rb (see Sec. 10.2.3).

### 10.3.4 Fragmentation of Nuclear DNA

Stimulation of apoptotic pathways results in activation of endonucleases, such as caspase-activated DNase (CAD), that degrade the cellular DNA into fragments of various sizes. Upon agarose gel electrophoresis, DNA fragments from apoptotic cells reveal a distinctive ladder pattern consisting of multiples of an approximately 180 base pair periodicity that reflects nucleosome spacing (Fig. 10.8*A*).

Assays of DNA ladders are relatively insensitive and not suitable for assessing apoptosis in individual cells.

A more appropriate method to identify individual apoptotic cells based on their nuclear DNA fragmentation is the use of the TUNEL [terminal transferase (TdT)-mediated dUTP nick end-labeling] assay (Fig. 10.8*B*). In this assay TdT catalyzes a template-independent addition of fluorescein labeled-dUTP to the 3′hydroxyl termini of double- and single-stranded DNA. The incorporated fluorescein can then be visualized with a flow cytometer and/or a fluorescence microscope (Fig. 10.8*C*).

## 10.4 APOPTOSIS AND CANCER

Dysregulation of cellular pathways resulting in attenuation or enhancement of apoptosis can lead to diseases such as cancer, autoimmunity, or neurodegenerative disorders (Johnstone et al., 2002). Understanding the cascade of events leading to apoptosis may facilitate the design of more effective therapies for human diseases associated with defective apoptosis.

Tumorigenesis is a multistep process in which acquired mutations result in dysregulation of crucial cellular pathways including apoptosis, cell cycle, and repair of DNA damage (Hanahan and Weinberg, 2000). Loss of expression of the pro-apoptotic genes *caspase-8* or *Apaf-1*, and overexpression of the anti-apoptotic *Bcl-2* gene are among the defects of apoptosis associated with human cancers (Table 10.2). The loss of *CASPASE-8* expression has been found frequently in neuroblastomas and is associated with amplification of the oncogene *N-myc* (Teitz et al., 2000). *APAF-1* expression is frequently silenced in human melanomas (Soengas et al., 2001). In contrast, *BCL-2* is overexpressed in various types of tumors including human follicular B-cell lymphomas (Mullauer et al., 2001). The importance of defective apoptosis in cancer is also demonstrated by the fact that several human tumor suppressor genes (such as *P53* and *PTEN*) and oncogenes (such as *AKT*) play important roles in the regulation of apoptosis.

Most current cancer therapies are based on damaging cellular DNA by irradiation or in response to chemotherapeutic drugs. These treatments lead to cell death that may be mediated by apoptosis as well as by necrosis. Because markers of apoptosis are seen frequently after treatment of cells or tumors with radiation and anticancer drugs, it has often been assumed that these agents induce the process of apoptosis and that one of the causes of therapeutic resistance is diminished ability to undergo apoptosis (see Chap. 18, Sec. 18.2.8). However, as indicated in Chapter 14, Section 14.3.1 and Chapter 17, Section 17.2.3, the key property of effective therapeutic agents is that they should cause loss of reproductive integrity of cancer cells, assayed most easily by assessing their ability to generate progeny in a colony-forming assay. Several studies have

A

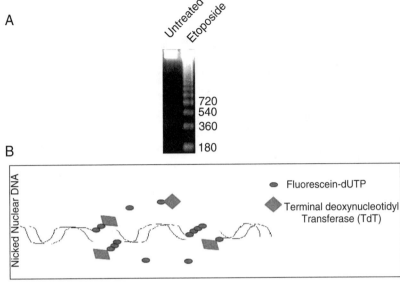

B

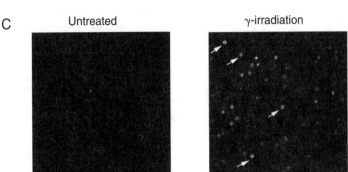

Fluorescein-dUTP

Terminal deoxynucleotidyl Transferase (TdT)

C      Untreated                    γ-irradiation

**Figure 10.8.** (*A*) DNA fragmentation of apoptotic thymocytes in response to treatment with etoposide (24 h). DNA fragments in multiples of 180 bp (Ladder) are observed when genomic DNA extracted from etoposide-treated cells (apoptotic) is run on agarose gels. (*B*) Schematic representation of the principle of the TUNEL [terminal transferase (TdT)-mediated dUTP nick end-labeling] assay for identifying apoptotic cells. TdT catalyzes the addition of fluorescein labeled-dUTP to the 3'hydroxyl termini of double- and single-stranded DNA present in apoptotic cells. The incorporated fluorescein can then be visualized with a flow cytometer or a fluorescence microscope as shown in (*C*). TUNEL assay was performed on spleen sections from untreated or γ-irradiated mice. Apoptotic nuclei (arrows) are seen in the spleen from irradiated but not control mice.

**Table 10.2.** Examples of Apoptotic Genes Involved in Human Cancer

| Gene | Role in Cancer |
| --- | --- |
| *P53* | The most commonly mutated gene in human cancer |
| *RB* | Mutated or nonfunctional in various cancers. Loss of Rb triggers p53 dependent and independent apoptosis |
| *PTEN* | Mutated or altered expression in cancers. Regulates Akt activation |
| *BAK* | Mutated or decreased expression in some tumors |
| *BAX* | Mutated or decreased expression in some tumors |
| *APAF-1* | Mutated or transcriptionally silenced in melanoma |
| *CASPASE-8* | Mutated or transcriptionally silenced in neuroblastoma with *N-myc* amplification |
| *FAS (CD95)* | Mutated or downregulated in lymphoid and solid tumors |
| Trail receptors *DR4 and DR5* | Mutated in metastatic breast cancers |
| *BCL-2* | Frequently overexpressed in cancer |
| *IAPs* | Frequently overexpressed in cancer |
| *MDM2* | Overexpressed in some tumors |
| *AKT* | Frequently amplified in solid tumors |
| *FLIP* | Overexpressed in some cancers |

Dysregulation of various apoptotic and anti-apoptotic genes has been shown to be associated with cancer development or metastasis (Johnstone et al., 2002).

indicated that loss of cell survival indicated by these assays is not well correlated with apoptosis (Brown and Wouters, 1999). Thus apoptosis may sometimes represent a pathway by which cells that are already dead (in the sense of having lost their ability for indefinite reproduction) undergo lysis, rather than a primary mechanism that mediates killing by anticancer agents.

New therapeutic modalities, including monoclonal antibodies or antisense oligonucleotides, have been developed with the aim of stimulating apoptosis of cancer cells (Reed, 2002). Thus, antisense to *Bcl-2* as well as small molecules inhibiting Bcl-2 function, are in development or being tested for therapy of various types of tumors. Similarly, recombinant adenoviruses expressing *p53* are being evaluated against various cancers, including head and neck cancer, colorectal cancer, and ovarian cancer.

## 10.5 SUMMARY

The genetic pathways that regulate apoptosis have been elucidated in the roundworm *C. elegans* and more recently in mammals. These studies have revealed a regulated cascade of caspase activation that leads to cleavage of key cellular proteins and a loss of integrity of the mitochondrial membrane. Taken together these events lead to commitment to cell death. This process shows cell type specificity and exquisite regulation during development and postdevelopment, and in human disorders such as cancer and autoimmunity. Future studies are aimed at the identification of the remaining apoptotic players, and establishing the functional interactions of the various pro-apoptotic and anti-apoptotic molecules. In addition, the mechanisms for necrosis remain unclear. A major challenge is to take advantage of our rapidly expanding knowledge of cell death to design better therapies for patients who suffer from diseases such as cancer and autoimmune disorders.

## REFERENCES

Ashkenazi A: Targeting death and decoy receptors of the tumour-necrosis factor superfamily. *Nat Rev Cancer* 2002; 2:420–430.

Brown JM, Wouters BG: Apoptosis, p53, and tumor cell sensitivity to anticancer agents. *Cancer Res* 1999; 59:1391–1399.

Cory S, Adams JM: The Bcl2 family: regulators of the cellular life-or-death switch. *Nat Rev Cancer* 2002; 2:647–656.

Deveraux QL, Reed JC: IAP family proteins—suppressors of apoptosis. *Genes Dev* 1999; 13:239–252.

Earnshaw WC, Martins LM, Kaufman SH: Mammalian caspases: structure, activation, substrates, and functions during apoptosis. *Annu Rev Biochem* 1999; 68:383–424.

Frisch SM, Screaton RA: Anoikis mechanisms. *Curr Opin Cell Biol* 2001; 13:555–562.

Gross A, McDonnell JM, Korsmeyer SJ: BCL-2 family members and the mitochondria in apoptosis. *Genes Dev* 1999; 13:1899–1911.

Hakem R, Hakem A, Duncan GS: Differential requirement for caspase 9 in apoptotic pathways in vivo. *Cell* 1998; 94:339–352.

Hanahan D, Weinberg RA: The hallmarks of cancer. *Cell* 2000;100:57–70.

Hengartner MO: The biochemistry of apoptosis. *Nature* 2000; 407:770–776.

Johnstone RW, Ruefli AA, Lowe SW: Apoptosis: a link between cancer genetics and chemotherapy. *Cell* 2002; 108:153–164.

Leist M, Jaattela M: Four deaths and a funeral: from caspases to alternative mechanisms. *Nat Rev Mol Cell Biol* 2001; 2: 589–598.

Li K, Li Y, Shelton JM: Cytochrome c deficiency causes embryonic lethality and attenuates stress-induced apoptosis. *Cell* 2000; 101:389–399.

Metzstein MM, Stanfield GM, Horvitz HR: Genetics of programmed cell death in C. elegans: past, present and future. *Trends Genet* 1998; 14:410–416.

Moroni MC, Hickman ES, Denchi EL: Apaf-1 is a transcriptional target for E2F and p53. *Nat Cell Biol* 2001; 3:552–558.

Mullauer L, Gruber P, Sebinger D: Mutations in apoptosis genes: a pathogenetic factor for human disease. *Mutat Res* 2001; 488:211–231.

Nagata S: Fas ligand-induced apoptosis. *Annu Rev Genet* 1999; 33:29–55.

Ranger AM, Malynn BA, Korsmeyer SJ: Mouse models of cell death. *Nat Genet* 2001; 28:113–118.

Reed JC: Apoptosis-based therapies. *Nat Rev Drug Discov* 2002; 1:111–121.

Robles AI, Bemmels NA, Foraker AB: APAF-1 is a transcriptional target of p53 in DNA damage-induced apoptosis. *Cancer Res* 2001; 61:6660–6664.

Soengas MS, Capodieci P, Polsky D: Inactivation of the apoptosis effector Apaf-1 in malignant melanoma. *Nature* 2001; 409:207–211.

Teitz T, Wei T, Valentine MB: Caspase 8 is deleted or silenced preferentially in childhood neuroblastomas with amplification of MYCN. *Nat Med* 2000; 6:529–535.

Van Cruchten S, Van Den Broeck W: Morphological and biochemical aspects of apoptosis, oncosis and necrosis. *Anat Histol Embroyl* 2002; 31:214–223.

Yoshida H, Kong YY, Yoshida R: Apaf1 is required for mitochondrial pathways of apoptosis and brain development. *Cell* 1998; 94:739–750.

Zheng TS, Hunot S, Kuida K: Caspase knockouts: matters of life and death. *Cell Death Differ* 1999; 6:1043–1053.

Zimmermann KC, Bonzon C, Green DR: The machinery of programmed cell death. *Pharmacol Ther* 2001; 92:57–70.

Zou H, Henzel WJ, Liu X: Apaf-1, a human protein homologous to C. elegans CED-4, participates in cytochrome c-dependent activation of caspase-3. *Cell* 1997; 90:405–413.

# 11

# Tumor Progression and Metastasis: Cellular, Molecular, and Microenvironmental Factors

*Rama Khokha, Evelyn Voura, and Richard P. Hill*

## 11.1 TUMOR PROGRESSION AND HETEROGENEITY

### 11.1.1 Tumor Progression

Cancer is not a static disease. In some tumors (e.g., melanoma, colon cancer, cervical cancer) there appears to be an orderly progression from benign tissue to premalignant lesion to frank malignancy. In other tumors, premalignant lesions are rarely identified, although it is likely the tumor passed through less malignant stages before detection. The pathologic and clinical criteria for degree of progression are often specific to a given type of tumor but, in general, tumors that are confined to a local site are at the benign end of the spectrum, progressing to locally invasive tumors. Tumors that have spread beyond the local site and have seeded metastases represent the malignant end of the spectrum. Increasing numbers and kinds of genetic abnormalities, often specific for the tumor type, accompany tumor progression (Chaps. 4 and 7).

About fifty years ago, Foulds defined tumor progression as "the acquisition of permanent, irreversible qualitative changes in one or more characteristics of a neoplasm" that cause the tumor to become more autonomous and malignant (for reviews, see Heppner and Miller, 1998; Klein, 1998). In 1986, Nowell proposed that such changes arise because cancer cells tend to be genetically unstable and described a conceptual model

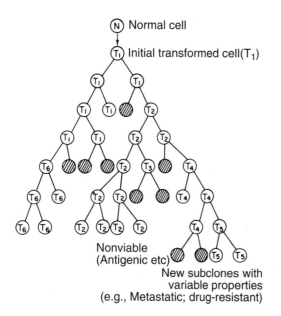

**Figure 11.1.** Schematic illustration showing the clonal evolution of tumors. New subclones arise by mutation. Many of these may become extinct (indicated by shading) but others may have a growth advantage and become dominant. All of the subclones (indicated by $T_2$ to $T_6$) may share common clonal markers, but many of them have new properties leading to heterogeneity.

to explain the process of tumor progression (Fig. 11.1). The key features of this model are the generation of variant (mutant) cells within a tumor and the selection and outgrowth of the more autonomous cells to become dominant subclones in the population, leading to progression of the tumor to increasing malignancy. More recent studies have confirmed the genetic instability of malignant cells (see Chap. 5, Sec. 5.2). It has been demonstrated that the growth and development of various cells within a tumor are subject to constraints associated with interactions among the cells and with the extracellular environment (reviewed by Heppner and Miller, 1998). Thus, the normal homeostatic mechanisms that control cell proliferation (see Chap. 9) in the body are not completely lost in a tumor, but rather the cells may become increasingly less responsive to them. These findings are consistent with the original concepts of Foulds that there are many different paths to malignancy. Tumors are thus evolving cell populations with properties that continue to change as they grow.

### 11.1.2 Molecular Genetics of Tumor Progression

Genetic instability of tumor cells may arise as a result of genetic and/or epigenetic changes (Balmain et al., 2003). Epigenetic changes such as methylation of cytosine bases in DNA or modifications to chromatin structure (by acetylation or phosphorylation) can modify the

expression of genes and are important mechanisms for silencing genes during normal differentiation (Verma and Srivastava, 2002). Genetic changes may occur by point mutation, deletion, gene amplification, chromosomal translocation, or other mechanisms (see Chap. 4, Sec. 4.2 and Chap. 5, Sec. 5.1). A cell is continually exposed to both external and internal stresses, such as reactive oxygen species, that may cause DNA damage, and there are inherent errors made by DNA polymerases whenever DNA is being replicated. Normally such damage is either repaired by the various DNA repair mechanisms in the cell (see Chap. 5, Sec. 5.4) or damaged cells undergo apoptosis (Chap. 10). However, these mechanisms are not perfect, leading to a natural frequency of mutation in cells.

Many cancer cells appear to have an increased frequency of mutation due both to deficiencies in their ability to repair lesions in DNA and/or decreased activation of apoptosis, so that mutated cells may survive and proliferate. For example, the breast-cancer–related genes *BRCA1/2* are linked with repair of DNA strand breaks (see Chap. 5, Sec. 5.4.5). As a result, cells in breast cancers with these mutations have a deficiency in repair of DNA damage. Oxidative lesions and deficiencies of mismatch repair have also been demonstrated in tumor cells, particularly those from patients with non-polyposis colon cancer (see Chap. 2, Sec. 2.3.3 and Chap. 5, Sec. 5.4.2). A deficiency in mismatch repair [also referred to as *replication error repair* (RER)] can result in up to a 1000-fold increase in the mutation frequency. Failures in DNA repair are likely to allow mutation or alteration in the expression of the many oncogenes and tumor suppressor genes that have been associated with different human cancers (see Chap. 7).

The finding that the *p53* gene is mutated or inactivated in a high percentage of human cancers is consistent with its role in controlling the response of cells to DNA damage (see Chap. 5, Sec. 5.6 and Chap. 7, Sec. 7.4.2). Normal p53 participates in cellular signaling that leads to cessation of proliferation of cells that have sustained damage to their DNA, or to cell death by apoptosis (Chap. 5, Sec. 5.5 and Chap. 10, Sec. 10.2.4). In human cancers, mutations have been observed primarily in the DNA binding region of the p53 protein (80 to 90 percent within exons 5 to 8); such binding is required for its function as a transcription factor (see Chap. 4, Sec. 4.5.4). Up to seven mutation hotspots have been identified. These hotspots probably occur in cancer cells because of the importance of these regions to the function of the protein (see Chap. 7, Sec. 7.4.2). These regions may also be more difficult to repair or they may be particularly vulnerable to a specific carcinogenic insult, as in skin cancers induced by ultraviolet (UV) radiation (see Chap. 3, Sec. 3.5.5). There is recent evidence that the hypoxic microenvironment that occurs in many solid tumors (see Chap. 15, Sec. 15.4 and Chap. 18, Sec. 18.3.2) may allow the selective survival of cells with p53 mutations, thus contributing to progressive changes in the malignant phenotype (Graeber et al., 1996).

That multiple changes must occur in cells during tumor development and progression is well illustrated by the model established by Vogelstein and colleagues to describe the changes that occur in the progression of colon cancer (see Chap. 2, Sec. 2.3.3 and Fig. 2.10, and Chap. 19, Sec. 19.3 and Fig. 19.9; Kinzler and Vogelstein, 1996). This model provides a paradigm for multistep carcinogenesis that is being applied to many other cancers (e.g., breast, pancreatic, bladder, and lung; Lakhani, 2001; Mao, 2001; Al-Sukhun and Hussain, 2003; Schneider and Schmid, 2003). A molecular description of tumor progression envisages that cancers will progress as a result of a series of genetic changes that have features that are similar between cancers, but also because of specific changes that may be unique to specific types of cancer. The advent of microarray technology (see Chap. 4, Sec. 4.4.4) is enabling rapid genetic analysis of genes turned on or off during disease progression. Such studies have detected large numbers of changes. For example, a recent analysis identified changes in expression of over 110 genes associated with progression in colon cancers (Agrawal et al., 2002). An integrin binding protein, osteopontin, was the gene that was most consistently associated with progression. Overexpression of osteopontin has also been associated with progression and metastases in breast, lung, and prostate cancer (Tuck and Chambers, 2001).

As a result of genetic and epigenetic changes, cells within animal and human tumors demonstrate considerable heterogeneity in their properties. This heterogeneity extends to almost any property that can be assessed and includes morphology, karyotype, surface markers, biochemical pathways, cell proliferation, metastatic ability, and sensitivity to therapeutic agents. The generation of cells within a cancer that have the ability to disseminate and form metastases represents its most malignant characteristic. Tumors that have metastasized are generally more difficult to treat successfully than those that have not spread, making it important to clarify how cancer cells metastasize and to determine the underlying genetic and molecular causes of metastasis. As described in the following sections, metastases probably arise from a small subset of cells within a primary tumor, so that histologic or biochemical characterization of the whole tumor may not give a reliable estimate of the propensity to metastasize. This property of tumors has made it difficult to determine the cellular and molecular properties necessary for metastatic spread because the bulk of the tumor population may not reflect the properties of the individual cells responsible for the metastases.

## 11.2 METASTASIS

### 11.2.1 The Spread of Cancer

Cancer cells can spread along tissue planes and into various tissue spaces and cavities, but the two major routes of metastatic spread are via lymphatic vessels and/or blood vessels. Indeed, for the purpose of clinical staging, metastases are subdivided into two groups: those in regional lymph nodes, which are usually regarded as having disseminated via the lymphatic circulation, and those that arise at more distant sites and organs, which have usually spread via the blood vascular system (Fig. 11.2). Different types of tumors have different patterns of spread. Tumors of the head and neck and uterine cervix, for example, usually spread initially to regional lymph nodes and, only when more advanced, to distant sites; thus, localized therapy that includes treatment of regional nodes can be curative. In contrast, tumors of the breast can spread early to distant sites, as well as to local lymph nodes. Involvement of axillary lymph nodes at the time of primary treatment for breast cancer is correlated with the presence of distant metastases, but about 25 percent of patients with no evidence of lymph node disease at the time of primary treatment are later found to have distant metastases. Most tumors appear to have few functional lymphatics (Jain et al., 2002), although there is evidence for their presence and possibly, growth into the periphery of tumors (Cassella and Skobe, 2002). Thus, the routes of spread may reflect invasion into lymphatics at the periphery of the tumor or into blood vessels within the tumor. Histologic detection of a high density of new blood vessels (angiogen-

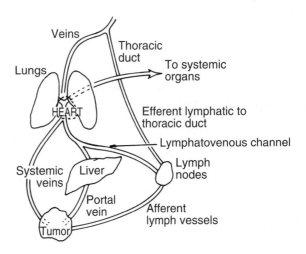

**Figure 11.2.** The major routes by which cancer cells can spread from a primary tumor are through the lymphatic or blood vessels. These two systems are interconnected as illustrated. The vascular drainage for tumors of the gastrointestinal tract is usually via the portal circulation, whereas for tumors at other sites in the body, drainage is via the systemic veins. (Adapted from Sugarbaker, 1981.)

**Table 11.1.** Clinical Metastasis to Specific Target Organs

| Primary Tumor | Common Distant Secondary Sites |
|---|---|
| Clear-cell carcinoma of the kidney | Lung, bone, adrenal |
| Gastrointestinal carcinomas | Liver |
| Prostatic carcinoma | Bone |
| Small-cell carcinoma of the lung | Brain, liver, bone marrow |
| Melanoma in the skin | Liver, brain, bowel |
| Melanoma in the eye | Liver |
| Neuroblastoma | Liver, adrenal |
| Carcinoma of breast | Bone, brain, adrenal, lung, liver |
| Follicular carcinoma of thyroid | Bone, lung |

esis, see Chap. 12, Sec. 12.3) in breast and other tumors has been reported to be associated with poor prognosis and increased likelihood that the patient will develop metastases, but this is not a universal finding (Hasan et al., 2002). These vessels provide nutrients for further growth of the tumor and may provide access to the circulation, thereby facilitating metastasis. Recent studies have also suggested that the tumor microenvironment, in particular hypoxia (see Chap. 15, Sec. 15.4 and Chap. 12, Sec. 12.3.3), may induce angiogenesis and other changes in gene expression that can enhance a more aggressive tumor-cell phenotype and increase the likelihood of metastases (Rofstad, 2000; Subarsky and Hill, 2003).

## 11.2.2 Organ Preference

Clinical observations have indicated that metastases from certain types of tumors tend to occur in specific target organs (see Table 11.1). While lungs, liver, lymph nodes, bone, and brain are the most common sites of spread, observation of the spread of breast cancer to specific sites led Paget (1989) to propose the soil-and-seed hypothesis. This hypothesis postulated that differential tumor-cell/host-organ interactions occur that are more or less favorable for metastatic development. The alternate, although not mutually exclusive, model is that organ preference can be explained largely on the basis of hemodynamic considerations: that is, the number of metastases that develop in an organ is related to the number of tumor cells delivered to that organ by the blood and the number that are arrested in the capillaries. The specificity of metastasis formation likely relates to both aspects because circulating cancer cells need first to arrest in the small vessels of an organ (and perhaps extravasate) but will grow only if the organ pro-

vides a suitable growth environment for the particular tumor cells.

Organ specificity of metastatic development is observed in rodent tumor models. Tumor cell populations that form a large number of metastatic deposits in one organ (e.g., the lung following intravenous injection of the cells) are not necessarily capable of doing so in another (e.g., the liver following intraportal injection). Furthermore, populations of tumor cells that have enhanced ability to form metastases in specific organs can be isolated by serially selecting cells from metastases in these organs. Cells forming metastases preferentially in the lung will home to a lung lobe even when it is transplanted ectopically into a subcutaneous site; such cells do not form metastases in other organs that are transplanted ectopically. The classic example of serial selection is the isolation of the B16F10 cell population from B16 mouse melanoma cells by Fidler (1973). The procedure (Fig. 11.3) involved serial passage of the cells through animals, with selection at each stage for cells that had formed lung metastases. The cells forming lung metastases were grown in culture to expand their number before being reinjected into animals. After ten such passages, a population of cells was obtained (termed B16F10 cells) that was about ten times as efficient at forming *experimental* lung metastases after intravenous injection as the starting B16F1 cell population. Interestingly, these cells were not more capable of forming *spontaneous* metastasis when implanted at a lo-

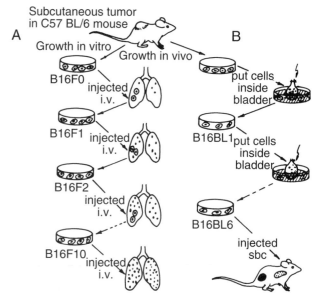

**Figure 11.3.** Procedures used for selecting highly metastatic cell populations from B16 melanoma cells. The B16F10 cells were selected by passing the cells ten times through the lungs of mice, while the B16BL6 cells were selected by requiring them to invade six times through the walls of mouse bladders. sbc = subcutaneous.

cal site, suggesting that selecting for increased ability to grow in lung does not affect the invasive properties necessary for initial escape from the primary tumor. Selection for B16 melanoma cells with increased spontaneous metastatic ability (B16BL6) was achieved by selecting for cells which could invade through the wall of the mouse bladder (see Fig. 11.3). Other investigators have also been successful, using similar approaches, in selecting cell populations from a number of rodent tumors that have enhanced experimental metastatic ability in a variety of organs including lung, liver, ovary, and brain. However, such selection procedures do not always yield cells with increased metastatic ability (Ling et al., 1985; Stackpole et al., 1991), leading to the suggestion that some properties that contribute to metastatic ability may not be stably maintained within the tumor cell population during the selection procedures and may function only transiently to promote metastasis.

The organ-specificity of metastatic human tumor cells has been tested in immune-deficient hosts [e.g., athymic *nude* mice or SCID (severe combined immune deficient) mice]. These studies have demonstrated that the local site of growth of an implanted tumor may influence its capacity to seed spontaneous metastases and that tumors transplanted into orthotopic sites (tissue of the same pathologic type as the tumor) are more likely to seed metastases (locally to lymph nodes or distantly to other organs) than tumors grown in ectopic sites (Radinsky, 1995; Fujihara et al., 1998). A refinement to these models is the transplantation of human tissue (e.g., fetal bone) into SCID mice to generate (so-called) SCID-hu models. When human tumor cells are implanted locally or injected intravascularly into such mice, they show similar organ preference for metastasis to that seen in clinical practice and the metastases occur preferentially in the human tissue rather than the same murine tissue (Shtivelman and Namikawa, 1995; Nemeth et al., 1999).

Chemokines (molecules used by leukocytes to home to specific organs) may play an important role in organ specificity of metastasis. Muller and colleagues (2001) reported that human breast cancer cells have high expression of the chemokine receptors CXCR4 and CCR7, while their respective ligands (CXCL12 and CCL21) were highly expressed in organs in which breast cancer cells have a high propensity to form metastases (lung, liver, regional lymph nodes, and bone marrow). Neutralization of the CXCL12/CXCR4 interaction significantly impaired formation of metastasis by a human breast cancer cell line in lung and lymph nodes in an experimental system.

The homing of metastatic cells to specific organs may also involve some of the specific molecular signatures that have been identified on the vasculature using the technique of phage display. Phage display libraries are mixtures of phage containing DNA sequences that code for the expression of random peptides on their surface. These libraries can be used to screen for binding of these peptides to a particular cellular receptor or other protein in vitro or they can be injected into animals to screen for peptides that bind to proteins expressed by a particular organ or tumor. The phage that express peptide(s) that bind to the organ of interest can then be isolated, amplified in vitro and reinjected into animals to enrich and refine the selection of the specific peptide(s) involved. The encoded peptide can be identified from the DNA sequence in the isolated phage. A wide heterogeneity of specific molecular differences has been demonstrated on vasculature and lymphatics in tumors and normal tissues using this technique (Ruoslahti, 2002, 2004). The identified peptides can be used for tissue-specific targeting in vivo and such peptides have been reported to be able to block tumor growth and metastasis (Lei et al. 2002).

## 11.3 STEPS IN THE METASTATIC PROCESS

### 11.3.1 Detachment from the Primary Tumor

The sequential steps in metastasis formation are shown in Figure 11.4. Some of the types of molecules involved in these various steps are also indicated to illustrate the multiple roles that similar molecules may play in this process. Detachment or shedding of cells into blood or lymphatic vessels may occur as a result of prior invasion of the tumor mass into vessels or because the abnormal vasculature of some tumors may permit passage of cells into the circulation. Recent studies with human melanoma cells have demonstrated that the tumor cells can sometimes form vascular channels (i.e., mimic endothelial cells) and in this way may gain ready access to the vascular space (Hendrix et al., 2002). Detachment of cancer cells from the primary tumor mass may involve decreased expression of adhesion molecules (e.g., cadherins) involved in the homotypic adhesion of cells to one another as well as increased protease expression (Secs. 11.5 and 11.6). Kim and colleagues (1998) used a developing chicken embryo to demonstrate that tumor cells injected into one part of the embryo require metalloproteinases to invade through the tissue, enter the bloodstream, and metastasize to other locations. Detachment of cells may also depend on the expression of motility factors (e.g., Hepatocyte Growth Factor/ Scatter Factor, autotoxin, or autocrine motility factor), which are glycoproteins that have been found to promote cell movement through interactions with cell surface molecules linked to the Rho/Rac/Cdc42 GTPase intracellular signaling system (Trusolino and Comoglio, 2002; Chap. 8, Sec. 8.3.4). These molecules may also play a role in extravasation (see Sec. 11.3.4).

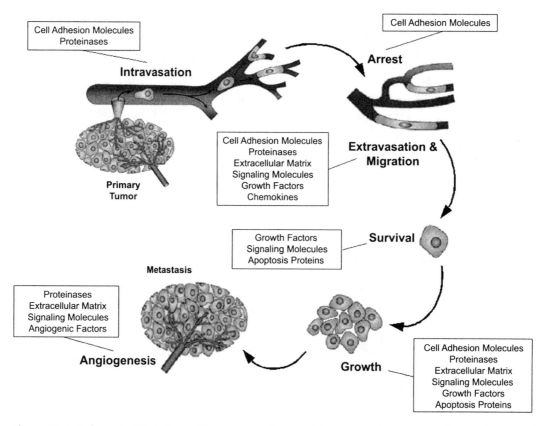

**Figure 11.4.** Schematic illustration of the sequential steps of the metastatic process and an indication of the various types of molecules thought to be involved at each stage. (Figure courtesy of R. Cairns modified from Chambers et al 2002.)

## 11.3.2 Tumor Cell Arrest

Experimental studies in which radiolabeled tumor cells were injected into the systemic or portal veins indicated that the majority of cells are arrested initially in the lung or liver capillaries, respectively. This finding has been confirmed by studies using intravital videomicroscopy (IVVM), a technique that permits dynamic study of events in the metastatic process (Fig. 11.5; Chambers et al., 2002; MacDonald et al., 2002). In this procedure, an anesthetized mouse is placed on the stage of an inverted microscope, with an organ for study (e.g., liver, muscle) surgically exposed so that the organ is viewed from below. Oblique fiberoptic illumination, provides sufficient contrast to permit clear views of the microcirculation of the organ. Steps in the metastatic process can be observed and quantified at various times during and following injection of cancer cells (fluorescently labeled to permit unambiguous identification) into the feeding blood vessels. Cells from most solid tumors are large relative to capillaries and thus tend to lodge in the first capillary bed encountered. This physical arrest is accompanied by deformation of the tumor cell in pro-

portion to the blood pressure in the particular organ (little cellular deformation occurs in low-pressure organs such as liver, and larger deformation in high-pressure organs, such as muscle; Fig. 11.6).

Experiments with radiolabeled cells suggested that most cells are lost from this initial site of arrest over the first few hours due to rapid cell death, based on the observation of the rapid loss of radioactivity from the site of arrest. This conclusion was not supported by IVVM, at least for metastasis to mouse liver, lung, and chick embryo chorioallantoic membrane. In these organs the vast majority of injected cells remained intact and succeeded in extravasating over the first 24 h or so after injection. The reason(s) for these apparently contradictory results remains unclear but may relate to the toxicity of the radiolabel. Recent work using genes encoding markers such as green fluorescent protein (GFP) or luciferase, transfected into the tumor cells, has demonstrated that these markers can be used for direct visualization of the growth of the tumor and its metastases in situ (Adams et al., 2002; Hoffman, 2002), and may provide an alternative way to study the fate of arrested cells.

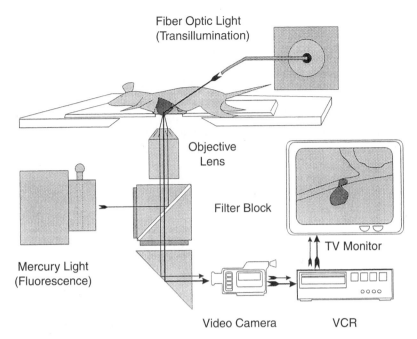

Fiber Optic Light
(Transillumination)

Objective
Lens

Filter Block

Mercury Light
(Fluorescence)

TV Monitor

Video Camera

VCR

**Figure 11.5.** Schematic diagram of intravital videomicroscopy procedure for studying steps of metastasis in vivo. Fluorescently labeled tumor cells are injected into the circulation of an experimental animal (chick embryo, mouse). At various times after injection, organs are exposed and placed intact on a coverslip over the objective lens of an inverted microscope. Lighting is provided by oblique transillumination using a fiber optic source, and/or episcopic fluorescent illumination. Images are viewed using a videocamera and monitor, and are recorded for subsequent analysis. The technique can be used for observing the fate of the injected tumor cells in chick chorioallantoic membrane, mouse liver (insert), or other organs. (Modified from Chambers et al., 1995.)

### 11.3.3 Surviving Host Defense Mechanisms

Immunologic mechanisms (see Chap. 20, Secs. 20.4 and 20.5) are involved in defense against development of metastases from experimental tumors and possibly also from human tumors. Tumors induced in animals by chemical carcinogens or viruses or resulting from exposure to UV light can be highly immunogenic and, although they grow locally, they rarely metastasize. Cytotoxicity mediated by T lymphocytes inhibits metastases by such tumor cells and immunosuppressive procedures can increase the metastatic ability of the tumor cells.

Many tumors have been reported to express tumor-associated antigens (TAAs) but the immune system develops tolerance or a state of anergy in relation to these TAAs (see Chap. 20, Sec. 20.5.3), so that the tumor cells are not killed by immune effector cells. There is evidence that some human tumors may elicit weaker immunologic responses mediated by various cytokines and by nonspecific effector cells such as natural killer (NK) cells (Chap. 20, Sec. 20.4.1). These processes might inhibit metastasis formation. Using transplanted rodent tumor cells, Hanna (1984) showed that there is an inverse correlation between the activity of NK cells in the

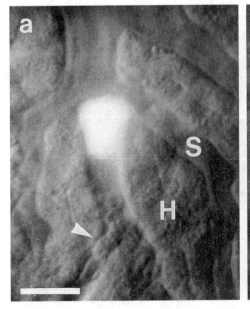

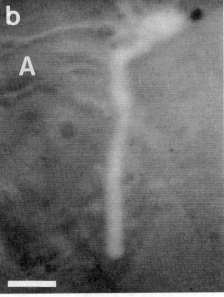

**Figure 11.6.** Initial arrest of fluorescently labeled cancer cells in mouse liver (*a*) and cremaster muscle (*b*). In liver, cells are arrested by size restriction on entering a liver sinusoid (S) from the terminal portal venule, and are only slightly deformed by the portal pressure; H, hepatocyte. In muscle, cells are also arrested by size restriction in vessels, but are deformed considerably by the higher blood pressure in this organ; A, arteriole. Bar, 20 $\mu$m. (Modified from Morris et al., 1993; Photo courtesy of E.E. Schmidt.)

host animal and the metastatic ability of injected tumor cells. Studies by Greenberg and colleagues (1987) demonstrated that NK cells acted in the first few days after intravenous injection of H-*ras*–transformed fibroblasts into mice by regulating seeding and early growth of metastases. Experiments with human tumor cells growing in immunocompromised mice have also indicated that NK cells can play a role in the reduction of metastases, and studies in patients have been supportive of such an effect (Brittenden et al., 1996). Approaches to inducing a more aggressive immune response to tumor cells are discussed in Chapter 20 (Sec. 20.5) and Chapter 21 (Secs. 21.3 and 21.4).

One mechanism of host defense is to induce apoptosis in tumor (foreign) cells in the circulation. Owen-Schaub and coworkers (1998) have demonstrated that expression of the apoptosis-inducing Fas receptor (see Chap. 10, Sec. 10.2.6) on the surface of a murine melanoma cell line may inhibit metastasis formation. The number of experimental metastases which formed in normal C3H mice, following intravenous injection of cells from two different sublines, was lower for cells of the subline expressing a high level of Fas on their surface, believe to be because of the expression of Fas ligand in the lungs of the mice. This difference was abolished, with all the mice showing similar levels of metastases, when the cells from the two sublines were injected into C3H mice that were knocked out for the gene for Fas ligand and hence were not expressing it in their lungs. It has been suggested that many tumor cells die in the vasculature by apoptosis prior to extravasation (Wong et al., 2001), possibly triggered by endothelial nitric oxide production (Carretero et al., 2001). Successful metastasis, therefore, may hinge on survival by overcoming apoptotic stimuli produced in the host organ as well as cytotoxicity induced by immune cells.

## 11.3.4 Extravasation of Tumor Cells

Following the arrest of cells in the microcirculation, they may extravasate. The basic concepts of tumor cell attachment to and invasion through endothelial cell monolayers (reviewed by Orr et al., 2000) and their basement-membrane–like matrix are illustrated in Figure 11.7. Tumor cells extend filopodia into the endothelial cell junctions, allowing access to the basement membrane. These projections, referred to as *invadopodia*, permit ready interaction of adhesion molecules with the endothelium and the basement membrane. Proteolytic digestion is thereby localized to the invasive front of the tumor cell and is critical for invasion. These interactions precipitate further molecular interactions between tumor cells and the endothelium and basement membrane. These complex interactions thus facilitate extravasation and invasion of the underlying extracellular matrix (Werb, 1997; Voura et al., 2001; Egeblad and Werb, 2002). As tumor cells penetrate the endothelium, the endothelial cells respond by changing shape to make room for the migrating tumor cell, but maintain adhesive contacts with the tumor cell during the process. The endothelium then closes in over the fully migrated tumor cells and re-establishes a continuous monolayer. Subsequent adhesion to, and migration through, the underlying basement membrane involves tumor cell interaction with matrix components such as laminin, fibronectin, vitronectin, type IV collagen, and proteoglycans. Binding to these molecules is mediated by cell-surface adhesion molecules such as integrins (Sec. 11.5.1) and invasion is further mediated by proteolysis of the matrix proteins (see Sec. 11.6).

Several groups have reported in vivo studies of extravasation using IVVM. Chambers and colleagues observed that the majority of arrested cells seem to be able

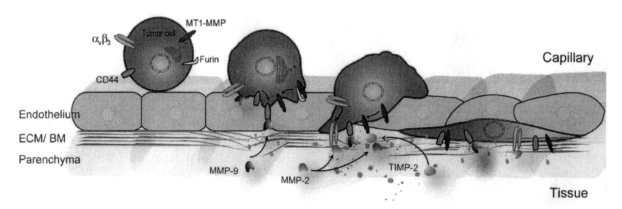

**Figure 11.7.** A model for the process of the transendothelial migration by a tumor cell into the tissue parenchyma. Migration is associated with active but focal matrix cleavage that results from redistribution and colocalization of cell adhesion molecules and metalloproteinases on the tumor cell surface and at the tumor cell-matrix interface.

to extravasate, even cells with reduced proteolytic capability or nonmalignant fibroblasts, suggesting that this process is not a major barrier to the metastatic process. Following extravasation, a fraction of the cells preferentially migrated through the tissue and adhered to the outer surface of arterioles, where they began to proliferate (see MacDonald et al., 2002). Other IVVM studies, however, found that extravasation was a formidable barrier to metastasis, and tumor cells were observed to proliferate intravascularly (Al-Mehdi et al., 2000; Ito et al., 2001). Yet others observed that tumor cell extravasation was dependent on cell adhesion molecules and could occur in precapillary vessels upon stimulation of the endothelial cells by inflammatory growth factors (Orr et al., 2000). The process of extravasation is probably influenced both by the type of tumor cell and the molecules expressed by the endothelium in the organ of metastasis. Extravasation is an active process requiring the participation of proteolysis and cell adhesion and involves both the endothelium and the tumor cells themselves.

### 11.3.5 Establishment of New Growth

The regulation of growth of tumor cells after extravasation is complex. The appropriateness of the microenvironment in a *specific* organ for a *particular* tumor cell is an important factor determining whether tumor growth will occur. Cells are known to require specific growth factors for proliferation (see Chap. 8, Sec. 8.2), but cellular interactions with the extracellular matrix (ECM) are also important. A number of soluble organ-derived factors have been identified that show some specificity for the stimulation of in vitro proliferation of tumor cells which preferentially metastasize to that particular organ. For example, melanoma cells that metastasize to brain may respond to neurotrophins produced by normal brain cells (Nicolson and Menter, 1995). In vivo, transgenic mice overexpressing tissue inhibitor of metalloproteinase 1 (TIMP-1), developed fewer metastases in brain following intravenous injection of fibrosarcoma cells than were observed in wild-type mice, but in the same mice the liver showed no change in the extent of metastases following injection of T-cell lymphoma cells. However, the livers in transgenic mice expressing reduced levels of TIMP-1 showed far greater metastases than livers in wild-type mice. Thus, the modulation of TIMP-1 levels altered the ability of the metastatic tumor cells to grow in different organs (Kruger et al., 1997; Kruger et al., 1998). Recent studies have also implicated specific molecular interactions in the ability of tumor cells to form bone metastases (Orr et al., 2000).

Tumor cells are less dependent on exogenous growth factors than normal cells, and there is evidence that the more autonomous the cells, the more capable they are of forming tumors in animals. For many tumor cells, lack of dependence on an exogenously produced growth factor is a result of autocrine production of such factors and/or modification of response to such factors. For example, during progression of melanoma, a switch from a requirement for exogenously supplied growth factors to independence from this requirement has been reported. Similarly, there is evidence that as tumor cells progress to greater malignancy, they may switch from being growth inhibited to being growth-stimulated by transforming growth factor $\beta$ (TGF-$\beta$; Wright et al., 1993; Lu and Kerbel, 1994). Recent work has also demonstrated that proteases can act to release growth factors from binding proteins in the blood (e.g., insulin-like growth factor-IGF) or in the extracellular matrix [e.g., fibroblast growth factor (FGF) or vascular endothelial growth factor (VEGF)], thus providing another mechanism by which increased protease activity may enhance metastatic ability of tumor cells (Egeblad and Werb, 2002).

Growth of a metastasis requires that the tumor cells induce angiogenesis (growth of new blood vessels). Several growth factors, particularly basic FGF and VEGF, are angiogenic and stimulate endothelial cell growth and morphologic differentiation (see Chap. 12, Sec. 12.2). Without such angiogenesis, a tumor would be unable to grow larger than about a millimeter in diameter because of limited diffusion of essential nutrients to the tumor cells. Factors that can suppress the formation of metastases by preventing their angiogenesis may be generated by the primary tumor leading to dormancy of metastases (Holmgren et al., 1995; Chap. 12, Sec. 12.4.1). Studies with IVVM have indicated that many tumor cells may not initiate growth at the new site, even though they have extravasated, or that they may only form micrometastases that do not continue to grow. These cells may die later or may remain in the tissue for long periods. Mechanisms which may trigger such dormant cells to start growth at later times are poorly understood.

### 11.3.6 Metastatic Inefficiency

The establishment of metastases by tumor cells appears to be a very inefficient process. Blood samples taken from cancer patients during or just after surgery often contain large numbers of tumor cells, yet the patients do not always develop metastatic disease. Glaves and colleagues (1988) took samples of blood from the renal vein in eleven patients just prior to surgery for renal cell carcinoma and estimated that tumor cells were being released at rates of $10^7$ to $10^9$ cells per day. Two of the patients had no evidence of metastatic disease 30 and 55 months after the surgery. Similarly, patients with peritoneovenous shunts for malignant ascites have shown no evidence that release of large numbers of tumor cells into the blood increases the number of metastases. Studies in animals have shown that many viable tumor cells are released into the circulation but that few circulating cells are able to form metastases. In experimental metastasis (or colonization) assays, tumor cells are injected directly into the arterial or venous blood circulation and allowed to disseminate and arrest at various sites. The choice of injection route will determine the organ in which the cells are most likely to be arrested (usually the first-pass organ). This assay allows direct quantitation of the number of tumor nodules formed in relation to the number of cells injected (seeded) into the first-pass organ. It is rare that more than 1 percent of injected cells form tumor nodules. More commonly, the efficiency is two or more orders of magnitude lower.

The inefficiency of the metastatic process leads naturally to the question of whether metastasis is a random or a specific process. A small subpopulation of the cells in a tumor might express properties that give the cells a higher probability of being able to form metastases, or all tumor cells might have an equal probability of forming metastases, but only a few manage to survive through the various stages of the process. There is substantial evidence that specific cellular properties are associated with the formation of metastases, including the observation of organ preference and the isolation of specific gene products associated with metastasis (see Secs. 11.2.2 and 11.7). In contrast, support for the random nature of the metastatic process derives from studies that have failed to demonstrate that cells obtained from metastases are consistently more metastatic than cells from the parent tumor (Weiss, 1990). Such a result would be expected if cells from metastases were ex-

pressing a stable phenotype that predisposed them to form metastases. A possible explanation for these observations is that critical cellular properties that lead to metastases can be expressed only transiently (i.e., be unstable) and that both random and specific elements are involved in the metastatic process.

Fidler and Kripke (1977) cloned B16 melanoma cells by plating them in vitro at limiting dilution so that any growth could be expected to originate from a single cell. A number of clones were isolated and expanded in culture and the cells were tested for their ability to form experimental metastases (see Fig. 11.8). Variability in metastatic ability for cells from a single clone was found to be much less than that observed when different clones were compared. These results indicated wide heterogeneity in metastatic ability between the different clones, and limited experiments in which subclones were isolated and retested suggested that the individual clones bred true in terms of metastatic ability. These findings were initially interpreted as indicating the presence of pre-existing metastatic variants within a cell population. However, the finding that the metastatic properties of such clonal populations tends to be quite unstable has cast doubt on this interpretation. Because tumor cell populations are genetically unstable, the cells may rapidly become heterogeneous in their phenotypic properties during the growth of the clone. Nevertheless, clonal heterogeneity of metastasis formation is still consistent with the concept that specific phenotypes are associated with metastasis formation, even though these phenotypes may be only transiently expressed (Hill et al., 1986). Such changes might occur by differing metabolic or cell cycle states, by random epigenetic events, or by other physiologic variations associated with the growth of a tumor (Weiss, 1990). As the tumor grows, new genetic or epigenetic events may

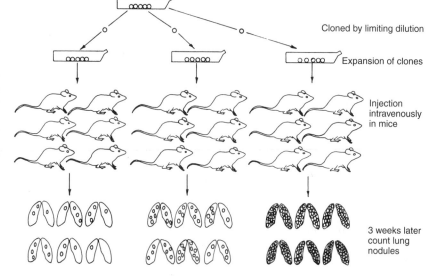

**Figure 11.8.** Clonal heterogeneity is demonstrated by establishing a series of clones from a tumor cell population and, after expansion, testing them for metastatic ability. Although there is some variability in the number of nodules observed in different animals injected with cells from the same clone, there is much greater variability between the clones.

Cloned by limiting dilution

Expansion of clones

Injection intravenously in mice

3 weeks later count lung nodules

occur leading to preferential growth of new variants giving tumor progression and increased malignancy. Thus, some of the multiple properties necessary for a cell to metastasize may be relatively stably expressed while others may be expressed only transiently. Some of the steps in the metastatic process are likely to occur fairly rapidly and hence may not require stable expression of a predisposing phenotype.

The many steps required for metastasis formation may be responsible for the inefficiency of the process. Alternatively, one specific property may represent a rate-limiting step that controls the frequency of metastasis formation. Such a rate-limiting property may vary for different tumors (or even different cells from the same tumor). Because assays for metastasis usually measure only whether metastatic tumors are present or not at the end of the assay, they cannot determine which properties may be critical during the course of the process. This concern has been addressed using IVVM as discussed above (see Secs. 11.3.2 and 11.3.4) and various in vitro assays, which clarify the nature of the molecular processes that occur during the formation of metastases.

## 11.4 THE EXTRACELLULAR MATRIX AND TUMOR MICROENVIRONMENT

Many mammalian cells are in contact with an ECM whose composition and structure is specific to the location and developmental stage. Epithelial cells, for example, have specialized lateral, apical, and basal borders. Interactions with the basement membrane are instrumental for the formation, maintenance, and polarized differentiated state of the epithelial tissue. The basement membrane, a specialized form of ECM, is composed of laminin, collagen type IV (and VII), entactin/nidogen, and heparan sulfate proteoglycan (HSPG), as well as smaller amounts of fibronectin, vitronectin, and chondroitin sulfate proteoglycans (Fig.

11.9). There are at least seven forms of laminin that are found in tissue-specific basement membranes.

In contrast to epithelial cells, mesenchymal cells are not attached to each other or to a basement membrane but are surrounded by an ECM of quite different composition. Typical components of this ECM are the interstitial collagens types I to III, elastin, proteoglycans, fibronectin, and vitronectin. Other specialized tissue-specific ECM molecules include tenascin, thrombospondin, and osteopontin. The ECM proteins interact to form a highly organized three-dimensional matrix, providing an adhesive environment for cells and other molecules such as growth factors. Cell interaction with the ECM is essential for growth and survival, and the ECM can also regulate the differentiation of a variety of cell types. Depriving cells of such interactions results in the induction of a subtype of apoptosis called anoikis (see Chap. 10, Sec. 10.4) in epithelial and endothelial cells (Boudreau et al., 1995), or in cell-cycle arrest in fibroblasts (Fang et al., 1996). Transformed cells are often defective in secreting fibronectin and laying down an organized matrix. A common property of malignant cells is their ability to survive and proliferate independently of interactions with an ECM.

The ECM provides the structural elements that together with cell-cell communication, stabilize the cellular microenvironment through interactions with various cell adhesion molecules (see Sec. 11.5). These latter molecules then interact with specific signal transduction pathways (see Chap. 8, Sec. 8.3.3). Growth factors are soluble, or embedded within the matrix, and in close proximity to their cell surface receptors, which facilitates cell signaling (Chap. 8, Secs. 8.2 and 8.3). Within this complex milieu are also the extracellular, plasma membrane-bound and ECM-bound proteinases and proteinase inhibitors (see Sec. 11.6). Normally, a balance exists in the biochemical activities of these various molecular entities, which is often disrupted within the tumor cell microenvironment. Aberrant proteolysis is an important means of upsetting this balance and can

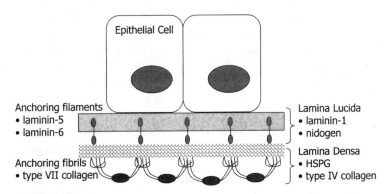

**Figure 11.9.** Schematic representation of the interaction of an epithelial cell with the specialized extracellular matrix called the *basement membrane*. The depicted proteins that constitute the lamina lucida, lamina densa, and the anchoring molecules are mostly synthesized by the endothelial cells. Basement membranes are especially rich in collagen type IV. (Modified from *Electronic Textbook of Dermatology*, Peter Marinkovich, Stanford University Medical Center, www.telemedicine.org/blister.htm dejfig.)

**Figure 11.10.** Proteolytic degradation in the tumor-stromal microenvironment. Proteinases are contributed by multiple cell types (epithelial cells, fibroblasts, and inflammatory cells). Proteolysis causes ECM cleavage to remove the physical barrier to cell migration, releases growth factors (GFs) sequestered within the matrix, and releases cryptic fragments and modifies cell adhesion molecules (CAMS) to allow cell dissociation and facilitate motility. Proteolysis also processes growth factors and cytokines at the tumor cell surface to initiate signal transduction, proliferation, and angiogenesis.

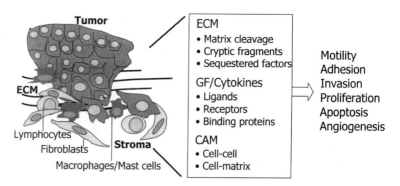

exert a ripple effect on multiple classes of molecules during tumor progression and metastasis (see Fig. 11.10). Proteolysis is influenced by and localized via cell adhesion molecules (CAMS), and it in turn acts on an array of substrates including the ECM, cell adhesion molecules, growth factors and cytokines, their receptors and binding proteins. For example, increased matrix metalloproteinase (MMP)-mediated activity influences cell adhesion by cadherins, and cadherin loss can promote a so-called epithelial-to-mesenchymal transition in phenotype leading to more aggressive cancers. Matrix metalloproteinases and their inhibitors [tissue inhibitors of metalloproteinases (TIMPs)] can alter the bioavailability of potent growth factors such as VEGF and IGF-II, with effects extending through the receptor tyrosine kinases activated by these molecules (see Chap. 8, Sec. 8.2). As well, MMPs have the ability to modulate *fas*-mediated cell death signals (see Chap. 10, Sec. 10.2.6). Upon proteolytic cleavage, fragments of ECM molecules can also act as stimulators or inhibitors of angiogenesis within the tumor (see Chap. 12, Sec. 12.4.1).

There is strong evidence that cellular interactions with the ECM, mediated by adhesion molecules capable of initiating intracellular signaling cascades, play a critical role in controlling cell behavior (see Sec. 11.5 and Chap. 8, Sec. 8.2). Similarly, proteinases can play roles in excess of those associated with invasion, causing, for example, disruption of ECM interactions with cells and releasing and/or activating growth factors bound to ECM molecules or released in latent forms (see Sec. 11.6). Thus, differences in adhesive or proteolytic activity can play a role in the facilitation of interstitial movement of cells and their success in initiation of new growths. Components of the ECM can interact with growth factors, especially basic fibroblast growth factor (bFGF) and TGF-β. Basic FGF binds to heparin and to heparan sulfate proteoglycans (HSPG) via the glycoaminoglycan moiety of HSPG, and can be released by heparitinase or plasmin. Release of bFGF by plasmin may be important because cancer cells often produce plasminogen activator that can convert plasminogen in serum to plasmin. Transforming

growth factor β binds to proteoglycans such as betaglycan and decorin, but the interactions occur via the protein cores of these proteoglycans. Fibronectin can also bind TGF-β.

During tumor invasion and metastasis, intimate interactions occur between cell-surface proteins on the tumor cells and the ECM proteins leading to expression and secretion of proteinases. These proteinases then degrade the ECM components, allowing invasion of the tumor cells through the basement membrane (Fig. 11.7). Degraded components of the ECM (e.g., fibronectin fragments) can trigger further induction of proteinase genes, resulting in a positive feedback loop that facilitates invasion and proliferation (Egeblad and Werb, 2002). Cell adhesion molecules and proteinases putatively involved in tumor progression and metastasis are discussed in more detail in Sections 11.5 and 11.6. It is increasingly recognized that the roles played by these various molecules in metastasis extends beyond those traditionally assigned (see Fig. 11.4).

## 11.5 CELL ADHESION MOLECULES

The cell-cell and cell-ECM interactions during invasion and metastasis depend upon several classes of molecules expressed on the cell surface, including integrins and cadherins, and the ligands that bind to these molecules. Cell adhesion molecules (CAMs) are transmembrane proteins with extracellular and intracellular domains, and some are anchored in the plasma membrane by an L-terminal glycophosphatidyl-inositol moiety. The generic structures of some of the major types of CAMs are shown in Figures 11.11 to 11.13 and are discussed below. Other CAMs, not discussed below, include the tetraspanins, transmembrane adaptor proteins, that are expressed on lymphocytic cells and are involved in their migration in tissue during inflammatory responses. The level of expression of members of the tetraspanin family has been reported to correlate with tumor cell invasiveness, ability to form metastases, and poor clinical outcome (Sauer et al., 2003).

While originally named and identified for cell adhesion, it is now clear that CAMs have multiple functions,

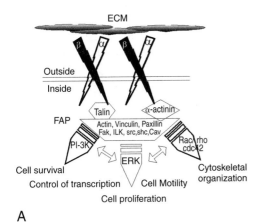

A

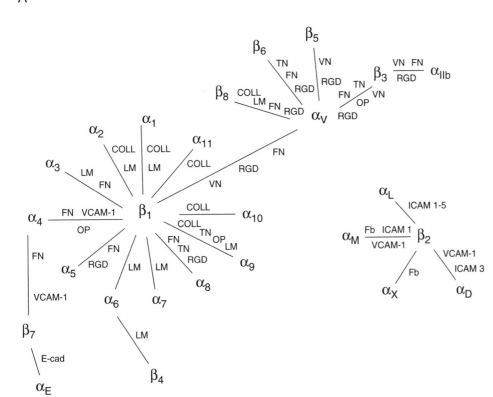

B

**Figure 11.11.** (*A*) Schematic diagram of integrin receptors with linkage to their major downstream signal transduction pathways. An integrin receptor contains two subunits ($\alpha$ and $\beta$) which cross the plasma membrane and the cytoplasmic tail of the $\beta$ subunit links to the actin cytoskeleton and components of the focal adhesion plaque (FAP) as shown. The interaction of the integrins with the components of the FAP can lead to signaling through various different intracellular signaling pathways to influence cell survival, cell growth and cell motility. Cav, caveolin; ECM, extracellular matrix; FAK, focal adhesion kinase; ILK, integrin-linked kinase; PI-3K, phosphatidylinositol-3-kinase pathway; ERK, ERK-MAP-kinase pathway. (*B*) Schematic representation of the various $\alpha\beta$ heterodimers in the integrin receptor family and some of their ECM ligands. Coll, collagen; E-cad, E-cadherin; Fb, fibrinogen; FN, fibronectin; ICAM, intracellular adhesion molecule; LM, laminin; OP, osteopontin: RGD, arginine-glycine-aspartic acid binding motif; TN, tenascin; VCAM, vascular cell adhesion molecule; VN, vitronectin. (Modified from Juliano, 2002; Hynes, 2002; van der Flier and Sonnenberg, 2001.)

including a major role in signaling from outside to inside a cell and vice versa (see Chap. 8, Sec. 8.3.3). The formation and breaking of adhesive bonds between tumor cells and their environment during steps in metastasis provides information to the cell about its environment and may lead to changes in the expression of specific genes that determine tumor cell proliferation, invasion, or other processes.

## 11.5.1 Integrins

Integrins are expressed in all cell types and are involved in the regulation of cellular functions during embryonic development, wound healing, inflammation, homeostasis, bone resorption, apoptosis, cell proliferation, tumor cell growth, and metastasis. They make up a family of widely expressed transmembrane receptors for proteins of the ECM, such as fibronectin, laminin, vitronectin, and collagens, as well as for other plasma membrane proteins. These adhesion molecules are obligate heterodimers, comprising noncovalently associated $\alpha$ and $\beta$ subunits, each of which spans the plasma membrane and typically possesses a short cytoplasmic domain (Fig. 11.11*A*). Receptor diversity and versatility in ligand binding is determined by the extracellular domains, through the specific pairing of 18 $\alpha$ and 8 $\beta$ subunits, to form a family of 24 recognized heterodimers (Fig. 11.11*B*; for review, see Hynes, 2002).

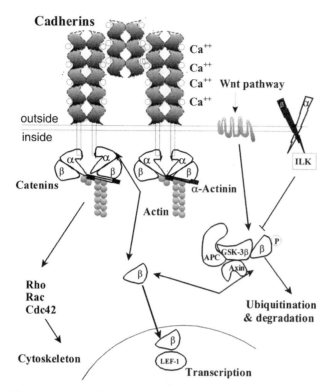

**Figure 11.12.** Schematic diagram of cadherin receptors and their linkage to the Rho/Rac/Cdc42 signaling pathway and to the Wnt signaling pathway through β-catenin. α, α-catenin; β, β-catenin; APC, adenopolyposis coli gene product; ILK, integrin-linked kinase. (Modified from Juliano, 2002.)

The cytoplasmic domain of the β subunit interacts directly with components of the actin cytoskeleton, such as α-actinin and talin, allowing its localization to focal adhesion plaques (FAPs) that form at points of contact between integrins and the ECM. Focal adhesion plaques represent the submembranous termini of actin stress fibers, indicating that integrins provide a structural bridge between the ECM and the actin cytoskeleton (Fig. 11.11A) (see also Chap. 8, Sec. 8.3.3). Integrins are also found at other contact points, where they might act to mediate cell migration. Focal adhesion plaques also contain a number of protein tyrosine kinases [such as the focal adhesion kinase p125 (FAK), integrin-linked kinase (ILK), and ser/thr kinases (such as protein kinase C)].

It is well established that integrins act as part of signal-transduction complexes that allow cells to sense (and respond to) their extracellular environment (Fig. 11.11A; for review see Juliano, 2002). Interactions occur through the focal adhesion plaques and through caveolin (Cav), a protein that is an integral part of cell surface structures called caveolae. One of the pathways involved is the Erk and c-Jun kinase (JNK) mitogen activated protein (MAP) kinase pathway (see Chap. 8, Sec. 8.2.6). Integrin activation of the Erk pathway is not sufficient in itself to push cells into cell cycle, but such activation may act to prolong and intensify signaling from growth factor receptors. There is also evidence that integrin-mediated signaling modulates the activity of the phosphatidylinositol-3 kinase (PI-3K) pathway that is

**Figure 11.13.** Schematic diagram of three further classes of the cell adhesion molecules.

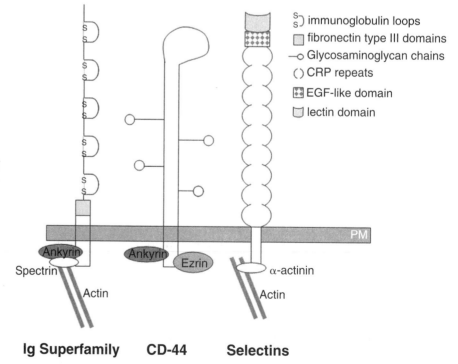

involved in cell survival and of the Rho/Rac/cdc42 small guanine nucleotide (GTP)ase signaling molecules, which are particularly important in regulation of the actin cytoskeleton (see Chap. 8, Sec. 8.3.4). The expression of integrin receptors is altered in malignant cells as compared with their normal counterparts, but the loss or gain of expression of a particular integrin has not been linked directly to malignant transformation. Rather, the changes in integrin expression seem to be specific to the tumor.

Integrins have been shown to be positive mediators of angiogenesis (see Chap. 12, Sec. 12.4.2). For example, migration of cultured endothelial cells on vitronectin and collagen was found to be mediated by $\alpha_v\beta_3$ and $\alpha_2\beta_1$ integrins, respectively. The expression of $\alpha_v\beta_3$ is increased in newly formed blood vessels, both in human wound granulation tissue and in chick chorioallantoic membranes treated with bFGF, a positive angiogenic factor. The addition of tumor fragments to chorioallantoic membranes also induced angiogenesis, which, along with tumor proliferation, was selectively inhibited by either an anti-$\alpha_v\beta_3$ monoclonal antibody or specific peptide inhibitors of $\alpha_v\beta_3$ (Brooks et al., 1996, 1998). This integrin has also recently been reported to enhance bone metastases in a human mammary Ca cell line (Pecheur et al., 2002).

## 11.5.2 Cadherins

Cadherins are intercellular adhesion receptors. Adherent junctions and desmosomes are the two major forms of intercellular junction required for maintenance of tissue architecture and for the differentiation of epithelial tissue. Distinct members of the cadherin family of cell adhesion receptors are principal constituents of each type of junction, mediating Ca-dependent adhesion between similar cells (Fig. 11.12). Many carcinomas display reduced intercellular adhesion and lose the characteristics of differentiated epithelium, suggesting a critical role for cadherins in the malignant progression of carcinoma. There are more than twenty recognized cadherins and protocadherins. E-cadherin (CDH1), the major epithelial cadherin, contains four conserved extracellular domains, a fifth extracellular domain possessing conserved cysteine residues, a transmembrane domain, and a cytoplasmic domain. Calcium binding sites lie between adjacent extracellular domains. The cytoplasmic domain associates with cellular proteins, catenins, which act to link cadherins to the actin cytoskeleton and to signal-transduction components and to form what has been called the cytoplasmic cell-adhesion complex (Cavallaro et al., 2002) (Fig. 11.12).

Evidence that cadherins are involved in the suppression of tumor invasion and metastasis derives from analyses of cadherin expression in tumors of variable differentiation status, from gene transfer experiments and from mutational analysis of cadherins in tumors. The role of the epithelial E-cadherin has been particularly well studied with respect to the influence of intercellular adhesion on tumor development. Expression of E-cadherin is low or absent in poorly differentiated, invasive tumors and various tumor-derived cell lines. Also, epithelial cells become invasive (as demonstrated in invasion assays using collagen gels and embryonic heart tissue) when intercellular adhesion is disrupted by anti–E-cadherin antibodies. Furthermore, reversion of an invasive phenotype was achieved by transfection of E-cadherin cDNA into a human breast carcinoma line and into highly invasive ras-transformed cell lines derived from canine kidney and murine mammary tumors. Reduced or absent E-cadherin expression in poorly differentiated or high-grade tumors has been reported for squamous-cell carcinoma of the head and neck, female genital tract tumors, and carcinomas of the stomach, bladder, breast (particularly lobular type), colon, and lung. Mechanisms of reduced E-cadherin levels in tumor cells have been attributed to mutations/deletions, altered transcription due to hypermethylation or chromatin rearrangements, mutations in $\beta$-catenin, aberrant phosphorylation of components of the cytoplasmic cell-adhesion complex, or to expression of the DNA binding protein Snail, which represses gene expression (Cavallaro et al., 2002).

In contrast to E-cadherin, increased levels of N-cadherin (CDH2) are correlated with cellular invasiveness (Nieman et al., 1999; Hazan et al., 2000). N-cadherin has been shown to link different N-cadherin expressing cell types (Navarro et al., 1998) and interacts with $\beta_1$-integrins through intracellular signals (Arregui et al., 2000), which further suggests an importance of this cadherin to metastatic invasion. A switch between expression of E- and/or P-cadherin (CDH3) to expression of N-cadherin in tumor cells may play an important role in tumor progression (Cavallaro et al., 2002). Expression of a dominant-negative N-cadherin mutant protein, lacking the extracellular domain, which leads to reduced E-cadherin expression in the intestinal crypts of transgenic mice, results in the development of multiple intestinal adenomas. These lesions are similar to those resulting from a germline mutation of the murine adenomatous polyposis coli (APC) homolog in the Min mouse model of multiple intestinal neoplasia (Su et al., 1992) (see also Chap. 2, Sec. 2.3.3). Both E-cadherin– and N-cadherin–mediated cell-cell interactions have been linked to elevated levels of the cyclin-dependent kinase inhibitor p27, which promotes cell cycle arrest (see Chap. 9, Sec. 9.3). Disruption of cadherin-catenin complexes leads to disruption of the cytoskeleton and this may affect signal-transduction because there is evidence that cytoskeletal proteins can act as a scaffold for the components of signal transduction pathways (Juliano, 2002). Cellular components that connect cadherin function to cytoskeletal organization and may play an important role in metastasis are the small GTPases of the Rho/Rac/Cdc42 family. These proteins are known to have a role in controlling the actin cytoskeleton and can modulate cadherin function (Price and Collard, 2001). Both RhoC and Tiam-1 have been reported to play a role in invasion and metastasis (Cavallaro and Christofori, 2001).

An important connection between cadherins, catenins, and tumor progression was made with the observation that the APC tumor suppressor protein and $\beta$-catenin form physiologic complexes (see Fig. 11.12; Juliano, 2002). E-cadherin and APC have overlapping binding sites within the internal repeat domain of $\beta$-catenin, and each of these complexes associates with $\alpha$-catenin through the N-terminal domain of $\beta$-catenin. APC protein and $\beta$-catenin form a complex with axin and GSK-3$\beta$, in which $\beta$-catenin can be phosphorylated by GSK-3$\beta$ and targeted for ubiquitin-mediated degradation (see Fig. 11.12 and Chap. 9, Sec. 9.2.1); this complex thereby acts to control the level of $\beta$-catenin in the cell. Besides binding APC and cadherins, $\beta$-catenin can also associate in the nucleus with the LEF-1/TCP transcription factors and upregulate genes involved with cell growth such as *Myc* and *cyclin D1*. Thus $\beta$-catenin can exist in three pools in the cell: bound to cadherins, in the cytoplasm bound to APC, and in the nucleus associated with the LEF-1/TCF family of transcription factors (see Fig. 11.12). Mutations in APC, which are associated with the formation of adenomas, cluster within the $\beta$-catenin binding region, yielding truncated APC peptides that are unable to bind to $\beta$-catenin. This reduces its degradation and increases its availability to diffuse to the nucleus and activate cell growth. Degradation of $\beta$-catenin is also disrupted if the activity of GSK-3$\beta$ is blocked by activation of the Wnt-signaling pathway (see Chap. 8, Sec. 8.4.1), or possibly through high activity of integrin-linked kinase (ILK).

### 11.5.3 Immunoglobulin Superfamily

Members of the immunoglobulin superfamily (Ig superfamily) are also involved in cell-cell adhesion. However, these interactions are independent of divalent cations such as Ca, in direct contrast to the adhesion mediated by cadherins. The nonlymphocyte members of this family typically express a number of immunoglobulin-related domains proximal to repeats of fibronectin type III domains (Fig. 11.13). This latter domain was first described in fibronectin, but it also occurs in cytokine receptors and in several ECM proteins. Well-characterized members of the Ig superfamily of CAMs include N-CAM, contactin, myelin-associated gly-

coprotein (MAG), DCC (deleted in colorectal carcinoma), CEA (carcinoembryonic antigen) intercellular adhesion molecules (I-CAMs), MUC-18, and vascular cell adhesion molecule (V-CAM). Some of these adhesion receptors mediate interactions between similar cells, in particular, those expressed in the nervous system, for example, N-CAM. Others are expressed on activated endothelial cells (I-CAM-1, I-CAM-2, and V-CAM) or on lymphocytes (I-CAMs). They mediate heterophilic interactions (i.e., those between different types of cell) and bind to integrin receptors on adjacent cells.

Allelic loss of *DCC*, a candidate tumor suppressor gene in a variety of carcinomas is consistent with DCC affecting late events in tumor formation and indicates that its tumor suppressor role is not restricted to colonic epithelium. Direct evidence for the role of *DCC* as a tumor suppressor gene has been obtained from transfection studies in human epithelial cells. Transformation of human papillomavirus-immortalized keratinocytes by nitrosomethylurea (NMU) results in allelic loss of *DCC*, with concomitant loss of DCC expression and the acquisition of a malignant phenotype (Klingelhutz et al., 1993). Transfection of a full-length cDNA for *DCC* into these NMU-transformed cells resulted in high levels of expression of the DCC protein and suppression of the malignant phenotype.

Another Ig protein family member, carcinoembryonic antigen (CEA) can function in epithelial cells to mediate Ca-independent, homotypic cell adhesion. CEA family members do not contain cytoplasmic or transmembrane domains but are anchored in the external plasma membrane by a C-terminal, glycophosphatidylinositol moiety. Carcinoembryonic antigen is overproduced in most colon carcinomas, as well as several other carcinomas, and 10- to 100-fold elevated serum levels of CEA indicate a poor prognosis in patients with adenocarcinomas of colon, breast, and lung. Carcinoembryonic antigen may contribute to tumor progression by prolonging cell survival in the presence of differentiation signals. Thus, CEA and DCC may play opposing roles in regulating growth and survival in epithelial cells (Juliano, 2002).

MUC-18 is overexpressed in human melanoma cell lines and it has been reported to correlate directly with more aggressive and metastatic disease. This has been related to loss of expression of the AP-2 transcription factor that controls the expression of a number of genes (including *E-cadherin*) associated with progression of human melanoma cells (Bar-Eli, 1999).

### 11.5.4 Selectins

Selectins (L, E, and P) are a small family of lectin-like adhesion receptors that play a major role in leukocyte adherence to endothelial cells and platelets during inflammatory processes. Their structure (see Fig. 11.13) consists of a lectin-like amino-terminal attached to an EGF-type domain and various numbers of consensus repeats (CRPs). They are anchored to the membrane with a single transmembrane region followed by a short cytoplasmic tail. The major structural difference between the selectins lies in the number of CRPs (Juliano, 2002; Patel et al., 2002). The expression of P- and E-selectins can be rapidly upregulated on the surface of endothelial cells and platelets (P-selectin) during an inflammatory response. Selectins can act as signaling molecules and they can trigger the activation of $\beta_2$-type integrins (Juliano, 2002). They can also play a role in the arrest of tumor cells. Intravital videomicroscopy studies in liver indicated that the site of arrest of intravenously injected (mesenteric vein) B-16 tumor cells was altered by prior treatment with the inflammatory cytokine IL-1; from the liver sinusoids, where they arrested mechanically, to the presinusoidal venules where they adhered to the vessel wall mediated by induced selectin expression on the endothelial cells. Treatment of endothelial cell layers with IL-1 in vitro caused increased adhesion of tumor cells, and activation of endothelial cells in vivo can result in increased formation of experimental metastasis (Orr et al., 2000).

Endothelial cell activation caused by the inflammatory effects of reactive oxygen intermediates, produced by chemotherapeutic drugs or radiation and possibly by the tumor cells, can also increase metastases. Some tumor cells express the selectin ligand, sialyl Lewis X, which may assist in their interaction with endothelial cells or platelets to form thrombi. Some cancer patients have increased platelet counts and thrombi formed around tumor cells in the circulation that might assist in their arrest in capillary beds and possibly protect them prior to extravasation. Treatment with anticoagulants can decrease metastasis formation in experimental metastasis assays but there is little evidence that this is important for spontaneous metastases in human cancers. Clinical trials of heparin, warfarin or other anticoagulants have been largely negative (Hejna et al., 1999; see also Chap. 17, Sec. 17.3.4).

## 11.5.5 CD44 Hyaluronate-Binding Proteins

CD44 is a cell-surface glycoprotein identified as the major receptor mediating cellular interactions with hyaluronate, a glycosaminoglycan component of the extracellular matrix. Its principal physiological functions are in the aggregation, migration, and activation of cells, and these occur through the adhesive qualities of the molecule. CD44 is widely expressed and exists in multiple forms with variable glycosylation. The N-terminal extracellular region mediates binding to hyaluronate. All CD44 isoforms contain a cytoplasmic domain, which may link CD44 to actin filaments through interactions with ankyrin, ezrin, and moesin (see Fig. 11.13). Alternative splicing of the mRNA to produce these variable isoforms is regulated in a tissue-specific manner or by antigen activation in lymphocytes. Recent evidence suggests that some metalloproteinases can form a complex with CD44 on the surface of cells and MMP-9 bound to CD44 has been reported to activate latent TGF-$\beta$, which is implicated in angiogenesis and tumor aggressiveness (Stamenkovic, 2000).

CD44 is overexpressed by many tumors, and the expression of CD44 and variants of CD44 have been correlated with clinical outcome in several human malignancies, although these findings are not consistent among various published studies (reviewed in Sneath and Mangham, 1998). The metastasis-promoting ability of one particular isoform (CD44v) was demonstrated by transfection of the cDNA for this particular isoform, which codes for a 162 amino acid insertion in the extracellular domain, into rat pancreatic carcinoma cells (Günthert et al., 1991). In contrast, primary colon carcinomas and carcinoma cell lines demonstrated very low expression of another isoform known as CD44H, whereas there is high expression found in normal colonic mucosa. Transfection of a cDNA for CD44H into the colon carcinoma cells restored CD44H expression and inhibited the tumor-forming potential of these cells. CD44 has been reported to be expressed at the invading edges of murine carcinoma cells and levels of CD44 decrease as the degree of cellular spreading increases (Ladeda et al., 1998). Furthermore, CD44 expression on melanoma cells is required for migration on type IV collagen and for invasion of the basement membrane (Knutson et al., 1996).

## 11.5.6 Gap Junctions

Gap junctions are formed when clusters of six connexin proteins assemble to form a connexon and this connexon associates with a connexon on a neighboring cell. Common connexin proteins include connexins 26, 37, 40, and 43. Recent studies have suggested a role for gap junctions, and the resulting communication, during metastasis. The transfection of connexin cDNA has been found to increase the invasive properties of cultured tumor cells (Graeber and Hulser, 1998). Melanoma cells have been shown to form connexin-43 and connexin-26-mediated gap junctions with endothelial cells in an adhesion-dependent fashion (Ito et al., 2000). Moreover, higher levels of connexin 43 were observed in melanoma cells with greater metastatic ability and this correlated with increased dye transfer from tumor cells to vascular endothelial cells in vitro (El-Sabban and Pauli, 1991).

Gap junctions may facilitate metastasis by mediating the transfer of metabolites between the interacting cells. One metabolite that might mediate these effects is 12(S)-hydroxyeicosatetraenoic acid [12(S)-HETE], a lipoxygenase metabolite of arachadonic acid, which is expressed by tumor cells and reported to correlate with the degree of experimental metastasis (reviewed by Tang and Honn, 1999). Melanoma cells were induced by 12(S)-HETE to spread on fibronectin and this involved the phosphorylation of focal adhesion kinase. In addition, tumor cell production of 12(S)-HETE was increased upon contact with the endothelium. 12(S)-HETE can also cause a rearrangement of the cytoskeleton and retraction of microvessel endothelial cells. This retraction is accompanied by a redistribution of adhesion molecules away from cell-cell contacts to the non-contact cell surfaces, resulting in increased $\alpha_v\beta_3$ surface accumulation that has been implicated in the adhesion of tumor cells to the endothelium. Using cultured human keratinocytes it was found that interaction of integrin $\alpha_3\beta_1$ with laminin 5 increased the assembly and function of connexin-43–containing gap junctions (Lampe et al., 1998), suggesting that gap junctions and the resulting intercellular communication might influence tumor cell metastasis.

## 11.6 PROTEOLYTIC ENZYMES AND THEIR INHIBITORS

A series of tissue barriers (e.g., basement membrane, interstitial connective tissue) are traversed by tumor cells during metastasis by processes involving proteolytic breakdown. Members of the four classes of naturally occurring proteinases (serine proteinases, cysteine proteinases, aspartic proteinases, and MMPs; Table 11.2) have been associated with increased aggressiveness of tumor cells, and functionally implicated during metastasis. Matrix metalloproteinases, including membrane type (MT)-MMPs, and serine proteinases are believed to be the major enzymes responsible for ECM

degradation (reviewed by Werb, 1997; Egeblad and Werb, 2002). These diverse proteinases have distinct structures, specific binding sites for substrates (Fig. 11.14A) and most have endogenous inhibitors. Therefore, any approach to controlling proteolysis as a cancer therapy must account not only for the opposing activities of proteinases and their inhibitors, but also for the concerted enzymatic action, involving diverse proteinases, that is required to degrade the matrix barriers, and allow tumor cells to invade the interstitial space as is illustrated in Figure 11.14B. Furthermore, proteinases can be contributed by multiple cell types within the tumor stromal environment (see Fig. 11.10).

### 11.6.1 Serine-, Cysteine- and Matrix Metalloproteinases and Their Inhibitors

Plasminogen activators [urokinase type (uPA) and tissue type (tPA)], which act on circulating plasminogen to release plasmin, have long been associated with malignant cells. The serine proteinase activity of plasminogen and plasmin are localized to the cell surface by the uPA receptor, which also associates with integrins and can bind to vitronectin in the ECM (reviewed by Werb, 1997). The MMPs bind two zinc ions: one is present in the active site and the other associates with the pro-peptide to stabilize the inactive state (reviewed in Egeblad and Werb, 2002). The ADAM (a disintegrin and metalloproteinase) proteinases are unique in that they possess both adhesion and proteolytic domains (reviewed by Werb, 1997). Various ADAMs have been correlated with cancer progression, and ADAMs (as well as MMPs) participate in the cleavage and activation of growth factors and cytokines at the cell membrane (see Egeblad and Werb, 2002). Proteinases, as exemplified by the MMPs and plasminogen, are often secreted in a latent form, and subsequently activated. For instance, MMPs can be autocatalyzed, activated by another MMP or by serine proteinases (Mazzieri et al., 1997), or activated by proprotein convertases. The interactions between different classes of proteinases gen-

**Table 11.2.** Proteinases in Specific Catalytic Classes

| Catalytic Type | Numbers (Human/Mouse) | Associated with Malignancy | Specific Inhibitors | Substrates |
|---|---|---|---|---|
| Cysteine | 143/153 | Cathepsins B, L, H | Kininogens, Cystatins, Stefins | ECM |
| Aspartic | 21/27 | Cathepsin D | Not known | ECM |
| Metallo | 186/197 | MMPs 2,3,7,9,11,13,14 | TIMPs | ECM, GFs/cytokines |
| Serine | 176/227 | uPA, tPA | PAIs | Plasminogen, latent MMPs |

(from Puente et al., 2003)

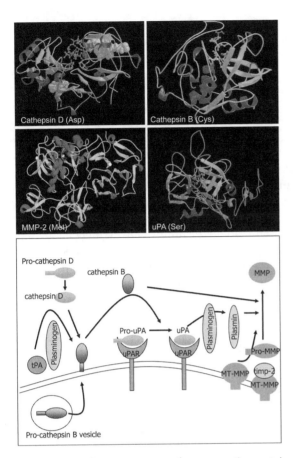

**Figure 11.14.** Tertiary structures of an aspartic proteinase (cathepsin D), cysteine proteinase (cathepsin B), matrix metalloproteinase (MMP-2, gelatinase A), and the kringle domain of a serine proteinase (urokinase plasminogen activator). Catalytic residues are shown in ball-and-stick representation for cathepsin D, cathepsin B, gelatinase A, and uPA. The distinct structures highlight the requirement for individual endogenous inhibitors, as well as the need to develop specific synthetic inhibitors as cancer therapeutics. The bottom panel illustrates a proteinase cascade linking these distinct classes of proteinases. Cathepsin B, typically a lysosomal protease, can be activated pericellularly by cathepsin D upon its own autoactivation. Cathepsin B then participates in the cell surface activation of uPA which in turn converts plasminogen into plasmin. Plasmin, cathepsin B, as well as a ternary complex of MMPs assembled at the cell surface, can activate MMP-2. [Top panel modified from the proteinase database (http://merops.sanger.co.uk) and bottom panel from Rao, 2003. (See color plate.)

erate complex proteolytic cascades as shown in Figure 11.14*B*.

Cathepsins are papain-like cysteine proteases that were presumed to be restricted to intracellular lysosomal proteolysis. However, they are found outside the cell during pathological conditions and their presence in body fluids is a poor prognostic indicator for several cancers. Slight structural differences between the eleven cathepsins are responsible for differences in substrate specificity, and for inhibition by their endogenous

inhibitors, the cystatins, kininogens, and stefins. Cathepsins B, H, and L are associated with tumor progression (see Lah et al., 1998; Turk et al., 2000). An imbalance between the cathepsins and their inhibitors occurs during tumor progression and may be responsible for direct digestion of the ECM or activation of other proteolytic enzymes such as uPA.

As for the cathepsins, inhibitors of the other proteinases are produced by both malignant and normal cells. Examples of these inhibitors are plasminogen activator inhibitors (PAI-1 and PAI-2) and tissue inhibitors of metalloproteinases (TIMPs). Under physiologic conditions a balance between activated proteinases and their inhibitors keeps proteolysis under strict control, but when malignant cells invade tissues, this balance is disrupted, allowing uncontrolled invasion. Downregulation of TIMP-1 activity in murine fibroblasts, using transfected antisense RNA (see Chap. 4, Sec. 4.3.10), was found to confer invasive capacity and ability to form metastatic tumors in nude mice (Khokha et al., 1989). Also increased levels of TIMP-1 or TIMP-2 reduce the invasive and metastatic ability of malignant cells and TIMP-1 provides increased resistance to metastatic colonization of organs (Kruger et al., 1998).

The relationship of advanced malignancy with increased proteolytic activity (such as that arising from increased MMP or decreased TIMP expression) is not always clear. For example, increased MMP activity during cancer progression can be associated with a favorable prognosis, as is the case of MMP-12 in colon cancer, and increased TIMP expression has been identified to be a poor prognostic indicator in many studies (reviewed in Egeblad and Werb, 2002). These contrasting scenarios and the recognition that proteolysis influences basic cellular processes including cell division, differentiation, dissociation, and cell death (Hojilla et al., 2003) highlight the complexity of the proteolytic balance and how changes in this balance play out in cancer progression. Cancer studies using genetic mouse models of MMPs and TIMPs have documented that proteolysis affects the early as well as the late stages of cancer progression (Egeblad and Werb, 2002).

Synthetic inhibitors of MMPs have been tested in the clinic but have not proven beneficial as cancer therapeutics for reasons that remain unclear. One difficulty is our current inability to assess their activity at the various stages of the metastatic process in vivo (Coussens et al., 2002).

### 11.6.2 Membrane Localization and Activation of Cellular Proteinases

Proteolysis must function at the tumor cell surface to facilitate degradation of the ECM during metastasis.

Extracellular proteinases, transmembrane proteinases, cell surface molecules, and intracellular factors all contribute to generating pericellular zones of proteolysis (see Fig. 11.14*B*). Mechanisms currently known to underlie the proteolytic activation at the cell membrane include the activation of plasmin by uPA and its receptor, and the activation of MMP-2 within a trimolecular complex generated by MT1-MMP, MMP-2, and TIMP-2 (Hernandez-Barrantes et al., 2000; Hofmann et al., 2000a; Overall et al., 2000). MT1-MMP, a transmembrane MMP associated with tumor progression, has been observed on the leading edge of migrating cells. For the cell surface activation of MMP-2 in the trimolecular complex, MT1-MMP must itself be activated by furin or other activators (Yana and Weiss, 2000). Mature furin can cycle between the Golgi and the cell surface and activate MT1-MMP at both locations (reviewed by Rozanov et al., 2001).

The integrin $\alpha_v\beta_3$ provides another means of localizing active MMP-2 to the cell surface (reviewed by Ivaska and Heino, 2000). Colocalization of these molecules was first observed on angiogenic blood vessels and on the tumor invasive front. In addition, the $\alpha_2\beta_1$ integrin can be involved in the cell surface localization of MMP-2. The association of pro-MMP-2 with $\alpha_2\beta_1$ integrin-bound collagen appears to provide a reserve of the enzyme for subsequent activation of the trimolecular complex described above (reviewed by Ellerbroek and Stack, 1999). CD44, the hyaluronate receptor (see Sec. 11.5.5), also provides a means of anchoring active MMP-9 to the cell surface of breast cancer and melanoma cells (Yu and Stamenkovic, 1999). CD44 levels correlate with invasiveness and it has been localized with active MMP-9 to invadopodia (Bourguignon et al., 1998; Kim et al., 1998). The association of CD44 with hyaluronic acid has also been shown to increase MMP-2 secretion (Zhang et al., 2002) and CD44 has been found to recruit MMP-7 and direct MT1-MMP localization to the cell membrane (Mori et al., 2002; Yu et al., 2002). These findings highlight the complex spatial coordination of enzymatic activity and adhesion molecules, which bring about controlled activation of MMPs and ultimately digestion of the ECM at the leading edge of invasive tumor cells.

## 11.7 METASTASIS-ASSOCIATED GENES

The evidence that metastatic properties of cells are heritable, at least in the short term, suggests that genetic changes may be involved. The question of whether metastatic phenotypes are dominant or recessive was initially studied using cell hybrids with a variety of different fusion partners. These studies suggested that some nonmetastatic cells are able to acquire metastatic properties by fusing with normal cells, possibly as a result of

modified immunogenicity, but more usually the hybrid cells were found to be depressed in their metastatic ability. A number of different groups have attempted to identify genes controlling metastatic behavior using techniques such as subtractive hybridization of cDNA libraries, differential display, and DNA microarray analysis (see Chap. 4, Secs. 4.3.3 and 4.4.4) using pairs of metastatic and nonmetastatic cell lines. A small number of genes has been identified (see Table 11.3). An extension of the cell hybrid technique involving the transfer of individual chromosomes by a process known as microcell-mediated chromosomal transfer (MMCT), has also identified a number of genes that suppress the metastatic ability of tumor cells. Using this technique, metastasis-suppressor activity has been identified on chromosomes 1, 6, 7, 8, 11, 12, 16, and 17, but only a few of the genes involved (see Table 11.3) have yet been identified (Yoshida et al., 2000; Debies and Welch, 2001).

The first group of genes in Table 11.3 consists of metastasis-suppressor genes. Strictly defined, these are genes whose products reduce the metastatic behavior of tumor cells without affecting their tumorigenic capacity. However, only a few of the genes in the list have been investigated in enough detail to be certain that they conform to the second part of this definition. The *nm-23* (*NME-1*) gene was the first metastasis-suppressor gene isolated and it has a number of isoforms. Inverse correlations between expression levels and metastatic potential have been observed in breast cancer and melanoma but increased expression has been correlated with metastasis in colon cancer. NME-1 has nucleoside diphosphate kinase (NDPK) activity as well as serine autophosphorylation and histidine kinase activity. The NDPK activity has been dissociated from the antimetastatic activity but the role of the other two potential cell signaling activities remains unclear. The *KAI-1* gene is a member of the tetraspanin (TM4SP) family of adhesion molecules that play a role in lymphocyte differentiation and function. It has been reported to have a p53 binding site in its promotor and the loss of KAI-1 correlated with loss of p53. Loss of expression is implicated in metastases in cancers of the prostate, breast, and colon and in melanoma. KiSS-1 appears to be involved in cell signaling because a post-translationally modified version of this protein, called metastatin, has been reported to bind to a G-protein coupled receptor (Axor12) and preliminary evidence suggests that activation of this receptor can alter signaling through focal adhesion kinase (FAK; see Sec. 11.5.1). MKK4 is also a molecule associated with signaling through the stress-activated protein kinase pathway (SAP-K; see Chap. 8, Sec. 8.2.6), and both these molecules may act to increase the likelihood that a tumor cell will be able to initiate growth at a new (meta-

**Table 11.3.** Metastasis-associated Genes

| Gene Identified | Protein Function/Homology |
|---|---|
| Metastasis-suppressor genes | |
| nm-23 | NDP kinase, transcription factor, signal transduction |
| KAI-1 | CD-82, membrane glycoprotein |
| KiSS-1 | Signal transduction (SH3 binding domain) |
| BrMS 1 | Cell communication |
| MKK4 | Stress-induced signal transduction |
| Maspin | Serine-proteinase inhibitor, modulation of integrin expression, inhibitor of angiogenesis |
| Metastasis-enhancing genes | |
| Ras | Signaling molecule (MAP kinase pathway) |
| MEK1 | Signaling molecule (MAP kinase pathway) |
| Stromelysin-3 | Metalloproteinase (MMP-II) |
| S110A4 (mts-1) | Calcium binding protein |
| Osteopontin | Component of ECM |
| MTA-1 | Histone remodelling (?) |
| Rho/Rac GTPases | Signal transduction, cytoskeletal |
| CXCR4/CCR7 | Chemokine/chemokine receptor |

identified *osteopontin* as the gene most consistently upregulated in relation to tumor progression (Agrawal et al., 2002). This gene has also been identified as a marker for more advanced stages of breast, lung and prostate cancer and may have a number of roles including acting as an integrin binding protein in the ECM (Tuck and Chambers, 2001). High levels of osteopontin in the serum have also been reported to correlate with increased levels of hypoxia and poorer treatment outcome in head and neck tumors (Le et al., 2003).

Proteins encoded by oncogenes have often been implicated in metastasis. Early work demonstrated that some nonmetastatic tumor cell lines and some immortalized (nontumorigenic) fibroblast cell lines could be converted into metastatic tumor cell lines by transfection with activated oncogenes (see Chambers and Tuck, 1993). Most of these studies involved the H-*ras* oncogene transfected into cells such as NIH/3T3 or (see Chap. 7, Sec. 7.3.2) C₃H10T1/2 cells, both immortalized fibroblast lines. It was demonstrated that the level of expression of the p21 (Ras) protein was correlated with metastatic ability, both by testing clonal isolates with different p21 expression and by transfecting the *Ras* gene attached to an inducible promoter. The H-*Ras* gene was also implicated when transfection of DNA from human tumors into NIH/3T3 cells was found capable of inducing tumorigenicity and metastatic ability. Other oncogenes that can induce a metastatic phenotype in immortalized fibroblasts include v-*src* and v-*mos*, while mutant forms of *myc* and *p53* can cause cells that are already tumorigenic to become metastatic.

Transfection of the H-*ras* oncogene can cause pleiotropic changes in cells. Particularly important in the metastatic process may be those changes associated with increased protease secretion. Transfection of the *E1A* oncogene (see Chap. 6, Sec. 6.2.2) from adenovirus 2 into H-*ras*–transformed NIH/3T3 cells can reduce the metastatic ability of such cells and their secretion of collagenase type IV activity (MMPs 2 and 9). This effect is consistent with the transactivating activity (ability to influence the expression of other genes) of E1A. It was also found that the cells had increased levels of *nm23* mRNA. Su and colleagues (1993) reported that transfection with the *Ras* oncogene caused metastatic behavior and reduced expression of nm23 in rat embryo fibroblasts. There were also changes in other metastasis-related genes, including MMPs, TIMPs, and osteopontin. The *ras* oncogene can also upregulate the expression of VEGF in malignant cells, thus potentially facilitating angiogenesis (Rak et al., 2000; see Chap. 12, Sec. 12.3.2).

Genetically modulated (transgenic or gene-deficient) mice (see Chap. 4, Sec. 4.3.12) have become a common tool used to study the role of individual genes involved in tumor induction and progression (for review, see

static) site. Breast metastasis suppressor 1 (BrMS 1) is frequently altered in late-stage breast cancers. Low levels of expression occur in metastatic breast cancer cell lines and re-expression of the protein following transfection restores gap junctional communication. The protein is primarily found in the nucleus of cells and recent data suggest that it may be part of a histone deacetylase complex. Clinical and experimental information about the genes listed in the first part of Table 11.3, has been reviewed recently (Yoshida et al., 2000; Debies and Welch, 2002; Meehan and Welch, 2003).

The second group of genes listed in Table 11.3 has been reported to enhance metastasis. For most of these genes the linkage (if any) between enhanced metastasis and enhanced tumorigenicity is unclear. Some are likely to be involved in stimulating cell growth at the new site, while others may be involved in invasion or other stages of the metastatic process. A study that used DNA array analysis to investigate gene expression as a function of stage of progression in biopsy specimens of premalignant and early and late stages of colon cancer

Herzig and Christofori, 2002). A widely studied model has been the knockout of the *p53* gene. Such knockout mice are viable but develop a high incidence of lymphomas and sarcomas at an early age (6 to 12 months). Breast cancer models include transgenic animals carrying the *Neu* gene or the polyoma middle T antigen (*PyMT*) gene driven by the mouse mammary tumor promotor that is quite specific for the mammary gland. These mice develop mammary tumors within the first 3 months (*PyMT*) or 6 to 9 months (*Neu*) of age and develop lung metastases. Another widely studied model is the Min mouse that has an inactivated *APC* gene. This mouse develops intestinal polyps similar to the human familial adenomatous polyposis (FAP) syndrome. Crossing this mouse with one knocked out for the mismatch repair genes *MSH2* or *MLH1* was found to accelerate the development of intestinal tumors (see Chap. 2, Sec. 2.3.3). Introduction of an *E-cadherin* mutation in mice carrying an *APC* mutation also enhanced tumor initiation, but surprisingly did not affect tumor progression (Smits et al., 2000). Another example of combining genetic alterations that can affect metastasis is the cross of *PyMT* mice with mice knocked out for the gene for *Mgat5*, a glucosaminyltransferase enzyme involved in a specific type of glycosylation of cell surface proteins. The high incidence of metastatic mammary tumors in *PyMT* mice is reduced in the knockout mice (Granovsky et al., 2000), presumably because the specific glycosylations play a role in cell-cell or cell-matrix interactions.

Gene expression profiling such as microarray analysis (see Chap. 4, Sec. 4.4.4) has also been used to search for patterns of gene expression associated with tumor progression. A study of breast cancer identified a group of seventy genes expressed in the primary tumor that formed a profile that could predict the likelihood that patients would develop distant disease (van't Veer et al., 2002). In a retrospective analysis this profile was claimed to outperform predictions based on histological and clinical criteria to select early stage patients who need adjuvant chemotherapy, and thereby avoid exposing those who do not need such treatment to the toxicity involved. Such predictions remain to be tested prospectively. Another study identified an expression profile involving 128 genes that distinguished between primary tumors and metastases of a range of different types of adenocarcinomas (Ramaswamy et al., 2003). This group of genes was refined down to a group of seventeen genes that retained a broad ability to predict outcome in a range of tumor types (lung, breast, and prostate adenocarcinomas and medulloblastoma, but not lymphoma). However, there is considerable variability between the genes identified by different groups of investigators. None of seventeen genes identified by Ramaswamy and colleagues is listed in Table 11.3 and the role of the products of the seventeen genes in the metastatic process remains to be identified. These authors have suggested that their finding that gene expression patterns associated with metastasis are widely expressed in the cells of primary tumors (otherwise they would not be detected in such analyses) challenges the ideas discussed earlier in this chapter that metastases arise from rare cells within the primary tumor that have the ability to metastasize. This interpretation has been disputed on the grounds that multiple interactions are involved in the metastatic process and different stages of the process may be involved (Fidler and Kripke, 2003; Hunter and Welch, 2003). There are many large ongoing studies that seek to relate gene expression profiles, obtained by microarray analysis, with patient prognosis. Such studies illustrate both the power of these types of analyses (many genes involved in metastasis can be identified simultaneously) but also their drawback (a large amount of work remains to be done to identify the specific roles of the many genes identified before their significance can be assessed).

## 11.8 SUMMARY

The development of a cancer is a multistep process that progresses through benign and premalignant changes to a frank malignancy. It involves a number of genetic or epigenetic changes that may be very extensive in a late stage cancer. The development of metastatic potential is viewed as one of the late stages of the process of tumor progression and metastases are the major cause of death in cancer patients. Evidence for organ-site specificity in the development of metastases from particular types of primary tumors has been collected from humans and experimental animals. Despite this evidence for specificity in metastatic development, metastasis is an inefficient process and may depend on random survival factors associated with traversing the various stages of the metastatic process.

Several major steps are involved in the process of metastasis, including the ability to go into and out of blood vessels, to survive in the circulation, and to arrest and grow at a new site. Extensive studies have identified a range of properties (particularly those relating to cell adhesion, secretion of proteolytic enzymes, and initiation of a new growth) that are involved in this process. Cellular interactions with the extracellular matrix are mediated through cellular adhesion molecules, such as integrins and cadherins. The formation and breakdown of adhesive bonds between tumor cells and their environment during metastasis provides information to the cell (via signaling) about its environment. This can lead to changes in gene expression and determine cell proliferation, invasion, and other processes. Proteolytic enzymes, such as the families of serine proteinases and metalloproteinases, play important roles in the breakdown of extracellular matrix components to enhance the invasive properties of tumor cells, and release and/or activate growth factors that assist the growth of tumor cells at a new metastatic site.

The identification of specific cellular or genetic properties that characterize all metastatic cells has proven elusive. Rather it appears that many different cellular changes are capable of producing phenotypes that increase the ability of tumor cells to form metastases and that these may be specific to different cancer types. A number of metastasis-associated genes have been identified and these range from adhesion molecules to proteineases to cell signaling molecules that ultimately stimulate cell proliferation and survival. High throughput analyses using microarrays is increasing the identification of genes involved in metastasis. The mechanisms by which these molecules modify metastatic ability remains to be determined for most of these genes.

# REFERENCES

Adams JY, Johnson M, Sato M, et al: Visualization of advanced human prostate cancer lesions in living mice by a targeted gene transfer vector and optical imaging. *Nature Med* 2002; 8:891–897.

Agrawal D, Chen T, Irby R, et al: Osteopontin identified as lead marker of colon cancer progression, using pooled sample expression profiling. *J Natl Cancer Inst* 2002; 94: 513–521.

Al-Mehdi AB, Tozawa K, Fisher AB, et al: Intravascular origin of metastasis from the proliferation of endothelium-attached tumor cells: a new model for metastasis. *Nature Med* 2000; 6:100–102.

Al-Sukhun S, Hussain M: Current understanding of the biology of advanced bladder cancer. *Cancer* 2003; 15 (Suppl 8):2064–2075.

Arregui C, Pathre P, Lilien J, et al: The nonreceptor tyrosine kinase Fer mediates cross-talk between N-cadherin and $\beta_1$-integrins. *J Cell Biol* 2000; 149:1263–1273.

Balmain A, Gray J, Ponder B. The genetics and genomics of cancer. *Nature Genet* 2003; 33(Suppl):238–244.

Bar-Eli M: Role of AP-2 in tumor growth and metastasis of human melanoma. *Cancer Metastasis Rev* 1999; 18:377–385.

Boudreau N, Sympson CJ, Werb Z, Bissell MJ. Suppression of ICE and apoptosis in mammary epithelial cells by extracellular matrix. *Science* 1995; 267:891–893.

Brittenden J, Heys SD, Ross J, Eremin O: Natural killer cells and cancer. *Cancer* 1996; 77:1226–1243.

Bourguignon LY, Gunja-Smith Z, Lida N, et al: CD44v(3,8-10) is involved in cytoskeleton-mediated tumor cell migration and matrix metalloproteinase (MMP-9) association in metastatic breast cancer cells. *J Cell Physiol* 1998; 176: 206–215.

Brooks PC, Stromblad S, Sanders LC, et al: Localization of matrix metalloproteinase MMP-2 to the surface of invasive cells by interaction with integrin $\alpha_v\beta_3$. *Cell* 1996; 85: 638–693.

Brooks PC, Silletti S, von Schalscha TL, et al: Disruption of angiogenesis by PEX, a noncatalytic metalloproteinase fragment with integrin binding activity. *Cell* 1998; 92: 391–400.

Carretero J, Obrador E, Esteve JM, et al: Tumoricidal activity of endothelial cells. Inhibition of endothelial nitric oxide production abrogates tumor cytotoxicity induced by hepatic sinusoidal endothelium in response to B16 melanoma adhesion in vitro. *J Biol Chem* 2001; 276:25775–25782.

Cassella M, Skobe M. Lymphatic vessel activation in cancer. *Ann NY Acad Sci* 2002; 979; 120–130.

Cavallaro U, Christofori G: Cell adhesion in tumor invasion and metastasis: loss of the glue is not enough. *Biochim Biophys Acta* 2001; 1552:39–45.

Cavallaro U, Schaffhauser B, Christofori G: Cadherins and tumour progression: is it all in a switch? *Cancer Lett* 2002; 176:123–128.

Chambers AF, Groom AC, MacDonald IC: Metastasis: dissemination and growth of cancer cells in metastatic sites. *Nat Rev Cancer* 2002; 2:563–572.

Chambers AF, MacDonald IC, Schmidt EE, et al: Steps in tumor metastasis: new concepts from intravital videomicroscopy. *Cancer Metastasis Rev* 1995; 14:279–301.

Chambers AF, Tuck AB: *Ras*-responsive genes and tumor metastasis. *Crit Rev Oncol* 1993; 4:95–114.

Coussens LM, Fingleton B, Matrisian LM: Matrix metalloproteinase inhibitors and cancer: trials and tribulations. *Science* 2002; 295:2387–2392.

Debies MT, Welch DR. Genetic basis of human breast cancer metastasis. *J Mammary Gland Biol Neoplasia* 2001; 6:441–451.

Ellerbroek SM, Stack MS: Membrane associated matrix metalloproteinases in metastasis. *BioEssays* 1999; 21:940–949.

El-Sabban ME, Pauli BU: Cytoplasmic dye transfer between metastatic tumor cells and vascular endothelium. *J Cell Biol* 1991; 115:1375–1382.

Egeblad M, Werb Z: New functions for the matrix metalloproteinases in cancer progression. *Nat Rev Cancer* 2002; 2:163–176.

Fang F, Orend G, Watanabe N, et al: Dependence of cyclin E-CDK2 kinase activity on cell anchorage. *Science* 1996; 271:499–502.

Fidler IJ: Selection of successive tumour lines for metastasis. *Nat New Biol* 1973; 242:148–149.

Fidler IJ, Kripke ML: Metastasis results from preexisting variant cells within a malignant tumor. *Science* 1977; 198:893–895.

Fidler IJ, Kripke ML. Genomic analysis of primary tumors does not address the prevalence of metastatic cells in the population. *Nat Genetics* 2003; 34:23.

Fujihara T, Sawada T, Hirakawa K, et al: Establishment of lymph node metastatic model for human gastric cancer in nude mice and analysis of factors associated with metastasis. *Clin Exp Metastasis* 1998; 16:389–398.

Glaves D, Huben RP, Weiss L: Haematogenous dissemination of cells from human renal adenocarcinomas. *Br J Cancer* 1988; 57:32–35.

Graeber S, Hulser D: Connexin transfection induces invasive properties in HeLa cells. *Exp Cell Res* 1998; 243:142–149.

Graeber TG, Osmanian C, Jacks T, et al: Hypoxia-mediated selection of cells with diminished apoptotic potential in solid tumours. *Nature* 1996; 379:88–91.

Granovsky M, Fata J, Pawling J, et al: Suppression of tumor growth and metastasis in Mgat5–deficient mice. *Nature Med* 2000 6:306–312.

Greenberg AH, Egan SE, Jarolin L, et al: Natural killer cell regulation of implantation and early lung growth of H-*ras*-transformed 10T1/2 fibroblasts in mice. *Cancer Res* 1987; 47:4801–4805.

Günthert U, Hofmann M, Rudy W, et al: A new variant of glycoprotein CD44 confers metastatic potential to rat carcinoma cells. *Cell* 1991; 65:13–24.

Hanna, N: Role of natural killer cells in host defense against cancer metastasis. In Nicolson GL, Milas L, eds. *Cancer Invasion and Metastasis: Biologic and Therapeutic Aspects.* New York: Raven Press, 1984:309–319.

Hasan J, Byers R, Jayson GC. Intra-tumoral microvessel density in human solid tumours. *Br J Cancer* 2002; 86:1566–1577.

Hazan RB, Phillips GR, Qiao RF, et al: Exogenous expression of N-cadherin in breast cancer cells induces cell migration, invasion, and metastasis. *J Cell Biol* 2000; 148:779–790.

Hejna M, Raderer M, Zielinski CC. Inhibition of metastases by anticoagulants. *J Natl Cancer Inst* 1999; 91:22–36.

Hendrix MJC, Seftor REB, Seftor EA, et al: Transendothelial function of human metastatic melanoma cells: role of the microenvironment in cell-fate determination. *Cancer Res* 2002; 62:665–668.

Hernandez-Barrantes S, Toth M, Bernardo MM, et al: Binding of active (57 kDa) membrane type 1-matrix metalloproteinase (MT1-MMP) to tissue inhibitor of metalloproteinase (TIMP)-2 regulates MT1-MMP processing and pro-MMP-2 activation. *J Biol Chem* 2000; 275:12080–12089.

Herzig M, Christofori G. Recent advances in cancer research: mouse models of tumorigenesis. *Biochim Biophys Acta* 2002; 1602:97–113.

Heppner GH, Miller FR: The cellular basis of tumor progression. *Int Rev Cytology* 1998; 177:1–56.

Hill RP, Young SD, Cillo C, Ling V: Metastatic cell phenotypes: quantitative studies using the experimental metastasis assay. *Cancer Rev* 1986; 5:118–151.

Hoffman R. Green fluorescent protein imaging of tumour growth, metastasis and angiogenesis in mouse models. *Lancet Oncol* 2002; 3:546–556.

Hofmann UB, Westphal JR, van Kraats, AA, et al: Expression of integrin alpha(v)beta(3) correlates with activation of membrane-type matrix metalloproteinase-1 (MT1-MMP) and matrix metalloproteinase-2 (MMP-2) in human melanoma cells in vitro and in vivo. *Int J Cancer* 2000; 87:12–19.

Hojilla CV, Mohammed FF, Khokha R: Matrix metalloproteinases and their tissue inhibitors direct cell fate during cancer development. *Br J Cancer* 2003; 89:1817–1821.

Holmgren L, O'Reilly MS, Folkman J: Dormancy in micrometastases: balanced proliferation and apoptosis in the presence of angiogenic suppression. *Nature Med* 1995; 1:149–153.

Hunter K, Welch DR, Liu ET: Genetic background is an important determinant of metastatic potential. *Nat Genetics* 2003; 34:23–24.

Hynes RO: Integrins: bidirectional, allosteric signaling molecules. *Cell* 2002; 111:673–687.

Ito A, Kotoh F, Kataoka TR, et al: A role for heterologous gap junctions between melanoma and endothelial cells in metastasis. *J Clin Invest* 2000; 105:1189–1197.

Ito S, Nakanishi H, Ikehara Y, et al: Real-time observation of micrometastasis formation in the living mouse liver using a green fluorescent protein gene-tagged rat tongue carcinoma cell line. *Int J Cancer* 2001; 93:212–217.

Ivaska J, Heino J: Adhesion receptors and cell invasion: mechanisms of integrin-guided degradation of extracellular matrix. *Cell Mol Lif Sci* 2000; 57:16–24.

Jain RK, Munn LL, Fukumura D: Dissecting tumour pathophysiology using intravital microscopy. *Nat Rev Cancer* 2002; 2:266–276.

Juliano RL: Signal transduction by cell adhesion receptors and the cytoskeleton: functions of integrins, cadherins, selectins, and immunoglobulin-superfamily members. *Annu Rev Pharmacol Toxicol* 2002; 42:283–323.

Khokha R, Waterhouse P, Yagel S, et al: Anti-sense RNA-induced reduction in murine TIMP levels confers oncogenicity in Swiss 3T3 cells. *Science* 1989; 243:947–950.

Kim J, Yu W, Kovalski K, Ossowski L: Requirement for specific proteases in cancer cell intravasation as revealed by a novel semiquantitative PCR-based assay. *Cell* 1998; 94:353–362.

Kinzler KW, Vogelstein B: Lessons from hereditary colorectal cancer. *Cell* 1996; 87:159–170.

Klein G: Foulds' dangerous idea revisited: the multistep development of tumors 40 years later. *Adv Cancer Res* 1998; 72:1–23.

Klingelhutz AJ, Smith PP, Garrett LR, McDougall JK. Alteration of the DCC tumor-suppressor gene in tumorigenic HPV-18 immortalized human keratinocytes transformed by nitrosomethylurea. *Oncogene* 1993; 8:95–99.

Knutson JR, Iida J, Fields GB, et al: CD44/chondroitin sulfate proteoglycan and $\alpha_2\beta_1$ integrin mediate human melanoma cell migration on type IV collagen and invasion of basement membranes. *Mol Biol Cell* 1996; 7:383–396.

Kruger A, Fata JE, Khokha R. Altered tumor growth and metastasis of a T-cell lymphoma in Timp-1 transgenic mice. *Blood* 1997; 90:1993–2000.

Kruger A, Sanchez-Sweatman OH, Martin DC, et al: Host TIMP-1 overexpression confers resistance to experimental brain metastasis of a fibrosarcoma cell line. *Oncogene* 1998; 16:2419–2423.

Ladeda V, Aguirre Ghiso J, Bal de Kier Joffe E: Function and expression of CD44 during spreading, migration and invasion of murine carcinoma cells. *Exp Cell Res* 1998; 242:515–527.

Lah TT, Kos J: Cysteine proteinases in cancer progression and their clinical relevance for prognosis. *Biol Chem* 1998; 379:125–130.

Lakhani SR: Molecular genetics of solid tumours: translating research into clinical practice. What we could do now: breast cancer. *Mol Pathol* 2001; 54:281–284.

Lampe P, Nguyen B, Gil S, et al: Cellular interaction of integrin $\alpha_v\beta_1$ with laminin 5 promotes gap junction communication. *J Cell Biol* 1998; 143:1735–1747.

Le QT, Sutphin PD, Raychaudhuri S, et al: Identification of osteopontin as a prognostic plasma marker for head and neck squamous cell carcinomas. *Clin Cancer Res* 2003;9:59–67.

Lei H, An P, Song S, et al: A novel peptide isolated from a phage display library inhibits tumor growth and metastasis by blocking the binding of vascular endothelial growth factor to its kinase domain receptor. *J Biol Chem* 2002; 277:43137–43142.

Ling V, Chambers AF, Harris JF, Hill RP: Quantitative genetic analysis of tumor progression. *Cancer Metastasis Rev* 1985; 4:173–192.

Lu C, Kerbel RS: Cytokines, growth factors and the loss of negative growth controls in the progression of human cutaneous malignant melanoma. *Curr Opin Oncol* 1994; 6:212–220.

MacDonald IC, Groom AC, Chambers AF. Cancer spread and micrometastatic development: quantitative approaches for in vivo models. *BioEssays* 2002; 24:885–893.

Mao L: Molecular abnormalities in lung carcinogenesis and their potential clinical implications. *Lung Cancer* 2001; 34(Suppl 2):S27–34.

Mazzieri R, Masiero L, Zanetta L, et al: Control of type IV collagenase activity by components of the urokinase-plasmin system: a regulatory mechanism with cell-bound reactants. *EMBO J* 1997; 16:2319–2332.

Meehan WJ, Welch DR. Breast cancer suppressor 1: update. *Clin Exp Metastasis* 2003; 20: 45–50.

Mori H, Tomari T, Koshikawa N, et al: CD44 directs membrane-type 1 matrix metalloproteinase to lamellipodia by associating with its hemopexin-like domain. *EMBO J* 2002; 21:3949–3959.

Morris VL, MacDonald IC, Koop S, et al: Early interactions of cancer cells with the microvasculature in mouse liver and muscle during hematogenous metastasis: videomicroscopic analysis. *Clin Exp Metastasis* 1993; 11:377–390.

Muller A, Homey B, Soto H, et al: Involvement of chemokine receptors in breast cancer metastasis. *Nature* 2001: 410:50–56.

Navarro P, Ruco L, Dejana E: Differential localization of VE- and N-cadherins in human endothelial cells: VE-cadherin competes with N-cadherin for junctional localization. *J Cell Biol* 1998; 140:1475–1484.

Nemeth JA, Harb JF, Barroso U Jr, et al: Severe combined immunodeficient-hu model of human prostate cancer metastasis to human bone. *Cancer Res* 1999; 59:1987–1993.

Nicolson GL, Menter DG: Trophic factors and central nervous system metastasis. *Cancer Metastasis Rev* 1995; 14:303–321.

Nieman MT, Prudoff RS, Johnson KR, et al: N-cadherin promotes motility in human breast cancer cells regardless of their E-cadherin expression. *J Cell Biol* 1999; 147:631–643.

Nowell P: Mechanisms of tumor progression. *Cancer Res* 1986; 46:2203–2207.

Orr FW, Wang HH, Lafrenie RM, et al: Interactions between cancer cells and the endothelium in metastasis. *J Pathol* 2000; 190:310–329.

Overall CM, Tam E, McQuibban GA, et al; Domain interactions in the gelatinase A.TIMP-2.MT1-MMP activation complex. The ectodomain of the 44-kDa form of membrane type-1 matrix metalloproteinase does not modulate gelatinase A activation. *J Biol Chem* 2000; 275:39497–39506.

Owen-Schaub LB, van Golen KL, Hill LL, Price JE: Fas and Fas ligand interactions suppress melanoma lung metastasis. *J Exp Med* 1998; 188:1717–1723.

Paget S. The distribution of secondary growths in cancer of the breast. *Cancer Metastasis Rev* 1989;8:98–101.

Patel KD, Cuvelier SL, Wiehler S: Selectins: critical mediators of leukocyte recruitment. *Semin Immunol* 2002; 14:73–81.

Pecheur I, Peyruchaud O, Serre CM, et al: Integrin alpha(v)beta3 expression confers on tumor cells a greater propensity to metastasize to bone. *FASEB J* 2002; 16:1266–1268.

Price LS, Collard JG: Regulation of the cytoskeleton by Rho-family GTPases: Implications for tumour cell invasion. *Cancer Biol* 2001; 11:167–173.

Puente XS, Sanchez LM, Overall CM, Lopez-Otin C: Human and mouse proteases: a comparative genomic approach. *Nat Rev Genet* 2003; 4:544–558.

Radinsky R: Modulation of tumor cell gene expression and phenotype by the organ-specific metastatic environment. *Cancer Metastasis Rev* 1995; 14:323–338.

Rak J, Mitsuhashi Y, Sheehan C, et al: Oncogenes and tumor angiogenesis: differential modes of vascular endothelial growth factor up-regulation in ras-transformed epithelial cells and fibroblasts. *Cancer Res* 2000; 60:490–498.

Ramaswamy S, Ross KN, Lander ES, Golub TR: A molecular signature of metastasis in primary solid tumors. *Nat Genetics* 2003; 33: 49–54.

Rao JS: Molecular mechanisms of glioma invasiveness: the role of proteases. *Nat Rev Cancer* 2003; 3:489–501.

Rofstad EK: Microenvironment-induced cancer metastasis. *Int J Radiat Biol* 2000; 76:589–605.

Rozanov DV, Deryugina El, Ratnikov BI, et al: Mutation analysis of membrane type-1 matrix metalloproteinase (MT1-MMP). The role of the cytoplasmic tail Cys(574), the active site Glu(240), and furin cleavage motifs in oligomerization, processing, and self-proteolysis of MT1-MMP expressed in breast carcinoma cells. *J Biol Chem* 2001; 276: 25705–25714.

Ruoslahti E: Specialization of tumour vasculature. *Nat Rev Cancer* 2002; 2:83–90.

Ruoslahti E: Vascular zip codes in angiogenesis and metastasis. *Biochem Soc Trans* 2004; 32:397–402.

Sauer G, Kurzeder C, Grundmann R, et al: Expression of tetraspanin adaptor proteins below defined threshold values is associated with in vitro invasiveness of mammary carcinoma cells. *Oncol Rep* 2003; 10:405–411.

Schneider G, Schmid RM: Genetic alterations in pancreatic cancer. *Mol Cancer* 22; 15:2003.

Shtivelman E, Namikawa R: Species-specific metastasis of human tumor cells in the severe combined immunodeficiency mouse engrafted with human tissue. *Proc Natl Acad Sci USA* 1995; 92:4661–4665.

Smits R, Ruiz P, Diaz-Cano S, et al: E-cadherin and adenomatous polyposis coli mutations are synergistic in intestinal tumor initiation in mice. *Gastroenterology* 2000; 119: 1045–1053.

Sneath RJ, Mangham DC: The normal structure and function of CD44 and its role in neoplasia. *Mol Pathol* 1998; 51:191–200.

Stackpole CW, Alterman AL, Valle EF: B16 melanoma variants selected by one or more cycles of spontaneous metastasis to the same organ fail to exhibit organ specificity. *Clin Exp Metastasis* 1991; 9:319–332.

Stamenkovic I: Matrix metalloproteinases in tumor invasion and metastasis. *Semin Cancer Biol* 2000; 10:415–433.

Su LK, Kinzler KW, Vogelstein B et al: Multiple intestinal neoplasia caused by a mutation in the murine homolog of the APC gene. *Science* 1992; 256:668–670.

Su ZZ, Austin VN, Zimmer SG, Fisher PB: Defining the critical gene expression changes associated with expression and suppression of the tumorigenic and metastatic phenotype in Ha-ras-transformed cloned rat embryo fibroblast cells. *Oncogene* 1993; 8:1211–1219.

Subarsky P, Hill RP: The hypoxic tumour microenvironment and metastatic progression. *Clin Exp Metastasis* 2003; 20:237–250.

Sugarbaker EV: Patterns of metastasis in human malignancies. *Cancer Biol Rev* 1981; 2:235–278.

Tang K, Honn KV. 12(S)-HETE in cancer metastasis. *Adv Exp Med Biol* 1999; 447:181–191.

Trusolino L, Comoglio PM: Scatter-factor and semaphorin receptors: cell signaling for invasive growth. *Nat Rev Cancer* 2002; 4:289–300.

Tuck AB, Chambers AF: The role of osteopontin in breast cancer: clinical and experimental studies. *J Mammary Gland Biol Neoplasia* 2001; 6:419–429.

Turk B, Turk D, Turk V: Lysosomal cysteine proteases: more than scavengers. *Biochim Biophys Acta* 2000; 1477:98–111.

van der Flier A, Sonnenberg A: Function and interactions of integrins. *Cell Tissue Res* 2001; 305:285–298.

Van't Veer LJ, Dai H, van de Vijver MJ, et al: Gene expression profiling predicts clinical outcome of breast cancer. *Nature* 2002; 415:530–536.

Verma M, Srivastava S: Epigenetics in cancer: implications for early detection and prevention. *Lancet Oncol* 2002; 3:755–763.

Voura EB, Ramjeesingh RA, Montgomery AM, et al: Involvement of the integrin $\alpha_V\beta_3$ and the cell adhesion molecule L1 in the transendothelial migration of melanoma cells. *Mol Biol Cell* 2001; 9:2699–2710.

Weiss L: Metastatic inefficiency. *Adv Cancer Res* 1990; 54:159–211.

Werb Z: ECM and cell surface proteolysis: regulating cellular ecology. *Cell* 1997; 91:439–442.

Wong CW, Lee A, Shientag L, et al: Apoptosis: an early event in metastatic inefficiency. *Cancer Res* 2001; 61:333–338.

Wright JA, Turley EA, Greenberg AH: Transforming growth factor beta and fibroblast growth factor as promoters of tumor progression to malignancy. *Crit Rev Oncogen* 1993; 4:473–492.

Yana I, Weiss SJ: Regulation of membrane type-1 matrix metalloproteinase activation by proprotein convertases. *Mol Biol Cell* 2000; 11:2387–2401.

Yoshida BA, Sokoloff MM, Welch DR, Rinker-Schaeffer CW: Metastasis-suppressor genes: a review and perspective on an emerging field. *J Natl Cancer Inst* 2000; 92:1717–1730.

Yu Q, Stamenkovic I: Localization of matrix metalloproteinase 9 to the cell surface provides a mechanism for CD44–mediated tumor invasion. *Genes Dev* 1999; 13:35–48.

Yu WH, Woessner JF, McNeish JD, et al: CD44 anchors the assembly of matrilysin/MMP-7 with heparin-binding epidermal growth factor precursor and ErbB4 and regulates female reproductive organ remodeling. *Genes Dev* 2002; 16:307–323.

Zhang Y, Thant AA, Machida K, et al: Hyaluronan-CD44s signaling regulates matrix metalloproteinase-2 secretion in a human lung carcinoma cell line QG90. *Cancer Res* 2002; 62:3962–3965.

# 12

# Angiogenesis

*Celina Sturk and Daniel Dumont*

## 12.1 INTRODUCTION

Blood vessel growth is essential during normal development of the embryo in order to supply tissues and organs with adequate amounts of nutrients and oxygen, and to allow for adequate removal of metabolic waste. In the adult, however, the vasculature is generally quiescent with the exception of female reproductive organs and specific instances such as inflammation and wound healing following tissue damage. Because it is such an important process, blood vessel growth and regression are carefully regulated events. Disruption of this normal control can lead to a number of pathological states including rheumatoid arthritis, psoriasis, proliferative retinopathy, atherosclerosis, and tumor progression (Folkman, 1995). *Angiogenesis,* that is, the growth of new vessels from pre-existing, larger vessels, plays an important role in cancer progression and targeting of tumor vasculature provides an attractive avenue for novel anti-cancer therapies. These and other aspects of the involvement of angiogenesis in cancer progression will be discussed in this chapter.

## 12.1.1 Angiogenesis During Development

The vasculature is one of the first organ systems to form in the developing embryo. The first stage in vascular development involves differentiation of a common precursor cell, the *hemangioblast,* into the endothelial cells of the vessel wall and the hematopoietic cells of the blood (see Fig. 12.1). This de novo formation of a primitive vascular network is called *vasculogenesis.* Vasculogenesis may also occur in the adult: de novo vessel formation in the adult is believed to arise from circulating endothelial progenitor cells that are able to form endothelial channels (Asahara et al., 1999; Carmeliet, 2000).

Once a primary vessel plexus has been laid down, this immature and poorly functioning network must be remodeled into the complex vasculature seen in adult tissues. The term, angiogenesis, was originally used to describe the sprouting of new vessels from the pre-existing, larger ones, but now is used in a more general sense to include the pruning and remodeling of the primitive network. It also encompasses intercalated growth for in-

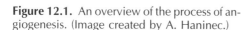
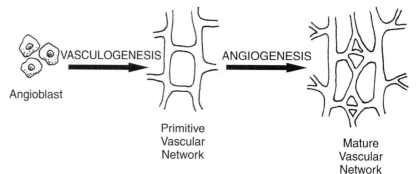

**Figure 12.1.** An overview of the process of angiogenesis. (Image created by A. Haninec.)

Primitive Vascular Network

Mature Vascular Network

creased luminal size or repair of a blood vessel, and intussusceptive growth for division of larger vessels into smaller ones (Carmeliet, 2000). Because these additional forms of angiogenesis most likely do not contribute significantly to tumor angiogenesis, they will not be described further.

*Vasodilation and Vascular Permeability*  Angiogenesis is a highly coordinated series of events beginning with vasodilation and an increase in vascular permeability, primarily in response to production of nitric oxide (see Fig. 12.2). Vascular endothelial growth factor (VEGF), originally termed vascular permeability factor (VPF), is an important mediator of angiogenesis and is transcriptionally upregulated in response to production of nitric oxide. Upregulation of VEGF contributes to vessel leakiness in part by causing redistribution of adhesion molecules such as platelet endothelial cell adhesion molecule (PECAM)-1 and vascular endothelial (VE)-cadherin (Conway et al., 2001). This increased vessel permeability allows for extravasation of plasma proteins into the extravascular space, laying down a matrix for the sprouting endothelial cells. Deregulated vessel permeability, however, is undesirable and can result in a pathological state. Therefore, there exists a naturally opposing ligand, angiopoietin-1 (Ang1) that can counteract the effects of VEGF on vessel permeability

(Thurston et al., 1999, 2000). This is just one example of the tightly controlled balance that must prevail in order for proper vascular development to occur.

*Basement Membrane Degradation*  In order for cells to migrate into the extracellular space, support cells (pericytes) must be loosened and attachment of endothelial cells to the surrounding matrix must be disrupted. Some of the enzymes activated during this time, including members of the matrix metalloproteinase family (MMPs; Chap. 11, Sec. 11.6), also aid in the release of growth factors from the matrix. Molecules released include basic fibroblast growth factor (bFGF), VEGF, and insulin-like growth factor-1 (IGF-1). These factors will in turn help to amplify the angiogenic signal. Another growth factor, Ang1 is also important at this stage as it has been shown to upregulate MMP2, 3, and 9 and downregulate tissue inhibitor of MMP (TIMP)-2 (Kim et al., 2000).

*Endothelial Proliferation and Migration*  Once a path has been cleared, proliferating endothelial cells loosely associate in a column, which protrudes into the extravascular space. A number of chemotactic molecules are involved at this step. Important roles for the VEGF, Ang1, and FGF signaling pathways have been established for endothelial cell proliferation and/or migra-

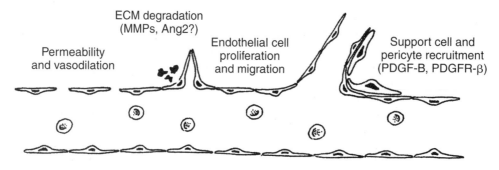

**Figure 12.2.** Steps involved in angiogenesis. (Image created by A. Haninec.) ECM = Extracellular matrix, MMP = Matrix metalloproteinase.

tion (Conway et al., 2001). Integrins and Eph/Ephrin receptor-ligand pairs have also been shown to be involved in cell migration via endothelial cell-cell interactions (Gale and Yancopoulos, 1999; Eliceiri and Cheresh, 2001).

Endothelial tubules usually develop initially as cords lacking a lumen. Lumen formation is a process that is not well understood, but the angiopoietins and VEGFs appear to play a role as they have an effect on lumen size. VEGF has several isoforms (see Sec. 12.2.1) and that action appears to be isoform specific as VEGF165 and 121 and their respective receptors increase lumen diameter, whereas VEGF 189 has the opposite effect (Conway et al., 2001). Circulating endothelial progenitor cells probably are also involved at this stage of angiogenesis through their ability to incorporate into new vessels (Crosby et al., 2000) and their contribution to increased vessel sprouting through release of growth factors (Bautz et al., 2000). Several endogenous inhibitors of lumen formation also exist, perhaps the most well known being thrombospondin-1 (TSP-1).

*Support Cell Recruitment and Vessel Fusion*  Mature blood vessels require recruitment of support cells, such as pericytes (for small vessels) and smooth muscle cells for large vessels. This process helps stabilize the new vessel and plays a role in inhibiting continued endothelial cell proliferation. The support layer also provides endothelial survival signals to protect against vascular regression (Carmeliet, 2000). Gene knockout studies (Chap. 4, Sec. 4.3.12) have elucidated a role for platelet-derived growth factor (PDGF)-B, PDGF receptor (PDGFR)-$\beta$ and Ang1, in recruitment of pericytes to vasculature. Disruption of this recruitment leads to abnormal vessel morphology and network structure (Suri et al., 1996; Hellstrom et al., 1999). For larger arteries, the addition of a thick muscularized coat confers viscoelastic properties and vasomotor (neuromuscular) control of vessel diameter. A new basal lamina is also formed around the vessel for support. The final stages of new capillary growth where vessels fuse to form closed loops and deliver circulation to newly vascularized areas are, however, poorly understood.

### 12.1.2 Physiological Angiogenesis

During development, the vascular network is laid down and endothelial cells subsequently become quiescent in most tissues. Endothelial cells may be the longest-lived cells outside the nervous system and in the normal adult, only about 0.01 percent of endothelial cells undergo division. Tissues that continue to undergo angiogenesis in the adult include female reproductive organs, organs undergoing physiological growth, or tissue that is undergoing repair. Study of angiogenesis under

physiological conditions can provide insight into mechanisms of tumor angiogenesis.

*Female Reproductive System*  Tissues of the female reproductive system, including the ovary and the uterus, continually undergo growth and regression. For example, during its growth phase (which lasts 8 to 10 days), the corpus luteum can double in size and in cell number every 60 to 70 hours. The corpus luteum is one of the most angiogenic tissues known and about 50 to 85 percent of the proliferation that occurs is localized to the microvasculature (Reynolds et al., 2002).

A large number of angiogenic growth factors are found in the corpus luteum including the angiopoietins, epidermal growth factor (EGF), fibroblast growth factors (FGFs), insulin-like growth factors (IGFs), nerve growth factor, transforming growth factors (TGFs), tumor necrosis factors (TNFs), and VEGFs. Vascular endothelial growth factor and FGF appear to play key roles in induction of angiogenesis. Several factors regulate production of angiogenic molecules in the female reproductive system. These include hormones, such as luteinizing hormone, which may regulate levels of VEGF in the corpus luteum, and estrogen, which has been shown to cause upregulation of VEGF and FGF-2, leading to increased angiogenesis. Levels of oxygen and nitric oxide can also regulate VEGF production. Knockout mice (Chap. 4, Sec. 4.3.12) that lack VEGF, or the VEGF receptors (VEGFR1, or VEGFR2) display defects in fetal and placental angiogenesis. Furthermore, antibodies against VEGF used in animal models of ovarian cancer have been successful in arresting tumor development (Geva and Jaffe, 2000).

*Wound Healing*  Wound healing begins immediately following tissue damage. Tissue injury results in production of two growth factors, FGF-1 and FGF-2, and creates a hypoxic environment, leading to upregulation of VEGF (see Sec. 12.3.3). Subsequently, components of the extracellular matrix (ECM) are degraded in response to release of specific enzymes, and fragments of collagen, fibronectin, and elastin are released. These fragments recruit peripheral blood monocytes to the site of injury where they become activated macrophages. Macrophages release a number of cytokines that further stimulate angiogenesis. Some of the growth factors stimulate production of plasminogen activator and procollagenase by endothelial cells, which in turn activate molecules involved in degradation of the basement membrane. This degradation allows for endothelial cell proliferation and migration into the extracellular space in response to the various angiogenic factors being expressed.

Throughout the process of wound healing, a dynamic interaction exists between the endothelial cells, the angiogenic growth factors, and the ECM. An important mediator of new vessel morphology is the $\alpha_v\beta_3$ integrin, which is believed to be important for allowing endothelial cell migration into the fibrin/fibrinogen rich clot. The $\alpha_v\beta_3$ integrin localizes to the tip of the sprouting endothelial cells and there is evidence that the ECM in the wound can also influence angiogenesis by modulating the levels of $\alpha_v\beta_3$ on the surface of the endothelial cells. Growth factors such as VEGF and FGF provide continual mitogenic signals to allow capillary extension. Transforming growth factor $\beta$ (TGF-$\beta$) may be involved in the subsequent laying down of the provisional matrix, and in formation of capillary tubes (Tonnesen et al., 2000).

Critical information has been gained regarding the interaction of the endothelial cells of the developing vessel with the surrounding ECM through study of neovascularization in wound healing. Furthermore, because generation of stroma in tumors is similar to that in wound healing, understanding neovascularization in this setting may lead to advances in tumor therapy

## 12.2 MECHANISMS OF ANGIOGENESIS

### 12.2.1 Vascular Endothelial Growth Factor

While the process of neovascularization is complex and involves a variety of growth factors and cytokines and their respective receptors, VEGF signaling appears to be central to vessel formation during development and in tumors (Ferrara, 2002). Vascular endothelial growth factor is a dimeric glycoprotein; the VEGF family comprises five members whose effects are primarily mediated via the VEGF receptors (VEGFRs) 1 to 3 along with the newly identified neuropilin coreceptors.

*VEGF-A (VEGF)* VEGF-A, normally referred to as VEGF, is the best characterized of the VEGF ligands. Alternative exon splicing of mRNA from a single gene gives rise to five isoforms, which range in length from 121 to 206 amino acid residues: VEGF 121, VEGF 145, VEGF165, VEGF189, and VEGF206. VEGF165 is the most predominant of the human isoforms. An amino terminal peptide sequence in all five isoforms mediates binding to the receptors VEGFRs 1 and 2, while the carboxy region of the larger isoforms mediates binding to heparin-sulfate proteins of the ECM (Keyt et al., 1996). VEGF121 is acidic and does not bind heparin. VEGF189 and VEGF206 are very basic and have a high affinity for binding heparin; they are therefore primarily sequestered to the ECM after secretion. VEGF165 has intermediate affinity for heparin and can be found both bound to ECM and in soluble fractions. Differential binding of the various VEGF isoforms to heparin affects their bioavailability, which encourages isoform specific angiogenic responses. The heparin bound molecules

can also be made available under certain conditions by enzymatic cleavage (e.g., by plasmin) to release soluble forms that are bioactive.

Vascular endothelial growth factor has been shown to be a potent angiogenic factor in a number of in vivo models, and more recently adenoviral delivery of VEGF was also shown to induce lymphangiogenesis (Nagy et al., 2002). Although highly mitogenic, VEGF also acts as a survival factor for endothelial cells both in vitro and in vivo via stimulation of the PI-3K/Akt pathway (Chap. 8, Sec. 8.2.7) and by upregulation of anti-apoptotic factors such as Bcl-2 and A1 (Chap. 10, Sec. 10.2.1; Gerber et al., 1998a; Gerber et al., 1998b). The role of VEGF in promoting survival of endothelial cells in vivo, however, has been shown to be restricted to the developing vasculature of neonatal mice or to newly formed, immature vessels in tumors (Benjamin et al., 1999; Gerber et al., 1999). It is believed that recruitment of pericytes to the sprout is an important step in liberating the endothelium from dependence on VEGF.

The importance of this signaling pathway is exemplified in a knockout model for VEGF-A. $VEGF^{-/-}$ mice die in utero at about embryonic day 9. Defects are observed in formation of blood islands implicating this molecule in early stages of vasculogenesis. Surprisingly, even loss of one allele leads to embryonic death (embryonic day 11 to 12) and suggests an essential role for regulation of VEGF levels during blood vessel development (Carmeliet et al., 1996).

*VEGF-B*  Also able to undergo alternative exon splicing, VEGF-B is a basic ligand and a member of the VEGF family that is able to bind VEGFR-1 and neuropilin-1. There are two VEGF-B isoforms, VEGF-B167, a soluble peptide, and VEGF-B189, which is bound to the ECM (Olofsson et al., 1996). This growth factor can exist as a homodimer or it can heterodimerize with VEGF-A. VEGF-B is most highly expressed in muscle. Subcutaneous injection of VEGF-B165 into nude mice demonstrated that this ligand can promote angiogenesis in vivo via its receptor, VEGFR-1 (Silvestre et al., 2003). Furthermore, mice null for VEGF-B demonstrate defects in vascularization of the embryonic heart (Bellomo et al., 2000). VEGF-B and VEGF-C promotors lack putative binding sites for hypoxia-induced factors and therefore are not upregulated in response to hypoxic conditions (see Sec. 12.3.3).

*VEGF-C*  VEGF-C was the first member of the VEGFR-3/Flt-4 ligand family to be discovered. While VEGFR-3 is expressed in embryonic endothelium, its expression becomes restricted postnatally to the cells of the lymphatics and some venules (Jussila and Alitalo, 2002). Tissue-specific overexpression of VEGF-C in the mouse results in a specific lymphangiogenic effect which can promote tumor metastasis (Mandriota et al., 2001). VEGF-C can also stimulate capillary angiogenesis in vitro and in vivo which may be due in part to its ability to also activate VEGFR-2 (Cao et al., 1998).

*VEGF-D* VEGF-D is also recognized by VEGFR-2 and VEGFR-3 and has been shown to stimulate lymphangiogenesis (Karkkainen and Petrova, 2000). This growth factor may also lead to an angiogenic response as demonstrated by adenoviral gene transfer of VEGF-D in rabbit hind-limb skeletal muscle (Rissanen et al., 2003). VEGF-C and VEGF-D undergo additional cell-associated proteolytic processing following secretion: this modification increases their affinity for VEGFR-3 and also allows binding to VEGFR-2.

*VEGF-E* The VEGF viral homologs are collectively referred to as VEGF-E. A member of this family was identified from the genome of the Orf virus, a para-poxvirus that induces proliferative skin lesions in goats, sheep and humans. VEGF-E appears to have a similar function to VEGF-A in in vitro assays of proliferation, migration, and tubule formation. However, unlike VEGF-A, it is able to bind VEGFR-2 but not VEGFR-1. It is also able to stimulate angiogenesis in vivo (Meyer et al., 1999).

*Placental Growth Factor (PlGF)* Placental growth factor (PlGF) is able to potentiate a VEGF-mediated response. Three isoforms arise from alternative splicing of the *PlGF* gene: PlGF 1, PlGF2, and PlGF3 (Cao et al., 1997). Placental growth factor can homodimerize, resulting in low levels of biological activity, or it can heterodimerize with VEGF, giving rise to intermediate activity between PlGF and VEGF homodimers. VEGF/PlGF heterodimers can elicit intramolecular cross talk between VEGFR1/2 heterodimers (Autiero et al., 2003). Placental growth factor is able to bind VEGFR-1 but not VEGFR-2 (Park et al., 1994) and while it is not mitogenic on its own, it can potentiate the VEGF response where limited VEGF-A is available. Placental growth factor is involved in physiological angiogenesis through its ability to induce revascularization of ischemic tissues (De Falco et al., 2002).

The phenotype of the $PlGF^{-/-}$ mouse provides evidence that this growth factor is also important for pathological angiogenesis in the adult. $PlGF^{-/-}$ mice are healthy and fertile, indicating that PlGF is not essential during development. Further studies, however, revealed subsequent defects in angiogenesis in these mice including impaired tumor growth, collateralization in ischemic conditions, angiogenesis in ischemic retinopathy, plasma extravasation, and wound healing of skin (De Falco et al., 2002; Carmeliet et al., 2001).

### 12.2.2 Vascular Endothelial Growth Factor Receptors

Vascular endothelial growth factor receptors comprise a family of receptor tyrosine kinases (RTKs) (see Chap. 8, Sec. 8.2.2) that possess seven characteristic immunoglobulin-like domains that form the extracellular region (Fig. 12.3). While VEGFR-1 and VEGFR-2 are expressed primarily on endothelial cells, the third family member, VEGFR-3 is mainly expressed in lymphatic vessels. Vascular endothelial growth factors can also bind to a number of coreceptors, the neuropilins, which seem to be involved in modulating binding to the primary VEGFR receptors.

*VEGFR-1* VEGFR-1, also known as Flt-1 (Fms-like tyrosine kinase) has similarities to c-Fms, c-Kit, and PDGFR, and binds with high affinity to VEGF and to PlGF. Although both VEGF and PlGF bind VEGFR-1, they elicit distinct phosphorylation patterns and profiles of gene expression.

Mice that are deficient in *VEGFR-1* die at approximately embryonic days 8 to 9 and fail to form an organized vascular network. There appears to be an overgrowth of endothelial cells which is postulated to be due to an increase in the mesenchymal to hemangioblast cell transition, and thus the aberrant vasculature may be a secondary effect (Fong et al., 1999). Molecular mechanisms behind these observations are not well understood.

The idea that the extracellular domain of VEGFR-1 may simply act as a sink for VEGF (so that it is unable to signal via other VEGFRs) arose when it was shown that deletion of the VEGFR-1 cytoplasmic domain resulted in normal, fertile mice that simply harbored a slight defect in macrophage migration (Hiratsuka et al., 1998). Furthermore, it was shown that an excess of the soluble form of VEGFR-1, sFlt-1, blocks tumor formation and metastasis (Goldman et al., 1998).

Evidence for a direct role for VEGFR-1 in angiogenic signaling pathways comes from the observation that deletion of the VEGFR-1 cytoplasmic domain or inhibition of this domain using VEGFR-1 antagonists, impairs angiogenesis in tumors (Hiratsuka et al., 2001). Evidence for VEGFR-1/VEGFR-2 receptor cross talk also highlights the possible importance of VEGFR-1 signaling in tumor angiogenesis (Autiero et al., 2003).

*VEGFR-2* The VEGFR-2 receptor, also known as kinase-insert-domain containing receptor (KDR), is homologous to the fetal liver kinase-1 (Flk-1) receptor in mice. In the developing embryo VEGFR-2 expression is localized to endothelial cells and is highest in regions of vasculogenesis (Quinn et al., 1993). $VEGFR-2^{-/-}$ knockout mice die *in utero* at about embryonic day 9 due to defects in hematopoietic and endothelial cell development indicating that VEGFR-2 may be a marker of early stages of vasculogenesis (Shalaby et al., 1995).

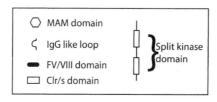

| MAM domain |
| IgG like loop |
| FV/VIII domain |
| Clr/s domain |

Split kinase domain

**Figure 12.3.** Schematic diagram illustrating the structure of receptors for vascular endothelial growth factor (VEGF).

| VEGF121 | VEGF121 | VEGF-C | VEGF145 | Semaphorin | Semaphorin |
| VEGF165 | VEGF145 | VEGF-D | VEGF165 | VEGF165 | VEGF165 |
| VEGF-B | VEGF165 | | VEGF189 | PlGF-2 | |
| PlGF-1 | VEGF-C | | PlGF-2 | VEGFB | |
| PlGF2 | VEGF-D | | VEGF-B167 | | |
| | VEGF-E | | | | |

VEGFR-1 (Flt-1)  VEGFR-2 (Flt-1)  VEGFR-3 (Flt-4)  Heparin-Sulfate Proteoglycan  Neuropilin-1  Neuropilin-2

*VEGFR-3 and Neuropilin*  VEGFR-3 (or Flt-4) is primarily expressed in the lymphatic endothelium in adult tissue, and, together with its ligands VEGF-C and VEGF-D, has been implicated in lymphangiogenesis (see Sec. 12.2.1).

Early studies established that there existed additional receptors for VEGF on select tumor and endothelial cells. The neuropilins, -1 (NRP1) and -2 (NRP2), originally described as receptors for members of the class-3 semaphorin subfamily, were shown to bind VEGF in an isoform-specific manner. VEGF165 binds both neuropilins, while VEGF145 is able to bind NRP2 but not NRP1, and VEGF121 is not able to bind either of the neuropilins (reviewed in Neufeld et al., 2002). A strong role for NRP1 in vascular development comes from knockout studies that show that NRP1 null mice display severe vascular and neuronal abnormalities (Kawasaki et al., 1999). In contrast, mice lacking NRP2 are viable and do not display cardiovascular defects; their phenotype is characterized by neuronal, and to a lesser degree, peripheral lymphatic abnormalities (Yuan et al., 2002). Interestingly, mice lacking both NRP1 and NRP2

display more severe vascular defects than either NRP1 or NRP2 single knockouts indicating a role for both these receptors in embryonic vascular development (Takashima et al., 2002). In the presence of VEGFR-2, binding of NRP1 by VEGF enhanced VEGFR-2 mediated signaling. Neuropilin-1 is believed to act as a coreceptor for VEGF by binding and presenting it to VEGFR-2. This hypothesis may explain the increased mitogenic potential of VEGF165 as compared to VEGF121. Furthermore, there is no detectable signaling downstream of NRP1 as is normally seen when it is bound by the semaphorins. Other genetic studies were able to determine that VEGF/NRP1 signaling, but not Sema/NRP1, is required for angiogenesis (Gu et al., 2003). These discoveries suggest overlapping mechanisms of neurogenesis and vessel formation.

### 12.2.3 Angiopoietins and Tie Receptors

While VEGF plays a pivotal role in vascular formation, it must work in combination with other factors. The angiopoietins are a family of ligands for the Tie family of

RTKs. This family of RTKs, which includes Tie-1 and Tie-2 (Tek), are primarily expressed in endothelial cells, although they may also be found on hemopoietic precursor cells.

There are four members of the angiopoietin family: Ang1, Ang2, Ang3, and Ang4. All the angiopoietins bind Tie-2, leaving Tie-1 as an orphan receptor. These four members appear to have opposing actions on endothelial cells because Ang1 and Ang4 act as receptor agonists, while Ang2 and Ang3 act as context-dependent antagonists (Ward and Dumont, 2002). Mouse Ang3 and human ANG4 represent the mouse and human counterparts for the same gene locus but they have evolved to become quite different from one another; they are more divergent than the mouse and human counterparts of Ang1 and Ang2 (Valenzuela et al., 1999).

The angiopoietins share a conserved structure comprising an N-terminal region responsible for oligomerization and a C-terminal fibrinogen-like domain involved in receptor mediated interactions (Procopio et al., 1999). Recently it has been shown that both Ang1 and Ang2 have two specific N-terminal domains, one of which is responsible for receptor dimerization while the other is required for formation of higher order multimers (Davis et al., 2003). An Ang1 tetramer appears to be the minimum structure required for activation of the receptor. Both Ang1 and Ang2 are secreted proteins; Ang1 has a widespread distribution while Ang2 is predominantly expressed in endothelial cells. Furthermore, Ang1, but not Ang2, can be sequestered by the ECM, which may play a role in determining different signaling targets for these ligands (Xu and Yu, 2001). The angiopoietins are not mitogenic but mediate other cellular processes important for angiogenesis such as cell migration, cell survival, and tubule formation.

Tie-2 deficient mice die between embryonic days 9 and 13 due to vascular abnormalities. These include a lack of normal sprouting and remodeling of the primary capillary plexus leading to incomplete development of the heart and head regions. Furthermore, there is a noticeable decrease in endothelial cell number and lack of recruitment of pericytes to the nascent vessels (Dumont et al., 1994). The phenotype of Ang1 deficient mice is similar to that of Tie-2 deficient mice, although somewhat less severe, implying that additional angiopoietins may contribute to Tie-2 signaling. Mice engineered to overexpress Ang1 display a modest increase in vessel number but a marked increase in vessel size: this is in contrast to VEGF overexpression which primarily results in an increase in vessel number. Concurrent overexpression of both these ligands results in an increase in both vessel number and size. In these studies Ang1 was shown to counter vessel leakiness induced either by VEGF or inflammatory agents, suggesting that a balance between Ang1 and VEGF may regulate normal vascular permeability (Thurston et al., 2000).

Overexpression of Ang2 in embryonic endothelium results in a phenotype very similar to that produced in Tie-2 and Ang1 knockout mice, suggesting that Ang2 can act as an antagonist of Tie-2 signaling (Maisonpierre et al., 1997). High levels of Ang2 have been observed at sites of vascular remodeling in vessels in the ovary or in highly vascularized tumors in humans and in animals (Holash et al., 1999). This observation has led to the hypothesis that Ang2 may act to destabilize vessels during vascular remodeling, allowing either for vessel regression in the absence of growth factor stimulation, or in neovascularization in the presence of angiogenic factors such as VEGF.

While the role of Tie-2 and the angiopoietins has been well documented in development, their role in tumor growth and metastasis is poorly understood. Immunohistochemical analysis has demonstrated that expression of Tie-1, Tie-2, Ang1, and Ang2 is elevated in some but not all tumors indicating that these receptors may play a role in specific tumor micorenvironments (Kaipainen et al., 1994; Peters et al., 1998). Inhibition of Tie-2 signaling, using a soluble extracellular domain of the receptor, has been shown to inhibit angiogenic growth and metastases in tumor bearing mice, supporting a role for this receptor in tumor angiogenesis (Lin et al., 1998; Siemeister et al., 1999).

### 12.2.4 The Ephrins

The Eph receptors are the largest known family of RTKs to date. Their respective ligands, the ephrins, appear to be just as numerous and are unique in that they are tethered to the cell membrane in order to elicit signaling via the Eph receptors. This distinctive feature of the Eph/ephrin signaling mechanism allows for bidirectional signal transduction to occur.

Originally characterized in the nervous system, the ephrins were shown to be important for embryonic patterning and neuronal targeting. Their role in angiogenesis became apparent when ephrin-B2 and EphB4 null mice were found to display lethal defects in early stages of angiogenesis. Their phenotype is similar to those seen in the Tie-1 and Ang1 deficient mice, and includes lethality due to cardiac defects, disrupted capillary remodeling, and a lack of recruitment of support cells to endothelial cells (Wang et al., 1998; Adams and Klein, 2000). These two molecules may play a role in venous versus arteriole identity as ephrin-B2 appears to be specifically expressed in arterial vessels, while EphB4 is found in vessels of venous origin. Ephrin-B2 is expressed in highly vascularized tissues, such as in the female reproductive organs and in tumors but angiogenic responses such as tubule formation, cell migration, and proliferation appear to be cell type specific.

Ephrin-A1 is expressed in the developing vasculature of the embryo, and in vitro studies have shown that it is involved in endothelial cell migration and tubule formation (McBride and Ruiz, 1998; Myers et al., 2000). Ephrin-A1 and its receptor, EphA2, are co-expressed in tumor vasculature. Furthermore, soluble EphA receptors were shown to disrupt endothelial cell migration in vitro as well as in vivo, supporting a role for these molecules in tumor angiogenesis and progression (Brantley al., 2002).

## 12.3 TUMOR ANGIOGENESIS

Tumors require nutrients to grow and viable cells are usually within 100 to 200 micrometers of a capillary blood vessel. During tumor formation, a disruption in the balance between production of pro- and anti-angiogenic molecules occurs. This is sometimes referred to as the *angiogenic switch* (Fig. 12.4) and allows continued proliferation and growth of tumor cells (Hanahan et al., 1996; Bergers and Benjamin, 2003). A number of factors appear to contribute to a change in the balance of pro- versus anti-angiogenic signals during tumor development (Fig. 12.4). These include oncogene-driven production of growth factors by tumor cells, changes in the tumor microenvironment, the recruitment of progenitor endothelial cells from bone marrow, and the downregulation of natural inhibitors of angiogenesis.

### 12.3.1 Morphology of Tumor Vessels

Tumor vasculature is very distinct from that seen in normal tissue (Bergers and Benjamin, 2003). Blood vessels in tumors are tortuous, dilated, and have an irregular shape. They can be dead-ended and leaky due to the high levels of VEGF present in tumors and due to changes in perivascular cell numbers and associations. While the normal vessel wall consists of endothelial and

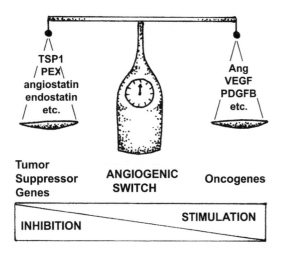

**Figure 12.4.** The angiogenic switch. (Image created by A. Haninec.)

support cells, tumor vasculature can sometimes harbor tumor cells as part of the vessel (Folberg et al., 2000). Some tumors may also recruit endothelial precursor cells from the bone marrow (Lyden et al., 2001), although the number of cells incorporated is low. Tumor vasculature also lacks the characteristic organizational patterns of capillaries, arteries, and venules observed in normal tissues. Moreover, in normal tissue, vessel organization is determined by the oxygen and metabolic needs of the tissue, whereas many tumors have excess capillary growth. Because of these structural differences, blood flow in tumors is often slow and may be intermittent.

### 12.3.2 Growth Factors and Oncogenes

The concept of a tumor angiogenesis factor, or TAF, that diffuses into the microenvironment and initiates the generation of tumor blood vessels was first proposed in 1971 by Dr. Judah Folkman. Shortly thereafter, a factor from the FGF family of proteins was discovered to have a mitogenic effect on endothelial cells. Since then, myriad angiogenic molecules, such as VEGF, FGF, and angiopoietin, have been shown to play a critical role in angiogenesis (Table 12.1). However, the molecular mechanisms that stimulate angiogenesis during tumor growth are not as well understood as those that occur during development, perhaps because expression of angiogenic growth factors in tumors is quite variable.

Tumor formation is a multistep process whereby acquisition of a malignant phenotype results from the accumulation of mutations in oncogenes and/or in tumor suppressor genes (Chaps. 7 and 11, Sec. 11.1). Oncogene driven upregulation of a number of growth factors (VEGF, bFGF, IL-8, PlGF, TGF-$\beta$, PD-ECGF, pleiotrophin, and others), and downregulation of angiogenic inhibitors [Thrombospondin-1 (TSP-1), maspin, interferon-$\alpha$, etc.], are believed to play a role in tumor angiogenesis (Kerbel and Folkman, 2002).

Ras proteins are very often upregulated in human tumors and are responsible for control of signaling cascades which most likely play a role in angiogenesis (Chap. 8, Sec. 8.2.5; Arbiser et al., 1997; Rak et al., 2000). Constitutive expression of H-ras in rat intestinal epithelial cells leads to acquisition of a malignant phenotype in vivo (Buick et al., 1987). Development of tumors (greater than 1 mm in diameter) would not be possible under avascular conditions and the cells were postulated to have acquired an angiogenic phenotype as a result of the sustained H-ras expression. Conditioned media from these cells cultured in vitro was also able to sustain growth of primary endothelial cells (Rak et al., 1995) suggesting that altered signaling in these cells leads to production of factors that promote endothelial cell survival. It has since been shown that Ras

**Table 12.1.** Molecules That Stimulate Angiogenesis

| Factor | Properties | Receptor |
|---|---|---|
| Vascular endothelial growth factor/vascular permeability factor (VEGF/VPF) | Endothelial mitogen, survival factor, and permeability inducer produced by many types of tumor cells | VEGFR2 VEGFR1 (both present on activated endothelium) |
| Placental growth factor (PlGF) | Weak endothelial mitogen | VEGFR1 |
| Basic fibroblast growth factor (bFGF/FGF-2) | Endothelial mitogen, angiogenesis inducer, and survival factor; inducer of VEGFR-2 expression | FGFR1-4 |
| Acidic fibroblast growth factor (aFGF/FGF-1) | Endothelial mitogen and angiogenesis inducer | FGFR1-4 |
| Fibroblast growth factor 3 | Endothelial mitogen and angiogenesis inducer | FGFR1-4 |
| Fibroblast growth factor-4 (FGF-4/Hst/K-FGF) | Endothelial mitogen and angiogenesis inducer | FGFR1-4 |
| Transforming growth factor $\alpha$ (TGF-$\alpha$) | Endothelial mitogen and angiogenesis inducer of VEGF expression | EGFR |
| Epidermal growth factor (EGF) | Weak endothelial mitogen; inducer of VEGF expression | EGFR |
| Hepatocyte growth factor/scatter factor (HGF/SF) | Endothelial mitogen and angiogenesis inducer | c-MET |
| Transforming growth factor $\beta$ (TGF-$\beta$) | In vivo-acting angiogenesis inducer or endothelial growth inhibitor; inducer of VEGF expression | TGF-$\beta$ R I, II, II |
| Tumor necrosis factor $\alpha$ (TNF-$\alpha$) | In vivo-acting angiogenesis inducer, endothelial mitogen (low concentrations) or inhibitor (high concentrations); inducer of VEGF expression | TNFR-55 (TNFR-75?) |
| Platelet-derived growth factor (PDGF) | Mitogen and motility factor for endothelial cells and fibroblasts; in vivo angiogenesis inducer | PDGFR |
| Granulocyte colony-stimulating factor (G-CSF) | In vivo-acting angiogenesis-inducing factor with some mitogenic activity for endothelial cells | G-CSFR |
| IL-8 | Endothelial mitogen, survival factor and inducer of MMP production and tube formation in vitro | CXCR1 CXCR2 |
| Pleiotrophin | Angiogenesis-inducing pleiotrophic growth factor | Proteoglycan |
| Thymidine phosphorylase (tP)/platelet-derived endothelial cell growth factor (PD-ECGF) | In vivo-acting angiogenesis factor | The mode of action remains unclear |
| Angiogenin | In vivo-acting angiogenesis inducer with RNAse activity | 170-kDa angiogenin receptor |
| Proliferin | 35-kDa angiogenesis-inducing protein in mouse | Unknown |
| Angiopoietin-1 | Endothelial survival factor, angiogenesis inducer, and anti-permeability factor | Tie2 |
| Angiopoietin-2 | Context dependent agonist/antagonist of Tie-2 | Tie2 |
| Ephrin-B2 | Allows venous vs. arterial identity; endothelial cell migration, tubule formation | EphB4 |
| Ephrin-A1 | Stimulates endothelial cell migration and tubule formation | EphA2 |

transformation upregulates VEGF protein and mRNA expression levels (Grugel et al., 1995; Rak et al., 1995). Treatment of the conditioned media with anti-VEGF antibodies was found to neutralize the observed activity on cultured human endothelial cells, consolidating a link between Ras oncogenic properties and upregulation of the potent angiogenic factor VEGF.

Levels of Ras expression are also important in determining whether a tumor will acquire angiogenic potential (reviewed in Hahn and Weinberg, 2002). Cells that express low levels of H-ras and that had been transformed with SV40 early region and human telomerase reverse transcriptase (*hTERT*) develop small, avascular tumors in nude mice presumably due to inability to induce neovascularization. This inability to recruit a tumor vasculature was overcome by exogenous addition of VEGF or by higher levels of oncogenic Ras. In this system, transfection with Ras was also shown to inhibit the angiogenic inhibitor TSP-1 (Watnick et al., 2003). These studies highlight the importance of both the *ras* oncogene and the angiogenic inhibitor TSP-1 in regulation of tumor angiogenesis. Several other oncogenes, including *c-myc, v-src, c-jun,* and *Id1* have been shown to repress TSP-1, while tumor suppressors, such as *p53* and *PTEN,* activate TSP-1 (reviewed in Lawler, 2002).

Many other oncogenes and tumor suppressor genes have been implicated in angiogenesis. For example, transfection of the *bcl-2* oncogene into tumor cells results in an increase in VEGF expression (Fernandez et al., 2001). Activation of tumor suppressor genes, such as *p53,* can also reduce tumor angiogenesis. Mechanisms include upregulation of TSP1, degradation of the $\alpha$-subunit of hypoxia inducible factor 1 (HIF-1$\alpha$) (see Chap. 15, Sec. 15.4.2), suppression of transcription of VEGF, and downregulation of bFGF-binding protein (Dameron et al., 1994; Ravi et al., 2000; Sherif et al., 2001).

## 12.3.3 The Tumor Microenvironment

Tumors are known to contain regions of hypoxia (Chap. 15, Sec. 15.4). In tumors, VEGF expression is upregulated in areas surrounding necrotic foci, suggesting a means by which the hypoxic environment created by the growing tumor mass may be upregulating angiogenic factors to increase their supply of oxygen (Plate et al., 1992; Shweiki et al., 1992). Study of the VEGF sequence has revealed the presence of a consensus binding sequence for HIF-1$\alpha$. HIF-1$\alpha$ is a transcriptional regulator that is activated in response to hypoxic conditions (see Chap. 15, Sec. 15.4.2); it can increase transcription of VEGF mRNA as well as stabilize the mRNA by associating with a HIF-1 binding site in the VEGF promoter region (Stein et al., 1998). Vascular endothelial growth factor signaling is also en-

hanced by hypoxia-induced upregulation of the receptors, VEGFR-1 and VEGFR-2 (Waltenberger et al., 1996; Gerber et al., 1997). Hypoxia-inducible factors have been shown to upregulate production of other angiogenic factors such as nitric oxide, PlGF, and Ang2 (Semenza, 1998; Kelly et al., 2003).

## 12.3.4 Circulating Endothelial Cells

Bone marrow is rich in tissue-specific stem and progenitor cells including hematopoietic and endothelial precursors. Emerging evidence suggests that a small subpopulation of these cells can mobilize to the circulation and contribute to angiogenesis, both during development and in the adult. In the case of tumorigenesis, the tumor can secrete factors, such as VEGF, that promote mobilization of circulating endothelial progenitor cells (CEPs) to sites of neovascularization (reviewed in Rafii et al., 2002). Collaboration between CEPs and hematopoietic cells co-recruited to the vascular bed aids in differentiation and incorporation of CEPs into the tumor vasculature. This process, however, is poorly understood. Molecules such as matrix metalloproteinases (specifically MMP-9), as well as cytokines released from bone-marrow derived stromal cells, are believed to be involved in CEP and hematopoietic cell recruitment to the vasculature (Heissig et al., 2002; Rafii and Lyden, 2003).

## 12.3.5 Lymphangiogenesis in Tumors

The lymphatics are a network of vessels that collect bloodless fluid, proteins, and cells (such as immune cells) that have extravasated from tissue and drain it back into the venous system. The lymphatic vessels also provide a route by which malignant cells can travel to reach the lymph nodes and can enter the bloodstream causing metastatic progression (Chap. 11, Sec. 11.2.1). Lymphatic vessels are lined with endothelial cells and have a layer of smooth muscle cells for support. However, the lymphatics are more leaky than blood vessels. Study of the lymphatic system has been hindered by the lack of lymphatic specific markers, which distinguish these vessels.

Both Prox-1, a transcription factor, and VEGFR-3 are molecules believed to play a role in establishment of the lymphatic system during development. VEGFR-3 and its ligand VEGF-C are co-expressed at sites of lymphatic sprouting in the embryo and in disease, including cancer (Kukk et al., 1996; Kim and Dumont, 2003). In vitro VEGF-C can induce proliferation, migration, survival, and sprouting of lymphatic endothelial cells, and in transgenic mice engineered to overexpress this ligand, lymphatic vessel hyperplasia is observed (Jeltsch et al., 1997). Furthermore, when the transgenic mice were induced to form tumors, metastatic growth occurred in areas surrounding the lymphatic vessels and the tumors were able to metastasize to the lymph nodes. In contrast, mice lacking the *VEGF-C* transgene did not develop such metastases (Mandriota et al., 2001).

VEGF-D has also been shown to play a role in metastatic spread of tumors, and its expression appears to increase tumor growth rate and angiogenesis (Stacker et al., 2001). These additional effects may occur via increased processing of VEGF-D, allowing for binding to and activation of VEGFR-2 receptors.

## 12.4 INHIBITORS OF ANGIOGENESIS

A novel approach to anticancer therapy has been the targeting of vascular cells that support the tumor rather than the actual tumor cells (Kerbel and Folkman, 2002). The attraction to these therapies has been the hope that targeting of the relatively stable endothelial cells of the tumor vasculature will diminish the possibility of acquiring drug resistance.

Angiogenic inhibitors can be classified into two broad categories based on their mode of action: direct and indirect (Fig. 12.5). Direct inhibitors, such as Vitaxin™ and angiostatin (see Table 12.2), inhibit endothelial cell function directly by preventing cell migration, proliferation, or evasion of cell death. Indirect inhibitors of angiogenesis block expression or activity of tumor derived factors that are responsible for inducing an angiogenic response; many of these targets are proteins produced by oncogenes. Therefore, therapies originally designed to target oncogenic products may also play an indirect role in inhibition of angiogenesis. For example, the RAS farnesyltransferase inhibitors (Chap. 17, Sec. 17.6.2) block oncogenic pathways responsible for upregulating VEGF and downregulating the angiogenic inhibitor, TSP-1 (Brunner et al., 2003).

Some molecules have the ability to inhibit angiogenesis by both direct and indirect mechanisms. For example, interferon-α (IFN-α) inhibits both tumor-cell production of bFGF (a pro-angiogenic factor) and suppresses endothelial cell migration. This agent has limited activity against kidney cancer and melanoma.

### 12.4.1 Endogenous Inhibitors of Angiogenesis

The concept that tumors secrete specific angiogenic inhibitors was suggested by observations showing that removal of a patient's primary tumor may lead to growth of metastases. Because of the rapid rate at which these tumors progress upon removal of the primary lesion, their growth was proposed to be regulated by angiogenic inhibitors released into the circulation by the primary tumor, hence preventing further progression of the metastases.

A number of endogenous inhibitors of angiogenesis have been discovered, including angiostatin and endostatin (see Table 12.2). Angiostatin and endostatin are proteolytic fragments of the larger extracellular matrix proteins, plasminogen, and collagen XVIII, respectively. Angiostatin binds ATP synthase on the surface of human endothelial cells (Moser et al., 1999). Angiostatin and endostatin may shrink or inhibit growth of some mouse tumors (reviewed in Dell'Eva et al., 2002).

Another endogenous angiogenic inhibitor is PEX. PEX is formed by the proteolysis of matrix metalloprotease-2 (MMP-2) and has been shown to inhibit vascular growth by preventing MMP-2 from interacting with the integrin $\alpha_v\beta_3$ found on the endothelial cell surface. Matrix metalloprotease-2 contributes to the angiogenic process in a positive manner by degradation of the extracellular matrix (see Sec. 12.1.1 and Chap. 11, Sec. 11.6).

Thrombospondin-1 is an extracellular matrix glycoprotein and was the first naturally occurring inhibitor of angiogenesis to be discovered (Good et al., 1990). Thrombospondin-1 has been shown to inhibit MMP-9, an extracellular matrix metalloproteinase responsible for release of VEGF sequestered in the ECM (Rodriguez-Manzaneque et al., 2001). It has also been shown to directly inhibit angiogenesis by inhibiting

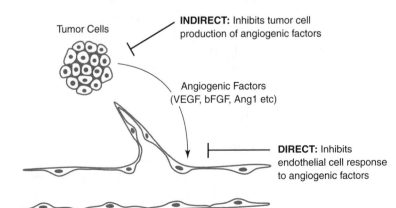

**Figure 12.5.** Direct and indirect inhibitors of angiogenesis. (Image created by A. Haninec.)

**Table 12.2.** Inhibitors of Angiogenesis

| Inhibitor | Mechanism of Action |
|---|---|
| **Endogenous** | |
| PEX<br>TIMP-1, -2, -3, -4 | Block endothelial and tumor cell invasion by inhibiting MMPs |
| Angiostatin<br>Endostatin | Proteolytic fragments of larger extracellular matrix proteins (plasminogen/collagen XVIII) that inhibit endothelial cell proliferation, angiogenesis, and tumor growth |
| Thrombospondin-1 (TSP-1) | Extracellular matrix glycoprotein able to inhibit endothelial cell migration, proliferation, and cell survival |
| INF-$\alpha$, -$\beta$, and -$\gamma$ | Inhibit endothelial cell migration and proliferation. INF-$\alpha$ inhibits bFGF |
| **Pharmacological** | |
| Thalidomide | Teratogen that inhibits angiogenesis in vivo |
| Batimastat<br>Marimastat<br>AG3340 | MMP inhibitors (MMPIs) that block endothelial and tumor cell invasion |
| LM609<br>Vitaxin™<br>RGD containing peptides | Block endothelial cell adhesion and induce endothelial cell apoptosis |
| SU5416<br>Soluble Flt-1<br>VEGF antibodies (Bevacizumab) | Inhibit angiogenesis and tumor growth by interfering with VEGF activity |
| SU6668, SU011248, BAY43-9006 | Broad spectrum small molecule inhibitors of the tyrosine kinase activity of VEGFR, PDGFR, and other receptors |
| TNP-470 | Synthetic analog of fumagillin that blocks endothelial cell proliferation |

CD36 found on the surface of endothelial cells (Dawson et al., 1997). In vitro, TSP-1 inhibits angiogenesis and affects endothelial cell motility, adhesion, and growth and has been found to induce apoptosis of endothelial cells (Armstrong et al., 2003). In vivo studies using TSP-1 knockout in mice that are prone to mammary tumors demonstrated increased tumor burden and vessel density. Mice engineered to overexpress TSP-1 in the mammary gland displayed a delay or reduction of tumor growth in ~20 percent of the animals (Rodriguez-Manzaneque et al., 2001). Several oncogenes, including *ras, c-myc, v-src,* and *c-jun,* have been shown to repress TSP-1 while tumor suppressors, such as *p53* and *PTEN,* activate TSP-1 (reviewed in Lawler, 2002) implying that, in addition to controlling proliferation of the tumor cells, these oncogenes and tumor suppressors also modulate angiogenesis balance (see Sec. 12.3.2).

Endogenous angiogenic inhibitors probably contribute to maintenance of the normal quiescent state of endothelial cells and to control transient angiogenic responses. These molecules represent potential candidates for use in anti-angiogenic therapies.

### 12.4.2 Pharmacological Inhibitors of Angiogenesis

Interferon-$\alpha$ is made in mammalian cells as a response to viral infection but can also be synthesized for pharmacologic use. It was found to inhibit endothelial cell migration in vitro, and was subsequently shown to inhibit angiogenesis in vivo (Brouty-Boye et al., 1980; Sidky et al., 1987; Dvorak and Gresser, 1989). These antiangiogenic properties are conferred, at least in part, by indirect downregulation of bFGF expression (Singh et al., 1995). In humans, IFN-$\alpha$ has been used successfully to treat rare tumors where angiogenesis is primarily mediated by bFGF (such as hemangiomas, angioblastomas, and giant-cell tumors) but has limited efficacy for other tumor types such as melanoma and kidney cancer.

The anti-inflammatory (and teratogenic) drug thalidomide was found to inhibit bFGF and VEGF induced angiogenesis during corneal vascularization and in animal tumors (D'Amato et al., 1994; Verheul et al., 1999). This compound was subsequently shown to be effective in patients with multiple myeloma (Singhal et al., 1999). Thalidomide has been shown to suppress production of the angiogenic molecule TNF-$\alpha$, but probably possesses alternative anti-angiogenic mechanisms as other, more potent inhibitors of TNF-$\alpha$ have little or no effect on tumor angiogenesis.

Several chemotherapeutic agents have been found to possess anti-angiogenic effects and their activity may depend on dose and schedule. Conventional cytotoxic chemotherapy has traditionally been administered at maximum tolerated doses followed by intervals of nontreatment (see Chaps. 16 and 17). Anti-angiogenic agents, however, usually work best when given to maintain a constant level of the inhibitor in the circulation without a period of rest that would allow for revascularization (Kisker et al., 2001). Optimization of the anti-angiogenic properties of these chemotherapy drugs may therefore require more frequent administration of lower doses of the drug, a process called *metronomic therapy*. Several anti-cancer drugs, including cyclophosphamide and vinblastine, have activity in tumor-bearing mice when used in this way, especially if combined with other anti-angiogenic drugs (Browder et al., 2000; Klement et al., 2000).

Improved understanding of the molecular mechanisms underlying angiogenesis has allowed for the design of compounds that can interfere with this process. These agents include modulators of proteolytic enzymes responsible for degradation of the extracellular matrix, inhibitors of endothelial cell proliferation and survival, and molecules that block growth-factor activity (including VEGF signaling).

Regulation of the proteolytic MMPs appears to be lost during tumor growth and metastasis, and may contribute to angiogenic activity (see Chap. 11, Sec. 11.6). Increased MMP activity has been shown in a number of tumor types and there is a positive correlation between levels of MMPs and tumor aggressiveness (reviewed in Pavlaki et al., 2003). This finding has led to the evaluation of synthetic MMP inhibitors (MMPIs), which function by competing with MMP substrates at the MMP catalytic site. These agents have been evaluated in clinical trials but have shown minimal therapeutic benefit (Zucker et al., 2000; Hidalgo and Eckhardt, 2001).

The integrins $\alpha_V\beta_3$ and $\alpha_V\beta_5$ are important for vascular development. $\alpha_V\beta_3$ is an attractive candidate for anti-angiogenic therapy as it is prominently expressed on proliferating vascular endothelial cells in tumors, while being minimally expressed on resting endothelium (Eliceiri and Cheresh, 2001; Rupp and Little, 2001). Inhibition of $\alpha_V\beta_3$ using monoclonal antibodies, such as LM609, or low-molecular weight antagonists, such as RGD-containing peptides, inhibits neovascularization in some in vivo models (Brooks et al., 1994). The monoclonal antibody, Vitaxin™ is the humanized form of LM609 and has shown promise in shrinking solid tumors in phase II clinical trials without harmful side effects (Brower, 1999).

Many strategies have been used in the design of angiogenic inhibitors that interfere with the production or secretion of angiogenic factors (primarily VEGF and FGF-2) or that disrupt binding of these molecules to their respective receptors. Anti-VEGF antibodies, soluble VEGF receptors, or dominant negative VEGFR-2 have proven promising in interfering with angiogenesis and tumor growth in animal models (Ferrera, 1999). SU5416 is an inhibitor of VEGF induced VEGFR-2

phosphorylation and is being evaluated in clinical trials for Kaposi's sarcoma, colorectal cancer, and von Hippel-Lindau disease (Brower, 1999). Other small molecules, such as SU011248 and BAY43-9006, inhibit VEGFR and other tyrosine kinase receptors and are showing promising activity against human kidney cancer. Bevacizumab (Avastin) is a monoclonal anti-VEGF antibody that has been shown to reduce VEGF levels in in vitro and in vivo models, and has been shown to inhibit tumor growth in mice. Bevacizumab is also being evaluated in clinical trials and has been shown to prolong survival when used to treat metastatic colorectal cancer (Hurwitz et al., 2004).

Because of the inherent instability of tumor cells and their ability to switch to production of an alternate cytokine should another become unavailable, inhibition of a single growth factor or receptor may not always prove to be effective. Thus development of inhibitors, which blocks VEGF, FGF-2, and PDGF receptors, may provide additional benefits in the clinic.

### 12.4.3 Approaches to Tumor Therapy Through Inhibition of Angiogenesis

The initial evaluation of anti-angiogenic therapy in clinical trials has been disappointing, and more innovative approaches may be required to obtain useful anticancer effects. Compounds that inhibit angiogenesis probably need to be administered to maintain a constant level in the circulation for a long period of time. Also, monitoring the effectiveness of anti-angiogenic therapy may require different methods from those used for cytotoxic chemotherapy. Tumor regression, as a result of anti-angiogenic therapy, is usually slow whereas chemotherapy generally induces rapid tumor regression.

A potential problem for use of anti-angiogenic therapies is the development of resistance of tumor cells to apoptosis because inhibition of tumor vasculature might lead to a hypoxic environment that selects for cells which overexpress anti-apoptotic proteins (Graeber et al., 1996). However, a study conducted using the angiogenic inhibitor TNP-470 demonstrated that in vivo administration of this drug was able to overcome the anti-apoptotic advantage conferred by overexpression of BCL-2. Furthermore, this agent was shown to inhibit tumor growth (Yanase et al., 1993).

The targeting of signaling circuits in both stromal (including endothelial) and tumor cell populations represents a logical progression in the search for effective anticancer therapies. One example is the use of xenografts treated with vinblastine, and DC101, a neutralizing monoclonal antibody targeting VEGFR-2. With individual treatment using either agent, transient regression of xenografts and inhibition of tumor angiogenesis was seen. However, when used together these compounds induced sustained regression of large, established tumors. No toxicity or drug resistance was observed (Klement et al., 2000).

Another study where chemotherapeutic drugs and angiogenesis inhibitors have been combined involves targeting of endoglin, a transmembrane endothelial receptor that binds to members of the TGF-$\beta$ superfamily and their protein complexes. Endoglin is expressed in tumor-associated angiogenic vascular endothelium. The use of antibodies targeting the endoglin receptor, in conjunction with cyclophosphamide, inhibited angiogenesis and induced regression of MCF-7 human breast cancer xenografts (Takahashi et al., 2001).

The use of multiple anti-angiogenic compounds to target proteins involved in different stages of tumor progression may be promising. A mouse model for pancreatic B-cell carcinoma demonstrates this principle. The mice develop tumors in a stepwise fashion, allowing the study of therapeutic agents at various stages of tumor progression. Studies have shown that the VEGF receptor inhibitor SU5416 targets early stage, premalignant lesions but does not have an effect on late stage, well-vascularized tumors. VEGFR must therefore play an important role in early stages of angiogenesis. A second compound (SU6668) is a broad tyrosine kinase inhibitor: it is somewhat selective for PDGFRs and to a lesser extent, VEGFRs. This second agent results in pericyte detachment from the endothelial cells of the vasculature and has been shown to be more effective in blocking growth of late, end-stage tumors. Because the mouse model chosen expresses PDGFR exclusively in the pericytes of the tumor, this may be a valuable target for antitumor therapy. When these therapies were used in combination there was a greater effect on tumors of all stages than if either compound was used independently (Bergers et al., 2003). This is an example of new directions for anti-angiogenic therapy.

## 12.5  SUMMARY

This chapter presents some of the key aspects of angiogenesis. While an increasingly large number of molecules appear to be involved in neovascularization, the importance of key players, such as VEGF, bFGF, and angiopoietin, is becoming apparent as we learn more about the molecular mechanisms governing this carefully regulated and balanced process. Disruption of the angiogenic balance can have a large impact on normal biological functions. Induction of the angiogenic switch can lead to a number of pathological states, including tumor growth and metastasis. Understanding the molecular basis for this complex process is important in the search for novel anticancer therapies. Some anti-angiogenic agents, such as bevecizumab, are now being

used in the clinic, but for the most part these therapies have not lived up to the high expectations originally set for them. A better understanding of how to administer and combine these therapies should lead to strategies that will be more effective in halting tumor growth and progression.

## REFERENCES

Adams RH, Klein R: Eph receptors and ephrin ligands. Essential mediators of vascular development. *Trends Cardiovasc Med* 2000; 10:183–188.

Arbiser JL, Moses MA, Fernandez CA, et al: Oncogenic H-ras stimulates tumor angiogenesis by two distinct pathways. *Proc Natl Acad Sci USA* 1997; 94:861–866.

Armstrong LC, Bornstein P: Thrombospondins 1 and 2 function as inhibitors of angiogenesis. *Matrix Biol* 2003; 22:63–71.

Asahara T, Takahashi T, Masuda H, et al: VEGF contributes to postnatal neovascularization by mobilizing bone marrow-derived endothelial progenitor cells. *EMBO J* 1999; 18:3964–3972.

Autiero M, Waltenberger J, Communi D, et al: Role of PlGF in the intra- and intermolecular cross talk between the VEGF receptors Flt1 and Flk1. *Nat Med* 2003; 9:936–943.

Bautz F, Rafii S, Kanz L, Mohle R: Expression and secretion of vascular endothelial growth factor-A by cytokine-stimulated hematopoietic progenitor cells. Possible role in the hematopoietic microenvironment. *Exp Hematol* 2000; 28:700–706.

Bellomo D, Headrick JP, Silins GU, et al: Mice lacking the vascular endothelial growth factor-B gene (Vegfb) have smaller hearts, dysfunctional coronary vasculature, and impaired recovery from cardiac ischemia. *Circ Res* 2000; 8:86:E29–E35

Benjamin LE, Golijanin D, Itin A., et al: Selective ablation of immature blood vessels in established human tumors follows vascular endothelial growth factor withdrawal. *J Clin Invest* 1999; 103:159–165.

Bergers G, Benjamin LE: Tumorigenesis and the angiogenic switch. *Nat Rev Cancer* 2003; 3:401–410.

Bergers G, Song S, Meyer-Morse N, et al: Benefits of targeting both pericytes and endothelial cells in the tumor vasculature with kinase inhibitors. *J Clin Invest* 2003; 111:1287–1295.

Brantley DM, Cheng N, Thompson EJ, et al: Soluble Eph A receptors inhibit tumor angiogenesis and progression in vivo. *Oncogene* 2002; 21:7011–7026.

Brooks PC, Montgomery AM, Rosenfeld M, et al: Integrin alpha v beta 3 antagonists promote tumor regression by inducing apoptosis of angiogenic blood vessels. *Cell* 1994; 79:1157–1164.

Brouty-Boye D, Zetter BR: Inhibition of cell motility by interferon. *Science* 1980; 208:516–518.

Browder T, Butterfield CE, Kraling BM, et al: Antiangiogenic scheduling of chemotherapy improves efficacy against experimental drug-resistant cancer. *Cancer Res* 2000; 60:1878–1886.

Brower V: Tumor angiogenesis—new drugs on the block. *Nat Biotechnol* 1999; 17:963–968.

Brunner TB, Hahn SM, Gupta AK, et al: Farnesyltransferase inhibitors: an overview of the results of preclinical and clinical investigations. *Cancer Res* 2003 Sep 15;63:5656–5668.

Buick RN, Filmus J, Quaroni A: Activated H-ras transforms rat intestinal epithelial cells with expression of alpha-TGF. *Exp Cell Res* 1987; 170:300–309.

Cao Y, Ji WR, Qi P, et al: Placenta growth factor: identification and characterization of a novel isoform generated by RNA alternative splicing. *Biochem Biophys Res Commun* 1997; 235:493–498.

Cao Y, Linden P, Farnebo J, et al: Vascular endothelial growth factor C induces angiogenesis in vivo. *Proc Natl Acad Sci USA* 1998; 95:14389–14394.

Carmeliet P, Ferreira V, Breier G: Abnormal blood vessel development and lethality in embryos lacking a single VEGF allele. *Nature* 1996; 380:435–439.

Carmeliet P: Mechanisms of angiogenesis and arteriogenesis. *Nat Med* 2000; 6:389–395.

Carmeliet P, Moons L, Luttun A, et al: Synergism between vascular endothelial growth factor and placental growth factor contributes to angiogenesis and plasma extravasation in pathological conditions. *Nat Med* 2001; 7:575–583

Conway EM, Collen D, Carmeliet P: Molecular mechanisms of blood vessel growth. *Cardiovasc Res* 2001; 49:507–521.

Crosby JR, Kaminski WE, Schatteman G, et al: Endothelial cells of hematopoietic origin make a significant contribution to adult blood vessel formation. *Circ Res* 2000; 87:728–730.

D'Amato RJ, Loughnan MS, Flynn E, Folkman J: Thalidomide is an inhibitor of angiogenesis. *Proc Natl Acad Sci USA* 1994; 91:4082–4085.

Dameron KM, Volpert OV, Tainsky MA, Bouck N: Control of angiogenesis in fibroblasts by p53 regulation of thrombospondin-1. *Science* 1994; 265:1582–1584.

Davis S, Papadopoulos N, Aldrich TH, et al: Angiopoietins have distinct modular domains essential for receptor binding, dimerization and superclustering. *Nat Struct Biol* 2003; 10:38–44.

Dawson DW, Pearce SF, Zhong R, et al: CD36 mediates the in vitro inhibitory effects of thrombospondin-1 on endothelial cells. *J Cell Biol* 1997; 138:707–717.

De Falco S, Gigante B, Persico MG: Structure and function of placental growth factor. *Trends Cardiovasc Med* 2002; 12:241–246.

Dell'Eva R, Pfeffer U, Indraccolo S, et al: Inhibition of tumor angiogenesis by angiostatin: from recombinant protein to gene therapy. *Endothelium* 2002; 9:3–10.

Dumont DJ, Gradwohl G, Fong GH, et al: Dominant-negative and targeted null mutations in the endothelial receptor tyrosine kinase, tek, reveal a critical role in vasculogenesis of the embryo. *Genes Dev* 1994; 8:1897–1909.

Dvorak HF, Gresser I: Microvascular injury in pathogenesis of interferon-induced necrosis of subcutaneous tumors in mice. *J Natl Cancer Inst* 1989; 81:497–502.

Eliceiri BP, Cheresh DA: Adhesion events in angiogenesis. *Curr Opin Cell Biol* 2001; 13:563–568.

Fernandez A, Udagawa T, Schwesinger C, et al: Angiogenic potential of prostate carcinoma cells overexpressing bcl-2. *J Natl Cancer Inst* 2001; 93:208–213.

Ferrara N: Vascular endothelial growth factor: molecular and biological aspects. *Curr Top Microbiol Immunol* 1999; 237:1–30.

Ferrara N: VEGF and the quest for tumour angiogenesis factors. *Nat Rev Cancer* 2002; 2:795–803.

Folberg R, Hendrix MJ, Maniotis AJ: Vasculogenic mimicry and tumor angiogenesis. *Am J Pathol* 2000; 156:361–381.

Folkman J: Angiogenesis in cancer, vascular, rheumatoid, and other disease. *Nat Med* 1995; 1:27–31.

Fong GH, Zhang L, Bryce DM, Peng J: Increased hemangioblast commitment, not vascular disorganization, is the primary defect in flt-1 knock-out mice. *Development* 1999; 126:3015–3025.

Gale NW, Yancopoulos GD: Growth factors acting via endothelial cell-specific receptor tyrosine kinases: VEGFs, angiopoietins, and ephrins in vascular development. *Genes Dev* 1999; 1:1055–1066.

Gerber H-P, Condorelli F, Park J, Ferrara N: Differential transcriptional regulation of the two vascular endothelial growth factor receptor genes. Flt-1, but not Flk-1/KDR, is up-regulated by hypoxia. *J Biol Chem* 1997; 272:23659–23667.

Gerber HP, Dixit V, Ferrara N: Vascular endothelial growth factor induces expression of the antiapoptotic proteins Bcl-2 and A1 in vascular endothelial cells. *J Biol Chem* 1998a; 273:13313–13316.

Gerber HP, Hillan KJ, Ryan AM, et al: VEGF is required for growth and survival in neonatal mice. *Development* 1999; 126:1149–1159.

Gerber HP, McMurtrey A, Kowalski J: VEGF regulates endothelial cell survival by the PI3–kinase/Akt signal transduction pathway. Requirement for Flk-1/KDR activation. *J Biol Chem* 1998b; 273:30366–30343.

Geva E, Jaffe RB: Role of vascular endothelial growth factor in ovarian physiology and pathology. *Fertil Steril* 2000; 74:429–438.

Goldman CK, Kendall RL, Cabrera G, et al: Paracrine expression of a native soluble vascular endothelial growth factor receptor inhibits tumor growth, metastasis, and mortality rate. *Proc Natl Acad Sci USA* 1998; 95:8795–8800.

Good DJ, Polverini PJ, Rastinejad F, et al: A tumor suppressor-dependent inhibitor of angiogenesis is immunologically and functionally indistinguishable from a fragment of thrombospondin. *Proc Natl Acad Sci USA* 1990; 87:6624–6628.

Graeber TG, Osmanian C, Jacks T, et al: Hypoxia-mediated selection of cells with diminished apoptotic potential in solid tumours. *Nature* 1996; 379:88–91.

Grugel S, Finkenzeller G, Weindel K, et al: Both v-Ha-ras and v-raf stimulate expression of the vascular endothelial growth factor in NIH 3T3 cells. *J Biol Chem* 1995; 270:25915–25919.

Gu C, Rodriguez ER, Reimert DV, et al: Neuropilin-1 conveys semaphorin and VEGF signaling during neural and cardiovascular development. *Dev Cell* 2003; 5:45–57.

Hahn WC, Weinberg RA: Rules for making human tumor cells. *N Engl J Med* 2002; 347:1593–1603.

Hanahan D, Christofori G, Naik P, Arbeit J: Transgenic mouse models of tumour angiogenesis: the angiogenic switch, its molecular controls, and prospects for preclinical therapeutic models. *Eur J Cancer* 1996; 32A:2386–2393.

Heissig B, Hattori K, Dias S, et al: Recruitment of stem and progenitor cells from the bone marrow niche requires MMP-9 mediated release of kit-ligand. *Cell* 2002; 109: 625–637.

Hellstrom M, Kalen M, Lindahl P, et al: Role of PDGF-B and PDGFR-beta in recruitment of vascular smooth muscle cells and pericytes during embryonic blood vessel formation in the mouse. *Development* 1999; 126:3047–3055.

Hidalgo M, Eckhardt SG: Development of matrix metalloproteinase inhibitors in cancer therapy. *J Natl Cancer Inst* 2001; 93:178–193.

Hiratsuka S, Maru Y, Okada A, et al: Involvement of Flt-1 tyrosine kinase (vascular endothelial growth factor receptor-1) in pathological angiogenesis. *Cancer Res* 2001; 61:1207–1213.

Hiratsuka S, Minowa O, Kuno J, et al: Flt-1 lacking the tyrosine kinase domain is sufficient for normal development and angiogenesis in mice. *Proc Natl Acad Sci USA* 1998; 95:9349–9354.

Holash J, Maisonpierre PC, Compton D, et al: Vessel cooption, regression, and growth in tumors mediated by angiopoietins and VEGF. *Science* 1999; 284:1994–1998.

Hurwitz H, Fehrenbacher L, Novotny W, et al: Bevacizumab plus irinotecan, fluorouracil and leucovorin for metastatic colorectal cancer. *N Engl J Med* 2004; 350:2335–2342.

Jeltsch M, Kaipainen A, Joukov V, et al: Hyperplasia of lymphatic vessels in VEGF-C transgenic mice. *Science* 1997; 276:1423–1425.

Jussila L, Alitalo K: Vascular growth factors and lymphangiogenesis. *Physiol Rev* 2002; 82:673–700.

Kaipainen A, Vlaykova T, Hatva E, et al: Enhanced expression of the Tie receptor tyrosine kinase messenger RNA in the vascular endothelium of metastatic melanomas. *Cancer Res* 1994; 54:6571–6577.

Karkkainen MJ, Petrova TV: Vascular endothelial growth factor receptors in the regulation of angiogenesis and lymphangiogenesis. *Oncogene* 2000; 19:5598–5605.

Kawasaki T, Kitsukawa T, Bekku Y: A requirement for neuropilin-1 in embryonic vessel formation. *Development* 1999; 126:4895–4902.

Kelly BD, Hackett SF, Hirota K, et al: Cell type-specific regulation of angiogenic growth factor gene expression and induction of angiogenesis in nonischemic tissue by a constitutively active form of hypoxia-inducible factor 1. *Circ Res* 2003; 93:1074–1081.

Kerbel R, Folkman J: Clinical translation of angiogenesis inhibitors. *Nat Rev Cancer* 2002; 2:727–739.

Keyt BA, Berleau LT, Nguyen HV: The carboxyl-terminal domain (111–165) of vascular endothelial growth factor is critical for its mitogenic potency. *J Biol Chem* 1996; 271: 7788–7795.

Kim H, Dumont DJ: Molecular mechanisms in lymphangiogenesis: model systems and implications in human disease. *Clin Genet* 2003; 64:282–292.

Kim I, Kim HG, So J-N, et al: Angiopoietin-1 regulates endothelial cell survival through the phosphatidylinositol 3′-kinase/Akt signal transduction pathway. *Circ Res* 2000; 86: 24–29.

Kisker O, Becker CM, Prox D, et al: Continuous administration of endostatin by intraperitoneally implanted osmotic pump improves the efficacy and potency of therapy in a mouse xenograft tumor model. *Cancer Res* 2001; 61:7669–7674.

Klement G, Baruchel S, Rak J: Continuous low-dose therapy with vinblastine and VEGF receptor-2 antibody induces sustained tumor regression without overt toxicity. *J Clin Invest* 2000; 105:R15–R24.

Kukk E, Lymboussaki A, Taira S, et al: VEGF-C receptor binding and pattern of expression with VEGFR-3 suggests a role in lymphatic vascular development. *Development* 1996; 122:3829–3837.

Lawler J: Thrombospondin-1 as an endogenous inhibitor of angiogenesis and tumor growth. *J Cell Mol Med* 2002; 6:1–12.

Lin P, Buxton JA, Acheson A, et al: Antiangiogenic gene therapy targeting the endothelium-specific receptor tyrosine kinase Tie2. *Proc Natl Acad Sci USA* 1998; 95:8829–8834.

Lyden D, Hattori K, Dias S, et al: Impaired recruitment of bone-marrow-derived endothelial and hematopoietic precursor cells blocks tumor angiogenesis and growth. *Nat Med* 2001; 7:1194–1201

Maisonpierre PC, Suri C, Jones PF, et al: Angiopoietin-2, a natural antagonist for Tie2 that disrupts in vivo angiogenesis. *Science* 1997; 277:55–60.

Mandriota SJ, Jussila L, Jeltsch M: Vascular endothelial growth factor-C-mediated lymphangiogenesis promotes tumour metastasis. *EMBO J* 2001; 20:672–682.

McBride JL, Ruiz JC: Ephrin-A1 is expressed at sites of vascular development in the mouse. *Mech Dev* 1998; 77:201–204.

Meyer M, Clauss M, Lepple-Wienhues A, et al: A novel vascular endothelial growth factor encoded by Orf virus, VEGF-E, mediates angiogenesis via signalling through VEGFR-2 (KDR) but not VEGFR-1 (Flt-1) receptor tyrosine kinases. *EMBO J* 1999; 18:363–374.

Moser TL, Stack MS, Asplin I, et al: Angiostatin binds ATP synthase on the surface of human endothelial cells. *Proc Natl Acad Sci USA* 1999; 96:2811–2816.

Myers C, Charboneau A, Boudreau N: Homeobox B3 promotes capillary morphogenesis and angiogenesis. *J Cell Biol* 2000; 148:343–351.

Nagy JA, Vasile E, Feng D, et al: Vascular permeability factor/vascular endothelial growth factor induces lymphangiogenesis as well as angiogenesis. *J Exp Med* 2002; 196: 1497–1506.

Neufeld G, Cohen T, Shraga N, et al: The neuropilins: multifunctional semaphorin and VEGF receptors that modulate axon guidance and angiogenesis. *Trends Cardiovasc Med* 2002; 12:13–19.

Olofsson B, Pajusola K, von Euler G, et al: Genomic organization of the mouse and human genes for vascular endothelial growth factor B (VEGF-B) and characterization of a second splice isoform. *J Biol Chem* 1996; 271:19310–19317.

Park JE, Chen HH, Winer J, et al: Placenta growth factor. Potentiation of vascular endothelial growth factor bioactivity, in vitro and in vivo, and high affinity binding to Flt-1 but not to Flk-1/KDR. *J Biol Chem* 1994; 269:25646–25654.

Pavlaki M, Zucker S: Matrix metalloproteinase inhibitors (MMPIs): the beginning of phase I or the termination of phase III clinical trials *Cancer Metastasis Rev* 2003; 22: 177–203.

Peters KG, Coogan A, Berry D, et al: Expression of Tie2/Tek in breast tumour vasculature provides a new marker for evaluation of tumour angiogenesis. *Br J Cancer* 1998; 77:51–56.

Plate KH, Breier G, Weich HA, Risau W: Vascular endothelial growth factor is a potential tumour angiogenesis factor in human gliomas *in vivo. Nature* 1992; 359:845–848.

Procopio WN, Pelavin PI, Lee WM, Yeilding NM: Angiopoietin-1 and -2 coiled coil domains mediate distinct homooligomerization patterns, but fibrinogen-like domains mediate ligand activity. *J Biol Chem* 1999; 274:30196–30201.

Quinn TP, Peters KG, De Vries C, et al: Fetal liver kinase 1 is a receptor for vascular endothelial growth factor and is selectively expressed in vascular endothelium. *Proc Natl Acad Sci USA* 1993; 90:7533–7537.

Rafii S, Lyden D, Benezra R, et al: Vascular and haematopoietic stem cells: novel targets for anti-angiogenesis therapy? *Nat Rev Cancer* 2002; 2:826–835.

Rafii S, Lyden D: Therapeutic stem and progenitor cell transplantation for organ vascularization and regeneration. *Nat Med* 2003; 9:702–712.

Rak J, Mitsuhashi Y, Bayko L, et al: Mutant ras oncogenes upregulate VEGF/VPF expression: implications for induction and inhibition of tumor angiogenesis. *Cancer Res* 1995; 55:4575–4580.

Rak J, Yu JL, Klement G, Kerbel RS: Oncogenes and angiogenesis: signaling three-dimensional tumor growth. *J Investig Dermatol Symp Proc* 2000; 5:24–33.

Ravi R, Mookerjee B, Bhujwalla ZM, et al: Regulation of tumor angiogenesis by p53–induced degradation of hypoxia-inducible factor 1alpha. *Genes Dev* 2000; 14:34–44.

Reynolds LP, Grazul-Bilska AT, Redmer DA: Angiogenesis in the female reproductive organs: pathological implications. *Int J Exp Pathol* 2002; 83:151–163.

Rissanen TT, Markkanen JE, Gruchala M, et al: VEGF-D is the strongest angiogenic and lymphangiogenic effector among VEGFs delivered into skeletal muscle via adenoviruses. *Circ Res* 2003; 92:1098–1106.

Rodriguez-Manzaneque JC, Lane TF, Ortega MA, et al: Thrombospondin-1 suppresses spontaneous tumor growth and inhibits activation of matrix metalloproteinase-9 and mobilization of vascular endothelial growth factor. *Proc Natl Acad Sci USA* 2001; 98:12485–12490.

Rupp PA, Little CD: Integrins in vascular development. *Circ Res* 2001; 89:566–572.

Semenza GL: Hypoxia-inducible factor 1: master regulator of $O_2$ homeostasis. *Curr Opin Genet Dev* 1998; 8:588–594.

Shalaby F, Rossant J, Yamaguchi TP, et al: Failure of blood-island formation and vasculogenesis in Flk-1–deficient mice. *Nature* 1995; 376:62–66.

Sherif ZA, Nakai S, Pirollo KF, et al: Downmodulation of bFGF-binding protein expression following restoration of p53 function. *Cancer Gene Ther* 2001; 8:771–782.

Shweiki D, Itin A, Soffer D, Keshet E: Vascular endothelial growth factor induced by hypoxia may mediate hypoxia-initiated angiogenesis. *Nature* 1992; 359:843–845 .

Sidky YA, Borden EC: Inhibition of angiogenesis by interferons: effects on tumor- and lymphocyte-induced vascular responses. *Cancer Res* 1987; 47:5155–5161.

Siemeister G, Schirner M, Weindel K, et al: Two independent mechanisms essential for tumor angiogenesis: inhibition of human melanoma xenograft growth by interfering with either the vascular endothelial growth factor receptor pathway or the Tie-2 pathway. *Cancer Res* 1999; 59:3185–3191.

Silvestre JS, Tamarat R, Ebrahimian TG, et al: Vascular endothelial growth factor-B promotes in vivo angiogenesis. *Circ Res* 2003; 93:114–123.

Singh RK, Gutman M, Bucana CD, et al: Interferons alpha and beta down-regulate the expression of basic fibroblast growth factor in human carcinomas. *Proc Natl Acad Sci USA* 1995; 92:4562–4566.

Singhal S, Mehta J, Desikan R, et al: Antitumor activity of thalidomide in refractory multiple myeloma. *N Engl J Med* 1999; 341:1565–1571.

Stacker SA, Caesar C, Baldwin ME, et al: VEGF-D promotes the metastatic spread of tumor cells via the lymphatics. *Nat Med* 2001; 7:186–191.

Stein I, Itin A, Einat P, et al: Translation of vascular endothelial growth factor mRNA by internal ribosome entry: implications for translation under hypoxia. *Mol Cell Biol* 1998; 18:3112–3119.

Suri C, Jones PF, Patan S, et al: Requisite role of angiopoietin-1, a ligand for the TIE2 receptor, during embryonic angiogenesis. *Cell* 1996; 87:1171–1180.

Takahashi N, Haba A, Matsuno F, Seon BK: Antiangiogenic therapy of established tumors in human skin/severe combined immunodeficiency mouse chimeras by anti-endoglin (CD105) monoclonal antibodies, and synergy between anti-endoglin antibody and cyclophosphamide. *Cancer Res* 2001; 61:7846–7854.

Takashima S, Kitakaze M, Asakura M, et al: Targeting of both mouse neuropilin-1 and neuropilin-2 genes severely impairs developmental yolk sac and embryonic angiogenesis. *Proc Natl Acad Sci USA* 2002; 99:3756–3662.

Thurston G, Rudge JS, Ioffe E, et al: Angiopoietin-1 protects the adult vasculature against plasma leakage. *Nat Med* 2000; 6:460–463.

Thurston G, Suri, Smith K, et al: Leakage-resistant blood vessels in mice transgenically overexpressing angiopoietin-1. *Science* 1999; 286:2511–2514.

Tonnesen MG, Feng X, Clark R: Angiogenesis in wound healing. *Investig Dermatol Symp Proc* 2000; 5:40–46.

Valenzuela DM, Griffiths JA, Rojas J, et al: Angiopoietins 3 and 4: diverging gene counterparts in mice and humans. *Proc Natl Acad Sci USA* 1999; 96:1904–1909.

Verheul HM, Panigrahy D, Yuan J, D'Amato RJ: Combination oral antiangiogenic therapy with thalidomide and sulindac inhibits tumour growth in rabbits. *Br J Cancer* 1999; 79:114–118.

Waltenberger J, Mayr U, Pentz S, Hombach V: Functional upregulation of the vascular endothelial growth factor receptor KDR by hypoxia. *Circulation* 1996; 94:1647–1654.

Wang HU, Chen ZF, Anderson DJ: Molecular distinction and angiogenic interaction between embryonic arteries and veins revealed by ephrin-B2 and its receptor Eph-B4. *Cell* 1998; 3:741–753.

Ward NL, Dumont DJ: The angiopoietins and Tie2/Tek: adding to the complexity of cardiovascular development. *Semin Cell Dev Biol* 2002, 1:19–27.

Watnick RS, Cheng YN, Rangarajan A, et al: Ras modulates Myc activity to repress thrombospondin-1 expression and increase tumor angiogenesis. *Cancer Cell* 2003; 3:219–231.

Xu Y, Yu Q: Angiopoietin-1, unlike angiopoietin-2, is incorporated into the extracellular matrix via its linker peptide region. *J Biol Chem* 2001; 276:34990–34998.

Yanase T, Tamura M, Fujita K, et al: Inhibitory effect of angiogenesis inhibitor TNP-470 on tumor growth and metastasis of human cell lines in vitro and in vivo. *Cancer Res* 1993; 53:2566–2570.

Yuan L, Moyon D, Pardanaud L, et al: Abnormal lymphatic vessel development in neuropilin 2 mutant mice. *Development* 2002; 129:4797–4806.

Zucker S, Cao J, Chen WT: Critical appraisal of the use of matrix metalloproteinase inhibitors in cancer treatment. *Oncogene* 2000; 19: 6642–6650.

# 13

# Imaging in Oncology

*Michael D. Sherar*

## 13.1 INTRODUCTION

Medical imaging is important for the diagnosis, staging, and monitoring of response to treatment in patients with cancer. The vast majority of procedures produce anatomic images based on endogenous contrast between human tissues. These images can be captured as a still image or monitored over time to understand the kinetics of a biological process.

Newer imaging methods, termed *functional and molecular imaging*, can provide information about the physiology, biochemistry, protein expression, and genetics of tissues. For clarity, *functional* imaging refers to studies that map changes in tumor or normal tissue function that are based on the interaction of many biochemical or physiological events, whereas *molecular* imaging refers to studies of single molecules that may be important in experimental or clinical oncology. For the purposes of this chapter, we shall restrict *molecular imaging* to those techniques capable of providing information in vivo within tumor and normal cells.

## 13.2 TECHNOLOGIES FOR ANATOMIC IMAGING AND STAGING OF TUMORS

### 13.2.1 Computed Tomography

Computed tomography (CT) scanning is based on the measurement of the amount of x-ray attenuation as x-rays pass through different tissues within the body (i.e., bone and soft tissues have different attenuation coefficients due to variable x-ray interactions within these tissues). Normally, the detection of x-rays after transmission through the body results in an image projected onto a two-dimensional plane and captured as a film or data file. This is the case with standard projection x-ray imaging used for chest x-rays (which can detect primary or secondary lung tumors) and mammography (to detect breast cancers), in which the solid tumor has a different attenuation coefficient from surrounding normal lung or breast tissues, respectively. In CT scanning, a cross-sectional image is obtained by exposure to a thin beam of x-rays throughout a 360° rotation, with a detector on the opposite side of the body to the source. The x-ray attenuation coefficients can be calculated as a function of the spatial location in the two-dimensional cross-sectional slice and are represented by different shades on a gray scale (termed *Hounsfield units*) within a computerized image. The administration of contrast agents that have a higher x-ray attenuation than the surrounding tissue can allow improved contrast, for example, in bowel or bladder, and the vasculature within tissues can be highlighted by injection of intravenous contrast material (Fig. 13.1). Both standard x-ray imaging and CT scanning provide only anatomical information.

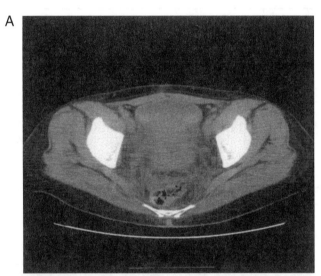

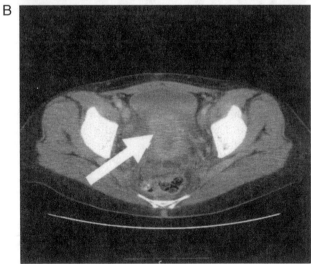

**Figure 13.1.** (*A*) Axial CT scan of the pelvis of a patient with carcinoma of the cervix. (*B*) Contrast enhanced image taken at 60 seconds after injection of x-ray contrast. The tumor (arrow) shows good enhancement due to uptake of the contrast agent.

## 13.2.2 Nuclear Medicine and Bone Scans

Nuclear medicine uses the introduction of radioactive agents into the body for the purposes of diagnosis or therapy (see Chap. 15, Sec. 15.2.3). Radioactive isotopes used for diagnostic imaging emit high-energy photons. The most commonly used radiopharmaceutical is technetium (Tc-99m, half-life ~6 hours) which produces 140 kiloelectronvolt photons. Technetium can be attached to biologically active compounds for cancer imaging. The photons can be detected by a large sodium iodide (NaI) crystal within the body scanner, which transforms the high-energy photons into light signals (scintillation) that are then detected using a photomultiplier tube. A spatial resolution of approximately 3 millimeters is achieved by placing a collimator between the patient and the NaI crystal to eliminate photons that are not traveling parallel to the collimator leaves.

Nuclear medicine imaging is used commonly for detecting the presence of metastatic disease to the bone. In one example, Tc-99m methylene diphosphonate (MDP) is injected intravenously into the patient and whole body imaging (lasting ~45 minutes) is undertaken 3 hours after the injection. The MDP is absorbed by and bound to bone matrix as a result of the osteoblastic activity caused by metastatic deposits. Any process that results in increased osteogenic activity or blood perfusion to bone will be detected, including infection, fracture, and metabolic disorders, so the scan must be interpreted with knowledge of the patient's clinical history.

Single photon emission computed tomography (SPECT) combines nuclear medicine imaging with CT reconstruction to render a three-dimensional display. Unlike conventional nuclear medicine imaging where the detector is static, the SPECT detector is rotated around the patient to give many views. Computed tomographic reconstruction methods are then used to create a three-dimensional image of the distribution of the radionucleotides in the body. Single photon emission computed tomography can also be used to quantify pharmacokinetics of a biologic tracer within the body using dynamic imaging techniques known as dSPECT (Celler et al., 2000).

Radionucleotides used for conventional scintigraphy and SPECT, such as Tc-99m, can be obtained from medical radionucleotides generators that do not require nuclear reactors or particle accelerators. As such, they provide a low cost and convenient method of radionucleotides delivery. However the radionucleotides produced by these generators are isotopes of atoms not found in most biochemical processes. Isotopes of nuclei commonly found in the body (e.g., carbon, nitrogen, oxygen, and fluorine) can be produced using a particle accelerator (usually a cyclotron) and then incorporated into agents that interact within intracellular metabolic pathways. Positron emission tomography (PET) can then be used to image the distribution of biochemicals labeled with isotopes of these common atoms.

### 13.2.3 Positron Emission Tomography

Positron emission tomography scanning is based on the detection of a radioactive tracer compound that emits a positron. The positron will, almost immediately, and without traveling more than a few microns, interact with an electron, resulting in the production of two 511 kev photons traveling in opposite directions. The photon pair is detected simultaneously by a ring of detectors surrounding the body in what is called an *emission scan*. This coincidence detection of photon pairs can be used to calculate the concentration of the injected tracer throughout a two-dimensional (2D) slice. The patient can be scanned in the third dimension to create a three-dimensional (3D) map of the tracer concentration. A second scan must be performed that uses an external tracer source. This *transmission scan* is used to correct the map formed by the emission scan for differences in photon attenuation throughout the body (Fig. 13.2A and B).

The main advantage of PET imaging is that high-resolution 3D images of radionucleotide distribution can be obtained that are specific to a particular biochemical pathway (e.g., glucose metabolism). However, PET scanning has some major disadvantages: imaging is restricted to positron-emitting radionucleotides which have short half-lives (i.e., minutes to hours); production of PET radionucleotides requires the use of a cyclotron, a very expensive particle accelerator; and sophisticated chemistry must be performed to incorporate the positron emitter into a biologically active compound (see Table 13.1 for a list of PET radionucleotides).

The tracer used most often in PET scanning is [18F]-fluorodeoxyglucose or FDG. Like glucose, FDG is phosphorylated in the cell by hexokinase but FDG-6-phosphate is not metabolized further and is trapped within the cell. The concentration of FDG in the cell is therefore a surrogate marker for the rate of glucose phosphorylation. The specific uptake of FDG is computer analyzed for a specific region of interest and reflected in an increased intensity on the resulting PET scan. [18F]-fluorodeoxyglucose uptake and retention is greater in many tumors than in normal tissues, so that PET scanning is a highly sensitive method for localizing and imaging tumors (Fig. 13.2C), in monitoring the response of tumors to treatment, (Fig. 13.2D and E). A

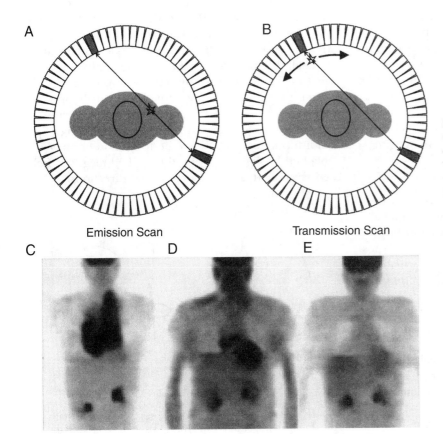

Emission Scan    Transmission Scan

**Figure 13.2.** Positron emission tomography (PET). (*A*) An emission scan is used for the detection of two 511 kiloelectronvolt photons produced by a positron/electron annihilation event. The annihilation event takes place within the patient and is detected by a 360° ring of detectors surrounding the patient. (*B*). A transmission scan then uses an external photon source for correction of the emitted information due to the attenuation by the various tissues within the body. (*C*) FDG-PET images of a patient with Hodgkin's disease in the mediastinum before (*C*), after first cycle (*D*), and at completion of (*E*) chemotherapy. Note clearance of disease from the mediastinum following chemotherapy.

**Table 13.1.** Radionucleotides Used in Positron Emission Tomography

| Radionucleotide | Half-Life | Imaging Application(s) |
| --- | --- | --- |
| Carbon-11 | 20 min | Metabolism, amino acids, tumor receptors |
| Fluorine-18 | 110 min | Glucose and chemotherapy drug analogs |
| Iodine-122 | 4 min | Blood flow |
| Iodine-124 | 4 day | Vascular growth, apoptosis |
| Iron-52 | 8 h | Bone marrow |
| Nitrogen-13 | 10 min | For vascular perfusion |
| Oxygen-15 | 120 sec | As $H_2O$ or CO for vascular perfusion |
| Rubidium-82 | 1 min | Vascular perfusion |
| Copper-64 | 13 h | Intratumoral hypoxia |

limitation of FDG imaging is that FDG has increased uptake within areas of inflammation, which confounds the image and its interpretation. The specificity and sensitivity (see Chap. 22, Sec. 22.2) of PET scanning is being actively investigated in relation to MRI and CT for diagnosis and staging.

A large number of other positron emitters can be used to develop tracers to investigate physiological and pathological processes (see Table 13.1). These include: [$^{11}$C]-thymidine as a marker for DNA synthesis, labeled estrogen and progesterone analogs for imaging receptor concentration, and imaging of hypoxia using a variety of copper, oxygen, or fluorine labeled compounds. Most probes have been targeted at proteins, but halogen labeling (F, Br, or I) of antisense oligonucleotides may allow imaging of mRNA within tissues (Tavitian, 2000). The major challenge is to achieve high enough sensitivity in PET imaging to detect the signal from labeled mRNA due to its very low copy number as compared to translated proteins in order to track transcription and translation using non-invasive imaging.

### 13.2.4 Magnetic Resonance Techniques

Magnetic resonance imaging (MRI) is based on magnetization of tissues when a patient is placed in a large externally applied magnetic field contained within the MRI scanner. Protons (and other atomic nuclei possessing a magnetic moment) within tissues oscillate, or *precess*, in this magnetic field (B) at a frequency (*v*) given by:

$$v = \gamma B$$

where the proportionality constant, $\gamma$, is called the gyromagnetic ratio (see Fig. 13.3). $\gamma$ is specific for each nucleus and depends on the magnetic moment of the nucleus.

The precession frequency of protons in a 1.5 tesla (T) magnetic field (i.e., the field strength of most clin-

ical scanners) is 64 megahertz giving an imaging resolution of approximately 1 millimeter. By applying a radiofrequency (RF) pulse of energy at this frequency, the angle at which the protons are precessing around the magnetic field lines can be changed, most commonly to 90° or at right angles to the magnetic field lines. Once the pulse is switched off, the angle of precession gradually returns to normal. The time taken for the return to normal (the T1 signal) is one factor that can provide contrast between tissues due to the variation in the biochemical environment experienced by the protons. Similarly, when the atoms are flipped into the transverse plane (180° to the magnetic field), the phase of their precession can be synchronized. Again, when the RF is switched off, the phase synchronicity gradually disappears. The time for the dephasing to occur (the T2 signal) is commonly used to optimally distinguish soft tissues in the body. Different RF-pulse sequences can be applied to give images with contrast that depend on T1 and T2 with a variety of weightings. Spatial information that allows the formation of images is obtained by slightly varying the applied magnetic field across the body in three orthogonal directions.

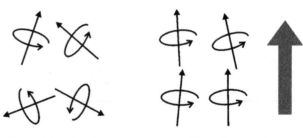

Normal (randomly arranged) magnetic nuclei.

Aligned magnetic nuclei under magnetic field (gray arrow).

**Figure 13.3.** Alignment of magnetic spins in the externally applied magnetic field in MRI. The spins precess around the applied magnetic field.

Magnetic resonance imaging has become a standard technique for diagnosis and staging of cancer due to the excellent soft tissue contrast and resolution, particularly for imaging the brain, head and neck, and pelvic region of the body (see Fig. 13.4).

Magnetic resonance spectroscopy imaging (MRSI) can be used to image metabolites in tissue. The frequency of precession of the atomic spins of nuclei around the magnetic field in the MRI scanner is dependent on the local biochemical environment. For example, the atomic spins nuclei of phosphorus atoms will precess at slightly different rates for a number of phosphorus-containing proteins. By applying radiofrequency energy during MRSI, the relative absorption of energy of the different biochemical species can be measured and expressed as nuclear magnetic resonance spectra (MRS) (chemical shift spectra) within tissues.

Examples of $^1H$ (proton) MRS are shown in Figure 13.5 for normal and cancerous brain tissues. Of particular interest here is the ratio of citrate to choline that can be calculated from these spectra within defined voxels or tissue locales. A map of the concentration of the molecules can then be overlaid on the anatomical im-

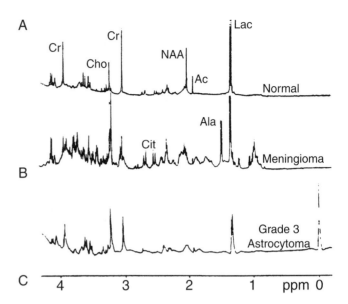

**Figure 13.5.** Chemical shift spectra of normal and cancerous brain tissues with identified biochemical species (e.g., Cho, choline; Lac, lactate; Cit, citrate; Ala, alanine; Ac, Acetate; Cr, Creatine; NAA, N-acetyl aspartate). The area under each peak can be used to quantify the concentrations of individual chemicals which together with spatial localization forms the basis of MRSI. Note the relative amount of citrate-to-choline is different between normal and tumor tissues.

age. Using this analysis, the citrate-to-choline ratio was found to be altered in tumors as compared to normal tissues, due to the relative proliferation of cells and the corresponding metabolic rates.

The absorption of RF energy in the magnetic field as a function of frequency by atoms such as $^{31}P$, $^{19}F$, $^{23}Na$ can also be imaged using MRSI. However, the signal strength is usually much weaker than for $^1H$ because the natural abundance of these elements in tissue is much lower than hydrogen. Phosphorus spectroscopy is informative because of its importance in many biochemical pathways and its presence in bone, both of which can be used to distinguish primary and metastatic tumors from surrounding normal tissues.

The signal-to-noise ratio for all types of MRI, including MRSI, is improved with the use of higher magnetic field strengths. Three-tesla magnets are now common and are particularly useful for MRSI. Much higher field magnets, including those of 7 tesla for human imaging and those up to 12 tesla for small animal studies, are now also available.

Although MRSI can image the distribution of individual molecular species, it is restricted to imaging abundant metabolites. New approaches that may allow the imaging of molecules at much lower concentrations involve the use of contrast agents. Contrast agents can be synthesized by incorporating gadolinium or iron into molecular probes that reflect a tumor's inherent biology or genetics. Even with the introduction of contrast agents, amplification strategies are often required to al-

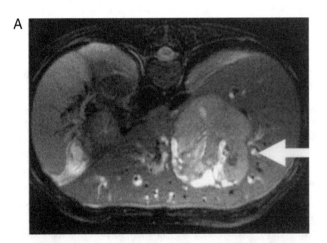

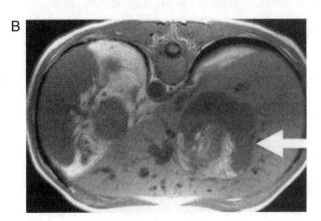

**Figure 13.4.** T1 (A) and T2 (B) weighted images of multiple liver metastases (arrows) of melanoma demonstrating different contrast.

low detection by MRI. One amplification strategy involves the attachment of a transferrin receptor to a membrane-bound receptor of interest, which, when activated, translocates to within the cell and traps the iron providing a better image of cells within tissues.

A new class of paramagnetic contrast agents that can be activated to change their magnetic properties by a molecule of interest has recently been developed (Louie et al., 2000). These agents usually incorporate a gadolinium ion that is physically shielded by the molecular structure from surrounding water so that it cannot affect the local magnetic field experienced by the water and therefore does not affect contrast. The contrast agent is constructed such that the target molecule of interest, when it interacts with the agent, changes the structure to uncover the gadolinium ion, resulting in association with surrounding water and a change in signal. The high specificity of such an approach may allow molecules with very low tissue concentrations to be mapped with MRI.

### 13.2.5 Ultrasound

Standard B-mode ultrasound imaging is based on the reflection of very high frequency sound signals (in the megahertz range) from tissue interfaces. The ultrasound source, usually a piezoelectric crystal, generates a short ultrasound pulse that penetrates the tissue and is reflected by structures with different mechanical properties. An image is formed by time-gating the signals scattered back to the transducer. The scattering of ultrasound by tumor and normal tissues is often different, leading to tissue contrast in the ultrasound image. Ultrasound imaging has become an important tool in visualizing tumors, particularly in the soft tissue of the abdomen where both the ultrasound transmission and soft-tissue interface is optimal (see Fig. 13.6). Ultrasound does not pass sufficiently through bone to allow its use for imaging bony structures.

An important application in cancer diagnosis uses *Doppler ultrasound*, which measures the Doppler shift in frequency when the ultrasound scatters from moving objects, such as red blood cells in the vasculature. The ultrasound frequency employed in standard high-resolution scanners is in the 5-to-20 megahertz range, leading to Doppler shifts due to blood flow in the 1 kilohertz range. This technique can be used to measure blood flow in large vessels and has been used to visualize tumor versus normal tissues, and to diagnose blood clots which interrupt blood flow. The method can be adapted to visualize flow in smaller vessels.

### 13.2.6 In Vivo Optical Imaging

Optical imaging techniques that rely on fluorescence, reflectance, or bioluminescence as contrast mechanisms can be used to provide images of specific mole-

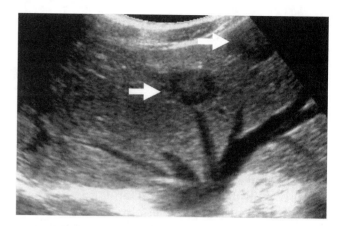

**Figure 13.6.** Transverse ultrasound image through the liver shows a tree of large blood vessels and hypoechoic liver metastases (arrows) from nasopharyngeal cancer. (Courtesy of Martin E. O'Malley, MD, Department of Medical Imaging, University Health Network and Mount Sinai Hospital, University of Toronto.)

cules or complexes in vivo. In general, these techniques are restricted to the imaging of small animals or superficial targets in humans, due to the relatively short penetration depth of light in tissue.

Fluorescence imaging involves exposure of a target tissue containing fluorescent molecules to a source of light of specific wavelength—the *absorption spectra*. The fluorescent molecules are excited to a higher energy state by the light and then relax to a lower energy state through a different energy transition, thereby emitting light of a different *emission* spectra (i.e., color) which is detected using a CCD (charge-coupled device) camera. Most biological molecules of interest are not naturally fluorescent and therefore must be labeled with exogenous fluorescent contrast agents such as infrared fluorescent probes or green fluorescent protein (GFP). Bioluminescence imaging is based on biochemical reactions involving the luciferase gene. This approach has been common in imaging individual cells which express the luciferase gene with a specialized microscope and is now possible in vivo with the development of bioluminescence cameras.

For experimental oncology, high-resolution optical images can be obtained in small animals using intravital microscopy (Jain et al., 2002). The live animal is placed such that the region bearing the tumor or area of interest is exposed. Images of a single plane in the live tumor can be obtained using a confocal laser scanning microscope (CLSM) or a multiphoton laser scanning microscope (MPLSM). The CLSM accepts light originating from a single plane in the tumor using a pinhole that is placed in the path to the lens. In the MPSLM, fluorescence is activated in one plane only using a focused infrared laser, and the excitation that is detected for the image only occurs at the focal spot of the laser. If the focal area is scanned in two dimensions, an image of fluorescence at a constant depth in the tumor is produced. These techniques have been used to visualize experimental angiogenesis and metastasis in vivo (see Chap. 11, Sec. 11.3.2).

## 13.3 FUNCTIONAL AND MOLECULAR IMAGING

### 13.3.1 Blood Flow, Angiogenesis, and Hypoxia

The vascular tree that develops in tumors is quite different in organization from the normal vasculature. Tumor vasculature is often characterized by spatial heterogeneity, abnormal arteriovenous shunts, transient flow, and leaky vessels. These differences may be useful predictors of tumor aggressiveness and response to therapy (see Chap. 12, Sec. 12.4.3).

Measurement of blood flow within a tumor may provide a useful surrogate marker for hypoxia. Hypoxia has been linked to both genetic instability and resistance to radiation therapy (see Chap. 15, Sec. 15.4). In addition, if tumor blood flow is compromised, the effectiveness of systemically applied therapy may be reduced. The absolute rate of blood flow through a tissue cannot be measured with medical imaging techniques. However, CT- and MRI-based methods have been developed based on measuring the appearance and disappearance of contrast agents following a bolus intravenous injection.

The mathematical analysis of signals and their relationship to tracer kinetics is similar for CT and MRI. The injected tracer flows through the vasculature with some escaping into the tissue compartment through the vessel walls. The amount of tracer that is detected at a particular location/image voxel is dependent on the tracer that previously entered the voxel locale and the amount of tracer that is washed out from the voxel locale, either through the tissue or blood compartment. From measurements of the signal changes caused by in-

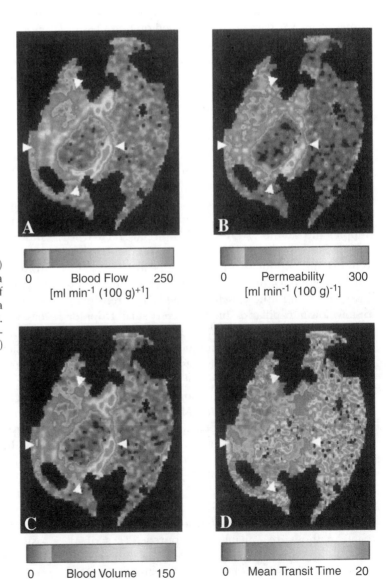

**Figure 13.7.** Functional CT perfusion maps of (A) blood flow, (B) microvessel permeability surface area product, (C) blood volume, and (D) mean transit of blood time as measured in a VX-2 tumor grown in a rabbit thigh (arrowheads mark the tumor boundary). Note the vascular rim (A,B,C) and the long blood transit time in the core (D). (From Purdie et al., 2001.) (See color plate.)

jection of a bolus of tracer into a local artery and the signal changes in the perfused tissue, four parameters can be calculated: blood flow, blood volume, mean transit time, and vessel permeability (see Fig. 13.7). The accuracy of the method is limited by the models and their assumptions, but can correlate well with more invasive techniques (e.g., injection and imaging of intravascular microspheres; Purdie et al., 2001).

Magnetic resonance imaging can be used in a similar way to measure perfusion, although an extra step is required. The vascular contrast agent used in MRI, most often Gd-PTA, causes a change in relaxation time due to its high magnetic susceptibility compared with blood or tissue. *Gradient-echo MR* techniques are used to measure the MR signal with and without contrast (the ratio of which is used to calculate the concentration of contrast agent). The time-dependent concentration at each location can then be used as input into a similar mathematical model of washout as described above for CT to determine blood kinetic parameters. Most perfusion studies using MR have been performed on brain tissue. This simplifies the mathematics because the contrast agent can be assumed to remain in the blood compartment due to the blood-brain barrier.

Clinical MRI studies (e.g., Hawighorst et al., 1997) have demonstrated correlations between perfusion, microvessel density measured by histology, and measures of tumor aggressiveness such as lymph node involvement. Due to the very good resolution of MRI, perfusion imaging can be used in experimental tumor models to monitor angiogenesis (Dennie et al., 1998) and anti-angiogenic therapies.

Blood flow can also be measured directly using Doppler ultrasound as the signal is directly related to flow. However, quantification of perfusion with ultrasound is difficult due to a number of factors. These include dependence on the angle of incidence of the ultrasound beam to the vessels and the lack of sensitivity to slow flow in capillaries due to the very small Doppler frequency shift produced. With the development of high frequency Doppler techniques, accurate quantification of flow in much smaller vessels is possible.

In addition to measurement of perfusion, more direct molecular events in the angiogenic process can be followed in vivo. These include MR imaging of endothelial integrin levels using liposomes filled with a paramagnetic material (Sipkins et al., 1998), radiolabeled analogs of a urokinase plasminogen activator receptor agonist, and radiolabeled TGF-$\beta$ (Bredow et al., 2000) (see Chaps. 8 and 11).

No imaging method is available for directly and noninvasively measuring oxygen tension in tissues, but surrogate methods are available. One approach (described above) is to correlate blood flow imaging with the hypoxic state of tissues based on the fact that acute and chronic hypoxia are related to a lack of blood flow.

However, no studies have directly linked blood flow imaging to the fraction of hypoxic cells within tumors.

Additional approaches to indirect imaging of oxygen using MRI include: (1) BOLD (blood oxygen level dependent)-imaging, and (2) $^{19}F$ imaging following perfluoro-carbon injection. BOLD imaging exploits the natural paramagnetization difference between oxy- and de-oxyhemoglobin, which represent well- and poorly-oxygenated blood, respectively. The increase in paramagnetization upon deoxygenation leads to an inhomogeneity in the local magnetic field, which in turn causes a decrease in the T2 relaxation time. T2-weighted images can then be used to image perfusion changes that cause a change in oxygenation and this technique is being investigated as a potential marker of intratumoral hypoxia. The second approach is based on the T1 signal relaxation time of $^{19}F$, which is dependent on the local oxygen tension (Mason et al., 1996). A major challenge with this method is achieving high enough tissue concentrations of $^{19}F$ to give a sufficient signal-to-noise ratio for tissue oximetry.

Electron paramagnetic resonance (EPRI) techniques are sensitive to oxygen concentration and can give spatial information on oxygen tension within tissues. Measurements of oxygen tension in tissue are now possible with the availability of water soluble and biologically compatible paramagnetic agents whose excitation is oxygen dependent (Ardenkjaer-Larsen et al., 1998).

Magnetic resonance imaging techniques based on the Overhauser effect (OMRI) couple MRI with EPR to give sensitive tissue oximetry combined with anatomical mapping. Electron paramagnetic resonance contrast in the MR image is achieved by including an RF pulse sequence that elicits the Overhauser effect. This effect is based on the excitation of a paramagnetic contrast agent using RF energy as in EPRI. However, the excited contrast agent also causes an increase in the MR signal from the surrounding water molecules. OMRI-based oximetry has been studied in animal tumors and shown good agreement with polarographic oxygen measurements using an Eppendorf electrode (Fig. 13.8; Krishna et al., 2002; see Chap. 15, Sec. 15.4.3). Useful spatial ($\sim1$ mm) and temporal (2 min) resolution can be achieved with this method. The main challenge in extending this technique to imaging in humans is the relatively high RF power required, which could cause local heating.

Other approaches to tissue oxygenation using nuclear imaging have been based on molecules that are activated to bind in hypoxic tissues. Hypoxia imaging using standard nuclear imaging or SPECT has been demonstrated using $^{125}I$-labeled iodoazomycin arabinoside (IAZA; Urtasun et al., 1996) as well as PET imaging using $^{18}F$ labeled fluoromisonidazole (FMISO; Rasey et al., 1996) and $^{18}F$-fluoroerythronitroimidazole (FETNIM; Lehtio et al., 2001). Given that most of the imaging methods

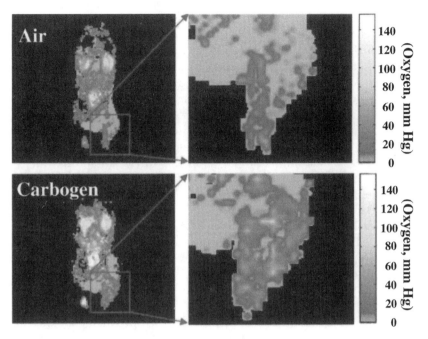

**Figure 13.8.** The Overhauser effect and MRI used to produce tissue oxygenation ($pO_2$) images of a C3H mouse with a 1-cm diameter squamous cell carcinoma tumor during air breathing (upper) and carbogen breathing (lower). The expanded tumor region (right) shows $pO_2$ heterogeneity. (Reprinted from Krishna et al., 2002.) (See color plate.)

described indirectly probe oxygenation, it is useful to calibrate them against other standard biological or physical measurements. One approach is to perform in vivo or in vitro radiosensitivity assays on the same tumors that are imaged by a specific technique (Kavanagh et al., 1996). Another approach is to use the Eppendorf $pO_2$ probe, a needle-based microelectrode that measures oxygen tension directly in human tumors (see Chap. 15, Sec. 15.4.3).

### 13.3.2 Tumor Biochemistry

[$^{18}$F]-fluorodeoxyglucose/positron emission tomography imaging is based on altered glucose uptake into cells as discussed in Section 13.2.3. However, FDG metabolism can vary considerably depending on tissue and cell type. It is also complicated by other factors including endogenous levels of adenosine triphosphate (ATP), insulin, hexokinase, oxygen, and cell cycle status.

The uptake of radiolabeled metabolites and subsequent imaging using PET or SPECT is being studied. Carbon-labeled thymidine ([$^{11}$C]-thymidine) was first studied as an imaging agent, because of the four bases incorporated into DNA, thymidine is the only base not to be incorporated in RNA, and the background signal due to RNA synthesis can therefore be avoided. This method is analogous to the use of tritiated thymidine to study cell proliferation (see Chap. 9, Sec. 9.4.2). Use of labeled thymidine suffers from the fact that rapid metabolism removes most of the injected compound before incorporation into DNA and the distribution of labeled metabolites makes interpretation and quantification of images difficult. Solutions to this problem have included the development of a modified mathematical uptake model that takes into account labeled

metabolites, the use of long half-life tracers that can be imaged after labeled metabolites have cleared the tissue (e.g., [$^{124}$I]IUdR or [$^{76}$Br]BudR), or the use of labeled thymidine analogs that are resistant to metabolism.

### 13.3.3 Imaging of Receptors

Receptors for hormones and growth factors are potential targets for molecular imaging that might be used to assess the heterogeneity of receptor expression in tumors. Nuclear imaging, particularly PET, has the sensitivity to detect radiolabeled steroid receptors at physiologic concentrations. Several halogenated estrogens, progesterones, and androgens (usually labeled with $^{18}$F due to the long half-life) have been developed for the imaging of receptor status in breast and prostate cancers (Mankoff et al., 2000). Uptake of $^{18}$F-fluoroestradiol (FES) in breast tumors, as measured using PET, correlates well with conventional ligand binding assays of estrogen receptor concentration (Mintun et al., 1988; Chap. 19, Sec. 19.2). This imaging method was able to predict for response to tamoxifen hormone therapy in estrogen receptor positive metastatic breast cancer (Dedashti et al., 1999).

### 13.3.4 Gene Expression

Magnetic resonance imaging, PET, and optical imaging have been used to map the expression of genes in tumors of animals, and more recently, in cancer patients. One goal of this work is to develop noninvasive techniques for monitoring gene therapy and the distribution of gene expression when constructs are introduced systemically in host animals or patients. The first studies using PET were aimed at mapping the expression of *HSV1-tk*, a gene from the herpes simplex virus that can activate the drug gancyclovir into a cytotoxin in mice (Tjuvajev et al., 1998). HSV1-tk expression was imaged by injecting radioactive-labeled FIAU (2-fluoro-2'-deoxy-5-iodo-1-β-D-arabinofuranosyluracil). The enzyme product of HSV-tk acts by adding phosphate groups to thymidine, which in turn converts FIAU into a form that is trapped in cells. The uptake of FIAU is then proportional to the level of expression of HSV-tk. This is an example of imaging protein function within cells and tumors using an amplification strategy. Positron emission tomography images in rats, mice, and humans have demonstrated the feasibility of this technique for monitoring gene therapy (Jacobs et al., 2001; Yaghoubi et al., 2001).

It is also possible to use PET to monitor endogenous genes using a similar technique. The same gene, HSV-tk, can be linked to a DNA fragment that is controlled by an endogeneous gene. In a study of this type, HSV-tk was linked to a *p21^{WAF}* sequence activated by the p53 tumor suppressor protein following DNA damage (e.g., due to chemotherapy). The activity of p53 intracellular signaling after treatment with BCNU (which damages the DNA) was then imaged in a rat tumor model (Fig. 13.9; Doubrovin et al., 2001).

Imaging of gene expression by MR is being developed with the promise of higher resolution than can be obtained with PET (Louie et al., 2000). The methods are based on the activation of contrast agents by gene products in which activation of the gene leads to removal of sugar residues on the contrast agent, making it more amenable to visualization by MR methods. Imaging of gene expression using B-galactosidase activation of MRI contrast agents will allow genes with a *lacZ* marker to be mapped in three dimensions with living organisms.

As introduced in Section 13.2.6, optical imaging has been developed that allows visualization of fluorescently tagged endogenous genes whose distribution of expression within tumor or normal tissues can be imaged using CCD cameras. An early demonstration of this technology involved the attachment of the *luciferase* gene to a DNA sequence that is activated by dimethylsulfide. When this chemical was injected into the mice, the *luciferase* gene was expressed producing a molecule that fluoresces in the visible spectrum.

### 13.3.5 Drug and Biological Agents

Pharmacokinetics has traditionally been studied by examining blood or tissue samples at different times af-

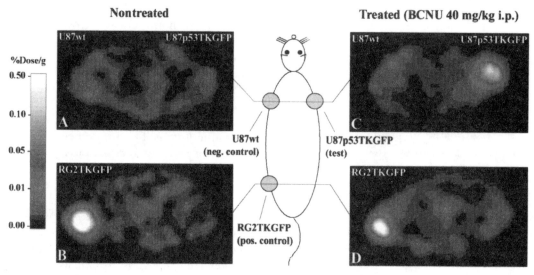

**Figure 13.9.** Positron emission tomography imaging of endogenous p53 activation using the HSV-tk reporter. Positron emission tomography images through the shoulder (*A* and *C*) and pelvis (*B* and *D*) of two rats are shown. A nontreated animal is shown on the left, and a BCNU-treated (to promote p53 activity) animal is shown on the right. Both animals had three subcutaneous tumor xenografts expressing mutant *p53* (test) in the right shoulder, wild-type *p53* (negative control) in the left shoulder, and a tumor line which constituitively expresses the HSV-tk reporter (positive control) in the left thigh. The nontreated animal on the left shows localization of radioactivity only in the positive control tumor (left thigh); the test and negative control tumors are at background levels. The BCNU-treated animal on the right shows significant localization of radioactivity in the test tumor (right shoulder) and in the positive control (left thigh), but no radioactivity above background in the negative control (left shoulder). (From Doubrovin, 2001.) (See color plate.)

ter injection of a drug (see Chap. 16, Sec. 16.1). A more detailed pharmokinetic study might be possible using molecular imaging techniques with either PET or MRSI because, in theory, 3D-volumetric data are available. Most work in this area has been performed with 5-[$^{18}$F]-fluorouracil (5-[$^{18}$F]U), which is a radioactively-labeled version of the anticancer drug 5-FU. The same preparation is used with PET imaging because the fluorine isotope is a positron emitter.

The isotopes of platinum $^{191}$Pt, $^{193m}$Pt, $^{195m}$Pt, and $^{197}$Pt emit $\gamma$-rays that can be imaged using standard $\gamma$-camera techniques or SPECT (see Sec. 13.2.2), allowing the imaging of cisplatin and related drugs. Most studies have used $^{191}$Pt, which can be produced in a cyclotron, or $^{195m}$Pt, which requires production in a nuclear reactor. Both suffer from relatively poor production efficiency and in vivo the active metabolites cannot be differentiated from nonactive drug. Consequently, an image of total platinum is produced. To distinguish signals from different metabolites, multicompartment pharmacokinetic models have been employed (Dowell et al., 2000), although these may give inaccurate results due to variations in the model parameters from animal to animal or patient to patient.

### 13.3.6 Cell Death and Apoptosis

Traditional endpoints for evaluating apoptosis have been based on techniques used on tissue sections, and it has been difficult to develop noninvasive endpoints in vivo (see Chap. 10, Sec. 10.3). New methods for imaging apoptosis in vivo have now been developed using MRSI, radionucleotide or PET imaging, and high-frequency ultrasound. High-frequency ultrasound is exquisitely sensitive to the process of apoptosis; experiments demonstrated that the condensation and fragmentation of DNA during the process of apoptosis leads to a large increase in scattering of high frequency ultrasound by apoptotic cells as compared to normal cells (Fig. 13.10, Czarnota et al., 1999). Although the individual cells are not resolvable in the B-scan images, areas containing as few as 5 percent apoptotic cells may be detectable against a background of normal cells (Kolios et al., 2002). One limitation of high-frequency ultrasound is the relatively poor penetration; on the order of 1 centimeter at 30 to 50 megahertz, which limits the noninvasive detection of apoptosis to superficial tumors or those body cavities where a probe can be introduced.

Magnetic resonance imaging technology is being developed to detect apoptosis noninvasively within deeper tissues in humans. In vitro studies have indicated that $^1$H MRS may detect an increase in intracellular triglycerides and free fatty acids that are associated with membrane changes during apoptosis (Blankenberg et al., 1996; Hakukami et al., 1999). Changes in lipid metabolism during apoptosis have also been detected using $^{31}$P MRS, including changes in the level of phosphocholine, perhaps due to breakdown of sphingomyelin (Adebodun and Post, 1994; Willliams et al., 1998; Ronen et al., 1999). However, these changes are quite cell-type dependent and a limitation for human studies is the poor sensitivity of MRSI to detect small fractions of apoptotic cells that might occur in tumors.

Molecules associated with apoptotic breakdown in the cell can be radiolabeled in order to image their function in vivo. Annexin V, which binds to phosphatidylserine (PS) on the cell surface, can be used as a surrogate marker for apoptosis (see Chap. 10, Sec. 10.3.1). Annexin V has been labeled with a variety of radioactive isotopes for PET, SPECT, or conventional nuclear imaging (Blankenberg and Strauss, 2001). Some of these agents have been used in the clinic to study apoptosis in the central nervous system, the heart, and bone.

### 13.4 SUMMARY

The development of anatomic, functional and molecular imaging has provided important insights into tumor

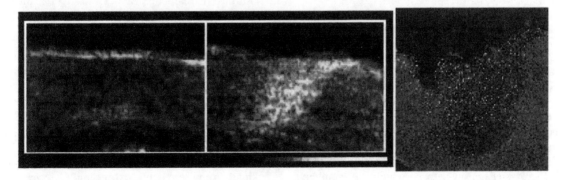

**Figure 13.10.** High-frequency ultrasound images of apoptosis in response to photodynamic therapy (PDT) in rat brain. *Left*: untreated; *middle*: 24 hours after PDT; *right*: TUNEL assay of same region. High-frequency ultrasound images are 4 mm × 4 mm. (See color plate.)

physiology and staging. As these methods mature they will add to the tools available for management of cancer patients, including the distribution and activity of systemic agents in patients, and the planning of radiotherapy. Molecular imaging is now providing a window into tumor function at the molecular level. As the role of genes and proteins in tumor physiology are discovered, their study in vivo is likely to develop rapidly as creative labeling of the target molecules or genes for MR, PET, and optical imaging becomes common.

## REFERENCES

Adebodun F, Post JF: $^{31}$P NMR characterization of cellular metabolism during dexamethasone induced apoptosis in human leukemic cell lines. *J Cell Physiol* 1994; 158:180–186.

Ardenkjaer-Larsen JH, Laursen I, Leunbach I, et al: EPR and DNP properties of certain novel single electron contrast agents intended for oximetric imaging. *J Magn Reson* 1998; 133:1–12.

Blankenberg FG, Storrs RW, Naumovski L, et al: Detection of apoptotic cell death by proton nuclear magnetic resonance spectroscopy. *Blood* 1996; 87:1951–1956.

Blankenberg FG, Strauss HW: Will imaging of apoptosis play a role in clinical care? A tale of mice and men. *Apoptosis* 2001; 6:117–123.

Bredow S, Lewin M, Hofmann B, et al: Imaging of tumour neovasculature by targeting the TGF-beta binding receptor endoglin. *Eur J Cancer* 2000; 36:675–681.

Celler A, Farncombe T, Bever C, et al: Performance of the dynamic single photon emission computed tomography (dSPECT) method for decreasing or increasing activity changes. *Phys Med Biol* 2000; 45:3525–3543.

Czarnota GJ, Kolios MC, Abraham J, et al: Ultrasound imaging of apoptosis: high-resolution non-invasive monitoring of programmed cell death in vitro, in situ and in vivo. *Br J Cancer* 1999; 81:520–527.

Dehdashti F, Flanagan FL, Mortimer JE, et al: Positron emission tomographic assessment of "metabolic flare" to predict response of metastatic breast cancer to antiestrogen therapy. *Eur J Nucl Med* 1999; 26:51–56.

Dennie J, Mandeville JB, Boxerman JL, et al: NMR imaging of changes in vascular morphology due to tumor angiogenesis. *Magn Reson Med* 1998; 40:793–799.

Doubrovin M, Ponomarev V, Beresten T, et al: Imaging transcriptional regulation of p53–dependent genes with positron emission tomography in vivo. *Proc Natl Acad Sci USA* 2001; 98:9300–9305.

Hakumaki JM, Poptani H, Sandmair AM, et al: $^1$H MRS detects polyunsaturated fatty acid accumulation during gene therapy of glioma: implications for the in vivo detection of apoptosis. *Nat Med* 1999; 5:1323–1327.

Hawighorst H, Knapstein PG, Weikel W, et al: Angiogenesis of uterine cervical carcinoma: characterization by pharmacokinetic magnetic resonance parameters and histological microvessel density with correlation to lymphatic involvement. *Cancer Res* 1997; 57:4777–4786.

Jacobs A, Voges J, Reszka R, et al: Positron-emission tomography of vector-mediated gene expression in gene therapy for gliomas. *Lancet* 2001; 358:727–729.

Jain RK, Munn LL, Fukumura D: Dissecting tumour pathophysiology using intra-vital microscopy. *Nat Rev Cancer* 2002; 2:266–276.

Kavanagh MC, Sun A, Hu Q, Hill RP. Comparing techniques of measuring tumor hypoxia in different murine tumors: Eppendorf pO2 Histograph, [3H]misonidazole binding and paired survival assay. *Radiat Res* 1996; 145:491–500.

Kolios MC, Czarnota GJ, Lee M, et al: Ultrasonic spectral parameter characterization of apoptosis. *Ultrasound Med Biol* 2002; 28:589–597.

Krishna MC, English S, Yamada K, et al: Overhauser enhanced magnetic resonance imaging for tumor oximetry: coregistration of tumor anatomy and tissue oxygen concentration. *Proc Natl Acad Sci USA* 2002; 99:2216–2221.

Lehtio K, Oikonen V, Gronroos T, et al: Imaging of blood flow and hypoxia in head and neck cancer: initial evaluation with [(15)O]H(2)O and [(18)F]fluoroerythronitroimidazole PET. *J Nucl Med* 2001; 42:1643–1652.

Louie AY, Huber MM, Ahrens ET, et al: In vivo visualization of gene expression using magnetic resonance imaging. *Nat Biotechnol* 2000; 18:321–325.

Mintun MA, Welch MJ, Siegel BA, et al: Breast cancer: PET imaging of estrogen receptors. *Radiology* 1988; 169:45–48.

Purdie TG, Henderson E, Lee TY: Functional CT imaging of angiogenesis in rabbit VX2 soft-tissue tumour. *Phys Med Biol* 2001; 46:3161–3175.

Rasey JS, Koh WJ, Evans ML, et al: Quantifying regional hypoxia in human tumors with positron emission tomography of [18F]fluoromisonidazole: a pretherapy study of 37 patients. *Int J Radiat Oncol Biol Phys* 1996; 36:417–428.

Ronen SM, DiStefano F, McCoy CL, et al: Magnetic resonance detects metabolic changes associated with chemotherapy-induced apoptosis. *Br J Cancer* 1999; 80:1035–1041.

Sipkins DA, Cheresh DA, Kazemi MR, et al: Detection of tumor angiogenesis in vivo by alphaVbeta3–targeted magnetic resonance imaging. *Nature Med* 1998; 4:623–626.

Tavitian B: In vivo antisense imaging. *Q J Nucl Med* 2000; 44:236–255.

Tjuvajev JG, Avril N, Oku T, et al: Imaging herpes virus thymidine kinase gene transfer and expression by positron emission tomography. *Cancer Res* 1998;58:4333–4341.

Urtasun RC, Parliament MB, McEwan AJ, et al: Measurement of hypoxia in human tumours by non-invasive SPECT imaging of iodoazomycin arabinoside. *Br J Cancer* 1996; 27(Suppl):S209–S212.

Williams SN, Anthony ML, Brindle KM: Induction of apoptosis in two mammalian cell lines results in increased levels of fructose-1,6-bisphosphate and CDP-choline as determined by $^{31}$P MRS. *Magn Reson Med* 1998; 40:411–420.

Yaghoubi S, Barrio JR, Dahlbom M, et al: Human pharmacokinetic and dosimetry studies of [(18)F]FHBG: a reporter probe for imaging herpes simplex virus type-1 thymidine kinase reporter gene expression. *J Nucl Med* 2001; 42:1225–1234.

# 14

# Molecular and Cellular Basis of Radiotherapy

*Robert G. Bristow and Richard P. Hill*

## 14.1 INTRODUCTION

Since their discovery by Roentgen more than a century ago, x-rays have played a major role in modern medicine. The first recorded use of x-rays for the treatment of cancer occurred within about 1 year of their discovery. Subsequently there has been intensive study of x-rays and other ionizing radiations, and their clinical application to cancer treatment has become increasingly sophisticated. This chapter and Chapter 15 review the biological effects of ionizing radiation and the application of that knowledge to cancer treatment.

The present chapter begins with a review of the physical properties of ionizing radiations, their interactions within the cell (membrane, cytoplasm, and nucleus), and the molecular and cellular processes that ensue. The effect of energy deposition in tissue is discussed with emphasis on the pathways that control cellular proliferation following exposure to ionizing radiation. Finally, various genetic and epigenetic factors known

to influence the relative radiosensitivity of normal and tumor cells are described in the context of using molecular targets for designing treatment and predicting response to radiotherapy.

## 14.2 INTERACTION OF RADIATION WITH MATTER

### 14.2.1 Types of Radiation, Energy Deposition, and Measurements of Radiation Dose

X- and $\gamma$-rays constitute part of the continuous spectrum of electromagnetic (EM) radiation that includes radio waves, heat, and visible and ultraviolet (UV) light (see Fig. 14.1). All types of EM radiation can be considered as moving packets (quanta) of energy called *photons*. The amount of energy in each individual photon defines its position in the electromagnetic spectrum. For example, x- or $\gamma$-ray photons carry more energy than heat or light photons and are at the high energy end of the EM spectrum. Individual photons of

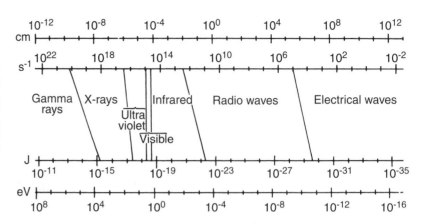

**Figure 14.1.** Electromagnetic spectrum showing the relationship of photon wavelength in centimeters (cm) to its frequency in inverse seconds ($s^{-1}$) and to its energy in joules (J) and electron volts (eV). The various bands in the spectrum are indicated. Slanted lines between bands indicate the degree of overlap in the definition of the various bands.

x-rays are sufficiently energetic that their interaction with matter can result in the complete displacement of an electron from its orbit around the nucleus of an atom. Such an atom (or molecule) is left with a net (positive) charge and is thus an ion; hence the term *ionizing radiation.* Typical binding energies for electrons in biological material are in the neighborhood of 10 electron volts. Thus, photons with energies greater than 10 electron volts are considered to be ionizing radiation, while photons with energies of 2 to 10 electron volts are in the UV range and are nonionizing. An interaction that transfers energy, but does not completely displace an electron, produces an "excited" atom or molecule and is called an *excitation.*

X-rays are produced when accelerated electrons hit a tungsten target and then decelerate emitting a spectrum of *bremsstrahlung* radiation. The resulting spectrum is filtered to produce a clinically useful beam with minimal x-ray scatter from the axis of the central beam. When x-ray photons interact with tissue, they give up energy by one of three processes: the photoelectric effect, the Compton effect, or pair production. In the energy range most widely used in radiotherapy (100 keV to 25 MeV), the Compton effect is the most important mechanism leading to deposition of energy in tissue. This energy-transfer process involves a billiard-ball type of collision between the photon and an outer orbital electron of an atom, with partial transfer of energy to the electron and scattering of the photon into a new direction. The electron (and the photon) can then undergo further interactions, causing more ionizations and excitations, until its energy is dissipated. All three of the interaction processes mentioned above result in the production of energetic electrons that, in turn, lose energy by exciting and ionizing target atoms and molecules and setting more electrons in motion.

Modern clinical radiotherapy uses ionizing radiation to treat cancer patients and can be delivered to tissues by external beam radiotherapy using linear accelerators (i.e., high energy x-rays and electron beams), $^{60}$Co sources ($\gamma$-rays produced by radioactive decay due to unstable nuclei), or charged particle accelerators. Clinical radiotherapy can also be given using *brachytherapy,* which delivers highly localized radiation dose from within an organ or tissue using implanted wires or "seeds" containing radioisotopes such as $^{125}$I, $^{198}$Au, or $^{103}$Pd that undergo radioactive decay (see Chap. 15).

Due to their initial attenuation within the first few millimeters of tissue, low energy x-ray beams (50 to 250 keV) deposit their energy at or just below the skin surface, and are therefore used typically to treat skin cancers or skin metastases. In contrast, high energy x-ray beams (18 or 25 MeV) are less attenuated by the skin surface (i.e., are "skin sparing") and deposit most of their energy at a greater depth within the body.

Charged particles can also be used for clinical radiotherapy and include electrons, light particles (such as protons) and heavy particles (such as carbon or argon ions). Typically, electron beams are used to treat clinical tissues or tumors that require a uniform dose distribution from the outer skin surface to a point at depth within the body, while particle beams have been used for high-precision dose delivery at depth in the body. Neutrons have also been used in radiotherapy. They have no charge and deposit energy by collision with nuclei, particularly hydrogen nuclei (protons), thereby transferring their energy to create moving charged particles (protons and electrons) capable of both ionization and excitation.

Radiation dose is measured in terms of the amount of energy (joules) absorbed per unit mass (kg) and is quoted in grays (1 Gy is equivalent to 1 J/kg). It is not the total amount of energy absorbed that is critical for the biologic effect of ionizing radiation. For example, a whole body dose of 8 Gy would result in the death (due to bone marrow failure) of many animals, including humans, yet the amount of energy deposited, if evenly distributed, would cause a temperature rise of only 1 to $3 \times 10^{-3}$ °C. It is the size and localized nature of the individual energy deposition events caused by ionizing radiations that is the reason for their efficacy in damaging biological systems.

## 14.2.2 Linear Energy Transfer and Energy Absorption

The deposition of energy in matter by moving charged particles is chiefly a result of electrical field interactions. As a charged particle moves through matter, it transfers energy by a series of interactions that occur at random. Thus, particles lose energy along their track (i.e., their range) proportional to their energy. The particle's energy loss $dE$, along a portion of this track $dx$, is also dependent on its velocity $v$, charge $Z$, and the electron density of the target $\rho$ as indicated by Eq. (14.1):

$$\frac{dE}{dx} \, \alpha \, \frac{Z^2 \rho}{v^2} \qquad (14.1)$$

The efficiency with which different types of ionizing radiation cause biological damage varies, even though photons, charged particles, and neutrons ultimately all set electrons in motion. The important difference between different types of radiation is the average density of energy loss *along* the path of the particle. The average energy lost by a particle over a given track length is known as the *linear energy transfer* (LET). The units of LET are given in terms of energy lost per unit pathlength (e.g., keV/μm). Some representative values of LET for different particles are given in Table 14.1. From Eq. (14.1), it can be seen that as a particle slows down, it loses energy more and more rapidly and reaches a maximum rate of energy loss (the Bragg peak) just before it comes to rest (Fig. 14.2). The LET of a charged particle thus varies along the length of its track.

The biological effect of a dose of radiation depends on its LET; it is therefore necessary to know the LET at each point in an irradiated volume to predict the biological response accurately. When *low-LET* radiation (e.g., 6-MeV photons) is used to irradiate tissue, electrons are set in motion in the tissue. Due to their small mass (1/1860 of the mass of a proton), they are easily deflected and their track through the tissue is tortuous. Each electron track has a Bragg peak at its termination and a range of LET values along its track, but both the initiation and termination points of the electron tracks occur at random in the tissue, so that the LET spectrum is similar at all depths. A similar result occurs if the irradiation is with a primary electron beam. In contrast, if a beam of monoenergetic heavier-charged particles (e.g., *high-LET* protons: He or Ne nuclei) is used

**Table 14.1.** Linear Energy Transfer (LET) of Various Radiations

| Radiation | LET (keV/μm) |
|---|---|
| Photons | |
| $^{60}$Co (~1.2 MeV) | 0.3 |
| 200-keV x-ray | 2.5 |
| Electrons | |
| 1 MeV | 0.2 |
| 100 keV | 0.5 |
| 10 keV | 2 |
| 1 keV | 10 |
| Charged particles | |
| Proton 2 MeV | 17 |
| Alpha particle 5 MeV | 90 |
| Carbon ion 100 MeV | 160 |
| Neutrons | |
| 2.5 MeV | 15–80 |
| 14.1 MeV | 3–30 |

to irradiate the tissue, the tracks of the particles are much straighter because their much larger mass reduces the chance of significant deflection. The Bragg peak then occurs at a similar depth in the tissue for all particles. Thus, there is a region in the tissue where a relatively large amount of energy is deposited. This feature of irradiation with high-LET particles makes them

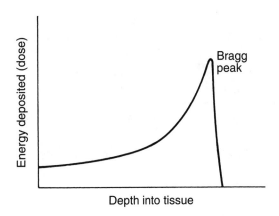

**Figure 14.2.** Schematic illustration of the energy deposition by a charged particle along its track in tissue. The particle has a high velocity at the left-hand side of the figure, but as it loses energy, it slows down until it comes to rest in the region of the Bragg peak.

potentially attractive for radiotherapy because the beam can be designed to deposit most of its energy within a deep-seated tumor (Chap. 15, Sec. 15.2.4).

### 14.2.3 Radiation Damage Within the Cell

The interactions leading to energy deposition in tissue occur very rapidly and generate chemically reactive free electrons and free radicals (molecules with unpaired electrons). Many different molecules in cells will be altered either as a result of *direct* energy absorption or as a result of energy transfer from one molecule to another, giving rise to *indirect* effects (see Fig. 14.3A). Most of the energy deposited in cells is absorbed initially in water (because the cell is about 80 percent water), leading to the rapid (i.e., within $10^{-14}$ to $10^{-4}$ s) production of reactive radical intermediates (oxidizing and reducing) which, in turn, can interact with other molecules in the cell (indirect effect). The [OH$^\bullet$] radical, an oxidizing agent, is probably the most damaging. The cell contains naturally occurring thiol compounds such

as glutathione and cysteine, whose structures contain sulfhydryl (SH) groups that can react chemically with the free radicals to decrease their damaging effects. Other antioxidants include the vitamins C and E and intracellular manganese superoxide dismutase (MnSOD). The intracellular levels of thiols and antioxidative molecules may differ between normal and tumor tissues and their manipulation may offer a clinical strategy to protect normal tissues from radiotherapy-induced damage. One example is the use of the drug amifostine (a thiol-containing compound) to protect against radiotherapy-induced xerostomia (i.e., dry mouth after irradiation of salivary glands; see Chap. 15, Sec. 15.5.8).

The random nature of the energy deposition events means that radiation-induced changes can occur in any molecule in a cell. Biochemical processes in cells, such as DNA, RNA, or protein synthesis, respiration, or other metabolic processes can be inhibited by irradiation but this usually requires quite large doses of radiation of the order of 10 to 100 Gy. DNA is a major target of ionizing radiation because of its biological importance to

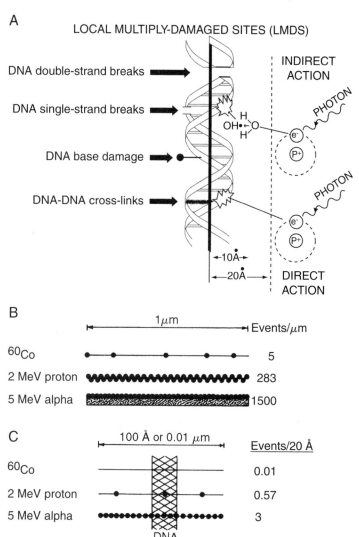

**Figure 14.3.** (A) Direct and indirect effects of ionizing radiation on DNA. In the indirect model, chemically reactive free electrons are produced during ionization and interact with water molecules in close proximity (i.e., 10-20 Angstroms) to the DNA helix. These free radicals, such as the hydroxyl radical, OH$^\bullet$, can react chemically with DNA to produce DNA damage. In the direct model, absorption of the reactive free electron occurs directly within the DNA causing localized damage without an intermediate free radical step. Indirect and direct damage can lead to clusters of DNA single-strand and double-strand breaks, DNA base damage, DNA-DNA or DNA-protein cross-links. These can occur as Local Multiply-Damaged Sites (LMDS). (Adapted from Hall, 2000). (B) and (C) The frequency of primary energy-loss events along the tracks of various radiations of widely differing linear energy transfer; (B) Schematic diagram of primary energy-loss events over a distance of 1 $\mu$m. (C) Primary energy-loss events over 0.01 $\mu$m or 100 Å dependent on type of radiation. The cross-hatched region represents the dimensions of a DNA double helix.

the cell. Even relatively small amounts of DNA damage can lead to cell lethality. Ward (1994) has described focal areas of DNA damage that arise because of the clustering of ionizations within a few nanometers of the DNA. These "local multiply-damaged sites" (LMDS; see Fig. 14.3) include combinations of DNA single- or double-strand breaks in the sugar-phosphate backbone of the molecule, alteration or loss of DNA bases, and formation of crosslinks (between the DNA strands or between DNA and chromosomal proteins). It has been estimated that approximately $10^5$ ionizations can occur within the cell per Gy of absorbed radiation dose, leading to approximately 1000 to 3000 DNA-DNA or DNA-protein crosslinks, 1000 damaged DNA bases, 500 to 1000 single-strand DNA breaks and 25 to 50 double-strand DNA breaks (i.e., the vast majority of the ionization events do not cause DNA damage; see Fig. 14.3B and C). Most of these DNA lesions can be repaired by a variety of DNA repair pathways (described in detail in Chap. 5, Sec. 5.3) probably acting together to repair clustered LMDS-associated lesions. High-LET irradiation causes an increase in both the number and complexity of DNA-clustered lesions which are often more difficult to repair.

The results from a number of assays of double-strand breaks in DNA suggest that cell survival following radiation is correlated with the residual level of DNA double-strand breaks (Nunez et al., 1996). Evidence to support damage to DNA as a crucial type of cellular damage in relation to cell killing is outlined in Table 14.2. A number of techniques—such as velocity sedimentation, filter elution, assays for chromosomal damage, and

DNA electrophoresis—have been used to study specific DNA lesions caused by radiation (Whitaker et al., 1991; Fairbairn et al., 1995). Two techniques, fluorescence in situ hybridization (FISH; see Chap. 4, Sec. 4.4.1) and premature chromosome condensation (PCC), allow the quantification of single- or double-strand breaks (ssb or dsb) manifest as chromatid breaks or aberrant chromosomal forms following doses of ionizing radiation as low as 1 Gy (Sasai et al., 1994). Other techniques, such as pulsed-field gel electrophoresis (PFGE) or the Comet assay (Fig. 14.4A) (Fairbairn et al., 1995) can facilitate the separation and quantitation of large DNA fragments secondary to single- or double-strand DNA breaks following radiation damage (Table 14.3). Other assays use the rejoining of DNA-dsbs induced within DNA-containing plasmids by DNA restriction enzymes (i.e., I-SceI) to measure the fidelity of DNA-dsb repair (see Fig. 14.4B).

Ionizing radiation leads to rapid phosphorylation of a nucleosomal histone protein, H2AX (γH2AX is the phosphorylated form) that can be quantified as an intracellular marker of DNA double-strand breaks (Rogakou; 1998; Fig. 14.5 and Chap. 5, Fig. 5.10). This early event precedes the action of repair enzymes involved in homologous recombination and nonhomologous end-joining of these breaks (see Chap. 5, Secs. 5.3.5 and 5.3.6). Nuclear foci, each containing thousands of γH2AX molecules covering about 2 megabases of DNA surrounding the break, can be detected using antibody staining and fluorescence microscopy. Foci of γH2AX are believed to recruit repair enzymes to sites of DNA damage (Paull et al., 2000). The number of γH2AX foci has been directly correlated to the number of DNA-dsbs in [125]IUdR-treated cells (Sedelnikova et al., 2002) as each [125]I decay yields a DNA-dsb and each DNA-dsb yielded a visible γH2AX focus. It is probable that residual nuclear foci at late times following irradiation (>12 hrs) represent nonrepaired DNA double-strand breaks that lead to subsequent cell lethality (MacPhail et al., 2003).

The reactive oxygen species induced by ionizing radiation can also interact with proteins in the cell membrane, some of which may be involved in signal transduction. This can lead to apoptosis in certain cell types (e.g., endothelial cells) by activation in the membrane of a ceramide-sphingomyelin pathway (Fuks et al., 1995). Furthermore, pre-incubation of cells with agents capable of altering either protein function or lipid peroxidation within the cell membrane can also modify the level of radiation-induced apoptosis (Fuks et al., 1995). Overall, the cellular response to ionizing radiation is mediated both by the direct damage to DNA and a complex interaction between a number of proteins located within the plasma membrane, cytoplasm, and nucleus of the cell. These responses determine the type and extent of cell death in irradiated cells (see Sec. 14.3.2).

**Table 14.2.** Evidence Supporting DNA as a Critical Target for Radiation-induced Lethality

1. Microbeam irradiation demonstrates the cell nucleus to be much more sensitive than the cytoplasm.

2. Radioisotopes with short-range emissions (e.g., $^3$H, $^{125}$I) incorporated into the DNA cause cell killing at much lower absorbed doses than those incorporated into the cellular cytoplasm.

3. Incorporation of thymidine analogues (e.g., IUdR or BUdR) into DNA modifies cellular radiosensitivity.

4. The level of chromatid and chromosomal aberrations following ionizing radiation correlates well with cell lethality.

5. The number of unrepaired DNA double-strand breaks correlates with cell lethality following ionizing radiation in many cells.

6. For different types of radiation, cell lethality correlates best with the level of radiation-induced DNA double-strand breaks rather than with other types of damage.

7. The extreme radiosensitivity of some mutant cells is due to defects in DNA repair (see Chap. 5, Secs. 5.3 and 5.5).

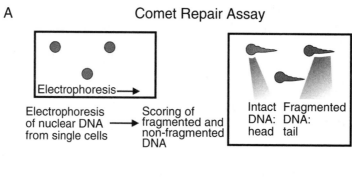

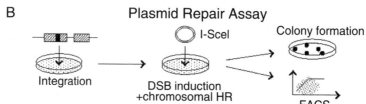

**Figure 14.4.** Assays to quantify the rejoining and repair of DNA double-strand breaks. (*A*) DNA rejoining assays are based on the determination of the ratio of fragmented (i.e., containing DNA breaks) to non-fragmented DNA (without DNA breaks) as a function of time following irradiation. An example of such an assay is the Comet assay. In this assay, irradiated single cells are immobilized in a thin agarose film on a microscope slide and then undergo either neutral pH lysis (to measure DNA double-strand breaks) or alkaline pH lysis (to measure DNA single-strand breaks) to remove cellular protein, but not DNA. The remaining cellular DNA is then subjected to electrophoresis and stained to allow for the relative quantification of fragmented DNA (i.e., DNA containing breaks which migrates away from the cell nucleus and appears as the Comet-like "tail") versus non-fragmented DNA (i.e., intact DNA still contained within the cell nucleus which appears as the Comet "head"). This reflects the relative number of DNA breaks at a given time point. (*B*) To assess the fidelity of DNA double-strand repair by homologous (HR) or non-homologous (NHEJ) recombination, cells can be initially transfected with pathway-specific plasmid reporter constructs. These constructs contain DNA sequences encoding for either a drug resistance or fluorescence (e.g., a green-fluorescent protein [GFP]) gene. However, these genes have been rendered non-functional on the basis of an intervening DNA sequence that prevents transcription. The intervening gene sequence can be removed by a secondary transfection of a DNA restriction enzyme (e.g., I-SceI) which creates DNA double-strand breaks at either end of the DNA insert. Successful and error-free recombination of the remaining gene segments within the chromosome can then be quantified by determining the number of drug resistant or fluorescent cells using colony-based or flow cytometric assays (FACS). (Modified from Willers et al., 2002.)

## 14.2.4 Genetic Instability, Chromosomal Damage, and Bystander Effects

Many human cancer cells contain chromosomal rearrangements including translocations, deletions, and amplifications. DNA double-strand breaks can lead to chromosomal rearrangements at the first mitosis after exposure to ionizing radiation and the type of aberration (i.e., chromosomal vs. chromatid types of rearrange-ments) (see Fig. 14.6) will reflect the cell cycle phase at the time of irradiation. Chromosome rearrangements can also be observed many days after irradiation. Pathways for rejoining of DNA double-strand breaks in mammalian cells, include homologous recombination (HR) and nonhomologous end-joining (NHEJ; see Chap. 5, Secs. 5.3.5 and 5.3.6, and Sec. 14.4.3), but it is unclear which factors determine whether an induced break will or will not lead to a chromosomal rearrangement.

**Table 14.3.** Assays for the Detection of DNA Damage Following Ionizing Radiation

| Assay | Dose Range[a] | Technique | Limitations |
|---|---|---|---|
| 1. Sucrose velocity sedimentation | ssb > 5 Gy<br>dsb > 15 Gy | Larger DNA fragments sediment to a greater extent. | Insensitive to clinically-relevant low radiation doses |
| 2. Filter elution | ssb > 1 Gy (alkaline elution)<br>dsb > 5 Gy (neutral elution) | Smaller DNA fragments elute more quickly through a filter of defined pore size. | Uncertain effects of DNA conformation, cell cycle, cell number, and lysis |
| 3. Nucleoid sedimentation | ssb 1–20 Gy | Irradiated cells show altered DNA supercoiling within nucleus. | Uncertain which DNA lesion(s) are being detected. |
| 4. Pulse-field gel electrophoresis (PFGE) | dsb > 5–10 Gy | Allows for resolution of DNA-dsb, which can be quantified by relative migration within the gel. | Uncertain effects of DNA conformation. High number of cells in S phase may bias results of assay. |
| 5. Comet assay | ssb > 1 Gy (alkaline lysis)<br>dsb > 2 Gy (neutral lysis) | Following lysis, individual nuclei are subjected to agarose gel electrophoresis. The DNA that moves out of the nucleus (head) to form the "tail" of the comet is quantitated to provide a measure of DNA damage. | Requires image analysis system to quantify DNA damage. Increased numbers of cells in S phase may bias assay. |
| 6. Fluorescence in situ hybridization (FISH) | Doses >1 Gy | Chromosome-specific probes, which can be detected with a fluorescent ligand, are used to identify radiation-induced translocations. | May be difficult to interpret in tumor cells that contain translocations prior to irradiation. |
| 7. Premature chromosome condensation (PCC) | Doses >1 Gy | An irradiated interphase cell is fused to a mitotic cell. The chromosomes in the interphase cell undergo premature condensation, allowing radiation-induced chromosome damage to be scored. | May be difficult to interpret in tumor cells that contain chromosome aberrations prior to irradiation. |
| 8. $\gamma$-H2AX Intranuclear Foci | Doses >0.05 Gy | Immunofluorescence microscopy or flow cytometry using an antibody to $\gamma$-H2AX phosphoprotein. | Requires image analysis system. No standard for size or type of foci to count as DNA breaks. |

[a]ssb, single-strand breaks; dsb, double-strand breaks.

*Source:* Adapted from Whitaker et al. (1991).

Examination of the breakpoints in very large deletions often show that novel chromosomal fragments are derived from multiple chromosomal sites of radiation damage in the same cell. This indicates that they can arise as a result of complex interactions between a number of damaged sites in the cellular DNA (Singleton et al., 2002). Furthermore, if a cell does survive and goes on to proliferate after irradiation, delayed chromosomal instability can be observed in its clonal descendants. Factors that perpetuate the unstable phenotype in irradiated cells include the continued production of reactive oxygen species (Huang et al., 2003). Such species or other factors may be released from an irradiated cell and cause damage to neighboring nonirradiated cells

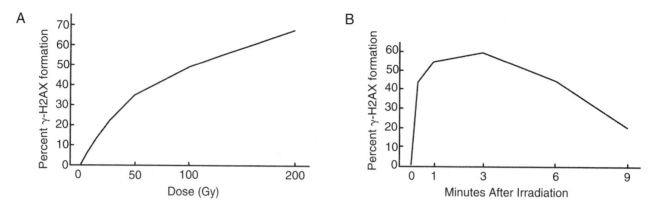

**Figure 14.5.** Histone biomarkers of ionizing radiation-induced DNA damage. When cells are irradiated, the H2AX histone protein becomes phosphorylated at residue serine-139. This histone phosphoform is then known as γ-H2AX. The presence of γ-H2AX in a cell is detected following irradiation by western blotting or immunohistochemistry using γ-H2AX-specific antibodies. Shown in (*A*) is the percentage of γ-H2AX in Chinese Hamster Ovary (CHO) cells at 30 minutes following irradiation as a function of radiation dose; the phosphorylation is linear up to doses of ~20 Gy. H2AX phosphorylation can also be visualized using immunohistochemistry (see Fig. 5.10). (*B*) Percentage of γ-H2AX as a function of time following 200 Gy in CHO cells. γ-H2AX forms within minutes of irradiation and is maximal at 10-30 minutes. (Redrawn from Rogakou et al., 1998.)

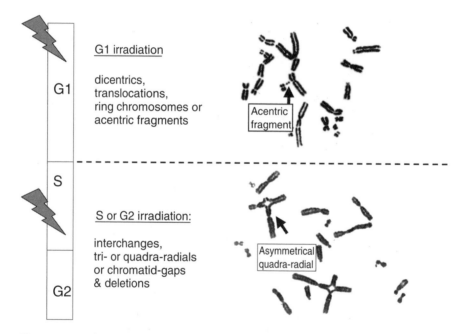

**Figure 14.6.** Chromosome- and chromatid-type aberrations following ionizing radiation. Radiation-induced chromosomal damage occurs as distinct structural aberrations dependent on the cell cycle phase during which irradiation occurred. If a cell is irradiated during the G1 or early S phase when only one chromosomal homolog exists, a non-repaired DNA break can lead to dicentric chromosomes, reciprocal translocations, chromosomal rings and acentric DNA fragments. In contrast, irradiation in late S and G2 phase (when the sister chromatids have duplicated) can lead to chromatid-type aberrations in the form of chromatid interchanges, tri- or quadra-radials or chromatid deletions (examples courtesy of William F. Morgan, University of Maryland, Baltimore, USA). The type of aberrations may also reflect defects in DNA repair pathways that are preferential to a certain cell cycle phase. For example, cells which have defects in non-homologous end-joining (NHEJ) may acquire increased chromosomal-type aberrations during irradiation of cells in the G1 phase and similarly, cells defective in homologous recombination (HR) may acquire chromatid-type aberrations following irradiation in the S and G2 phase. (Adapted from Steel, 2002.)

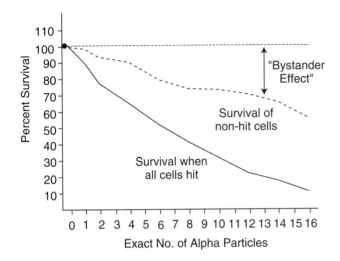

**Figure 14.7.** The radiation bystander effect. Direct single-cell irradiation of V79 cells with alpha-particles can be accomplished using a specialized targeting microbeam irradiator facility in which the irradiation and fate of single cells can be tracked post-irradiation. Using this system, it was observed that cells that were not targeted by the alpha particles can also be killed (i.e., they do not form colonies). This phenomenon is termed the *radiation bystander effect* and may be secondary to factors released by irradiated cells into the surrounding media. In the plot shown, direct cell kill increases with increasing alpha-particle traversal following single cell irradiation. However, the death of non-irradiated cells also increases as a function of dose. The difference between an expected survival of 100% for non-irradiated cells and the actual survival observed, reflects the extent of cell kill by the bystander effect. (Adapted from Hall and Hei, 2003.)

(e.g., *bystander* cells). For example, transfer of media from irradiated unstable cell clones to a nonirradiated cell population can lead to cell death in some of the nonirradiated cells within 24 hours. Similarly, targeting of 10 to 30 percent of a cellular population with high-LET irradiation using a microbeam can lead to cell death in the nontargeted surrounding cells within the same culture dish (Belyakov et al., 2003; Nagasawa et al., 2003; see also Fig. 14.7). These data are consistent with clinical studies that have shown chromosomal changes in circulating peripheral lymphocytes in patients who received only localized radiotherapy. This *indirect (bystander) effect* of radiation has implications for assessment of radiation risk and for health risks associated with radiation exposure (see Chap. 3, Sec. 3.5) as the total cell kill within an irradiated cell population may be greater than that calculated simply on the basis of the number of cells that were directly irradiated.

### 14.2.5 Ultraviolet Radiation and DNA Damage

Ultraviolent irradiation can also cause damage to cells. In contrast to ionizing radiation, UV radiation (wavelength 200 to 400 nm) deposits energy in selected molecules. The energy absorbed, in the range of 3 to 10 electron volts per photon, is not enough to ionize these molecules, but it is enough to put them in a short-lived excited state and make them chemically reactive. In DNA in aqueous solution, absorption of photons with a wavelength in the range 200 to 300 nm results in the excitation of pyrimidine bases (thymine or cytosine) that can react with water (to form pyrimidine hydrates) or with a neighboring pyrimidine to give rise to pyrim-

idine dimers of the cyclobutane type (thymine-thymine, cytosine-thymine, or cytosine-cytosine) as well as other linkages. Dimers formed in DNA are chemically stable, but the pyrimidine hydrates are unstable and can dehydrate, resulting in the restoration of the original pyrimidine or, in the case of cytosine, a deaminated derivative. Reaction of excited pyrimidines with other molecules such as amino acids can occur, and there is evidence for DNA-protein crosslinks in cells exposed to UV irradiation. Because of its chemical stability, the lesion that has been most extensively monitored in biological systems is the cyclobutane pyrimidine dimer. Pyrimidine dimers can be quantitated in mammalian cells by a variety of techniques and, at doses of biological interest, their production is linear with dose. Pyrimidine dimers appear to be formed at equal rates in all phases of the cell cycle. However, their repair may be influenced by gene transcription (see below).

When asynchronous populations of mammalian cells are exposed to UV irradiation and their colony-forming ability is determined, a survival curve (see Sec. 14.3.1) that is qualitatively similar to curves for ionizing radiation is obtained. The relative effectiveness of different wavelengths of UV light to inactivate cell colony-forming ability has a close correspondence to the absorption spectrum of DNA. This spectrum is identical to the action spectrum for dimer formation. Surviving cells respond to a second dose of UV radiation as if they had not been exposed to the first dose if they are allowed to progress through their DNA synthesis phase between the doses of fractionated radiation (Rauth, 1986). For many but not all cell lines, late S-phase cells are most resistant to UV radiation and there is increasing sensitivity through G1-to-early-S phase. UV-induced photoproducts play an important role in skin cancers induced by sun exposure (see Chap. 3, Sec. 3.5.5).

Cells possess mechanisms for removing pyrimidine dimers and UV-induced photoproducts which involves both the transcription-coupled, and genome-wide, repair subpathways of nucleotide excision repair (NER; see Chap. 5, Sec. 5.3.4). UV-induced lesions also initiate cell cycle checkpoint pathways leading to G1 and G2 arrest following UV irradiation (Chap. 5, Sec. 5.4). Patients with the disorders xeroderma pigmentosum (XP), Cockayne syndrome (CS), and trichothiodystrophy (TTD) have an increased sensitivity to UV that leads to increased skin tumor formation and accelerated aging in affected patients (see Chap. 5, Sec. 5.2).

## 14.3 CELL DEATH RESPONSES TO IONIZING RADIATION

### 14.3.1 In Vitro and In Vivo Assays for Cell Survival

Inhibition of the continued reproductive ability of cells is an important consequence of the molecular and cellular responses to radiation. It occurs at relatively low doses (a few grays) and it is the major aim of clinical radiotherapy. A tumor is controlled if its stem cells (i.e., clonogenic cells) are prevented from continued proliferation. A cell that retains unlimited proliferative capacity after radiation treatment is regarded as having *survived* the treatment, while one that has lost the ability to generate a clone or *colony* is regarded as having been killed, even though it may undergo a few divisions or remain intact in the cell population for a substantial period. Colony formation following irradiation is an im-

portant end point for radiobiologists and radiation oncologists, as it relates to a cell's ability to repopulate normal or tumor tissues following exposure to ionizing radiation. In the assay that is used most often to assess colony formation, cells grown in culture are irradiated either before or after preparation of a suspension of single cells and plated at low density in tissue-culture dishes. Following irradiation, the cells are incubated for a number of days, and those that retain proliferative capacity divide and grow to form discrete colonies of cells (Fig. 14.8A). After incubation, the colonies are fixed and stained so that they can be counted easily.

Cells that do not retain proliferative capacity following irradiation (i.e., are killed) may divide a few times but form only very small abortive colonies. If a colony contains more than 50 cells (i.e., derived from a single cell by at least six division cycles), it is usually capable of continued growth and can be regarded as having arisen from a surviving cell. The plating efficiency (PE) of the cell population is calculated by dividing the number of colonies formed by the number of cells plated. The ratio of the PE for the irradiated cells to the PE for control cells is calculated to give the fraction of cells surviving the treatment (*cell survival*). If a range of radiation doses is used, then these cell-survival values can be plotted to give a *survival curve*, such as the ones shown in Figures 14.9 and 14.10. Cells taken directly from animal or human tumors can also be grown in culture, allowing the in vitro assay method to be extended to the study of the radiation sensitivity of tumor cells treated in vivo (see Fig. 14.8B). Untreated cells rarely have a PE of 1 (more usually it is 0.5 to 0.8 for cells passed for many generations and much lower for cells derived from spontaneous tumors).

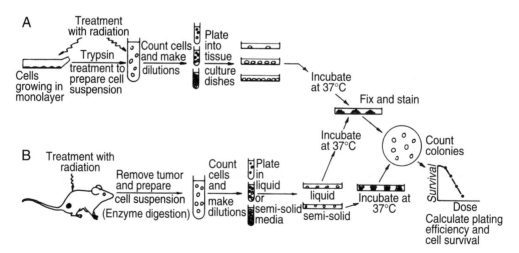

**Figure 14.8.** Schematic diagram of in vitro plating assays to assess cell survival. (*A*) Assay for the radiation sensitivity of cells growing in culture. (*B*) In vivo–in vitro assay for the sensitivity of tumor cells grown and irradiated in vivo.

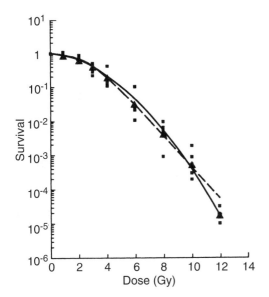

**Figure 14.9.** Survival data for a murine melanoma cell line treated with low-LET radiation. The survival is plotted on a logarithmic scale against dose plotted on a linear scale. The data from five independent survival experiments are shown as the small squares, with the geometric mean value at each dose shown as the large triangles. The survival curves shown are the result of fitting the data to target theory or linear-quadratic models (see Appendix 14.1). (Adapted from Bristow et al., 1990.)

The techniques described above have been used to obtain survival curves for a wide range of malignant and normal cell populations. In general, for low-LET radiation (e.g., x- or γ-rays), these curves have the shape(s) illustrated in Figure 14.9, where cell survival is plotted on a log scale as a function of dose, which is plotted on a linear scale. At low doses, there is evidence of a shoulder region; but at higher doses, the curve either becomes steeper and straight so that survival decreases exponentially with dose (dashed line) or appears to be continually bending downward on the semilogarithmic plot (solid line). The accuracy of the data obtained is usually such that either shape could fit the data adequately over the first few decades of survival.

The difference in survival curves for x- or γ-rays (low-LET) and for fast-neutron (high-LET) irradiation is illustrated in Figure 14.10. In general, both the slope and the shoulder of the survival curve are reduced for higher LET radiation. The biological effectiveness of different types of radiation can be characterized by a parameter known as the *relative biological effectiveness* (RBE). The RBE is defined as the ratio of the dose of a standard type of radiation to that of the test radiation that gives the same biological effect. The standard type of radiation is usually taken as 200- or 250-kilovolt (peak) x-rays. Cobalt 60 γ-rays are also used as a standard for comparison studies, although their RBE rela-

tive to 250-kilovolt (peak) x-rays is about 0.9. Because the shoulder of the survival curve is reduced for high-LET radiation, the RBE varies with the dose or the survival level at which it is determined (see Fig. 14.10; Barendsen, 1968).

Many different mathematical models have been used to produce equations that can fit survival-curve data within the limits of experimental error. Two of the more commonly used models are the *target-theory* and *linear-quadratic* models of cell survival (explained in detail in Appendix 14.1) from which parameters ($D_0$, $D_q$ and $n$, or $\alpha$ and $\beta$) can be obtained to describe the shape of the low-dose and high-dose regions of cell survival curves. Such descriptions are useful when comparing cellular radiosensitivity among a variety of cell types or when the shape of the survival curve is altered following treatment with drugs or changes in the environment (e.g., hypoxia). From these models, it has been observed that there is greater variation in the low-dose or shoulder region of the radiation survival curves obtained for mammalian cells as compared to the variation in the slopes of the high-dose region of the curves (see Chap. 15, Sec. 15.3.2).

Nonclonogenic assays have also been used to estimate the relative radiosensitivity of cells, although assays that measure short-term growth or apoptosis (see Sec. 14.3.2) often do not correlate with the longer-term clonogenic assay. Assays for apoptosis may predict clonogenic survival within some cancer cell lines e.g.,

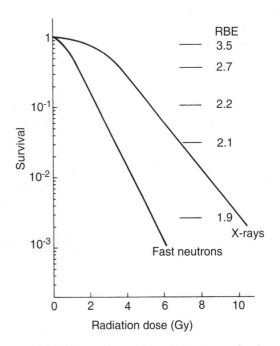

**Figure 14.10.** Comparison of survival curves for low-LET (x-ray) and high-LET (fast-neutron) irradiation. The RBE is calculated as indicated in the text and varies at different levels of survival.

neuroblastoma, lymphoma, and testicular, as these cell types tend to die uniformly by apoptosis following irradiation. Assays that evaluate cellular growth for a short period (e.g., 24 to 48 h) following radiation, include the *MTT assay* that determines cellular viability by colorimetric assessment of the reduction of a tetrazolium compound. They are of limited value for radiosensitivity studies because it is rarely possible to assess more than one decade of cell kill and they usually do not correlate with the clonogenic assay. At present, clonogenic survival remains the gold standard for determining the radiosensitivity of cells in vitro.

Methods have also been developed for assessing the ability of cells to form colonies in vivo. One of these is the spleen-colony method, which has been used to assess both the radiation and drug sensitivity of bone marrow stem cells (McCulloch and Till, 1962). In this assay bone marrow from treated animals is injected into irradiated hosts and colonies from surviving bone marrow stem cells can be then counted in the spleen. In an analogous method, the lung-colony assay, tumor cells from treated animals are injected intravenously and form colonies in the lungs of syngeneic mice (Hill and Bush, 1969). Other colony-forming assays have been developed to study the radiation response of stem cells in situ in certain proliferative tissues, including skin, gas-

trointestinal tract, testis, cartilage, kidney, and certain tumors (see Chap. 15, Sec. 15.5.1).

### 14.3.2 Radiation-induced Cell Death: Apoptosis, Mitotic Catastrophe, and Terminal Growth Arrest

Many types of cells do not show morphological evidence of radiation damage until they attempt to divide. The morphology of the cell at the time of cell lysis following irradiation can be apoptotic or necrotic (see Chap. 10, Sec. 10.1). Following doses of less than about 10 Gy, lethally-damaged cells may: (1) undergo a permanent (terminal) growth arrest (senescence) such as that observed for fibroblasts, (2) undergo interphase death or lysis during radiation-induced apoptosis, or (3) undergo up to four abortive mitotic cycles and then finally undergo cell lysis as a result of mitotic catastrophe (see Fig. 14.11). The clonogenic radiation survival curve represents the total or cumulative cell death within an irradiated cell population as a result of all types of cell death. The biochemical and morphologic differences observed for cells undergoing these types of cell death can be related to clonogenic cell kill to determine the dominant mode of radiation-induced cell death for a given cell type.

**Figure 14.11.** Mechanisms of cell death following exposure to ionizing radiation. Cells can undergo apoptosis (top figure), mitotic catastrophe (middle figure) or terminal cell arrest (bottom figure) following irradiation. The extent to which one mode of cell death is dominant over another is dependent on cell type, radiation dose and the cell's microenvironment (e.g., relative oxygenation and availability of growth factors) (Figures courtesy of Gillian Bromfield, University of Toronto, Toronto, Canada and reproduced from Sato et al., 2000, with permission). Each type of cell death has a unique morphology and timing following irradiation as described in Section 14.3.2 and can be quantified by specific methods: apoptotic cells show condensed chromatin bodies; mitotic catastrophe cells show multiple tubulin spindles and centrosomes; terminally-arrested cells express SA-β-galactosidase (see Fig. 14.12). Although the majority of human epithelial tumor cells respond to ionizing radiation by undergoing mitotic arrest and/or terminal growth arrest, the accumulation of all death events by these three mechanisms reflects the final cell kill as measured by a long-term clonogenic assay. (See color plate.)

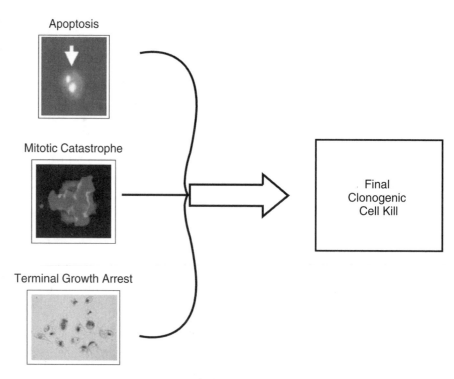

For the majority of normal and tumor cells, death secondary to mitotic catastrophe accounts for most of the cell kill following irradiation. However, in some radiosensitive cells and the cancers that arise from them—notably lymphocytes, spermatocytes, thymocytes, and salivary gland epithelium—irradiation causes the cells to undergo an early (within a few hours) interphase death. This death is associated with the biochemical and morphologic characteristics of apoptosis (i.e., cell membrane blebbing, the formation of nuclear apoptotic bodies, and specific DNA fragmentation patterns). Depending on the type of cell, the intracellular target(s) for the induction of the apoptotic response may be either the cell membrane or the DNA or both. The reasons why some cell types undergo extensive radiation-induced apoptosis within a few hours after irradiation, while others do not, remain to be elucidated, but may relate to the relative expression and function of proteins which trigger an apoptotic response. For ex-

ample, in hematopoietic cells, radiation can lead to up-regulation of genes (such as *Fas, Bax,* and *Caspase-3),* which can facilitate apoptosis and/or downregulation of genes, (such as *Bcl-2),* which act to prevent apoptosis (see Chap. 10, Kitada et al., 1996).

The involvement of the cell membrane in triggering radiation-induced apoptosis is supported by the observation that ionizing radiation can initiate a sphingomyelin-dependent signaling pathway within the cell membrane of endothelial cells which, in turn, can induce apoptosis in the absence of DNA damage (Ruiter et al., 1999; Kolesnick and Fuks, 2003). Ceramide is generated from sphingomyelin (SM) by the action of acid sphingomyelinase (ASM), or by de novo synthesis coordinated through the enzyme ceramide synthase. In the radiation response, ceramide serves as a second messenger in initiating apoptosis, while some of its metabolites block apoptosis (Fig. 14.12A). In certain cells, such as endothelial, lymphoid and hematopoietic

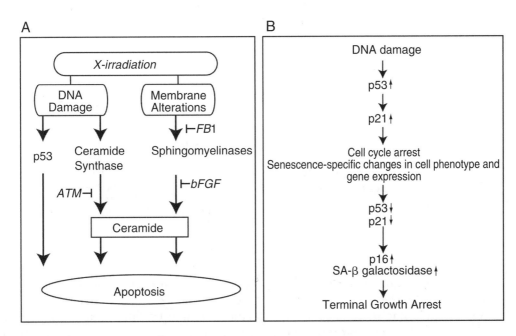

**Figure 14.12.** (*A*) Exposure of cells to ionizing radiation can elicit a biochemical response in the plasma membrane in which ceramide acts as a second messenger to initiate apoptosis. Ceramide is generated from sphingomyelin by the action of acidic-sphingomyelinase (ASM). Radiation-induced ceramide then activates stress- or mitogen-activated protein kinase (SAPK/MAPK) pathways resulting in apoptosis in selected tissues, such as the vascular endothelium. As discussed in Chapter 15, Section 15.5.2, growth factors (such as basic fibroblast growth factor-bFGF) can antagonize this pathway and prevent this radiation damage. Radiation-induced apoptosis can also occur via p53-dependent and p53-independent mechanisms following damage directly to the DNA. The latter pathway is ATM-dependent leading to increased expression of ceramide through ceramide synthase. This pathway can be antagonized by fumonisin B1 (FB1), an inhibitor of ceramide synthase. (Modified from Kolesnick and Fuks, 2003.) (*B*) In cells irradiated with lethal doses, ionizing radiation can also induce a terminal growth arrest leading to a senescent-like morphology. This can occur in both normal cells (e.g., fibroblasts) and tumor cells. Initial attempts at p53-dependent reversible cell cycle arrest are followed by the activation of the terminal arrest pathway when the amount of DNA damage it is beyond repair. At these later times post-irradiation, cells acquire a senesecent-like morphology (i.e., increasing granularity within the nucleus) and may express increased levels of p16[INK4A] and SA-$\beta$-galactosidase (both markers of senescent cells). (Modified from Roninson, 2003.)

cells, ceramide mediates apoptosis, while in others ceramide may serve only as a co-signal or play no role in the death response. The ceramide-mediated apoptotic response to radiation can be inhibited by basic fibroblast growth factor or by genetic mutation of *ASM*. Radiation-induced crypt damage, organ failure, and death from the gastrointestinal syndrome were reduced when endothelial apoptosis in the supporting vasculature was inhibited pharmacologically by intravenous basic fibroblast growth factor (bFGF) (Chapter 15, Section 15.5.1) or genetically by deletion of the acid sphingomyelinase gene (Paris et al., 2001). The release and/or effect of growth factors in irradiated normal tissues is further discussed in Chapter 15, Section 15.5.2. Altering the apoptotic response of tumor cells may be one strategy to sensitize tumors to radiotherapy. Some tumors may evade radiation therapy-induced apoptosis by carrying *p53* gene mutations or by lacking p53 expression or function; restoration of wild-type p53 function using gene therapy may potentiate radiation cell kill (reviewed in Ma et al., 2003).

Induction of apoptosis following irradiation appears insufficient to account for the therapeutic effect of radiation in solid epithelial tumors. The level of radiation-induced apoptosis does not correlate with eventual clonogenic cell survival as measured by colony-forming assays (Aldridge et al., 1995; Brown and Wouters, 2001; Bromfield et al., 2003). The other modes of cell death shown in Figure 14.11 (i.e., mitotic catastrophe and/or terminal growth arrest) account for this difference. Most tumor cell lines have retained the capacity of normal cells to undergo accelerated senescence after irradiation, and although the cell-cycle-related *p53* and *p21^{Waf1}* genes (see Sec. 14.4.2) act as positive regulators of treatment-induced senescence, they are not required for this response in tumor cells (Chang et al., 2000). Senescent or terminal-arrested cells are metabolically active but do not proliferate and do not form colonies following irradiation. They eventually die, days to weeks following irradiation, by necrosis. This may explain the relatively slow resolution, yet ultimate cure, of some tumors following radiotherapy (Bromfield et al., 2003; Roninson, 2003). Treatments which may differentially increase terminal arrest in tumor cells may sensitize these cells to the effects of radiotherapy. Differentiation agents (e.g., retinoids) have been used to induce a senescence-like phenotype and can radiosensitize both breast cancer and head and neck cancer cells in vitro and in vivo (reviewed in Ma et al., 2003).

### 14.3.3 Cellular Repair of Radiation Damage

The repair of cellular damage between radiation doses is the major mechanism underlying the clinical obser-

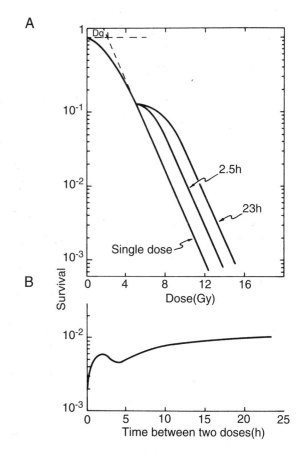

**Figure 14.13.** Illustration of the repair of sublethal damage that occurs between two radiation treatments. (*A*) Survival curves for a single-dose treatment or for treatments involving a fixed first dose followed, after 2.5 or 23 h of incubation (at 37°C), by a range of second doses. (*B*) Pattern of survival observed when two fixed doses of irradiation are given with a varying time interval of incubation (at 37°C) between them. (Adapted from Elkind and Sutton, 1960.)

vation that a larger total dose can be tolerated when the radiation dose is fractionated. Elkind and Sutton (1960) showed that the shoulder of the survival curve for Chinese hamster cells reflects the accumulation of *sublethal damage* that can be repaired (Fig. 14.13). When the cells were incubated at 37 °C for 2.5 hours between the first and second radiation treatments, the original shoulder of the survival curve was partially regenerated, and it was completely regenerated when the cells were incubated for 23 hours between the treatments (Fig. 14.13*A*). When the interval between two fixed doses of radiation was varied (Fig. 14.13*B*), there was a rapid rise in survival as the interval was increased from zero (single dose) to about 2 hours. This was followed by a decrease before the survival rose again to a maximum level after about 12 hours. *Repair of sublethal damage* (SLDR) accounts for the early rise in survival. Because cells that survive radiation tend to be synchronized in the more

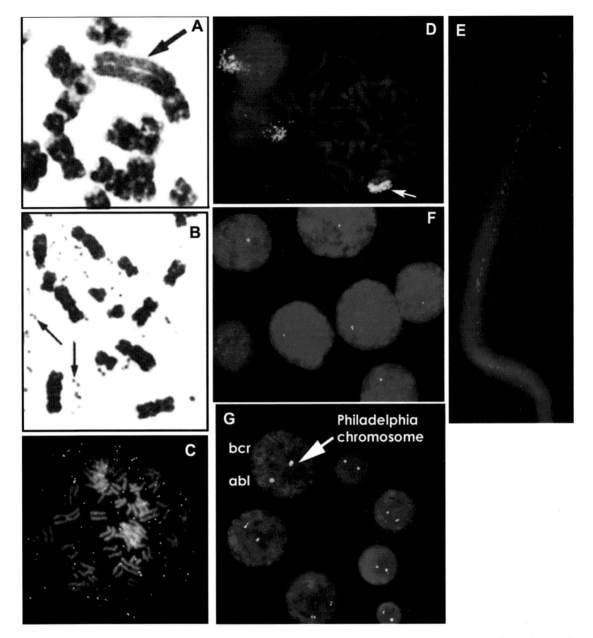

**Figure 4.14.** Analysis of oncogene rearrangements in tumors by conventional cytogenetics and FISH analysis. (*A*) An abnormally long chromosome (*arrow*). The extended region of this chromosome has no identifiable bands and is called a *homogeneously staining region* (HSR). (*B*) Multiple paired dots of chromatic material. These chromosomal abnormalities are called *double minutes* (DM). Both HSRs and DMs are associated with gene amplification. DMs are extrachromosomal circular DNA containing a few copies of the oncogene. HSRs are integrated multiple tandem repeats of the oncogene. (*C*) Metaphase preparation from a neuroblastoma that has N-*myc* amplification on DMs (green dots) detected by FISH. (*D*) A metaphase from another neuroblastoma that has N-*myc* amplification and an HSR. In this FISH preparation, the additional N-*myc* signals can be seen to decorate the HSR (*arrow*), the HSR is also apparent as clusters of yellow signal in the interphase nuclei. (*E*) A HSR in a neuroblastoma cell line with gene amplification of N-*myc*. In this preparation, the HSR has been stretched so that, in the extended form, multiple N-*myc* signals can be seen as a linear array. (Courtesy of Ajay Pandita, Pathology Department, University of Toronto.) (*F*) Interphase nuclei from a neuroblastoma with DMs. The bright pink dots within each nucleus are the FISH signals from the N-*myc* oncogene, which is known to be amplified to 50–100 copies per cell in this patient's tumor. In addition the single green dot indicates the loss of one copy of chromosome region 1p36. (*G*) Interphase cytogenetic analysis of a leukemia to identify the Philadelphia chromosome using FISH with the *bcr* and *abl* probes. The *abl* probe has been labeled with a red fluorochrome (*black dot*) and the *bcr* with a green fluorochrome (*shaded dot*). When the Philadelphia chromosome is present in a nucleus, both the red and green signals become superimposed, producing one strong yellow signal (*white dot*). If the nucleus does not have this abnormality, two red signals and two green signals will be present.

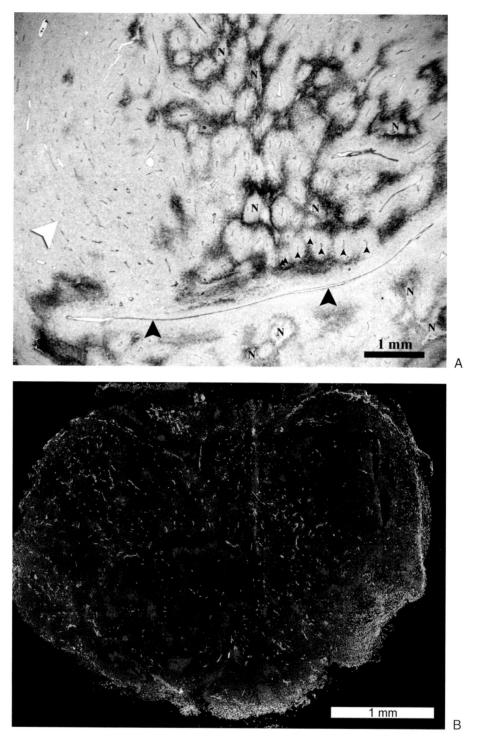

**Figure 15.11.** Tumor Hypoxia. Panel (*A*) shows a section of a high grade human soft tissue sarcoma (rhabdomyosarcoma, pleomorphic) showing hypoxic regions (dark brown membraneous CA IX staining) distant from blood vessels (reddish-brown CD31 staining). Small black arrowheads point to blood vessels at the center of tumor cords with peripheral CA IX staining. Large black arrowheads point to one long blood vessel in the plane of the section. Necrotic regions are labeled with an N. The large white arrowhead points to a well-vascularized region with no hypoxia (and absence of CA IX staining). This picture illustrates the cordlike structure which is associated with (chronic) hypoxia in regions of many tumors. (Courtesy of Dr. K. Maseide, University of Toronto, Toronto, Canada.) Panel (*B*) shows staining for EF5 (red) in a complete section through a human pancreatic tumor xenograft growing in a SCID mouse. The blood vessels are stained for CD31 (green) and regions close to functional blood vessels are indicated by the blue staining for Hoechst 33342 that was injected into the mouse a few minutes before the animal was killed and the tumor was removed. Brightish staining in the bottom right edge of the figure is an artifact. (Courtesy of Dr. David Hedley and Ms Nhu-An Pham, University of Toronto, Toronto, Canada.)

cells, ceramide mediates apoptosis, while in others ceramide may serve only as a co-signal or play no role in the death response. The ceramide-mediated apoptotic response to radiation can be inhibited by basic fibroblast growth factor or by genetic mutation of *ASM*. Radiation-induced crypt damage, organ failure, and death from the gastrointestinal syndrome were reduced when endothelial apoptosis in the supporting vasculature was inhibited pharmacologically by intravenous basic fibroblast growth factor (bFGF) (Chapter 15, Section 15.5.1) or genetically by deletion of the acid sphingomyelinase gene (Paris et al., 2001). The release and/or effect of growth factors in irradiated normal tissues is further discussed in Chapter 15, Section 15.5.2. Altering the apoptotic response of tumor cells may be one strategy to sensitize tumors to radiotherapy. Some tumors may evade radiation therapy-induced apoptosis by carrying *p53* gene mutations or by lacking p53 expression or function; restoration of wild-type p53 function using gene therapy may potentiate radiation cell kill (reviewed in Ma et al., 2003).

Induction of apoptosis following irradiation appears insufficient to account for the therapeutic effect of radiation in solid epithelial tumors. The level of radiation-induced apoptosis does not correlate with eventual clonogenic cell survival as measured by colony-forming assays (Aldridge et al., 1995; Brown and Wouters, 2001; Bromfield et al., 2003). The other modes of cell death shown in Figure 14.11 (i.e., mitotic catastrophe and/or terminal growth arrest) account for this difference. Most tumor cell lines have retained the capacity of normal cells to undergo accelerated senescence after irradiation, and although the cell-cycle-related *p53* and *p21^Waf1* genes (see Sec. 14.4.2) act as positive regulators of treatment-induced senescence, they are not required for this response in tumor cells (Chang et al., 2000). Senescent or terminal-arrested cells are metabolically active but do not proliferate and do not form colonies following irradiation. They eventually die, days to weeks following irradiation, by necrosis. This may explain the relatively slow resolution, yet ultimate cure, of some tumors following radiotherapy (Bromfield et al., 2003; Roninson, 2003). Treatments which may differentially increase terminal arrest in tumor cells may sensitize these cells to the effects of radiotherapy. Differentiation agents (e.g., retinoids) have been used to induce a senescence-like phenotype and can radiosensitize both breast cancer and head and neck cancer cells in vitro and in vivo (reviewed in Ma et al., 2003).

### 14.3.3 Cellular Repair of Radiation Damage

The repair of cellular damage between radiation doses is the major mechanism underlying the clinical obser-

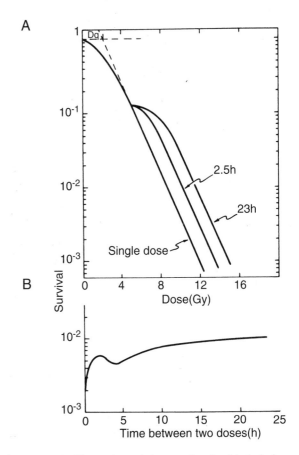

**Figure 14.13.** Illustration of the repair of sublethal damage that occurs between two radiation treatments. (*A*) Survival curves for a single-dose treatment or for treatments involving a fixed first dose followed, after 2.5 or 23 h of incubation (at 37°C), by a range of second doses. (*B*) Pattern of survival observed when two fixed doses of irradiation are given with a varying time interval of incubation (at 37°C) between them. (Adapted from Elkind and Sutton, 1960.)

vation that a larger total dose can be tolerated when the radiation dose is fractionated. Elkind and Sutton (1960) showed that the shoulder of the survival curve for Chinese hamster cells reflects the accumulation of *sublethal damage* that can be repaired (Fig. 14.13). When the cells were incubated at 37 °C for 2.5 hours between the first and second radiation treatments, the original shoulder of the survival curve was partially regenerated, and it was completely regenerated when the cells were incubated for 23 hours between the treatments (Fig. 14.13*A*). When the interval between two fixed doses of radiation was varied (Fig. 14.13*B*), there was a rapid rise in survival as the interval was increased from zero (single dose) to about 2 hours. This was followed by a decrease before the survival rose again to a maximum level after about 12 hours. *Repair of sublethal damage* (SLDR) accounts for the early rise in survival. Because cells that survive radiation tend to be synchronized in the more

For the majority of normal and tumor cells, death secondary to mitotic catastrophe accounts for most of the cell kill following irradiation. However, in some radiosensitive cells and the cancers that arise from them—notably lymphocytes, spermatocytes, thymocytes, and salivary gland epithelium—irradiation causes the cells to undergo an early (within a few hours) interphase death. This death is associated with the biochemical and morphologic characteristics of apoptosis (i.e., cell membrane blebbing, the formation of nuclear apoptotic bodies, and specific DNA fragmentation patterns). Depending on the type of cell, the intracellular target(s) for the induction of the apoptotic response may be either the cell membrane or the DNA or both. The reasons why some cell types undergo extensive radiation-induced apoptosis within a few hours after irradiation, while others do not, remain to be elucidated, but may relate to the relative expression and function of proteins which trigger an apoptotic response. For ex-

ample, in hematopoietic cells, radiation can lead to up-regulation of genes (such as *Fas, Bax,* and *Caspase-3*), which can facilitate apoptosis and/or downregulation of genes, (such as *Bcl-2*), which act to prevent apoptosis (see Chap. 10, Kitada et al., 1996).

The involvement of the cell membrane in triggering radiation-induced apoptosis is supported by the observation that ionizing radiation can initiate a sphingomyelin-dependent signaling pathway within the cell membrane of endothelial cells which, in turn, can induce apoptosis in the absence of DNA damage (Ruiter et al., 1999; Kolesnick and Fuks, 2003). Ceramide is generated from sphingomyelin (SM) by the action of acid sphingomyelinase (ASM), or by de novo synthesis coordinated through the enzyme ceramide synthase. In the radiation response, ceramide serves as a second messenger in initiating apoptosis, while some of its metabolites block apoptosis (Fig. 14.12A). In certain cells, such as endothelial, lymphoid and hematopoietic

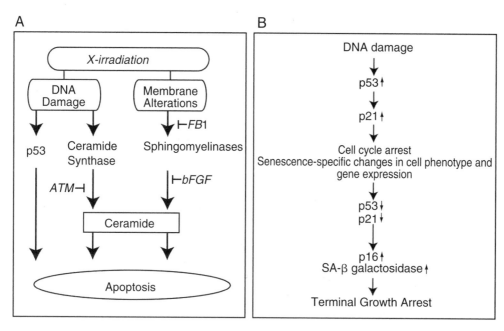

**Figure 14.12.** (A) Exposure of cells to ionizing radiation can elicit a biochemical response in the plasma membrane in which ceramide acts as a second messenger to initiate apoptosis. Ceramide is generated from sphingomyelin by the action of acidic-sphingomyelinase (ASM). Radiation-induced ceramide then activates stress- or mitogen-activated protein kinase (SAPK/MAPK) pathways resulting in apoptosis in selected tissues, such as the vascular endothelium. As discussed in Chapter 15, Section 15.5.2, growth factors (such as basic fibroblast growth factor-bFGF) can antagonize this pathway and prevent this radiation damage. Radiation-induced apoptosis can also occur via p53-dependent and p53-independent mechanisms following damage directly to the DNA. The latter pathway is ATM-dependent leading to increased expression of ceramide through ceramide synthase. This pathway can be antagonized by fumonisin B1 (FB1), an inhibitor of ceramide synthase. (Modified from Kolesnick and Fuks, 2003.) (B) In cells irradiated with lethal doses, ionizing radiation can also induce a terminal growth arrest leading to a senescent-like morphology. This can occur in both normal cells (e.g., fibroblasts) and tumor cells. Initial attempts at p53-dependent reversible cell cycle arrest are followed by the activation of the terminal arrest pathway when the amount of DNA damage it is beyond repair. At these later times post-irradiation, cells acquire a senesecent-like morphology (i.e., increasing granularity within the nucleus) and may express increased levels of p16[INK4A] and SA-β-galactosidase (both markers of senescent cells). (Modified from Roninson, 2003.)

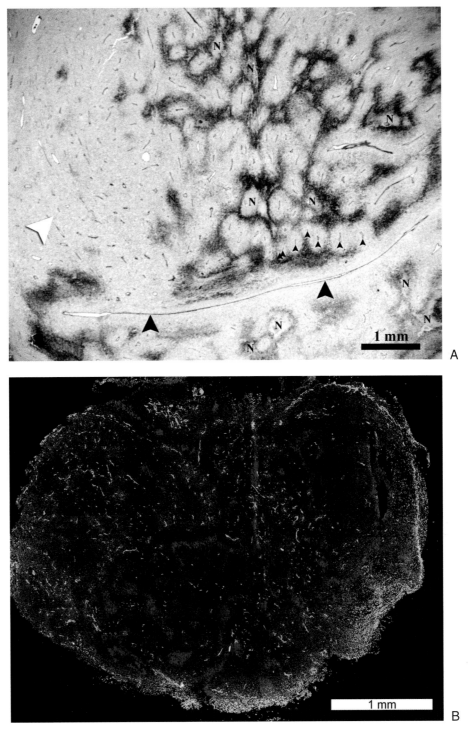

**Figure 15.11.** Tumor Hypoxia. Panel (*A*) shows a section of a high grade human soft tissue sarcoma (rhabdomyosarcoma, pleomorphic) showing hypoxic regions (dark brown membraneous CA IX staining) distant from blood vessels (reddish-brown CD31 staining). Small black arrowheads point to blood vessels at the center of tumor cords with peripheral CA IX staining. Large black arrowheads point to one long blood vessel in the plane of the section. Necrotic regions are labeled with an N. The large white arrowhead points to a well-vascularized region with no hypoxia (and absence of CA IX staining). This picture illustrates the cord-like structure which is associated with (chronic) hypoxia in regions of many tumors. (Courtesy of Dr. K. Maseide, University of Toronto, Toronto, Canada.) Panel (*B*) shows staining for EF5 (red) in a complete section through a human pancreatic tumor xenograft growing in a SCID mouse. The blood vessels are stained for CD31 (green) and regions close to functional blood vessels are indicated by the blue staining for Hoechst 33342 that was injected into the mouse a few minutes before the animal was killed and the tumor was removed. Brightish staining in the bottom right edge of the figure is an artifact. (Courtesy of Dr. David Hedley and Ms Nhu-An Pham, University of Toronto, Toronto, Canada.)

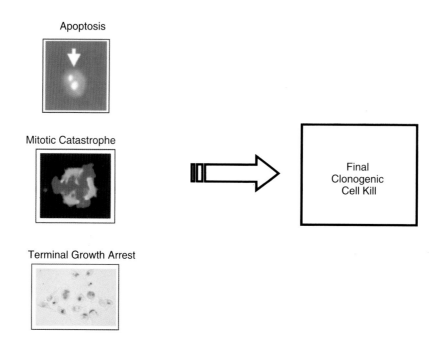

**Figure 14.11.** Mechanisms of cell death following exposure to ionizing radiation. Cells can undergo apoptosis (top figure), mitotic catastrophe (middle figure) or terminal cell arrest (bottom figure) following irradiation. The extent to which one mode of cell death is dominant over another is dependent on cell type, radiation dose and the cell's microenvironment (e.g., relative oxygenation and availability of growth factors) (Figures courtesy of Gillian Bromfield, University of Toronto, Toronto, Canada and reproduced from Sato et al., 2000, with permission). Each type of cell death has a unique morphology and timing following irradiation as described in Section 14.3.2 and can be quantified by specific methods: apoptotic cells show condensed chromatin bodies; mitotic catastrophe cells show multiple tubulin spindles and centrosomes; terminally-arrested cells express SA-$\beta$-galactosidase (see Fig. 14.12). Although the majority of human epithelial tumor cells respond to ionizing radiation by undergoing mitotic arrest and/or terminal growth arrest, the accumulation of all death events by these three mechanisms reflects the final cell kill as measured by a long-term clonogenic assay.

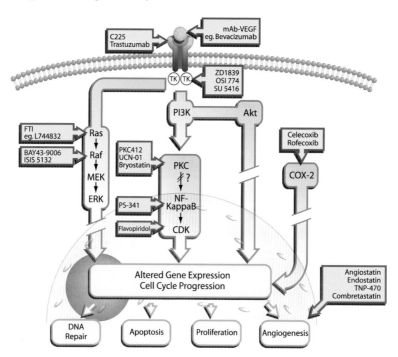

**Figure 14.23.** Pathways involved in tumor cell radioresistance amenable to molecular targeting in addition to radiotherapy. A number of oncogenic pathways are abnormal in radioresistant tumor cells leading to abnormal cell proliferation, DNA repair, cell death responses or angiogenesis. Specific agents that target these pathways have been used in preclinical and clinical studies as a means of overcoming this resistance. In this figure, pathways relating to increased radioresistance in vitro and in vivo are presented as altered growth factor (i.e., EGFR, VEGF) PI-3K/PTEN-AKT and RAS-RAF intracellular signaling and abnormalities in angiogenesis. Selected agents can lead to radiosensitization by blocking receptors with competing antibodies or inhibiting intracellular signaling cascades. These approaches are discussed in more detail in Section 14.4.4. (Reproduced with permission from Ma et al., 2003.)

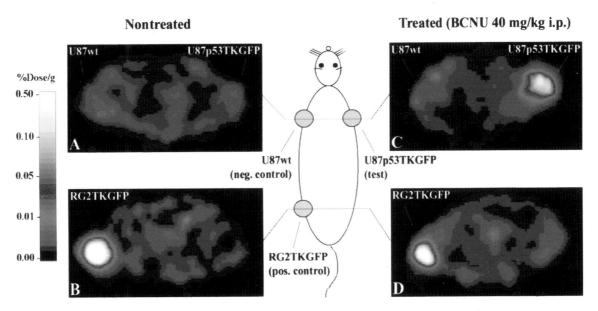

**Figure 13.9.** Positron emission tomography imaging of endogenous p53 activation using the HSV-tk reporter. Positron emission tomography images through the shoulder (*A* and *C*) and pelvis (*B* and *D*) of two rats are shown. A nontreated animal is shown on the left, and a BCNU-treated (to promote p53 activity) animal is shown on the right. Both animals had three subcutaneous tumor xenografts expressing mutant *p53* (test) in the right shoulder, wild-type *p53* (negative control) in the left shoulder, and a tumor line which constituitively expresses the HSV-tk reporter (positive control) in the left thigh. The nontreated animal on the left shows localization of radioactivity only in the positive control tumor (left thigh); the test and negative control tumors are at background levels. The BCNU-treated animal on the right shows significant localization of radioactivity in the test tumor (right shoulder) and in the positive control (left thigh), but no radioactivity above background in the negative control (left shoulder). (From Doubrovin, 2001.)

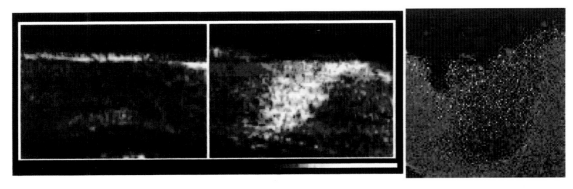

**Figure 13.10.** High-frequency ultrasound images of apoptosis in response to photodynamic therapy (PDT) in rat brain. *Left*: untreated; *middle*: 24 hours after PDT; *right*: TUNEL assay of same region. High-frequency ultrasound images are 4 mm × 4 mm.

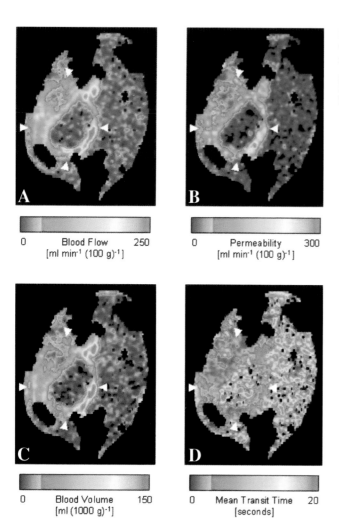

**Figure 13.7.** Functional CT perfusion maps of (A) blood flow, (B) microvessel permeability surface area product, (C) blood volume, and (D) mean transit of blood time as measured in a VX-2 tumor grown in a rabbit thigh (arrowheads mark the tumor boundary). Note the vascular rim (A,B,C) and the long blood transit time in the core (D). (From Purdie et al., 2001.)

0    Blood Flow    250
[ml min⁻¹ (100 g)⁻¹]

0    Permeability    300
[ml min⁻¹ (100 g)⁻¹]

0    Blood Volume    150
[ml (1000 g)⁻¹]

0    Mean Transit Time    20
[seconds]

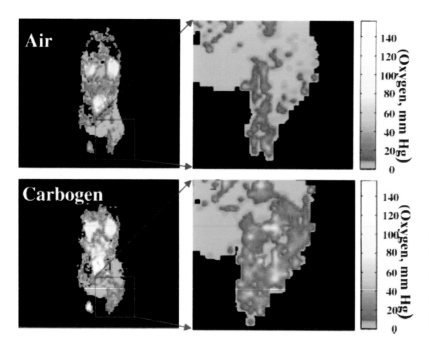

**Figure 13.8.** The Overhauser effect and MRI used to produce tissue oxygenation (pO₂) images of a C3H mouse with a 1-cm diameter squamous cell carcinoma tumor during air breathing (upper) and carbogen breathing (lower). The expanded tumor region (right) shows pO₂ heterogeneity. (Reprinted from Krishna et al., 2002.)

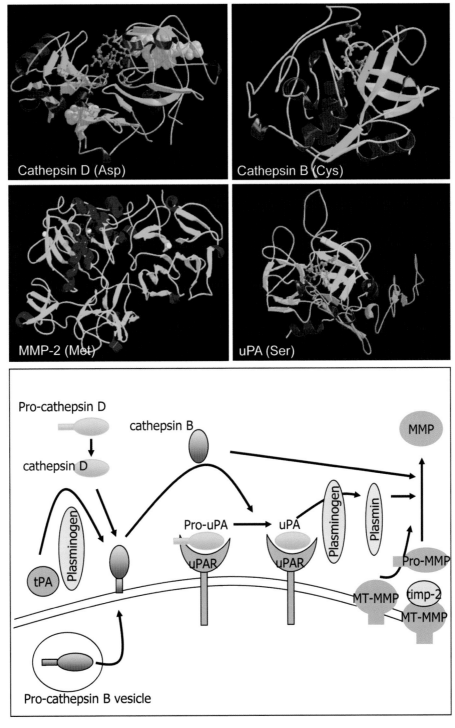

**Figure 11.14.** Tertiary structures of an aspartic proteinase (cathepsin D), cysteine proteinase (cathepsin B), matrix metalloproteinase (MMP-2, gelatinase A), and the kringle domain of a serine proteinase (urokinase plasminogen activator). Catalytic residues are shown in ball-and-stick representation for cathepsin D, cathepsin B, gelatinase A, and uPA. The distinct structures highlight the requirement for individual endogenous inhibitors, as well as the need to develop specific synthetic inhibitors as cancer therapeutics. The bottom panel illustrates a proteinase cascade linking these distinct classes of proteinases. Cathepsin B, typically a lysosomal protease, can be activated pericellularly by cathepsin D upon its own autoactivation. Cathepsin B then participates in the cell surface activation of uPA which in turn converts plasminogen into plasmin. Plasmin, cathepsin B, as well as a ternary complex of MMPs assembled at the cell surface, can activate MMP-2. [Top panel modified from the proteinase database (http://merops.sanger.co.uk) and bottom panel from Rao, 2003.

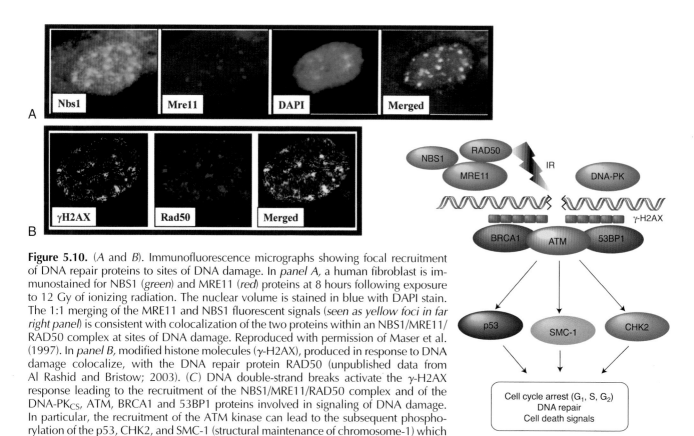

**Figure 5.10.** (*A* and *B*). Immunofluorescence micrographs showing focal recruitment of DNA repair proteins to sites of DNA damage. In *panel A,* a human fibroblast is immunostained for NBS1 (*green*) and MRE11 (*red*) proteins at 8 hours following exposure to 12 Gy of ionizing radiation. The nuclear volume is stained in blue with DAPI stain. The 1:1 merging of the MRE11 and NBS1 fluorescent signals (*seen as yellow foci in far right panel*) is consistent with colocalization of the two proteins within an NBS1/MRE11/RAD50 complex at sites of DNA damage. Reproduced with permission of Maser et al. (1997). In *panel B,* modified histone molecules (γ-H2AX), produced in response to DNA damage colocalize, with the DNA repair protein RAD50 (unpublished data from Al Rashid and Bristow; 2003). (*C*) DNA double-strand breaks activate the γ-H2AX response leading to the recruitment of the NBS1/MRE11/RAD50 complex and of the DNA-PK$_{CS}$, ATM, BRCA1 and 53BP1 proteins involved in signaling of DNA damage. In particular, the recruitment of the ATM kinase can lead to the subsequent phosphorylation of the p53, CHK2, and SMC-1 (structural maintenance of chromosome-1) which control the cell cycle checkpoints in the G1, S, and G2 phases of the cell cycle, leading to DNA repair and/or activation of cell death. (Adapted after Abraham, 2001.)

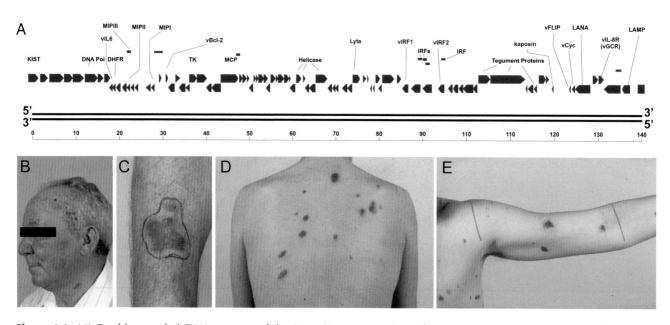

**Figure 6.6.** (*A*) Double-stranded DNA genome of the Kaposi's sarcoma virus. The genome contains 87 open reading frames (ORFs) coding for latency proteins, reactivation proteins, and structural proteins. Host genes that help the virus evade immune surveillance and inhibit apoptosis have been acquired from chromosomes through a process of molecular piracy. These genes include vFLIP, vBcl-2, v-cyclin, interferon response factors (IRFs), and membrane cofactor protein (MCP), KIST, vIL6, MIP chemokines, LANA, vIL-8R (vGCR), and LAMP. (*B-E*) Skin lesions associated with Kaposi sarcoma. Lesions present as red blotches on the skin due to the infection of spindle cells. Angiogenesis occurs in the surrounding tissue. *Panels B and C* are examples of endemic or Mediterranean Kaposi's sarcoma, while panels D and E illustrate epidemic or AIDS-related Kaposi sarcoma. (Photographs courtesy of Dr. Fei-Fei Liu, Ontario Cancer Institute.)

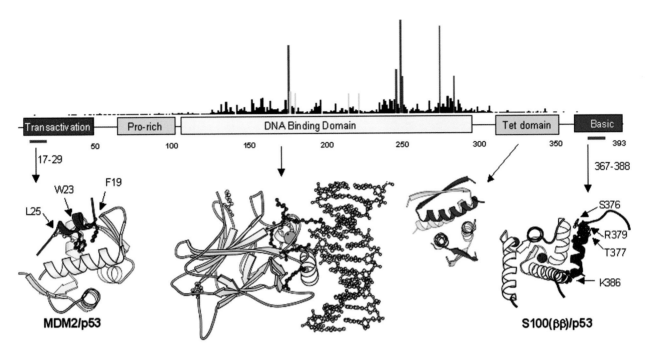

**Figure 4.20.** Linear schematic of p53 outlining the different functional and structural domains. The primary sequence of p53 is represented as a horizontal line with domains shown as *colored rectangles* with residue numbers underneath. The frequency of cancer-associated mutations at each amino acid residue is indicated as a histogram above the primary sequence. Hotspot mutations are colored in *red* (R248, R273, R175), in *blue* (G245, R282, R249), and in *yellow* (C176, H179, Y220, and F212). The corresponding residues are colored in the same manner and drawn in *ball-and-stick* representation in the x-ray crystal structure of the DNA binding domain bound to DNA and zinc ion (*blue sphere*) shown in the lower central panel. Most of these hotspot mutations result in disruption of amino acid side chains either directly involved in DNA binding, or in supporting either the helix or loops that interact with DNA. Those more distal from the DNA interface have an overall destabilizing effect on the domain. The *lower left panel* shows the x-ray structure of Mdm2 (*cyan*) bound to a p53-derived peptide (*red*) from the transactivation domain. The three hydrophobic residues (F19, W23, and L25) on one face of the p53 helix responsible for the interaction with Mdm2 are shown in *ball-and-stick* representation. The NMR-derived structure of the tetramerisation domain revealed a dimer of dimers (*yellow/blue and yellow/pink*). The NMR-derived structure of the complex between S100(ββ) and a peptide derived from the basic regulatory domain of p53 (*dark blue*) revealed the manner in which posttranslational phosphorylation by protein kinase C (at residues S376 and T377) and acetylation by p300 (at residues R379 and K386) are blocked by the interaction. Calcium ions in S100(ββ) are represented by the *red spheres*.

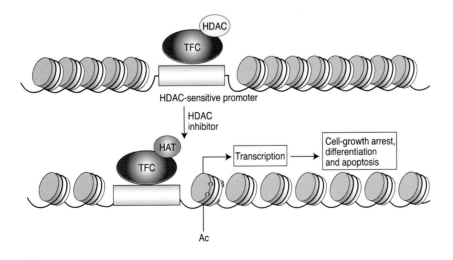

**Figure 5.2.** Action of histone deacetylase inhibitors (HDAC inhibitors). With inhibition of histone deacetylases (HDACs), histones are acetylated, and the DNA that is tightly wrapped around deacetylated histone cores relaxes. Accumulation of acetylated histones in nucleosomes leads to increased transcription of a subset of genes (for example, *p21*$^{WAF}$) which, in turn, leads to downstream effects that result in cell-growth arrest, differentiation, and/or apoptotic cell death and as a consequence, inhibition of tumor growth. Ac, acetyl group; HAT, histone acetyltransferase, TFC-transcription factor complex. (Reproduced with permission from Marks et al., 2001.)

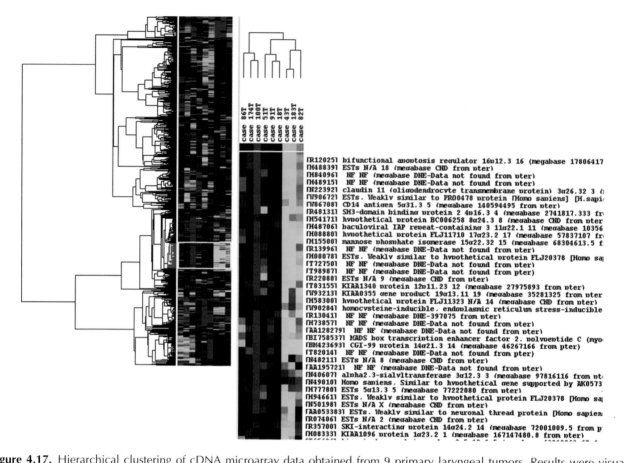

**Figure 4.17.** Hierarchical clustering of cDNA microarray data obtained from 9 primary laryngeal tumors. Results were visualized using Tree view software, and include the dendogram (clustering of samples) and the clustering of gene expression, based on genetic similarity. Tree view represents 946 genes that best distinguish these two groups of samples. Genes whose expression is higher in the tumor sample relative to the reference sample are shown in *red*; those whose expression is lower than the reference sample are shown in *green*; and no change in gene expression is shown in *black*. (Courtesy of Patricia Reis and Shilpi Arora, The Ontario Cancer Institute and Princess Margaret Hospital, Toronto.)

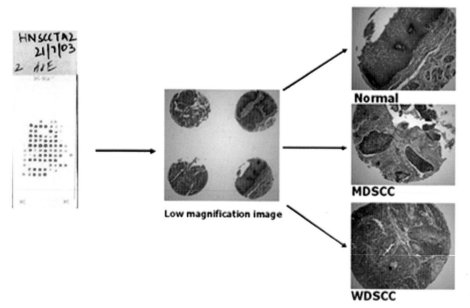

**Figure 4.18.** Hematoxylin & Eosin stained tissue array slide. This slide contains approximately 100 tissue spots, including control tissues, oral squamous cell carcinoma, and adjacent normal tissues. All samples are spotted in duplicate. MDSCC is moderately differentiated squamous cell carcinoma. WDSCC is well-differentiated squamous cell carcinoma. (Courtesy of Shilpi Arora, The Ontario Cancer Institute and Princess Margaret Hospital, Toronto.)

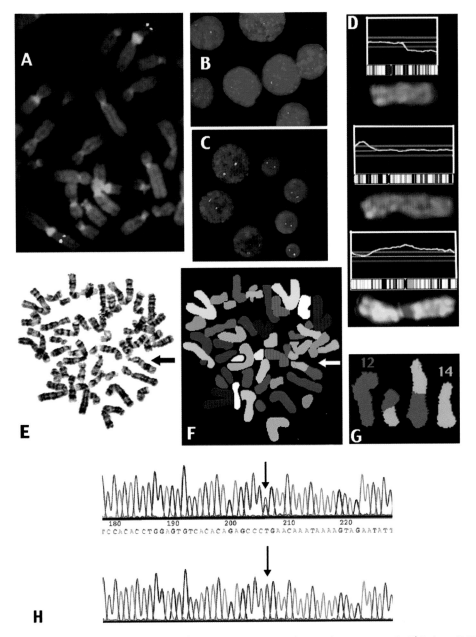

**Figure 4.16.** (*A*) Example of FISH mapping of a single copy genomic probe to chromosome 1. This is a DAPI (*blue counter-stain*) banded normal metaphase preparation showing the location of positive signals (*yellow signals*) obtained with a cosmid probe containing an insert size of 40 kilobases of DNA from a gene on chromosome 1. A positive FISH signal is present on each chromatid of both pairs of chromosome 1 at band 1q25. (*B*) MYCN amplification in nuclei from neuroblastoma detected by FISH with a MYCN probe (*magenta speckling*) and a deletion of the short arm of chromosome 1. The signal (*pale blue/green*) from the remaining normal chromosome 1 is seen as a single spot in each nucleus. (*C*) Detection of a Philadelphia chromo-some in interphase nuclei of leukemia cells. All nuclei contain one green signal (BCR gene), one pink signal (ABL gene), and an intermediate fusion yellow signal because of the 9;22 chromosome translocation. (*D*) The comparative genomic hybridiza-tion analysis profile from a neuroblastoma cell line. Chromosome 1 shows an overall gain of DNA indicated by an increase in the level of green signal (*bottom panel*). In this cell line most of chromosome 1 was trisomic. Chromosome 2 has a strong green signal at band 2p24 due to amplification (50 copies/cell) of MYCN in the cell line (*middle panel*). The long arm of chromo-some 6 shows a loss (deletion) of DNA and a shift toward the red signal (*top panel*). (*E-G*) SKY analysis of blood lymphocytes from a patient with a translocation. (*E*) One of the aberrant chromosomes can be seen by classic G-banding (*arrow*); (*F*) the same metaphase spread has been subjected to SKY; and (*G*) the 12;14 reciprocal translocation is identified. (*H*) Automated se-quencing of BRCA2, the hereditary breast cancer predisposition gene. Each colored peak represents a different nucleotide. The *lower panel* is a sequence of a wild-type DNA sample. The sequence of a mutation carrier in the upper panel contains a dou-ble peak (*indicated by an arrow*) in which the nucleotide T in intron 17 located at 2 bp downstream of the 5′ end of exon 18 is converted to a C. This mutation results in aberrant splicing of exon 18 of the BRCA2 gene. The presence of a T nucleotide, in addition to the mutant C, implies that only one copy of the two BRCA2 genes is mutated in this sample (see Sec. 4.3.9 for details).

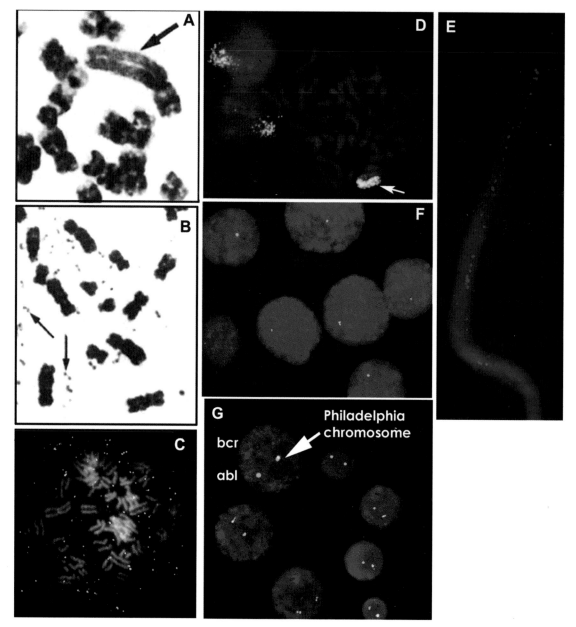

**Figure 4.14.** Analysis of oncogene rearrangements in tumors by conventional cytogenetics and FISH analysis. (*A*) An abnormally long chromosome (*arrow*). The extended region of this chromosome has no identifiable bands and is called a *homogeneously staining region* (HSR). (*B*) Multiple paired dots of chromatic material. These chromosomal abnormalities are called *double minutes* (DM). Both HSRs and DMs are associated with gene amplification. DMs are extrachromosomal circular DNA containing a few copies of the oncogene. HSRs are integrated multiple tandem repeats of the oncogene. (*C*) Metaphase preparation from a neuroblastoma that has N-*myc* amplification on DMs (green dots) detected by FISH. (*D*) A metaphase from another neuroblastoma that has N-*myc* amplification and an HSR. In this FISH preparation, the additional N-*myc* signals can be seen to decorate the HSR (*arrow*), the HSR is also apparent as clusters of yellow signal in the interphase nuclei. (*E*) A HSR in a neuroblastoma cell line with gene amplification of N-*myc*. In this preparation, the HSR has been stretched so that, in the extended form, multiple N-*myc* signals can be seen as a linear array. (Courtesy of Ajay Pandita, Pathology Department, University of Toronto.) (*F*) Interphase nuclei from a neuroblastoma with DMs. The bright pink dots within each nucleus are the FISH signals from the N-*myc* oncogene, which is known to be amplified to 50–100 copies per cell in this patient's tumor. In addition the single green dot indicates the loss of one copy of chromosome region 1p36. (*G*) Interphase cytogenetic analysis of a leukemia to identify the Philadelphia chromosome using FISH with the *bcr* and *abl* probes. The *abl* probe has been labeled with a red fluorochrome (*black dot*) and the *bcr* with a green fluorochrome (*shaded dot*). When the Philadelphia chromosome is present in a nucleus, both the red and green signals become superimposed, producing one strong yellow signal (*white dot*). If the nucleus does not have this abnormality, two red signals and two green signals will be present.

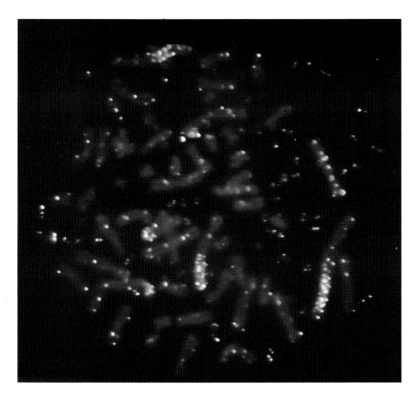

**Figure 18.8.** Fluorescent in situ hybridization analysis of *MRP1*. The normal cellular locus of the *MRP1 (ABCC1)* gene encoding the 190 kilo-Dalton ABC drug efflux pump, MRP1, is chromosome 16p13.1. However, in many drug-resistant cell lines, *MRP1* has been amplified. The figure shows a metaphase spread of a highly drug-resistant lung cancer cell which contains approximately 100 copies of *MRP1*. Note that the fluorescently labeled MRP1 probe has hybridized to several homogeneously staining regions (HSRS) and multiple double minute chromosomes (DMINS). (With permission from Slovak et al., 1993.)

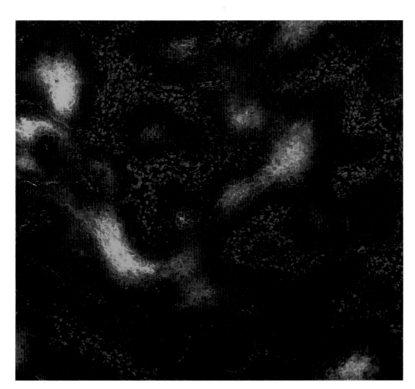

**Figure 18.16.** Three-color photomicrograph of a section of the 16C mouse mammary tumor generated with a Zeiss Axiovert fluorescent microscope showing immunostaining of blood vessels using anti-CD31 (red), hypoxic regions using anti-EF5 (green) and the distribution of fluorescent doxorubicin (blue) 20 minutes after intravenous injection. Bar = 100 μm. Unpublished data of Primeau and Tannock.

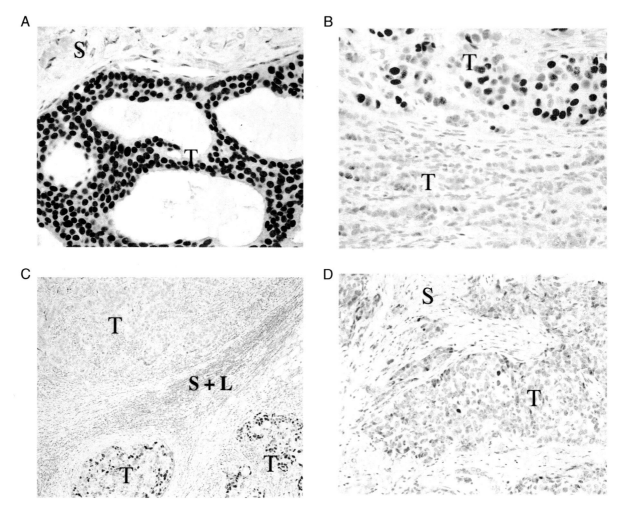

**Figure 19.8.** Immunohistograms illustrating heterogeneity of human breast cancer biopsy samples. Brown staining represents ER-$\alpha$ positivity. T, invasive breast cancer; S, stromal and connective tissue elements; L, lymphocytes. (A) Homogenous expression of ER-$\alpha$ within an invasive breast cancer, with negative adjacent vessels and stroma. (B) Moderate heterogeneity of expression of ER-$\alpha$ within an invasive breast cancer, with strong expression within solid nests of tumor cells in the upper field and weak or negative expression within less cohesive clusters of tumor cells in the lower field. Stromal and lymphocytic elements are negative for ER-$\alpha$. (C) Marked heterogeneity of expression of ER-$\alpha$ within an invasive tumor metastatic to an axillary lymph node. In the upper part of the section one metastatic component is homogenously ER-$\alpha$ negative and in the lower section, the other component is moderate to high ER-$\alpha$ positive. These two different elements are separated in this field of view by a band of fibrous stroma and infiltrating lymphocytes. (D) Marked heterogeneity of ER-$\alpha$ expression within an invasive breast cancer with sporadic ER-$\alpha$ positive invasive breast cancer cells within a predominantly ER-$\alpha$ negative invasive tumor.

resistant phases of the cell cycle, their subsequent progression (inevitably into more sensitive phases) leads to a reduction in survival at 4 hours. Continued repair and repopulation explain the increases in survival at later times. This pattern of SLDR has been demonstrated for a wide range of cell lines.

The repair capacity of the cells of many tissues in vivo has been demonstrated using cell-survival and functional assays in vivo. An increase in total dose is required to give the same level of biological damage when a single dose ($D_1$) is split into two doses (total dose $D_2$) with a time interval between them (see Fig. 14.14). The difference in dose ($D_2$-$D_1$) is a measure of the repair by the cells in the tissue.

The capacity of different cell populations to undergo SLDR is reflected by the width of the shoulder on their survival curve, that is, the $D_q$ or $D_2$-$D_1$ value. Survival curves for bone marrow cells or cells derived from the radiosensitive disorders AT (ataxia telangiectasia) and NBS (Nijmegen Breakage Syndrome) (or cells which lack DNA-repair enzymes) have no shoulder and demonstrate little or no evidence of cellular repair (Fig. 14.15A). Recent data suggest that AT and NBS cells may also have increased residual DNA double-strand breaks following irradiation, suggesting a subtle defect in DNA-dsb repair (Fig. 14.15B). Other cells (e.g., jejunal crypt cells) can demonstrate a large repair capacity ($D_2$-$D_1$ value of 4 to 5 Gy; Fig. 14.14A).

To maximize SLDR capacity in tissues, cells can be irradiated under low-dose rate conditions, as in brachytherapy (see Chap. 15, Sec. 15.2.3). The effect of radiation on tissues and cells for the same dose differs widely for exposure over a short time (acute irradiation) or for continuous irradiation over an extended period of time (irradiation given at a low-dose rate). Dose rates above about 1 Gy per minute can be regarded as acute (single-dose) treatment. As the total dose of x- or $\gamma$-rays is delivered at decreasing dose rates,

the DNA damage in the cell (i.e., yield of chromosome aberrations and DNA-double strand breaks) progressively diminishes due to its ability to repair the damage during the treatment (Cornforth et al., 2002). As a result, the shape of the radiation survival curve changes from one exhibiting pronounced curvature at high-dose rates to one approaching linearity at low-dose rates (Fig. 14.16A).

The magnitude of the *dose-rate sparing effect* may be calculated as the relative survival under conditions of low-dose rate irradiation compared to survival under conditions of acute-dose rate irradiation. Cell lines with a greater capacity to repair sublethal damage will demonstrate a large dose-sparing effect relative to those cells that have limited capacity to repair the damage. If the dose rate is low enough, the cells will continue to divide and repopulate without activating cell cycle checkpoints (see Chap. 5, Sec. 5.5). This process of cell cycle redistribution leads to a relative radiosensitization of the entire population (see Chap. 15, Sec. 15.6.3). Most of the effect of cellular repair occurs in the range of dose rates of 1.0 to 0.01 Gy per minute (Ruiz de Almodovar et al., 1994). Below about 0.1 Gy per minute, the effects of cell cycle progression (redistribution and the G2 block; see Sec. 14.4.2) become apparent; below about 0.01 Gy per minute, the effects of cell repopulation will start to become evident as the radiation damage is not severe enough to trigger cell cycle arrest. At lower dose rates, the processes of repair and cellular repopulation within the cell culture predominate (Fig. 14.16B).

Cell survival can also be increased by holding cells after irradiation under conditions of suboptimal growth such as low temperature, nutrient deprivation, or high cell density. The latter conditions may reflect those experienced by G0/G1 populations of cells in growth-deprived regions of tumors (Malaise et al., 1989). The increased survival is due to the repair of *potentially lethal*

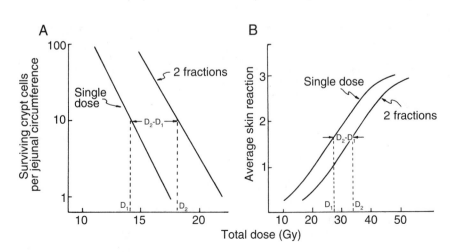

**Figure 14.14.** Repair of radiation damage in vivo. (A) Survival curves for murine intestinal crypt cells $\gamma$-irradiated in situ with a single dose or with two equal fractions given 3 h apart. (Modified from Withers et al., 1974.) (B) Average skin reaction following x-irradiation of mouse skin with a single dose or two fractions given 24 h apart.

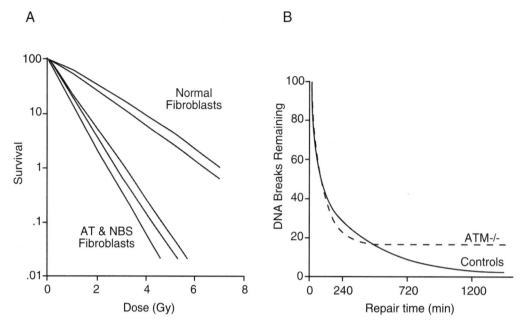

**Figure 14.15.** Radiosensitivity and DNA rejoining defects in cells derived from *ataxia telan-giectasia (AT)* or *Nijmegen Breakage Syndrome (NBS)* patients. In addition to aberrant cell cycle checkpoints, subtle DNA double-strand break repair defects are associated with the AT and NBS disorders. Shown in (*A*) is the relative radiation survival for normal diploid fibroblasts versus that of AT or NBS fibroblasts. Note increased radiosensitivity following clinically relevant doses of 1 to 2 Gy. Shown in (*B*) are the DNA double-strand break rejoining curves (based on pulse-field gel electrophoresis) for AT cells relative to normal cells. The number of DNA double-strand breaks remaining is plotted against time following irradiation. Although the two sets of data initially have similar rates of DNA rejoining, the AT cells have increased numbers of residual DNA double-strand breaks relative to controls at later times post-irradiation. (Modified from Girard et al., 2000.)

*damage* (PLDR), which usually results in a change in the slope of the cell-survival curve. Such repair may contribute to increased radiation survival observed in vivo for some transplantable cell lines when compared to the radiosensitivity of the same cells growing in vitro (Weichselbaum et al., 1983).

### 14.3.4 Adaptive Radiation Responses and Low-dose Hyperradiosensitivity

Following very low doses of radiation, mammalian cells may have an inducible radioprotective response that acts both in vitro and in vivo. This so-called *adaptive*

**Figure 14.16.** (*A*) Survival curves for HeLa cells treated with gamma-radiation at different continuous (low) dose rates. (Redrawn from Mitchell et. al., 1979.) (*B*) Schematic diagram to illustrate the influence on the survival curve following continuous low-dose rate irradiation, of the processes of repair, redistribution and the G2 block, and repopulation. (Redrawn from Hall, 2000.)

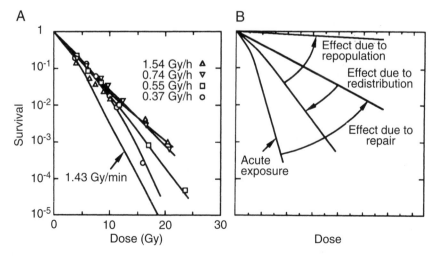

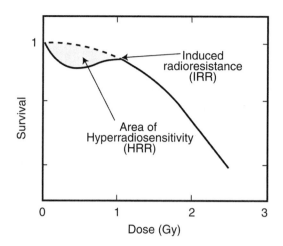

**Figure 14.17.** Low-dose hyperradiosensitivity (HRR). Following very low doses of ionizing radiation (e.g., 0.01 to 0.3 Gy), selected mammalian cells may have an inducible radioprotective response (i.e., induced radioresistance or IRR) that can be triggered at a certain threshold dose. The figure illustrates the difference in the expected (dashed line) and observed (solid line) survival in cells that show an initial hypersensitivity (HRS) followed by induced radioresistance (IRR) at doses greater than ~0.3 Gy. (Modified from Skov, 1999.)

*response* appears to be triggered by a threshold level of radiation damage (Joiner et al., 2001). For example, some mammalian cells appear to be hypersensitive to very low doses of ionizing radiation (0.01 to 0.3 Gy) as compared with higher radiation doses (see Fig. 14.17). Following doses of radiation above about 1 Gy, this hyperradiosensitivity (HRS) is not observed. Two hypotheses have been proposed for increased survival at doses above 0.3 Gy: (1) there is an inducible damage-sensing threshold (IRR; induced radioresistance) for triggering faster or more efficient DNA repair, and (2) the low dose injury induces changes in DNA structure or organization that facilitates constitutive repair. An adaptive radiation response is observed in rodents for irradiated normal skin and kidney cells. For example, the use of multiple radiation fractions of less than 1 Gy can decrease the total dose required for the same biological effect in vivo by a factor of 2 to 4 (relative to that required with fractions of 2 Gy). It has been argued that differences in the radiosensitivity of human tumor cells might be explained in part by the variation in the adaptive response observed for different human tumor cell lines (Lambin et al., 1996). A recent in vivo study using ultrafractionated treatment of tumors, derived from human tumor cell line that demonstrated HRS in vitro, failed to demonstrate any evidence that HRS influenced sensitivity in vivo (Krause et al., 2003). However, there are many other factors that could have influenced this result, including effects on tumor cell proliferation during treatment, as discussed in Chapter 15 (Sec. 15.6.2).

## 14.4 MOLECULAR AND CELLULAR RESPONSES TO IONIZING RADIATION

### 14.4.1 Genomic and Proteomic Studies of Irradiated Cells

Cellular damage following ionizing radiation can affect the expression of a number of genes involved in the response of cells to stress. Induction of the expression of early-response genes by ionizing radiation can be initiated by damage to the plasma membrane or to nuclear DNA (Criswell et al., 2003). Some early-response genes, such as the early growth response factor (*EGR*-1) contain radiation-responsive regulatory domains in their promoter regions that can facilitate their rapid induction by ionizing radiation (Hallahan et al., 1995). These sequences might be used in radiation-induced gene-therapy vectors to drive expression of suicide genes within an irradiated field for tumor therapy (Fig. 14.18). Synthetic enhancers of gene expression designed for use with radiation utilize short motifs of sequence CC(A/T)₆GG (i.e., radiation-responsive CArG elements) derived from the *EGR1* gene (Dalta et al., 1992; Maples et al., 2002). Such constructs can be responsive to radiation at doses of 1 to 5 Gy. These tumor-targeting vectors might be used in clinical situations where the irradiation volume of normal tissue can be tightly controlled using conformal radiotherapy planning (see Chap. 15, Sec. 15.2.2) and have shown early promise in animal models (Weichselbaum et al., 2002; Mauceri et al., 1996).

Irradiation can also modify intracellular signaling through modification of the activity of tyrosine kinases, MAP-kinases, SAP-kinases, and Ras-associated proteins (see Chap. 8, Sec. 8.2) (Schmidt-Ullrich et al., 2003; Dent et al., 2003; Ruiter et al., 1999). An example is the activation of the c-Abl pathway which phosphorylates Rad51, a DNA repair protein, at sites of DNA damage (see Chap. 5, Sec. 5.3.5). Other genes induced by radiation include those encoding cell cycle related proteins [e.g., growth arrest after DNA damage *(GADD)*, *p34^cdc2*, *cyclin B, p53*], growth factors, and cytokines [e.g., platelet-derived growth factor *(PDGF)*, transforming growth factor beta *(TGF-β)*, basic fibroblast growth factor *(bFGF)*, tumor necrosis factor *(TNF)*], and enzymes (e.g., plasminogen activator). Liberation of inflammatory cytokines such as TGF-α and interleukin-1 (IL-1) by cells following radiation damage may lead to a continuing cascade of cytokine production, which may be responsible for the acute inflammation and late-onset fibrosis observed in some irradiated tissues (see Chap. 15, Sec. 15.5.3).

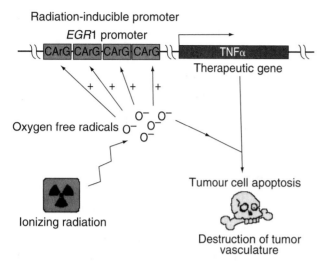

**Figure 14.18.** Radiation-induced gene expression as the basis for gene therapy. Ionizing radiation induces the expression of a number of radiation-responsive genes. This may be exploited to regulate the expression of exogenous therapeutic genes during gene therapy. For example, the promoter of the early growth response gene *(EGR1)* contains radiation-inducible CArG DNA sequences allowing for the expression of *EGR1* within minutes of irradiation. These dose-responsive promoter elements can be linked to DNA sequences that encode for genes whose products are toxic to the cell. In the example shown, *EGR1*-promoter sequences have been linked to the tumor necrosis factor *(TNF-alpha)* gene to create a construct that expresses TNF-alpha in a radiation-dose dependent manner. By expressing this construct in tumor cells and then giving localized experimental radiotherapy, it was shown that increased tumor and endothelial cell killing occurred within the irradiated tumor volume compared to that expected for radiation alone. (Reproduced with permission from Weichselbaum et al., 2002.)

Approaches using cDNA microarrays (see Chap. 4, Sec. 4.4.4) have led to the discovery that radiation-induced gene expression can be cell-type specific. Activation of some genes is dose dependent, while others are activated specifically at either low (i.e., 1 to 3 Gy) or high doses (i.e., 10 Gy) (Amundson et al., 2003; Chaudhry et al., 2003; Tusher et al., 2001; Khodarev et al., 2001). Furthermore, gene expression following a given radiation dose can be substantially higher when tumor cells are irradiated in vivo rather than in culture. Biopsies from human tumors have demonstrated that differences in radiation-induced gene expression are greater between patients' tumors than within the tumor of a given patient (Hartmann et al., 2002). This observation supports the concept that molecular profiling of individual tumors and normal tissues may be able to predict radiation response.

The majority of proteins involved in DNA repair undergo posttranslational modification or protein-protein interactions following irradiation. Because such modifications would not be detected using cDNA microarray analyses (see Chap. 4, Sec. 4.4.4), which detect al-

teration of mRNA expression, proteomic analyses of tissue samples or sera may be additionally useful in tracking molecular radioresponse in patients.

## 14.4.2 Cell Cycle Sensitivity and DNA Damage Checkpoints

Mammalian cells respond to ionizing radiation by delaying their progression through the cell cycle. Such delays could allow for the repair of DNA damage in cells prior to undergoing DNA replication or mitosis and is thought to prevent genetic instability in future cell generations (Harwell and Kastan, 1994). Early kinetic studies reported a rapid decrease in the mitotic index in an irradiated cell population, as both lethally damaged and surviving cells ceased to enter mitosis, while cells already in mitosis continued their cell cycle progression. After a period of time, which depends on both the cell type and the radiation dose, surviving cells re-enter mitosis (Fig. 14.19); this time is known as the *mitotic delay.* Mitotic delay appears to be due largely to a block of cell cycle progression in G2 phase, although cells in G1 and S phases are also delayed in their progression, albeit to a lesser extent. There is approximately 3–4 hours of G2 delay per 1 Gy in a diploid cell. Cells may continue to experience delays in their progression through the next and subsequent cell cycles. As a result of radiation-induced delays in the cell cycle, cell populations can be partially synchronized by irradiation.

Cells in different phases of the cell cycle have different radiosensitivities (Terasima and Tolmach, 1961; Bernhard et al., 1999). This is illustrated for Chinese hamster cells by the survival curves shown in Figure 14.20*A*. If a single radiation dose is given to cells in different phases (i.e., a vertical cut is taken through the curves in Fig. 14.20*A*), then a pattern of cell survival as a function of cell cycle position is obtained (Fig. 14.20*B*). Figure 14.20 shows that Chinese hamster cells in late S phase have the highest probability of survival after radiation (i.e., are the most resistant), and that cells in G2/M phases are the most sensitive. Although many cell lines appear to have a resistant period in S phase and a sensitive period in G2 phase following irradiation in vitro, other cell lines have different patterns of sensitivity throughout the cell cycle. Some oncogene-transfected cells (e.g., overexpressing the *ras* oncogene) show increased resistance in the G2 phase, whereas other cells, including DNA repair-deficient cells, show similar sensitivity throughout all phases of the cell cycle. The pattern of radiosensitivity throughout the cell cycle can be different for the same tumor cells growing in vivo or in vitro, indicating the influence of cell-cell interactions on cell survival (Keng et al., 1984).

The molecular biology of the mammalian cell cycle and its response to DNA damage (including that from ionizing radiation) has been discussed in detail in Chap-

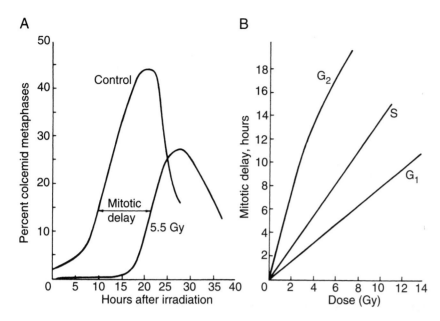

**Figure 14.19.** The effects of radiation on the progression of cells into mitosis after the treatment. (*A*) At time zero, the cells are placed in medium containing colcemid, a drug that arrests cells in mitosis, and the percentage of cells that accumulate in mitosis is plotted as a function of time. The decline in the curves at late times is a result of cells escaping the drug-induced block or dying. The mitotic delay due to a radiation dose of 5.5 Gy displaces the curves for the radiation-treated cells to the right. (*B*) Cells are irradiated when in different phases of the cell cycle and the mitotic delay observed is plotted as a function of radiation dose. (Adapted from Elkind and Whitmore, 1967.)

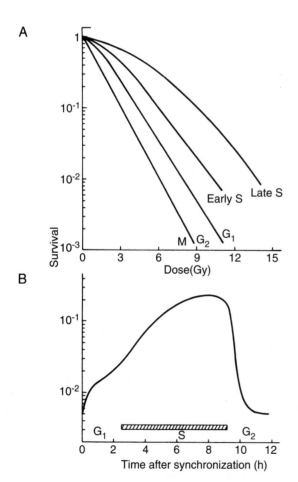

**Figure 14.20.** The effect of position in the cell growth cycle on cellular radiosensitivity. (*A*) Survival curves for Chinese hamster cells irradiated in different phases of the cell cycle. (*B*) Cells were selected in mitosis and irradiated with a fixed dose as a function of time of incubation after synchronization. The pattern of cell survival reflects the changing cellular sensitivity as the cells move through the cell cycle.

ter 5, Section 5.5 and Chapter 9, Section 9.2. The ATM (ataxia telangiectasia mutated) protein plays a role in initiating checkpoint pathways in all three cell cycle phases (reviewed in Shiloh, 2003). G1 cell cycle arrest following irradiation centers on an intact ATM-p53/Cdc25A pathway and decreased activity of cyclin D and E complexes (see Fig. 14.21). This leads to continued hypophosphorylation of the Rb protein at the G1/S interface and blocking of the initiation of DNA replication. The radiation-induced G1 arrest is abrogated in cells that lack functional p53, ATM, or Rb proteins (Fei and El-Deiry, 2003; Cuddihy and Bristow, 2004). Most data suggest that cells having altered p53 protein function (and an abrogated G1 checkpoint) acquire relative radioresistance in comparison with those cells having normal p53 protein function (reviewed in Bristow et al., 1996). The radioresistant phenotype has been correlated with the level of expression of mutant p53 protein in transformed cells. Acquired radioresistance may also result from the inactivation of normal p53 function by viral proteins such as the HPV-E6 protein, which can bind to and degrade the normal p53 protein (Tsang et al., 1995). The S-phase checkpoint is controlled though ATM-mediated phosphorylation of the BRCA1, NBS1, SMC1, and FANCD2 proteins which modify the activity of transcription factors (i.e., E2F) and replication proteins (RPA, PCNA) during S phase and DNA replication (Fei and El-Deiry, 2003).

Molecular alterations that have been associated with the onset and duration of the G2 delay following radiation treatment include: (1) decreased expression or stability of the cyclin-B protein; (2) inhibitory phosphorylation of the p34$^{cdc2}$ protein after inactivation of the Cdc25C phosphatase following radiation-induced activation of Chk1 kinase; and (3) cytoplasmic sequestration

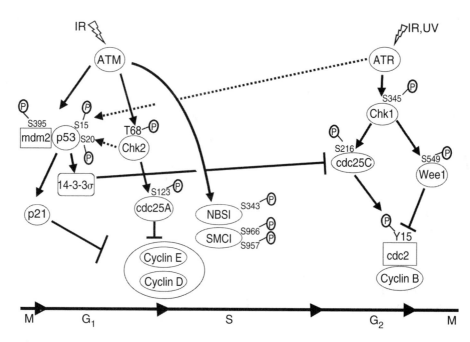

**Figure 14.21.** Summary of effects of ionizing radiation on cell cycle progression and checkpoint control. DNA damage imparted by ionizing radiation (IR) or ultraviolet radiation (UV) preferentially activates the PI-3K-like kinases ATM, and ATR, respectively. Thereafter a series of phosphorylations determines the extent of reversible G1, S and G2 cell cycle arrests in response to sub-lethal DNA damage. ATM can phosphorylate p53 directly on serine 15 and indirectly on serine 20, via Chk2. Other modifications allow p53 to become fully stabilized with an increased protein half-life due to acquired resistance to mdm2-mediated proteosomal degradation; Mdm-2 is itself a target of the ATM kinase. One of the main transcriptional targets of stabilized p53 is the p21$^{WAF}$ gene, which encodes an inhibitor of cyclin-dependent kinases. The p21$^{WAF}$ protein can bind to both cdk4/cyclin D and cdk2/cyclin E complexes, causing a cell cycle block in late G1 and early S phases, respectively. A second more rapid G1 checkpoint can be facilitated directly by Chk2 through the Cdc25A kinase. An intra-S checkpoint is mediated by an ATM-mediated post-translational modification of the NBS1 and SMC1 proteins. p53 has also been implicated in the G2 checkpoint through its upregulation of the 14-3-3σ gene. The 14-3-3 proteins bind and sequester Cdc25C, whose activity is required for the G2 to M transition. In order for Cdc25C to bind 14-3-3σ, it must be phosphorylated by the Chk1 kinase, a target of ATR. Chk1 also phosphorylates and activates the protein kinase Wee1 which helps to maintain the cdc2/cyclin B complex in an inactive form and delays entry into mitosis providing a G2 arrest. (Modified from Cuddihy and Bristow, 2004.)

of the cyclin-B protein, thereby preventing the formation of nuclear cyclin-B-p34$^{cdc2}$ complexes (Maity et al., 1994; Metting and Little, 1995; Fletcher et al., 2002; Iliakis et al., 2003). Cells lacking ATM or ATR-Chk1 function exhibit a defective G2 checkpoint after irradiation (Fig. 14.21). The G2 arrest following exposure to ionizing radiation probably allows damaged chromosomes to be repaired prior to mitosis, since DNA repair activity has been detected during the radiation-induced G2 delay and been related to cellular radiosensitivity (Kao et al., 2001; Nagasawa et al., 1994; Xu et al., 2002).

Tumor cells often exhibit an aberrant G1 cell cycle checkpoint while the G2 cell cycle checkpoint remains intact. There have been attempts to develop drugs that abrogate the G2 checkpoint (i.e., caffeine, methylxanthines, UCN-01) in tumor cells to potentiate the cyto-

toxicity of ionizing radiation over that of normal cells. These drugs lead to the induction of premature mitosis and mitotic catastrophe in the treated cells and UCN-01 preferentially sensitizes p53-mutated, radioresistant tumor cells to ionizing radiation. Identification of the targets of caffeine and UCN-01 (i.e., ATM/ATR and Chk1, respectively) has allowed the development of this class of agent for the radiosensitization of tumors (Tenzer and Pruschy, 2003). A number of these agents are currently being tested in combination with radiotherapy in clinical trials (Ma et al., 2003).

### 14.4.3 Molecular Repair of DNA Damage

The molecular components of DNA repair pathway(s) have been described in Chapter 5 (Sec. 5.4). Data from a number of studies indicate that the base excision repair (BER) and DNA-dsb repair pathways are involved in repairing the majority of ionizing radiation-induced DNA damage. For DNA-dsb repair, the main pathways of repair include homologous recombination (HR), which is maximally operational during the S phase and G2 phase, and nonhomologous end joining (NHEJ), which is operational during G1 phase (Jackson, 2002; Valerie and Povirk, 2003).

There is no simple relationship between expression of DNA repair genes or proteins and the relative radiosensitivity among unselected normal or tumor cells (Tenzer and Pruschy, 2003). However, in defined cell models, DNA repair capacity can influence cellular radiosensitivity as indicated by the extreme radiosensitivity of cells from some patients with DNA repair deficiency syndromes such as ataxia telangiectasia and the Nijmegen breakage syndrome (see Chap. 5, Sec. 5.4 and

Sec. 14.3.3). Similarly, isogenic cells defective in the expression of the BRCA1 and BRCA2 proteins can have decreased HR-related repair of DNA-dsbs and decreased radiation cell survival (Powell and Kachnic, 2003). A reduced capacity for repair of DNA double-strand breaks is also observed among x-ray–sensitive mutant Chinese hamster ovary (CHO) cells and among radiosensitive fibroblasts derived from severe combined immunodeficient mice (SCID) in which deficient NHEJ was correlated to a lack of DNA-PKcs kinase expression (Jeggo, 2002). Indeed, mouse cells made deficient for NHEJ (i.e., mouse knockouts for *DNA-PKcs* or *Ku70* genes) have exquisite radiosensitivity and defective rejoining of DNA-dsbs (Fig. 14.22).

The understanding of the relationship between deficient DNA repair and radiosensitivity has led to strategies designed to radiosensitize tumor cells. In human fibroblasts, small silencing RNAs (siRNA) have been

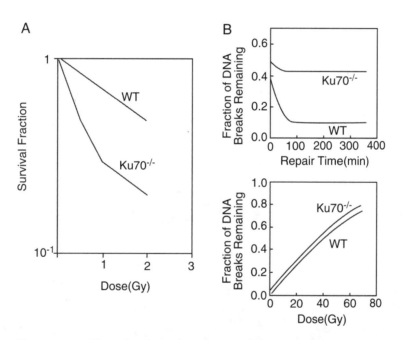

**Figure 14.22.** The role of non-homologous end-joining (NHEJ) in DNA double-strand break repair and cellular radiosensitivity. (*A*) The Ku70 protein with the Ku80 and DNA-PKcs proteins form an important DNA-PK complex which initially catalyzes the repair of DNA-double-strand breaks (see Chap. 5; Sec. 5.4 for details). As shown in (*A*), cells that are deficient in NHEJ proteins (e.g., *Ku70*−/− fibroblast cells) show radiosensitivity relative to normal wild-type (WT) cells. This is also true for Ku80- and *DNA-PKcs*-deficient cells. This increased radiosensitivity is a result of a reduced capacity for DNA break rejoining such that NHEJ-deficient cells have increased residual DNA breaks following irradiation leading to increased cell killing. This is illustrated in (*B*, upper panel) where the number of remaining DNA double-strand breaks at 400 minutes following irradiation is increased in *Ku70*−/− cells relative to WT cells. This is consistent with a DNA rejoining defect in the Ku70−/− cells. Note that the induction of DNA double-strand breaks is similar between the two types of cells (*B*, lower panel, showing the number of DNA breaks induced for a given dose measured immediately following irradiation). This confirms that the NHEJ defect is associated with differences in DNA rejoining rather than differences in initial DNA damage. (Modified from Ouyang et al., 1997.)

used to decrease endogenous DNA-PKcs or ATM expression and result in a reduced capacity for repair of radiation-induced chromosome breaks and an increased yield of acentric chromosome fragments. These chromosomal rearrangements are associated with increased radiation cell killing. Similarly, antisense RNA or specific pharmacological approaches (i.e., drugs which inhibit the function of the Rad51 DNA repair protein by altering the expression of the c-abl oncoprotein following irradiation) have been used to ablate DNA repair protein expression with resulting radiosensitization (Collis et al., 2003; Slupianek et al., 2002). Inhibitors of DNA repair appear to be a promising area of development and may have clinical value if the repair of DNA-dsbs in tumor tissues is reduced preferentially to that in normal tissues following irradiation (i.e., improve the therapeutic ratio; see Chap. 15, Sec.15.5.7).

Finally, DNA repair and telomerase activity have been linked (see Chap. 5, Sec. 5.5.3) and altered telomerase activity is frequently associated with the malignant phenotype. Telomeres are important structures which interact with the repair proteins MRE11 and KU70 to affect DNA repair and chromosomal stability following irradiation. Both telomere length and telomere function have been suggested to be possible determinants of chromosomal radiosensitivity (Bouffler et al., 2001). For example, mice that are deficient in telomerase are relatively radiosensitive secondary to an increased rate of

apoptosis and terminal growth arrest in irradiated intestinal and stromal tissues, respectively (Finnon et al., 2001; Goytisolo et al., 2000; Wong et al., 2000). Additionally, an inverse correlation between telomere length and chromosomal radiosensitivity has been observed in lymphocytes from breast cancer patients and normal individuals (McIlrath et al., 2001).

### 14.4.4 Oncogenes, Tumor Suppressor Genes, and Growth Factors

Aberrant expression of oncogenes or tumor suppressor genes may increase the intrinsic cellular radioresistance of human and rodent cells (Haffty and Glazer, 2003). For example, increased radiation survival has been observed in selected cell lines following the transfection of a single oncogene, such as activated *Ras*, *Src*, or *Raf* (Kasid et al., 1996; McKenna et al., 1990). This has led to studies designed to radiosensitize tumor cells by the inhibition of oncogene function using inhibitors of intracellular signaling pathways (see Fig. 14.23) or antisense techniques (or siRNA) to decrease oncogene overexpression (Peng et al., 2002; Ma et al., 2003; Kasid and Dritschilo, 2003).

When the *Ras* oncogene undergoes mutation, it is permanently activated in the GTP-bound signaling state, providing proliferative signals in the absence of growth factor ligands, leading to altered cell growth,

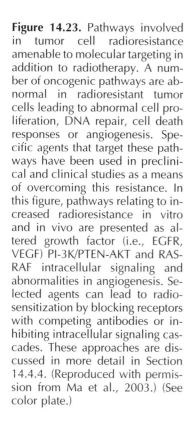

**Figure 14.23.** Pathways involved in tumor cell radioresistance amenable to molecular targeting in addition to radiotherapy. A number of oncogenic pathways are abnormal in radioresistant tumor cells leading to abnormal cell proliferation, DNA repair, cell death responses or angiogenesis. Specific agents that target these pathways have been used in preclinical and clinical studies as a means of overcoming this resistance. In this figure, pathways relating to increased radioresistance in vitro and in vivo are presented as altered growth factor (i.e., EGFR, VEGF) PI-3K/PTEN-AKT and RAS-RAF intracellular signaling and abnormalities in angiogenesis. Selected agents can lead to radiosensitization by blocking receptors with competing antibodies or inhibiting intracellular signaling cascades. These approaches are discussed in more detail in Section 14.4.4. (Reproduced with permission from Ma et al., 2003.) (See color plate.)

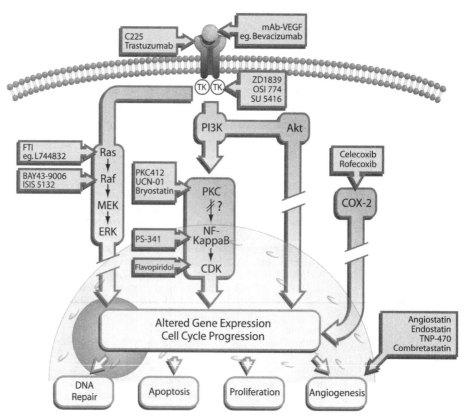

transformation, and occasionally radioresistance (see Chap. 8, Sec. 8.2.5). However, increased radioresistance is more commonly observed in cells transfected with an activated *Ras* gene in combination with a nuclear co-operating oncogene, such as *c-Myc* or mutant *p53* (Bristow et al., 1996; McKenna et al., 1990). Inhibitors of *RAS* protein prenylation or function (farnesyl transferase inhibitors) have been reported to enhance radiation-induced cytotoxicity among preclinical models of human breast, lung, colon, and bladder cancer cells expressing mutated *H-* or *K-RAS* genes (Gupta et al., 2001). Although improvements in *RAS*-pathway specificity are required for future development of farnesyl transferase inhibitors, at least one early clinical trial has shown success with minimal toxicity using these drugs in combination with radiotherapy in the treatment of advanced lung, and head and neck cancers (Hahn et al., 2002).

Downstream to *RAS*, the *RAF-MEK-ERK* and phosphatidylinositol-3 kinase *(PI-3K)-AKT/PKB* pathways are two separate signaling pathways that have been linked to tumor radioresistance. Using antisense oligonucleotides against human *RAF* increased radiosensitivity has been observed in a human squamous cancer cell line (SQ-20B). Inhibitors of *PI-3K* signaling such as LY294002 and wortmannin enhanced the response to radiation in lung, bladder, colon, breast, HNSCC, and cervical cancer cells. There are limited studies reporting the in vivo antitumor activity of wortmannin and LY294002, although the target specificity of these agents is uncertain as they can also inhibit other important PI-3K-related proteins (ATM, ATR, and DNA-PKcs) in normal tissues.

The radiosensitivity of cells may be influenced by the addition of exogenous growth factors or hormones in receptor-positive cells before or after irradiation. The insulin-like growth factor-1 receptor (IGF-1R) is a cell surface receptor with tyrosine kinase activity which has been linked to increased radioresistance. IGF-1R is expressed at low levels in AT cells; this may in part contribute to the radiosensitivity of AT cells, because reintroduction of IGF-1R, or addition of exogenous IGF, can increase their radioresistance. Tyrosine kinase activity of the epidermal growth factor receptor (EGFR) is increased following cellular exposure to ionizing radiation and addition of exogenous EGF to cells in culture render them relatively radioresistant (Kwok and Sutherland, 1991). Both EGFR and the related HER-2/neu receptor are overexpressed in a wide variety of epithelial tumors (head and neck squamous cell cancers (HNSCC), gliomas, breast, lung, colorectal, and prostate cancers) and this overexpression has been associated with poor clinical outcome following radiotherapy (Harari and Huang, 2001). Targeting EGF and HER-2/neu receptor signaling using monoclonal antibodies or specific inhibitors of EGFR or HER-2 leads to radiosensitization in vitro and in vivo. These drugs are being tested in randomized, multicenter clinical trials (Ma et al., 2003).

The translation of preclinical to clinical testing for molecular-based therapies is limited by a number of factors including the appropriate scheduling and toxicity of the agent, the interpatient and intratumoral variability of the expression of the molecular target and molecular cross-talk amongst parallel intracellular signaling pathways. These limitations might be bypassed by simultaneous determination of multiple pathways using genomic and proteomic analyses as the basis for selection of the best molecular agents to be combined with radiation treatments (Ma et al., 2003).

## 14.5 SUMMARY

Ionizing radiation causes damage to cells and tissues by depositing energy as a series of discrete events. Different types of radiation have different abilities to cause biological damage because of the different densities of the energy deposition events produced. The relative biological effectiveness of densely ionizing (high-LET) radiation is greater than that of low-LET radiation. Radiation can cause damage to any molecule in a cell, but damage to DNA is most crucial in causing cell lethality expressed by loss of proliferative potential. Depending on cell type, cells may die by a permanent (terminal) growth arrest, undergo interphase death or lysis during radiation-induced apoptosis, or undertake up to four abortive mitotic cycles before mitotic catastrophe. Radiation may also cause delays in the progression of cells through the cell cycle. The molecular events relating to G1- and G2-phase cell cycle arrest following ionizing radiation appear to involve ATM, p53, and cyclin-cdc complexes that are associated with cell cycle regulation.

Several assay procedures have been developed for assessing the clonogenic capacity of both normal and malignant cells, and these have been used to obtain radiation survival curves for a wide range of different cell types. For x- and γ-rays, survival curves for most mammalian cells have a shoulder region at low doses, while at higher doses the survival decreases approximately exponentially with dose. No systematic differences are observed between normal and malignant cells. The slope of the high-dose region of the survival curve is quite similar for most mammalian cells, but there are differences in the clinically relevant, low-dose shoulder region that may reflect differences in repair capacity.

Various factors can influence the response of cells to radiation treatment. These include LET, cell cycle position, DNA repair, growth factors, and certain oncogenes. Following treatment with low-LET radiation, cells can repair some of their damage over a period of a few hours; thus, if the treatment is prolonged or fractionated, it is less effective than if given as a single acute dose. The accurate and timely rejoining of DNA double-strand breaks may be correlated to the relative radiation survival of both normal and tumor cells. Cells in S phase are often more resistant than cells in the G2/M phases, but there is variability between cell types. There is an association between the aberrant expression of Ras, Raf, and p53 proteins and cellular response to ionizing radiation. Future treatments involving radiation will utilize targeted drugs which increase tumor radiosensitivity by interfering with the G1, S, and G2 cell cycle checkpoints, or by modifying intracellular signaling following DNA damage. Genomic and proteomic assays may be used to delineate the most appropriate molecular targets for radiosensitization within tumors of selected groups of patients.

## REFERENCES

Aldridge DR, Arends MJ, Radford IR: Increasing the susceptibility of the rat 208F fibroblast cell line to radiation-induced apoptosis does not alter its clonogenic survival dose-response. *Br J Cancer* 1995; 71:571–577.

Amundson SA, Bittner M, Fornace AJ Jr: Functional genomics as a window on radiation stress signaling. *Oncogene* 2003; 22:5828–5833.

Barendsen GW: Responses of cultured cells, tumours and normal tissues to radiations of different linear energy transfer. *Curr Top Radiat Res* 1968; 4:293–356.

Belyakov OV, Folkard M, Mothersill C, et al: A proliferation-dependent bystander effect in primary porcine and human urothelial explants in response to targeted irradiation. *Br J Cancer* 2003; 88:767–774.

Bernhard EJ, McKenna WG, Muschel RJ: Radiosensitity and the cell cycle. *Cancer J Sci Am* 1999; 5:194–204.

Bouffler SD, Blasco MA, Cox R, Smith PJ: Telomeric sequences, radiation sensitivity and genomic instability. *Int J Radiat Biol* 2001; 77:995–1005.

Bristow RG, Hardy PA, Hill RP: Comparison between in vitro radiosensitivity and in vivo radioresponse of murine tumor cell lines. I: parameters of in vitro radiosensitivity and endogenous cellular glutathione levels. *Int J Radiat Oncol Biol Phys* 1990; 18:133–145.

Bristow RG, Benchimol S, Hill RP: The p53 gene as a modifier of intrinsic radiosensitivity: implications for radiotherapy. *Radiother Oncol* 1996; 40:197–223.

Bristow RG, Hill RP: Comparison between in vitro radiosensitivity and in vivo radioresponse in murine tumor cell lines. II: in vivo radioresponse following fractionated treatment and in vitro/in vivo correlations. *Int J Radiat Oncol Biol Phys* 1990; 18:331–345.

Bromfield GP, Meng A, Warde P, Bristow RG: Cell death in irradiated prostate epithelial cells: role of apoptotic and clonogenic cell kill. *Prostate Cancer Prostatic Dis* 2003; 6:73–85.

Brown JM, Wouters BG: Apoptosis: mediator or mode of cell killing by anticancer agents? *Drug Resist Updat* 2001; 4:135–136.

Chang BD, Watanabe K, Broude EV, et al: Effects of p21Waf1/Cip1/Sdi1 on cellular gene expression: implications for carcinogenesis, senescence, and age-related diseases. *Proc Natl Acad Sci USA* 2000; 97:4291–4296.

Chaudhry MA, Chodosh LA, McKenna WG, Muschel RJ: Gene expression profile of human cells irradiated in G1 and G2 phases of cell cycle. *Cancer Lett* 2003; 195:221–233.

Collis SJ, Swartz MJ, Nelson WG, DeWeese TL: Enhanced radiation and chemotherapy-mediated cell killing of human cancer cells by small inhibitory RNA silencing of DNA repair factors. *Cancer Res* 2003; 63(7):1550–1554.

Cornforth MN, Bailey SM, Goodwin EH: Dose responses for chromosome aberrations produced in noncycling primary human fibroblasts by alpha particles, and by gamma rays delivered at sublimiting low dose rates. *Radiat Res* 2002; 158(1):43–53.

Criswell T, Leskov K, Miyamoto S, et al: Transcription factors activated in mammalian cells after clinically relevant doses of ionizing radiation. *Oncogene* 2003; 22:5813–5827.

Cuddihy AR, Bristow RG: The p53 protein family and radiation sensitivity: Yes or No? *Cancer Metastasis Rev* 2004; 23(3–4):237–257.

Datta R, Rubin E, Sukhatme V, et al: Ionizing radiation activates transcription of the EGR1 gene via CArG elements. *Proc Natl Acad Sci USA* 1992; 89:10149–10153.

Dent P, Yacoub A, Fisher PB, et al: MAPK pathways in radiation responses. *Oncogene* 2003; 22:5885–5896.

Elkind MM, Sutton H: Radiation response of mammalian cells growth in culture: I. Repair of x-ray damage in surviving Chinese hamster cells. *Radiat Res* 1960; 13:556–593.

Elkind MM, Whitmore GF: *The Radiobiology of Cultured Mammalian Cells.* New York: Gordon and Breach; 1967.

Fairbairn DW, Olive PL, O'Neill KL: The comet assay: a comprehensive review. *Mutat Res* 1995; 339:37–59.

Fei P, El-Deiry WS: P53 and radiation responses. *Oncogene* 2003; 22:5774–5783.

Finnon P, Wong HP, Silver AR, et al: Long but dysfunctional telomeres correlate with chromosomal radiosensitivity in a mouse AML cell line. *Int J Radiat Biol* 2001; 77:1151–1162.

Fletcher L, Cheng Y, Muschel RJ: Abolishment of the Tyr-15 inhibitory phosphorylation site on cdc2 reduces the radiation-induced G(2) delay, revealing a potential checkpoint in early mitosis. *Cancer Res* 2002; 62:241–250.

Fuks Z, Haimovitz-Friedman A, Kolesnick RN: The role of the sphingomyelin pathway and protein kinase C in radiation-induced cell kill. *Imp Adv Oncol* 1995; 19–31.

Girard PM, Foray N, Stumm M, et al: Radiosensitivity in Nijmegen Breakage Syndrome cells is attributable to a repair defect and not cell cycle checkpoint defects. *Cancer Res* 2000; 60:4881–4888.

Goytisolo FA, Samper E, Martin-Caballero J, et al: Short telomeres result in organismal hypersensitivity to ionizing radiation in mammals. *J Exp Med* 2000; 192:1625–1636.

Gupta AK, Bakanauskas VJ, Cerniglia GJ, et al: The Ras radiation resistance pathway. *Cancer Res* 2001; 61:4278–4282.

Haffty BG, Glazer PM: Molecular markers in clinical radiation oncology. *Oncogene* 2003; 22:5915–5925.

Hahn SM, Bernhard EJ, Regine W, et al: A Phase I trial of the farnesyltransferase inhibitor L-778,123 and radiotherapy for locally advanced lung and head and neck cancer. *Clin Cancer Res* 2002; 8:1065–1072.

Hall EJ: *Radiobiology for the Radiobiologist.* 5th Ed., Lippincott, Williams & Wilkins. Philadelphia; 2000.

Hall EJ, Hei TK: Genomic instability and bystander effects induced by high-LET radiation. *Oncogene* 2003; 22:7034–7042.

Hallahan DE, Dunphy E, Virudachelam S, et al: C-Jun and egr-1 participate in DNA synthesis and cell survival in response to ionizing radiation. *J Biol Chem* 1995; 270;30303–30309.

Harari PM, Huang SM: Radiation response modification following molecular inhibition of epidermal growth factor receptor signaling. *Semin Radiat Oncol* 2001; 11:281–289.

Hartmann KA, Modlich O, Prisack HB, et al: Gene expression profiling of advanced head and neck squamous cell carcinomas and two squamous cell carcinoma cell lines under radio/chemotherapy using cDNA arrays. *Radiother Oncol* 2002; 63:309–320.

Hartwell LH, Kastan MB: Cell cycle control and cancer. *Science* 1994; 266:1821–1828.

Hill RP, Bush RS: A lung-colony assay to determine the radiosensitivity of cells of a solid tumour. *Int J Radiat Biol* 1969; 15:435–444.

Huang L, Snyder AR, Morgan WF: Radiation-induced genomic instability and its implications for radiation carcinogenesis. *Oncogene* 2003; 22:5848–5854.

Iliakis G, Wang Y, Guan J, Wang H: DNA damage checkpoint control in cells exposed to ionizing radiation. *Oncogene* 2003; 22:5834–5847.

Jackson SP: Sensing and repairing DNA double-strand breaks. *Carcinogenesis* 2002; 23:687–696.

Jeggo PA: The fidelity of repair of radiation damage. *Radiat Prot Dosimetry* 2002; 99:117–122.

Joiner MC, Marples B, Lambin P, et al: Low-dose hypersensitivity: current status and possible mechanisms. *Int J Radiat Oncol Biol Phys* 2001; 49:379–389.

Kao GD, McKenna WG, Yen TJ: Detection of repair activity during the DNA damage-induced G2 delay in human cancer cells. *Oncogene* 2001; 20:3486–3496.

Kasid U, Dritschilo A: RAF antisense oligonucleotide as a tumor radiosensitizer. *Oncogene* 2003; 22:5876–5884.

Kasid U, Suy S, Dent P, et al: Activation of Raf by ionizing radiation. *Nature* 1996; 382:813–816.

Keng PC, Siemann DW, Wheeler KT: Comparison of tumour age response to radiation for cells derived from tissue culture or solid tumours. *Br J Cancer* 1984; 50:519–526.

Khodarev NN, Park JO, Yu J, et al: Dose-dependent and independent temporal patterns of gene responses to ionizing radiation in normal and tumor cells and tumor xenografts. *Proc Natl Acad Sci USA* 2001; 98:12665–12670.

Kitada S, Krajewski S, Miyashita T, et al: Gamma-radiation induces upregulation of Bax protein and apoptosis in radiosensitive cells in vivo. *Oncogene* 1996; 12:187–192.

Kolesnick R, Fuks Z: Radiation and ceramide-induced apoptosis. *Oncogene* 2003; 22:5897–5906.

Krause M, Hessel F, Wohlfarth J, et al: Ultrafractionation in A7 human malignant glioma in nude mice. *Int J Radiat Biol* 2003; 79:377–383.

Kwok TT, Sutherland RM: Differences in EGF related radiosensitisation of human squamous carcinoma cells with high and low numbers of EGF receptors. *Br J Cancer* 1991; 64:251–254.

Lambin P, Malaise EP, Joiner MC: Might intrinsic radioresistance of human tumour cells be induced by radiation? *Int J Radiat Biol* 1996; 69:279–290.

Ma BB, Bristow RG, Kim J, Siu LL: Combined-modality treatment of solid tumors using radiotherapy and molecular targeted agents. *J Clin Oncol* 2003; 21(14):2760–2776.

MacPhail SH, Banath JP, Yu TY, et al: Expression of phosphorylated histone H2AX in cultured cell lines following exposure to X-rays. *Int J Radiat Biol* 2003; 79:351–358.

Maity A, McKenna WG, Muschel RJ: The molecular basis for cell cycle delays following ionizing radiation: a review. *Radiother Oncol* 1994; 31:1–13.

Malaise EP, Deschavanne PJ, Fertil B: The relationship between potentially lethal damage repair and intrinsic radiosensitivity of human cells. *Int J Radiat Biol* 1989; 56:597–604.

Marples B, Greco O, Joiner MC, Scott SD: Molecular approaches to chemo-radiotherapy. *Eur J Cancer* 2002; 38:231–239.

Mauceri HJ, Hanna NN, Wayne JD, et al: Tumor necrosis factor alpha (TNF-alpha) gene therapy targeted by ionizing radiation selectively damages tumor vasculature. *Cancer Res* 1996; 56:4311–4314.

McCulloch EA, Till JE: The sensitivity of cells from normal mouse bone marrow to gamma radiation in vitro and in vivo. *Radiat Res* 1962; 16:822–832.

McIlrath J, Bouffler SD, Samper E, et al: Telomere length-abnormalities in mammalian radiosensitive cells. *Cancer Res* 2001; 61:912–915.

McKenna WG, Weiss MC, Endlich B, et al: Synergistic effect of the v-myc oncogene with H-ras on radioresistance. *Cancer Res* 1990; 50:97–102.

Metting NF, Little JB: Transient failure to dephosphorylate the cdc2-cyclin B1 complex accompanies radiation-induced G2-phase arrest in HeLa cells. *Radiat Res* 1995; 143:286–292.

Mitchell JB, Bedford JS, Bailey SM: Dose-rate effects in mammalian cells in culture III. Comparison of cell killing and cell proliferation during continuous irradiation for six different cell lines. *Radiat Res* 1979; 79:537–551.

Nagasawa H, Huo L, Little JB: Increased bystander mutagenic effect in DNA double-strand break repair-deficient mammalian cells. *Int J Radiat Biol* 2003; 79:35–41.

Nagasawa H, Keng P, Harley R, et al: Relationship between gamma-ray-induced G2/M delay and cellular radiosensitivity. *Int J Radiat Biol* 1994; 66:373–379.

Nunez MI, McMillan TJ, Valenzuela MT, et al: Relationship between DNA damage, rejoining and cell killing by radiation in mammalian cells. *Radiother Oncol* 1996; 39:155–165.

Ouyang H, Nussenzweig A, Kurimasa A, et al: Ku70 is required for DNA repair but not for T cell antigen receptor gene recombination in vivo. *J Exp Med* 1997; 186:921–929.

Paull TT, Rogakou EP, Yamazaki V, et al: A critical role for histone H2AX in recruitment of repair factors to nuclear foci after DNA damage. *Curr Biol* 2000; 10:886–895.

Paris F, Fuks Z, Kang A, et al: Endothelial apoptosis as the primary lesion initiating intestinal radiation damage in mice. *Science* 2001; 293:293–297.

Peng Y, Zhang Q, Nagasawa H, et al: Silencing expression of the catalytic subunit of DNA-dependent protein kinase by small interfering RNA sensitizes human cells for radiation-induced chromosome damage, cell killing, and mutation. *Cancer Res* 2002; 62:6400–6404.

Peretz S, Jensen R, Baserga R, Glazer PM: ATM-dependent expression of the insulin-like growth factor-I receptor in a pathway regulating radiation response. *Proc Natl Acad Sci USA* 2001; 98:1676–1681.

Powell SN, Kachnic LA: Roles of BRCA1 and BRCA2 in homologous recombination, DNA replication fidelity and the cellular response to ionizing radiation. *Oncogene* 2003; 22:5784–5791.

Rauth AM: The induction and repair of ultraviolet light damage in mammalian cells. In Burns FJ, Upton AC, Silini G, eds. *Radiation Carcinogenesis and DNA Alterations*. New York: Plenum Press; 1986:212–226.

Rogakou EP, Pilch DR, Orr AH, et al: DNA double-stranded breaks induce histone H2AX phosphorylation on serine 139. *J Biol Chem* 1998; 273: 5858–5868.

Roninson IB: Tumor cell senescence in cancer treatment. *Cancer Res* 2003; 63:2705–2715.

Ruiter GA, Zerp SF, Bartelink H, et al: Alkyl-lysophospholipids activate the SAPK/JNK pathway and enhance radiation-induced apoptosis. *Cancer Res* 1999; 59:2457–2463.

Ruiz de Almodovar JM, Bush C, Peacock JH, et al: Dose-rate effect for DNA damage induced by ionizing radiation in human tumor cells. *Radiat Res* 1994; 138:S93–S96.

Sasai K, Evans JW, Kovacs MS, Brown JM. Prediction of human cell radiosensitivity: comparison of clonogenic assay with chromosome aberrations scored using premature chromosome condensation with fluorescence in situ hybridization. *Int J Radiat Oncol Biol Phys* 1994; 30:1127–1132.

Sato N, Mizumoto K, Nakamura M, et al: A possible role for centrosome overduplication in radiation-induced cell death. *Oncogene* 2000; 19:5281–5290.

Schmidt-Ullrich RK, Contessa JN, Lammering G, et al: ERBB receptor tyrosine kinases and cellular radiation responses. *Oncogene* 2003; 22:5855–5865.

Sedelnikova OA, Rogakou EP, Panyutin IG, Bonner WM: Quantitative detection of (125)IdU-induced DNA double-strand breaks with gamma-H2AX antibody. *Radiat Res* 2002; 158:486–492.

Shiloh Y: ATM and related protein kinases: safeguarding genome integrity. *Nat Rev Cancer* 2003; 3:155–168.

Singleton BK, Griffin CS, Thacker J: Clustered DNA damage leads to complex genetic changes in irradiated human cells. *Cancer Res* 2002; 62:6263–6269.

Skov KA: Radioresponsiveness at low doses: hyper-radiosensitivity and increased radioresistance in mammalian cells. *Mutation Research* 1999; 430:241–253.

Slupianek A, Hoser G, Majsterek I, et al: Fusion tyrosine kinases induce drug resistance by stimulation of homology-dependent recombination repair, prolongation of G(2)/M phase, and protection from apoptosis. *Mol Cell Biol* 2002; 22:4189–4201.

Steel GG (ed.): *Basic Clinical Radiobiology*. 3rd Ed. Arnold, London. 2002.

Tenzer A, Pruschy M: Potentiation of DNA-damage-induced cytotoxicity by G2 checkpoint abrogators. *Curr Med Chem Anti-Canc Agents* 2003; 3:35–46.

Terasima T, Tolmach LJ: Changes in the x-ray sensitivity of HeLa cells during the division cycle. *Nature* 1961; 190:1210–1211.

Tsang NM, Nagasawa H, Li C, Little JB: Abrogation of p53 function by transfection of HPV16 E6 gene enhances the resistance of human diploid fibroblasts to ionizing radiation. *Oncogene* 1995; 10:2403–2408.

Tusher VG, Tibshirani R, Chu G: Significance analysis of microarrays applied to the ionizing radiation response. *Proc Natl Acad Sci USA* 2001; 98:5116–5121.

Valerie K, Povirk LF: Regulation and mechanisms of mammalian double-strand break repair. *Oncogene* 2003; 22: 5792–5812.

Ward JF: The complexity of DNA damage: relevance to biological consequences. *Int J Radiat Biol* 1994; 66:427–432.

Weichselbaum RR, Kufe DW, Hellman S, et al: Radiation-induced tumour necrosis factor-alpha expression: clinical application of transcriptional and physical targeting of gene therapy. *Lancet Oncol* 2002; 3:665–671.

Weichselbaum RR, Little JB: Repair of potentially lethal X ray damage and possible applications to clinical radiotherapy. *Int J Radiat Oncol Biol Phys* 1983; 9:91–96.

Whitaker SJ, Powell SN, McMillan TJ: Molecular assays of radiation-induced DNA damage. *Eur J Cancer* 1991; 27: 922–928.

Willers H, Xia F, Powell SN: Recombinational DNA repair in cancer and normal cells: The challenge of functional analysis. *J Biomed Biotechnol* 2002; 2:86–93.

Withers HR, Mason K, Reid BO, et al: Response of mouse intestine to neutrons and gamma rays in relation to dose fractionation and division cycle. *Cancer* 1974; 34:39–47.

Wong KK, Chang S, Weiler SR, et al: Telomere dysfunction impairs DNA repair and enhances sensitivity to ionizing radiation. *Nat Genet* 2000; 26:85–88.

Xu B, Kim ST, Lim DS, Kastan MB: Two molecularly distinct G(2)/M checkpoints are induced by ionizing irradiation. *Mol Cell Biol* 2002; 22:1049–1059.

## APPENDIX 14.1 THE TARGET-THEORY AND LINEAR-QUADRATIC MODELS OF RADIATION CELL SURVIVAL

### Appendix 14.1.1 Target Theory

The target-theory model of cell survival was based on the hypothesis that a number of critical targets had to be inactivated for cells to be killed. Cell killing by radiation is now recognized to be more complex, but the equation and parameters derived from the model are still used to describe the shape of cell survival curves. The number of targets ($dN$) inactivated by a small dose of radiation ($dD$) should be proportional to the initial number of targets $N$ and $dD$, so that

$$dN \, \alpha \, N \cdot dD \quad \text{or} \quad dN = -\frac{N \cdot dD}{D_0} \quad \text{(Appendix Eq. 14.1)}$$

where $1/D_0$ is a constant of proportionality and the negative sign is introduced because the number of active targets $N$ decreases with increasing dose. This equation can be integrated to give

$$N = N_0 \cdot e^{-D/D_0} \quad \text{(Appendix Eq. 14.2)}$$

where $N_0$ is the number of active targets present at zero dose. If it is assumed that cells contain only a single target that must be inactivated for them to be killed, then the fractional survival ($S$) of a population of cells is represented by

$$S = \frac{N}{N_0} = e^{-\frac{D}{D_0}} \quad \text{(Appendix Eq. 14.3)}$$

where $N_0$ and $N$ are the initial and final number of cells surviving following a radiation dose $D$, respectively, and $D_0$ is a constant. This also represents the probability that any individual cell will survive the radiation dose $D$. Appendix Eq. (14.3) gives a *single-hit, single-target* survival curve that is a straight line on a semilogarithmic plot originating at a surviving fraction of 1 at zero dose (Appendix Fig. 14.1, line *a*). Survival curves of this shape have been obtained for viruses and bacteria, for radiosensitive normal and malignant cells (i.e., cells in the bone marrow or lymphoma cells), and for many types of cells treated with high-LET radiation. The term $D_0$ represents the dose required to reduce the surviving fraction to 37 percent and is a measure of the slope of the line. It can be shown mathematically that the radiation dose required to kill 90 percent of the initial number of cells, termed the $D_{10}$ value, is equivalent to $2.3 \times D_0$ (where 2.3 is the natural logarithm of 10).

If it is assumed that a cell contains $n$ identical targets, *each of which* must be inactivated (by a single hit) to

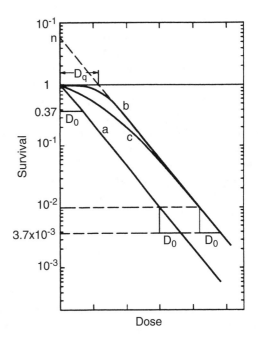

**Appendix Figure 14.1.** Survival curves defined by the single-hit and multitarget models of cell killing discussed in the text. *Curve a:* Single-hit (single-target) survival curve defined by Appendix Eq. (14.3). *Curve b:* Multitarget survival curve defined by Appendix Eq. (14.4). *Curve c:* Composite (two-component) survival curve resulting from both multitarget and single-hit components. Also shown is how the parameters $D_0$, $n$, and $D_q$ can be derived from the survival curves.

cause cell death, then the *multitarget, single-hit* cell survival equation can be represented by

$$S = \frac{N}{N_0} = 1 - (1 - e^{-D/D_0})^n \quad \text{(Appendix Eq. 14.4)}$$

Again, this equation represents the probability that any individual cell will survive a dose $D$. A plot of this equation leads to a survival curve with a shoulder at low doses and a straight-line section at higher doses on a semilogarithmic plot, as shown in Appendix Figure 14.1, line *b*. The parameters $D_0$, $n$, and $D_q$ can be determined for this curve as shown. At doses that are large compared to $D_0$ (i.e., $D >> D_0$), Appendix Eq. (14.4) reduces to $S = n \exp(-D/D_0)$, which is similar to Appendix Eq. (14.3). The straight-line part of the survival curve thus extrapolates to a value $n$ at zero dose and has a slope defined by $D_0$. As indicated previously, the $D_0$ value is the dose required to reduce cell survival from $S$ to $0.37S$ in the *straight-line region* of the survival curve. The quasi-threshold dose, $D_q$, is the dose at which the extrapolated straight-line section of the survival curve crosses the dose axis (survival = 1) and quantitatively describes the size of the shoulder. It can be calculated by $D_q = D_0 \ln n$. For this model, the size of the shoulder is regarded as giving an indication of the repair capacity of the cells. Typical values of $D_0$ for mammalian cells are in the range 1–2 Gy. Values for $n$ or $D_q$ vary widely for different cells (see Chap. 15, Sec. 15.3.2).

One limitation of Appendix Eq. (14.4) is that it predicts that a certain amount of damage must be accumulated in a cell before it is killed—i.e., that, at very low doses, the survival curve should be parallel to the dose axis or have an initial slope of zero. This is contrary to much experimental data, which indicate that, for cell populations irradiated with x- or $\gamma$-rays, the survival curve often has a finite initial slope (Appendix Fig. 14.1, curve $c$).

## Appendix 14.1.2 The Linear-Quadratic Model

The linear-quadratic model of cell kill is based on the idea that multiple lesions, induced by radiation, interact in the cell to cause cell killing. The lesions that interact could be caused by a single ionizing track, giving a direct dependence of cell killing on dose, or by two or more separate tracks, giving a dependence of lethality on higher powers of dose. The assumption that two lesions must interact to cause cell killing gives an equation that can fit most experimental survival curves quite adequately, at least over the first few decades of survival, and is given by

$$S = N/N_0 = e^{-(\alpha D + \beta D^2)} \qquad \text{(Appendix Eq. 14.5)}$$

The parameters $\alpha$ and $\beta$ are assumed to describe the probability of the interacting lesions being caused by energy-deposition events due to a single charged-particle track or by two independent tracks, respectively. The linear-quadratic equation defines a survival curve that is concave downward on a semilogarithmic plot and never becomes strictly exponential. However, the curvature is usually small at high doses. The $\alpha$ com-

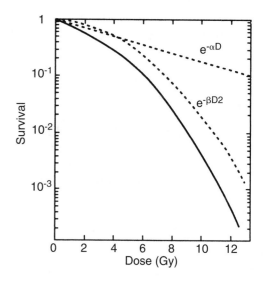

**Appendix Figure 14.2.** Survival curve (*solid line*) as defined by the linear-quadratic model of cell killing, Eq. (14.5). The curves defined by the two components of the equation are shown separately as the dashed lines.

ponent can be regarded as describing cell inactivation by nonrepairable damage, while the $\beta$ component describes cell inactivation by accumulation of repairable damage (see Appendix Fig. 14.2). The values for $\alpha$ and $\beta$ vary considerably for different types of mammalian cells both in vitro and in vivo. Typical values of $\alpha$ are in the range 1 to $10^{-1}$ Gy and of $\beta$ in the range $10^{-1}$ to $10^{-2}$ Gy.

Alternative equations similar to the linear-quadratic equation can be derived by making various biological assumptions, for example, concerning the capacity of cells to repair radiation damage and the effect of radiation treatment on that capacity. It should be stressed that a good fit of a given equation to the survival data does not validate the underlying biological assumptions of the model.

# 15

# The Scientific Basis of Radiotherapy

*Richard P. Hill and Robert G. Bristow*

## 15.1 INTRODUCTION

The dose of radiation that can be delivered to a tumor is limited by the damage caused to surrounding normal tissues and the consequent risk of complications. Whether a certain risk of developing complications is regarded as acceptable depends both on the function of the tissue(s) and the severity of the damage involved. This risk must be compared to the probability of benefit (i.e., eradicating the tumor) in order to determine the overall gain from the treatment. This gain can be estimated for an average group of patients but it may vary for individual patients depending on the particular characteristics of their tumors and the normal tissues at risk. The balance between the probabilities for tumor control and normal tissue complications gives a measure of the therapeutic ratio of a treatment (see Sec. 15.5.7). The therapeutic ratio can be improved either by increasing the effective radiation dose delivered to the tumor relative to that given to surrounding normal tissues or by increasing the biological response of the tumor relative to that of the surrounding normal tissues.

Increasing the dose to a tumor requires improvement in the physical aspects of radiation therapy. The introduction of high-energy x- and $\gamma$-ray treatment machines has allowed an increase in the effective dose of radiation to deep-seated tumors without increasing the dose to normal tissues. Further improvements are occurring with the use of more sophisticated treatment methods, allowing for *conformal* and *stereotactic* treatments. These new methods limit the volume of normal tissues irradiated to high doses and allow escalated doses to the tumor. The empiric development of multifractionated treatments is an example of exploiting biological factors to improve the therapeutic ratio. Exploration of ways to exploit the oxygen effect to cause greater tumor cell killing, to modify existing fractionation schedules, or to protect against the normal tissue effects of irradiation may offer further improvements. Biological factors that may influence the outcome of radiation therapy and their exploitation to improve therapy are discussed in this chapter.

## 15.2 PRINCIPLES OF CLINICAL RADIOTHERAPY

### 15.2.1 Radiotherapy Dose

As discussed in Chapter 14, radiotherapy involves both *external beam radiotherapy* and *brachytherapy;* treatment choice depends on the type of tumor and location within the body. The dose of radiation is determined by the intent of the therapy (i.e., curative or palliative), the volume of tumor, the relative radiosensitivity of the tumor cells and expected toxicity to the surrounding normal tissues. Other factors taken into consideration relate to the condition of the patient, including age or health problems that might increase the side effects of radiotherapy (e.g., connective tissue disorders, such as scleroderma). The acute and chronic side effects that may occur following local radiotherapy are directly linked to the normal structures and tissues within the irradiated volume (see Table 15.1); these effects increase with the volume of the tissue irradiated and with the size of the dose per fraction. For example, head and neck irradiation can lead to altered swallowing or a dry mouth (xerostomia), while irradiation of pelvic structures may lead to nausea or a change in bladder and bowel function. Whole body radiotherapy, which is sometimes given in

addition to chemotherapy during bone marrow transplantation, can lead to nausea and vomiting, decreased blood counts, and altered humoral and cell-mediated immune responses (see Sec. 15.5).

Most curative radiotherapy regimens consist of daily treatments or fractions in the range of 1.8 to 3 Gy per day over a period of 5 to 8 weeks. The intent is to achieve local control of the tumor to prevent further local tissue destruction, organ failure, and the seeding of secondary metastases. Using modern planning techniques (see Sec. 15.2.2), doses up to about 75–80 Gy to the tumor can usually be achieved without causing severe side effects. There are substantial data to indicate that increased radiotherapy dose is associated with increased local control (Armstrong, 2002; Suit, 2002). Typically, the dose to normal tissues is limited so that severe complications occur in no more than 5 percent of the population after a period of 5 years (known as the $TD_{5/5}$ value). However, this dose limit may be increased if radiotherapy is the only curative treatment option for the patient. Palliative radiotherapy is given (when the disease is regarded as incurable) in order to achieve better pain control, to control bleeding, or to prevent tissue destruction or ulceration. These radiotherapy treatments are usually of short duration and consist of 1 to 3 fractions of 5 to 8 Gy or 5 to 10 fractions of 3 to 4 Gy.

### 15.2.2 Radiotherapy Planning and Dose Delivery

Conformal radiotherapy employs *three-dimensional treatment planning* using a series of specific radiation beams given from different angles to maximize tumor dose while minimizing normal tissue irradiation. This planning uses magnetic resonance imaging (MRI) or computed tomography (CT) scans or other imaging to lo-

**Table 15.1.** Severe Acute and Chronic Side Effects of Radiotherapy[a]

| Irradiation Site | Tissues at Risk | Acute Effect | Chronic Effect[b] |
|---|---|---|---|
| Brain | Brain; neural structures (eye, brain stem) | Hair loss | Cognitive dysfunction and decreased visual acuity |
| Head and neck | Oral mucosa, salivary glands, skin | Oral inflammation (mucositis), xerostomia (dry mouth), erythema (skin redness) | Permanent xerostomia, decreased ability to open mouth (trismus), dental caries, skin fibrosis |
| Thorax | Esophageal mucosa, lung, skin | Esophagitis, pneumonitis | Lung fibrosis, esophageal stricture, skin fibrosis |
| Abdomen | Intestine, pancreas, liver, spleen, kidneys | Nausea, hepatitis, diarrhea | Renal compromise, liver fibrosis, intestinal obstruction |
| Pelvis | Bladder, rectum, prostate | Increased urinary frequency and dysuria, diarrhea | Bladder or rectal bleeding or rectal ulceration, impotence |

[a]Acute and chronic (late) effects will be idiosyncratic to the patient, the total dose, the dose fractionation, and the irradiation volume.

[b]Severe chronic effects observed in less than 5 percent of population at 5 years.

calize the tumor and critical normal tissues (see Chap. 13). The energy, type and number of radiation beams and their orientation are then chosen. Successful delivery is tracked during treatment using verification images. The extent of the tumor is defined as the *gross tumor volume* (GTV), but the final radiation plan will deliver the maximum dose to a slightly larger radiation volume (the *planning target volume*, PTV). The PTV accounts for microscopic disease just beyond the detectable edge of the tumor, for body or organ movement, and for issues pertaining to the physics of the radiation beam (see Fig. 15.1A). Special techniques and markers are sometimes used to track organ movement within the body (e.g., movement of a lung tumor during normal breathing), thereby during daily treatments the accurate targeting of the radiation dose maintaining.

Recent improvements in radiotherapy planning involve the use of *intensity modulated radiation therapy* (IMRT) in which a computerized algorithm is used to design optimal beam orientations and intensities. With IMRT, the radiation beam is shaped using special collimators that move during the time of irradiation. The beams are differentially regulated within the area of irradiation so that there are relatively low- and high-dose volumes of irradiation. The combination of multiple beams allows for better dose distributions resulting in a decreased volume of normal tissue in the high-dose region (PTV).

For small anatomically accessible tumors, such as those involving the head and neck, cervix, or brain, high doses of finely localized irradiation can be delivered through the use of brachytherapy (discussed in Sec. 15.2.3) or stereotactic radiosurgery. The latter uses highly focused irradiation beams of charged particles (e.g., proton beams; see Sec. 15.2.4), γ-rays, or high-energy x-rays precisely targeted to the tumor site.

Determination of the relationship between normal tissue response and dose is often confounded by the nonuniform dose distribution within the normal organs. However, a dose-volume histogram (DVH) can be generated as part of a modern radiotherapy plan for each exposed organ in a patient (see Fig. 15.1B). Several models have been proposed for predicting normal tissue response to radiotherapy using such histograms. However, the quality of clinical data available to validate such predictions is rarely sufficient to alter radiotherapy practice. Nonetheless, in prostate cancer radiotherapy, for example, DVH plots can be used to illustrate that the volume of the anterior rectum irradiated to high doses is directly correlated to late complications within the rectum. One important complexity with IMRT plans is that increased volumes of normal tissue are exposed to low doses and this raises concerns as to the potential for increased radiation-induced second malignancies (see Chap. 3, Sec. 3.5).

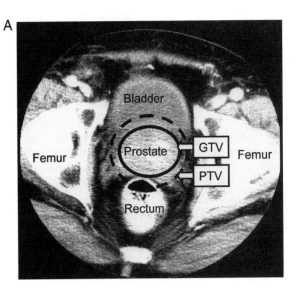

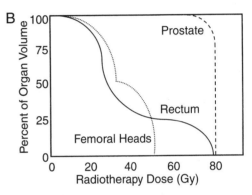

**Figure 15.1.** Radiotherapy planning volumes. (*A*) Cross-section of a male pelvis derived from a computed tomographic (CT) scan for use in planning of radiotherapy for prostate cancer. In this illustrative case, the entire prostate gland will be irradiated as the tumor target and denoted as the gross target volume (GTV). The planning target volume (PTV) will include the GTV plus a further margin for microscopic tumor cells and patient and organ motion. Note that the PTV partially encompasses normal tissues such as the bladder anteriorly and the rectum posteriorly. (*B*) A dose volume distribution (DVH) which plots the percent of organ volume (y-axis) receiving different doses of radiation (x-axis). In this case, the radiotherapy plan was designed to deliver 80 Gy to the prostate gland, whereas the normal tissues, such as the rectum and femoral heads, receive much lower doses. The dose received by a particular volume of an organ (e.g., 25% of the rectum received a dose of approximately 60 to 65 Gy) can be used to correlate normal tissue dose to complications of radiotherapy.

## 15.2.3 Brachytherapy, Radionucleotides, and Radioimmunotherapy

Interstitial or intracavitary low-dose rate irradiation sources placed into or beside the tumor (known as brachytherapy) are used either alone or in combination with external beam radiotherapy for accessible tumors such as those of the cervix, prostate, head and neck, breast, bladder, lung, esophagus, and some sarcomas. Close to the implanted brachytherapy source the dose is high and tumor cell killing will be high. At increasing distance from the source, normal cell killing will be less due to lower dose rates and a decreased total dose over the duration of treatment (see Fig. 15.2). The cellular effects of continuous low-dose rate irradiation (described in Chap. 14, Sec. 14.3.3) are similar to those of reducing fraction size, and allow for cellular repair in normal tissues (see Sec. 15.6.1). Computer-controlled brachytherapy systems can deliver radiation doses as short pulses (pulsed-dose brachytherapy) delivered by a high-dose rate source traveling along a catheter track within the tumor. Radiobiological modeling suggests that the acute and late reactions are similar to traditional (continuous) brachytherapy if the gaps between pulses are less than 1 hour (Brenner and Hall, 1991).

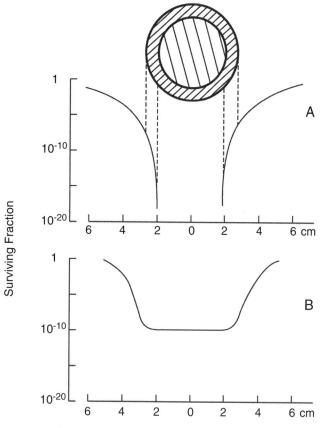

**Figure 15.2.** (*A*) Variation of cell kill around a point source of radiation during brachytherapy. The source gives 0.87 cGy/min at 2 cm (i.e., 75 Gy in 6 days); there are $10^9$ cells/g of tissue. The inner hatched area indicates the volume within which the surviving fraction is predicted to be below $10^{-20}$. The surrounding outer hatched area indicates the volume where the survival is between $10^{-20}$ and $10^{-6}$, which is the critical region for tumor control. (*B*) The type of profile expected using external beam radiotherapy. (Redrawn from Steel, 2002.)

The use of injected radionucleotides to treat cancer is based on their selective uptake by certain tumors so that local irradiation may lead to death of the tumor cells. Examples are $^{131}$I to treat well-differentiated thyroid cancer, radiolabeled somatostatin analogues for the treatment of neuroendocrine tumors, and $^{89}$Sr to treat bone metastases mainly in prostate cancer.

The conjugation of radionucleotides to specific antibodies or to agents that bind to receptors on cancer cells allows targeted radiotherapy to tumors expressing the relevant antigens or receptors and is termed *radioimmunotherapy*. Optimal radionucleotides are those emitting $\alpha$-particles and short-range electrons resulting in the killing of cells within a radius of 1 to 3 cell diameters of the bound isotope (e.g., indium-111). In animal models, radioimmunotherapy was found to kill disseminated solid tumor cells and small metastases when targeting differentiation antigens (e.g., CD20 or CD21) on lymphomas, somatostatin receptors on neuroendocrine tumors, or epidermal growth factor receptors on certain breast cancers. However, in patients this approach has been limited by the lack of specific uptake in tumor cells when compared to normal cells and the attendant difficulty of accurate dosimetry and treatment planning. Newer approaches utilizing tumor-specific antigens or liposomes filled with radionucleotides may improve this treatment modality (Carlsson, 2003)

### 15.2.4 High Linear Energy Transfer Radiotherapy

The use of *high-LET (linear energy transfer)* radiations can contribute to improvements in the therapeutic ratio in a number of different ways. First, particle beams, because much of their energy is deposited in tissue at the end of particle tracks (i.e., in the region of the Bragg peak, see Chap. 14, Sec. 14.2.2), can give improved depth-dose distributions for deep-seated tumors. Neutron beams are not useful in this regard because they do not demonstrate a Bragg peak and depth-dose distributions are similar to those for low-LET radiation (Fig. 15.3). The oxygen enhancement ratio is also reduced for high LET radiation (see Sec. 15.4.1 and Fig. 15.4*A*), so that hypoxic cells are protected to a lesser degree. The variation in radiosensitivity with position in the cell cycle (see Chap. 14, Sec. 14.4.2) is also reduced for high-LET radiation. Finally, cells exhibit reduced capacity for repair following high-LET radiation relative to that following low-LET radiation. This property leads to increased relative biological effectiveness (RBE; see Chap. 14, Sec. 14.3.1 and Fig. 15.4*A*) for high-LET radiations.

A comparison of various radiations with different LET in relation to their potential physical or biological

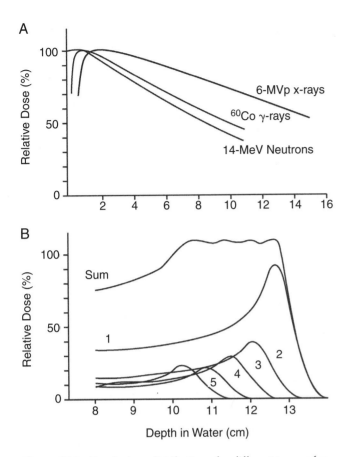

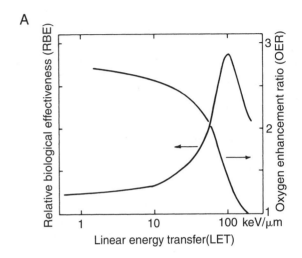

high-LET radiation is that because late-responding tissues demonstrate greater repair capacity than early-responding tissues (see Secs. 15.7.1 and 15.7.2), the reduction in repair capacity following high-LET irradiation will result in relatively higher RBE values for late-responding tissues.

Clinical studies using high-LET radiation have been most extensive with fast neutrons. Neutron therapy has

**Figure 15.3.** Depth-dose distributions for different types of radiation. (*A*) The energy deposited decreases as a function of depth into the body for both $^{60}$Co γ-rays, 6-MeV X-rays (after the initial build-up region) and for 14-MeV neutrons. The vertical scale relates to the three types of radiation independently and does not provide an intercomparison. (*B*) For protons the energy deposition increases with depth to a peak (the Bragg peak) at a depth that depends on the energy of the protons; importantly the dose falls off precipitously beyond the peak. By inserting absorbers in front of the primary proton beam (1) the peak will occur at different depths as indicated (2–5). This results in a spreading of the peak region (Sum) and allows adjustment to the beam, so that the spread peak covers the whole depth of the tumor but falls off rapidly beyond the tumor. (Modifed from Steel, 2002.)

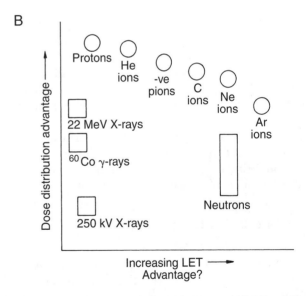

**Figure 15.4.** (*A*) Illustration of the dependence of the RBE (*left-hand axis*) and the OER (*right-hand axis*) on the LET of the radiation. The actual value of the RBE depends on the level of biological damage being examined. (*B*) Schematic comparison of the possible therapeutic advantage of using different types of radiation. The vertical axis represents the advantage due to improved depth-dose distribution. The horizontal axis represents increasing LET, which may give an advantage for the treatment of some tumors but not others. (Adapted from Raju, 1980.)

therapeutic advantages is shown in Figure 15.4*B*. The vertical axis represents the potential gain due to improved depth-dose distribution, while the horizontal axis represents potential gain due to the biological aspects of increased LET. The expected gains with protons are largely confined to improved dose distribution, while for neutrons any gains are likely to be related to the biological factors. Negative pions and accelerated ions can give both advantages, but they have had only limited clinical application because they are very expensive to produce and only a few places in the world have suitable facilities. One potential difficulty in using

been associated with an increase in complications, particularly subcutaneous fibrosis, and randomized trials have not demonstrated therapeutic gain (Fowler, 1988; Raju, 1996). Similarly, randomized results with pion therapy also failed to suggest any clinical advantage compared to photons (Pickles, 1995). In contrast results with protons have demonstrated an advantage for treatment of tumors, such as choroidal melanomas and skull-base tumors, that require precise treatment of a highly localized lesion and proton therapy might improve outcome in other tumor sites (Suit, 2002). High-energy photons (x- or γ-rays) deliver doses that decrease exponentially with depth, whereas protons show a rapid fall-off distal to a specific depth (Fig. 15.3$B$). This can lead to increased dose to the tumor and decreased normal tissue dose when compared with x- or γ-rays. Proton therapy planning can also be combined with IMRT planning techniques to give finely contoured dose distributions, but cost limitations (i.e., the requirement for a cyclotron or synchrotron) currently preclude proton therapy as a common approach to radiotherapy.

There has been interest, particularly for treatment of brain tumors, in *boron neutron capture therapy* (BNCT), in which compounds enriched with $^{10}$B are administered prior to irradiation with a thermal neutron beam (Barth, 2003; Nakagawa et al., 2003). Neutrons interact preferentially with the $^{10}$B atoms in the tumors, and, a fission reaction produces high-energy charged particles ($^{7}$Li and $^{4}$He) resulting in tumor cell killing. For an improved therapeutic ratio with BNCT, relatively high concentrations of $^{10}$B must be achieved in the tumor, with low concentrations in normal tissues. New boronated compounds and new strategies for delivering the compounds have improved the differential concentrations achievable in tumors and surrounding normal tissues with encouraging results (Barth et al., 2003). However, the depth-dose distribution for the thermal neutron beam is relatively poor and this remains a limitation in the clinical use of this treatment approach.

### 15.2.5 Combining Radiotherapy with Other Cancer Treatments

Radiotherapy is used increasingly with other cancer treatments including surgery, hormone therapy, and chemotherapy. Combining radiotherapy with surgery can improve outcome by sterilizing microscopic or residual disease within, and just beyond, the surgical bed. Alternatively, surgery can be used as salvage therapy in cases where the use of radiotherapy alone was not sufficient to control the tumor. Examples of novel molecular targeting agents that can inhibit an oncogenic signaling pathway or reactivate a tumor suppressor gene pathway to sensitize tumor cells to radiotherapy were described in Chapter 14 (Sec. 14.4.4). Concomitant

chemoradiotherapy or hormone radiotherapy is used in locally advanced cancers that would not be cured by either therapy alone, including advanced head and neck, lung, prostate, and cervical cancers. Important interactions between radiation and chemotherapy in tumor and normal tissues are reviewed in Chapter 17 (Sec. 17.5).

### 15.3 TUMOR CONTROL FOLLOWING RADIOTHERAPY

#### 15.3.1 Dose Response and Tumor Control Relationships

The emphasis in Chapter 14 on the molecular and cellular effects of radiation treatment reflects the belief that the response of tumors can be understood largely in terms of the response of the cells within those tumors. Tumor response to radiation treatment can be assessed by techniques that do not measure tumor cell survival directly (Fig. 15.5). One such endpoint is growth delay that is determined by measuring the size of untreated and irradiated tumors as a function of time to generate growth curves (Fig. 15.5$A$). The delay in growth is the difference in time for treated and untreated tumors to grow to a defined size. The time difference is a measure of tumor response and can be plotted as a function of radiation dose, as shown in Figure 15.5$B$. The shape and position of this curve will be different for different treatments. The curve shown in Figure 15.5$B$ has a change in slope, consistent with the presence of a fraction of hypoxic cells in the tumor (see Sec. 15.4.2). At higher radiation doses, some tumors will be permanently controlled. If groups of animals receive different radiation doses to their tumors, the percentage of controlled tumors can be plotted as a function of dose to give a dose-control curve as shown in Figure 15.5$C$.

Intrinsic to tumor growth is the concept that tumors contain a fraction of cells that have unlimited proliferative capacity (i.e., tumor stem cells, see Chap. 9, Sec. 9.4.4). To achieve tumor control, all the tumor stem cells must be killed. For a simple model, which assumes that the response of a tumor to radiation depends on the individual responses of the cells within it, the dose of radiation required to control a tumor only depends on: (1) the radiation sensitivity of the stem cells and (2) their number. From a knowledge of the survival curve for the cells in a tumor, it is possible to predict the expected level of survival following a given single radiation dose. A simple calculation, using Eq. 14.4 in Appendix 14.1 (Chap. 14) and typical survival curve parameters for well-oxygenated cells ($D_0 = 1.3$ Gy, $D_q = 2.1$ Gy), indicates that a single radiation dose of 26 Gy might be expected to reduce the probability of survival of an individual cell to about $10^{-8}$. For a tumor con-

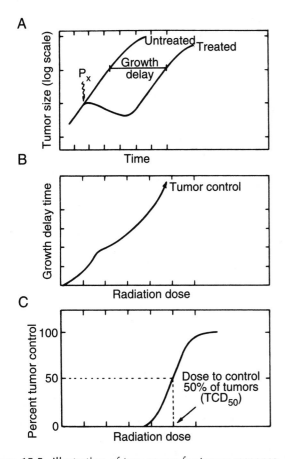

**Figure 15.5.** Illustration of two assays for tumor response. In (A), growth curves for groups of treated and untreated tumors are shown and the measurement of growth delay indicated. Growth delay is plotted as a function of radiation dose in (B). At large doses some of the tumors may not regrow and the percentage of controlled tumors can be plotted as a function of dose as in (C).

taining $10^8$ stem cells, this dose would thus leave, on average, one surviving cell. Because of the random nature of radiation damage there will be statistical fluctuation around this value. The statistical fluctuation expected from random cell killing by radiation follows a Poisson distribution; the probability ($P_n$) of a tumor having $n$ surviving cells when the average number of cells surviving is $a$ is given by:

$$P_n = (a^n e^{-a})/n! \qquad (15.1)$$

For tumor control, the important parameter is $P_0$ which is the probability that a tumor will contain no surviving stem cells (i.e., $n = 0$). From Eq. (15.1):

$$P_0 = e^{-a} \qquad (15.2)$$

so for $a = 1$, as in the example above, the probability of control would be $e^{-1} = 0.37$. Different radiation

doses will, of course, result in different values of $a$. For example, for identical tumors each containing $10^8$ cells, a dose that reduces the survival level to $10^{-9}$ will give $a = 0.1$ (i.e., 10 cells surviving in 100 tumors) with an expected probability of control of $e^{-0.1} = 0.90$. From such calculations, it is possible to construct a theoretical tumor control versus dose curve, which shows a sigmoid relationship (Fig. 15.6, solid lines).

The central solid curve in Figure 15.6 represents a group of identical tumors each containing $10^8$ tumor stem cells. For tumors containing $10^7$ or $10^9$ stem cells, the curves will be displaced (to smaller or larger doses, respectively) by a dose sufficient to reduce survival by a factor of 10. These dose-control curves illustrate the concept that the dose of radiation required to control a tumor depends on the number of stem cells that it contains.

The above discussion assumes that the tumor stem cells exhibit uniform radiosensitivity within a tumor that reflects their radiosensitivity in vitro. However, as discussed in Section 15.4, the microenvironment of the cells in the tumor can affect their sensitivity to radiation. This is well documented for hypoxia but there may also be interactions of the cells with the extracellular matrix (ECM) and/or interactions with growth factors, such as transforming growth factor $\beta 1$ (TGF-$\beta 1$), which may influence cellular sensitivity and tumor response (Ewan et al., 2002). Interactions between the tumor cells and the ECM might also influence cellular signaling such as the EGFR/MEK/ERK pathway that can affect cellular sensitivity to radiation (Chap. 14, Sec. 14.4.4). As discussed in Sections 15.5.1 and 15.5.2, there is increasing evidence that vascular damage and the induction of inflammatory cytokines play an important role in the responses of normal tissues to radiation treatment. The role that such factors may play in tumor re-

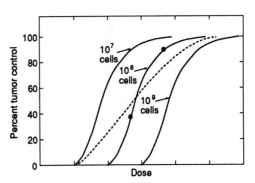

**Figure 15.6.** Percentage tumor control plotted as a function of dose for single radiation treatments. Theoretical curves for groups of tumors containing different numbers of tumor stem cells are shown. The points on the curve labeled "$10^8$ cells" are derived as discussed in the text. The composite curve (dashed) was obtained for a group containing equal proportions from the three individual groups.

sponse is largely unexplored. However, radiation-induced apoptosis of microvascular endothelial cells in the tumor might play a role in its response to radiation treatment (Garcia-Barros et al., 2003).

The terms *radiosensitive* and *radioresistant* have been used to describe, respectively, tumors that regress rapidly or slowly after radiation treatment. This can be misleading because the rate of regression may not correlate with the ability to cure a tumor with tolerable doses of radiation. A better term to describe a tumor that regresses rapidly after treatment is *radioresponsive*. The rate of response of a tumor depends on the proliferative rate of its cells because most tumor cells express their radiation damage when they attempt mitosis (Chap. 14, Sec. 14.3.2). Thus, a tumor that contains a large proportion of proliferating cells will tend to express radiation damage to its cells early and will regress rapidly. Although radioresponsive, the tumor may contain surviving stem cells that will be responsible for its recurrence.

**Table 15.2.** Values of the Surviving Fraction at 2 Gy for Human Tumor Cell Lines

| Tumor Cell Type[a] | Number of Lines | Mean Survival at 2 Gy (Range) |
|---|---|---|
| 1. Lymphoma<br>Neuroblastoma<br>Myeloma<br>Small-cell lung cancer<br>Medulloblastoma | 14 | 0.20 (0.08–0.37) |
| 2. Breast cancer<br>Squamous cell cancer<br>Pancreatic cancer<br>Colorectal cancer<br>Non–small-cell<br>    lung cancer | 12 | 0.43 (0.14–0.75) |
| 3. Melanoma<br>Osteosarcoma<br>Glioblastoma<br>Hypernephroma | 25 | 0.52 (0.20–0.86) |

[a]Tumor types are grouped (1–3) approximately in decreasing order of their likelihood of local control by radiation treatment. (Modified from Deacon et al., 1984.)

### 15.3.2 Predicting the Response of Tumors

Even tumors of the same size and histopathological type are likely to vary in their proportion of stem cells. Thus, a dose-control curve for a group of human tumors will be a composite of ones similar to those shown in Figure 15.6; the slope of the composite dose-control curve will be less than that for the individual groups of tumors (Fig. 15.6, dashed line). Fractionation of the radiation treatment (see Sec. 15.6) and heterogeneity in the radiosensitivity of tumor stem cells will also result in a decrease in the slope of the dose-control curve. Thus, the slope of the dose-control curve derived from a clinical study is likely to be shallow due to tumor heterogeneity. It is therefore desirable to seek a way of assigning the tumors to more homogeneous groups, so that patients with differences in prognosis can be identified. This is a major motivation for attempts to develop predictive assays.

Studies of a wide range of cell lines derived from human tumors have shown intrinsic variations in radiation sensitivity (see Table 15.2). Survival curves can vary considerably even for cells of similar histopathological types (see Fig. 15.7). It is the size of the shoulder of the curves that varies most widely. Even small differences in the shoulder region can be important because they are magnified during the multiple fractionated daily doses of 1.8 to 2 Gy given in clinical radiotherapy. Figure 15.7A illustrates the variability in cell survival curves for cell lines derived from different human melanomas (Fertil and Malaise, 1981). Survival following a dose of 2 Gy varies from about 0.2 to 0.9 (Fig. 15.7B). Consider a tumor for which survival following a dose of 2 Gy is 0.8. Assuming that each fraction of a multiple-dose

treatment is equally effective, and that there is no cell proliferation between dose fractions (an assumption that ignores some of the issues to be discussed in Sec. 15.6), the survival following thirty fractions of 2 Gy would be $(0.8)^{30} = 10^{-3}$. In contrast, for a tumor in which the survival following 2 Gy is 0.6, survival after 30 fractions would be $(0.6)^{30} = 2 \times 10^{-7}$. Thus, small differences in survival at low doses can translate into very large differences during a course of fractionated treatment. Estimates of the surviving fraction following a dose of 2 Gy for different human tumor cell lines growing in culture may be grouped according to histopathological type and compared with the likelihood that such tumors will be controlled by radiation treatment (Table 15.2). There is a trend toward higher levels of survival at 2 Gy for the cells from tumor groups expected to be less radiocurable.

The concept that tumor response for an individual patient can be predicted has been tested using the survival following 2 Gy of radiation (or another parameter that reflects radiosensitivity at clinically relevant low doses) to predictive for the outcome of fractionated radiotherapy treatment. Using the cell-adhesive matrix (CAM) growth assay, Girinsky and colleagues (1994) reported that increased survival in the low-dose region of the radiation survival curve was associated with decreased local control and survival in patients treated with radiation for head and neck cancer or cervical cancers. Using a clonogenic assay for cells from primary human cervix tumor biopsies grown in soft agar, West and coworkers (1997) found that patients with tumors containing radioresistant cells (SF2 > median) had sig-

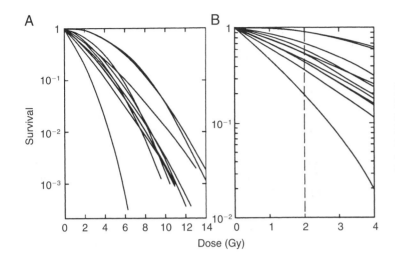

**Figure 15.7.** (*A*) Survival curves for a number of different human melanoma cell lines. The lines were drawn to be continuously curving and conform to the linear-quadratic model (see Chap. 14, Appendix 14.1). (*B*) The low-dose region of the curves is illustrated, demonstrating the range of survival values at 2 Gy. (Adapted from Fertil and Malaise, 1981.)

nificantly worse local control and survival than those with more tumors containing radiosensitive cells (SF2 < median; see Fig. 15.8) and similar results were reported for head and neck cancers (Bjork-Eriksson et al., 2000). However, other groups have not reported confirmatory results. Furthermore, the widespread application of such assays is limited by technical problems: for example the soft agar assay required 5 to 6 weeks before scoring and measurements could not be obtained in 25 to 30 percent of tumors. Other potential limitations of such assays are: (1) they do not account for microenvironmental factors influencing radiosensitivity in vivo (see Sec. 15.4) and (2) tumors may contain clonogenic subpopulations of different intrinsic radiosensitivity.

Other proposed predictive assays have evaluated radiation-induced apoptosis or senescence within solid tumors, or the expression of genes or proteins which relate to cell cycle control, cell death, and DNA repair. Data from murine tumors suggest that the levels of pretreatment apoptosis correlate with radiation-induced apoptosis, and predict tumor responses (Meyn et al., 1993). However, the use of pretreatment apoptotic index (determined from characteristic morphological features on histological sections) as a predictive assay in a number of (small) clinical studies has given variable results. It is uncertain whether larger studies will confirm the predictive value of the apoptotic index given the limited correlation with cell death as assessed by a colony forming assay (see Chap. 14, Sec. 14.3.2).

## 15.4 HYPOXIA AND RADIATION RESPONSE

### 15.4.1 The Oxygen Effect and Radiosensitivity

The biological effects of radiation on cells are enhanced by oxygen. There is some uncertainty about exact mechanisms but $O_2$ can interact with radicals formed by radiation, resulting in products which cause damage to DNA that is more difficult for the cell to repair. For this effect oxygen must be present in the cells at the time of or within a few milliseconds of the radiation exposure. Cells irradiated in the presence of air are about three times more sensitive than cells irradiated under conditions of severe hypoxia (see Fig. 15.9*A*). The sensitizing effect of different concentrations of oxygen is shown in Figure 15.9*B*. At very low levels of oxygen the cells are resistant but, as the level of oxygen increases, their sensitivity rises rapidly to almost maximal levels at oxygen concentrations above about 35 micromoles per liter (equivalent oxygen partial pressure 25 mmHg). The oxygen concentration at which the sensitizing effect is one half of maximum (the $K_m$ value) varies

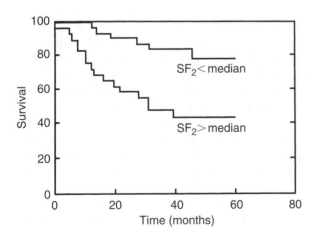

**Figure 15.8.** Actuarial survival in patients with cervical cancer treated by radical radiotherapy as a function of intrinsic radiosensitivity of tumors stratified as above or below the median survival following 2 Gy ($SF_2$) of 0.41. Survival and local control (not shown) are significantly worse for patients with $SF_2 > 0.41$. (Redrawn from Levine et al, 1995.)

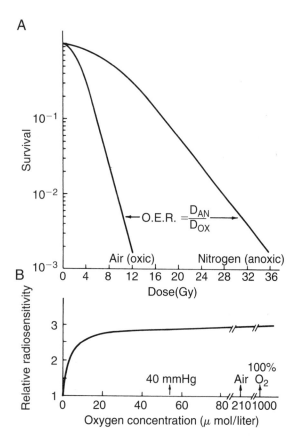

**Figure 15.9.** Effect of oxygen as a radiosensitizer. (*A*) Survival curves obtained when cells are treated with low-LET radiation in the presence (air) or absence (nitrogen) of oxygen. The oxygen enhancement ratio (OER) is calculated as indicated ($D_{OX}$ = dose in air, $D_{AN}$ = dose in nitrogen) and as described in the text. (*B*) The relative radiosensitivity of cells is plotted as a function of oxygen concentration in the surrounding medium to illustrate the dependence of the sensitizing effect on oxygen concentration. (Adapted from Chapman et al, 1974.)

among cell lines but is usually in the region of 5 to 17 micromoles per liter (3 to 10 mmHg equivalent partial pressure).

The degree of sensitization afforded by oxygen is characterized by the oxygen enhancement ratio (OER), which is defined (see Fig. 15.9*A*) as the ratio of doses required to give the same biological effect in the absence or the presence of oxygen. For doses of x- or $\gamma$-radiation greater than about 3 Gy, the OER for a wide range of cell lines in vitro and for most tissues in vivo is in the range of 2.5 to 3.3. For x- or $\gamma$-ray doses less than 3 Gy (i.e., in the shoulder region of the survival curve), the OER is reduced in a dose-dependent manner (Palcic and Skarsgard, 1984). A reduction of the OER at low doses is clinically important because the individual treatments of a fractionated course of radiation are usually 2 Gy or less. The OER is also dependent on the type of

radiation, declining to a value of 1 for radiation with linear energy transfer values greater than about 200 keV/$\mu$m (see Fig. 15.4).

### 15.4.2 Tumor Hypoxia

The cells in a tumor are influenced both by their interactions with the ECM (see Chap. 11, Sec. 11.4), and by the microenvironment of solid tumors, which is characterized by regions of nutrient deprivation, low extracellular pH, high interstitial fluid pressure (IFP), and hypoxia. The oxygen concentration (pO$_2$) in most normal tissues ranges between 10 and 80 mmHg, depending on the tissue type, whereas tumors often contain regions where the pO$_2$ is less than 5 mmHg. These conditions in solid tumors are due primarily to the abnormal vasculature that develops during tumor angiogenesis (see Chap. 12, Sec. 12.3). The blood vessels in solid tumors have highly irregular architecture, and may have an incomplete endothelial lining and basement membrane, which makes them more leaky than vessels in normal tissues. The leakiness of tumor blood vessels and a lack of functional lymphatic vessels is believed to be responsible for the increased IFP in tumors (Jain et al., 2002). A proportion of tumor cells may lie in hypoxic regions beyond the diffusion distance of oxygen where they are exposed to chronically low oxygen tensions (see Figs. 15.10 and 15.11*A*, which illustrate the tumor cord model). Tumor cells may also be exposed to shorter (often fluctuating) periods of (acute) hypoxia due to intermittent flow in individual blood vessels (see Fig. 15.10). Tumor hypoxia has been found to be heterogeneous both within and among tumors, even those of identical histopathological type, and it does not correlate simply with standard prognostic factors such as tumor size, stage, and grade (Vaupel et al., 2001).

Studies with both extrinsic and intrinsic markers of hypoxia (see Sec. 15.4.3; Bussink, 2003) have shown that hypoxic cells can occur close to blood vessels, presumably due to fluctuation in blood flow in individual vessels resulting in regions of hypoxia for short periods of time (minutes to hours). Studies involving the intravenous injection of diffusible fluorescent dyes as markers of functional blood vessels and measurements of microregional blood flow and tissue oxygenation have given direct evidence for this effect in experimental tumors (Dewhirst, 1998). Acute and chronic hypoxia can coexist in the same tumor and hypoxic regions in tumors are often diffusely distributed throughout the tumor (see Fig. 15.11*B*) and rarely concentrated only around a central core of necrosis.

Hypoxia may play an important role in treatment outcome for many tumor types and hypoxia can affect the metastatic ability of some tumor cells (for review see

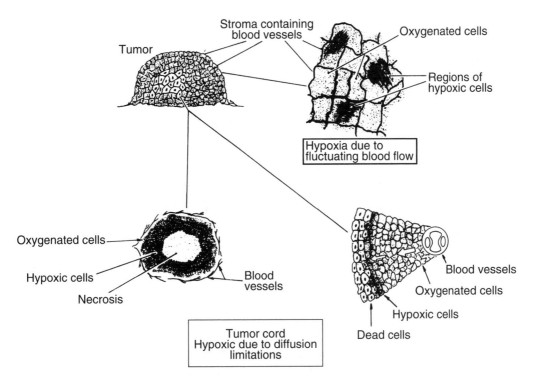

**Figure 15.10.** Schematic illustration of two possible models for the development of hypoxia in tumors. Hypoxia may arise as a result of fluctuating blood flow (as illustrated in the diagram on the upper right) or as a result of diffusion limitations in the tumor cord model (inward or outward diffusion from vessels as illustrated in the lower two diagrams).

Rofstad, 2000; Subarsky and Hill, 2003). This is probably due to altered gene expression associated with exposure to hypoxia. The expression of as much as 1.5 percent of the genome may be modified by exposure to hypoxia. Many of these genes are involved in cellular functions such as anaerobic respiration and include glycolytic enzymes and cell membrane proteins such as glucose transporters (e.g., GLUT-1) and enzymes that control carbonate levels (e.g., carbonic anhydrase IX, CA-IX). Genes that modify the oxygen carrying capacity of blood (e.g., erythropoietin) or increase vascularity, such as angiogenic growth factors like vascular endothelial growth factor (VEGF, see Chap. 12, Sec. 12.2.1) are also upregulated, as are survival factors and invasive factors (Semenza, 2003).

Many of the genes upregulated by hypoxia contain a hypoxia response element (HRE) in their promotor region that is responsive to the transcription factor, hypoxia-inducible factor 1 (HIF-1). HIF-1 is expressed at increased levels in cells exposed to hypoxia and is often overexpressed in tumors. It is a heterodimeric basic helix-loop-helix transcription factor (Chap. 8, Sec. 8.2.8) and is composed of two subunits, HIF-1$\alpha$ and HIF-1$\beta$ (also called ARNT). HIF-1$\beta$/ARNT is stably expressed in cells but the HIF-1$\alpha$ protein is unstable in the presence of oxygen, because it can be hydroxylated on specific proline residues and ubiquitinated in the presence of the von Hippel-Lindau (VHL) protein, thereby targeting it for degradation by the proteosomal pathway (see Chap. 9, Sec. 9.2.1). Under hypoxic conditions HIF-1$\alpha$ is not hydroxylated, cannot bind to VHL, and hence increases in the cell, allowing it to migrate to the nucleus, bind to HIF-1$\beta$ and initiate transcription. HIF-1 may also act in concert with other transcription factors to modify the expression of genes. Cells expressing activated oncogenes (such as *Ras* or *src*) demonstrate increased expression of angiogenic factors such as VEGF under hypoxic conditions. There is also evidence that signaling pathways, such as the PI-3K/AkT or MEK-ERK pathways) (see Chap. 8, Sec. 8.2), can increase the expression of HIF-1 responsive genes by enhancing the transcriptional activity of HIF-1. While increases in HIF-1 during hypoxic exposure appear to occur in all cell types, these secondary effects are cell-type specific (Semenza, 2003).

Prolonged exposure to hypoxia can lead to cell death by apoptosis. Cells that have a mutated p53 gene have been found to acquire genetic resistance to hypoxia-mediated apoptosis (Graeber et al., 1996; see also Chap. 18, Sec. 18.3.2). This suggests that hypoxia may pro-

A

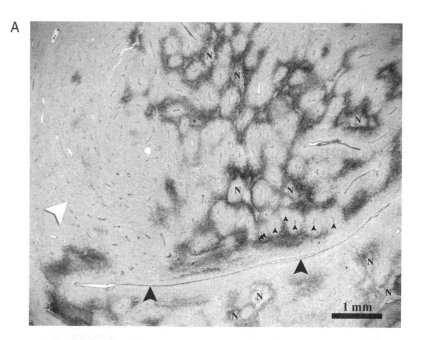

**Figure 15.11.** Tumor Hypoxia. Panel (*A*) shows a section of a high grade human soft tissue sarcoma (rhabdomyosarcoma, pleomorphic) showing hypoxic regions (dark brown membraneous CA IX staining) distant from blood vessels (reddish-brown CD31 staining). Small black arrowheads point to blood vessels at the center of tumor cords with peripheral CA IX staining. Large black arrowheads point to one long blood vessel in the plane of the section. Necrotic regions are labeled with an N. The large white arrowhead points to a well-vascularized region with no hypoxia (and absence of CA IX staining). This picture illustrates the cord-like structure which is associated with (chronic) hypoxia in regions of many tumors. (Courtesy of Dr. K. Maseide, University of Toronto, Toronto, Canada.) Panel (*B*) shows staining for EF5 (red) in a complete section through a human pancreatic tumor xenograft growing in a SCID mouse. The blood vessels are stained for CD31 (green) and regions close to functional blood vessels are indicated by the blue staining for Hoechst 33342 that was injected into the mouse a few minutes before the animal was killed and the tumor was removed. Brightish staining in the bottom right edge of the figure is an artifact. (Courtesy of Dr. David Hedley and Ms Nhu-An Pham, University of Toronto, Toronto, Canada.) (See color plate.)

B

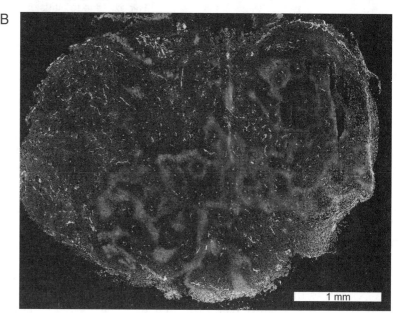

mote tumor progression by selecting for cells with p53 mutations (see Chap. 11, Sec. 11.1). Other studies suggest that the cells which are exposed to a hypoxic tumor environment are more likely to develop genomic instability and acquire mutant genotypes (Reynolds et al., 1996). There is also evidence that exposure to hypoxia may reduce the functionality of DNA repair proteins, such as MSH-2, that are involved in mismatch repair (see Chap. 5, Sec. 5.3.3). These observations suggest that cells growing within hypoxic regions of tumors constitute an important target for cancer treatment.

Evidence that cells in the hypoxic regions of tumors are viable and capable of regrowing the tumor is pro-

vided by analysis of cell survival curves. For most tumors the terminal slope of such curves is characteristic of that for hypoxia cells (see Fig. 15.12). The proportion of viable hypoxic cells in tumors can be estimated (see Fig. 15.12) from the ratio ($S_{air}/S_{anox}$) of the cell survival obtained for tumors in air-breathing animals irradiated with a large dose to the cell survival obtained for tumors irradiated with the same dose under anoxic conditions (e.g., tumor blood supply clamped or animal killed prior to the irradiation). It is assumed that the tumors made deliberately anoxic contain 100 percent hypoxic cells and that the radiation survival curve for the naturally occurring hypoxic cells is the same as that

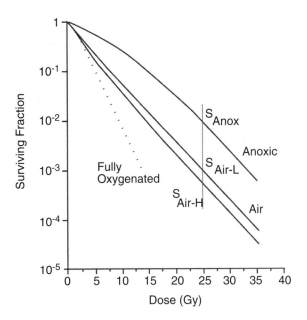

**Figure 15.12.** The influence of a subpopulation of hypoxic cells on the survival curve obtained for an irradiated tumor. The four curves shown are for a well-oxygenated population of cells (dotted line), two curves derived from tumors irradiated under air-breathing conditions and a curve for tumors irradiated under anoxic conditions. The two curves for irradiation under air-breathing conditions are for tumors in animals with high (H) or low (L) hemoglobin levels. The hypoxic fraction can be estimated by taking the ratio of the survival obtained under air-breathing conditions ($S_{air}$) to that obtained under anoxic conditions ($S_{anox}$) at a dose level where the survival curves are parallel, as illustrated. For the tumors in animals with a high hemoglobin this value is about 0.06 (6%) and for the tumors in animals with low hemoglobin it is about 0.12 (12%). (Modified from Hill et al., 1971.)

for the cells made deliberately anoxic. Most experimental tumors treated in air-breathing animals contain a proportion of hypoxic cells, in the range 10 to 20%. These proportions represent the cells that are maximally resistant to irradiation (radiobiologically hypoxic). There will also be a substantial proportion of cells in tumors which are at intermediate oxygen levels. Many techniques have provided evidence that hypoxic cells exist in human tumors, and may affect the outcome of radiation therapy (see Sec. 15.4.3). As illustrated in Figure 15.12, the response of tumors to large single doses of radiation is dominated by the presence of hypoxic cells within them, even if only a very small fraction of the tumor cells are hypoxic. Immediately after a dose of radiation, the proportion of the surviving cells that is hypoxic will be elevated. However, with time, some of the surviving hypoxic cells may gain access to oxygen and hence, become more sensitive to a subsequent radiation treatment. This process of reoxygenation can result in a substantial increase in the sensitivity of tumors during fractionated treatment and is discussed in more detail in Section 15.6.4.

### 15.4.3 Measuring Hypoxia in Tumors

Techniques to determine oxygenation in individual tumors are listed in Table 15.3 (see also Chap. 13, Sec. 13.3.1). The most commonly used method in human tumors has been the commercially available polarographic oxygen electrodes (the Eppendorf oxygen electrode. These electrodes can measure microregional $pO_2$ (estimated to be in a volume equivalent to about 500 cells) in multiple locations giving a distribution of values. Measurements of tumor $pO_2$ using this technology have revealed wide $pO_2$ variations both within and between tumors (see Fig. 15.13A and B). Results from clinical studies in cervix (see Fig. 15.13C) and head and neck carcinomas treated by radiotherapy or radiotherapy and chemotherapy indicate that hypoxic tumors (median $pO_2$ value < 5 to 10 mm Hg) have a worse prognosis both in terms of disease-free and overall survival (for review, see Milosevic et al., 2004). Similar results have been obtained for soft tissue sarcoma in smaller studies. The data suggest that the hypoxia measurements can predict for distant metastases as well as local failure. The oxygen electrode has the disadvantage that it is invasive and it is difficult to distinguish between measurements made in viable versus nonviable tissue regions. Studies with intrinsic markers of hypoxia (such as HIF-1$\alpha$, GLUT-1, and CA-IX; see Sec. 15.4.2) have the advantage that they can be applied to existing tissue blocks for retrospective analysis of previous clinical studies (see Fig. 15.11A). Increased levels of these markers have been associated with poorer treatment outcome in different tumor types (Bussink et al., 2003). The most commonly used extrinsic markers are pimonidazole and EF-5 (see Fig. 15.11B), which have provided further evidence for substantial heterogeneity in hypoxia both within and between tumors, but only one study has linked results with these agents to treatment outcome (Kaanders, Wijffels, et al., 2002). Further studies are required to establish whether these extrinsic markers will be reliable predictors of tumor hypoxia and treament outcome. The correlations between measured $pO_2$ values, and/or between extrinsic and intrinsic markers have not been very consistent.

### 15.4.4 Increasing Oxygen Delivery to Tumors

Because hypoxic cells represent a radiation-resistant subpopulation in tumors that is not present in most normal tissues, the therapeutic ratio might be improved by techniques to reduce the influence of hypoxic cells on tumor response. Clinical studies have demonstrated the negative effect of anemia on prognosis (Fyles et al., 2000), and in many centers, blood transfusions are used to maintain patients at normal hemoglobin levels during treatment. A small randomized study in patients

**Table 15.3.** Assays for Intratumoral Hypoxia

| Technique | Principle | Advantages | Disadvantages |
|---|---|---|---|
| Histomorphometric assays | Measures distance between blood vessels and zones of necrosis. Measures vascular density. | Simple. Can be applied on archived tissue. Can be combined with cryospectrophotometry to measure hemoglobin saturation within frozen tissue section. | Indirect measure of tumor oxygenation. Does not take into account perfusion in blood vessels. |
| Oxygen electrode measurements | $pO_2$ electrode is stepped through tissue and electrode signals are converted to $pO_2$ values. | Provides real-time measure of tissue oxygenation with multiple sampling. Precalibrated probe does not consume oxygen. This allows for measurements of $pO_2$ over time in the same location. | Invasive. Does not differentiate $pO_2$ values in necrotic vs viable regions or between tumor and normal tissue. $pO_2$ electrode consumes oxygen, preventing measurements over time in same location. |
| Luminescent probe | Probe is inserted into the tissue and interrogated with light pulses to measure lifetime of luminescence, which is proportional to $O_2$ concentration. | | |
| DNA strand-break assays | Comet assay to measure DNA strand breaks in irradiated tumor cells. Hypoxic cells exhibit fewer breaks. | Direct assay to measure DNA damage in cells under hypoxia conditions in situ. | Invasive and indirect. Requires rapid preparation of a cell suspension from a tissue biopsy post-irradiation. Subject to sampling errors. |
| Extrinsic hypoxic cell markers | Preferential binding/ uptake by hypoxic cells of radioactive or fluorescent compounds (e.g., nitroimidazoles). Imaged by MRS, PET, SPECT, or fluorescence microscopy. | Detection of the hypoxic cells is noninvasive with external scanning procedures. Microscopy analysis can visualize the hypoxic cells at the cellular level. | Requires the injection or ingestion of the marker drug. Binding can be affected by metabolic factors and diffusion limitations. Microscopic analysis subject to sampling error. |
| Intrinsic hypoxic cell markers | Antibody staining of proteins upregulated in cells by hypoxic exposure (e.g., HIF-1$\alpha$, CA-IX, GLUT-1, VEGF) | Markers can be assessed in archived tissue. | Markers may be upregulated by factors other than hypoxia. Uniform fixation of tissue important for reliable quantitation. Subject to sampling error. |
| Imaging of blood oxygenation and flow | MRI–BOLD (blood oxygen level dependent) imaging or functional MRI or CT using contrast agents introduced into the blood. Near-infrared light spectroscopy. Measures $HbO_2$ saturation by absorption at different wavelengths. | Noninvasive. | Does not measure tumor oxygenation directly. Relatively poor spatial resolution. |

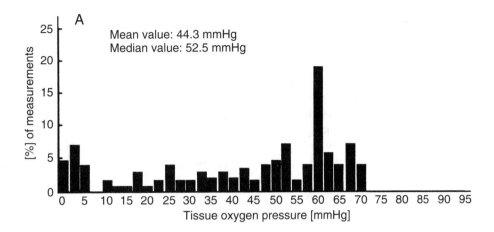

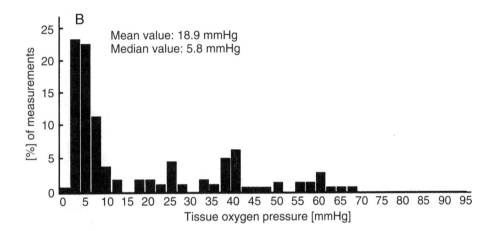

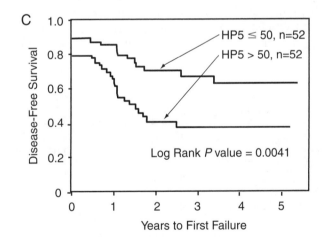

**Figure 15.13.** Distribution of tumor $pO_2$ in two human cervix carcinomas as measured by the Eppendorf oxygen electrode. Each distribution represents 160 individual measurement points in the tumor. Tumor in (A) is less hypoxic and shows fewer regions with low $pO_2$ measurements than tumor in (B). (Courtesy of Fyles et al., unpublished.) Panel (C) shows results for cancer of the cervix treated with radiotherapy and demonstrates that patients with tumors with a higher degree of hypoxia (HP5 > 50%) have poorer disease-free survival. HP5 is the percentage of $pO_2$ measurements in the tumor that were below 5 mm Hg. (Redrawn from Fyles, Milosevic, et al, 2002.)

with carcinoma of the cervix showed improvement of local control with blood transfusions (Bush, 1986). The administration of erythropoietin has been used to correct anemia in some centers (Siedenfeld et al., 2001) but there is little evidence that it can improve local control or disease-free survival following radiotherapy (Henke et al., 2003). Experimental studies have suggested that low arterial oxygen tensions may also influence tumor response by affecting the level of hypoxia. Carbon monoxide in cigarette smoke reduces the oxygen carrying and unloading capacity of the blood and may result in reduced tumor oxygenation. Patients with head and neck cancer who continue to smoke during radiotherapy have been found to have decreased local control and survival after radiation treatment (Browman et al., 1993), although similar results in cervix cancer did not reach statistical significant (Fyles, Voduc, et al., 2002).

Oxygen delivery to tumor cells may be increased by giving animals or patients oxygen under hyperbaric conditions (200 to 300 kPa) during radiation treatment. An increase in the dissolved oxygen concentration in blood plasma should result in greater diffusion of oxygen into the hypoxic regions. Studies with animal tumors have demonstrated that the use of hyperbaric oxygen (HPO) will indeed sensitize them to radiation. Clinical studies with HPO as an adjuvant to radiation therapy have demonstrated significant improvement in local tumor control and survival for patients with cancers of the head and neck and cervix (see Table 15.4), but this has not been observed in the limited studies of tumors at other sites (Overgaard and Horsman, 1996).

Other possible strategies for improving tumor oxygenation include the use of a combination of nicotin-amide, which has been shown to increase tumor perfusion, and carbogen (95% $O_2$ and 5% $CO_2$) breathing. This combination (called ARCON therapy) has been reported to improve outcome in head and neck cancers treated with radiation therapy (Kaanders, Bussink, et al., 2002). Paradoxically, there is evidence in animal tumor models that treatment with anti-angiogenesis agents (see Chap. 12, Sec. 12.4) can improve oxygenation in some tumors, possibly due to regularization of the vasculature. Studies combining such agents with radiation treatment of experimental tumors have indicated improved treatment response (Lee et al., 2000; Kozin et al., 2001). It remains uncertain whether these improved responses are due to improved oxygenation or to factors such as direct tumor cell kill induced by the anti-angiogenesis treatment.

### 15.4.5 Hypoxic Cell Sensitizers and Cytotoxins

An alternative approach to reduce the influence of tumor hypoxia involves the use of drugs that mimic the radiosensitizing properties of oxygen. These drugs, known as *hypoxic-cell radiosensitizers,* must diffuse to all parts of a tumor to be effective. Development of radiosensitizers was based on the idea that the radiosensitizing properties of oxygen are due to its electron affinity and that other electron-affinic compounds might act as sensitizers. A family of compounds, the nitromidazoles, has been found to contain members (Fig. 15.14) that can sensitize hypoxic cells both in vitro and in animal tumors. The most extensively studied of these compounds is misonidazole, which can sensitize hypoxic cells in vitro in a dose-dependent fashion and does not sensitize oxygenated cells. The extent of the

**Table 15.4.** Summary of Clinical Trials Testing Sensitization of Hypoxic Cells

| Sensitizing Agent | Number of Trials | Significant Benefit | Non-significant Trend for Benefit | No Benefit |
|---|---|---|---|---|
| Hyperbaric Oxygen | 15 | 3 | 6 | 6 |
| Misonidazole | 39 | 4 | 4 | 31 |

| Tumor Site | Number of Patients (Trials) | Percentage Local Control | | p Value |
|---|---|---|---|---|
| | | Radiation Alone | Radiation Plus Sensitizer | |
| Head and neck cancer | 4064 (22) | 40.6% | 47.2% | 0.00002 |
| Cervical cancer | 2292 (12) | 59.6% | 61.2% | 0.014 |

The upper part of the table gives results from individual trials while the lower part gives the results of a meta-analysis of all the suitable data (using HPO or hypoxic-cell radiosensitizers).

*Sources:* Top, adapted from Dische (1989); bottom, data from Overgaard and Horsman (1996).

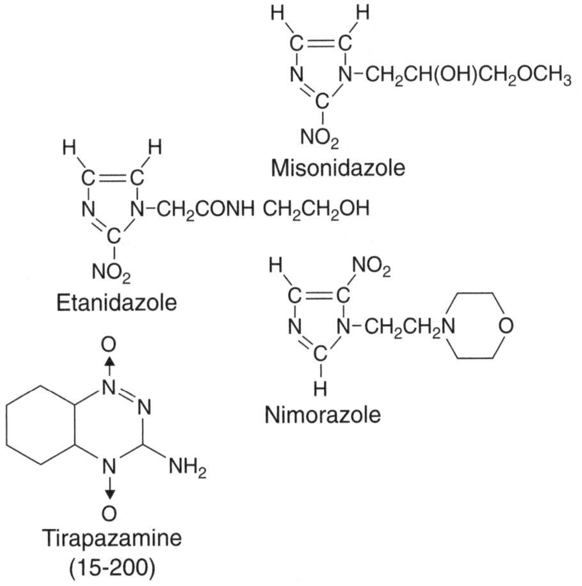

**Figure 15.14.** Structures of some hypoxic cell radiosensitizers that have been studied in clinical trials, and of the bioreductive agent, tirapazamine, that is of current clinical interest. The numbers in parentheses show an approximate range of the ratios of tirapazamine concentrations to produce equal cell kill for aerobic and hypoxic cells for a variety of different tumor cell lines.

sensitization can be assessed in terms of a sensitizer enhancement ratio (SER) that is analogous to the OER discussed in Section 15.4.1. Sensitizer enhancement ratios depend on the drug concentration in the tumor at the time of radiation. There is a good correspondence between the values obtained for tumors and the results from in vitro studies. If misonidazole is combined with fractionated radiation doses, the SER is reduced both because of reoxygenation occurring between the fractions (see Sec. 15.6.4) and because lower individual doses of the drug must be given as fractionated treatment.

A large number of sensitizers have been investigated, and nine have reached clinical evaluation. Overall, results from the trials using misonidazole have been disappointing (see Table 15.4), possibly because the dose of misonidazole was limited by a dose-dependent peripheral neuropathy. Studies using drugs that are less toxic, such as etanidazole and nimorazole, revealed conflicting results. Whereas nimorazole has been associated with improved tumor control in head and neck cancer in the Danish Head and Neck Cancer Study (DAHANCA) trial (Overgaard et al., 1998), a benefit was not demonstrated in two multicenter trials for head and neck cancer using etanidazole (Lee et al., 1995; Eschwege et al., 1997). Although most trials with nitroimidazoles have failed to demonstrate a significant

benefit, a recent meta-analysis of results from over 7000 patients included in fifty randomized trials (see Table 15.4) indicated a small but significant improvement in local control and survival, with most of the benefit attributed to an improved response in patients with head and neck cancer (Overgaard and Horsman, 1996). This suggest the lack of clinical benefit in most of the individual trials may be due to the small numbers of patients included, rather than lack of the biologic importance of tumor hypoxia.

Another approach to reducing the influence of hypoxia on the radiation response of tumors is to use (bioreductive) drugs that are toxic under hypoxic conditions. Complementary effects of radiation (against aerobic cells) and of drug (against hypoxic cells) might then increase the therapeutic ratio. The principal bioreductive drug of current clinical interest is tirapazamine (Brown, 1999), a benzotriazine di-N-oxide (see Fig. 15.14). Tirapazamine is cytotoxic to hypoxic cells at oxygen concentrations up to about 10 $\mu$M/L (equivalent partial pressure of $\sim$6 mmHg). Under hypoxia, it is metabolized to an oxidizing radical that produces DNA damage including double-strand breaks, probably by interacting with topoisomerases. In the presence of oxygen, the radical is converted (by oxidation) back to the parent compound. The drug also interacts with the chemotherapeutic agent cisplatin to increase its toxicity (see also Chap. 17, Sec. 17.5.4 and Chap. 18, Sec. 18.3.2). Tirapazamine is being evaluated in clinical trials and has shown efficacy in a phase III trial with cisplatin in non–small-cell carcinoma of the lung (von Pawel et al., 2000) and in early studies with advanced head and neck cancers treated with combination radiation and cisplatin therapy (Rischin et al., 2001).

## 15.5 NORMAL TISSUE RESPONSE TO RADIOTHERAPY

### 15.5.1 Cellular and Tissue Responses

Radiation treatment can cause loss of function in normal tissues. In renewal tissues, such as bone marrow or the gastrointestinal tract, loss of function may be correlated with loss of proliferative activity of stem cells. In other tissues, loss of function may occur through damage to more mature cells and/or through damage to supporting stroma and vasculature. Traditionally the effects of radiation treatment on normal tissues have been divided, based largely on functional and histopathological endpoints, into early (or acute) responses, which occur within a few weeks of radiation treatment, and late responses that may take many months or years to develop. Acute responses occur primarily in tissues with rapid cell renewal where cell division is required to maintain the function of the organ. Because many cells

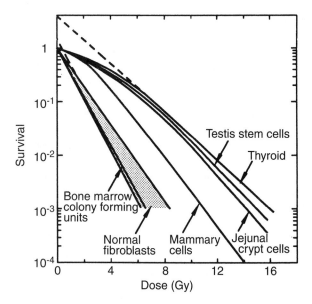

**Figure 15.15.** Survival curves for cells from some normal tissues. Most of the curves are for cells from rodent tissues and the curves were produced using in vivo or in situ clonogenic assays. The range of survival curves for normal human fibroblasts are for cultured cell strains. (Modified from Hall, 1988.)

express radiation damage during mitosis, there is early death and loss of cells killed by the radiation treatment. Late responses tend to occur in organs whose parenchymal cells divide infrequently (e.g., liver or kidney) or rarely (e.g., central nervous system or muscle) under normal conditions. Depletion of the parenchymal cell population due to entry of cells into mitosis, with the resulting expression of radiation damage and cell death, will thus be slow. Damage to the connective tissue and vasculature of the organ may lead to progressive impairment of its circulation. If the damage to the circulation is severe enough, secondary parenchymal cell death may occur due to nutrient deprivation. The loss of functional cells may induce other parenchymal cells to divide, causing further cell death as they express their radiation damage. The end result may be functional failure of the organ involved. *Consequential late effects* may also occur where severe early reactions have led to impaired tissue recovery and/or development of infection.

The radiosensitivity of the cells of a number of normal tissues can be determined directly using in situ assays. Survival curves obtained for the cells of different normal tissues in mice and rats are shown in Figure 15.15. Considerable variability in sensitivity is apparent and as with tumor cells, most of the difference appears to be in the shoulder region of the survival curve. The crudest functional assay for normal tissue damage is the determination of the dose of radiation given either to the whole body or to a specific organ that will cause

lethality in 50 percent of the treated animals within a specified time ($LD_{50}$). The relationship between lethality and single radiation dose is usually sigmoidal in shape, and some experimentally derived relationships for different normal tissues are shown in Figure 15.16.

Dose-response relationships for normal tissues are generally quite steep and well defined. For study of the response of individual organs, one widely used approach is to define a level of functional deficit and to determine the percentage of irradiated animals that express at least this level of damage following different radiation doses. An example of such dose-response curves for the rat spinal cord using forelimb paralysis as the endpoint is shown in Figure 15.17. This approach also results in sigmoidal dose-response curves similar to the percent lethality curves shown in Figure 15.16. Similar results have been reported for specific functional deficits in many other tissues (e.g. increased breathing rate in lung, reduced flexibility due to increased fibrosis in subcutaneous tissue).

Increased cytokine and chemokine expression has been observed within hours after irradiation when there are no apparent functional or histopathological changes, and may recur and/or persist in cycles over many months (Rubin et al., 1995; Chiang et al., 1997). This cyclic expression has been documented most clearly in lung (see Fig. 15.18) and brain tissue. Early increases in cytokine expression can occur after low doses of radiation (~1 Gy) but longer-term changes have been observed after larger doses (5 to 25 Gy). The cytokines involved include pro- and anti-inflammatory

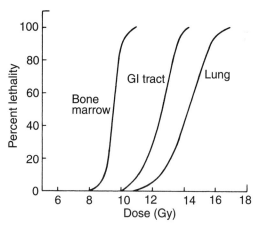

**Figure 15.16.** Three different curves indicating percentage lethality plotted as a function of radiation dose for the same strain of mouse. The "bone marrow" and "GI tract" curves were obtained using whole body irradiation and assessing lethality prior to day 30 or prior to day 7, respectively, because death due to damage to the gastrointestinal tract occurs earlier than that due to bone marrow failure. The curve labeled "lung" was obtained by assessing lethality 180 days after local irradiation to the thorax.

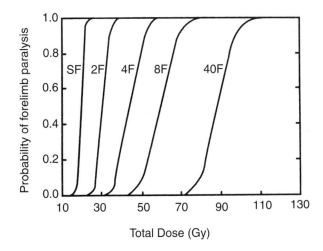

**Figure 15.17.** Dose-response curves for forelimb paralysis following fractionated radiation treatments to the rat spinal cord. The fractions (F) were given once daily to allow for complete repair of radiation damage between fractions. SF, single fraction. (Redrawn from Wong et al., 1992.)

factors such as tumor necrosis factor (TNF-$\alpha$), interleukin 1 (IL-1$\alpha$ and IL-1$\beta$), and transforming growth factor (TGF-$\beta$). In specific tissues they may include other growth factors that are associated with collagen deposition, fibrosis, inflammation, and aberrant vascular growth (Stone et al., 2003). These inflammatory factors may induce production of damaging radicals such as reactive oxygen species independently of those caused directly by the radiation treatment. The interplay among these various factors (cell killing, cytokine production, vascular damage) in producing the overall tissue damage remains poorly understood and is likely to vary from one organ to another.

### 15.5.2 Acute Tissue Responses

Acute radiation responses occur mainly in renewal tissues and have been related to death of critical cell populations such as the stem cells in the crypts of the small intestine, in the bone marrow, or in the basal layer of the skin. These responses occur within 3 months of the start of radiotherapy but are not usually limiting for fractionated radiotherapy because of the ability of the tissue to undergo rapid repopulation to regenerate the parenchymal cell population. Radiation-induced cell death in normal tissues generally occurs when the cells attempt mitosis; thus the tissue tends to respond on a time scale similar to the normal rate of loss of functional cells in that tissue and the demand for proliferation of the supporting stem cells. Radiation-induced apoptosis has also been detected in many cells and tissues, such as lymphoid, thymic, and hematopoietic cells, spermatogonia, and intestinal crypts. In lymphoid and

myeloid tissue a substantial fraction of the functional cells can die by apoptosis and, thus, this mode of death plays an important role in the temporal response of these tissues to irradiation. In the crypts of the small bowel there is a small fraction of stem cells that die by apoptosis, but the majority die a mitosis-linked death and the significance of radiation-induced apoptosis is unclear (Potten, 1998).

Endothelial cells in the vasculature supporting the crypts and villi of the small intestine of mice are also prone to radiation-induced apoptosis, and these cells can be protected by treatment of the animal with basic fibroblast growth factor (Paris et al., 2001). This treatment also protected the animals against radiation-induced gastrointestinal injury, suggesting that dysfunction of the vasculature can reduce the ability of the crypts to regenerate. Radiation-induced apoptosis in endothelial cells occurs via activation of the ceramide pathway rather than as a direct result of DNA damage (see Chap. 14, Sec. 14.3.2), thus, inhibition of this pathway might protect the gastrointestinal tract against radiation damage (Kolesnick and Fuks, 2003).

Following irradiation of skin, there is early erythema within a few days of irradiation and this is believed to be related to the release of 5-hydroxytryptamine by mast cells, increasing vascular permeability. Similar mechanisms may lead to the early nausea and vomiting observed following irradiation of the intestine. Expression of further acute skin reactions (moist desquamation and ulceration) depends on the relative rates of cell loss and cell proliferation of the basal cells, and they occur more rapidly in murine (7 to 10 d) than in human skin (2 to 3 wk). The extent of these reactions and the length of time for recovery depend on the dose received and the volume (area) of skin irradiated, because early re-

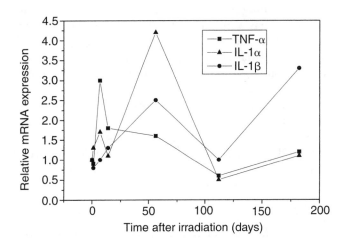

**Figure 15.18.** Relative mRNA levels for various cytokines in lung tissue at different times after irradiation (12.5 Gy) of the lung of C3H mice. (Redrawn from Johnston et al, 1995,1996.)

covery depends on the number of surviving basal cells that are needed to repopulate the tissue. Erythema in human skin occurs at single doses greater than about 7 Gy, while moist desquamation and ulceration occur after single doses of 20 to 25 Gy. Increased cytokine levels have also been observed in skin and plasma following large doses of irradiation.

### 15.5.3 Late Tissue Responses

Late tissue responses occur in organs whose parenchymal cells normally divide infrequently and hence do not express mitosis-linked death until later times when called upon to divide. They also occur in tissues that manifest early reactions, such as skin/subcutaneous tissue and intestine, but the nature of these reactions (subcutaneous fibrosis, intestinal stenosis) is quite different from the early reactions in these tissues. Late responses (usually regarded as those which occur more than 3 months after treatment) usually limit the dose of radiation that can be delivered to a patient during radiotherapy. The nature and timing of late reactions depends on the tissue involved and can be expressed as diminished organ function. For example, radiation-induced nephropathy leads to symptoms of hypertension, increased creatinine and blood urea nitrogen levels. However, one common late reaction is the slow development of tissue fibrosis that occurs in many tissues (e.g., subcutaneous tissue, muscle, lung, gastrointestinal tract), often a number of years after radiation treatment. Radiation-induced fibrosis appears to be associated with the aberrant and prolonged expression of the growth factor TGF-$\beta$ following irradiation (Hakenjos et al., 2000; Martin et al., 2000). This growth factor can stimulate proliferation of fibroblasts and their differentiation into fibrocytes that produce collagen. Transforming growth factor $\beta$ also plays a major role in wound healing and the development of late radiation reactions has similarities to the healing of chronic wounds (Denham and Hauer-Jensen, 2002).

Apoptosis has also been observed within hours after irradiation of a number of late responding normal tissues in rodents, such as the salivary glands (Stephens et al., 1991), pulmonary and brain endothelial cells (Fuks et al., 1994; Pena et al., 2000) and spinal cord (Li et al., 1996). For example, in rat spinal cord it has been reported that endothelial cell apoptosis following irradiation initiates the disruption of the blood/spinal cord barrier, which may be an early lesion leading to the development of white matter necrosis and myelitis (Li et al., 2003). Apoptotic endpoints, however, have often not correlated with clonogenic survival or functional or histopathological endpoints, and the relevance of apoptosis in radiation-induced late normal tissue damage remains to be established.

The lung is an important site of late radiation damage. There are two types of reactions: pneumonitis that occurs within 2 to 6 months after irradiation, and fibrosis which usually occurs more than 1 year after irradiation. If severe these reactions can cause increases in tissue density on lung scans and increases in breathing rate. Measuring changes in breathing rate has been used extensively to determine the dose-response relationship for radiation-induced lung damage in rats and mice, particularly the development of pneumonitis. Studies in rodents have documented that there is a rapid induction of inflammatory cytokines in lung after irradiations, but the relationship between this induction and the later development of functional symptoms is unclear (see Fig. 15.18). Studies in lung cancer patients have related prolonged increases in TGF-$\beta$ levels in plasma following radiotherapy to the likelihood of developing lung fibrosis (Anscher et al., 1998; Marks et al., 2003). In rodents, genetic factors can influence the development of pneumonitis and fibrosis following lung irradiation, although these factors do not affect the radiosensitivity of lung cells directly (Franko et al., 1996; Haston et al., 2002). Genetic variability may help to explain interpatient differences in response to lung irradiation.

The dose required to cause a functional impairment in lung depends on the volume of lung irradiated, with small volumes being able to tolerate quite large doses. This effect is due to the functional reserve of the lung because imaging with CT scans or plain x-ray films demonstrates that the irradiated region has sustained severe damage and will develop fibrosis. Studies in rodents, using the dose required to cause an increased breathing frequency in 50% of animals ($ED_{50}$) as an endpoint, have defined a relationship between $ED_{50}$ and volume irradiated which is not linear with dose and which indicates that the base of the lung is more sensitive than the apex (Travis et al., 1997). Similar findings have been reported for measurements of DNA damage in fibroblasts from irradiated lungs (Khan et al., 2003). The underlying mechanisms may relate to the functional reserve in different regions of the lung and/or to the extent of cytokine production following irradiation of different regions of the lung. There is also evidence for regional effects following irradiation of human lung (Yorke et al., 2002).

### 15.5.4 Whole Body Irradiation

The response of animals to single dose whole body irradiation can be divided into three separate syndromes (hematological, gastrointestinal, and neurovascular) that manifest following different doses and at different times after irradiation (Mettler and Voelz, 2002; Dainiak et al., 2003). The neurovascular syndrome occurs following large doses of radiation ($>20$ Gy) and usually results in rapid death (hours to days) due to cardiovascular and neurological dysfunction. The gastrointestinal syndrome occurs after doses greater than about 5 to 12 Gy, and in rodents, doses at the upper end of this range usually result in death at about 1 week after irradiation due to severe damage to the mucosal lining of the gastrointestinal tract; this causes a loss of the protective barrier with consequent infection, loss of electrolytes and fluid imbalance. Intensive nursing with antibiotics, fluid, and electrolyte replacement can prevent early death from this syndrome in human victims of radiation accidents, but these patients may die later due to damage to other organs. The hematopoietic syndrome occurs at doses in the range of 2 to 8 Gy in humans (3 to 10 Gy in rodents) and is caused by severe depletion of blood elements due to killing of precursor cells in the bone marrow (see Chap. 9, Sec. 9.4.3). This syndrome causes death in rodents (at the higher dose levels) between about 12 to 30 days after irradiation and somewhat later in larger animals, including humans. Death can sometimes be prevented by bone marrow transplantation (BMT) and cytokine therapy (e.g., GM-CSF, G-CSF, stem cell factor) provided that the radiation dose is not too high ($<10$ Gy) when damage to other organs (e.g., gastrointestinal tract) may become lethal. There are substantial differences in the doses required to induce death from the hematopoietic syndrome (i.e., $LD_{50}$ value) between different species of animals and even between different strains of the same species. The $LD_{50}$ value for humans has been estimated at 4 to 7 Gy depending on the available level of supportive care (excluding BMT). Following doses greater than about 2 Gy, humans will develop early nausea and vomiting within hours of irradiation (prodromal syndrome), which may be controlled with 5-hydroxy-tryptamine antagonists.

### 15.5.5 Retreatment Tolerance

Although tissues may repair damage and regenerate after irradiation, previously irradiated tissues may have a reduced tolerance for subsequent radiation treatments, indicating the presence of residual injury. For early-responding tissues there is almost complete recovery in a few months so that a second high dose of radiation can be tolerated. For late-responding tissues the extent of residual injury depends on the level of the initial damage and is tissue dependent. There is substantial recovery in skin, mucosa, spinal cord, and lung over a period of 3 to 6 months, but kidney, heart, and bladder show little evidence of recovery (Stewart, 1999; Nieder et al., 2000). Clinical studies have demonstrated that retreatment to high doses with curative intent is

possible depending on the tissues involved but usually entails increased risk of normal tissue damage.

### 15.5.6 Predicting Normal Tissue Response

Patients receiving identical radiation treatments may experience differing levels of normal tissue injury; thus predictive assays might be useful in identifying those patients at greater risk of experiencing the side effects of radiotherapy. The enhanced radiosensitivity of patients with ataxia telangiectasia (AT) and Nijmegen breakage syndrome (NBS; see Chap. 5, Sec. 5.2) supports a genetic contribution to individual variability in radiosensitivity. Studies of breast cancer patients have also shown individual correlation of acute and late skin reactions in one treatment field with those in a different treatment field (Bentzen et al., 1993). Several studies have quantitated the in vitro radiosensitivity of fibroblasts and peripheral lymphocytes as a potential predictive assay for normal tissue damage. These studies have shown variations in the radiosensitivity of fibroblasts from individual patients, but have been inconsistent in predicting late radiation fibrosis (Russell and Begg, 2002). While large differences in radiosensitivity, such as those observed in AT patients, are sufficient to cause discernible differences in late normal tissue effects, the differences in radiosensitivity of normal cells between most patients may not be sufficient to override the effects of the other factors, such as cytokine induction and the response of the tissue stroma and vasculature, that also influence the development of normal tissue damage.

### 15.5.7 Therapeutic Ratio

The therapeutic ratio is ill defined numerically. The concept is illustrated in Figure 15.19, which shows theoretical dose-response curves for tumor control and normal tissue complications as described in Sections 15.3.1 and 15.5.1. Tumor-control curves tend to be shallower than those for normal tissue response because of heterogeneity as discussed in Section 15.3.1. The therapeutic ratio is often defined as the percentage of tumor cures that are obtained at a given level of normal tissue complications (i.e., by taking a vertical cut through the two curves at a dose that is clinically acceptable, e.g., at 5% complications after 5 years, to give the $TD_{5/5}$ value). An approach more in keeping with the definition of other ratios, such as relative biological effectiveness (RBE) and oxygen enhancement ratio (OER), is to define the therapeutic ratio in terms of the ratio of radiation doses $D_n/D_t$ required to produce a given percentage of complications and tumor control (usually 50%). It is then a measure of the horizontal displacement between the two curves. It remains imprecise, however, because it depends on the shape of the dose-response curves for tumor control and normal tissue complications.

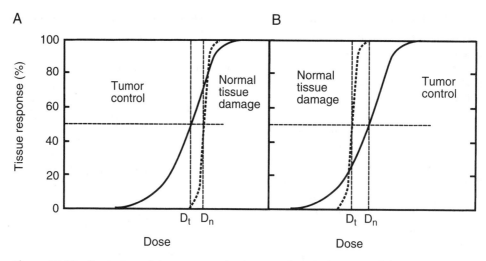

**Figure 15.19.** Illustration of the concept of a therapeutic ratio in terms of dose-response relationships for tumor control and normal tissue damage. See the text for discussion of the two parts of the figure.

The curves shown in Figure 15.19*A* depict a situation in which the therapeutic ratio is favorable because the tumor-control curve is displaced to the left of that for normal tissue damage. The greater this displacement, the more radiocurable the tumor. Because the tumor-control curve is shallower than that for normal tissue damage, the therapeutic ratio tends to be favorable only for low and intermediate tumor-control levels. If the two curves are close together (see Fig. 15.19*B*) or the curve for tumor control is displaced to the right of that for complications, the therapeutic ratio is unfavorable because a high level of complications must be accepted to achieve even a minimal level of tumor control.

### 15.5.8 Radioprotection

One potential mechanism to improve the therapeutic ratio is to protect normal tissue selectively from radiation damage. Many agents can protect against radiation damage to cells in culture. These include agents that can scavenge radiation-produced radicals, such as dimethyl sulfoxide (DMSO) or the superoxide dismutase enzymes (SODs), and those that can donate a hydrogen atom back to a radical site created on a macromolecule such as DNA, including the nonprotein sulfhydryls, glutathione, and cysteine. Because of the short lifetimes of radiation-induced radicals, these agents have to be present in the cell at the time of the irradiation. They are equally effective for tumor and normal cells in vitro; thus, specificity in vivo depends largely on preferential uptake (or presence) of such agents into the normal tissue. One agent that appears to fulfill this criterion is amifostine (WR2721), a phosphorothioate compound that is converted into a sulfhydryl-containing compound in vivo by the action

of alkaline phosphatases. This compound was shown to protect a variety of normal tissues with variable, mostly small, protection of tumors in animal models (for review, see Lindegaard and Grau, 2000). Studies in patients (head and neck and lung cancers) have shown substantial protection of normal tissue, including salivary gland, lung, and mucosa, without detectable change in tumor response (Brizel et al., 2000; Antonadou et al., 2003). The selective uptake of this compound in normal tissue is believed to be due to poor penetration from tumor blood vessels and reduced levels of alkaline phosphatase in tumors.

Another strategy for radioprotection is the use of gene therapy with a viral vector designed to induce expression of manganese superoxide dismutase (MnSOD). This approach is being used in the esophagus and lung by administering the vector topically or as an inhalant. It has been reported to provide protection for the lung and oral mucosa in rodents with no protection for the tumor growing in the lung (Greenberger et al., 2003). Presumably the viral vector can be effectively adsorbed through the mucosa or lung surface but cannot penetrate effectively into the tumor. Clinical trials of this strategy are in progress.

A third approach to achieving protection of normal tissue is to block the development of late radiation effects with treatment given after the end of the radiation (Moulder, 2003). The use of steroids after irradiation to prevent lung injury is an example, although this treatment appears to delay the development of symptoms rather than prevent them. This approach has been investigated experimentally, particularly for the prevention of late effects in lung and kidney. Studies in rodents have demonstrated that expression of angiotension converting enzyme (ACE) is increased in lung and kidney at late times after irradiation. Agents which block ACE activity (e.g., captopril) or agents which block directly the action of angiotensin II have been found to protect lung and kidney from the development of radiation-induced fibrosis and nephropathy respectively. Only in kidney has it been demonstrated clearly that reduced functional damage can be sustained after the end of the drug treatment (Moulder et al., 2003). Initial studies have suggested that the extent of subcutaneous fibrosis in patients may be reduced by direct injections of agents, such as α-tocopherol that can block the action of reactive oxygen radicals, into the fibrotic region (Delanian et al., 2003).

## 15.6 RADIOTHERAPY FRACTIONATION

It is generally accepted that the therapeutic ratio is improved by fractionating radiation treatments. Many of the underlying biological effects occurring during fractionated radiation treatment have been identified, and the improvement of the therapeutic ratio may be explained in terms of the biological response of tissue. The most important biological factors influencing the responses of tumors and normal tissues to fractionated treatment are often called the "five Rs": radiosensitivity, repair, repopulation, redistribution, and reoxygenation. Radiosensitivity has been discussed in detail in Section 15.3.2. The other four Rs are described below.

### 15.6.1 Repair

The molecular and cellular mechanisms underlying the repair of radiation damage are discussed in Chapter 5 and 14 (Secs. 5.4 and 14.3.3 and 14.4.3). The shoulder on a survival curve after single radiation doses is indicative of the capacity of the cells to accumulate and repair radiation damage. If multiple doses are given with sufficient time between the fractions for repair to occur (4 to 24 h, depending on the cells or tissue involved) survival curves for cells treated with fractionated irradiation will be similar to those illustrated in Figure 15.20. The dashed lines in this figure represent the effective survival curves for different fractionated treatments. The effective slope depends on the size of the individual dose fractions, becoming shallower as the fraction size is reduced. This effect is also illustrated by the dose-response curves shown in Figure 15.17 for forelimb paralysis of rats following irradiation with different numbers of fractions to the spinal cord, where the curves for higher numbers of fractions are displaced to higher total doses.

The single dose survival curve for most cells has a finite initial slope apparently due to a (single-hit) nonrepairable damage component (Chap. 14, Appendix 14.1), so there is a limit below which further reduction of the fraction size will no longer reduce the effective

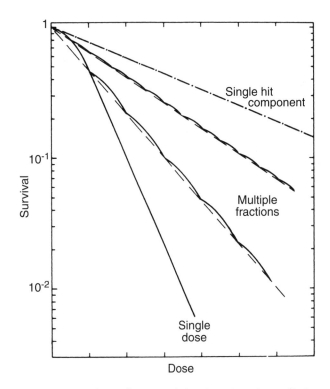

**Figure 15.20.** The influence of fractionating the radiation treatment on the shape of cell survival curves. When repair occurs between the fractions, the shoulder of the survival curve is repeated for every fraction. The curve labeled "single-hit component" is discussed in the text.

slope of the survival curve (see Fig. 15.20). At this limit, essentially all the repairable damage is being repaired between each fraction so that the cell killing is due almost entirely to nonrepairable events. The fraction size at which this limit is reached is likely to be different for different cell populations.

When the size of the individual dose fractions is such that the survival is represented by the curvilinear shoulder region of the survival curve, as for most dose fractions used clinically, then repair will be maximal when equal-sized dose fractions are given. Thus, if a certain total dose is given with unequal fraction sizes, it would be expected to produce more damage than the same total dose given in equal fraction sizes.

### 15.6.2 Repopulation

In both tumors and in normal tissues, proliferation of surviving cells may occur *during the course* of fractionated treatment. Furthermore, as cellular damage and cell death occur during the course of the treatment, the tissue may respond with an increased rate of cell proliferation. The effect of this cell proliferation during treatment, known as repopulation, will be to increase the number of cells during the course of the treatment and reduce the overall response to irradiation. This ef-

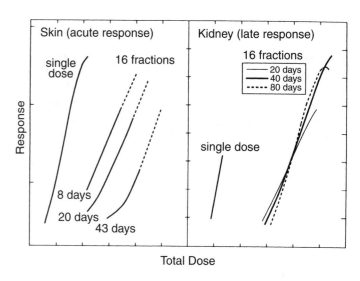

**Figure 15.21.** Illustration of the effect of repopulation during fractionated treatment of skin or kidney. Treatment was a single dose or sixteen equal fractions given in different overall times as indicated. Acute skin response was assessed using a numerical scoring technique and kidney response was determined by reduction in EDTA clearance. For acute skin reactions, extending the time over which a course of sixteen fractions is given results in an increase in the total dose required for a given level of effect. In contrast, for late response of kidney there is no change in the isoeffective dose for sixteen fractions regardless of whether the treatment is given over 20 or 80 days. (Modified from Denekamp, 1986.)

fect is most important in early-responding normal tissues (e.g., skin, gastrointestinal tract) or in tumors whose stem cells are capable of rapid proliferation; it will be of little consequence in late-responding, slowly proliferating tissues (e.g., kidney), which do not suffer much early cell death and hence do not produce an early proliferative response to the radiation treatment. This effect of repopulation is illustrated in Figure 15.21. Regenerative responses are important in reducing acute responses during prolonged treatments, such as those involving a period without irradiation (split-course treatment).

Repopulation is likely to be more important towards the end of a course of treatment, when sufficient damage has accumulated (and cell death occurred) to induce a regenerative response. This appears to be true for tumors as well as for normal tissues. Evidence that accelerated repopulation can occur in human tumors during a course of fractionated therapy is shown in Figure 15.22. Here the total dose required to give 50 percent control of head and neck cancers is plotted as a function of the overall duration of the fractionated treatment. For overall times less than about 3 to 4 weeks, there is little change in the dose required for 50 percent tumor control; at longer times, however, there is a substantial increase in the total dose required as the duration of treatment increases. This observation suggests that the initial part of the fractionated therapy has resulted in increased proliferation of the surviving tumor stem cells, which for head and neck tumors becomes apparent at 3 to 4 weeks after the start of the treatment. The data are consistent with an (accelerated) doubling time of about 4 days for the clonogenic tumor cells, compared to a median volume doubling time of about 2 to 4 months for unperturbed tumor growth (see Chap. 9, Sec. 9.4.1).

Repopulation of tumor cells during a conventional course of radiotherapy is believed to be an important

factor influencing local tumor control in patients with head and neck or cervical cancer. It has been estimated that local control is reduced by approximately 0.5% for each day that overall treatment time is prolonged. Repopulation provides the biological rationale for accelerated fractionated radiation therapy (see Sec. 15.7.4). Overall treatment time would be expected to be less important for slower-growing tumors such as prostate or breast cancer.

The potential doubling time ($T_{pot}$) is a measure of the rate at which new tumor cells are added to the tumor cell population (see Chap. 9, Sec. 9.4.2). Values of $T_{pot}$ for human tumors vary quite widely, but the me-

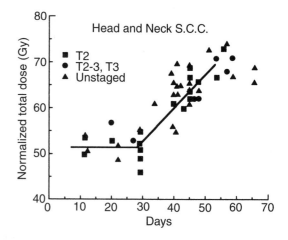

**Figure 15.22.** Estimated total doses of fractionated irradiation required to achieve 50 percent probability of tumor control for squamous cell carcinomas of the head and neck (various stages) plotted as a function of the overall treatment time. Each point is for a different group of patients and is obtained from published results. The actual doses used to treat the different groups of patients were normalized to a standard schedule of 2 Gy per fraction using the technique described in Section 15.7.3. (Modified from Withers et al., 1988.)

dian is in the range 4 to 5 days (Begg, 1995). The $T_{pot}$ value can be estimated for human tumors by taking a tumor biopsy a few hours after injection of bromo-deoxyuridine, which is taken up by S-phase cells, and detected subsequently in the cells by flow cytometry or from histological sections (Wilson et al., 1995). The pretreatment $T_{pot}$ has been suggested as a measure of the proliferative rate of the surviving tumor cells following radiotherapy and has been evaluated as a predictive assay. A trend for an adverse treatment outcome associated with short $T_{pot}$ has been reported in patients with head and neck cancer and cervical cancer (Begg, 1995) and $T_{pot}$ was initially thought to predict for the repopulation potential of tumors during therapy. However, subsequent studies have not confirmed its utility (Begg et al., 1999; Wilson, 2003) and the development of better assays of tumor cell proliferation during therapy are required.

## 15.6.3 Redistribution

Variation in the radiosensitivity of cells in different phases of the cell cycle results in the cells in the more resistant phases being more likely to survive a dose of radiation (see Chap. 14, Sec. 14.2). Two effects can make the cell population more sensitive to a subsequent dose of radiation. Some of the cells will be blocked in the G2 phase of the cycle (see Chap. 14, Sec. 14.2), which is usually a sensitive phase. Some of the surviving cells will redistribute into more sensitive parts of the cell cycle. Both effects will tend to make the whole population more sensitive to fractionated treatment as compared with a single dose. Because redistribution inevitably involves cell proliferation, the survival will also be influenced by repopulation, which reduces the effect of redistribution. Both redistribution and repopulation are important primarily in proliferating cell populations. Also, not all cell lines show large differences in radiosensitivity between cells in different cell cycle phases, and the effect of redistribution will be correspondingly less for these types of cells. In many normal tissues (and probably in some tumors), stem cells can be in a resting phase (G0) but can be recruited into the cell cycle to repopulate the tissue (see Chap. 9, Sec. 9.4). There is some evidence that cells in cycle are slightly more sensitive to radiation than G0 cells, possibly because G0 cells may repair more potentially lethal damage (Chap. 14, Sec. 14.3.3). Recruitment of resting cells into the proliferative cycle during the course of fractionated treatment, therefore, may tend to increase the sensitivity of the whole population. Neither recruitment nor redistribution would be expected to have much influence on late responses that occur predominantly as a result of injury to tissues in which the rate of proliferation is low.

## 15.6.4 Reoxygenation

The response of tumors to large single doses of radiation is dominated by the presence of hypoxic cells within them, even if only a very small fraction of the tumor stem cells are hypoxic (see Sec. 15.4.2). Immediately after a dose of radiation, the proportion of the surviving cells that is hypoxic will be elevated. However, with time, some of the surviving hypoxic cells may gain access to oxygen and hence become *reoxygenated* and more sensitive to a subsequent radiation treatment. Reoxygenation can result in a substantial increase in the sensitivity of tumors during fractionated treatment. In Figure 15.23 it is shown that the survival curve following fractionated irradiation for a tumor containing 10 percent hypoxic cells that *do not* reoxygenate would be dominated at higher doses by the radioresistant hypoxic cells. In contrast, the survival curve for a reoxygenating tumor cell population lies close to the curve for a fully oxygenated population. This example considers only two populations of cells: those that are fully oxygenated and those that are fully radiobiologically hypoxic. However, there will also be many cells at intermediate oxy-

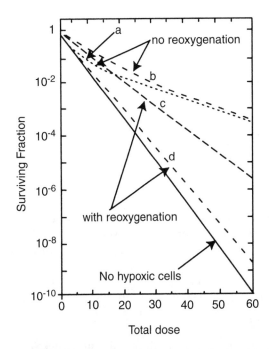

**Figure 15.23.** Theoretical survival curves calculated to illustrate the influence of reoxygenation on the level of cell killing in a tumor following treatment with 2 Gy fractions. It was assumed that the tumor initially had 10 percent hypoxic cells and either 90 percent well-oxygenated cells (*lines a and d*) or a proportion of well-oxygenated cells and cells at intermediate oxygen concentrations calculated using a radial diffusion model (*lines b and c*). It was assumed that reoxygenation was sufficient to maintain the same proportions of hypoxic cells among the surviving cells during the fractionated treatment. (Redrawn from Wouters and Brown, 1997.)

gen levels in tumors, and as seen in Figure 15.23, it is the cells at intermediate oxygen concentrations that may come to dominate the survival curve when reoxygenation occurs during fractionated treatment (Wouters and Brown, 1997).

Reoxygenation has been shown to occur in almost all rodent tumors that have been studied, but both the extent and timing of this reoxygenation are variable. Reoxygenation may result from increased or redistributed blood flow, reduced oxygen utilization by radiation-damaged cells, or rapid removal of radiation-damaged cells so that the hypoxic cells become closer to functional blood vessels. Measurements of the $pO_2$ in human tumors (using Eppendorf oxygen electrodes; see Sec. 15.4.3) during fractionated radiotherapy have demonstrated improved oxygen status in some tumors, suggesting reoxygenation (Dunst et al., 1999). However, these measurements do not distinguish between surviving cells and those already inactivated by the treatment. Even though there is no direct evidence for reoxygenation of surviving hypoxic cells in human tumors, it is probable that it is a major reason why fractionating treatment leads to an improvement in therapeutic ratio (as compared to single large doses) in clinical radiotherapy. Evidence that the oxygen status of tumors can predict treatment outcome following radiation therapy (see Sec. 15.4.3) suggests that reoxygenation is inadequate to eliminate the effects of hypoxia on treatment response for at least some tumors in man.

## 15.7 MODELING THE EFFECTS OF FRACTIONATION

### 15.7.1 Time and Dose Relationships

Repair and repopulation increase the total dose required to achieve a given level of biological damage (an isoeffect) in a course of fractionated radiation treatment. Redistribution and reoxygenation would be expected to reduce the total dose required for the isoeffect. Reoxygenation applies mostly to tumors (because they contain hypoxic cells), while repopulation and redistribution apply both to tumors and proliferating normal tissues. Repair is an important factor in the response of nearly all tissues.

It is often difficult to dissect the influence of the individual factors. The relative importance of repair and repopulation was addressed in studies of the response of pig skin to fractionated radiation (Fowler and Stern, 1963). Pig skin was chosen because it has a structure similar to that of human skin. The data, summarized in Table 15.5, show that the total radiation dose required to produce a given level of early skin reaction was substantially greater when the number of fractions was increased from five to twenty, but delivered over a constant time of 28 days; in contrast, an increase in the

**Table 15.5.** Single and Fractionated Doses Required for a Fixed Level of Acute Reaction in Pig Skin

| Number of Fractions | Overall Time (Days) | Total Dose (Gy) |
|---|---|---|
| 1 | <1 | 20 |
| 5 | 4 | 36 |
| 5 | 28 | 42 |
| 20 | 28 | ~60 |

*Source:* Adapted from Fowler and Stern (1963).

duration of treatment from 4 to 28 days when the fraction number (5) remained constant required a smaller increase in total dose. These results suggest that repair of sublethal damage between fractions is more important than repopulation over the course of a 4-week treatment. If the fractionated treatment had been extended to longer times, the contribution of repopulation would have been greater for the early skin reaction endpoint used in these studies.

That the biological effect of radiation depends on the fractionation schedule has important clinical implications for the planning of therapy. To obtain the maximum dose to a tumor while minimizing dose to surrounding normal tissue, the radiation oncologist will often use a number of overlapping radiation beams. The dose at any given location will be calculated by summing the doses given by the various individual beams, and the dose distribution will be represented by a series of isodose curves (like contours on a map) joining points that are expected to receive equal percentages of the dose at a particular point (usually within the tumor). These isodose lines must be viewed with caution because the same total dose may not give the same biological effect if the doses delivered by the individual beams are of unequal size and they are not given in close temporal sequence. For example, equal-sized dose fractions allow for maximum repair; thus, if different beams are delivered on different days, the surrounding normal tissues, that receive unequal contributions from different beams, would have less optimal repair capacity than the tumor where the contributions from the different beams are equal. The biological effect would then be different at different points on the same isodose line. This provides the radiobiological rationale for treating all fields daily when multiple fields are used to treat a tumor.

### 15.7.2 Isoeffect Curves

Different fractionation schedules that give the same level of biological effect can be presented in the form of an isoeffect curve. Isoeffect curves are generated by plotting the total radiation dose to give a certain bio-

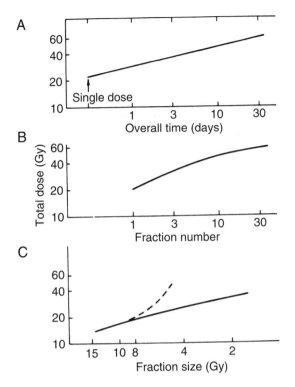

**Figure 15.24.** Isoeffect curves for fractionated treatments plotted in three different formats. (*A*) Line plotted by Strandqvist (1944) to define normal tissue tolerance and control of carcinoma of the skin and lip using the axes of total dose and overall treatment time. (*B*) Isoeffect curve for damage to pig skin plotted as total dose versus number of fractions. (Adapted from Fowler, 1971.) (*C*) Isoeffect curve for the crypt cells of the mouse intestine plotted as total dose versus fraction size using an inverted scale. The solid line is for fractions given 3 hours apart and the broken line for fractions given 24 hours apart. (Adapted from Withers and Mason, 1974.)

radiotherapy. This is discussed in more detail in Section 15.7.4.

### 15.7.3 The Linear Quadratic Equation and Models for Isoeffect

Most models of isoeffect relationships used clinically are based on the linear-quadratic (LQ) equation (Chap. 14; Appendix 14.1). In using the LQ model, it is assumed that each fraction has an equal effect, thus for a fractionated regime (*n* fractions of size *d*):

$$SF = [e^{-(\alpha d + \beta d^2)}]^n \qquad (15.3)$$

or

$$-\ln SF = n(\alpha d + \beta d^2) \qquad (15.4)$$

It is further assumed that if different fractionation regimes (e.g., $n_1$ fractions of size $d_1$ and $n_2$ fractions of size $d_2$) are isoeffective for a given tissue, they lead to the same surviving fraction (SF). Thus we have:

$$\text{Isoeffect } (E) = -\ln SF = n_1(\alpha d_1 + \beta d_1{}^2)$$
$$= n_2(\alpha d_2 + \beta d_2{}^2) \quad (15.4)$$

Eq. (15.4) can then be simplified to give:

$$n_1 d_1 / n_2 d_2 = (\alpha + \beta d_2)/(\alpha + \beta d_1) \qquad (15.5)$$

From this relationship and knowing the values of $n_1$, $d_1$, $n_2$, and $d_2$, the constant $\alpha/\beta$ can be determined for the

logical effect against the overall treatment time, fraction number, or fraction size as illustrated in Figure 15.24. Experimental studies performed mainly in rodents have established isoeffect curves for different normal tissues using endpoints of either early or late radiation damage. Some of these isoeffect curves are shown in Figure 15.25, with the broken lines representing early responses and the solid lines late responses. The isoeffect lines for late responses are steeper than those for early responses, that is, a larger increase in total dose is required to give the same level of late toxicity as the dose per fraction is reduced and the number of fractions increased. This implies a greater capacity for the repair of damage in tissues where it is expressed late than for damage in tissues where it is expressed early after radiation treatment. The reasons for this difference remain unknown. The observation that late-responding normal tissues demonstrate greater repair capacity than early-responding normal tissues is the radio-biological principle underlying altered fractionation schedules using multiple daily fractions in clinical

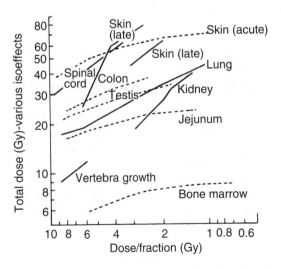

**Figure 15.25.** Isoeffect curves for a number of rodent tissues obtained using a variety of different cell survival or functional assays. The total dose required to obtain a fixed level of tissue damage is plotted as a function of the dose/fraction. The displacement of the curves on the vertical axis is a result of the fact that different isoeffective endpoints were used for the different tissues. (Modified from Thames et al., 1982.)

particular tissue and used in the equation to predict other isoeffective treatment schedules.

The parameter $\alpha/\beta$ has the units of dose (Gy) and is a measure of the shape of the survival curve (see Chap. 14, Appendix 14.1.2). The parameter $\alpha$ defines the initial slope of the survival curve; the larger the value of $\alpha$, the steeper the initial part of the curve. The parameter $\beta$ defines the curvature of the survival curve and a large value of $\beta$ implies more curvature. Thus, a large value of $\alpha/\beta$ implies a steep curve with little curvature (i.e., a small shoulder to the survival curve) and a small value of $\alpha/\beta$ implies a shallow curve with greater curvature (i.e., a large shoulder to the survival curve). Because the size of the shoulder of the survival curve is a measure of the repair capacity of the cells, this means that a small value of $\alpha/\beta$ is consistent with greater repair capacity and a steep isoeffect curve, whereas a large value of $\alpha/\beta$ is consistent with lesser repair capacity and a shallow isoeffect curve.

Data similar to those shown in Figure 15.25 have been used to derive $\alpha/\beta$ values for different normal tissues in rodents. In general, it is found that late-responding tissues have $\alpha/\beta$ values in the range 2 to 4 Gy (i.e., consistent with a steep isoeffect curve), while early-responding tissues have $\alpha/\beta$ values in the range 8 to 12 Gy (i.e., consistent with a shallow isoeffect curve). The limited data available for human tissues suggest values in the same ranges (Thames et al., 1990). Most tumors appear to have $\alpha/\beta$ values similar to or greater than those for early-responding tissues. One exception is prostate cancer, which may have an $\alpha/\beta$ value between 1 and 3 Gy (Brenner and Hall, 1999), suggesting a large repair capacity.

There is no consideration of the effect of treatment time in the LQ model. In practice, this is a limitation that applies to early normal tissue responses, which occur in proliferative tissues (and tumors), rather than to late normal tissue responses, which generally occur in tissues that have slowly proliferating parenchymal cell populations, and for which response to radiation is less influenced by the duration of fractionated treatment. An analysis of fractionation responses in human lung demonstrates an effect of treatment time for the induction of pneumonitis but not for fibrosis, suggesting that pneumonitis has some characteristics of an early response (Bentzen et al., 2000). In the LQ model, it is also assumed that there is complete repair between the fractions, and predictions from the model may lead to serious overdosing when the interfraction interval is too short or where repair of sublethal damage is slow.

### 15.7.4 Altered Fractionation Schedules

The higher capacity for repair of radiation damage in late-responding normal tissues (low $\alpha/\beta$ values) as compared with early-responding normal tissues and most tumors (high $\alpha/\beta$ values) can be exploited to obtain a therapeutic gain by reducing the fraction size below that used conventionally (from about 2 Gy to 1 to 1.5 Gy) and increasing the number of fractions. The increase in dose that can be tolerated at the isoeffective level of late normal tissue damage should be greater than that required to maintain the same level of tumor control (i.e., the tumor would receive a larger biologically effective dose and hence the control rate should be higher).

The larger number of fractions required must be given more than once per day if the treatment time is not to be prolonged. Such a treatment protocol is termed *hyperfractionation*. The intent of hyperfractionation is to reduce late effects while achieving the same or better tumor control and the same or slightly increased early effects. The time interval between the fractions must be sufficiently long to allow time for complete repair to occur. Repair kinetics have been estimated in a number of normal rodent tissues, and half-times for repair ranged from 0.5 hour in jejunum to 1 to 2 hours in skin, lung, and kidney. Thus, repair will be complete in most normal tissues after an interfraction interval of 6 to 8 hours. In the rodent spinal cord, it has been found that the effective repair half-time is greater than 2 hours, so repair is not complete even with an interfraction interval of 8 hours (Ang et al., 1992). Thus, an increase in late morbidity would be expected when multiple fractions per day are given to fields that include the spinal cord, as was observed by Dische and Saunders (1989) in patients given three fractions per day. An increase in early normal tissue reactions would be expected with hyperfractionation because the larger $\alpha/\beta$ value for early-responding tissues implies a smaller change in the amount of repair as fraction size is reduced relative to that occurring in late-responding tissues. The increase in dose that can be tolerated can be estimated as discussed in Section 15.7.3, but such calculations are limited by the low reliability of available estimates of $\alpha/\beta$ for human tissues.

The rationale for hyperfractionation does not consider reoxygenation. Because there is no change in overall treatment time, it is assumed that reoxygenation will not be much different than for a conventional fractionation scheme. Clinical trials evaluating a larger total dose delivered by hyperfractionation have reported an increase in local control with no difference in late normal tissue damage (see Horiot et al., 1992). These results support the hypothesis that an increase of total dose can be achieved by hyperfractionation without increasing the probability of late complications.

Shortening of the overall treatment time might also improve the therapeutic ratio because it will reduce the time for repopulation to occur in the tumor during treatment (Sec. 15.6.2). A similar effect might be achieved by blocking growth factors or their receptors, which are required for tumor cell proliferation (see Chap. 14, Sec. 14.4.4). The tolerance of late-responding normal tissues should be little affected because cell proliferation is slow within them. Reduced treatment time is achieved by giving more than one fraction per day with standard dose fractions of 1.8 to 2.5 Gy given 6 to 8 hours apart to allow for repair, a strategy called *accelerated fractionation*. Randomized trials of accelerated fractionation compared to conventional fractionation for treatment of head and neck cancer have provided evidence supporting the importance of repopulation as a cause of treatment failure. A combined hyperfractionated accelerated radiation therapy (CHART) study gave a reduced dose in the experimental arm of the study but maintained the same tumor control level, with a slight reduction in late morbidity (Dische et al., 1997). A second study, which gave a similar total dose in both arms, reported increased tumor control in the accelerated fractionation arm, but there was also increased late toxicity (Horiot et al., 1997). This increased toxicity was likely due to the short (4 h) interfraction interval, which was probably not sufficient to allow for complete repair between the fractions so that severe early reactions may have led to consequential late effects. The ARCON radiotherapy protocols mentioned in Section 15.4.4 involve accelerated radiotherapy combined with carbogen (95% oxygen plus 5% carbon dioxide) breathing and nicotinamide and are designed to limit repopulation and decrease the influence of hypoxia, since reoxygenation may be reduced during short treatment schedules. Phase I and II clinical trials have shown the feasibility and tolerability of ARCON, and have produced promising results in terms of tumor control in cancers of the head and neck and bladder (Kaanders, Bussink, et al., 2002). Factors relating to altered fractionation schedules are outlined in Table 15.6.

## 15.8 SUMMARY

Radiotherapy for cancer usually involves giving 25–40 individual dose fractions of about 2 Gy once daily, over a period of 5 to 8 weeks. These treatment schedules have been developed empirically and show a better therapeutic ratio than single doses because they give greater tumor control at tolerable levels of normal tissue damage. Improvements in therapeutic ratio have also been associated with the introduction of conformal and intensity modulated radiotherapy because these have allowed decreased normal tissue dose (and, hence, side effects) with dose escalation to tumor tissues. Other radiotherapy technologies that have improved the therapeutic ratio for some types of tumors through physical means include high-LET irradiation, brachytherapy, and stereotactic radiotherapy.

Studies with cells in culture and with animal models have identified biological factors (the "five Rs") that can influence response to fractionated treatment and hence, may affect therapeutic ratio. These are radiosensitivity, repair of radiation damage, repopulation of damaged tissues by proliferation of surviving cells, redistribution of proliferating cells through the cell cycle, and reoxygenation of hypoxic cells. Repair and repopulation are the reasons why cells and tissues can tolerate a larger total dose when it is fractionated. They occur both in tumors and normal tissues, although repopulation has a minor effect on the late radiation damage that occurs in slowly proliferating normal tissues. Repopulation by tumor cells during the latter part of conventional (5 to 7 week) fractionated treatments may play an important role in increasing the dose required for tumor control. Reoxygenation in tumors contributes to the improved therapeutic ratio obtained with fractionated treatment.

Both tumor and normal tissue responses to irradiation are complex. Radiation can kill individual tumor and normal cells directly and this can be expressed as mitosis-linked cell death or, in a few tissues, as early apoptosis. Particularly in normal tissues, there are also indirect effects, such as the induction of cytokines, that can influence early and late tissue effects. An example is the role of TGF-$\beta$ in radiation-induced fibrosis. Tumor control requires the killing of all the tumor stem cells but there is heterogeneity in cellular radiosensitivity in tumors due to microenvironmental factors such

**Table 15.6.** Summary of Normal Tissues Responses to Altered Schedules of Fractionated Radiation

| Normal Tissue Reaction | Acute | Late | Consequential |
|---|---|---|---|
| Tissues | Skin, oral mucosa, G.I. mucosa | Liver, kidney, spinal cord, lung or skin fibrosis, muscle | Skin, mucosa. |
| Time of onset | < 3 months | > 6 months | > 6 months |
| $\alpha/\beta$ values | ~ 8–12 Gy | ~ 2–4 Gy | ?? |
| Fractionation response | Hyperfractionated ⇔ Accelerated ⇑ | Hyperfractionated ⇓ Accelerated ⇔ | Hyperfractionated ⇓ Accelerated ⇑ |

⇔ no change, ⇑ increased effect, ⇓ decreased effect

as hypoxia and possibly also due to the development of resistant subpopulations as a result of genetic instability.

In clinical radiotherapy, different fractionated schedules that give an equal level of normal tissue response or tumor control can be expressed in the form of iso-effect relationships described by the parameters $\alpha$ and $\beta$ of the linear-quadratic model. Late-responding tissues tend to have smaller $\alpha/\beta$ values than early-responding tissues, implying greater capacity for repair of damage that leads to late effects. The difference in the isoeffect relationships for early and late damage implies that reducing fraction size will reduce damage to late-responding tissues to a greater extent than to early-responding tissues or tumors. A therapeutic gain might therefore be achieved by using hyperfractionation, where treatment with smaller dose fractions is given 2 or 3 times per day. Giving treatments more than once per day with the aim of reducing overall treatment time might also lead to a therapeutic gain if repopulation occurs more rapidly in the tumors than in the dose-limiting normal tissues.

The knowledge of biological factors that influence the response of tissues and tumors to fractionated irradiation has led to interest in prediction of treatment outcome for individual patients based on assays that assess intrinsic radiation sensitivity of tumor and normal cells, the proliferative capacity of the tumor cells and the extent of tumor hypoxia. Only measurements of tumor hypoxia have sufficient predictive power at present to be useful in planning cancer treatments. It is possible that evaluation of the expression of multiple genes in tumors using DNA microarrays or other techniques might lead to better predictive assays.

## REFERENCES

Ang KK, Jiang GL, Guttenberger HD, et al: Impact of spinal cord repair kinetics on the practice of altered fractionation schedules. *Radiother Oncol* 1992; 25:287–294.

Anscher MS, Kong FM, Andrews K, et al: Plasma transforming growth factor beta1 as a predictor of radiation pneumonitis. *Int J Radiat Oncol Biol Phys* 1998; 41:1029–1035.

Antonadou D, Throuvalas N, Petridis A, et al: Effect of amifostine on toxicities associated with radiochemotherapy in patients with locally advanced non-small-cell lung cancer. *Int J Radiat Oncol Biol Phys* 2003; 57:402–408.

Armstrong J: Three-dimensional conformal radiation therapy: evidence-based treatment of prostate cancer. *Radiother Oncol* 2002 ; 64:235–237.

Barth RF: A critical assessment of boron neutron capture therapy: an overview. *J Neurooncol* 2003; 62:1–5.

Barth RF, Yang W, Coderre JA: Rat brain tumor models to assess the efficacy of boron neutron capture therapy: a critical evaluation. *J Neurooncol* 2003; 62:61–74.

Begg AC: The clinical status of Tpot as a predictor? Or, why no tempest in the Tpot! *Int J Radiat Oncol Biol Phys* 1995; 32:1539–1541.

Begg AC, Haustermans K, Hart AA, et al: The value of pretreatment cell kinetic parameters as predictors for radiotherapy outcome in head and neck cancer: a multicentre analysis. *Radiother Oncol* 1999; 50:13–23.

Bentzen SM, Overgaard M, Overgaard J: Clinical correlations between late normal-tissue endpoints after radiotherapy: implications for predictive assays of radiosensitivity. *Eur J Cancer* 1993; 29A:1373–1137.

Bentzen SM, Skoczylas JZ, Bernier J: Quantitative clinical radiobiology of early and late lung reactions. *Int J Radiat Biol* 2000; 76:453–462.

Bjork-Eriksson T, West C, Karlsson E, Mercke C. Tumor radiosensitivity (SF2) is a prognostic factor for local control in head and neck cancers. *Int J Radiat Oncol Biol Phys* 2000; 46:13–19.

Brenner DJ, Hall EJ: Conditions for the equivalence of continuous to pulsed low dose rate brachytherapy. *Int J Radiat Oncol Biol Phys* 1991; 20:181–190.

Brenner DJ, Hall EJ: Fractionation and protraction for radiotherapy of prostate cancer. *Int J Radiat Oncol Biol Phys* 1999; 43;1095–1101.

Brizel DM, Wasserman TH, Henke M, et al: Phase III randomized trial of amifostine as a radioprotector in head and neck cancer. *J Clin Oncol* 2000; 18:3339–3345.

Browman GP, Wong G, Hodson I: Influence of cigarette smoking on the efficacy of radiation therapy in head and neck cancer. *N Engl J Med* 1993; 328:159–163.

Brown JM: The hypoxic cell: a target for selective cancer therapy—eighteenth Bruce F. Cain Memorial Award lecture. *Cancer Res* 1999; 59:5863–5870.

Bush RS: The significance of anemia in clinical radiation therapy. *Int J Radiat Oncol Biol Phys* 1986; 12:2047–2050.

Bussink J, Kaanders JH, van der Kogel AJ: Tumor hypoxia at the micro-regional level: clinical relevance and predictive value of exogenous and endogenous hypoxic cell markers. *Radiother Oncol* 2003; 67:3–15.

Carlsson J, Forssell Aronsson E, Hietala SO, et al: Tumour therapy with radionuclides: assessment of progress and problems. *Radiother Oncol* 2003; 66:107–117.

Chapman JD, Dugle DL, Reuvers AP, et al: Studies on the radiosensitizing effect of oxygen in Chinese hamster cells. *Int J Radiat Biol* 1974; 26:383–389.

Chiang CS, Hong JH, Stalder A: Delayed molecular responses to brain irradiation *Int J Radiat Biol* 1997; 72:45–53.

Dainiak N, Waselenko JK, Armitage J, et al: The hematologist and radiation casualties. *Hematology (Am Soc Hematol Educ Program)* 2003; 473–496.

Deacon J, Peckham MJ, Steel GG: The radioresponsiveness of human tumors and the initial slope of the cell survival curve. *Radiother Oncol* 1984; 2:317–323.

Delanian S, Porcher R, Balla-Mekias S, Lafaix JL: Randomized, placebo-controlled trial of combined pentoxifylline and tocopherol for regression of superficial radiation-induced fibrosis. *J Clin Oncol* 2003; 21:2545–2550.

Denekamp J: Cell kinetics and radiation biology. *Int J Radiat Biol* 1986; 49:357–380.

Denham JW, Hauer-Jensen M: The radiotherapeutic injury—a complex 'wound'. *Radiother Oncol* 2002; 63:129–145.

Dewhirst MW: Concepts of oxygen transport at the microcirculatory level. *Semin Radiat Oncol* 1998; 8:143–150.

Dische S: Hypoxic cell sensitizers: clinical developments. *Int J Radiat Oncol Biol Phys* 1989; 16:1057–1060.

Dische S, Saunders MI: Continuous, hyperfractionated, accelerated radiotherapy (CHART): an interim report upon late morbidity. *Radiother Oncol* 1989; 16:67–74.

Dische S, Saunders MI, Barrett A, et al: A randomised multi-centre trial of CHART versus conventional radiotherapy in head and neck cancer. *Radiother Oncol* 1997; 44:123–136.

Dunst J, Hansgen G, Lautenschlager C, et al: Oxygenation of cervical cancers during radiotherapy and radiotherapy + cis-retinoic acid/interferon. *Int J Radiat Oncol Biol Phys* 1999; 43:367–373.

Eschwege F, Sancho-Garnier H, Chassagne D, et al: Results of a European randomized trial of Etanidazole combined with radiotherapy in head and neck carcinomas. *Int J Radiat Oncol Biol Phys* 1997; 39:275–281.

Ewan KB, Henshall-Powell RL, Ravani SA, et al: Transforming growth factor-beta1 mediates cellular response to DNA damage in situ. *Cancer Res* 2002; 62:5627–5631.

Fertil B, Malaise EP: Inherent cellular radiosensitivity as a basic concept for human tumor radiotherapy. *Int J Radiat Oncol Biol Phys* 1981; 7:621–629.

Fowler JF: Experimental animal results relating to time-dose relationships in radiotherapy and the "ret" concept. *Br J Radiol* 1971; 44:81–90.

Fowler JF: What to do with neutrons in radiotherapy. *Radiother Oncol* 1988; 13:233–235.

Fowler JF, Stern BE: Dose-time relationships in radiotherapy and the validity of cell survival curve models. *Br J Radiol* 1963; 36:163–173.

Franko AJ, Sharplin J, Ward WF, Taylor JM: Evidence for two patterns of inheritance of sensitivity to induction of lung fibrosis in mice by radiation, one of which involves two genes. *Radiat Res* 1996; 146:68–74.

Fuks Z, Persaud RS, Alfieri A, et al: Basic fibroblast growth factor protects endothelial cells against radiation-induced programmed cell death in vitro and in vivo. *Cancer Res* 1994; 54:2582–2259.

Fyles AW, Milosevic M, Pintilie M, et al: Anemia, hypoxia and transfusion in patients with cervix cancer: a review. *Radiother Oncol* 2000; 57:13–19.

Fyles A, Voduc D, Syed A, et al: The effect of smoking on tumour oxygenation and treatment outcome in cervical cancer. *Clin Oncol (R Coll Radiol)* 2002; 14:442–446.

Fyles A, Milosevic M, Hedley D, et al: Tumor hypoxia has independent predictor impact only in patients with node-negative cervix cancer. *J Clin Oncol* 2002; 20:680–687.

Garcia-Barros M, Paris F, Cordon-Cardo C, et al: Tumor response to radiotherapy regulated by endothelial cell apoptosis. *Science* 2003; 300:1155–1159.

Graeber T, Osmanian C, Jacks T, et al: Hypoxia-mediated selection of cells with diminished apoptotic potential in solid tumours. *Nature* 1996; 379:88–91.

Greenberger JS, Epperly MW, Gretton J, et al: Radioprotective gene therapy. *Curr Gene Ther* 2003; 3:183–195.

Girinsky T, Bernheim A, Lubin R, et al: In vitro parameters and treatment outcome in head and neck cancers treated with surgery and/or radiation: cell characterization and correlations with local control and overall survival. *Int J Radiat Oncol Biol Phys.* 1994; 30:789–794.

Hakenjos L, Bamberg M, Rodemann HP. TGF-beta1-mediated alterations of rat lung fibroblast differentiation resulting in the radiation-induced fibrotic phenotype. *Int J Radiat Biol* 2000; 76:503–509.

Hall EJ: *Radiobiology for the Radiologist.* 3rd ed. Philadelphia: Lippincott; 1998.

Haston CK, Zhou X, Gumbiner-Russo L, et al: Universal and radiation-specific loci influence murine susceptibility to radiation-induced pulmonary fibrosis. *Cancer Res* 2002; 62:3782–3788.

Henke M, Laszig R, Rube C, et al: Erythropoietin to treat head and neck cancer patients with anemia undergoing radiotherapy: randomized, double-blind, placebo-controlled trial. *Lancet* 2003; 362:1255–1260.

Hill RP, Bush RS, Yeung P: The effect of anaemia on the fraction of hypoxic cells in an experimental tumour. *Br J Radiol* 1971; 44:299–304.

Horiot JC, Bontemps P, van den Bogeart W, et al: Accelerated fractionation (AF) compared to conventional fractionation (CF) improves locoregional control in the radiotherapy of advanced head and neck cancers: results of the EORTC 22851 randomized trial. *Radiother Oncol* 1997; 44:111–122.

Horiot JC, LeFur R, N'Guyen T, et al: Hyperfractionation versus conventional fractionation in oropharyngeal carcinoma: final analysis of a randomized trial of the EORTC cooperative group of radiotherapy. *Radiother Oncol* 1992; 25:231–241.

Jain RK, Munn LL, Fukumura D: Dissecting tumour pathophysiology using intravital microscopy. *Nat Rev Cancer* 2002; 2:266–276.

Johnston CJ, Piedboeuf B, Baggs R, et al: Differences in correlation of mRNA gene expression in mice sensitive and resistant to radiation-induced pulmonary fibrosis. *Radiat Res* 1995; 142:197–203.

Johnston CJ, Piedboeuf B, Rubi P, et al: Early and persistent alterations in the expression of interleukin-1 alpha, interleukin-1 beta and tumor necrosis factor alpha mRNA levels in fibrosis-resistant and sensitive mice after thoracic irradiation. *Radiat Res* 1996; 145:762–767.

Kaanders JH, Bussink J, van der Kogel AJ: ARCON: a novel biology-based approach in radiotherapy. *Lancet Oncol* 2002; 3:728–737.

Kaanders JH, Wijffels KI, Marres HA, et al: Pimonidazole binding and tumor vascularity predict for treatment outcome in head and neck cancer. *Cancer Res* 2002; 62:7066–7074.

Khan MA, Van Dyk J, Yeung IW, Hill RP: Partial volume rat lung irradiation; assessment of early DNA damage in different lung regions and effect of radical scavengers. *Radiother Oncol* 2003; 66:95–102.

Kolesnick R, Fuks Z: Radiation and ceramide-induced apoptosis. *Oncogene* 2003; 22:5897–5906.

Kozin SV, Boucher Y, Hicklin DJ, et al: Vascular endothelial growth factor receptor-2-blocking antibody potentiates radiation-induced long-term control of human tumor xenografts. *Cancer Res* 2001; 61:39–44.

Lee D-J, Cosmatos D, Marcial VA, et al: Results of an RTOG phase III trial (RTOG 85-27) comparing radiotherapy plus etanidazole (SR-2508) with radiotherapy alone for locally advanced head and neck carcinomas. *Int J Radiat Oncol Biol Phys* 1995; 32:567–576.

Lee CG, Heijn M, di Tomaso E, et al: Anti-vascular endothelial growth factor treatment augments tumor radiation response under normoxic or hypoxic conditions. *Cancer Res* 2000; 60:5565–5570.

Li YQ, Chen P, Haimovitz-Friedman A, et al: Endothelial apoptosis initiates acute blood-brain barrier disruption after ionizing radiation. *Cancer Res* 2003; 63:5950–5956.

Li YQ, Jay V, Wong CS: Oligodendrocytes in rat spinal cord undergo radiation-induced apoptosis. *Cancer Res* 1996; 56:5417–5422.

Lindegaard JC, Grau C: Has the outlook improved for amifostine as a clinical radioprotector? *Radiother Oncol* 2000; 57:113–118.

Marks LB, Yu X, Vujaskovic Z, et al: Radiation-induced lung injury. *Semin Radiat Oncol* 2003; 13:333–345.

Martin M, Lefaix J, Delanian S: TGF-beta1 and radiation fibrosis: a master switch and a specific therapeutic target? *Int J Radiat Oncol Biol Phys* 2000; 47:277–290.

Mettler FA Jr, Voelz GL: Major radiation exposure—what to expect and how to respond. *N Engl J Med* 2002; 346:1554–1561.

Meyn RE, Stephens LC, Ang KK, et al: Heterogeneity in apoptosis development among irradiated murine tumors of different histologies. *Int J Radiat Oncol Biol* 1993; 64:583–591.

Milosevic M, Fyles A, Hedley D, Hill R: The human tumor microenvironment: invasive (needle) measurement of oxygen and interstitial fluid pressure. *Semin Radiat Oncol* 2004; 14:249–258.

Moulder JE: Pharmacological intervention to prevent or ameliorate chronic radiation injuries. *Semin Radiat Oncol* 2003; 13:73–84.

Moulder JE, Fish BL, Cohen EP: ACE inhibitors and AT II receptor antagonists in the treatment and prevention of bone marrow transplant nephropathy. *Curr Pharm Des* 2003; 9:737–749.

Nakagawa Y, Pooh K, Kobayashi T, et al: Clinical review of the Japanese experience with boron neutron capture therapy and a proposed strategy using epithermal neutron beams. *J Neurooncol* 2003; 62:87–99.

Nieder C, Milas L, Ang KK: Tissue tolerance to reirradiation. *Semin Radiat Oncol* 2000; 10:200–209.

Overgaard J, Hansen HS, Overgaard M, et al: A randomized double-blind phase III study of nimorazole as a hypoxic radiosensitizer of primary radiotherapy in supraglottic larynx and pharynx carcinoma. Results of the Danish Head and Neck Cancer Study (DAHANCA) Protocol 5–85. *Radiother Oncol* 1998; 46:135–146.

Overgaard J, Horsman MR: Modification of hypoxia-induced radioresistance in tumors by the use of oxygen and sensitizers. *Semin Radiat Oncol* 1996; 6:10–21.

Palcic B, Skarsgard LD: Reduced oxygen enhancement ratio at low doses of ionizing radiation. *Radiat Res* 1984; 100:328–339.

Paris F, Fuks Z, Kang A, et al: Endothelial apoptosis as the primary lesion initiating intestinal radiation damage in mice. *Science* 2001; 293:293–297.

Pena LA, Fuks Z, Kolesnick RN: Radiation-induced apoptosis of endothelial cells in the murine central nervous system: protection by fibroblast growth factor and sphingomyelinase deficiency. *Cancer Res* 2000; 60:321–327.

Pickles T: Pion studies completed at TRIUMF, Vancouver Canada. *Particles News Letter* 1995; 16:11.

Potten CS, Grant HK: The relationship between ionizing radiation-induced apoptosis and stem cells in the small and large intestine. *Br J Cancer* 1998; 78:993–1003.

Raju, MR: *Heavy Particle Radiotherapy*. New York: Academic Press; 1980.

Raju, MR: Particle radiotherapy. *Radiat Res* 1996; 145:391–407.

Reynolds TY, Rockwell S, Glazer PM: Genetic instability induced by the microenvironment. *Cancer Res* 1996; 56:5754–5757.

Rischin D, Peters L, Hicks R, et al: Phase I trial of concurrent tirapazamine, cisplatin, and radiotherapy in patients with advanced head and neck cancer. *J Clin Oncol* 2001; 19:535–542.

Rofstad EK: Microenvironment-induced cancer metastasis. *Int J Radiat Biol* 2000; 76:589–605.

Rubin P, Johnston CJ, Williams JP, et al: A perpetual cascade of cytokines post-irradiation leads to pulmonary fibrosis. *Int J Radiat Oncol Biol Phys* 1995; 33:99–109.

Russell NS, Begg AC: Editorial: radiotherapy and oncology 2002: predictive assays for normal tissue damage. *Radiother Oncol* 2002; 64:125–129.

Semenza GL: Targeting HIF-1 for cancer therapy. *Nat Rev Cancer* 2003; 3:721–732.

Siedenfeld J, Piper M, Flamm C, et al: Epoietin treatment of anemia associated with cancer therapy: a systematic review and meta-analysis of controlled clinical trials. *J Natl Cancer Inst* 2001; 93:1204–1214.

Steel GG, ed: *Basic Clinical Radiobiology*: 3rd ed. London: Arnold; 2002.

Stephens LC, Schultheiss TE, Price RE, et al: Radiation apoptosis of serous acinar cells of salivary and lacrimal glands. *Cancer* 1991; 67:1539–1543.

Stewart FA: Re-treatment after full-course radiotherapy: is it a viable option? *Acta Oncol* 1999; 38;855–862.

Stone HB, Coleman CN, Anscher MS, McBride WH: Effects of radiation on normal tissue: consequences and mechanisms. *Lancet Oncol* 2003; 4:529–536.

Strandqvist M: Studien Uber die kumulative Wirkung der Rontgenstrahlen bei Fracktionierung. *Acta Radiologica* 1944; Suppl LV.

Subarsky P, Hill RP: The hypoxic tumour microenvironment and metastatic progression. *Clin Exp Metastasis* 2003; 20:237–250.

Suit H: The Gray Lecture 2001: coming technical advances in radiation oncology. *Int J Radiat Oncol Biol Phys* 2002; 53:798–809.

Thames HD, Withers HR, Peters LJ, Fletcher GH: Changes in early and late radiation responses with altered dose fractionation: Implications for dose-survival relationships. *Int J Radiat Oncol Biol Phys* 1982; 8:219–226.

Thames HD, Bentzen SM, Turesson I, et al: Time-dose factors in radiotherapy: a review of the human data. *Radiother Oncol* 1990; 19:219–235.

Travis EL, Liao ZX, Tucker SL: Spatial heterogeneity of the volume effect for radiation pneumonitis in mouse lung. *Int J Radiat Oncol Biol Phys* 1997; 38:1045–1054.

Vaupel P, Kelleher DK, Hockel M: Oxygen status of malignant tumors: pathogenesis of hypoxia and significance for tumor therapy. *Semin Oncol* 2001; 28(Suppl 8):29–35.

von Pawel J, von Roemeling R, Gatzemeier U, et al: Tirapazamine plus cisplatin versus cisplatin in advanced non-small-cell lung cancer: a report of the international CATAPULT I study group. Cisplatin and Tirapazamine in Subjects with Advanced Previously Untreated Non-Small-Cell Lung Tumors. *J Clin Oncol* 2000;18:1351–1359.

West CM, Davidson SE, Roberts SA, Hunter RD: The independence of intrinsic radiosensitivity as a prognostic factor for patient response to radiotherapy of carcinoma of the cervix. *Br J Cancer* 1997; 76:1184–1190.

Wilson GD, Dische S, Saunders MI: Studies with bromodeoxyuridine in head and neck cancer and accelerated radiotherapy. *Radiother Oncol* 1995; 36:189–197.

Wilson GD: Proliferation models in tumours. *Int J Radiat Biol* 2003; 79:525–530.

Withers HR, Mason KA: The kinetics of recovery in irradiated colonic mucosa of the mouse. *Cancer* 1974; 34:896–903.

Withers HR, Taylor JMG, Maciejewski B: The hazard of accelerated tumor clonogen repopulation during radiotherapy. *Acta Oncologica* 1988; 27:131–146.

Wong CS, Minkin S, Hill RP: Linear-quadratic model underestimates sparing effect of small doses per fraction in rat spinal cord. *Radiother Oncol* 1992; 23:176–184.

Wouters BG, Brown JM: Cells at intermediate oxygen levels can be more important than the "hypoxic fraction" in determining the response to fractionated radiotherapy. *Radiat Res* 1997; 147:541–550.

Yorke ED, Jackson A, Rosenzweig KE, et al: Dose-volume factors contributing to the incidence of radiation pneumonitis in non-small-cell lung cancer patients treated with three-dimensional conformal radiation therapy. *Int J Radiat Oncol Biol Phys* 2002; 54:329–339.

## BIBLIOGRAPHY

Hall EJ: *Radiobiology for the Radiologist*: 5th ed. Philadelphia: Lippincott; 2000.

Steel GG, ed: *Basic Clinical Radiobiology*: 3rd ed. London: Arnold; 2002.

Thames HD, Hendry JH: *Fractionation in Radiotherapy*. London: Taylor and Francis; 1987.

# 16

# Pharmacology of Anticancer Drugs

*Lillian L. Siu and Malcolm J. Moore*

## 16.1 GENERAL PRINCIPLES OF PHARMACOLOGY

In this chapter some general principles of pharmacology relevant to anticancer drug treatment are presented. The specific properties of the most important anticancer drugs in clinical use are then reviewed, with particular emphasis on their structure, mechanism of action, pharmacokinetics, and host toxicity. This chapter will emphasize cytotoxic drugs; a discussion of the properties of hormonal agents is provided in Chapter 19, while biological agents such as monoclonal antibodies are discussed in Chapter 21. However, this distinction is becoming blurred as many prototype anticancer drugs are now being synthesized to target specific molecules in cancer cells, and some of the promising new agents will be discussed briefly.

## 16.1.1 Pharmacokinetics

*Pharmacokinetics* is the study of the time course of drug and metabolite levels in different body fluids and tissues; it includes drug absorption, distribution, metabolism, and elimination. It can be considered as what the body does to the drug. The study of drug effect or response at the cellular level (what the drug does to the body) is known as *pharmacodynamics*. Alterations in drug pharmacokinetics may account for subsequent differences in drug effect or response.

At present most anti-cancer agents are given intravenously and thus drug absorption is not a therapeutic concern. Some drugs are given orally, which is convenient for patients, but introduces problems of compliance and a requirement for efficient absorption from the intestine. Only a proportion of an orally administered drug may be delivered into the circulation and become available for a potential therapeutic effect. The term *bioavailability* refers to the amount of drug that is available after oral administration divided by the amount available after intravenous administration. Factors influencing the bioavailability of a drug include patient compliance, dissolution of the capsule or tablet, absorption through the gastrointestinal mucosa, and first-pass metabolism in the liver. Problems seen in cancer patients, such as gastrointestinal obstruction, gastrointestinal mucosal damage from cancer therapy, and the use of other medications, can also affect bioavailability. Absorption of an oral anticancer agent (e.g., melphalan, capecitabine) may vary among patients receiving similar treatments, or within one patient from one course of treatment to another. This can account for some differences in toxicity, and possibly in tumor response.

The distribution of a drug within the body is governed by factors such as blood flow to different organs, diffusion, protein and tissue binding, and lipid solubility. In general, drugs with extensive binding to tissues (e.g., doxorubicin) or with high lipid solubility will tend to exhibit prolonged elimination phases because there is slow release of drug from tissues.

Metabolism takes place primarily in the liver and consists of oxidative and reductive reactions via the cytochrome P-450 system (phase I) and then conjugation (phase II; Chap. 3, Sec. 3.2.2). The phase II reactions lead to inactive metabolites that can be eliminated from the body by biliary or renal excretion. Phase I reactions can produce metabolites (e.g., doxorubicin) that retain therapeutic activity; for others (e.g., cyclophosphamide), metabolism is required for activation. Many anticancer drugs have active metabolites, and this introduces additional complexity into understanding the relationship between drug pharmacokinetics and effect. The activity of drug-metabolizing systems will influence drug effect. There are genetic polymorphisms of many of these enzymes (see Sec. 16.1.7 and Chap. 3, Sec. 3.2.3) as well as acquired changes due to hepatic impairment or the use of other medications. Simple tests of liver function, such as serum levels of bilirubin or transaminases, have not proved useful in predicting hepatic metabolic activity because the decline in activity of metabolizing enzymes varies in the setting of hepatic dysfunction.

Most drugs are eventually eliminated from the body by the kidney or through the biliary tract. Renal excretion can either be of the active drug (e.g., carboplatin) or of metabolites that have undergone phase II metabolism (e.g., doxorubicin). Impairment of renal function will influence drug clearance and may cause toxicity for drugs that are eliminated unchanged in the urine, such as carboplatin and methotrexate; dosage re-ductions proportionate to the decline in creatinine clearance (a common measure of kidney function) are usually required (Kintzel and Dorr, 1995). Several chemotherapy drugs are also toxic to the kidney (e.g., high-dose methotrexate and cisplatin), and combinations of these drugs with others that are eliminated by the kidney require extra caution and maintenance of a high urinary output.

Cancer therapy often involves the administration of several anticancer drugs to patients during a short interval of time, in addition to medications for relief of pain, nausea, and other symptoms. Interactions between drugs may influence each of the processes of absorption, metabolism, distribution, and excretion. There are examples where administration of one drug has been found to influence the disposition of another (e.g., excretion of methotrexate is inhibited by aspirin because both compete for transporters of weak acids in kidney tubules). However, possible interactions between anticancer drugs, and between such drugs and other medications have not been investigated extensively.

### 16.1.2 Pharmacokinetic Analyses

The concentration of most anticancer drugs can be measured in plasma or in the tissues of a patient. Phase I studies usually include pharmacokinetic analysis and more limited sampling may be undertaken in phase II and phase III studies. However, with the exception of protocols involving high-dose methotrexate, monitoring of drug concentration after administration of chemotherapy remains a research tool. If a drug is measured in plasma over time then a curve relating drug concentration to time can be defined. The area under the concentration/time curve (AUC) is a commonly used measure of total drug exposure; for drugs such as alkylating agents or cisplatin, the effect of the drug to cause killing of tumor cells or toxicity to normal tissues is related directly to the AUC. For other drugs, such as antimetabolites, taxanes, or topoisomerase I inhibitors, the duration of exposure above a threshold concentration may be more important than concentration, and weaker relationships between AUC and effect are seen.

The data generated from concentration/time profiles will characterize drug pharmacokinetics. Some of the important terms that can be derived from such modeling are listed in Table 16.1; these terms can be used to understand a drug's behavior in the body. Clearance is a measure of the rate of elimination of a drug from the body and is expressed as a volume from which the drug is totally eliminated in a unit of time, usually milliliters per minute. The two independent determinants of AUC are drug dose and clearance where

$$\text{Clearance} = \text{Dose/AUC} \quad \text{or} \quad \text{AUC} = \text{Dose/Clearance}$$

**Table 16.1.** Glossary of Terms Used Commonly in Pharmacokinetics

| Pharmacokinetic Term | Definition |
|---|---|
| AUC | Area under the plasma concentration/time curve from zero to infinity (also referred to as $C \times T$); determined by integrating drug concentration in plasma over time. |
| $C(t)$ | Drug concentration in plasma at time $t$. |
| Cl | Clearance. This is an indicator of the rate of elimination of the drug from the body. |
| Css | Steady state plasma drug concentration. |
| $t_{1/2}$ | Half-life. The time required for the drug concentration in plasma to decrease by half. $t_{1/2}\alpha$ distribution half-life; $t_{1/2}\beta$ elimination half-life. |
| $V_d$ | Volume of distribution. A hypothetical volume required to dissolve the total amount of drug at the same concentration as is found in blood immediately after injection. |

Thus, if the clearance of a drug declines (i.e., in the setting of renal or hepatic dysfunction), then, without an adjustment in the dose, the AUC and drug effect will increase. Similarly, individual variability in drug clearance will manifest as differences in AUC and in effect. The equation also demonstrates that if clearance remains constant then the AUC will increase proportionately to the dose. Clearance is usually independent of dose unless there is saturation of the drug metabolizing enzymes (this may occur, for example, following treatment with 5-fluorouracil) in which case the AUC will increase at a greater rate than dose and severe toxicity can result.

The volume of distribution ($V_d$) represents a *hypothetical* volume of body fluid that would be required to dissolve the total amount of drug at the same concentration as that found in plasma immediately after injection. A large $V_d$ (a value larger than the total volume of the body is possible) represents extensive binding of drug in tissue (e.g., vinca alkaloids). The half-life of a drug represents the time required for the drug concentration in plasma to decrease by half. Half-life is dependent upon both the rate of elimination of the drug (the clearance) and the volume of distribution, as indicated in the following equation:

Elimination half-life $(t_{1/2})$ = 0.693 $V_d$/Clearance

The half-life of a drug is prolonged in the setting of a large volume of distribution as well as a low clearance. Half-life is a useful parameter for designing treatment by continuous infusion because the time to reach a steady state concentration (Css) is approximately five half-lives. A continuous infusion of 5-fluorouracil, which has a half-life of 10 to 15 minutes, will reach a steady state (the time at which the amount of drug being eliminated by the body is equal to the amount being added, and thus the plasma concentration remains constant) within 50 to 75 minutes. Steady state concentration is determined solely by the rate of drug infusion and the clearance.

In the above discussion, it is the elimination or $\beta$ half-life that is important. Most drugs undergo rapid distribution to tissues and an initial shorter half-life that reflects the rate of distribution into other tissues ($t_{1/2}\alpha$) can be determined (Fig. 16.1). For some drugs there may also be a slow phase of delayed elimination (e.g., removal of cisplatin bound to plasma proteins) that may

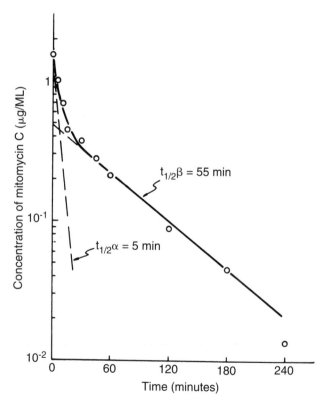

**Figure 16.1.** Plasma clearance curve for the drug mitomycin C. Initial and final plasma half-lives are referred to as $t_{1/2}\alpha$ and $t_{1/2}\beta$, respectively.

be apparent if plasma drug concentrations are measured for several days. The half-life of this third component of the plasma clearance curve is referred to as $t_{1/2}\beta$.

## 16.1.3 Pharmacodynamics

Once a drug is delivered by the bloodstream to the tissues and tumor there are several processes that will influence response. These include uptake of the drug into cells, intracellular metabolism, binding to molecular targets, and cellular mechanisms for overcoming drug-induced damage (see Chap. 18). Drug effects inside cells, and the mechanisms that the cell uses to try to circumvent or repair damage caused by them (Chap. 5, Sec. 5.3), vary widely among the different types of drugs; these factors are described for individual drugs in subsequent sections. Variability in any of these processes will influence response and will not be explicable on the basis of a pharmacokinetic analysis.

Most anticancer drugs have a low therapeutic index (i.e., a small difference between doses that cause antitumor effects and those that cause toxicity; Chap. 17, Sec. 17.3.5). Pharmacokinetic/pharmacodynamic modeling examines the relationship between a clinical endpoint, such as toxicity or response, and drug pharmacokinetics. This approach has the potential for identifying parameters that are important in clinical toxicity or response. Most of the work to date has explored relationships between toxicity and drug pharmacokinetics. The absence of a direct relationship between drug concentration in blood and tumor response or normal tissue toxicity has limited the practical utility of routine therapeutic drug monitoring (see also Sec. 16.1.4).

## 16.1.4 Dosing of Chemotherapy in the Individual

Most chemotherapeutic drugs have a narrow therapeutic index and are given at close to the maximum tolerated dose (MTD). There is a need to reduce interindividual variability in pharmacokinetics in order to have a consistent response and to minimize toxicity. This accounts for the use of intravenous rather than oral administration. Most drugs are dosed on the basis of body surface area (BSA) on the premise that the factors relevant in drug pharmacokinetics, such as cardiac output, body fat, and creatinine clearance, are all related to body size. Body surface area dosing is useful in interspecies comparisons as MTD remains relatively constant between different animals when expressed as milligrams per square meter, and it may have value in pediatric patients where there may be large ranges in body size. Many reports have questioned the convention of calculating the dose of chemotherapy in adults on the basis of BSA (Ratain, 1998). Analyses show no reduction in pharmacokinetic variability when compared to a standard dose or dose based upon body weight, and BSA dosing makes drug administration unnecessarily complex and more subject to error.

Factors within the individual that may account for variability in pharmacokinetics, toxicity, and response are still poorly understood. The usual approach is to use a standard starting dose (in mg/m$^2$) and then modify subsequent doses based upon the observed toxicity. An exception is the dosing of carboplatin, where a relationship between kidney function and clearance and toxicity of carboplatin has been demonstrated and the dose is calculated on the basis of the creatinine clearance. The approach to dose modification will also be influenced by the goals of therapy. In a setting where treatment is curative (e.g., testicular cancer), the drug doses are usually maintained despite severe toxicity, whereas in a palliative situation (e.g., 5-FU for advanced colon cancer) dose reductions are appropriate in the setting of even modest toxicity. The approach to dose reduction is usually empiric with fractional dose reductions of one or more of the drugs thought to be causing the toxicity. The efforts to better understand the variability in drug response and toxicity have been enhanced by the use of pharmacogenomics.

## 16.1.5 Regional Chemotherapy

Regional chemotherapy has been used to achieve higher tumor concentrations and to obtain a therapeutic advantage over systemic administration when treating disease localized to one region of the body. Most anticancer drugs have limited access to the central nervous system (CNS), and one form of regional chemotherapy has involved injection of drugs directly into the cerebrospinal fluid (CSF). Other uses of regional chemotherapy involve instillation of drugs into the bladder (for treatment of superficial bladder cancer), injection of drugs into the peritoneal cavity in patients with peritoneal malignant disease, or direct arterial infusion into limbs, liver, or other organs of the body. Regional administration offers a therapeutic advantage if the tumor exposure is higher than achievable with systemic administration, or if systemic exposure and toxicity can be reduced (Collins, 1984). Because the drug will eventually move into the systemic circulation, a pharmacological advantage is obtained if there is a low rate of drug exchange between the site of perfusion and the systemic circulation (e.g., intrathecal and intravesical therapy), or if the drug is rapidly metabolized and eliminated. The use of 5-fluorodeoxyuridine (5-FUdR) by intrahepatic infusion is based on the rapid removal of this drug from blood by the liver, resulting in a high exposure in the liver as compared with organs supplied by the systemic circulation. This treatment is more effective than systemic therapy in shrinking hepatic metastases, but has not been shown to increase the overall survival of patients who have liver metastases.

## 16.1.6 High-Dose Chemotherapy

An underlying principle for many of the drugs described in this chapter is that the higher the dose of drug, the greater the effect on the cancer (and the toxicity). When these agents are used in conventional chemotherapy regimens they are given at the maximally tolerated dose (MTD), the highest dose possible before serious toxicity occurs. For many of these drugs the dose limiting toxicity (DLT) is the effect on the bone marrow (i.e., myelosuppression) leading to a fall in white blood cells and platelets, with increased risk of infection and bleeding. This toxicity can be circumvented with the use of autologous (from the same individual) or allogeneic (from another individual) transplantation where either bone marrow or peripheral blood stem cells are re-infused after treatment to allow the bone marrow to reconstitute (see also Chap. 17, Sec. 17.4.1). The drugs used in these regimens are selected primarily on the basis of selective toxicity to bone marrow and tolerance by other organs; a dose escalation factor can be defined that represents the ratio of the MTD for toxicity other than myelosuppression, divided by the MTD. The drugs used most commonly in high-dose regimens are cyclophosphamide, ifosfamide, carboplatin, and etoposide. All have dose escalation factors in the range of 3 to 5. Many other drugs, such as the anthracyclines or the anti-metabolites, are not useful in this setting because of toxicity to other normal tissues such that their dose can only be escalated by a factor of 1.0 to 1.2. Clinical results with the higher dose regimens will depend upon the incremental cell kill and the sensitivity of the cancer to the two or three drugs being given. In general, these strategies have not been useful in cancers that are resistant to therapy at conventional doses, but have shown some benefit for drug-sensitive hematological cancers.

## 16.1.7 Pharmacogenomics or Pharmacogenetics

Pharmacogenomics and pharmacogenetics refer to the study of how genetic features of the patient (and their tumor) will influence response and toxicity. In the broadest sense, pharmacogenomics seeks to explain phenotypic differences in response on the basis of differences in the activity of genes that are involved in drug pharmacokinetics and are related to specific mutations or polymorphisms. In the past this was done by defin-

ing a particular phenotype following drug exposure (e.g., serious toxicity, second malignancy) and then looking for changes at the genetic level that might account for this phenotype. This could be due to determinants of drug pharmacokinetics, such as the function of drug metabolizing enzymes, to genetic factors that would influence response to therapy or even to genetic polymorphisms that might relate to the development of cancers.

The use of 5-FU in the treatment of colorectal cancer provides several examples of how pharmacogenomics can influence response. Dihydropyrimidine dehydrogenase (DPD) is the enzyme that breaks down 5-FU to an inactive metabolite, and there is now recognition of a genetic deficiency of DPD that under normal circumstances does not lead to any detectable problems. However, when patients with this deficiency are exposed to 5-FU, they experience overwhelming toxicity that relates to sustained concentrations of 5-FU (Diasio and Johnson, 2000). As well as the rare patients who are homozygous or heterozygous for loss of the active DPD allele, there is a six-fold range of expression of DPD within the normal population. The influence of this variability in DPD on alterations in 5-FU plasma concentrations, and in toxicity and response to the drug, is under investigation. One approach to overcome this variability is to use a much lower dose of 5-FU in combination with an inhibitor of DPD.

Another example of how genetic changes could influence response to 5-FU is provided by the study of genetic polymorphisms in the enzyme thymidylate synthase (TS), the target for 5-FU. There is good evidence that patients with a high expression of TS are unlikely to respond to 5-FU and that the variability in TS expression in tumors and normal tissue can be explained partially by genetic polymorphisms that alter gene expression. Most polymorphisms identified so far have differential expression in different races and sexes. The basis of the repeated observation that women have greater toxicity than men when treated with 5-FU is probably related to a sex-related difference in some aspect of 5-FU metabolism.

There are several other examples of genetic polymorphisms leading to alterations in drug toxicity that have been described—most of these relate to individual differences in drug metabolizing enzymes (Danesi et al., 2001). Thiopurine methyltransferase (TPMT) inactivates the antimetabolites 6-mercaptopurine (6-MP) and 6-thioguanine (6-TG). At least three mutant alleles of the TPMT gene lead to decreased function. Patients with mutant alleles are at increased risk of toxicity (due to decreased drug metabolism), have a greater likelihood of response, and may also be at greater risk for the development of secondary malignancies such as brain tumors (Lilleyman and Lennard, 1994).

Glutathione-S-transferase–pi (GST-Pi) is involved in the detoxification of a variety of anticancer drugs, most notably the alkylating and platinating agents (see Chap. 18, Sec. 18.2.4). Individuals with a mutation in the gene for GST-Pi that reduces its expression have increased toxicity from these agents and may also have improved survival. The main toxicity of irinotecan is diarrhea that is probably related to the concentration of the unconjugated form of the active metabolite SN-38 within the small bowel. Polymorphisms of UGT-1A1, the enzyme involved in conjugation of SN-38, have been identified and those leading to reduced rates of conjugation are associated with a higher risk of irinotecan toxicity. Polymorphisms in drug metabolizing enzymes may also have longer-term consequences. CYP17 (previously referred to as aromatase, see Chap. 19, Sec. 19.4.1) is involved in the metabolism of estrogenic compounds. Recent studies have demonstrated that the risk of developing second cancers (most notably endometrial cancer) in people using estrogen is dependent upon the particular CYP17 genotype.

The field of pharmacogenomics is expanding but has yet to affect day-to-day patient management such that individuals will have a genetic profile determined before the appropriate drugs and dosages are determined. The number of single nucleotide polymorphisms [SNPs] within the genome is enormous—already over two million have been identified and characterized. Single nucleotide polymorphisms that occur within the coding regions of drug metabolizing enzymes are being examined for their influence. Rapid advances in genetics have led to recent efforts to identify the genotypic variations and look for possible changes in phenotype. While the genetic basis of variability in metabolism of some drugs and response to them has been identified, it is probable that there are many other clinically important genetic polymorphisms that remain to be identified.

## 16.2 ALKYLATING AGENTS

Alkylating agents were the first nonhormonal agents introduced for the systemic therapy of cancer. They are chemically diverse drugs that act through the covalent bonding of alkyl groups (e.g.,—$CH_2Cl$) to intracellular macromolecules. In general they act through the generation of highly reactive, positively charged intermediates, which then combine with an electron-rich nucleophilic group such as an amino, phosphate, sulfhydryl, or hydroxyl moiety. Alkylating agents may contain either one or two reactive groups and are thus classified as monofunctional or bifunctional, respectively. Bifunctional alkylating agents have the ability to form crosslinks between biological molecules and are the most clinically useful of these agents.

Nucleophilic groups that are potential sites of alkylation occur on almost all biological molecules. Alkylation of bases in DNA appears to be the major cause of lethal toxicity. This is supported by a quantitative relationship between the concentration of drug that causes toxicity to cells and the production of lesions in DNA, such as single-strand breaks and crosslinks. Also, increased toxicity of alkylating agents has been found in mutant cells that are deficient in the enzymes required for repair of DNA (see Chap. 5, Sec. 5.2.2 and Chap. 18, Sec. 18.2.7). Interstrand crosslinking of DNA seems to be the major mechanism of cytotoxicity for bifunctional alkylating agents; these linkages prevent cell replication unless repaired. The cytotoxicity of monofunctional alkylating agents is probably related to single-strand breaks in DNA or to damaged bases. Mechanisms of resistance to alkylating agents include decreased transport across the cell membrane, increased intracellular thiol concentrations (e.g., glutathione; these compounds react with alkylating agents and thus reduce the likelihood of interaction with DNA), increased enzymatic detoxification of reactive intermediates, and alterations in DNA repair enzymes such as guanine-O$^6$-alkyltransferase (see Chap. 5, Sec. 5.3.1 and Chap. 18, Secs. 18.2.4 and 18.2.7). The nitrogen mustards are the most clinically useful alkylating agents; other alkylating compounds have been synthesized but few of them have roles in the first-line treatment of cancers.

Alkylating agents bind directly to DNA, and have limited cell cycle specificity (see Chap. 17, Sec. 17.2.4). The sensitivity to these drugs is dependent upon the area under the concentration curve and is relatively independent of the schedule of administration. Toxicities common to all agents of this class are myelosuppression, immunosuppression, hair loss, nausea and vomiting. Some alkylating agents have longer-term effects, such as infertility and carcinogenesis due to long-lasting DNA damage. Nitrogen mustard, melphalan, and the nitrosoureas have been associated with an increased incidence of acute myelogenous leukemia, and cyclophosphamide with the development of bladder tumors. The development of infertility and carcinogenesis depend both upon which alkylating agent is used, and the cumulative dose given.

### 16.2.1 Nitrogen Mustards

This family of drugs, derived from the prototype alkylating agent nitrogen mustard (or mechlorethamine), contains several drugs in common clinical use, including cyclophosphamide, ifosfamide, melphalan, and chlorambucil. The structures of these drugs are shown in Figure 16.2; each of them is bifunctional, with two chloroethyl groups that form the reactive electron-deficient groups responsible for alkylation of DNA.

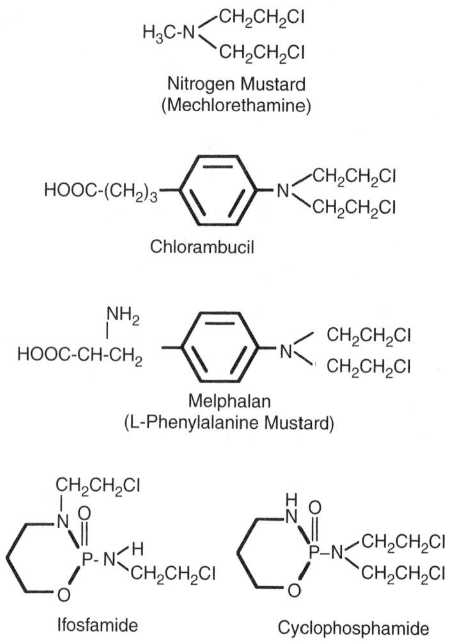

Nitrogen Mustard
(Mechlorethamine)

Chlorambucil

Melphalan
(L-Phenylalanine Mustard)

Ifosfamide                    Cyclophosphamide

**Figure 16.2.** Structure of clinically used alkylating agents of the nitrogen mustard family.

The most common site of alkylation of DNA by the nitrogen mustards is the N-7 position on the base guanine (Fig. 16.3). First, one of the chloroethyl side chains undergoes a first-order reaction, leading to release of a chloride ion and to formation of a highly reactive, positively charged intermediate. This intermediate may then bind covalently with the electronegative N-7 group on a guanine base, resulting in alkylation. Alkylation of guanine may lead to mispairing with thymine or to strand breakage. The second chloroethyl side chain of nitrogen mustard may undergo a similar reaction, leading to covalent binding with another base on the opposite strand of DNA and thus to formation of an interstrand crosslink.

In the 1940s mechlorethamine was the first anticancer agent to be used clinically. The original studies in malignant lymphoma were instituted based on observations of lymphoid aplasia in men exposed during war to the more reactive, but chemically similar, sulfur mustard gas. Following introduction of mechlorethamine, a large number of analogs were produced in an attempt to reduce the reactivity and improve the therapeutic ratio. These studies identified what are still the four most commonly used alkylating agents: cyclophosphamide, ifosfamide, melphalan, and chlorambucil (Fig. 16.2).

Although mechlorethamine is still used clinically as part of the four-drug MOPP (mechlorethamine, Oncovin [vincreatine], procarbazine, prednisone) protocol for Hodgkin's disease, the other nitrogen mustards have re-

placed it for the treatment of other tumors. The addition of ring structures to the nitrogen mustard molecule conveys increased stability, such that oral preparations of chlorambucil, melphalan, and cyclophosphamide are available.

Chlorambucil is a well-absorbed oral drug with a narrow spectrum of activity that is used mainly in slowly progressive neoplasms such as low-grade lymphomas and chronic lymphocytic leukemia. Oral melphalan is used for treatment of plasma cell myeloma and in some high-dose bone marrow transplantation protocols. Absorption of melphalan is variable and unpredictable; some patients with no effect after oral dosage have responded to the drug given intravenously. Detoxification is primarily through spontaneous hydrolysis, although increased toxicity is seen in patients with renal dysfunction, suggesting that elimination by the kidney also plays a role. Uptake of melphalan into cells is mediated by an amino acid active transport system, and resistance may occur because of changes in this transport system. Both chlorambucil and melphalan are almost equally toxic to cycling and noncycling cells and may lead to delayed and/or cumulative effects on bone marrow because of their toxicity to hematopoeitic stem cells.

Cyclophosphamide is the alkylating agent in widest clinical use and is part of treatment protocols for breast, lymphatic, gynecological, and pediatric tumors, in high-dose chemotherapy regimens, and for a number of autoim-

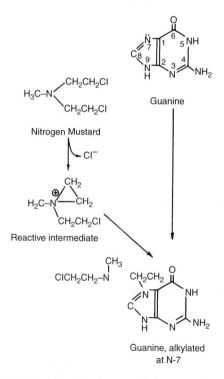

**Figure 16.3.** Reactions leading to alkylation at the N-7 position of guanine by nitrogen mustard.

mune diseases. The parent compound is inactive, requiring metabolism by hepatic mixed-function oxidases to form the alkylating intermediate phosphoramide mustard (Fig. 16.4). Hepatic microsomal enzymes metabolize cyclophosphamide to 4-hydroxycyclophosphamide, which exists in equilibrium with its acyclic isomer aldophosphamide. 4-hydroxycyclophosphamide enters cells and spontaneously decomposes to form phosphoramide mustard plus acrolein, or it is detoxified by aldehyde dehydrogenase to form inactive metabolites. Cyclophosphamide is well absorbed after oral administration. Elimination of the parent drug is initially by hepatic transformation to the active metabolites, and then most of the drug is eventually eliminated via renal excretion of inactive metabolites. The use of cyclophosphamide in patients with renal failure has not been associated with increased toxicity, as renal clearance of the parent compound and active metabolites is quite low. Cyclophosphamide induces cytochrome P-450 enzymes and will induce its own metabolism with repeated administration (Moore, 1991). This alters the rate but not the absolute amount of phosphoramide mustard formation, so no alteration in therapeutic ratio is likely to occur.

The dose of cyclophosphamide ranges from 100 to 200 milligrams per day given continuously by mouth, to 600 to 1000 milligrams per square meter given intravenously every 3 to 4 weeks. Very high doses are commonly used in preparation for bone marrow transplantation. The dose in this setting is limited by irreversible damage to the heart, which occurs with single dosages greater than 60 milligrams per kilogram (about 2500 mg/m²). The usual dose-limiting toxicity is myelosuppression, and cyclophosphamide causes a fall in granulocyte count with rapid recovery by 3 to 4

weeks after administration. There is relative sparing of stem cells and platelets, which may be due to the higher concentrations of aldehyde dehydrogenase (which inactivates the drug intracellularly) in early progenitor cells (Kastan et al., 1990). Cumulative toxicity to bone marrow is not commonly seen. Other toxicities of cyclophosphamide are common to many alkylating agents and include nausea, vomiting, hair loss, gonadal damage, and potential carcinogenicity. Acrolein appears to be the major cause of the bladder toxicity (hemorrhagic cystitis) that may occur with chronic usage or higher dosage of either cyclophosphamide or ifosfamide. The mechanism has a direct irritative effect on the bladder mucosa.

Ifosfamide is an analog of cyclophosphamide that differs in the presence of one chloroethyl group on the oxazaphosphorine ring (Fig. 16.2). It is used in the treatment of testicular cancer, sarcoma, and lung cancer. In animals, ifosfamide has a better ratio of activity to toxicity than cyclophosphamide, particularly when repeated daily doses are used. Although the metabolism of ifosfamide is similar to that of cyclophosphamide, there is less affinity for the microsomal mixed-function oxidases and more transformation by other pathways, including dechloroethylation. This alteration in metabolism is the reason why higher doses of ifosfamide are required and some differences in toxicity are seen. Hemorrhagic cystitis due to increased production of acrolein is more common with ifosfamide, such that all patients receiving the drug require coadministration of a sulfhydryl-containing compound such as 2-mercaptoethane sulfonate (Mesna), which conjugates with acrolein in the urinary tract and protects the bladder from damage. As Mesna is inactive in plasma, and is converted to its active form only in urine,

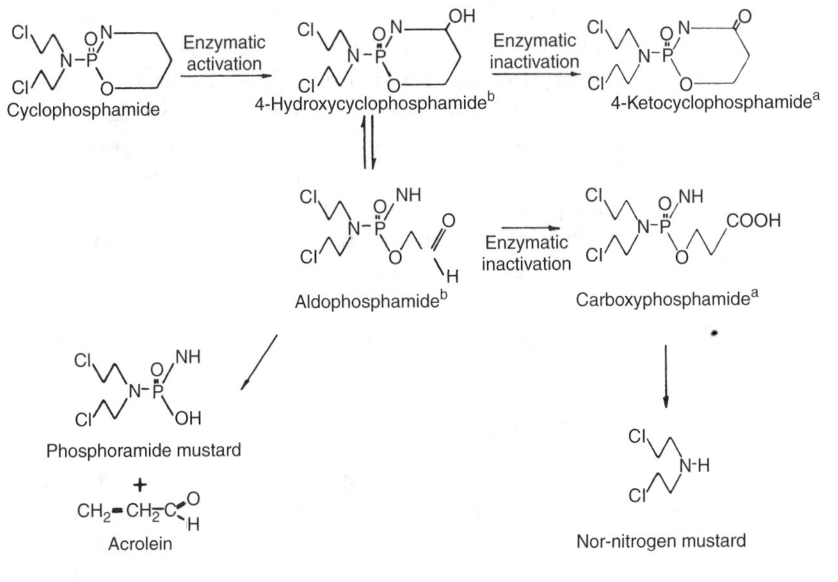

**Figure 16.4.** The metabolism of cyclophosphamide. [a]Major urinary metabolites; [b]transport forms. Phosphoramide mustard is an active alkylating agent, and acrolein is the probable cause of toxicity to the bladder.

it does not influence the cytotoxicity of cyclophosphamide or ifosfamide at other sites (Benvenuto et al., 1992). Neurotoxicity, manifesting as changes in mental status, may occur with higher doses of ifosfamide. This is not seen with cyclophosphamide and is probably related to the differences in metabolism and the formation of chlorethylacetaldehyde from ifosfamide. Other toxicities are similar to those observed with cyclophosphamide.

### 16.2.2 Nitrosoureas

The chloroethylnitrosoureas, BCNU (carmustine) and CCNU (lomustine), are lipid-soluble drugs that can penetrate into the CNS. The drugs are effective for treatment of experimental tumors but have found only limited clinical application, largely because normal tissue toxicity has limited the ability to achieve effective concentrations in vivo. They cause prolonged myelosuppression and are highly leukemogenic, probably because of direct effects on bone marrow stem cells.

BCNU resembles the nitrogen mustards in having two chloroethyl groups, whereas CCNU is a monofunctional agent with a single chloroethyl group. BCNU forms DNA interstrand crosslinks by chloroethylation of two nucleophilic sites on opposite DNA strands. CCNU is rapidly and completely absorbed after oral administration, but BCNU must be given intravenously. Both drugs undergo rapid tissue uptake and metabolism; the extent to which metabolites contribute to the toxicity of these agents is unknown.

BCNU and CCNU are used to treat some brain tumors and BCNU is also used in some high-dose programs for lymphatic cancers. Many other nitrosoureas have been synthesized, but only streptozotocin, a methylnitrosourea that has a direct toxic effect on pancreatic islet cells, has proven to be useful clinically. It is a component of first-line treatment regimens for pancreatic islet-cell tumors and other gastrointestinal endocrine tumors.

### 16.2.3 Other Alkylating Agents

Busulfan, an alkyl alkane sulfonate, has a different mechanism of alkylation to the nitrogen mustards, but also forms DNA crosslinkages and has selective effects on blood-forming cells. It is now used mainly in high-dose bone marrow transplantation regimens. Busulfan is eliminated via hepatic metabolism, and the higher doses of busulfan used in marrow transplantation may cause hepatic veno-occlusive disease in patients who metabolize the drug slowly.

Aziridines such as thio-TEPA are structurally similar to intermediate alkylating species of the nitrogen mustards but are less reactive. They have no unique advantages, but thio-TEPA has been used for intravesical treatment of superficial bladder cancer, and is occasionally used in the treatment of breast cancer and as intrathecal therapy of meningeal carcinomatosis.

Procarbazine is a synthetic derivative of hydrazine that was used in combination to treat lymphomas, including Hodgkin's disease. The drug undergoes extensive metabolism to produce alkylating species, although details of its metabolism and mechanism of action remain unclear. Due to its potential for causing leukemia, other alkylating agents have largely replaced it.

Dacarbazine (DTIC) was synthesized originally as an antimetabolite to inhibit purine biosynthesis, but is believed to function through formation of a metabolite with alkylating properties. The drug is occasionally used for treatment of sarcomas, Hodgkin's disease, and melanoma. It causes severe nausea and vomiting and the dose-limiting toxicity is myelosuppression. Temozolomide is an oral agent that contains a triazine that is thought to be the active component of dacarbazine. It has a simpler metabolism and undergoes spontaneous decomposition to an alkylating intermediate. This drug has some activity against malignant glioma and melanoma. Hexamethylmelamine is another oral triazine derivative that requires activation to an alkylating intermediate. It has demonstrated activity against ovarian cancer but has largely been replaced by cisplatin, cyclophosphamide, and paclitaxel.

## 16.3 PLATINATING AGENTS

The prototype agent is cisplatin (*cis*-diamminedichloroplatinum II; Fig. 16.5), a drug whose discovery followed an observation that an electric current delivered to bacterial culture via platinum electrodes led to inhibition of bacterial growth. The active compound was found to be cisplatin, and this compound was shown subsequently to exert broad cytotoxic activity in vitro. Cisplatin is one of the most useful anticancer agents and is part of first-line therapy for testicular, urothelial, lung, gynecological, and other cancers. It is also associated with substantial toxicity, which limits both the number of patients who are able to receive the drug, as well as the cumulative dose that can be given. There has been a major effort to identify other platinum analogs, either to reduce the toxicity while maintaining efficacy, or to expand the use of these compounds to tumors resistant to cisplatin. The two analogs in routine clinical usage are carboplatin and oxaliplatin (Table 16.2), with a number of other analogs undergoing clinical trials

### 16.3.1 Pharmacology

Platinum drugs can exist in a 2+ (II) or 4+ (IV) oxidation state, with four or six bonds respectively. All currently used platinum drugs are platinum II compounds

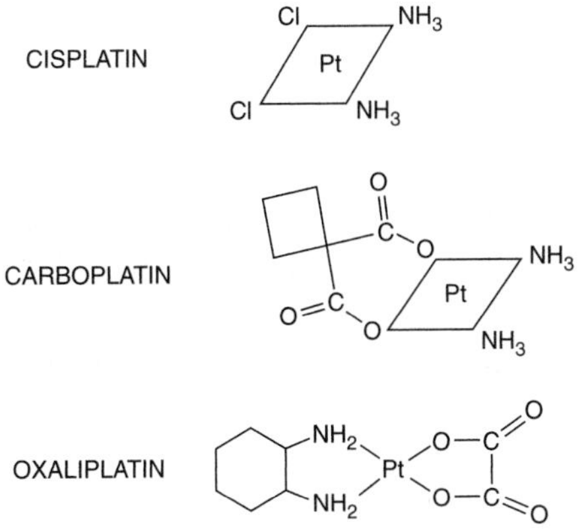

**Figure 16.5.** Structure of cisplatin, carboplatin, and oxaliplatin.

that exhibit a planar structure and have four attached chemical groups (Fig. 16.5). The nature of these groups dictates the efficacy and pharmacokinetics of the compound (Go and Adjei, 1999). Two of the groups are considered carrier groups and are chemically inert whereas the two leaving groups are available for substitution and reaction with molecules such as DNA.

Cisplatin acts by a mechanism that is similar to that of classic alkylating agents. The chlorine atoms are leaving groups that may be compared to those of nitrogen mustards (Fig. 16.2); these atoms may be displaced directly by nucleophilic groups of DNA or indirectly after chloride ions are replaced by hydroxyl groups through reaction of the drug with water. These reactions occur more readily in environments where the chloride concentration is low, such as within the cell. The preferred sites for binding of cisplatin to DNA are

the seven positions of the guanine and adenine bases (Eastman, 1987). The fact that structurally similar analogs, such as transplatin, will produce DNA binding but are devoid of cytotoxicity suggests that the stereochemistry of the compound is critical. Cisplatin binds to two sites on DNA and 95 percent of the binding produces intrastrand crosslinkages, usually between two adjacent guanine bases or adjacent guanine and adenine sites, with the remainder being interstrand guanine crosslinkages. The binding of platinum compounds to DNA is responsible for their cytotoxicity although the mechanism whereby this leads to cell death is not clear.

Carboplatin is an analog of cisplatin with substitution of a cyclobutanedicarboxylate for the chloride leaving groups (Fig. 16.5). This leads to a less reactive compound that also has less toxicity and either comparable or less efficacy to cisplatin. Oxaliplatin is one of a series of analogs with a substitution of a diaminocyclohexane (DACH) for the amine carrier groups (Fig. 16.5). The DACH analogs have a different efficacy profile to cisplatin and have shown effects in tumors resistant to cisplatin. The analogs carboplatin and oxaliplatin produce the same types of DNA adducts as cisplatin although a higher concentration of carboplatin is required to produce a comparable number of adducts to cisplatin (Blommaert et al., 1995). The adducts formed by oxaliplatin are more likely to cause cell death, probably because of the different three-dimensional structure that results from the DACH groups (Rixe et al., 1996).

The pharmacokinetic differences between cisplatin and its analogs are due to the differences in the leaving groups. Cisplatin is the most reactive and, following administration, it is rapidly and irreversibly bound

**Table 16.2.** Comparison of Platinum Agents

|  | Cisplatin | Carboplatin | Oxaliplatin |
|---|---|---|---|
| Dosage | 50 to 100 mg/m² q 3 weeks | 300 to 400 mg/m² q 3 weeks[a] | 85 to 130 mg/m² q 2 to 3 weeks |
| Toxicities |  |  |  |
| Myelosuppression | + | +++ | ++ |
| Nausea & vomiting | +++ | ++ | + |
| Nephrotoxicity | +++ | + | + |
| Neurotoxicity[b] | +++ | + | +++ |
| Ototoxicity | +++ | 0/+ | 0/+ |
| Efficacy |  |  |  |
| Bladder (urothelial cancer) | +++ | ++ | ++ |
| Colorectal cancer | 0 | 0 | ++ |
| Lung cancer | +++ | ++ | ++ |
| Ovarian cancer | +++ | +++[c] | ++[c] |
| Testicular cancer | ++++ | +++ | ? |

[a]Carboplatin is often dosed based on a desired AUC of 5 to 6 using the Calvert formula (Calvert et al., 1989).

[b]Both cisplatin and oxaliplatin will lead to a predictable cumulative peripheral sensory neuropathy although the manifestations are slightly different.

[c]Oxaliplatin has produced responses in cisplatin resistant tumors whereas carboplatin has not.

to plasma proteins, with greater than 90 percent of free cisplatin lost in the first 2 hours. Total cisplatin (free and bound drug) disappears more slowly from plasma, with a prolonged half-life of 2 to 3 days. Cisplatin is excreted mainly via the urine, and 15 to 30 percent of the administered dose is excreted during the first 24 hours. Carboplatin is more stable in plasma and is excreted primarily unchanged by the kidney. The clearance of carboplatin is predicted by creatinine clearance and the relationship between dose and renal function has been determined, leading to the definition of a model that can be used to predict the dose of carboplatin required to achieve a desired plasma AUC (Calvert et al., 1989). Similar to cisplatin, oxaliplatin also binds to plasma proteins although at a somewhat slower rate; it is also excreted primarily by the kidneys.

### 16.3.2 Resistance

Most tumors eventually become resistant to platinum. In general, resistance can be due either to reduced platinum-DNA adduct formation, or to increased repair or tolerance of the platinum-DNA adduct (Johnson et al., 1998; Boulikas and Vougiouka, 2003). In cell lines and experimental animals, resistance to cisplatin has been associated with decreased drug uptake although whether specific transporters exist is not clear. These drugs are not substrates for P-glycoprotein, MRP, or other ABC transporters (see Chap. 18, Sec. 18.2.3). Resistance has also been related to an increase in the binding of cisplatin to intracellular scavengers such as glutathione or metallothionein. In other models of drug resistance, the binding of cisplatin to DNA is not changed but there is an increase in the ability to repair the DNA adduct. Interestingly, testicular cancer, which is exquisitely sensitive to cisplatin, has a defect which prevents the repair of the cisplatin-DNA adduct. In other resistant lines the cell is seemingly more tolerant of the DNA adduct and either fails to undergo cell cycle arrest or apoptosis, or else can replicate around the adduct. Which, if any, of these mechanisms is most important in causing clinical drug resistance to cisplatin is not well understood.

### 16.3.3 Clinical Usage

Cisplatin causes little toxicity to bone marrow as a single agent, but can add to the toxic effects of other drugs, and may lead to anemia. Its major dose-limiting toxicities are nausea and vomiting, and damage to the kidney, to nerves, and to the ear, with resulting loss of hearing. Intravenous hydration and maintaining a rapid urine output during and after drug administration may minimize the effects on the kidneys; there is no known method for reducing the auditory or neurotoxicity. Cisplatin is usually given as a single dose of 50 to 100 milligrams per square meter every 3 or 4 weeks; fractionated dosage regimens such as 20 milligrams per square meter per day for 5 days are also used and may reduce the acute toxicity of the drug.

Carboplatin has comparable activity to cisplatin against ovarian and lung tumors but is less active against urothelial and testicular cancers (Table 16.2). Carboplatin has a better overall toxicity profile, which may make it preferable in palliative treatment regimens. There is minimal nephrotoxicity, and the drug causes less nausea and vomiting than cisplatin, but bone marrow suppression, and particularly thrombocytopenia, is the dose-limiting toxicity. Carboplatin is used in some high-dose regimens prior to stem cell transplantation because its toxicities other than myelosuppression are relatively mild. Oxaliplatin has shown anti-tumor activity in tumors that are resistant to cisplatin such as colorectal cancer; it has minimal renal toxicity, and causes less vomiting than cisplatin and no ototoxicity. Oxaliplatin causes a unique cumulative sensory neurotoxicity with a marked sensitivity to the cold, particularly in the oropharynx. While the platinum agents interact with DNA and cause strand crosslinkages, the propensity of these agents to cause second cancers or infertility is much less than for the alkylating agents.

## 16.4 ANTIMETABOLITES

Antimetabolites are drugs that interfere with normal cellular function, particularly the synthesis of DNA that is required for replication. Many of the clinically useful agents are purine (e.g., 6-thioguanine, 2-chlorodeoxyadenosine) or pyrimidine (e.g., 5-fluorouracil, cytosine arabinoside, gemcitabine) analogs that either inhibit the formation of the normal nucleotides or interact with DNA and prevent further extension of the new DNA strand, leading to inhibition of cell division. The antifolates (e.g., methotrexate) are not nucleoside analogs; they prevent the formation of reduced folates, which are required for the synthesis of DNA. Recently, specific inhibitors of critical enzymes required for DNA synthesis (e.g., thymidylate synthase) have been brought into clinical practice and a number of others are undergoing early clinical studies.

Most antimetabolites are cell cycle specific; their toxicity reflects effects on proliferating cells and is primarily seen in bone marrow and gastrointestinal mucosa (see Chap. 17, Secs. 17.2.4 and 17.4). As they do not interact directly with DNA, they do not cause the later problems of carcinogenesis seen with DNA-binding drugs like the alkylating agents. The effects of these drugs are dependent upon the schedule of administration. For many drugs the duration of exposure above a critical threshold required to inhibit an enzyme is more important than the peak concentration. Therefore,

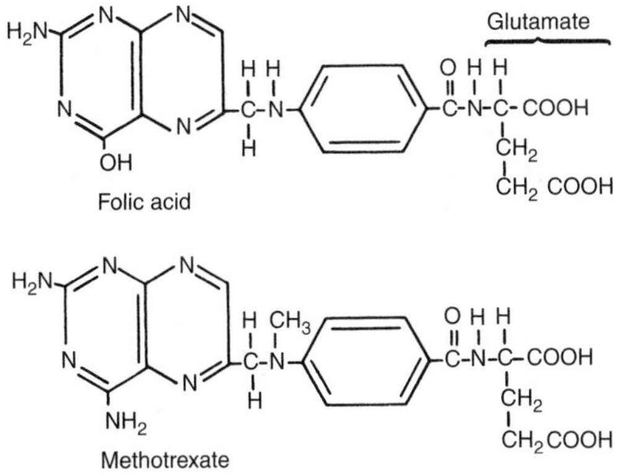

Folic acid

Methotrexate

**Figure 16.6.** Structure of folic acid and its analog methotrexate. Note that glutamate forms one end of these molecules and further glutamic acid molecules may be added to methotrexate within the cell.

while large doses may be tolerated if the drug is given as a single intravenous injection, a much lower dose is required if the drug is given repeatedly or by continuous infusion.

### 16.4.1 Methotrexate

Methotrexate is an analog of the vitamin folic acid (Fig. 16.6). Reduced folate is required for transfer of methyl groups in the biosynthesis of purines and in the conversion of deoxyuridine monophosphate (dUMP) to thymidine monophosphate (dTMP), a reaction catalyzed by thymidylate synthase. Reduced folate becomes oxidized in the latter reaction; its regeneration is dependent on the enzyme dihydrofolate reductase (DHFR) for reduction to its active form. Methotrexate is a competitive inhibitor of DHFR and thus prevents the formation of reduced folate (Fig. 16.7). The result of this inhibition may be cessation of DNA synthesis due to nonavailability of dTMP and/or purines, leading to cell death.

Methotrexate enters the cell primarily by active transport. However, drug uptake may be by passive diffusion at high drug concentration (>20 micromole per liter). Intracellular metabolism of methotrexate may lead to addition of glutamic acid residues to the initial glutamate residue of the drug (Fig. 16.6), a process known as *polyglutamation*. Methotrexate polyglutamates cannot be transported across the cell membrane, so their formation prevents efflux of the drug, and they appear to be more effective than methotrexate in inhibiting the activity of DHFR. The cytotoxic action of methotrexate depends critically on the duration of exposure of tissue to levels of drug above a certain threshold rather than on the peak levels of drug in the tissue. For many tissues, the threshold concentration for cytotoxicity appears to be in the range of $10^{-8}$ to $10^{-7}$ mole per liter. Methotrexate has selective toxicity for cells synthesizing

DNA, and prolonged treatment with the drug may expose more cells that enter this drug-sensitive phase of the cell cycle.

The toxicity of methotrexate may be reversed by administration of thymidine and exogenous purines or by a source of reduced folate ($FH_4$). These agents circumvent the effects of methotrexate by providing products of the interrupted metabolism (Fig. 16.7); they have been used clinically to reverse the activity of methotrexate following a defined period of exposure (usually 24 to 36 h) to methotrexate at high doses. Reduced folate in the form of 5-formyltetrahydrofolate (also known as leucovorin or folinic acid) has been used in many clinical protocols and has allowed the administration of doses of methotrexate that are increased by factors of 10 to 100 over conventional doses. The arguments put forward for such high-dose methotrexate treatment include (1) selective uptake by tumor cells, (2) better CNS penetration, and (3) lack of myelosuppression. This type of protocol may allow for frequent administration of methotrexate and retained therapeutic efficacy with little or no toxicity in many patients. However, responses to treatment are observed only rarely in patients who are refractory to conventional doses of methotrexate given without leucovorin rescue. Although toxicity is often lower with the use of high doses of methotrexate and leucovorin, an occasional patient may experience life-threatening toxicity, usually due to damage to the kidney or sequestration in fluid-filled spaces (e.g., ascites, pleural effusions) and consequent delayed clearance of drug.

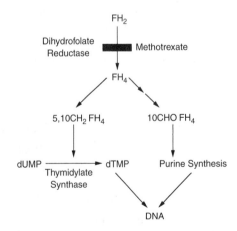

**Figure 16.7.** Influence of methotrexate on cellular metabolism. Through competitive inhibition of the enzyme dihydrofolate reductase, the drug depletes the pools of reduced folates ($FH_4$): 5,10-methylene tetrahydrofolate ($5,10CH_2FH_4$) and 10 formyltetrahydrofolate ($10CHOFH_4$). These reduced folates are required in the conversion of deoxyuridine monophosphate (dUMP) to deoxythymidine monophosphate (dTMP) and for purine synthesis, respectively. Interruption of these processes leads to inhibition of DNA synthesis.

Methotrexate can be given orally, intramuscularly, intravenously, and intrathecally (i.e., into the cerebrospinal fluid that surrounds the brain and spinal cord). It crosses the blood-brain barrier but achieves cytotoxic concentrations in the central nervous system only with intrathecal or high-dose intravenous administration. It accumulates in fluid-filled spaces such as pleural effusions, from which it is released slowly. The parent compound and hepatic metabolites such as 7-hydroxymethotrexate are excreted by the kidney. This excretion can be inhibited by the presence of weak organic acids such as aspirin or penicillin. Aspirin may also displace methotrexate from its binding site on plasma albumin, and these two effects of aspirin can increase the toxicity of methotrexate.

Most reports indicate that the pharmacokinetics of methotrexate can be described by an initial phase of drug disappearance from plasma, which has a half-life of 2 to 3 hours, and a final phase with a half-life of 8 to 10 hours. This terminal half-life may be prolonged in patients with poor kidney function. Enterohepatic circulation of methotrexate (i.e., circulation from liver to intestine to liver via the biliary tract and portal veins), which has been reported in some studies, may contribute to a slow third phase of elimination from plasma. Mechanisms which cause resistance to methotrexate include decreased uptake into cells, variant forms of DHFR, and increased production of DHFR because of gene amplification (see Chap. 18, Sec. 18.2).

Methotrexate has a wide spectrum of clinical activity and may be curative for women with choriocarcinoma, a tumor derived from fetal elements. Its major toxicities are myelosuppression and inflammation of the oral and gastrointestinal mucosa; these toxicities are usually observed within 5 to 7 days of administration, earlier than for many other drugs. Damage to kidneys may occur after high doses of methotrexate due to precipita-

tion of the drug in renal tubules; the risk of such toxicity may be minimized by maintaining a high output of alkaline urine to prevent precipitation. Rarer toxicities include damage to liver, lung, and brain, the latter occurring most frequently after intrathecal administration. In general, the drug is well tolerated compared with many other anticancer drugs.

### 16.4.2 5-Fluorouracil and Related Drugs

5-Fluorouracil (5-FU or FURa) is a drug that resembles the pyrimidine bases uracil and thymine, which are components of RNA and DNA, respectively (Fig. 16.8). The drug penetrates rapidly into cells, where it is metabolized to nucleoside forms by the addition of the sugars ribose or deoxyribose; these reactions are catalyzed by enzymes that normally act on uracil and thymine. Phosphorylation then leads to the active fluorinated nucleotides 5-FUTP and 5-FdUMP (Fig. 16.9). 5-FUTP can be incorporated into RNA in place of UTP (uridine triphosphate); this leads to inhibition of the nuclear processing of ribosomal and messenger RNA and may cause other errors of base pairing during transcription of RNA. 5-FdUMP inhibits irreversibly the enzyme thymidylate synthase, leading to depletion of dTMP (thymidine monophosphate), which is required for DNA synthesis.

The relative importance of the above mechanisms for toxicity of 5-FU are disputed. Separation of these effects may be achieved by administration of (1) 5-fluorodeoxyuridine (5-FUdR), another agent that is available for clinical use and that seems to act solely (after phosphorylation) to inhibit thymidylate synthase (Fig. 16.9), or (2) 5-FU together with thymidine, which should prevent any toxic effects from inhibition of thymidylate synthase. Both of these measures lead to toxicity for various types of cells. The relative impor-

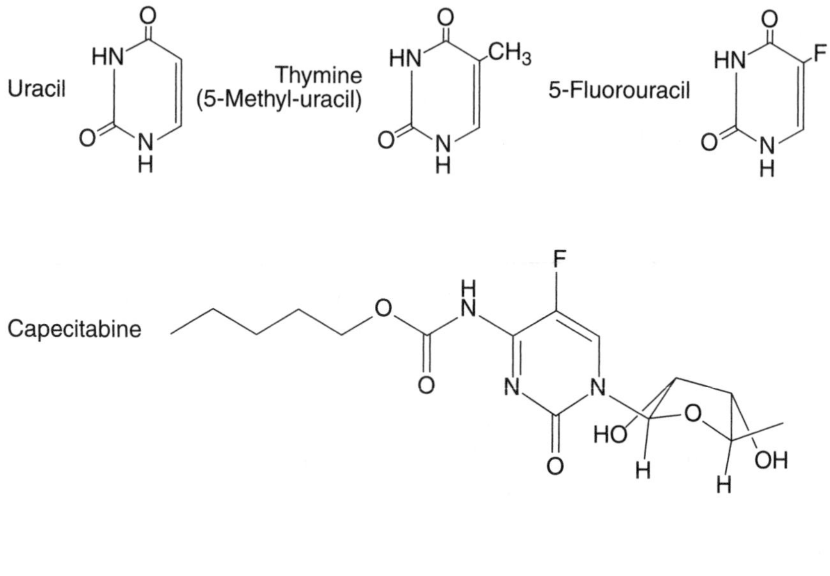

**Figure 16.8.** Structure of uracil, thymine, 5-fluorouracil, and capecitabine.

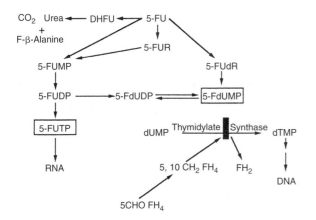

**Figure 16.9.** Metabolic activation of 5-fluorouracil (5-FU) leads to formation of 5-fluorodeoxyuridine monophosphate (5-FdUMP), which inhibits the enzyme thymidylate synthase, and 5-fluorouridine triphosphate (5-FUTP), which may be incorporated into RNA. Folinic acid (5-CHOFH$_4$) is metabolized to 5,10-methylene tetrahydrofolate (5,10CH$_2$FH$_4$), the cofactor that forms a ternary complex with 5-FdUMP and the enzyme thymidylate synthase. 5-FU is catabolized to dihydrofluorouracil (DHFU) and excreted as CO$_2$, urea, and α-fluoro-β-alanine (F-β-Alanine).

tance of the two mechanisms underlying cytotoxicity of 5-FU probably varies for treatment of different tumors and normal tissues. In cells where toxicity is due to interruption of DNA synthesis through inhibition of thymidylate synthase, the drug should have specificity for cells in the S phase of the cycle; when the major mechanism is incorporation of 5-FUTP into RNA, the effects may be independent of cell cycle phase.

Approximately 80 percent of 5-FU administered clinically is catabolized to the end products of CO$_2$, urea, and α-fluoro-β-alanine, mainly in the liver. The catabolism of 5-FU appears to be an important determinant of normal-tissue toxicity. If 5-FU is catabolized rapidly, then the exposure of both tumor and normal tissues to active metabolites of the drug will be decreased. About 3 percent of patients have a partial deficiency of the rate-limiting enzyme for elimination of 5-FU, dihydropyrimidine dehydrogenase (DPD), and are at risk for severe toxicity from the drug (Milano and Etienne, 1994; see also Sec. 16.1.7).

Inhibition of thymidylate synthase by FdUMP is dependent on the presence of the cofactor 5,10-methylenetetrahydrofolate, which combines with thymidylate synthase and FdUMP to form a covalent ternary complex (Fig. 16.9). The dissociation rate of this complex is decreased in the presence of excess cofactor (Moran and Keyomarsi, 1987). This led to experiments indicating that addition of the prodrug 5-formyltetrahydrofolate (folinic acid or leucovorin) increased the cytotoxicity of 5-FU (Fig. 16.9). Clinical studies have

demonstrated that this combination has greater activity in the treatment of patients with metastatic colorectal cancer than 5-FU alone.

5-Fluorouracil is most commonly used for treatment of breast and gastrointestinal cancer. The drug is usually given intravenously, because bioavailability after oral administration is variable. It is eliminated rapidly from plasma with a half-life of a few minutes. This agent demonstrates nonlinear pharmacokinetics due to a saturation of metabolism at higher peak concentrations, which may be seen when it is given by bolus injection but not when given by infusion. This difference in pharmacokinetic behavior under the two conditions of administration may explain why the dose-limiting toxicity differs for bolus injection and infusion. Major toxicity is to bone marrow and mucous membranes with the latter becoming dominant if the drug is given over 4 to 5 days by continuous infusion. Rarer toxicities include skin rashes, conjunctivitis (inflammation of the eye), and ataxia (loss of balance) due to effects on the cerebellum, and cardiotoxicity. Prolonged low-dose infusions of 5-FU can be administered with a decrease in some of the above forms of systemic toxicity, but they are associated with changes in sensation as well as with redness and peeling of the skin on the palms of the hands and the soles of the feet, referred to as palmarplantar erythrodysesthesia, also known as the hand–foot syndrome. There is limited evidence that this method of 5-FU administration results in improvement of antitumor effects when compared with 5-FU given by bolus injections.

Oral fluoropyrimidine derivatives such as capecitabine have been developed to provide a convenient route of administration, a fine control of dosing, and sustained drug exposure (Fig. 16.8). Capecitabine is absorbed unchanged from the gastrointestinal tract, metabolized in the liver by carboxylesterase to 5′-deoxy-5-fluorocytidine (5′-DFCR), which is then converted to 5′-deoxy-5-fluorouridine (5′-DFUR) by cytidine deaminase, mainly located in the liver and tumor tissue. Further metabolism of 5′-DFUR to the cytotoxic moiety 5-FU occurs at the site of the tumor by thymidine phosphorylase (TP), which has levels considerably higher in tumor tissues compared to normal tissues (Fig. 16.10). The toxicity profile of capecitabine is similar to that of prolonged low-dose infusions of 5-FU, with lower frequencies of myelosuppression and stomatitis (soreness in the mouth) but higher incidence of palmar-plantar erythrodysesthesia than intravenous bolus 5-FU. Capecitabine has demonstrated efficacy in breast and colorectal malignancies. Randomized phase III trials comparing capecitabine to intravenous 5-FU plus leucovorin have shown equivalent efficacy in terms of survival in metastatic colorectal cancer (Hoff et al., 2001; Van Cutsem et al., 2001).

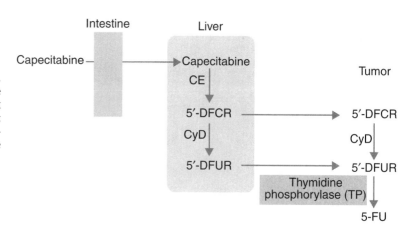

**Figure 16.10.** Enzymatic activation of capecitabine. Capecitabine is preferentially converted to the pharmacologically active 5-fluorouracil in target tumor tissue through a series of three metabolic steps. 5'-DFCR = 5'-deoxy-5-fluorocytidine; 5-DFUR = 5'-deoxy-5-fluorouridine; CyD = cytidine deaminase; CE = carboxylesterase

### 16.4.3 Thymidylate Synthase Inhibitors

Compounds designed specifically to inhibit thymidylate synthase (TS), by binding to the site for 5,10-methylene tetrahydrofolate, have been developed (Tourtoutoglou and Pazdur, 1996). These compounds deplete dTMP required for DNA synthesis. Two compounds are undergoing clinical development (Fig. 16.11). Raltitrexed (Tomudex) and premetrexed disodium (Alimta) are folate-based TS inhibitors with glutamic acid at one end of the molecule (similar to methotrexate) and can be polyglutamated for increased retention in cells and increased potency of TS inhibition. These agents require transport via the reduced folate carrier and are potent inhibitors of TS. In addition to targeting TS, premetrexed inhibits DHFR as well as glycinamide ribonucleotide formyltransferase (GARFT); the latter is a folate-dependent enzyme involved in purine synthesis. Due to its inhibitory activity against these three key fo-

late enzymes, premetrexed is known as a multitargeted antifolate agent, but its cytotoxicity is predominantly mediated through inhibition of TS (Adjei, 2000).

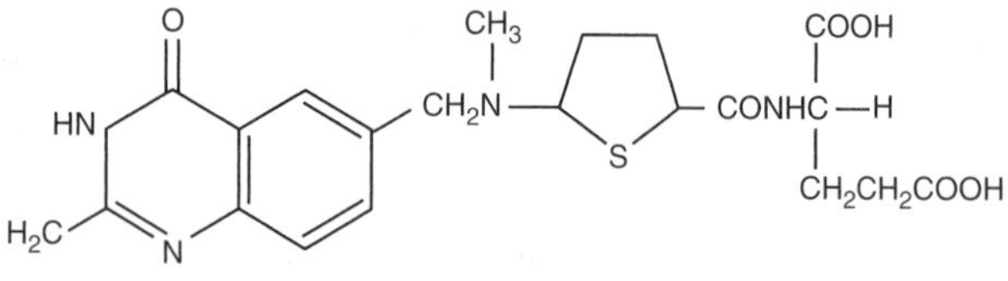

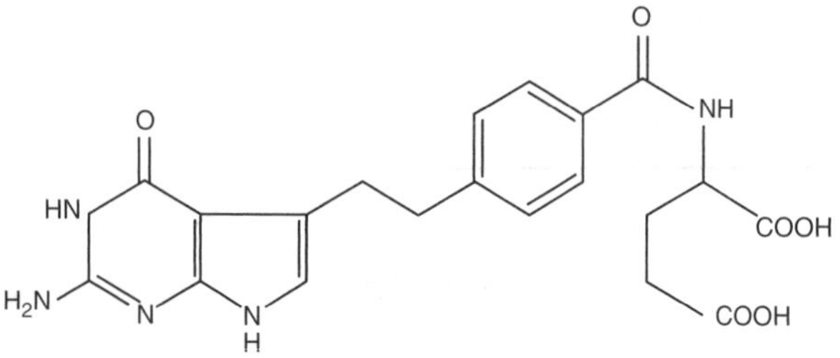

Both ralitrexed and premetrexed are administered intravenously. Renal excretion appears to be the major route of elimination for both agents. The clinical activity of ralitrexed appears comparable to that of 5-FU combined with leucovorin in metastatic colorectal cancer, and activity has also been seen in breast cancer. Ralitrexed has been associated with transient elevations in some liver-function tests. Premetrexed has demonstrated preliminary clinical activity in non–small-cell lung cancer, mesothelioma, and breast cancer, and clinical trials of premetrexed used with other cytotoxic agents such as gemcitabine and cisplatin are ongoing. The main clinical toxicities are myelosuppression, inflammation of the oral and gastrointestinal mucosa, and skin rash. Supplementation with oral folic acid and intramuscular vitamin B12 has been shown to reduce toxicities related to premetrexed (Scagliotti et al., 2003). The ultimate clinical utility of these compounds is yet to be defined.

### 16.4.4 Cytidine Analogs

Cytosine arabinoside (ara-C) differs from the nucleoside deoxycytidine only by the presence of a $\beta$-hydroxyl group on the 2-position of the sugar, so that the sugar moiety is arabinose instead of deoxyribose (Fig. 16.12). Ara-C penetrates cells rapidly by a carrier-mediated process shared with deoxycytidine and is phosphorylated to ara-CTP (Fig. 16.13). Ara-CTP is a competitive inhibitor of DNA polymerase, an enzyme necessary for DNA synthesis, and has similar affinity for this enzyme to the normal substrate dCTP. When ara-CTP binds to this enzyme, DNA synthesis is arrested and S-phase cells may die. Incorporation of ara-C into DNA also occurs and may contribute to its cytotoxic effects, possibly because of defective ligation or incomplete synthesis of DNA fragments, resulting in DNA chain termination.

Raltitrexed

Premetrexed

**Figure 16.11.** Stucture of the thymidylate synthase inhibitors raltitrexed (Tomudex) and premetrexed (Alimta).

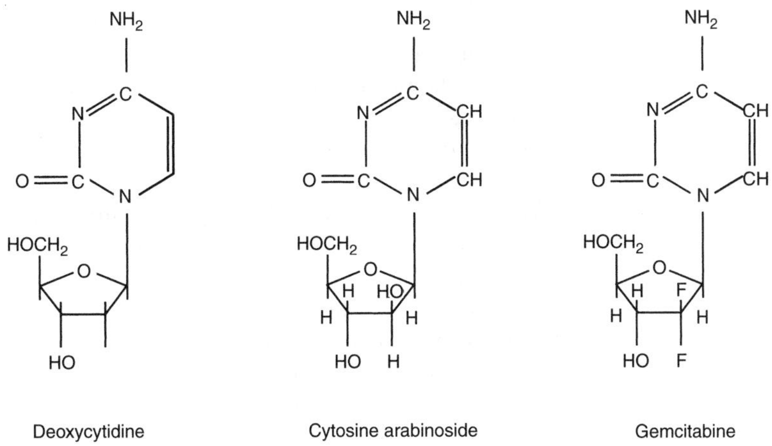

**Figure 16.12.** Structure of deoxycytidine and its analogs, cytosine arabinoside and gemcitabine.

Deoxycytidine          Cytosine arabinoside          Gemcitabine

The availability of ara-CTP for cytotoxic activity depends critically on the balance between the kinases that activate the drug and the deaminases that degrade it (Fig. 16.13). The activity of these enzymes varies greatly among different types of cells, leading to different rates of generation of ara-CTP. Resistance to the action of ara-C may occur by mutations that lead to deficiency in deoxycytidine kinase or to cells with an expanded pool of dCTP that competes with the active metabolite ara-CTP and regulates enzymes involved in activation and degradation of the drug. Ara-C is specific in its activity for cells synthesizing DNA. Because it is rapidly degraded in plasma with a half-life of 7 to 20 minutes, it must be given intravenously by frequent injections or by continuous infusion to kill cells as they pass from G1 phase to S phase of the cycle. The drug is used primarily for treatment of acute leukemia. Myelosuppression and gastrointestinal toxicity are the major side effects, but abnormal behavior and thought processes may also occur following high doses.

Gemcitabine (2'2'-difluorodeoxycytidine) is a cytosine analog with structural similarities to ara-C (Fig. 16.12). Unlike ara-C, gemcitabine has activity against a variety of solid tumors. Like ara-C, gemcitabine requires intracellular activation to its triphosphate derivative dFdCTP, which is incorporated into DNA and then inhibits DNA synthesis. Although gemcitabine is less effective than ara-C in DNA chain termination, a favorable pharmacokinetic characteristic of gemcitabine is the prolonged retention of its cytotoxic triphosphate in cells, with terminal elimination rates as long as 72 hours (Plunkett et al., 1995). Gemcitabine has other intracellular effects that may contribute to its cytotoxic activity: these include inhibition of ribonucleotide reductase; stimulation of deoxycytidine kinase, the enzyme responsible for its activation; and inhibition of cytidine deaminase, the primary enzyme responsible for its degradation (Huang et al., 1991). Through inhibition of ribonucleotide reductase, gemcitabine affects DNA synthesis by preventing the de novo biosynthesis of the deoxyribonucleoside triphosphate precursors. The drug is schedule dependent, with once-weekly administration providing a good therapeutic ratio. It also has radiosensitizer properties that may be associated with the depletion of deoxyadenosine triphosphate pools via the inhibition of ribonucleotide reductase (Shewach et al., 1994). In clinical studies, gemcitabine has activity against non–small cell lung cancer, pancreatic cancer, breast cancer, nasopharyngeal cancer, and bladder cancer. Toxicity is primarily myelosuppression.

### 16.4.5 Purine Antimetabolites

Many purine analogs have been synthesized, and a few of these have found application as antiviral agents (e.g., adenosine arabinoside, ara-A), immunosuppressive agents used in preservation of kidney and other organ

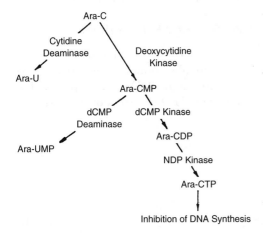

**Figure 16.13.** Metabolic activation and degradation of cytosine arabinoside (ara-C). Formation of the active metabolite ara-CTP depends on the balance between kinases that activate the drug and deaminases that degrade it.

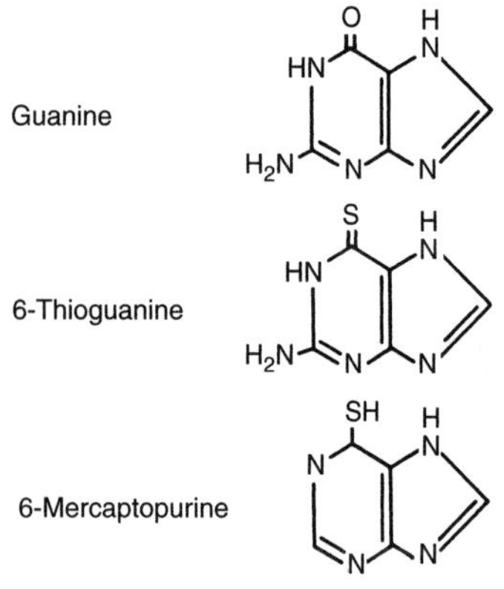

Guanine

6-Thioguanine

6-Mercaptopurine

**Figure 16.14.** Structure of guanine and the analogs 6-thioguanine and 6-mercaptopurine.

grafts (e.g., azathioprine), and as anticancer drugs [e.g., 6-mercaptopurine (6-MP) and 6-thioguanine (6-TG); Fig. 16.14]. Use of the last two of these drugs is limited to treatment of leukemia.

Like guanine, 6-MP and 6-TG are metabolized to deoxynucleotides by addition of the sugar-phosphate moiety and are incorporated into DNA. This mechanism presumably accounts for their selective toxicity for cells in DNA synthesis. Metabolites of the drugs may also inhibit purine and RNA synthesis; the relative importance of these mechanisms is unclear. Cross-resistance is usually observed between 6-MP and 6-TG, and drug-resistant mutant cells may have decreased activity of the enzyme HGPRT (hypoxanthine–guanine phosphoribosyltransferase), which is necessary for their activation. Alternative mechanisms that convey resistance probably involve increased degradation of the drugs and their metabolites. Recent studies of the clinical pharmacology of 6-MP have revealed a low bioavailability of drug when administered orally because of first-pass hepatic metabolism and wide patient-to-patient variability. The clinical toxicities of 6-MP include myelosuppression, mucositis, diarrhea, nausea, and vomiting.

Early analogs of adenine and its nucleoside derivative adenosine (Fig. 16.15) were limited by their rapid deamination by adenosine deaminase (ADA). Fludarabine (9-β-arabinofuranosyl-2-fluoroadenine monophos-

phate) is a derivative that is resistant to deamination and has activity against low-grade lymphomas, chronic lymphocytic leukemia, hairy cell leukemia, and Waldenstrom's macroglobulinemia (Keating et al., 1994). After administration, fludarabine is rapidly dephosphorylated to 2-fluoro-ara-A, which then is transported into cells and converted to the active triphosphate derivative. Mechanisms of cytotoxicity include inhibition of DNA polymerase and termination of DNA and RNA replication. Because 2-fluoro-ara-A is excreted primarily unchanged in the urine, dose reduction is necessary in the setting of renal insufficiency. The major toxicity of fludarabine is myelosuppression and immunosuppression.

2-Chlorodeoxyadenosine (2CdA; Fig. 16.15) is a potent chlorinated adenosine derivative that is resistant to deamination. It has a similar spectrum of clinical activity and toxicity to fludarabine. It is transported directly into cells, where the triphosphate 2-CdATP is formed by deoxycytidine kinase. While 2-CdATP can induce DNA breaks and inhibit replication, its mechanism of cytotoxicity in slowly proliferating cells is not well understood.

Deoxycoformycin (Fig. 16.15) is an inhibitor of adenosine deaminase (ADA) that has demonstrated activity against hairy cell leukemia and some indolent lymphomas. Why inhibition of the ability of cells to break down normal nucleosides should be cytotoxic is not understood, but accumulation of adenine nucleosides might lead to secondary inhibition of DNA synthesis. Most of the drug is excreted unchanged in urine and, as with fludarabine, dose reduction is necessary in the setting of renal insufficiency. The dose of deoxycoformycin required to maximally inhibit ADA leads to substantial toxicity. However, hairy cell leukemias have low ADA activity, and the lower dose of deoxycoformycin required to treat this disease has minimal toxicity.

## 16.5 TOPOISOMERASE INHIBITORS

DNA topoisomerases are ubiquitous nuclear enzymes that relax supercoiled double-stranded DNA to allow DNA replication and RNA transcription. Torsional strain is relieved via the formation of a single-strand

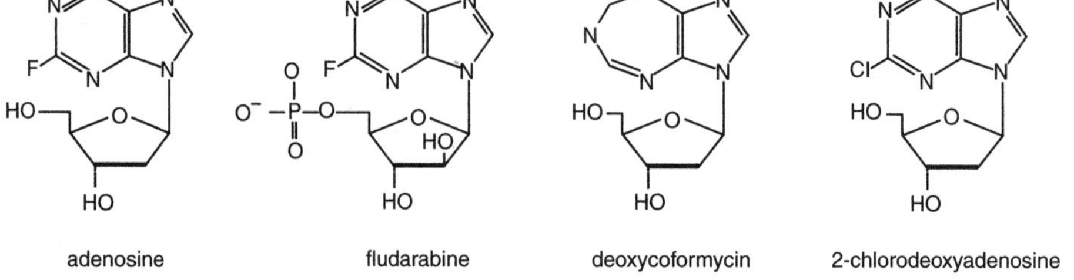

**Figure 16.15.** Structure of adenosine and the analogs fludarabine, deoxycoformycin, and 2-chlorodeoxyadenosine.

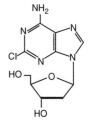

adenosine                fludarabine                deoxycoformycin                2-chlorodeoxyadenosine

nick (topoisomerase I) or a double-strand nick (topo-isomerase II), followed by swivelling of DNA at the nick(s) and subsequent religation (Fig. 16.16; see also Chap. 18, Sec. 18.2.6). Topoisomerase inhibitors bind to and stablize the DNA/topoisomerase cleavable complex, thus preventing the religation of DNA strands. Ir-reversible damage results when an advancing DNA replication fork encounters the drug-stabilized cleavable complex, ultimately leading to lethal double-stranded breaks and cell death.

Multiple mechanisms can lead to resistance to topo-isomerase inhibitors (see Chap. 18, Sec. 18.2.6). Topo-isomerase II inhibitors but not topoisomerase I inhibi-tors are substrates for P-glycoprotein, and have the classic multidrug resistance (MDR) phenotype. For both topoisomerase I and II inhibitors, the degree of cellular sensitivity to the drug correlates directly with the abundance of the target enzyme, such that more cleavable complexes and lethal DNA lesions are formed. Resistance can be due to either reduced topo-isomerase levels or to changes in the enzymes due to mutation.

### 16.5.1 Topoisomerase I Inhibitors

Camptothecin is an extract from the wood of the Chi-nese tree *Camptotheca acuminata* (Fig. 16.17). Camp-tothecin was found to be active in vivo against a murine leukemia, but phase I studies conducted in the early 1970s were terminated because of severe and unpre-

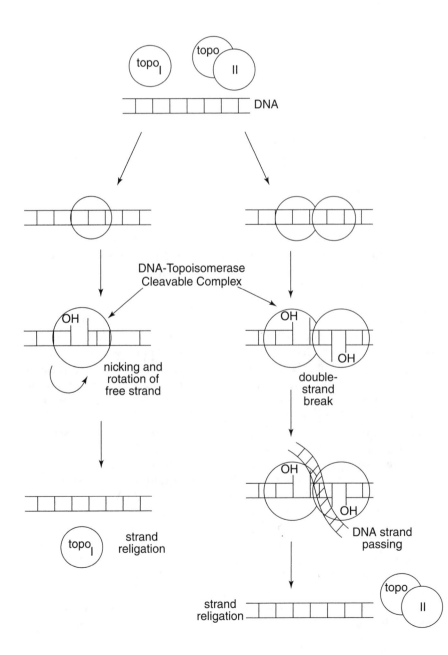

**Figure 16.16.** Topoisomerase I and II en-zymes form single-strand nicks, and dou-ble-strand nicks, respectively. Swiveling of supercoiled DNA then occurs at the nick(s), followed by religation to relieve torsional strain. Topoisomerase inhibitors bind to and stabilize the DNA-topoisom-erase cleavable complex, preventing the religation of DNA strands. Double-stranded breaks result when an advanc-ing DNA replication fork encounters the cleavable complex, and leads to cell death.

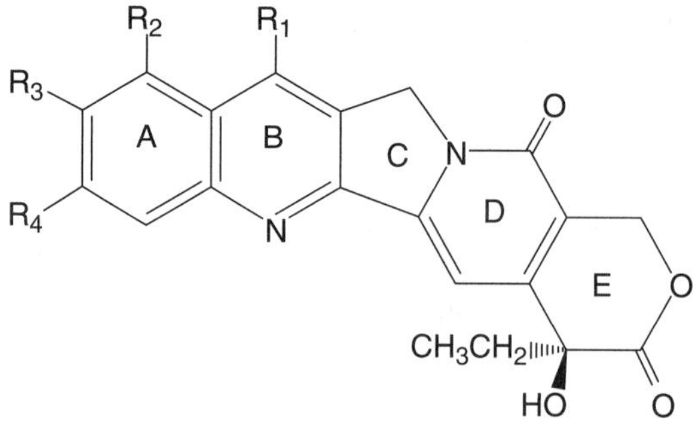

**Figure 16.17.** Structure of camptothecin and its derivatives: topotecan, irinotecan, and SN-38.

| Compound | Molecular weight | R$_1$ | R$_2$ | R$_3$ | R$_4$ |
|---|---|---|---|---|---|
| Camptothecin | 348 | –H | –H | –H | –H |
| Topotecan | 421 | –H | –CH$_2$N(CH$_3$)$_2$ | –OH | –H |
| Irinotecan | 587 | –CH$_2$CH$_3$ | –H | 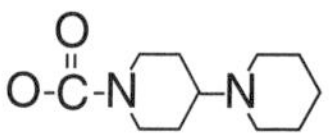 O-C-N⟨⟩-N⟨⟩ | –H |
| SN-38 | 392 | –CH$_2$CH$_3$ | –H | –OH | –H |

dictable toxicity, namely hemorrhagic cystitis and toxic gastroenteritis. Camptothecin affects only topoisomerase I activity; cells in S phase are very sensitive, possibly because the process of DNA replication requires topoisomerase I activity and because the topoisomerase-associated single-strand breaks are converted into double-strand breaks (Pommier, 1993). However, cytotoxicity is not restricted to cells in S phase, and the proportion of cells killed following an exposure to camptothecin has been demonstrated in vitro to exceed the S-phase fraction.

Several analogs of camptothecin have been synthesized. All camptothecins have a basic heterocyclic five-ring structure with a lactone moiety and an α-hydroxyl moiety on the E ring. For those agents under clinical development, substitutions on the A ring tend to increase the aqueous solubility while retaining cytotoxicity (topotecan and irinotecan; Fig. 16.17). All camptothecins can undergo a rapid, reversible, pH-dependent, nonenzymatic hydrolysis of the closed lactone ring to yield an open-ring carboxylate form. The carboxylate form is more water soluble than the lactone; it predominates at physiologic pH, but is much less active as an inhibitor of topoisomerase I.

*Topotecan* has activity in vitro and in vivo that is similar to that of camptothecin. It does not undergo any appreciable metabolism and is primarily eliminated unchanged by the kidneys. Therefore dose reduction in the setting of renal dysfunction is required. Topotecan can be given either intravenously or orally. Interest in the oral formulation has been stimulated by preclinical evidence of a better cell kill when this drug is given continuously. The dose-limiting toxicity in most clinical

studies is myelosuppression. Topotecan has promise as a treatment for ovarian cancer and small cell lung cancer (von Pawel et al., 1999; Gordon et al., 2001).

*Irinotecan (CPT-11)* requires esterification by serum and tissue carboxylesterases to an active metabolite SN-38 before becoming cytotoxic. SN-38 is 1000-fold more potent than irinotecan at inhibiting topoisomerase I activity (Kawato et al., 1991). Glucuronidation of SN-38 into its inactive glucuronide, SN-38G, and subsequent excretion of SN-38G into bile and intestines represent the major mechanisms of elimination for SN-38. Irinotecan has activity in vivo that is greater than or equal to that seen with camptothecin. Dose-limiting toxicity has consisted of both myelosuppression and diarrhea. Irinotecan can produce an early cholinergic syndrome consisting of abdominal cramps, early diarrhea, and diaphoresis that typically occurs acutely during or immediately after its infusion, and prompt resolution can be obtained with intravenous or subcutaneous atropine. Patients who experience this reaction may benefit from prophylactic atropine prior to subsequent irinotecan infusions. A second distinct type of diarrhea is associated with irinotecan, typically with a delayed onset. It tends to be more severe and protracted compared to the early-onset cholinergic-based diarrhea, and generally requires pharmacological and supportive measures in its management. A biliary index has been developed to estimate the relative exposures of SN-38 to SN-38G in the bile (i.e., high biliary concentrations of SN-38 are toxic), and the inability to form the less toxic SN-38G by glucuronidation may be associated with increased gastrointestinal toxicity from irinotecan therapy (Gupta et al., 1994). Irinotecan is approved for first-line therapy in metastatic colorectal cancer, where it has been shown to improve survival when used in combination with 5-FU and leucovorin (Douillard et al., 2000; Saltz et al., 2000). Other tumor types where irinotecan has demonstrated promising activity include small cell lung, gastric, esophageal, and gynecological cancers.

### 16.5.2 Epipodophyllotoxins

Etoposide (VP-16) and teniposide (VM-26) are semi-synthetic glycoside derivatives of podophyllotoxin, an antimitotic agent derived from the mandrake plant. Although podophyllotoxin binds to tubulin and inhibits its polymerization, etoposide and teniposide act through inhibition of DNA topoisomerase II (Van Mannen et al., 1988). These agents are substrates for P-glycoprotein, and drug resistance can thus be mediated by the MDR mechanism (see Chap. 18, Sec. 18.2.3). Etoposide (Fig. 16.18) is a widely used drug and is a component of first-line treatment regimens in small-cell lung cancer, testicular cancer, pediatric tumors, and malignant lymphomas. It also has activity against gastric cancer, non–small cell lung cancer, and acute leukemia. Teniposide has a more limited role in childhood hematologic cancer. Etoposide is markedly schedule dependent, with repeated daily doses providing greater activity than a single intravenous injection. Synergy between cisplatin and etoposide has been demonstrated in vitro, and these two drugs are commonly given together to patients with lung or testicular tumors (Eder et al., 1990).

Etoposide is usually given intravenously but can be given orally, with a bioavailability of approximately 50 percent and considerable interindividual variability. Following intravenous administration, etoposide is eliminated by hepatic glucuronidation and approximately 40 percent of the drug is excreted unchanged

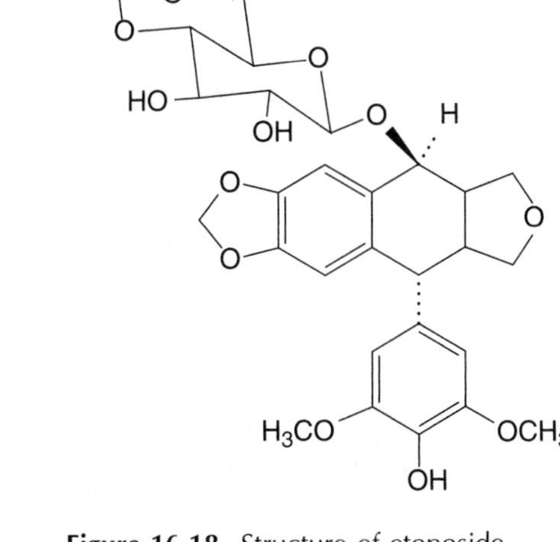

**Figure 16.18.** Structure of etoposide.

in the urine. The toxicity of etoposide at standard doses is myelosuppression and hair loss, with other effects being uncommon. This toxicity profile makes etoposide ideal for high-dose transplantation regimens, and at these higher doses (1.0 to $1.5 \, g/m^2$), mucositis becomes dose-limiting. An association between the use of etoposide and a secondary leukemia with a characteristic 11q23 translocation has been described (Winick et al., 1993). In contrast to secondary leukemias arising from use of alkylating agents which occur with a latency of up to 10 years, those arising from etoposide tend to occur sooner, with a median latent period of about 2 to 3 years after drug administration. Most cases of etoposide-induced secondary leukemias are monocytic and myelomonocytic (FAB M-4 and M-5) with no antecedent pancytopenia before the development of frank leukemia.

### 16.5.3 Anthracyclines and Anthracenediones

The original anthracycline, daunorubicin, is a product of a *Streptomyces* species isolated from an Italian soil sample in 1958. The drug had high activity against acute leukemia and remains a component of many current protocols for acute myelogenous leukemia. Modifications of the structure of daunorubicin led to the identification of doxorubicin, an analog with greater activity against many solid tumors and one of the most active anticancer drugs in current clinical practice (Fig. 16.19). The success of doxorubicin led to a major effort to synthesize other analogs, but of the hundreds developed and tested, only two are used currently; both have only marginal advantages. Idarubicin is an orally absorbed daunorubicin analog with similar activity against acute leukemia. Epirubicin differs from doxorubicin only in its three-dimensional configuration; it has equivalent activity and possibly less toxicity.

Several mechanisms may contribute to the cytocidal effect of doxorubicin and related drugs. These include interaction with topoisomerase II, DNA intercalation, formation of free radicals, and effects on the cell membrane. Doxorubicin can interact with topoisomerase II by binding directly with the enzyme and preventing resealing of topoisomerase II–induced DNA cleavage, ultimately leading to fatal DNA breaks. Doxorubicin can also intercalate between base pairs perpendicular to the long axis of the double helix, leading to partial unwinding of the DNA helix. However, much of the DNA is organized and folded into chromatin and may be protected from this type of drug interaction. Also, the concentration of doxorubicin required to intercalate into DNA and to cause inhibition of DNA and RNA polymerase cannot be achieved in vivo without excessive toxicity.

Doxorubicin may undergo metabolism of its quinone ring to a semiquinone radical (i.e., a group containing

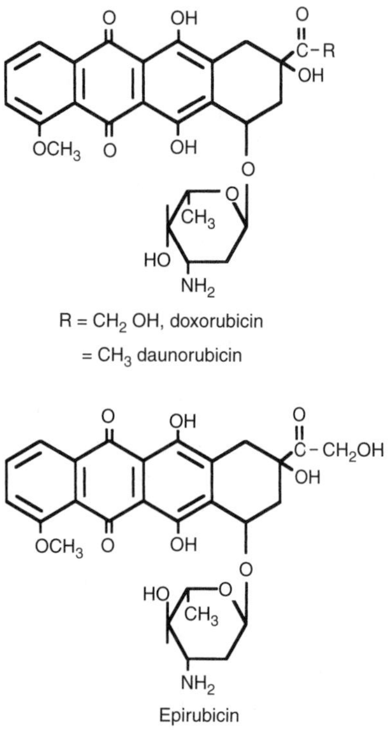

R = CH₂OH, doxorubicin

= CH₃ daunorubicin

Epirubicin

**Figure 16.19.** Structure of doxorubicin (Adriamycin), daunorubicin, and epirubicin.

an unpaired electron) that, in turn, reacts rapidly with oxygen to yield superoxide, $O_2^-$. The superoxide radical is known to undergo several reactions that can lead to cell death, including oxidative damage of cell membranes and DNA. There is evidence that free radical formation accounts for the cardiac toxicity of anthracyclines, but the contribution of free radicals to the killing of cancer cells is uncertain. Resistance to anthracyclines has been associated with an increase in the free radical scavenger system (glutathione and related compounds), but doxorubicin retains toxicity under hypoxic conditions, when superoxide radicals cannot be formed.

Doxorubicin and related drugs also bind to cell membranes and may kill cells through membrane-related effects. Tritton and Yee (1982) studied the effects of doxorubicin in vitro, when it was linked to beads, and demonstrated that the drug could cause cell death without being transported into the cell. However, others (Gieseler et al., 1994) have emphasized the relationship between cellular uptake and cytotoxicity, and that cell death correlates directly with the amount of DNA-bound anthracyclines.

With the exception of idarubicin, anthracyclines are administered intravenously, because oral absorption is poor. They are widely distributed in the body, with significant binding to plasma proteins and tissue. Plasma clearance after intravenous administration may be described by three exponential components with half-lives

in the ranges of 8 to 25 minutes, 1.5 to 10 hours, and 24 to 48 hours (Robert and Gianni, 1993). The second phase is attributed to metabolism of the drug in liver and the final phase to release of drug from tissue-binding sites. Doxorubicin is metabolized in the liver to doxorubicinol, which retains some cytotoxic activity, and to several other metabolites; the drug and its metabolites are excreted via the bile. Thus, dosage reduction is required for patients with hepatic dysfunction or biliary obstruction.

The acute toxicities of doxorubicin include myelosuppression, total loss of hair, nausea, vomiting, mucositis, and local tissue necrosis following leakage of drug at the injection site. Repeated administration is limited by a chronic irreversible cardiomyopathy that occurs with increasing frequency once a total dose of about 500 milligrams per square meter has been given. The mechanism of cardiotoxicity is probably related to damage to sarcoplasmic reticulum mediated by the formation of free radicals within cardiac muscle. Patients with pre-existing cardiac disease or those who have received mediastinal radiation are more likely to develop this problem. Cardiac toxicity appears to be more related to peak concentration of drug than to overall exposure, so that infusional or repeated lower dose administration will reduce the chances of its occurrence. Dexrazoxane, an iron-chelating agent, has been demonstrated to reduce cardiac toxicity without compromising efficacy when given concurrently with doxorubicin.

Mitoxantrone is an anthracenedione that differs from the anthracyclines in lacking the sugar and the tetracyclic ring. It is a synthetic drug with three planar rings that intercalates into DNA, with a preference for guanine-cytosine base pairs. It may also function as an inhibitor of topoisomerase II. This drug is used as an alternative to anthracyclines in the treatment of acute myelogenous leukemia and breast cancer. While generally less active than doxorubicin, it causes less nausea, vomiting, mucositis, and hair loss and has found a role in the palliative treatment of cancers of the breast and prostate.

## 16.6 ANTIMICROTUBULAR AGENTS

### 16.6.1 Vinca Alkaloids

The vinca alkaloids—vinblastine, vincristine, and vinorelbine—are naturally occurring or semisynthetic derivatives from the periwinkle plant. These compounds bind to the protein tubulin and inhibit its polymerization to form microtubules (Rowinsky and Donehower, 1996). Microtubules have several important cellular functions, including formation of the mitotic spindle responsible for separation of chromosomes, and structural and transport functions in axons of nerves. Microtubules are in a state of dynamic equilibrium, with continuous formation and degradation from cytoplas-

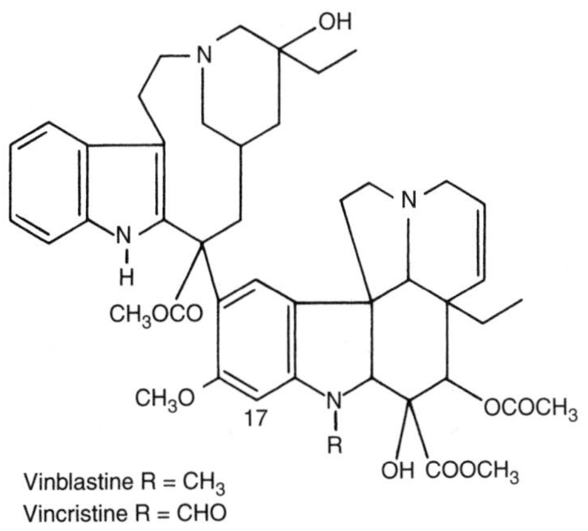

**Figure 16.20.** Structure of vinblastine and vincristine.

mic tubulin. This process is interrupted by treatment with vinca alkaloids, and lethally damaged cells may be observed to enter an abortive metaphase and then lyse. However, experiments with synchronized cells have demonstrated that maximum lethal toxicity for vinblastine and vincristine occurs when cells are exposed during the period of DNA synthesis (see Chap. 17, Sec. 17.2.4); presumably the morphologic expression of that damage is observed in the attempted mitosis.

Vincristine and vinblastine are structurally similar, differing only in a substitution on the central rings (Fig. 16.20). Vinca alkaloids have large volumes of distribution, indicating a high degree of tissue binding, and are eliminated mainly by hepatic metabolism and biliary excretion. Their plasma clearance is described by tri-exponential curves, with terminal half-lives of about 20 to 40 hours.

Despite similarities in their structures, these drugs differ in both their clinical spectra of activity and their toxicities. Vinblastine is an important drug in combination chemotherapy of testicular cancer, while vincristine is a mainstay of treatment for childhood leukemia. Both drugs have been combined with other cytotoxic agents to treat lymphomas or various solid tumors. Vinorelbine has been introduced more recently and has activity as a single agent against lung and breast cancers.

Vinblastine causes major toxicity to bone marrow, with some risk of autonomic neuropathy, leading to

constipation. The dose of vincristine is limited by its toxicity to peripheral nerves, and this damage relates to the duration of treatment as well as the total dose of vincristine used. This neurotoxicity probably occurs because of damage to the microtubules in axons. The dose-limiting toxicity of vinorelbine is myelosuppression. Neurotoxicity can occur but is less common than with vincristine, possibly due to a lower affinity for axonal microtubules. Table 16.3 summarizes some of the common toxic effects of the vinca alkaloids. Resistance to the vinca alkaloids is mediated primarily by the MDR mechanism (Chap. 18, Sec. 18.2.3), and by mutations or posttranslational modifications of the microtubules.

### 16.6.2 Taxanes

Paclitaxel (Taxol) and docetaxel (Taxotere) are plant alkaloids derived from the bark of the Pacific yew tree *Taxus brevifolia*, and the needles of the European yew tree *Taxus baccata*, respectively (Fig. 16.21). Paclitaxel was identified as an anticancer drug more than 25 years ago, but its clinical development was hampered by a limited drug supply, which depended on the bark of the relatively rare yew tree. Interest increased once it became apparent that the mechanism of action was unique and that there was evidence of activity in ovarian cancer. Docetaxel is a semisynthetic derivative of the needles of the yew tree.

Taxanes are anti-microtubular agents and bind to tubulin at a site different from that of the vinca alkaloids. In contrast to the vinca alkaloids, which inhibit the polymerization of tubulin into microtubules, taxanes are believed to inhibit microtubular disassembly, which then prevents the normal growth and breakdown of microtubules that is required for cell division (Rowinsky and Donehower, 1995). However, the classic view of vinca alkaloids depolymerizing microtubules and taxanes stabilizing microtubules has been challenged. Dumontet and Sikic (1999) suggest that both classes of agents may have a similar mechanism of action, involving the inhibition of microtubule dynamics.

The pharmacokinetics of paclitaxel and docetaxel are characterized by a large volume of distribution with extensive tissue binding, elimination by hepatic metabo-

**Table 16.3.** Comparison of Toxicity of the Vinca Alkaloids

| Drug | Myelosuppression | Neurotoxicity | Autonomic | Others |
|---|---|---|---|---|
| Vinblastine | +++ | + | ++ | Cramps or pains in jaw, pharynx, back, or limbs following injection. |
| Vincristine | + | +++ | + | Syndrome of inappropriate anti-diuretic hormone (SIADH) with associated hyponatremia (low serum sodium levels). |
| Vinorelbine | +++ | + | ++ | |

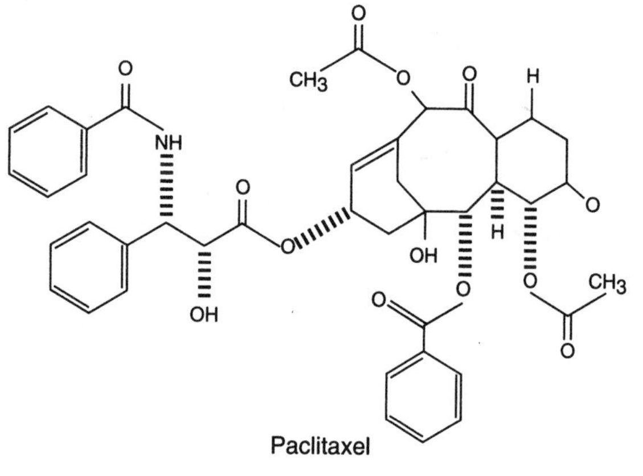

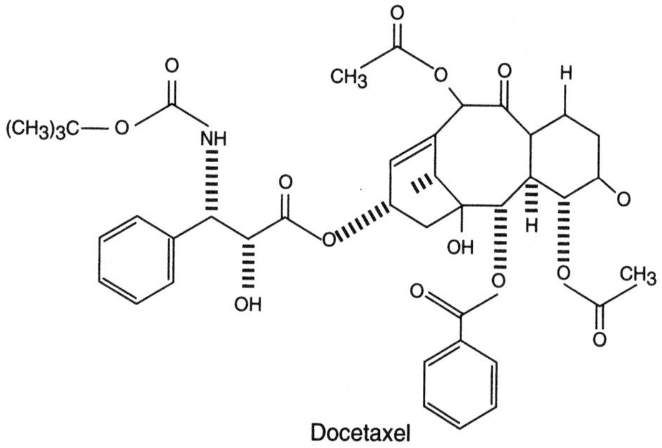

**Figure 16.21.** Structure of paclitaxel and docetaxel.

risk of infection. Both can cause hypersensitivity reactions with bronchial constriction, urticaria (hives), and hypotension. This problem has been reduced substantially by prophylactic treatment with steroids and histamine blockers. The vehicles in which the taxanes are formulated have been implicated as possible causes of the hypersensitivity reactions, but different vehicles have been used for paclitaxel (Cremophor EL) and for docetaxel (polysorbate 80). A sensory peripheral neuropathy can occur with repeated or high-dose administration. Docetaxel can also cause fluid retention and skin and nail changes with repeated usage. These drugs have activity against ovarian, breast, lung and prostate cancers and are being evaluated in patients with several other types of tumor.

## 16.7 MISCELLANEOUS DRUGS

### 16.7.1 Bleomycin

Bleomycin consists of a family of molecules with a complex structure; it is derived from fungal culture, the dominant active component being known as bleomycin A2 (Lazo and Chabner, 1996). Bleomycin causes DNA double-strand breaks through a complex sequence of reactions involving the binding of a bleomycin/ferrous iron complex to DNA. This binding leads to insertion of the drug between base pairs (intercalation) and unwinding of the double helix. A second step in the formation of DNA strand breaks may involve the reduction of molecular oxygen to superoxide or hydroxyl radicals, catalyzed by the bleomycin/ferrous iron complex. However, like doxorubicin, bleomycin retains some of its lethal activity under hypoxic conditions. Bleomycin may exert preferential toxicity in the G2 phase of the cell cycle, but it also has toxicity for slowly proliferating cells in plateau-phase cell culture. Bleomycin is a large molecule that crosses cell membranes slowly. Once within the cell, it can be activated or broken down by bleomycin hydrolase; cellular sensitivity to bleomycin has been found to correlate inversely with the concentration of this enzyme.

After intravenous injection, most of the administered drug is eliminated unchanged in the urine. Plasma clearance curves have two components with half-lives of about 0.5 hour and 4 to 8 hours, respectively. The major use of bleomycin is in combination with other drugs for the curative therapy of testicular cancer and lymphomas. Bleomycin has little toxicity to bone marrow but may cause fever, chills, and damage to skin and mucous membranes. The most serious toxicity is interstitial fibrosis of the lung leading to shortness of breath and death of some patients; its incidence is related to cumulative dose, age, renal function, and the use of other agents that may damage the lung, such as high oxygen concentrations or radiation therapy.

lism, and elimination half-lives of 10 to 12 hours (Sonnichsen and Relling, 1994). As hepatic elimination to inactive metabolites is mediated through cytochrome P-450 enzymes, agents that influence cytochrome P-450 can modify the clearance and toxicity of the taxanes; thus patients on anticonvulsants have demonstrated increased clearance and reduced toxicity. For paclitaxel, the severity of neutropenia correlates best with the duration that plasma concentration exceeds a critical threshold level ranging from 0.05 to 0.1 micromole per liter. Paclitaxel is generally given as a 3-hour infusion, although longer infusion schedules have better activity in vitro and are undergoing clinical testing. Both paclitaxel and docetaxel are substrates for P-glycoprotein, so that MDR plays a clinically important role in conferring resistance to the taxanes (see Chap. 18, Sec. 18.2.3). Alterations of microtubule structure resulting in altered microtubule dynamics and/or binding of the taxanes to tubulin may also contribute to drug resistance (Dumontet and Sikic, 1999).

Paclitaxel and docetaxel share many common toxicities. The dose-limiting toxicity is a noncumulative myelosuppression, mainly neutropenia, with increased

## 16.7.2 Mitomycin C

Mitomycin C is derived from a *Streptomyces* species and is a quinone-containing compound that requires activation to an alkylating metabolite by reductive metabolism. Because of the requirement for reductive metabolism, the drug is more active against hypoxic than aerobic cells, at least in tissue culture. Mitomycin C causes delayed and rather unpredictable myelosuppression. More seriously, the drug can produce kidney failure through a hemolytic-uremic syndrome, which is usually fatal and is probably due to small-vessel endothelial damage. Another potentially lethal effect is interstitial lung disease with progression to pulmonary fibrosis. The availability of equally active drugs with lower toxicities limits the clinical utility of mitomycin C. It is sometimes instilled into the bladder by a catheter to treat superficial bladder cancer and is also used with radiation therapy to treat cancer of the anal canal.

## 16.8 MOLECULAR TARGETED AGENTS

Advances in molecular biology have provided a better understanding of intricate cellular pathways that are critical to tumor formation and growth. A new era of anticancer drug development has arrived with the emergence of molecular targeted therapy, whereby DNA is no longer the principal therapeutic target, as is the case for most of the drugs discussed previously. Molecular targeted agents offer attractive therapeutic options due to the potential for greater specificity and less toxicity than is found for most cytotoxic agents described above. Aberrant expression or alterations in molecular targets tend to be present at higher frequencies in tumors than normal tissues, enabling specificity and selectivity with the novel agents. Some of the current approaches to molecular targeted therapy are described in Chapter 17, Section 17.6. Many drugs are under development and for most of them it is uncertain whether they will find a role in routine clinical practice. Monoclonal antibodies with therapeutic application are described in Chapter 21, Section 21.3.4, and below we describe briefly the important properties of other selected targeted agents.

**Imatinib (Gleevec)** is an orally available derivative of the 2-phenylaminopyrimidine series of protein tyrosine kinase inhibitors. Imatinib inhibits the tyrosine kinase of the constitutively active fusion product *BCR-ABL* arising from the Philadelphia (Ph) chromosome of chronic myelogenous leukemia (CML; Druker et al., 2001; see Chap. 7, Sec. 7.2.4 and Chap. 17, Sec. 17.6.2). Imatinib has led to a large increase in the rate of remission in CML as compared to treatment with chemotherapy and interferon (Hughes et al., 2003). A variety of mechanisms are involved in the development of resistance of CML to imatinib, and CML stem cells may be inher-

ently more resistant than their differentiated progency which constitute the bulk of disease (reviewed in Jones et al., 2004). Imatinib also inhibits the tyrosine kinase of c-kit (CD-117, stem cell factor), which is overexpressed in gastrointestinal stromal tumors (GIST), and is more effective than other agents in inducing remission of this disease (Demetri et al., 2002). Imatinib has inhibitory activity against the tyrosine kinase of the platelet-derived growth factor receptor (PDGFR), and studies evaluating its activity against this target are ongoing. Imatinib has been approved by the United States Food and Drug Administration (FDA) for the treatment of CML and GIST.

The recommended dosing of imatinib is 400 to 600 mg daily. Side effects from imatinib experienced in >10% of patients included nausea, diarrhea, edema, dermatitis, muscle cramps, fatigue, abdominal pain, headache, flatulence, vomiting, and dyspepsia. Imatinib is well absorbed after oral administration with $C_{max}$ achieved within 2 to 4 h post-dose. Mean absolute bioavailability is 98%, with a mean half-life in the circulation of approximately 20 hours. The mean plasma concentration increases with dose.

**Erlotinib (Tarceva) and gefitinib (Iressa)** are orally active, low molecular weight, synthetic quinazolines which are selective inhibitors of the EGFR tyrosine kinase (Chap. 8, Sec. 8.2.2). These agents cause diarrhea and an acneiform skin rash involving the face and upper trunk. Other toxicities are generally mild and consist of nausea and vomiting, elevation in bilirubin, headaches, and mucositis. These agents have elimination half-lives in the range of 24 hours. Phase II evaluations have shown modest activity in head and neck and gynecological malignancies. In patients with non–small-cell lung cancer (NSCLC), large randomized trials of erlotinib or gefitinib given in combination with cytotoxic chemotherapy demonstrated no survival benefit over chemotherapy alone (e.g., Giaccone et al., 2004). As single agents in patients with NSCLC who are refractory to one or two lines of chemotherapy these agents lead to symptomatic responses and may cause a modest increase in survival (Kris et al., 2003; Shepherd et al., 2004). The expression of EGFR has not been predictive of efficacy in the study of EGFR tyrosine kinase inhibitors, but recent data have shown that the presence of EGFR activation mutations correlate well with tumor response (Lynch et al., 2004; Paez et al., 2004). The monoclonal antibody cetuximab is another clinically approved agent that is directed against the EGFR, but acts by binding to the external domain of the receptor (see Chap. 21, Sec. 21.3.4).

**Bortezomib (PS341, Velcade)** is a dipeptide boronic acid derivative synthesized as a highly selective, potent, reversible inhibitor of the proteasome, which is involved in degradation and recycling of cellular proteins (Chap. 9, Fig. 9.4). Using the National Cancer Institute's in vitro screen, bortezomib showed cytotoxicity against a range of tumor cell lines and had antitumor activity in human prostate and lung cancer xenograft models (Adams et al., 1999; Teicher et al., 1999). Phase I evaluations of bortezomib using a schedule of twice weekly intravenous injections for 2 weeks, followed by a 1-week recovery period, every 3 weeks, have been conducted in patients with solid and hematological malignancies. Pharmacokinetic studies demonstrated that the mean elimination half-life after the first bortezomib dose varied from 9 to 15 h. The drug is metabolized by cytochrome P450-3A4, -2D6, -2C19, -2C9, and -1A2. Safety and efficacy were evaluated in a Phase II study of 202 patients wtih multiple myeloma who had received at least two prior therapies and had demonstrated disease progression on their most recent therapy. The overall response rate was 28% with complete responses in 5 of 188 evaluable patients (Bross et al., 2004). The drug is quite toxic and adverse events occurring in more than 30% of patients included fatigue and malaise, nausea and vomiting, diarrhea, decreased appetite, constipation, thrombocytopenia, peripheral neuropathy, fevers and anemia. The FDA has granted marketing approval for bortezomib for the treatment of multiple myeloma in patients who have disease progression after at least two prior therapies. Studies in patients with solid tumors, especially prostate cancer, are ongoing.

**Tipifarnib (Zarnestra),** a quinolone analog of imidazole, is an oral farnesyltransferase inhibitor, which inhibits signaling from the *RAS* oncogene (see Chap. 7, Sec. 7.3.2 and Chap. 17, Sec. 17.6.2). It has antiproliferative activity against pancreatic cell lines in vitro, and in nude mice tipifarnib inhibited growth of xenografts bearing mutated and wild-type *RAS* genes. Inhibition of proliferation, angiogenesis, and apoptosis was observed in different xenograft models (End et al., 2001). Tipifarnib has dose-limiting toxicities of myelosuppression and neurotoxicity. Phase II and III development of this agent in solid tumors has been largely disappointing: for example, a randomized phase III trial of tipifarnib plus gemcitabine versus placebo plus gemcitabine in patients with advanced pancreatic cancer showed no survival benefit (Van Cutsem et al., 2004). However, the use of tipifarnib in hematological malignancies, particularly those of myeloid origin, appears more promising.

The optimal ways to incorporate molecular targeted therapy into clinical practice remains uncertain. In the setting of locally advanced disease, addition of molecular targeted agents to a definitive therapeutic modality such as radiotherapy or surgery might augment tu-

mor control; for example, by inhibition of repopulation of surviving tumor cells during fractionated radiotherapy (Chap. 15, Sec. 15.6.2). Some agents have demonstrated additive or synergistic effects when administered concurrently with radiotherapy in preclinical models. Use of such agents as adjuvant therapy after radiation or surgery is appealing, given that they are most likely to be effective against a minimal tumor burden. For patients with advanced stages of cancer, some agents discussed above have led to tumor responses and good palliation for some patients. However, most molecular targeted agents are cytostatic and are unlikely to cause shrinkage of large tumors. They might add to the beneficial effects of conventional cytotoxic agents, although careful attention to scheduling will be needed because a cytostatic agent may decrease the efficacy of a cycle-dependent cytotoxic drug.

## 16.9 SUMMARY

Anticancer drugs are grouped for convenience into categories based on their mechanism of action or derivation. The intracellular effects that lead to cell death following administration of these drugs are varied and complex, but most of them cause damage to DNA, either directly or indirectly. Several anticancer drugs have been introduced in the past few years. These include not only analogs of previously existing drugs, such as vinorelbine or gemcitabine, but also new categories of agents with different cellular targets and novel mechanisms of action, such as the taxanes and the camptothecin derivatives. With increased understanding of aberrant molecular pathways in cancer cells, emphasis in drug development has now shifted to molecular targeted agents.

The efficacy of anticancer drugs depends on drug concentration and time of exposure, which in turn depend on absorption, metabolism, distribution, and excretion. An understanding of the basic components of the pharmacology of these drugs is essential if we are to use them effectively and safely. New advances in the field of pharmacogenomics provide further insights to explain inter-patient differences in toxicity and response to chemotherapeutic drugs. Ultimately the delivery of systemic therapy may be tailored and customized to molecular properties of the tumor and of the patient.

## REFERENCES

Adams J, Palombella VJ, Sausville EA, et al: Proteasome inhibitors: a novel class of potent and effective antitumor agents. *Cancer Res* 1999; 59:2615–2622.

Adjei AA: Pemetrexed: a multitargeted antifolate agent with promising activity in solid tumors. *Ann Oncol* 2000; 11: 1335–1341.

Benvenuto JA, Ayele W, Legha SS, et al: Clinical pharmaco-kinetics of ifosfamide in combination with N-acetylcys-teine. *Anticancer Drugs* 1992; 3:19–23.

Blommaert F, van Kijk-Knijnenburg H, Dijt F, et al: Forma-tion of DNA adducts by the anticancer drug carboplatin: different nucleotide sequence preferences in vitro and in cells. *Biochemistry* 1995; 34:8474.

Boulikas T, Vougiouka M: Cisplatin and platinum drugs at the molecular level. (Review.) *Oncol Rep* 2003; 10:1663–1682.

Bross PF, Kane R, Farrell AT, et al: Approval summary for bortezomib for injection in the treatment of multiple myeloma. *Cancer Res* 2004; 10:3954–3964.

Calvert AH, Newell DR, Gumbrell LA, et al: Carboplatin dos-age: prospective evaluation of a simple formula based on renal function. *J Clin Oncol* 1989; 7:1748.

Collins JM: Pharmacologic rationale for regional drug deliv-ery. *J Clin Oncol* 1984; 2:498–504.

Danesi R, DeBraud R, Fogli S, et al: Pharmacogenetic deter-minants of anti-cancer drug activity and toxicity. *Trends Pharm Sci* 2001; 22:420–426.

Demetri GD, von Mehren M, Blanke CD, et al: Efficacy and safety of imatinib mesylate in advanced gastrointestinal stromal tumors. *N Engl J Med* 2002; 347:472–480.

Diasio RB, Johnson MR: The role of pharmacogenetics and pharmacogenomics in cancer chemotherapy with 5-fluo-rouracil. *Pharmacology* 2000; 61:199–203.

Douillard JY, Cunningham D, Roth AD, et al: Irinotecan com-bined with fluorouracil compared with fluorouracil alone as first-line treatment for metastatic colorectal cancer: a multicentre randomised trial. *Lancet* 2000; 355:1041–1047.

Druker BJ, Talpaz M, Resta DJ, et al: Efficacy and safety of a specific inhibitor of the BRC-ABL tyrosine kinase in chronic myeloid leukemia. *N Engl J Med* 2001; 344:1031–1037.

Dumontet C, Sikic BI: Mechanisms of action of and resistance to antitubulin agents: microtubule dynamics, drug trans-port, and cell death. *J Clin Oncol* 1999; 17:1061–1070.

Eastman A: The formation, isolation and characterization of DNA adducts produced by anticancer platinum com-plexes. *Pharmacol Ther* 1987; 34:155.

Eder JP, Teicher BA, Holder SA, et al: Ability of 4 potential topoisomerase II inhibitors to enhance the cytotoxicity of cisplatin in Chinese hamster ovary cells and in epipodo-phyllotoxin-resistant subline. *Cancer Chemother Pharmacol* 1990; 26:423–428.

End DW, Smets G, Todd AV, et al: Characterization of the an-titumor effects of the selective farnesyl protein transferase inhibitor R115777 in vivo and in vitro. *Cancer Res* 2001; 61:131–137.

Giaccone G, Herbst RS, Manegold C, et al: Gefitinib in com-bination with gemcitabine and cisplatin in advanced non-small-cell lung cancer: a phase III trial—INTACT 1. *J Clin Oncol* 2004; 22:777–784.

Gieseler F, Biersack H, Brieden T, et al: Cytotoxicity of an-thracyclines: correlation with cellular uptake, intracellular distribution and DNA binding. *Ann Hematol* 1994; 69(Suppl 1):S13–S17.

Go RS, Adjei AA: A review of the comparative pharmacology and clinical activity of cisplatin and carboplatin. *J Clin On-col* 1999; 17:409–422.

Gordon AN, Fleagle JT, Guthrie D, et al: Recurrent epithelial ovarian carcinoma: a randomized phase III study of pegy-lated liposomal doxorubicin versus topotecan. *J Clin On-col* 2001; 19:3312–3322.

Gupta E, Lestingi TM, Mick R, et al: Metabolic fate of irinote-can in humans: correlation of glucuronidation with diar-rhea. *Cancer Res* 1994; 54:3723–3725.

Hoff PM, Ansari R, Batist G, et al: Comparison of oral capecitabine versus intravenous fluorouracil plus leucov-orin as first-line treatment in 605 patients with metastatic colorectal cancer: results of a randomized phase III study. *J Clin Oncol* 2001; 19:2282–2292.

Huang P, Chubb S, Hertel LW, et al: Action of gemcitabine on DNA synthesis. *Cancer Res* 1991; 51:6110–6117.

Hughes TP, Kaeda J, Branford S, et al: Frequency of major molecular responses to imatinib or interferon alfa plus cy-tarabine in newly diagnosed chronic myeloid leukemia. *N Engl J Med* 2003; 349:1423–1432.

Johnson S, Ferry K, Hamilton T: Recent insights into platinum drug resistance in cancer. *Drug Resist Updat* 1998; 1:243.

Jones RJ, Matsui WH, Smith BD. Cancer stem cells: are we missing the target? *J Natl Cancer Inst* 2004; 96:583–585.

Kastan MB, Schlaffer E, Russo JE, et al: Direct demonstration of elevated aldehyde dehydrogenase in human hemato-poietic progenitor cells. *Blood* 1990; 75:1947–1950.

Kawato Y, Aonuma M, Hirota Y, et al: Intracellular roles of SN-38, a metabolite of the camptothecin derivative CPT-11, in the antitumor effect of CPT-11. *Cancer Res* 1991; 51: 4187–4191.

Keating MJ, O'Brien S, Plunkett W, et al: Fludarabine phos-phate: a new active agent in hematogic malignancies. *Semin Hematol* 1994; 31:28–39.

Kintzel PE, Dorr RT: Anticancer drug renal toxicity and elim-ination: dosing guidelines for altered renal function. *Can-cer Treat Rev* 1995; 21:33.

Kris MG, Natale RB, Herbst RS, et al: Efficacy of gefitinib, an inhibitor of the epidermal growth factor receptor tyrosine kinase, in symptomatic patients with non-small cell lung cancer: a randomized trial. *JAMA* 2003; 290:2149–2158.

Lazo JS, Chabner BA: Bleomycin. In Chabner BA, Longo DL, eds. *Cancer Chemotherapy and Biotherapy*. Philadelphia: Lip-pincott; 1996:263–275.

Lilleyman JS, Lennard L: Mercaptopurine metabolism and risk of relapse in childhood lymphoblastic leukemia. *Lancet* 1994; 343:1188.

Lynch TJ, Bell DW, Sordella R, et al: Activating mutations in the epidermal growth factor receptor underlying respon-siveness of non-small-cell lung cancer to gefitinib. *N Engl J Med* 2004; 350:2129–2139.

Milano G, Etienne MC: Dihydropyrimidine dehydro-genase (DPD) and clinical pharmacology of 5-fluorouracil (re-view). *Anticancer Res* 1994; 14:2295–2297.

Moore MJ: Clinical pharmacokinetics of cyclophosphamide. *Clin Pharmacokinet* 1991; 20:194–208.

Moran RG, Keyomarsi K: Biochemical rationale for the syn-ergism of 5–fluorouracil and folinic acid. *Natl Cancer Inst Monogr* 1987; 5:159–163.

Paez JG, Janne PA, Lee JC, et al: EGFR mutations in lung can-cer: correlation with clinical response to gefitinib therapy. *Science* 2004; 304:1497–1500.

Plunkett W, Huang P, Xu YZ, et al: Gemcitabine: metabolism, mechanisms of action, and self-potentiation. *Semin Oncol* 1995; 22(Suppl 11):3–10.

Pommier Y: DNA topoisomerases I & II in cancer chemotherapy. *Cancer Chemother Pharmacol* 1993; 32:103–112.

Ratain MJ: Body-surface area as a basis for dosing of anticancer agents: science, myth, or habit? *J Clin Oncol* 1998; 16:2297.

Rixe O, Ortuzar W, Alvarez M, et al: Oxaliplatin, tetraplatin, cisplatin, and carboplatin: spectrum of activity in drug-resistant cell lines and in the cell lines of the National Cancer Institute's anticancer drug screen panel. *Biochem Pharmacol* 1996; 52:1855–1865.

Robert J, Gianni L: Pharmacokinetics and metabolism of anthracyclines. *Cancer Surv* 1993; 17:219–252.

Rowinsky EK, Donehower RD: Paclitaxel. *N Engl J Med* 1995; 332:1004–1014.

Rowinsky E, Donehower R: In Chabner BA, Longo DL, eds. *Cancer Chemotherapy and Biotherapy.* Philadelphia: Lippincott; 1996:379–393.

Saltz LB, Cox JV, Blanke C, et al: Irinotecan plus fluorouracil and leucovorin for metastatic colorectal cancer. Irinotecan Study Group. *N Engl J Med* 2000; 343:905–914.

Scagliotti GV, Shin DM, Kindler HL, et al: Phase II study of pemetrexed with and without folic acid and vitamin B12 as front-line therapy in malignant pleural mesothelioma. *J Clin Oncol* 2003; 1:1556–1561.

Shepherd FA, Pereira J, Ciuleanu TE, et al: A randomized placebo-controlled trial of erlotinib in patients with advanced non-small cell lung cancer (NSCLC) following failure of 1st line or 2nd line chemotherapy. A National Cancer Institute of Canada Clinical Trials Group (NCIC CTG) Trial. *Proc Am Soc Clin Oncol* 2004; 23(abstract 7022).

Shewach DS, Hahn TM, Chang E, et al: Metabolism of 2'-2'-difluoro-2'deoxycytidine and radiation sensitization of human colon carcinoma cells. *Cancer Res* 1994; 54:3218–3223.

Sonnichsen DS, Relling MV: Clinical pharmacokinetics of paclitaxel. *Clin Pharmacokinet* 1994; 27:256–269.

Teicher BA, Ara G, Herbst R, et al: The proteasome inhibitor PS-341 in cancer therapy. *Clin Cancer Res* 1999; 5:2638–2645.

Touroutoglou N, Pazdur R: Thymidylate synthase inhibitors (review). *Clin Cancer Res* 1996; 2:227–243.

Tritton TR, Yee G: The anticancer agent Adriamycin can be actively cytotoxic without entering cells. *Science* 1982; 217:248–250.

Van Cutsem E, Twelves C, Cassidy J, et al: Oral capecitabine compared with intravenous fluorouracil plus leucovorin in patients with metastatic colorectal cancer: results of a large phase III trial. *J Clin Oncol* 2001; 19:4097–4106.

Van Cutsem E, van de Velde H, Karasek P, et al: Phase III trial of gemcitabine plus tipifarnib compared with gemcitabine plus placebo in advanced pancreatic cancer. *J Clin Oncol* 2004; 22:1430–1438.

Van Mannen JM, Retel J, de Vries J, Pinedo HM: Mechanism of action of antitumor drug etoposide: a review. *J Natl Cancer Inst* 1988; 80:1526–1533.

Von Pawel J, Schiller JH, Shepherd FA, et al: Topotecan versus cyclophosphamide, doxorubicin, and vincristine for the treatment of recurrent small-cell lung cancer. *J Clin Oncol* 1999; 17:658–667.

Winick NJ, McKenna RW, Shuster JJ, et al: Secondary acute myeloid leukemia in children with acute lymphoblastic leukemia treated with etoposide. *J Clin Oncol* 1993; 11:209–217.

# 17

# Cellular and Molecular Basis of Drug Treatment for Cancer

*Michael J. Boyer and Ian F. Tannock*

## 17.1 INTRODUCTION

Chemotherapy is used primarily as: (1) the major curative modality for a few types of malignancies, such as Hodgkin's disease and other lymphomas, acute leukemia in children, and testicular cancer in men; (2) palliative treatment for many types of advanced cancers; and (3) adjuvant treatment before, during, or after local treatment (surgery and/or radiotherapy) with the aim of both eradicating occult micrometastases and of improving local control of the primary tumor. Such treatments usually involve a combination of drugs. The most important factors underlying the successful use of drugs in combination are (1) the ability to combine drugs at close to full tolerated doses with additive effects against tumors and less than additive toxicities to normal tissues and (2) the expectation that drug combinations will include at least one drug to which the tumor is sensitive.

Since the first documented clinical use of chemotherapy in 1942, when the alkylating agent nitrogen mustard was used to obtain a brief clinical remission in a patient with lymphoma, about forty-five cytotoxic drugs or biological agents (excluding hormonal agents) have been licensed for use in North America, and several more are undergoing clinical trials. The pharmacology of many of these agents has been described in Chapter 16. In recent years, new types of anticancer agents have been developed. These include monoclonal antibodies (such as rituximab, trastuzumab and bevacizumab) which target a range of cell surface receptors, and small molecules that interact with various cell signaling pathways (e.g., imatinib). These newer agents represent a substantial shift in emphasis in anticancer drug therapy. In contrast to conventional cytotoxic agents, these drugs do not interact with DNA or interfere directly with its replication. Rather, they interfere with the function of normal cellular pathways that promote cell division (trastuzumab, imatinib) or contribute to immune-mediated cellular damage (rituximab). Other agents, such as those that inhibit angiogenesis (e.g., bevacizumab, see Chap. 12, Sec. 12.4.2) act indirectly to inhibit tumor growth.

This chapter deals with the scientific basis underlying the treatment of cancer by drugs. It introduces the biologic properties of important anticancer drugs, experimental methods used to determine their activity, their toxicity to normal tissues and the concept of therapeutic index, interactions between therapeutic agents, and some of the methods used to discover and design new drugs. The many causes of drug resistance will be reviewed in Chapter 18.

## 17.2 CELLULAR EFFECTS OF DRUGS

### 17.2.1 Assessment of Cell Damage

For cancer treatment to be effective, therapy must cause sufficient damage to the tumor cells such that they lose their capacity for indefinite proliferation, and therefore the ability to regenerate the tumor. Tumor cells that have this property of indefinite proliferation are known as *tumor stem cells* (Chap. 9, Sec. 9.4.4) and loss of reproductive integrity of tumor stem cells is the important goal of treatment. There is a high rate of cell death in untreated tumors (Chap. 9, Sec. 9.4.5) and many tumor cells (by virtue of differentiation and/or unknown genotypic and phenotypic changes) may have lost this capacity for reproduction and are destined to die in the absence of cancer treatment. Tumor cells with a limited capacity for proliferation may constitute the majority of cells in many tumors, and may or may not have morphological characteristics that enable them to be distinguished from the tumor stem cells that are the more important targets of therapy. For this reason, assays of cell damage that rely on morphological changes to cancer cells may give misleading information about the effects of cancer treatment.

In practice, the activity of drugs against the more important population of tumor stem cells is assessed by their ability to produce colonies of progeny of a defined minimum size when placed in an environment that allows them to proliferate. Thus, measurement of cell survival after drug treatment is analogous to that for radiation, and involves the use of a clonogenic assay (Chap. 14, Sec. 14.3.1). Other types of damage, leading to transient changes in cell metabolism and proliferation and loss of nonclonogenic cells, occur frequently after drug treatment. These effects, which can lead to normal-tissue toxicity (Sec. 17.4), may contrib-

ute to tumor remission (i.e., to transient changes in tumor volume) but not to cure.

An in vitro assay that could predict the responsiveness of human tumors to drugs would be very valuable. Such predictive assays would be analogous to those used in selecting antibiotics to treat bacterial infections, where sensitivity of the bacteria to a range of antibiotics can be assessed in culture. Several of the assays described below have been evaluated for their ability to predict the responsiveness of individual human tumors.

### 17.2.2 Nonclonogenic Assays

Colony-forming assays (see following section) are time consuming, and are limited by the environment in which colony formation is assessed. Nonclonogenic assays can be performed more rapidly and can easily be automated. Such assays apply to an unselected population of tumor cells, rather than solely to the important subpopulation of stem cells. However, they may correlate with the more important effects of drugs against tumor stem cells and therefore have potential use in screening for drug activity and for prediction of drug effects against human tumors. Some of the measures of cell damage that have been used in nonclonogenic assays of drug activity are listed in Table 17.1

If the assessment of toxicity is delayed for a few hours to days after drug exposure, thereby allowing for the expression of lethal damage and/or the proliferation of surviving cells, then exclusion of dye from intact cells or assessment of metabolic activity can give reasonable

**Table 17.1.** Nonclonogenic Assays Used to Assess Drug Activity

- Microscopic evidence of cell damage
- Damage to cell membranes, as measured by failure to exclude dyes such as trypan blue, or loss of radioactivity (e.g., $^{51}Cr$) from prelabeled cells
- Separation of live from dead cells by their ability to metabolize colored dyes such as tetrazolium blue (MTT assay) or sulforhodamine B
- Inhibition of cell growth under defined conditions, which may be assessed in multiple samples by automated methods (e.g., by the MTT assay)
- Impairment of macromolecular synthesis, usually assessed by measuring the uptake of $^3H$-thymidine into DNA, $^3H$-uridine into RNA, or $^3H$-amino acids into proteins
- Changes in proliferative parameters such as thymidine-labeling index or S-phase fraction assessed by flow cytometry
- Formation of micronuclei in cells
- Exchange of sister chromatids detected at mitosis as an assay of damage to DNA
- Assays of apoptosis (e.g., by the TUNEL or other assays)

correlations with a colony-forming assay (Scheithauer et al., 1986). The methyl thiazole tetrazolium (MTT) assay depends on the reduction of a tetrazolium-based compound to a blue formazan product by living but not dead cells (Carmichael et al., 1987). The amount of reduced product is quantified in an automated system using multiple tissue-culture wells in which cells have been exposed to a range of doses of the drugs under test. Another dye that has been found to be useful in quantifying cell number is sulforhodamine B (SRB), a pink anionic dye that binds to basic amino acids of fixed cells such that dye intensity is linearly related to the number of cells. These methods are being used in the screening of new agents and technical factors must be optimized for each cell type studied.

Following treatment with drugs, certain types of tumor cells may undergo apoptosis. Apoptosis can be quantified by various methods (e.g., by TUNEL staining; Chap. 10, Sec. 10.3) to provide an estimate of the number of cells undergoing apoptosis or an apoptotic index. This index generally increases after drug treatment of tumors, and the proportion of cells undergoing apoptosis may give a broad indication of drug effectiveness. However, there is evidence that radiation and drugs often kill cancer cells by mechanisms other than apoptosis. Even where apoptosis is an important mechanism leading to drug-induced cell death, it is a dynamic process whose assessment can be very dependent on the time after treatment that measurements are made (Potten, 1996).

Predictive assays employing a variety of the end points listed in Table 17.1 have been used to assess the effects of anticancer drugs against biopsies from human tumors since the early days of chemotherapy. Such tests have been quite successful in predicting clinical resistance to chemotherapy (i.e., if a drug had no effect in the assay, it had no therapeutic effect in the patient donating the biopsy). Unfortunately the assays have had less success in predicting those tumors that were sensitive to drugs. For example, an assay based on the efficacy of drugs to inhibit DNA synthesis did not lead to improvement in survival of patients with ovarian or lung cancer when drugs selected by the in vitro assay were compared with empirical treatment (or to no adjuvant therapy) in randomized clinical trials (Nissen et al., 1978).

A general problem with most of the nonclonogenic assays is that they provide a measure of cell death or damage that is quantified on a linear scale from 0 to 100 percent. Major effects of drugs against a tumor-cell population require reduction in cell survival by several orders of magnitude; this is measured most easily by observation of colony formation from serial dilutions of cells, as described below. Even when cell survival (assessed by colony formation) is less than 1 percent, many

of the cells in the population appear to be viable by morphologic or metabolic criteria at short intervals after treatment. For these reasons, many nonclonogenic assays of cell damage correlate poorly with loss of reproductive integrity as measured by a colony-forming assay.

### 17.2.3 Colony-Forming Assays and Cell Survival Curves

Colony-forming assays were described in Chapter 14, Section 14.3.1 as methods for assessment of the lethal effects of radiation. The same assays are often used for assessing the lethal effects of drugs against tumor cells (Table 17.2). An important difference is that even high doses of radiation may be delivered over a few seconds or minutes, whereas some drugs require exposures of several hours to exert lethal effects on cells. Metabolism of the drug to active or inactive products during the exposure period may thus influence cell survival, and the effectiveness of a drug is dependent on both its concentration and the duration of exposure. It is usual to relate cell survival after drug treatment to both the drug concentration (for a constant exposure time) and to the duration of exposure (at a constant drug concentration).

The simplest assay to assess drug-induced lethality is to treat cells in tissue culture with the drug to be tested, followed by plating of different dilutions of cells in Petri dishes. Colony-forming assays in culture may also be used to study drug effects in vivo by using tumors whose cells have the ability to generate colonies in vitro following removal and dissociation of the tumor. Assessment of colony formation after treatment of transplanted tumors in vivo allows for drug metabolism and other aspects of drug pharmacology to be assessed. Toxicity to colony-forming cells of the bone marrow can also be determined by removal and culture of marrow in the same experiment. The problem with these assays is that

**Table 17.2.** Assays Used to Quantitate Stem Cells After Drug Treatment

- Colony formation on plastic or glass in liquid medium
- Colony formation in semisolid medium such as dilute agar or methylcellulose
- Serial dilution of cells into multiwell plates to establish the minimum number of cells that will lead to growth
- Serial dilutions of tumor cells implanted into syngeneic animals to establish the $TD_{50}$ (i.e., the number of cells that lead to growth of tumors in 50% of animals)
- Formation of spleen colonies after intravenous injection of hematologic cells (either malignant or normal bone marrow stem cells) into irradiated mice
- Formation of metastatic lung colonies after intravenous injection of tumor cells into mice

cells are removed from their native environment. The results of the assays are therefore subject to the assumption that colony, forming ability in the new environment is a true reflection of reproductive ability that would be expressed if the tumor cells were left in their original environment.

Courtenay and colleagues (1976) and Hamburger and Salmon (1977) developed assays using semisolid agar and enriched media that support colony growth from cell suspensions derived from a variety of human tumors. These assays have been used to predict the responsiveness of individual human tumors to chemotherapy, but have several limitations relating to the suitability of the growth conditions and to factors such as preparing suspensions of single cells and the separation of residual clumps from colonies (Selby et al., 1983). About 70 percent of human tumors will generate sufficient colonies in appropriate medium to allow assessment of drug effects. As for nonclonogenic assays, these assays are quite good at predicting resistance to treatment, but they are less reliable in predicting drug sensitivity. The response rate (i.e., decrease in volume) of tumors in patients treated with drugs selected by predictive assays is higher than that in patients treated empirically (von Hoff et al., 1991). However, there has been no evidence that the assays lead to improved survival of patients, and they should not be used outside of a research setting (Samson et al., 2004; Schrag et al., 2004).

In colony-forming assays, the proportion of cells surviving treatment with some drugs is related exponentially to drug concentration. As in the analysis of radi-ation effects (Chap. 14, Sec. 14.3.1), cell survival curves are often plotted using a logarithmic axis for cell survival and a linear axis for either drug concentration (using a constant exposure time) or for exposure time to a constant drug concentration. Exponential survival curves are then represented by straight lines (Fig. 17.1A). Exponential cell survival curves are expected if cell lethality is due to an interaction between molecules of the drug and a molecular target in the cell. The relationship is then analogous to the interaction of ionizing events due to radiation with a molecular target (thought to be DNA).

Tumors and normal tissues contain cells that are heterogeneous with respect to proliferative rate and intrinsic drug sensitivity; the latter depends on many factors including drug uptake and retention and the proficiency for repair of drug-induced damage. In addition, limited diffusion of some drugs and changes in activity due to metabolism may lead to delivery of varying drug concentrations to cells within the population (Chap. 18, Sec. 18.3.3). Each of these factors may influence the shape of the cell survival curve after drug treatment, so that departures from an exponential relationship between cell survival and dose occur commonly (Fig 17.1B and C). As discussed in subsequent sections, the shape of the dose-survival relationship may give important clues to mechanisms underlying drug activity.

### 17.2.4 Cell Cycle Effects

Most cytotoxic drugs that have been selected for clinical use are more active against proliferating cells rather

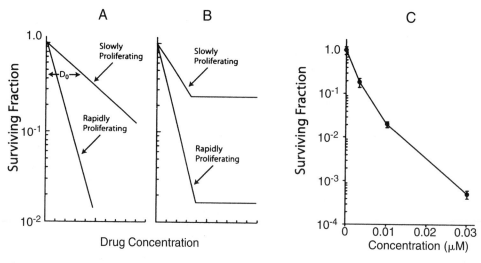

**Figure 17.1.** Model cell survival curves for rapidly and slowly proliferating cells generated following a short duration of exposure to varying concentrations of drugs (A) for drugs that are not cell-cycle–phase specific; (B) for drugs that are active in only certain phases of the cell cycle. (C) Experimentally determined cell survival curve for EMT-6 cells exposed to the drug mitoxantrone.

than tumor cells per se. This property explains their relatively low specificity for tumors and their common side effects against proliferating normal tissues such as bone marrow (see Sec. 17.4).

Two types of assay have been used to demonstrate the relative toxicity of anticancer drugs for rapidly proliferating and slowly proliferating cells of the same genetic origin. If tumor cells are adapted to grow in tissue culture, they will first grow exponentially when their concentration is initially low, but will proliferate more slowly when the cell number is such that the cells are now in contact (plateau phase). This enables both rapidly proliferating and slowly proliferating cells to be treated with drugs, and then to be re-plated to assess colony-forming ability. Most drugs have greater toxicity for exponentially growing cells than for plateau phase cells that are proliferating slowly (Fig. 17.1A). Exceptions to this include the nitrosoureas (BCNU, CCNU), bleomycin, and cisplatin, which show similar effects against proliferating and nonproliferating cells (Twentyman and Bleehan, 1975).

In the second method, known as the spleen colony assay, bone marrow or lymphoma cells from drug-treated or control mice are injected into irradiated genetically identical animals, where they will generate colonies in the spleen after a few days. The recipient animals are killed and these spleen colonies are counted to estimate the number of surviving stem cells. This assay has been used to compare the effects of drugs on the cell survival of slowly proliferating bone marrow precursors (CFU-S) with either rapidly proliferating murine lymphoma cells or with CFU-S that have been induced to proliferate (Bruce et al., 1969; Van Putten et al., 1972). Two basic shapes of survival curve can be obtained. For some drugs, including most of the alkylating agents and 5-fluorouracil, cell survival is exponentially related to dose, with most drugs having greater activity against proliferating cells (Fig. 17.1A). For other drugs, survival decreases exponentially at low drug doses, but with short exposure times there is no further decrease in survival above a threshold drug concentration, leading to a plateau in the cell survival curve (Fig. 17.1B). The plateau level of cell survival is always lower for rapidly proliferating cells. Drugs that show the latter pattern of survival are now known to act primarily at one phase of the cell cycle (see below); they include most of the antimetabolites such as methotrexate, cytosine arabinoside, 6-thioguanine, and 6-mercaptopurine, and tubulin-binding agents, such as vincristine and vinblastine. An increase in concentration of cell-cycle–specific drugs with a short exposure time gives no further cell kill once a threshold is exceeded because all cells in the drug-sensitive phase of the cycle are killed and those in the other phases of the cell cycle are not affected. An increase in exposure time with constant

drug concentration may allow more cells to enter the drug-sensitive phase, leading to an exponential relationship between cell survival and exposure time (Bruce et al., 1969). However, many drugs also inhibit the transit of surviving cells through the cell cycle (and hence their progression into the sensitive phase of the cycle).

For drugs that show an exponential relationship between cell survival and dose (Fig. 17.1A), the relative sensitivity of rapidly and slowly proliferating cells may be expressed as the ratio of doses required to achieve the same level of cell kill. Values of this ratio generally lie between 1.0 and 2.0 for alkylating agents, but cyclophosphamide has greater specificity for cycling cells with values in the range of 2.0 to 5.0 when tested using the spleen colony assay. Doxorubicin, 5-fluorouracil, and bleomycin also show marked selectivity for proliferating cells. Thus, the proliferative rate of the cell population being treated is a major determinant of drug activity.

Information about the activities of drugs at different phases of the cell cycle has been obtained by treatment of cells that have been synchronized in tissue culture (e.g., Donaldson et al., 1994). As cells progress in a cohort around the cell cycle, drug administration may be timed to treat a population that is enriched for cells in G1, S, G2, or mitotic phase. Alternative methods for studying drug effects involve separation of asynchronous cells on the basis of cell cycle phase either before or immediately after drug treatment, followed by assessment of colony formation. Techniques that have been used for this purpose include separation of cells on the basis of DNA content by flow cytometry (Chap. 9, Sec. 9.4.2) or separation by size or density using centrifugation (Donaldson et al., 1994).

Most drugs show variations in lethal toxicity around the cell cycle (Fig. 17.2). Many of the antimetabolites exert lethal toxicity only for cells that are synthesizing DNA, whereas methotrexate and doxorubicin have maximum toxicity for S-phase cells but have some activity during other phases of the cycle. Studies using thymidine labeling or flow cytometry have demonstrated that many of these drugs also inhibit the onset or continuation of DNA synthesis in cells that survive treatment. Such studies of nonlethal progression delay are always subject to problems of interpretation because of difficulty in recognizing surviving cells as opposed to lethally damaged cells prior to their lysis. Vincristine and vinblastine are known to disrupt formation of the mitotic spindle, leading to arrest of cells in mitosis. Experiments with synchronized cells have shown, however, that lethal effects of these drugs occur when cells are in S phase, presumably when formation of the mitotic spindle is initiated. Docetaxel and paclitaxel, which act to stabilize tubulin, have somewhat different cell cycle dependence: docetaxel is maximally toxic in S phase,

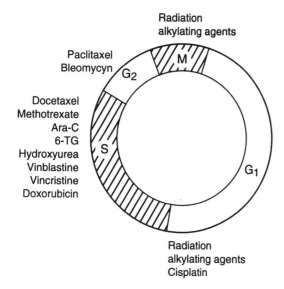

**Figure 17.2.** Phases of the cell cycle in which anticancer drugs show selective lethal toxicity. Ara-C, cytosine arabinoside; 6–TG, 6-thioguanine.

whereas paclitaxel shows increasing toxicity for cells as they progress from S phase through G2 phase to mitosis (Donaldson et al., 1994; Hennequin et al., 1995). Many alkylating agents (e.g., nitrogen mustard, melphalan) have a phase activity similar to that observed for radiation (Chap. 14, Sec. 14.4.2), with two peaks of maximum lethal activity—one near the G1/S phase boundary and one in G2/M phase. Cisplatin also appears to exert maximum lethal activity in late G1 phase.

The relative specificity of most drugs for one or more phases of the cell cycle leaves a partly synchronized population of surviving cells after treatment. Several investigators have proposed that such synchrony may allow scheduling of anticancer drugs to maximize killing of tumor cells by giving subsequent treatments when a large number of survivors are again in a drug-sensitive phase. In practice, the wide variation of cell cycle times observed in vivo leads to rapid loss of synchrony, and, together with heterogeneity of the tumor-cell population and of drug distribution, make optimal treatment scheduling difficult to apply. Furthermore, any such scheduling would need to avoid increased toxicity to critical normal tissues.

## 17.3 EFFECTS OF DRUGS AGAINST TUMORS

### 17.3.1 In Situ Assessment

The clonogenic assays described in the preceding sections have the advantage that they assess directly the reproductive death of cells after drug treatment. When used to study drug treatment in vivo, they require removal of tissue and production of a suspension of single cells, followed by study of colony formation in an environment that differs markedly from that in a tumor or normal tissue that is left in situ after treatment. These processes may: (1) add to cellular damage caused by drugs, (2) rescue cells that would have died in situ but are saved by removal into a tissue culture environment, and (3) bias the results by assessment only of cells that can proliferate in the new environment. Assays in situ avoid such problems, but do not usually provide a direct assessment of cell survival after drug treatment. In situ assays that have been used to assess the effects of drugs on tumors include the duration of animal survival after treatment or drug-induced delay in tumor growth. Revised attitudes to the ethics of animal experimentation have led to the discontinuation of experiments where animals die from the effects of transplanted tumors.

Comparison of tumor growth in treated and untreated animals is the preferred in situ method for assessing drug effects against solid tumors in animals (Fig. 17.3A). The determination of tumor shrinkage and delay of regrowth models the clinical assessment of tumor remission. It is relatively humane because animals can be killed painlessly before their (regrowing) tumors are sufficiently large to cause discomfort. The effect of drugs to cause delay in tumor growth is usually studied in groups of animals that received different doses of drugs. A dose-response curve can then be generated to relate drug dose with some measure of growth delay (e.g., the time for the tumor to grow to a fixed volume; Fig. 17.3B). Experiments with many drugs and tumors lead to regrowth curves after treatment that are parallel to (but displaced from) the growth curve for untreated controls. Under these conditions, the shape of the dose-response curve is independent of the endpoint selected as a measure of growth delay. Treatment with other drugs may lead to tumor regrowth that is slower than in controls, perhaps because of damage to blood vessels. Growth delay may then be due not only to lethal effects against tumor stem cells but also to the effect of the drug on other cells that may be present in the tumor as well as nonlethal effects that may lead to slower proliferation of tumor cells. Likewise, partial remission of human tumors after drug treatment does not necessarily imply major lethal effects of the drugs for the tumor cells.

The endpoints of growth delay and of excision followed by assessment of colony formation in vitro can both be used to study the responsiveness to drugs of human tumors that have been implanted into immune-deficient mice to generate xenografts. The most widely used host for xenografting of human tumors is the congenitally athymic nude mouse (so called because they lack fur). The nude mouse is not a perfect host because it may produce antibodies and also has large numbers of natural killer cells that may inhibit tumor growth (Chap. 20, Sec. 20.4.1). Alternative hosts include mice

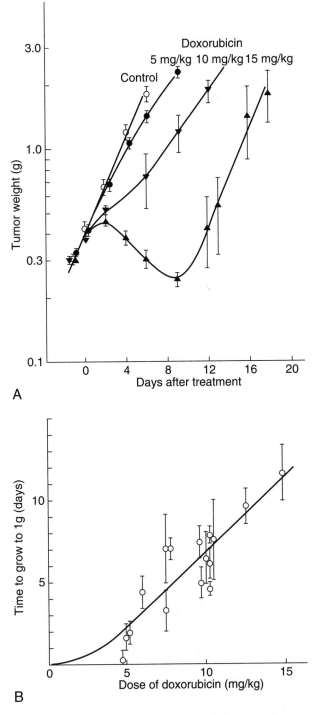

**Figure 17.3.** (A) Illustration of tumor growth curves for treatment of an experimental tumor with doxorubicin. Tumor weight was estimated by prior calibration with measurements of tumor diameter. Note that growth curves after drug treatment are not always parallel to the growth curve for controls and that interanimal variation may lead to large standard errors. (B) Dose-response curve relating drug dose to the time for tumors to grow from size at treatment (~0.4 g) to 1 gram. The curve was obtained from multiple experiments similar to that shown in Figure 17.3A. (Adapted from Tannock, 1982.)

with severe combined immune deficiency (SCID). These mice may be better recipients for transplanted human tissues and have allowed the establishment of grafts of lymphoid and hematopoietic tissues, as well as of solid tumors. In general, the generation of xenografts that grow at a relatively uniform rate requires either serial passaging of cells obtained from an original biopsy of a human tumor in immune-deficient mice or establishment of a tumor cell line in culture.

Xenografts possess the advantage that they may have characteristics similar to those of the human tumors from which they are derived (e.g., enzyme activities). They have been useful in assessing the activities of both new and established drugs against human tumors of varying origins and histologic types. There is a correlation between response of such xenografts to drugs and the clinical response of human tumors of the same histologic type to the same drugs, although this correlation is imperfect and most xenografted cell lines grow much faster than the human tumor from which they were derived. Xenografts grown using cell lines derived from common types of human tumor (e.g., breast, colon, lung) are used in the preclinical evaluation of new agents (see Sec. 17.6.1).

### 17.3.2 Relationship Between Tumor Remission and Cure

For most solid tumors the limit of clinical and/or radiologic detection is about 1 gram of tissue ($\sim 10^9$ cells). If therapy can reduce the number of malignant cells below this limit of detection, the patient will be described as being in complete clinical remission. Surgical biopsy of sites that were known to be involved with tumor previously may lower the limit of detection, but a pathologist is unlikely to detect sporadic tumor cells present at a frequency of less than 1 in 1000 normal cells. Therefore, even a surgically confirmed complete remission may be compatible with the remaining presence of a large number of tumor cells (up to $\sim 10^6$/g tissue). Tumor cure requires eradication of all tumor cells that have the capacity for tumor regeneration. The proportion of such stem cells among those of the tumor population is unknown, but clinical and even surgically confirmed complete remissions are compatible with the presence of a substantial residual population of tumor stem cells.

For some drugs the relationship between cell survival and dose is close to exponential (Sec. 17.2.3), so that a constant *fraction* of the cells (rather than a constant *number*) is killed by a given dose of drug. Drugs are usually given in sequential courses, with dosage and schedule limited by normal-tissue tolerance. Proliferation of surviving tumor cells (known as repopulation; Chap. 18, Sec. 18.3.4) will take place between courses so that the

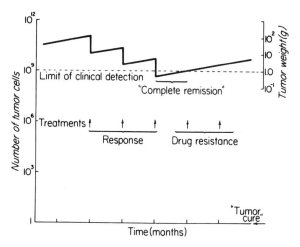

**Figure 17.4.** Illustration of the relationship between tumor remission and cure. In this hypothetical example, treatment of a human tumor starts when it has $10^{11}$ cells (at about 100 g), and each treatment, given at monthly intervals, kills 90 percent of the cells present. This course of therapy leads to complete disappearance of clinical tumor. Drug resistance then develops, and the tumor grows despite continued treatment. Note that despite the attainment of a complete clinical response, there are always at least $10^8$ viable cells present, and that the reduction in cell number is small compared with that required for cure.

number of tumor cells in a drug-sensitive tumor may change with time, as illustrated in Figure 17.4. In this example, each course of drug treatment kills 90 percent of the tumor cells, and starting from a large (~100 g) tumor, complete clinical remission is achieved after three courses. Note that a further six to ten courses (depending on the prevalence of tumor stem cells) would be required to achieve cure, if all cells in the population were equally sensitive. Realization of the need to continue aggressive treatment during complete remission led to success in the treatment of acute lymphoblastic leukemia in children and subsequently to cures in other tumors, such as lymphomas. Unfortunately, for most tumors, various types of drug resistance prevent eradication of all of the tumor cells (see Chap. 18) and the tumor regrows despite continued treatment, as shown in Figure 17.4.

### 17.3.3 Adjuvant Chemotherapy

Chemotherapy is often given to patients who have no overt evidence of residual cancer after local treatment with surgery or radiation. This strategy derives from past experience with similar patients who have shown a high rate of relapse (i.e., regrowth of tumor) from the presence of undetectable micrometastatic disease. Adjuvant chemotherapy is used widely in the clinic and has demonstrated an important effect to increase the probability of cure for some types of malignancy, including breast and colorectal cancer.

Several mechanisms may allow for increased curability of micrometastatic disease. Eradication of a smaller number of cells is more likely with a given dose of drug (see Fig. 17.4). Smaller tumors may have better perfusion of blood than larger tumors, allowing better access of drug to the tumor cells. A higher rate of cell proliferation due to better nutrition may also be important because rapidly proliferating cells are more sensitive to most anticancer drugs. Finally, drug-resistant cells are more likely to be present in larger tumors, thus reducing the chance of cure (Chap. 18, Sec. 18.2.1).

Despite the multiple mechanisms supporting the use of adjuvant treatment, as well as the definitive evidence of benefit for transplanted tumors in mice where chemotherapy can often lead to cures of microscopic but not established tumors (Fig. 17.5), it is disappointing that adjuvant chemotherapy has not been more beneficial to patients. This may be because transplanted tumors in mice are poor models for slowly growing and heterogeneous tumors in humans. A model to estimate the reduction in survival of tumor cells due to adjuvant chemotherapy for breast cancer has been proposed by Withers (1991). In this model (Fig. 17.6), it is assumed that in a large population of patients who are destined to develop disease recurrence, the distribution of cells after surgery (plus or minus adjuvant chemotherapy) ranges from 1 cell to $10^9$ cells (the limit of *clinical detection*). If adjuvant chemotherapy leads to an increase in 10-year recurrence-free survival for node-positive women with breast cancer from about 30 percent to about 45 percent, as suggested by various clinical trials, this model suggests a fractional reduction in cell survival due to chemotherapy of at most 100-fold (Fig. 17.6). This reduction of two logs in cell survival is a relatively small step on the road to cure. Further improvements in the probability of cure due to adjuvant

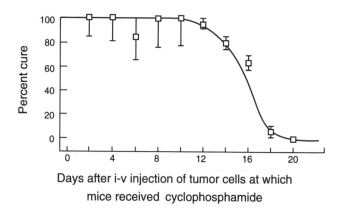

**Figure 17.5.** Result of an experiment in which mice were treated at different times after intravenous injection of Lewis lung tumor cells. Therapy is curative only if it is started early, when the number of tumor cells is low. (Adapted from Hill and Stanley, 1977.)

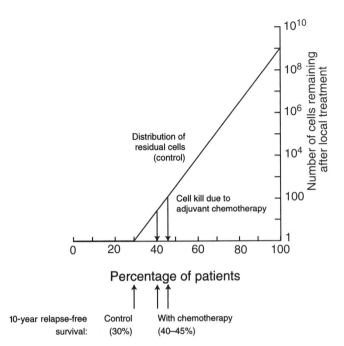

**Figure 17.6.** A model for the distribution of number of cells that remain after local treatment of patients with node-positive breast cancer, about 70 percent of whom will relapse within 10 years. The distribution is assumed to be exponential from 1 cell to $10^9$ cells (lower limit of clinical detection). If adjuvant chemotherapy increases 10-year relapse-free survival by 15 percent, as found in various clinical trials, the fractional cell survival due to this treatment is reduced about 100-fold. (Adapted from Withers, 1991.)

chemotherapy will require more active drugs in order to increase the fractional cell kill.

Adjuvant chemotherapy is sometimes started in patients before treatment of the primary tumor with surgery or radiation—a strategy that has been termed *neoadjuvant chemotherapy*. This approach is attractive because observation of the primary tumor during initial therapy may give an indication of responsiveness to the drugs used. Also, it has been shown that cancer cells may be spread into the bloodstream during surgery (Chap. 11, Sec. 11.3.1), so that chemotherapy given immediately prior to surgery might kill circulating cells and prevent seeding of metastases. However, administration of many drugs to animals has been found to increase the chance of metastasis to the lungs from circulating tumor cells (e.g., Iwamoto et al., 1992). This effect is largest after treatment with cyclophosphamide, when the frequency of metastasis after intravenous injection of tumor cells may be increased by a factor of 100 to 1000, but smaller effects have been observed following treatment with several other anticancer drugs. There is also some evidence that drug treatment may increase spontaneous metastasis from transplanted tumors, although this is not a universal finding. The mechanisms underlying these effects appear to include

drug-induced damage to endothelial cells, which may facilitate the trapping of tumor cells in small blood vessels, and drug-induced changes in malignant cells, which may increase their ability to metastasize (McMillan and Hart, 1986).

Neoadjuvant chemotherapy given before radiation therapy has been observed to cause initial shrinkage of tumors in some sites (e.g., head and neck cancer) without improvement in survival as compared with radiation treatment alone. It has been pointed out by Withers and colleagues (1988) that tumor shrinkage induced by drug therapy might stimulate proliferation of the surviving tumor cells. If this increased proliferation occurs earlier than would normally occur during the subsequent radiation therapy, it could increase the effective number of target tumor cells that must be sterilized by radiation and decrease the probability of tumor control (Chap. 15, Sec. 15.6.2; see also Fig. 17.12).

### 17.3.4 Drugs That Inhibit Metastasis

The complex process by which tumor cells may leave the primary tumor and metastasize to secondary sites has been described in Chapter 11, Section 11.2. While the drugs described in this chapter and Chapter 16 have the potential to kill cancer cells, including those in secondary sites and in the circulation, some agents have been developed specifically to inhibit the metastatic process.

Metastasis depends on the arrest of circulating tumor cells, and many anticoagulant drugs have been assessed for their ability to inhibit metastases (see systematic review by Hejna et al., 1999). There have been consistent effects to reduce metastases in animal systems by heparin, warfarin, and inhibitors of platelet aggregation (prostacyclin and dipyridamole), but there is only limited information from clinical trials. One large trial of the use of warfarin in patients with lung, colon, head and neck, and prostate cancer led to little or no improvement in survival (Zacharski et al., 1984). One of the more promising agents is the prostacyclin analog cicaprost, which has a longer half-life than prostacyclin. This agent inhibits tumor-cell induced platelet aggregation, tumor-cell adhesion to endothelial cells and to the subendothelial matrix, and endothelial cell retraction; it has pronounced antimetastatic action for a series of spontaneously metastasizing rodent tumors (Schneider et al., 1996).

Invasion of tumor cells, both from the primary tumor into the circulation and from the circulation into a secondary site, provides an alternative target for antimetastatic therapy. Invasion requires breakdown of the matrix that surrounds tumor cells or normal cells in the secondary site. Matrix metalloproteinases (MMPs) play a key role in these processes, and also in cell adhesion and others mechanisms that lead to formation of metastases (see Chap. 11, Secs. 11.4 and 11.6.1). For this reason a number of synthetic inhibitors of MMPs have been evaluated in clinical trials. The trials of these agents used to treat advanced cancer have been disappointing, but they were not specifically designed to study effects on formation of metastases (Zucker et al., 2000).

Increased understanding of the molecular pathways involved in tumor formation and progression is leading to evaluation of new biological agents that inhibit specific steps in these pathways (see Sec. 17.6). One promising agent that is a powerful inhibitor of metastases in rodent models is a ruthenium-containing agent called NAMI-A (Sava et al., 2003). This agent appears to inhibit the MEK/ERK signaling pathway (Chap. 8, Sec. 8.2.6) leading to down-regulation of *c-myc* gene expression (Pintus et al., 2002)

A major limitation to the clinical use of therapy to prevent metastasis formation is the presence of microscopic metastases prior to detection and treatment of the primary tumor. Prevention of secondary metastases (i.e., metastases from metastases) might be useful in palliation, but the potential for increased cure through the use of antimetastatic agents is limited to patients in whom metastases are seeded after diagnosis and prior to eradication of the primary tumor. Tumor cells are known to enter the circulation at the time of surgery, but seeding at the time of surgery is probably the sole source of metastases for only a small proportion of patients.

### 17.3.5 The Concept of Therapeutic Index

In addition to their anti-tumor effects, all anti-cancer drugs are toxic to normal tissues. It is this toxicity that limits the dose of drugs that can be given to patients. The relationship between the probability of a biologic effect of a drug and the administered dose is usually described by a sigmoid curve (Fig. 17.7). If the drug is to be useful, the curve describing the probability of anti-tumor effect (e.g., complete clinical remission) must be displaced toward lower doses as compared with the curve describing the probability of major toxicity to normal tissues (e.g., myelosuppression leading to infection). Therapeutic index (or therapeutic ratio) may be defined from such curves as the ratio of the dose required to produce a given probability of toxicity and the dose required to give a defined effect against the tumor (see also Chap. 15, Sec. 15.5.7). Therapeutic index in Figure 17.7 might be represented by the ratio of the drug dose required for a 5 percent level of probability of severe toxicity (sometimes referred to as Toxic Dose-05 or TD-05) to that required for 50 percent probability of anti-tumor effect (i.e., Effective Dose 50 or ED-50). Any stated levels of probability might be used. The appropriate endpoints of tumor response and toxicity

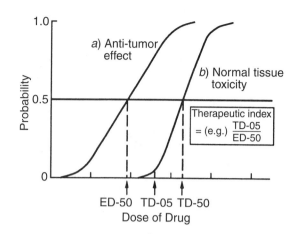

**Figure 17.7.** Schematic relationships between dose of a drug and the probability of a given measure of antitumor effect (curve A), and the probability of a given measure of normal tissue toxicity (curve B). The therapeutic index might be defined as the ratio of doses to give 50 percent probabilities of normal tissue damage and anti-tumor effects. However, if the endpoint for toxicity is severe (e.g., sepsis due to bone marrow suppression), it would be more appropriate to define the therapeutic index at a lower probability of toxicity (e.g., TD-05/ED-50).

will depend on the limiting toxicity of the drug and the intent of treatment (i.e., cure versus palliation). Improvement in the therapeutic index is the goal of experimental chemotherapy. However, although dose-response curves similar to those of Figure 17.7 have been defined in animals, they have rarely been obtained for drug effects in humans. They emphasize the important concept that any modification in treatment that leads to increased killing of tumor cells in tissue culture or animals must be assessed for its effects on critical normal tissues prior to therapeutic trials. These effects to cause normal tissue damage are summarized in the following section.

## 17.4 DRUG TOXICITY

Toxicity to normal tissues limits both the dose and frequency of drug administration. Many drugs cause toxicity because of their preferential activity against rapidly proliferating cells. Adult tissues that maintain a high rate of cellular proliferation include the bone marrow, intestinal mucosa, hair follicles, and gonads (Chap. 9, Sec. 9.4.3). Nausea, vomiting, fatigue, and carcinogenic effects are also common side effects of many drugs, while there are several drug-specific toxicities to other tissues of the body. The biological basis for toxic damage to normal tissues that may occur through a common mechanism is discussed below, whereas toxic effects specific for individual drugs are described in Chapter 16.

## 17.4.1 Bone Marrow

The pattern of cell proliferation and differentiation of hemopoietic cells in the bone marrow has been described in Chapter 9, Section 9.4.3. There is evidence for a pluripotent stem cell that under normal conditions proliferates slowly to replenish cells in the myelocytic, erythroid, and megakaryocytic lineages. Lineage-specific precursors proliferate more rapidly than stem cells, while the morphologically recognizable but immature precursor cells (e.g., myeloblasts) have a very rapid rate of cell proliferation. Beyond a certain stage of maturation, proliferation ceases and the cells mature into circulating blood cells.

The relationship between proliferation and maturation in bone-marrow precursor cells provides a plausible explanation for the observed fall and recovery of blood granulocytes that follows treatment with most anticancer drugs (Fig. 17.8). The effect of treatment will be to deplete the rapidly proliferating cells in the earlier part of the maturation series, with minimal effects against the more mature nonproliferating cells and against slowly proliferating stem cells. Blood counts may remain in the normal range while the more mature surviving cells continue to differentiate but will then fall rapidly at a time when the cells depleted earlier would normally have completed maturation. A substantial decrease in the number of mature cells is common for granulocytes because their lifetime is only 1 to 2 days, less common for platelets (lifetime of a few days), and rare for red blood cells (mean lifetime of about 120 days), but it may also be influenced by differences in the intrinsic sensitivities of their precursor cells for different drugs. The number of mature granulocytes usually decreases at 8 to 10 days after treatment with drugs such as cyclophosphamide or doxorubicin but may do so earlier for other drugs (e.g., vinblastine). The variation in time from treatment to the fall in peripheral blood counts for different drugs probably reflects their different effects on the rate of cell maturation.

When the peripheral granulocyte count falls, proliferation of stem cells is mediated by the production of growth factors (Chap. 9, Sec. 9.4.3), with subsequent recovery of the entire bone marrow population. Administration of growth factors (e.g., granulocyte colony-stimulating factor, or G-CSF) after chemotherapy has been shown to accelerate the reappearance of mature cells in the peripheral blood and to decrease the possibility of infection that can occur in the absence of mature granulocytes.

For many drugs (e.g., cyclophosphamide, doxorubicin; Fig. 17.8A), recovery of peripheral blood counts is complete at 3 to 4 weeks after therapy (or at 2 to 3 weeks if growth factors are given), and further treatment may be given with little or no evidence of residual damage to bone marrow. For other drugs, such as melphalan and nitrosoureas, recovery of mature granulocytes and platelets to normal levels is slower, usually requiring about 6 weeks after treatment (Fig. 17.8B). For such drugs, the bone marrow may be less tolerant of further treatment, indicating some latent damage. Drugs that produce prolonged myelosuppression tend to show only a small difference in effects against slowly and rapidly proliferating cells and may cause direct damage to slowly or nonproliferating stem cells. Thus recovery is delayed because of repopulation from a smaller number of bone marrow stem cells. Some of the damage may be permanent because of incomplete repopulation of the stem-cell pool.

There is experimental evidence that some drugs may damage stem cells and limit their ability to repopulate the bone marrow. Botnick and colleagues (1978, 1981) studied the proliferative potential of treated bone marrow by transplanting it serially into irradiated mice; they also studied the ability of treated bone marrow to regenerate stem cells by removing marrow at intervals

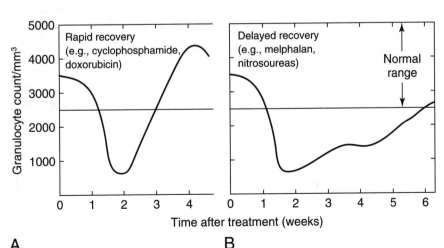

**Figure 17.8.** (A) Fall and rapid recovery of the peripheral granulocyte count after chemotherapy (e.g., with cyclophosphamide and/or doxorubicin). For most drugs the count falls to a nadir at 10 to 14 days after treatment, with complete recovery by 3 to 4 weeks. (B) Delayed and sometimes incomplete recovery is observed after treatment with wide field radiation and some drugs (e.g., melphalan, mitomycin C, and nitrosoureas).

after drug treatment and assessing its ability to form colonies in the spleens of irradiated mice. Busulfan and carmustine (BCNU) caused long-lasting defects in the ability of stem cells to repopulate; melphalan had an intermediate effect, while full and rapid recovery was observed after treatment with cyclophosphamide and 5-fluorouracil. These results are consistent with the clinical experience of bone marrow reserve following treatment of patients with the same drugs.

Recovery of blood counts after treatment with anticancer drugs is the usual determinant of the interval between courses of treatment. If myelosuppressive drugs are given when peripheral blood counts are low, they will not only delay recovery and increase the chance of infection and bleeding, but will also have a higher chance of depleting the stem-cell population, because it is likely to be proliferating rapidly. Drug administration can be repeated up to 1 week after initial treatment, before the decrease in mature granulocytes and platelets is observed; this schedule has been incorporated into several drug regimens where anticancer drugs are given on days 1 and 8 of a 21- or 28-day cycle. Some drugs cause only minimal toxicity to bone marrow (e.g., bleomycin and vincristine), probably because of intrinsic resistance of the precursor cells; they can be given when peripheral granulocyte and platelet counts are low following the use of myelosuppressive agents.

Red blood cells have a long lifetime, which usually prevents the rapid development of anemia following initiation of chemotherapy. However, repeated courses of chemotherapy cause repeated interruptions of red cell production so that the serum level of hemoglobin tends to decrease slowly, leading to anemia and contributing to fatigue. This effect can occur with all types of chemotherapy, but occurs more rapidly following the use of some drugs such as cisplatin. Injection of the growth factor erythropoietin can be used to stimulate production of red blood cells, thus minimizing the effects of chemotherapy to cause anemia and reducing the associated fatigue (Seidenfeld et al., 2001).

### 17.4.2 High-Dose Chemotherapy With Stem-Cell Transplantation

The dose of chemotherapy that can be administered to a patient is usually limited by toxicity to the bone marrow. A technique that can allow delivery of higher doses of chemotherapy involves replacement of bone marrow stem cells after drug treatment. Stem cells for transplantation may be derived from the bone marrow or peripheral blood of other individuals (allogeneic transplantation), when they are matched closely for histocompatibility (HLA) antigens with the recipient (Chap.

20, Sec. 20.2.2); or they may be the recipient's own stored stem cells that were harvested prior to chemotherapy (autologous transplantation). The underlying principle of high-dose chemotherapy is that drug resistance of tumor cells may be overcome by exposing them to higher concentrations of anticancer agents.

The most successful use of allogeneic stem-cell transplantation has been in the treatment of acute leukemia. Following initial chemotherapy to achieve a complete remission (when no leukemic cells can be detected), patients are subjected to high-dose chemotherapy and whole body irradiation aimed at eradicating subclinical disease. Then they are injected with HLA-matched stem cells, usually from a close relative. About 50 percent of recipients now survive long term if there is a suitable donor (Zittoun et al., 1995). Limitations include regrowth of leukemia despite high-dose chemotherapy, nonhematologic toxicity of the intensive treatment (e.g., to lungs and other organs), failure of the implant to regenerate, and graft-versus-host disease. This last syndrome occurs because immunologically competent stem cells are implanted into the host. Unless the patient has an identical twin, immunologic matching is always imperfect and the transplanted marrow will try to reject the host. This problem can lead to damage in multiple organs and, despite the use of immunosuppressive agents such as cyclosporin A, occasionally ends in death. However, the same immunologic effect may also translate into anti-leukemic activity, and patients who develop graft-versus-host disease have a lower relapse rate of their leukemia than those who do not.

Autologous stem-cell transplantation can lead to cure of some patients with lymphoma and drug-sensitive solid tumors (e.g., testicular cancers) which have recurred after conventional doses of chemotherapy. Autologous transplantation avoids graft-versus-host disease because the patient receives his or her own marrow. There has been considerable research into the role of high-dose chemotherapy with autologous stem-cell transplantation for patients with metastatic breast cancer or as adjuvant therapy in patients with breast cancer at high risk for recurrence. Randomized trials have not shown benefit from this approach.

A major limitation of high-dose chemotherapy with stem-cell transplantation is the toxicity of chemotherapy to organs other than bone marrow, especially liver, heart, lungs, and nervous system. Although drugs are selected (e.g., alkylating agents, carboplatin) whose major toxicity is to bone marrow, dose-limiting toxicity to other organs occurs commonly at about three to five times the dose that could be given in the absence of stem-cell transplantation. For most common solid tumors, this modest dose increment is unlikely to overcome drug resistance of the tumor cells, and the majority of patients cured with high-dose chemotherapy have chemosensitive tumors, such as lymphoma or testicular cancer.

Another problem may be the re-implantation of undetected tumor cells that had invaded the bone marrow prior to harvest from the patient. The use of hematopoietic stem cells obtained from the peripheral blood rather than bone marrow was initially thought to result in a lower likelihood of this problem, because even in the presence of bone marrow involvement by tumor there are relatively few tumor cells circulating in the peripheral blood (Franklin et al., 1996). In practice, however, contamination by tumor cells of the reinfused product may occur whatever method of collection is used.

The clinical significance of administering stem cells that are contaminated with tumor cells is not clear. Methods using monoclonal antibodies and/or the polymerase chain reaction (Chap. 4., Sec. 4.3.5) applied to tumor-specific genes are being used to increase the sensitivity of detection of contaminating tumor cells in bone marrow. Also, techniques that allow the selective removal (purging) of such cells (e.g., with the use of monoclonal antibodies) or the enrichment of stem cells have been developed. Although these methods have proven successful in reducing tumor cell contamination, the only randomized trial assessing this strategy has not demonstrated an improvement in disease-free or overall survival in patients with multiple myeloma undergoing high-dose chemotherapy (Stewart et al., 2001).

## 17.4.3 Toxicity of Drugs to Other Proliferative Tissues

Ulceration of the intestinal mucosa is a common dose-limiting toxicity when rodents are treated with anticancer drugs. It is due to interruption of the production of new cells (in the crypts of Lieberkuhn) that normally replace the mature cells continually being sloughed into the intestinal lumen from the villi (Chap. 9, Sec. 9.4.3). Damage to bone marrow is more commonly dose-limiting in humans, but mucosal ulceration may occur after treatment with several drugs, including methotrexate, 5-fluorouracil, bleomycin, and cytosine arabinoside; other drugs such as cyclophosphamide and doxorubicin may increase the severity of ulceration when used in combination with these drugs. Mucosal damage, resulting in mouth soreness and/or diarrhea, usually begins about 5 days after treatment, and its duration increases with the severity. Full recovery is usually possible if the patient can be supported through this period; recovery is analogous to that in the bone marrow, with repopulation from slowly proliferating stem cells.

Some drugs can also produce diarrhea without directly damaging the intestinal mucosa. For example, irinotecan can produce diarrhea soon after administration as a consequence of a direct cholinergic effect on the cells of the intestinal mucosa. This type of diarrhea may be prevented through the use of anti-cholinergic drugs. A second form of diarrhea, secretory in nature, may occur several days following administration of irinotecan, and may be due to damage to the mucosa coupled with cytokine release causing fluid secretion (Chap. 16, Sec. 16.5.1).

Partial or complete hair loss is common after treatment with many anticancer drugs and is due to lethal effects of drugs against proliferating cells in hair follicles; this usually begins about 2 weeks after treatment. Full recovery occurs after cessation of treatment, suggesting the presence of slowly proliferating precursor cells. In some patients, regrowth of hair is observed despite continued treatment with the agent that initially caused its loss. Regrowth of hair might reflect a compensating proliferative process that increases the number of stem cells or may represent the development of drug resistance in a normal tissue akin to that which occurs in tumors.

Spermatogenesis in men and formation of ovarian follicles in women both involve rapid cellular proliferation and are susceptible to the toxic effects of many anticancer drugs. Men who receive chemotherapy often have decreased production of sperm and consequent infertility. Testicular biopsy usually demonstrates a loss of germinal cells within the seminiferous tubules, presumably because of drug effects against these rapidly proliferating cells. Anti-spermatogenic effects may be reversible after lower doses of chemotherapy, but some men remain permanently infertile; it is now usual to recommend sperm banking for young men who undergo intensive chemotherapy for potentially curable malignancies such as Hodgkin's disease.

Chemotherapy given to premenopausal women often leads to temporary or permanent cessation of menstrual periods and to menopausal symptoms, and is accompanied by a fall in serum levels of estrogen. Reversibility of this effect depends on age, the types of drug used, and the duration and intensity of chemotherapy. Biopsies taken from the ovaries have shown failure of formation of ovarian follicles, sometimes with ovarian fibrosis. The pathologic findings are consistent with a primary effect of drugs against the proliferating germinal epithelium.

## 17.4.4 Determinants of Normal Tissue Toxicity

When chemotherapy is given to a patient, a drug dose is selected on the basis of early-phase clinical trials that have determined the *average* dose (usually per unit of body surface area) that gives some toxicity, but at an acceptable level. At this dose, there will be no detectable effects on normal tissues in a few patients, while severe, potentially lethal toxicity may be seen in others.

Multiple factors influence the distribution of drugs to tissues in the body (i.e., pharmacokinetics; Chap. 16, Sec. 16.1.1) and the response of normal cells to these drugs. Some patients have genetically determined traits that change drug metabolism or excretion, and the study of genetically determined factors that influence the probability of drug toxicity is known as pharmacogenetics. For example, patients who lack the enzyme dihydropyrimidine dehydrogenase (DPD), which catabolizes 5-fluorouracil show extreme sensitivity to this drug (Chap. 16, Sec. 16.4.2; Milano et al., 1999). Genetic abnormalities that give rise to the DPD deficient phenotype have been identified, and screening tests can identify susceptible individuals (Mattison et al., 2004). Changes in the activity of enzymes that metabolize other drugs, either genetically determined or induced by concomitant medications, may also have a profound effect on drug-induced toxicity.

Because lethal damage results most often from interaction of drugs with DNA, patients with deficiencies in DNA repair (Chap. 5, Sec. 5.2.2) are very sensitive to anticancer drugs, as they are to radiation. Heterozygotes for these defects (e.g., xeroderma pigmentosum or ataxia telangiectasia) may also be at high risk for severe toxicity if treated by chemotherapy. Predictive assays, based on assessing chromosomal damage in irradiated lymphocytes, are being developed that could allow identification of individuals who may exhibit extreme radio- (and possibly chemo-) sensitivity (Barber et al., 2000). However, the clinical utility of such tests will need to be evaluated carefully, given the low prevalence of the abnormalities being tested, although such individuals may be overrepresented among cancer patients (Chap. 5, Sec. 5.2).

### 17.4.5 Nausea, Vomiting, and Other Common Toxicities

Nausea and vomiting are frequent during the first few hours after treatment with many anticancer drugs and may be due to effects in several regions of the body. Drug-induced vomiting may occur because of direct stimulation of chemoreceptors in the brain stem, which then emit signals via connecting nerves to the neighboring vomiting center, thus eliciting the vomiting reflex. Major evidence for this mechanism comes from studies in animals, where induction of vomiting by chemotherapy is prevented by removal of the chemoreceptor zone. In addition to a central mechanism, some chemotherapeutic agents exert direct effects on the gastrointestinal tract that may contribute to nausea and vomiting. Several neurotransmitters, such as serotonin ($5HT_3$) and substance P are involved in transmitting signals involved in producing nausea and vomiting. Medications have been developed that inhibit nausea and vomiting after chemotherapy. The most effective of these are the serotonin antagonists (such as ondansetron, tropisetron, and granisitron), which block $5HT_3$ receptors, and the NK-1 receptor antagonists (such as aprepitant), which block substance P.

Fatigue and the possibility of cognitive dysfunction are being recognized increasingly as side effects of chemotherapy, especially in women who are receiving adjuvant chemotherapy for breast cancer and who do not have confounding effects due to metastatic disease (Schagen et al., 1999; Bower et al., 2000; Tannock et al., 2004). The mechanisms underling these effects are unknown; they may be mediated in part by changes in the levels of sex hormones and induction of menopausal symptoms, but are probably also due to direct effects of anti-cancer drugs on the brain.

### 17.4.6 Drugs as Carcinogens

Many anticancer drugs cause toxic damage through effects on DNA; they can also cause mutations and chromosomal damage. These properties are shared with known carcinogens (Chap. 3, Sec. 3.3.1), and patients who are long-term survivors of chemotherapy may be at an increased risk for developing a second malignancy. This effect has become apparent only under conditions where chemotherapy has resulted in long-term survival for some patients with drug-sensitive diseases (e.g., lymphomas, testicular cancer, myeloma, and carcinoma of the ovary) or where it is used as an adjuvant to decrease the probability of recurrence of disease following local treatment (e.g., breast cancer). Many of the second malignancies are acute leukemias, and their most common time of presentation is 2 to 6 years after initiation of chemotherapy. Increased incidence of solid tumors may also be observed after longer periods of follow-up.

Alkylating agents are the drugs most commonly implicated as the cause of second malignancy, and there is increased risk if patients also receive radiation. It is often difficult to separate an increase in the probability of second malignancy that may be associated with the primary neoplasm (e.g., in a patient with lymphoma) or with a shared etiologic factor, from that associated with treatment. Comparisons of the incidence of leukemia and other malignancies in clinical trials that randomize patients to receive adjuvant chemotherapy or no chemotherapy after primary treatment have given conclusive evidence of the carcinogenic potential of some drugs. The relative risk of leukemia in drug-treated, as compared with control patients, may be substantial; for example, the relative risk of leukemia was about 12 for 2000 patients receiving methyl-CCNU as adjuvant therapy for gastrointestinal cancer (Boice et al., 1983) and also for 19,000 women receiving adjuvant therapy (which included alkylating agents) for breast cancer (Fisher et al., 1985; Curtis et al., 1992). Leukemia is more common after treatment with alkylating agents that are damaging to bone marrow stem cells (e.g., melphalan, Sec. 17.4.1) than for cyclophosphamide.

Leukemia has been recognized as a complication of treatment with other agents. Cisplatin (and carboplatin), the anthracyclines, such as doxorubicin and epirubicin, and podophyllotoxins such as etoposide have all been identified as causes of treatment-related leukemia (Boshoff et al., 1995; Breslow et al., 1995; Travis et al., 1999). Leukemias that occur following treatment with these drugs have cytogenetic abnormalities distinguishing them from those that occur following alkylating agents (Pedersen-Bjergaard and Philip, 1991).

The risk of second solid tumors following treatment with chemotherapy is far lower than that of leukemia. Nonetheless, a 4.5-fold increase in the risk of transitional cell carcinoma of the urothelium has been demonstrated in patients who had received cyclophosphamide for the treatment of non-Hodgkin's lymphoma (Travis et al., 1995).

The absolute risk of second malignancy remains low and the risks of second malignancy are small compared with the potential benefits in treating patients with breast cancer or curable tumors such as Hodgkin's disease or testicular germ-cell tumors. However, care is needed in using carcinogenic drugs as adjuvant chemotherapy for malignancies where benefit is minimal.

## 17.5 TREATMENT WITH MULTIPLE AGENTS

### 17.5.1 Influence on Therapeutic Index

Patients are treated frequently with combination chemotherapy or with drugs and radiation therapy. When two or more agents are combined to give an improvement in the therapeutic index, this implies that the increase in toxicity to critical normal tissues is less than the increase in damage to tumor cells. Because the dose-limiting toxicity to normal tissues may vary for different drugs and for radiation, two agents may often be combined with only minimal reduction in doses as compared with those that would be used if either agent were given alone. Additive effects against a tumor with less than additive toxicity for normal tissue may then lead to a therapeutic advantage. Mechanisms by which different agents may give therapeutic benefit when used in combination have been classified by Steel and Peckham (1979) as follows: (1) independent toxicity, which may, for example, allow combined use of anticancer drugs at full dosage; (2) spatial cooperation, whereby disease that is missed by one agent (e.g., local radiotherapy) may be treated by another (e.g., chemotherapy); (3) protection of normal tissues; and (4) enhancement of tumor response.

The above mechanisms suggest guidelines for choosing drugs that might be given in combination. Most drugs exert dose-limiting toxicity for the bone marrow, but this is not the case for vincristine (dose-limiting neurotoxicity), cisplatin (nephrotoxicity), or bleomycin (mucositis and lung toxicity). These and some other drugs can be combined with myelosuppressive agents at close to full dosage and have contributed to the therapeutic success of drug combinations used to treat lymphoma and testicular cancer. Research on drug resistance (Chap. 18) has defined drugs that commonly (e.g., doxorubicin and vincristine) or rarely (e.g., doxorubicin and cyclophosphamide) demonstrate cross-resistance. Combination of non-cross-resistant drugs may contribute to therapeutic benefit, as, for example, in the combined use of doxorubicin and cyclophosphamide to treat many types of tumors. Nevertheless, most drug combinations in clinical use have evolved empirically through the combination of drugs that demonstrate some anti-tumor effects when used singly.

### 17.5.2 Synergy and Additivity: Isobologram Analysis

Claims are made frequently that two agents are synergistic, implying that the two agents given together are more effective than would be expected from their individual activities. Confusion has arisen because of disagreement as to what constitutes an expected level of effect when two non-interacting agents are combined. An appropriate definition must take into account the dose-effect relationship for each agent used alone rather than a simple summation or multiplication of individual effects. The use of multiple agents may lead to an increase in the therapeutic index, but it is rare that a claim for synergy of effects against a single population of cells can be substantiated.

The concepts of synergy and additivity between two agents can be understood by considering the level of cell survival after treatment of a single population of cells, either in a tumor or in a normal tissue (see Fig. 17.9). Suppose a given dose of agent A gives a surviving fraction of cells ($S_A$), that a surviving fraction ($S_B$) follows treatment with a given dose of agent B, and a combination of the agents gives a surviving fraction ($S_{AB}$). Claims for synergy are often made if $S_{AB}$ is less than the product $S_A \times S_B$. This conclusion is correct only if cell survival is exponentially related to dose for both agents. If the survival curves have an initial shoulder, as in Figure 17.9, then combined treatment will be expected to lead to a lower level of survival if, after treat-

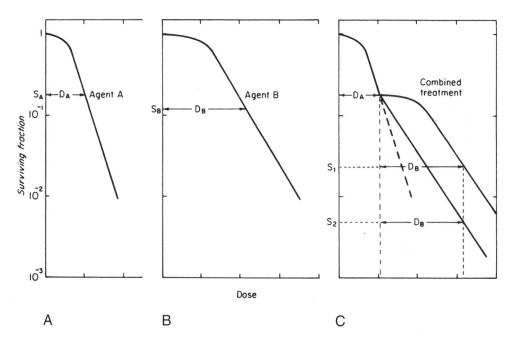

**Figure 17.9.** (*A* and *B*) Cell survival ($S_A$ or $S_B$) is indicated following treatment with either of two agents, A and B, each of which has a survival curve characterized by an initial shoulder followed by an exponential fall with increasing dose. (*C*) Survival ($S_{AB}$) after combined use of dose $D_A$ of agent A and dose $D_B$ of agent B will be equal to $S_1$ ($= S_A \times S_B$) if there is no overlap of damage, and the shoulder representing accumulation of sublethal damage is retained for the second agent. Survival after combined treatment ($S_{AB}$) will be equal to $S_2$ if cells have accumulated maximum sublethal damage from the first agent, A, and the shoulder of the curve is lost for the second agent, B.

ment with the first agent, A, the survival falls exponentially with dose (in the absence of a shoulder effect) for the second agent, B (Fig. 17.9*C*). The fallacy of defining this lower level of survival as a synergistic effect can be illustrated by replacing agent B with a second, equivalent dose of agent A given immediately after the first dose. The combined survival curve then follows that for agent A, with a survival level corresponding to a dose $2 \times D_A$ (Fig. 17.9*A*). If agent A has a survival curve with an initial shoulder, one would then conclude erroneously that agent A was synergistic with itself.

The above discussion implies that there is a range over which two agents can produce additive effects. Isobologram analysis provides a method for defining this range of additivity (Steel and Peckham, 1979). Dose-response curves are first generated for each agent used alone. These dose-response curves are then used to generate isoeffect plots (known as *isobolograms*). These curves relate the dose of agent A to the dose of agent B that would be predicted, when used in combination, to give a constant level of biological effect (e.g., cell survival) for the assumptions of (1) independent damage and (2) overlapping damage (Fig. 17.10). These curves define an envelope of additivity. If, when the two agents are given together, the doses required to give the same level of biological effect lie within the envelope, the interaction is said to be *additive*. If they lie between the lower isobologram and the axes (i.e., the combined effect is caused by lower doses of the two agents than predicted), the interaction is *supra-additive* or synergistic. If the required doses of the two agents in combination lie above the envelope of additivity (i.e., the effect is caused by higher doses than predicted), the interaction is *sub-additive* or antagonistic (Fig. 17.10).

Demonstration that two or more agents have a supra-additive or synergistic interaction has been used as a rationale for their inclusion in clinical protocols. This rationale is valid only if the interaction leads to a greater effect against the tumor as compared with that against limiting normal tissues (i.e., if it leads to an improvement in therapeutic index; Sec. 17.3.5). It is theoretically possible that antagonistic agents (sub-additive interaction) could improve therapeutic index provided that there was greater antagonism of toxic effects for normal tissues as compared to toxicity for the tumor, or they have non-overlapping toxicities.

### 17.5.3 Modifiers of Drug Activity

Some drugs with little or no toxicity for tumor cells may modify the action of anticancer drugs to produce increased anti-tumor effect or protection of normal tis-

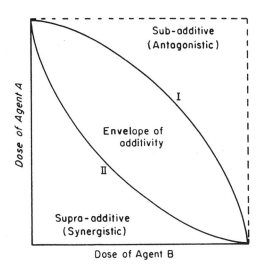

**Figure 17.10.** Isobologram relating the doses of two agents that would be expected to give a constant level of biologic effect when used together. It was generated from dose-response curves for each agent separately. Assumptions about overlap or nonoverlap of damage (Fig. 17.9) lead to the generation of two isobologram curves (I and II) that describe an envelope of additive interaction. Experimental data falling outside this envelope may indicate synergistic or antagonistic interactions, as shown. (Adapted from Steel and Peckham, 1979.)

sue. Examples of interactions that might lead to therapeutic benefit through increased anti-tumor effects include: (1) the use of doxorubicin with agents such as verapamil, cyclosporin A, or their analogs (which inhibit multidrug resistance; Chap. 18, Sec. 18.2.3); and (2) use of folinic acid with 5-fluorouracil, which may provide a necessary cofactor for inhibition of the target enzyme thymidilate synthase (Chap. 16, Sec. 16.4.2).

Alternatively, reduction of the toxic effects of chemotherapy against bone marrow may be achieved by co-administration of growth factors such as granulocyte colony-stimulating factor (G-CSF), which can stimulate earlier recovery of mature granulocytes after bone-marrow suppression by chemotherapy, or after stem cell transplantation (Secs. 17.4.1 and 17.4.2). Granulocyte colony-stimulating factor is used commonly in situations where reduction in dosage of chemotherapy might lead to a decrease in the probability of cure or long-term survival of patients. Erythropoietin stimulates the production of erythrocytes, and is used to prevent or treat chemotherapy-induced anemia.

Growth factors are also being developed to protect against the effects of chemotherapy (and radiotherapy) on other body systems. For example, keratinocyte growth factor (KGF) can stimulate proliferation of the oral and gastrointestinal mucosa, and is effective in decreasing mucosal injury in animals that receive chemotherapy (Farrell et al., 1998). Initial clinical trials have demonstrated that KGF may decrease the rate of oral mucositis induced by chemotherapy or radiotherapy.

Two other agents that may protect normal tissues from damage due to chemotherapy are dexrazoxane and amifostine. Dexrazoxane is a pro-drug whose active form chelates iron. Because complexes between iron and anthracyclines, such as doxorubicin, appear to mediate cardiac toxicity but not anti-tumor effects, dexrazoxane may decrease cardiac toxicity of these drugs and increase their therapeutic index (Speyer et al., 1988; Venturini et al., 1996). Amifostine is a pro-drug that is converted to a sulfhydryl-containing active form. Amifostine is localized selectively in normal tissues, probably because of increased activity of the activating enzyme alkaline phosphatase on the membranes of normal cells. Therefore, it may offer selective protection against a variety of drugs (and radiation, see Chap. 15, Sec. 15.5.8) that damage cells by producing reactive intermediates which bind to sulfhydryl groups (Kemp et al., 1996). There remain concerns, however, that these agents might also provide some protection of tumor cells from drug effects. The crucial test for all modifiers is the demonstration in well-designed clinical trials that higher doses of chemotherapy given with the modifier improve therapeutic index as compared to lower doses of chemotherapy used alone (Phillips and Tannock, 1998).

### 17.5.4 Drugs and Radiation

Many patients receive treatment with drugs and radiation, and there is increasing evidence that concurrent treatment with radiation and drugs such as cisplatin leads to improvement in therapeutic index in a variety of cancer sites such as the head and neck and uterine cervix.

Mechanisms of interaction between drugs and radiation at the cellular level may be evaluated from cell survival curves for radiation obtained in the presence or absence of the drug (Fig. 17.11). Drugs may influence the survival curve in at least three ways: (1) the curve may be displaced downward by the amount of cell kill caused by the drug alone; (2) the shoulder on the survival curve may be lost, suggesting an inability to repair radiation damage in the presence of the drug; and (3) the slope of the exponential part of the survival curve may be changed, indicating sensitization or protection by the drug. Most drugs influence survival curves according to the first two patterns; this corresponds to the limits of additivity defined in Section 17.5.2, where sublethal damage may be independent or overlapping. The third pattern, leading to a change in slope of the dose-response curve, defines agents that are radiation sensitizers or protectors (Chap. 15, Secs. 15.4.5 and 15.5.8). Sensitization of this type has been reported inconsistently for cisplatin and for prolonged exposure to 5-FU after radiation.

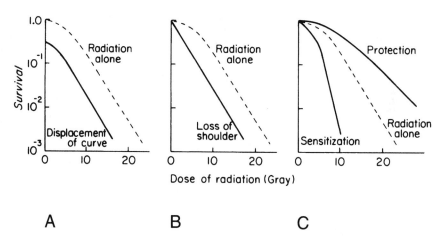

**Figure 17.11.** Possible influences of drug treatment on the relationship between radiation dose and cell survival: (*A*) displacement of curve; (*B*) loss of shoulder, indicating effects of drug on the repair of sublethal radiation damage; (*C*) change in the slope of the curve, indicating sensitization or protection.

Improvement in therapeutic index from use of drugs and radiation requires selective effects to increase damage to tumor cells as compared to those in normal tissues. One mechanism by which combined treatment with radiation and drugs leads to therapeutic advantage arises when radiation is used to provide effective treatment for sites of bulky disease (usually the primary tumor) and drugs are used to treat metastatic sites containing smaller numbers of cells. This spatial cooperation (Sec. 17.5.1) requires no interaction of the two modalities but involves different dose-limiting toxicities. There are also mechanisms whereby the combined use of radiation and drugs might be used to obtain therapeutic advantage for treatment of a primary tumor. Some properties of cells that might be exploited to give therapeutic advantage for the combined use of radiation and drugs are listed in Table 17.3.

Genetic instability in tumors often leads to the presence of subclones, which coexist in the tumor with different levels of sensitivity to drugs and to radiation (Chap. 11, Sec. 11.1). When therapy is applied, any resistant cells that are present will have a selective survival advantage and will determine tumor response: thus, heterogeneity in therapeutic response may tend to make tumors more resistant to treatment than normal tissues. Combined treatment with radiation and drugs might then lead to improved therapeutic index if radiation can eradicate small populations of drug-resistant cells, or if drugs can eliminate populations that are relatively resistant to radiation therapy. This cooperative effect requires that mechanisms of resistance to the two therapeutic agents are independent. Mechanisms (other than hypoxia) that convey clinical resistance to radiotherapy remain poorly understood, but probably include enhanced ability to repair damage to DNA, increased levels of SH compounds such as glutathione (or of associated GST enzymes) that scavenge free radicals (especially in hypoxic cells), and decreased ability to undergo apoptosis (Chap. 14, Sec. 14.3.2). These mechanisms may also convey resistance to some anticancer drugs, whereas many other mechanisms of drug resistance (Chap. 18) are unlikely to cause resistance to radiation. Resistance to any given drug may be caused by multiple mechanisms so that a radiation-drug combination that provides therapeutic advantage for one tumor may not do so for another if different mechanisms of drug resistance are dominant. Effective use of combined treatment would be facilitated by rapid pretreatment assays that give insight into mechanisms of resistance prior to initiation of therapy.

**Table 17.3.** Properties of Tumor Cells That Could Be Exploited to Provide Therapeutic Advantage from the Combined Use of Radiation and Drugs

| Property | Effect of Combined Treatment |
|---|---|
| Genetic instability of tumors, leading to drug and radiation resistance for different clones | Killing of drug-resistant cells by radiation, and radiation-resistant cells by drugs *if* mechanisms of resistance are independent |
| Differences in cell proliferation between tumor and normal tissue | Selective uptake of radiosensitizing nucleosides (e.g., IUdR) |
| Differences in repopulation during radiation treatment for tumor and normal tissue | Inhibition of repopulation by drugs could lead to therapeutic advantage *if* repopulation were faster in the tumor or if the drugs were selective inhibitors of tumor cell proliferation. |
| Environmental factors such as hypoxia and acidity, which are usually confined to tumors | Beneficial effects from drugs with selective toxicity for hypoxic and/or acidic cells |

Proliferation of surviving cells during a course of fractionated radiation (i.e., repopulation; Chap. 15, Sec. 15.6.2) acts to increase the total number of cells that must be killed. Anticancer drugs given *during* the course of fractionated radiation might be expected to inhibit repopulation (Fig.17.12*A*). Combined treatment may then convey therapeutic advantage if the rate of repopulation is greater for the tumor cells than it is for normal tissues within the radiation field. Greater specificity would be expected for agents that inhibit specifically the proliferation of tumor cells; this might be achieved through use of hormonal agents (tamoxifen, antiandrogens) used concurrently with radiation for treatment of breast or prostate cancer (Chap. 19, Sec. 19.4). Another possible strategy is to administer inhibitory growth factors (e.g., members of the TGF-$\beta$ family) or agents that block receptors for stimulatory growth factors such as epidermal growth factor receptor (EGFR) if they are expressed selectively on tumor cells. Promising results are being achieved in clinical trials with the monoclonal antibody cetaximab (C225) which inhibits signaling from the EGFR (see Sec. 17.6.2) used together with radiation therapy (Kim and Choy, 2004)

Repopulation during fractionated radiation therapy might also be influenced by prior treatment with neoadjuvant chemotherapy. Such chemotherapy may cause tumor shrinkage, followed by improved nutrition of surviving cells, with consequent stimulation of cell proliferation (Withers et al., 1988; Tannock, 1996). If there is increased repopulation of surviving cells during the subsequent course of fractionated radiation therapy, any advantage from initial shrinkage of the tumor caused by chemotherapy may be lost or reversed because of the decreased net effectiveness of subsequent radiation treatment (Fig. 17.12*B*).

A third mechanism that has potential for exploitation through combined use of radiation and drugs depends on the presence of a hypoxic microenvironment within solid tumors (Chap. 15, Sec. 15.4). A hypoxic environment conveys resistance to radiation because cell killing is dependent in part on the presence of oxygen. Drugs that have selective toxicity for hypoxic cells, such as tirapazamine, which requires bioreduction for activity, might therefore improve therapeutic index when used with radiation or with chemotherapy. Drugs that are activated under hypoxic conditions may also kill tumor cells in neighboring aerobic regions (Brown, 1999). Such drugs would be expected to have minimal effects against normal tissues, where adequate vasculature usually prevents development of a hypoxic microenvironment.

The effects of targeting hypoxic regions within tumors have been evaluated in clinical trials (Chap. 18, Sec. 18.3.2). In patients with advanced non–small cell lung cancer, the combination of tirapazamine and cisplatin resulted in survival that was superior to that obtained with cisplatin alone, with little additional normal tissue toxicity (von Pawel et al., 2000). A clinical study in patients with cancers of the head and neck also demonstrated that tirapazamine, in combination with cisplatin and radiation therapy, was safe to administer, and resulted in disappearance of tumor hypoxia as assessed with F[18] misonidazole positron emission tomography scans (Rischin et al., 2001).

Whenever radiation and drugs are used together or in sequence, there is potential for increased damage to

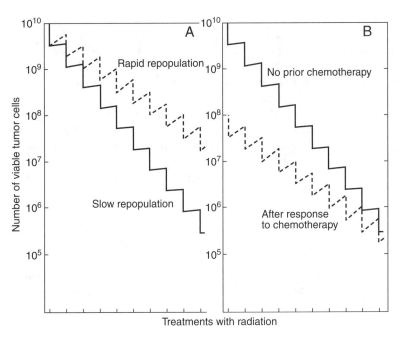

**Figure 17.12.** Schematic diagram illustrating the effect of repopulation in a tumor during a course of fractionated irradiation. Each radiation fraction is assumed to kill the same fraction of tumor cells. In (*A*) the effect of different rates of repopulation is illustrated; concurrent chemotherapy would be expected to reduce the rate of repopulation. In (*B*), it is assumed that prior chemotherapy kills 99 percent of the cells but induces accelerated repopulation by the survivors. Response to radiation treatment alone (*solid line*) or radiation treatment following the chemotherapy (*dashed line*) is illustrated. The accelerated repopulation induced by the prior drug treatment rapidly negates the extra cell kill achieved by the drug treatment. (Redrawn from Tannock, 1996, with permission.)

normal tissues in the radiation field. Some of the effects of combined treatment may lead to changes in function that occur months to years after treatment. Both clinical experience and studies in animals have shown that most anticancer drugs can increase the incidence of toxicity from radiation, sometimes in organs (e.g., the kidney) where the drugs alone rarely cause overt toxicity (Phillips and Fu, 1976; von der Maase, 1986). There is rather minimal information about the ability of drugs to increase the late effects of radiation on normal tissue in animal systems, even though these late effects are most often dose limiting (Chap. 15, Sec. 15.5.3). The effect of a drug on radiation toxicity to any organ may be expressed in terms of a dose-enhancement ratio (DER), which is the dose of radiation to produce a given effect when used alone divided by the dose of radiation that gives the same effect when combined with the drug. For acute effects of radiation on normal tissues of mice, typical values of DER range from 1.0 to 1.5, depending on the drug and normal tissue; maximum interaction occurs when drug and radiation are administered within a short time span (von der Maase, 1986). The therapeutic gain factor equals the ratio of DER for the tumor to the DER for the dose-limiting normal tissue in the radiation field. In experimental systems, this may vary widely depending on the drug used, the doses of drug and radiation, and the sequence. It is difficult to predict the dose schedules that are likely to lead to therapeutic gain in patients.

## 17.6 DISCOVERY AND DESIGN OF NEW ANTICANCER DRUGS

### 17.6.1 Screening for Activity of New Compounds

The synthesis and extraction of new compounds have led to a very large number of agents that might be considered for use as anticancer drugs. A major problem confronting cancer agencies and pharmaceutical companies is the selection for clinical testing of the compounds that have the highest probability of clinical activity. Ideally, the models chosen for screening should be rapid and simple (and inexpensive) and should have both a good chance of detecting clinically active agents (i.e., high sensitivity) and of excluding clinically inactive agents (i.e., high specificity).

The National Cancer Institute (NCI) in the United States employs screening methods that aim to detect clinically active drugs, particularly those with activity against the more common human tumors. Current assays depend on the initial assessment of drugs against a panel of sixty cell lines derived from a range of human tumors, using automated staining with the dye sulforhodamine B (SRB) to assess the number of viable cells after drug-induced damage (Sec. 17.2.2; Skehan et al., 1990; Boyd and Paull, 1995). The unique response pattern obtained within the screen for a new compound can be compared with the results of all other agents in a database, using the NCI's COMPARE computer program. This may assist in the identification of intracellular targets or mechanisms of action for a new agent, by comparison of its fingerprint with that of known agents (Weinstein et al., 1997). New agents that show activity in culture, and particularly those that appear to possess a novel mechanism of action, are then selected for further testing in mice, using the endpoint of growth delay to assess drug effects against a panel of human tumor cell lines that generate xenografts in nude mice. Promising drugs are tested against xenografts derived from common solid tumors, including those derived from colorectal and non–small-cell lung cancer, which demonstrate clinical resistance to most anticancer drugs currently available.

The source of new agents for testing in screening programs is changing. In the past, screening was undertaken on a wide range of compounds synthesized in the chemical and pharmaceutical industries, or extracted from natural sources. In recent years, a more rational approach has been pursued. The identification and characterization of some of the targets of existing anticancer agents has provided an opportunity for the rational design and subsequent development of new agents. Increasingly the source of these newer agents is the result of the application of combinatorial chemistry, which can be used to synthesize rapidly multiple different compounds based on a lead compound that is known to have biological activity. Combinatorial approaches have also been used to synthesize libraries of new compounds, unrelated to existing agents, that can then be subject to screening.

The identification of genes that are expressed selectively in malignant cells has allowed the development of agents that target their gene products. Computer-based approaches have been used to design small molecules that can interact specifically with these targets. For example, the crystal structures for several protein kinases have been obtained, and compounds have been designed to interact with the adenosine triphosphate (ATP) binding pocket of these kinases. One of these compounds (imatinib) is a potent inhibitor of the BCR-ABL tyrosine kinase.

If the crystal structures of potential targets for anticancer chemotherapy are not known, other techniques can be used to aid in the design of new drugs. Structure-activity studies examine systematically the effects of modification of a drug's structure on its properties and activity. This approach may be applied to lead compounds, which may have been discovered fortuitously or may themselves have been the product of a rational design process.

## 17.6.2 New Targets for Cancer Treatment

Conventional chemotherapeutic approaches have aimed to prevent cell growth at the level of DNA replication by inhibiting synthesis of DNA precursors, damaging the DNA template, or disrupting chromosomal segregation. These nonspecific approaches have resulted in drugs with limited tumor selectivity and poor therapeutic indices. Many of the biochemical and molecular changes that occur in malignancy are now better defined. As these processes are elucidated, they become potential targets for new therapeutic strategies (Fig. 17.13). In particular, knowledge of the products of oncogenes, and increased understanding of the processes of intracellular signaling, angiogenesis, and metastasis has provided the opportunity for novel therapeutic approaches. Some examples are given below.

*The RAS Oncogene*   The importance of the *RAS* oncogene in malignancy has been described in Chapter 7, Section 7.3.2. The existence of an oncogene that is mutated so commonly in human malignancy has prompted the search for methods of exploiting this abnormality therapeutically. The transforming activity of RAS proteins is dependent on their migration from the cytoplasm to the plasma membrane, an event that is facilitated by a series of posttranslational modifications. The first (and necessary) step in this process is the addition of a farnesyl group to a cysteine residue, which is catalyzed by the enzyme farnesyl transferase. Inhibitors of farnesyl transferase might thus act as anti-cancer agents. Several such compounds have been synthesized, using rational design techniques based on knowledge of the enzyme structure and its interaction with substrates (Patel et al., 1995). When tested in vivo, such compounds

are able to suppress the growth of tumors derived from *ras*-transfected cell lines (Kohl et al., 1994). Potent inhibitors of farnesylation are being tested in clinical trials: it is not clear how effective such approaches will be in human malignancy, where multiple genetic abnormalities often occur, although tumor response has been reported in such trials (Eskens et al., 2001; Karp et al., 2001; see also Chap. 16, Sec. 16.8).

An alternative approach to targeting RAS is inhibition of its downstream effectors. This strategy might be expected to have effects on other signaling pathways that share a common downstream cascade with RAS. Potential targets include MEK (MAP kinase kinase) or RAF-1 (Chap. 8, Secs. 8.2.5 and 8.2.6). Protein kinase inhibitors are available that interact specifically with these targets, and are now entering clinical trials.

*Protein tyrosine kinases* offer a target for a variety of novel anticancer strategies, including RAS-mediated signaling as described above. As described in Chapter 8, these enzymes play a central role in the generation of signals involved in proliferation and malignancy. The use of recombinant DNA techniques to inactivate kinase activity in vitro is associated with a loss of transforming potential (Snyder et al., 1985), suggesting that these enzymes may be a suitable target for anticancer drug development.

The first protein tyrosine kinase inhibitor to enter routine clinical use is imatinib (Gleevec; Chap. 16, Sec. 16.8). This drug was developed as an inhibitor of the tyrosine kinase that is the product of the *BCR-ABL* fusion gene. It also inhibits the tyrosine kinases of KIT, the product of the *c-kit* oncogene, and of the platelet-derived growth factor receptor. This agent, therefore,

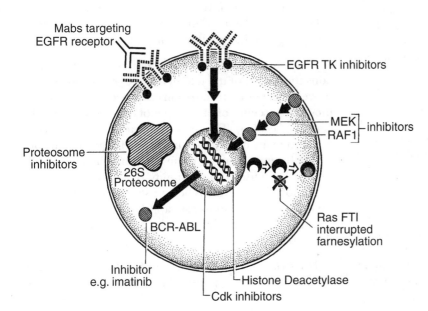

**Figure 17.13.** Schematic figure illustrating some of the molecular targets of new anticancer agents. EGFR = Epidermal Growth Factor Receptor. TK = Tyrosine Kinase, FTI = Farnesyl Transferase Inhibitor.

has activity in tumors that carry abnormalities in these genes and has found initial clinical application in the management of chronic myeloid leukemia (which express *BCR-ABL*) (see Chap. 7, Sec. 7.2.4) where it can induce remission in a large proportion of patients (O'Brien et al., 2003). It also has activity against gastrointestinal stromal tumors, the majority of which express c-kit.

Other new drugs inhibit tyrosine kinases associated with the family of human epidermal growth factor receptors. These small molecules enter cells and are able to inhibit the tyrosine kinase activity that results from heterodimerisation of human epidermal growth factor receptors (HER1 or EGFR). As discussed in Chapter 8, Section 8.2.2, there are four different HERs, and there is corresponding diversity in the agents that inhibit them. Some are able to inhibit tyrosine kinases associated with HER1–4, while others inhibit tyrosine kinases associated with HER1 only. Clinical trials of these agents have demonstrated that they possess activity in a range of tumor types, particularly those that express high levels of EGFR. Randomized trials are under way to define better the place of these agents in cancer treatment (see also Chap. 16, Sec. 16.8).

Tyrosine kinases are also associated with other types of receptors. For example, the vascular endothelial growth factor (VEGF) receptor relies on tyrosine kinase activity for downstream signaling, and molecules capable of specifically inhibiting this tyrosine kinase have been developed as part of an anti-angiogenic strategy (Chap. 12, Sec. 12.4).

*Monoclonal Antibodies Against Growth Factor Receptors* A different approach to interfering with intracellular signaling is to direct monoclonal antibodies against the extracellular portion of a growth factor receptor. This approach has been exploited in the development of trastuzumab, which has found clinical application in the management of breast cancer and cetuximab (C225), which has activity against colorectal cancers (see also Chap. 21, Sec. 21.3.4).

The human epidermal growth factor receptor 2 (HER-2) is amplified or overexpressed in approximately 25 percent of breast cancers. Overexpression is associated with more aggressive disease and a worse prognosis. In vitro experiments demonstrated that murine monoclonal antibodies directed against the extracellular domain of HER-2 were able to inhibit the growth of HER-2 overexpressing cell lines, but not of cells expressing normal amounts of the receptor. A humanized form of the most effective of these murine antibodies was developed, in an attempt to prevent the development of neutralizing antibodies, and thus allow long-term use in humans. This compound, trastuzumab, produces a pro-

longation in survival when used in conjunction with chemotherapy in women with HER-2 overexpressing metastatic breast cancer (Slamon et al., 2001).

*Angiogenesis* Tumor growth is dependent on its blood supply, and various inhibitors of angiogenesis are now in clinical trials. A range of approaches is being explored including: interfering with the function of the vascular endothelial growth factor receptor by using monoclonal antibodies such as bevacizumab or by inhibiting its tyrosine kinase activity with small molecules such as ZD6474 or SU5416; agents aimed at destroying tumor vasculature by preventing turnover of endothelial cells (e.g., combretastatin A); and through the use of endogenous inhibitors of angiogenesis such as angiostatin or endostatin. These approaches are described in more detail in Chapter 12, Section 12.4.

*Proteasome Inhibition* The 26S proteasome has as its major function the degradation of cellular proteins, including damaged, misfolded, and regulatory proteins (see Chap. 9, Fig. 9.4). Tumor cells require proteasome-dependent turnover of many cell cycle proteins in order to successfully complete mitosis, and proteasome inhibition has been shown to cause G2/M arrest followed by apoptosis (Adams et al., 1999). Proteasome inhibitors have been developed and are being evaluated in clinical trials (see also Chap. 16, Sec. 16.8).

*Histone deacetylase* catalyzes the removal of acetyl groups from lysine residues of nucleosomal histones. The acetylation status of histones is involved in the regulation of the transcriptional activity of some genes. Aberrant activity of histone deacetylase is associated with the development of some malignancies, and inhibitors of this enzyme (such as suberoylanilide hydroxamic acid) have been shown to induce apoptosis, as well as cellular differentiation in several cell lines (Marks et al., 2000). Clinical trials are under way with several agents that are inhibitors of histone deacetylase.

*Telomerase* is a ribonucleoprotein enzyme that maintains the length of the telomeres of chromosomes, thus preventing telomere attrition, a process that contributes to senescence of many types of cells (Axelrod, 1996; Chap. 5, Sec. 5.5). The presence of telomerase, which is active in many malignant tumors but few normal tissues (with the exception of germ cells and hematopoietic stem cells) raises the possibility of its therapeutic exploitation. Telomerase is being used as a target for gene therapy with an antisense approach (Chap. 4, Sec. 4.3.11), and specific inhibitors of the enzyme are being developed.

The *cyclins* are potential targets for therapeutic attack because they are responsible for control of the cell cycle. Details of the interactions between cyclins, the cyclin-dependent kinases (CDKs), and the retinoblastoma protein RB are presented in Chapter 9, Section 9.2.1. Expression of D-type cyclins usually follows stimulation of the cell by growth factors. Constitutive expression may be perceived by the cell as a signal that growth factors are present continuously, and this may be a step in malignant transformation. Consequently, inhibitors of the expression of D-type cyclins or of their interaction with other molecules, such as the CDKs, could have anticancer properties. First generation CDK inhibitors, such as UCN-01 and flavopirodol, have entered clinical trials, and second generation compounds, with greater specificity of CDKs (when compared to other kinases), are undergoing preclinical evaluation.

*Cellular Differentiation* In general, there is an inverse relationship between the degree of cellular differentiation and the rate of cell proliferation in tumors. Whether cells differentiate or proliferate depends on cell signaling pathways (described in Chap. 8). Although the mechanisms remain poorly understood, several agents have been shown to stimulate differentiation (and inhibit proliferation) of malignant cells in culture: these agents include retinoids, various cytokines, and analogs of vitamin D (Bollag, 1994). One agent that induces differentiation, all-trans retinoic acid, gives a high rate of complete clinical remission in the treatment of acute promyelocytic leukemia (APL). In this (rare) disease, the *retinoic acid receptor-α* gene is frequently rearranged and fused with another (*PML*) gene. Interaction of retinoic acid with this fusion product is the probable cause of differentiation and response in APL (Cornic et al., 1994). Unfortunately, retinoids have proven useful only in the management of APL, some skin cancers, and superficial bladder cancer, but research continues into agents that influence the balance between cell differentiation and proliferation in tumors.

Conventional cancer chemotherapy is based upon the concept of killing tumor stem cells in order to produce a cure. For many of the newer approaches to cancer control, cell kill is a less relevant endpoint. Inhibition of intracellular signaling may act to interfere with transformation and uncontrolled cell growth but may produce little or no cell killing. Similarly, inhibitors of angiogenesis (Chap. 12, Sec. 12.4) and stimulators of differentiation are unlikely to produce cell killing that could be measured by using traditional in vitro assays of anti-cancer drug activity. The effect of these agents may be to inhibit proliferation of tumor cells while cell death continues leading to gradual involution of the tumor. Toxicities of these agents are also likely to differ from those of current cytotoxic agents because a major goal is to achieve greater specificity for tumor cells by targeting molecular products that are specific to tumor cells. New assays and experimental models may be required to assess the therapeutic potential of these agents.

Likewise, novel approaches may be required to evaluate the role of new agents in clinical practice. In particular, the conventional approach of identifying a maximum tolerated dose based on normal tissue toxicity in a phase I trial and then evaluating the drug given at this dose in a phase II study may be suboptimal. Because the specific targets of many of these newer agents are known, it may be more useful to assess pharmacodynamic endpoints (such as enzyme inhibition, or interference in signaling pathways) in early phase trials. Dosing recommendations would then be based on the ability to inhibit molecular targets as well as on effects to cause normal tissue toxicity.

### 17.6.3 Directed Drug Delivery

A major limitation to the use of chemotherapy is lack of selectivity of most anticancer drugs for tumor cells. A potential method for increasing the therapeutic index is to direct drugs to tumor cells by linking them to a carrier. Several anticancer drugs have been linked to monoclonal antibodies directed against tumor-associated antigens, with occasional evidence of therapeutic effects in animal models, including human xenografts (e.g., Trail et al., 1993; Chap. 21, Sec. 21.3.4). Monoclonal antibodies or growth factors have also been linked to potent toxins such as *Pseudomonas* exotoxin, diphtheria toxin, and ricin (Pastan and Fitzgerald, 1991). The genes encoding these toxins have been cloned, and the DNA sequences encoding the different parts of the molecules that cause toxicity and binding to cells are known. This has made it possible to engineer chimeric molecules in which a tumor-binding ligand is conjugated to the toxic part of the molecule. Problems of specificity and toxicity have led to difficulties in applying these strategies in the clinic but activity has been described in patients with hairy-cell leukemia (Kreitman et al., 2001)

Another strategy is to conjugate an antibody that recognizes a tumor antigen to an enzyme that activates a nontoxic pro-drug within a tumor (Springer and Niculescu-Duvaz, 1997; Denny and Wilson, 1998). This strategy (ADEPT, or *antibody-dependent enzyme-activated pro-drug therapy*) overcomes the problem of limited delivery of conjugated drugs because a single enzyme molecule can activate many pro-drug molecules. Similar approaches have been developed using genes and viral vectors as the targeting agent. However, there are substantial problems in the clinical application of this therapeutic approach, with the large size of antibodies limiting the accessibility of the compounds to some tumor cells. In a small number of clinical trials these approaches have been shown to be feasible, but their utility has not yet been demonstrated (reviewed in Xu and McLeod, 2001).

A large body of research relates to the entrapment of anticancer drugs in liposomes (Gabizon, 1994; Mamot et al., 2003). Liposomes may be constructed of varying size and with positive, neutral, or negative charge; they may be single or multilayered; and the lipid composition may be varied to provide solid or fluid forms of the lipid membrane. In general, liposomes are taken up by reticuloendothelial cells in liver, spleen, and lungs, but they may also deliver relatively high concentrations of drug in tumors; their site of localization depends on the size of the liposomes and their membrane composition. There is particular interest in liposomes that contain polyethylene–glycol–derived phospholipids, which are sterically stabilized and may escape uptake by the reticuloendothelial system, leading to long circulation times. There is evidence that these stealth liposomes may localize in tumors (Gabizon, 1994; Sakakibara et al., 1996). Liposomes are also being used as vectors in approaches to gene therapy (Chap. 21, Sec. 21.2.3).

There are several mechanisms whereby drugs encapsulated in liposomes might lead to improvement in therapeutic index relative to free drug: (1) Slow, continuous release of the anticancer drug into the circulation; this may protect against organ-specific toxicity (e.g., cardiotoxicity due to doxorubicin) and/or lead to improvement in anti-tumor effects. (2) Fusion of liposomes with cell membranes, leading to efficient internal delivery of drugs; this may overcome drug resistance due to impaired uptake of free drug. (3) Selective localization of liposomes (especially small, sterically stabilized liposomes) in tumor tissue. Indeed, superior therapeutic effects of drugs encapsulated in liposomes, as compared with use of free drug, have been demonstrated in several animal models, including human tumor xenografts (e.g., Sakakibara et al., 1996). Randomized clinical trials have demonstrated that pegylated liposomal doxorubicin produces less toxicity, and has greater activity than doxorubicin (Northfelt et al., 1998) although other agents, such as liposomal cisplatin, have produced less encouraging results.

All carrier-mediated drug delivery systems involve large molecules, and there may be problems in delivering such large molecules to cells within a solid tumor. Even some free drugs may have difficulty in diffusing from blood vessels to tumor cells (Chap. 18, Sec. 18.3.3). For this reason, the clinical use of these approaches might be more successful against leukemias or as adjuvant treatment of micrometastases.

## 17.7 SUMMARY

A relevant endpoint for assessing lethal effects of most drugs on cells is loss of reproductive potential as measured by a colony-forming assay. Survival curves that relate colony-forming ability to drug concentration may be exponential or may demonstrate no further killing above a certain concentration if the drugs are cell-cycle-phase–specific. Most currently used chemotherapy drugs are more toxic to rapidly proliferating cells.

In situ assays of tumor response following drug treatment in animals include assessment of delay in tumor growth. Growth delay has been applied to the study of drug response of human tumor xenografts in immune-deficient mice. Automated assays of drug toxicity in culture are used for screening the activity of new agents, and promising drugs are tested against xenografts derived from drug-resistant human tumors. Attempts have been made to apply in vitro assays following drug treatment of cells obtained by biopsy from human tumors with the aim of prediction of clinical response. At present, several problems exist that necessarily limit the use of such assays to a research setting.

The toxicity of many drugs for bone marrow, intestine, hair follicles, and gonads is probably due to depletion of rapidly proliferating cells in these tissues, with subsequent recovery from slowly proliferating stem cells. However, some drugs may cause permanent damage to stem cell function. High-dose chemotherapy with stem cell transplantation provides a strategy to circumvent stem cell toxicity, but the dose of anticancer drugs is still limited by toxicity to other organs. Nausea and vomiting may occur through several mechanisms, and several drugs cause specific damage to organs such as heart, lung, or kidney. Many drugs cause damage to DNA, which may occasionally result in the induction of a second malignancy. Assays that can identify patients with genetically based defects having unusual sensitivity to anticancer drugs need to be further developed and tested for clinical utility.

Anticancer drugs are frequently used in combination with each other and with radiation. Analysis of interactions between different agents is complex and claims for synergy are rarely justified. Agents that modify the toxicity of anticancer drugs are leading to therapeutic benefit in selected situations. Mechanisms that may lead to therapeutic advantage from combined use of radiation and drugs include (1) spatial cooperation, whereby radiation is used to treat bulk disease and chemotherapy to treat metastases; (2) use of each modality to kill tumor cells that have developed resistance to the other, (3) inhibition by drugs of repopulation of surviving cells during fractionated radiotherapy, and (4) use of drugs that are selective for hypoxic cells that are resistant to radiation.

The molecular characterization of events that occur in cellular transformation to malignancy and in tumor progression is being used to identify new targets for anticancer agents. Such targets include the products of (mutated) oncogenes, other molecules involved in cell signaling or cell cycle control; enzymes such as telomerase and histone deacetylase; proteasomes responsible for intracellular protein degradation; and growth factors or their receptors that are essential for angiogenesis in tumors. These targets are expected to have greater selectivity for cancer cells than normal cells. Following identification of targets, computer-based drug design and combinatorial chemistry can now be used to synthesize new drugs for testing. Currently used cell survival assays may need to be refined for evaluation of newer agents directed against specific molecular targets, where chronic effects may be due to inhibition of the proliferation of tumor cells followed by gradual involution of the tumor as the natural processes of cell death continue.

## REFERENCES

Adams J, Palombella VJ, Sausville EA, et al: Proteasome inhibitors: a novel class of potent and effective antitumor agents. *Cancer Res* 1999; 59:2615–2622.

Axelrod N: Of telomeres and tumors. *Nature Med* 1996; 2:158–159.

Barber JB, Burrill W, Spreadborough AR, et al: Relationship between in vitro chromosomal radiosensitivity of peripheral blood lymphocytes and the expression of normal tissue damage following radiotherapy for breast cancer. *Radiother Oncol* 2000; 55: 179–186.

Boice JD Jr, Greene MH, Killen JY Jr, et al: Leukemia and preleukemia after adjuvant treatment of gastrointestinal cancer with semustine (methyl-CCNU). *N Engl J Med* 1983; 309:1079–1084.

Bollag W: Experimental basis of cancer combination chemotherapy with retinoids, cytokines, 1,25–dihydroxyvitamin D3, and analogs. *J Cell Biochem* 1994; 56:427–435.

Boshoff C, Begent RH, Oliver RT, et al: Secondary tumors following etoposide-containing therapy for germ cell cancer. *Ann Oncol* 1995; 6: 35–40.

Botnick LE, Hannon EC, Hellman S: Multisystem stem cell failure after apparent recovery from alkylating agents. *Cancer Res* 1978; 38:1942–1947.

Botnick LE, Hannon EC, Vigneulle R, Hellman S: Differential effects of cytotoxic agents on hematopoietic progenitors. *Cancer Res* 1981; 41:2338–2342.

Bower JE, Ganz PA, Desmond KA, et al: Fatigue in breast cancer survivors: correlates, and impact on quality of life. *J Clin Oncol* 2000; 18:743–753.

Boyd MR, Paull KD: Some practical considerations and applications of the National Cancer Institute in vitro anticancer drug discovery screen. *Drug Dev Res* 1995; 34:91–109.

Breslow NE, Takashima JR, Whitton JA, et al: Second malignant neoplasms following treatment for Wilm's tumor: a report from the national Wilms' Tumor Study Group. *J Clin Oncol* 1995; 13:1851–1859.

Brown JM: The hypoxic cell: a target for selective cancer therapy—eighteenth Bruce F. Cain Memorial Award Lecture. *Cancer Res* 1999; 59:5863–5870.

Bruce WR, Meeker BE, Powers WE, Valeriote FA: Comparison of the dose and time-survival curves for normal hematopoietic and lymphoma colony-forming cells exposed to vinblastine, vincristine, arabinosylcytosine, and amethopterin. *J Natl Cancer Inst* 1969; 42:1015–1023.

Carmichael J, DeGraff WG, Gazdar AF: Evaluation of a tetrazolium-based semiautomated colorimetric assay: assessment of chemosensitivity testing. *Cancer Res* 1987; 47: 936–942.

Cornic M, Agadir A, Degos L, Chomienne C: Retinoids and differentiation treatment: a strategy for treatment in cancer. *Anticancer Res* 1994; 14:2339–2346.

Courtenay VD, Smith IE, Peckham MJ, Steel GG: In vitro and in vivo radiosensitivity of human tumour cells obtained from a pancreatic carcinoma xenograft. *Nature* 1976; 263: 771–772.

Curtis RE, Boice JD Jr, Stovall M, et al: Risk of leukemia after chemotherapy and radiation treatment for breast cancer. *N Engl J Med* 1992; 326:1745–1750.

Denny WA, Wilson WR: The design of selectively-activated anti-cancer prodrugs for use in antibody-directed and gene-directed enzyme-prodrug therapies. *J Pharm Pharmacol* 1998; 50:387–394.

Donaldson KL, Goolsby GL, Wahl AF: Cytotoxicity of the anticancer agents cisplatin and taxol during cell proliferation and the cell cycle. *Int J Cancer* 1994; 57:847–855.

Eskens FA, Awada A, Cutler DL, et al: Phase I and pharmacokinetic study of the oral farnesyl transferase inhibitor SCH 66336 given twice daily to patients with advanced solid tumors. *J Clin Oncol* 2001; 19:1167–1175.

Farrell CL, Bready JV, Rex KL, et al: Keratinocyte Growth Factor protects mice from chemotherapy and radiation-induced gastrointestinal injury and mortality. *Cancer Res* 1998; 58:933–939.

Fisher B, Rockette H, Fisher ER, et al: Leukemia in breast cancer patients following adjuvant chemotherapy or postoperative radiation: the NSABP experience. *J Clin Oncol* 1985; 3:1640–1658.

Franklin WA, Shpall EJ, Archer P, et al: Immunocytochemical detection of breast cancer cells in marrow and peripheral blood of patients undergoing high-dose chemotherapy with autologous stem cell support. *Breast Cancer Res Treat* 1996; 41:1–13.

Gabizon AA: Liposomal anthracyclines. *Hematol Oncol Clin North Am* 1994; 8:431–450.

Hamburger AW, Salmon SE: Primary bioassay of human tumor stem cells. *Science* 1977; 197:461–463.

Hejna M, Raderer M, Zielinski CC: Inhibition of metastases by anticoagulants. *J Natl Cancer Inst* 1999; 91:22–36.

Hennequin C, Giocanti N, Favaudon V: S-phase specificity of cell killing by docetaxel (Taxotere) in synchronized HeLa cells. *Br J Cancer* 1995; 71:1194–1198.

Hill RP, Stanley JA: Pulmonary metastases of the Lewis lung tumor-cell kinetics and response to cyclophosphamide at different sizes. *Cancer Treat Rep* 1977; 61:29–36.

Iwamato Y, Fujita Y, Sugioka Y: VIGSR, a synthetic laminin peptide, inhibits the enhancement by cyclophosphamide of experimental lung metastasis of human fibrosarcoma cells. *Clin Exp Metastasis* 1992; 10:183–189.

Karp JE, Lancet JE, Kaufman SH, et al: Clinical and biologic activity of the farnesyltransferase inhibitor R115777 in adults with refractory and relapsed acute leukemias: a phase I clinical-laboratory correlative trial. *Blood* 2001; 97: 3361–3369.

Kemp G, Rose P, Lurain J, et al: Amifostine pretreatment for protection against cyclophosphamide-induced and cisplatin-induced toxicities: results of a randomized control trial in patients with advanced ovarian cancer. *J Clin Oncol* 1996; 14:2101–2112.

Kim DW, Choy H: Potential role for epidermal growth factor receptor inhibitors in combined-modality therapy for non-small-cell lung cancer. *Int J Radiat Oncol Biol Phys* 2004; 59(2Suppl):11–20.

Kohl NE, Wilson FR, Mosser SD, et al: Protein farnesyltransferase inhibitors block the growth of ras-dependent tumors in nude mice. *Proc Natl Acad Sci USA* 1994; 91:9141–9145.

Kreitman RJ, Wilson WH, Bergeron K, et al: Efficacy of the anti-CD22 recombinant immunotoxin BL22 in chemotherapy-resistant hairy-cell leukemia. *N Engl J Med* 2001; 345:241–247.

Mamot C, Drummond DC, Hong K, et al: Liposome-based approaches to overcome anticancer drug resistance. *Drug Resist Update* 2003; 6:271–279.

Marks PA, Richon VM, Rifkind RA: Histone deacetylase inhibitors: inducers of differentiation or apoptosis of transformed cells. *J Natl Cancer Inst* 2000; 92: 1210–1216.

Mattison LK, Ezzeldin H, Carpenter M, et al: Rapid identification of dihydropyrimidine dehydrogenase deficiency by using a novel 2-13C-uracil breath test. *Clin Cancer Res* 2004; 10:2652–2658.

McMillan TJ, Hart IR: Enhanced experimental metastatic capacity of a murine melanoma following pretreatment with anticancer drugs. *Clin Exp Metastasis* 1986; 4:285–292.

Milano G, Etienne MC, Pierrefite V, et al: Dihydropyrimidine dehydrogenase deficiency and fluorouracil-related toxicity. *Br J Cancer* 1999; 79:627—630.

Nissen E, Tanneberger S, Projan A, et al: Recent results of *in vitro* drug prediction in human tumour chemotherapy. *Arch Geschwulstforsch* 1978; 48:667–672.

Northfelt DW, Dezeube BJ, Thommes JA, et al: Pegylated-liposomal doxorubicin versus doxorubicin, bleomycin and vincristine in the treatment of AIDS-related Kaposi's sarcoma: results of a randomized phase III clinical trial. *J Clin Oncol* 1998; 16:2445–2451.

O'Brien SG, Guilhot F, Larson RA, et al: Imatinib compared with interferon and low-dose cytarabine for newly diagnosed chronic-phase chronic myeloid leukemia. *N Engl J Med* 2003: 348;996–1004.

Pastan I, Fitzgerald D: Recombinant toxins for cancer treatment. *Science* 1991; 254:1173–1177.

Patel DV, Schmidt RJ, Biller SA, et al: Farnesyl diphosphate-based inhibitors of ras farnesyl protein transferase. *J Med Chem* 1995; 38:2906–2921.

Pedersen-Bjergaard J, Philip P: Balanced translocations involving chromosome bands 11q23 and 21q22 are highly characteristic of myelodysplasia and leukemia following therapy with cytostatic agents targeting at DNA-topoisomerase II. *Blood* 1991; 78:1147–1148.

Phillips K-A, Tannock IF: Design and interpretation of clinical trials that evaluate agents that may offer protection from the toxic effects of cancer chemotherapy. *J Clin Oncol* 1998; 16:3179–3190.

Phillips TL, Fu KK: Quantification of combined radiation therapy and chemotherapy effects on critical normal tissues. *Cancer* 1976; 37:1186–1200.

Pintus G, Tadolini B, Posadino AM, et al: Inhibition of the MEK/ERK signaling pathway by the novel antimetastatic agent NAMI-A down regulates c-myc gene expression and endothelial cell proliferation. *Eur J Biochem* 2002; 269: 5861–5870.

Potten CS: What is an apoptotic index measuring? A commentary. *Br J Cancer* 1996, 74:1743–1748.

Rischin D, Peters L, Hicks R, et al: Phase I trial of concurrent tirapazamine, cisplatin and radiotherapy in patients with advanced head and neck cancer. *J Clin Oncol* 2001; 19: 535–542.

Sakakibara T, Chen FA, Kida H, et al: Doxorubicin encapsulated in sterically stabilized liposomes is superior to free drug or drug-containing conventional liposomes at suppressing growth and metastases of human lung tumor xenografts. *Cancer Res* 1996; 56:3743–3746.

Samson DJ, Seidenfeld J, Ziegler K, Aronson N: Chemotherapy sensitivity and resistance assays: a systematic review. *J Clin Oncol* 2004; 22:3618–3630.

Sava G, Zorzet S, Turrin C, et al: Dual action of NAMI-A in inhibition of solid tumor metastsis: Selective targeting of metastatic cells and binding to collagen. *Clin Cancer Res* 2003; 9:1898–1905.

Schagen SB, van Dam FSAM, Muller MJ, et al: Cognitive deficits after postoperative adjuvant chemotherapy for breast carcinoma. *Cancer* 1999; 85:640–650.

Scheithauer W, Clark GM, Moyer MP, von Hoff DD: New screening system for selection of anticancer drugs for treatment of human colorectal cancer. *Cancer Res* 1986; 46: 2703–2708.

Schneider MR, Schirner M, Lichtner RB, Graf H: Antimetastatic action of the prostacyclin analogue cicaprost in experimental mammary tumors. *Breast Cancer Res Treat* 1996; 38:133–141.

Schrag D, Garewal HS, Burstein HJ, et al: American Society of Clinical Oncology Technology Assessment: chemotherapy sensitivity and resistance assays. *J Clin Oncol* 2004; 22:3631–3638.

Seidenfeld J, Piper M, Flamm C, et al: Epoietin treatment of anemia associated with cancer therapy: a systematic review and meta-analysis of controlled clinical trials. *J Natl Cancer Inst* 2001; 93:1204–1214.

Selby P, Buick RN, Tannock I: A critical appraisal of the "human tumor stem cell assay." *N Engl J Med* 1983; 308:129–134.

Skehan P, Storeng R, Scudiero D, et al: New colorimetric cytotoxicity assay for anticancer-drug screening. *J Natl Cancer Inst* 1990; 82:1107–1112.

Slamon DJ, Leyland-Jones B, Shak S, et al: Use of chemotherapy plus a monoclonal antibody against HER2 for metastatic breast cancer that overexpresses HER2. *N Engl J Med* 2001; 344:783–792.

Snyder MA, Bishop JM, McGrath JP, Levinson AD: A mutation of the ATP binding site of pp60v-src abolishes kinase activity, transformation, and tumorigenicity. *Mol Cell Biol* 1985; 5:1772–1779.

Speyer JL, Green MD, Kramer E, et al: Protective effect of the bispiperazinedione ICRF-187 against doxorubicin-induced cardiac toxicity in women with advanced breast cancer *N Engl J Med* 1988; 319:745–752.

Springer CJ, Niculescu-Duvaz II: Antibody-directed enzyme prodrug therapy (ADEPT): a review. *Adv Drug Deliv Res* 1997; 26:151–172.

Steel GG, Peckham MJ: Exploitable mechanisms in combined radiotherapy-chemotherapy: the concept of additivity. *Int J Radiat Oncol Biol Phys* 1979; 5:85–91.

Stewart AK, Vescio R, Schiller G, et al: Purging of autologous peripheral-blood stem cells using CD34 selection does not improve overall or progression-free survival after high-dose chemotherapy for multiple myeloma: results of a multicenter randomized controlled trial. *J Clin Oncol* 2001; 19:3771–3779.

Tannock IF: Response of aerobic and hypoxic cells in a solid tumor to Adriamycin and cyclophosphamide and interaction of the drugs with radiation. *Cancer Res* 1982; 42:4921–4926.

Tannock IF: Treatment of cancer with radiation and drugs. *J Clin Oncol* 1996; 14:3156–3174.

Tannock IF, Ahles TA, Ganz PA, Van Dam FS: Cognitive impairment associated with chemotherapy for cancer: report of a workshop. *J Clin Oncol* 2004: 22:2233–2239.

Trail PA, Willner D, Lasch SJ, et al: Cure of xenografted human carcinomas by BR96–doxorubicin conjugates. *Science* 1993; 261:212–215.

Travis LB, Curtis RE, Glimelius B, et al: Bladder and kidney cancer following cyclophosphamide therapy for non-Hodgkin's lymphoma. *J Natl Cancer Inst* 1995; 87:524–530.

Travis LB, Holowaty EJ, Bergfeldt K, et al: Risk of leukemia after platinum-based chemotherapy for ovarian cancer. *N Eng J Med* 1999; 340:351–357.

Twentyman PR, Bleehen NM: Changes in sensitivity to cytotoxic agents occurring during the life history of monolayer cultures of a mouse tumour cell line. *Br J Cancer* 1975; 31:417–423.

Van Putten LM, Lelieveld P, Kram-Idsenga LKJ: Cell cycle specificity and therapeutic effectiveness of cytostatic agents. *Cancer Chemother Rep* 1972; 56:691–700.

Venturini M, Michelotti A, Del Mastro L, et al: Multicenter randomized controlled clinical trial to evaluate cardioprotection of dexrazoxane versus no cardioprotection in women receiving epirubicin chemotherapy for advanced breast cancer. *J Clin Oncol* 1996; 14:3112–3120.

von der Maase H: Experimental studies on interactions of radiation and cancer chemotherapeutic drugs in normal tissues and a solid tumour. *Radiother Oncol* 1986; 7:47–68.

von Hoff DD, Kronmal R, Salmon SE, et al: A Southwest Oncology Group study on the use of a human tumor cloning assay for predicting response in patients with ovarian cancer. *Cancer* 1991; 67:20–27.

von Pawel J, von Roemeling R, Gatzemeier U, et al: Tirapazamine plus cisplatin versus cisplatin in advanced non–small-cell lung cancer: a report of the International CATAPULT I Study Group. *J Clin Oncol* 2000; 18:1351–1359.

Weinstein JN, Myers TG, O'Connor PM, et al: An information intensive approach to the molecular pharmacology of cancer. *Science* 1997; 275: 343–349.

Withers HR: From bedside to bench and back. In Dewey WC, et al, eds. *Radiation Research: A Twentieth Century Perspective.* Vol II. *Congress Proceedings.* New York: Academic Press; 1991:26–31.

Withers HR, Taylor JMF, Maciejewski B: The hazard of accelerated tumor clonogen repopulation during radiotherapy. *Acta Oncol* 1988; 27:131–146.

Xu G, McLeod HL: Strategies for enzyme/prodrug cancer therapy. *Clin Cancer Research* 2001; 7:3314–3324.

Zacharski LR, Henderson WG, Rickles FR, et al: Effect of warfarin anticoagulation on survival in carcinoma of the lung, colon, head and neck, and prostate: Final Report of VA Cooperative Study #75. *Cancer* 1984; 53:2046–2052.

Zittoun RA, Mandelli F, Willemze R, et al: Autologous or allogeneic bone marrow transplantation compared with intensive chemotherapy in acute myelogenous leukemia. *N Engl J Med* 1995: 332:217–223.

Zucker S, Cao J, Chen WT: Critical appraisal of the use of matrix metalloproteinase inhibitors in cancer treatment. *Oncogene* 2000; 19:6642–6650.

# 18

# Drug Resistance

*Susan P.C. Cole and Ian F. Tannock*

## 18.1 INTRODUCTION

Many types of cancer that occur commonly in humans (e.g., colon cancer, most types of lung cancer) have a relatively low probability of response to treatment with anticancer drugs. Other human tumors (e.g., breast cancer, ovarian cancer, or small-cell cancer of the lung) often respond to initial treatment, but acquired resistance to further therapy usually prevents drug treatment from being curative. Resistance to chemotherapy may have multiple causes, and the most widely studied are genetically determined mechanisms that lead to resistance of the individual tumor cells. Sensitivity to drugs may differ widely among cell populations from tumors and normal tissues and also among the cells of a single tumor. The selection or induction of a drug-resistant subpopulation in human tumors is a major factor limiting the efficacy of clinical chemotherapy. Even if drug-resistant cells are present initially only at low frequency (e.g., one drug-resistant cell per $10^5$ drug-sensitive cells), their selective advantage during drug treatment will lead to their rapid emergence as the dominant cell population, giving the clinical impression of acquired resistance.

There is increasing recognition that factors other than those based on genetically determined mechanisms of resistance can lead to clinical resistance of human tumors to anticancer drugs. Transient changes in cellular phenotype may occur through what are known as epigenetic mechanisms: these mechanisms influence the levels of expression of genes (and hence of the proteins encoded by them) as compared to genetic mechanisms which refers to information transmitted on the basis of the DNA sequence of a gene.

The activity of many drugs is also dependent on the proliferative status of the cells, and for many of them on the phase of the cell cycle (Chap. 17, Sec. 17.2.4). Thus, a tumor may appear resistant if many of its constituent cells are nonproliferating or are spared in a drug-resistant phase of the cell cycle. Rapid proliferation of surviving tumor cells (repopulation) between courses of chemotherapy can counter the effects of cell killing and lead to effective resistance. Also, regardless of the intrinsic sensitivity of the constituent tumor cells, drugs can only exert lethal effects if they reach the cells in sufficient concentration to cause lethality. Thus, limited vascular access and the requirement to penetrate tissue from tumor blood vessels are additional potential causes of effective drug resistance.

This chapter provides a review of the various mechanisms that might lead to clinical resistance of human tumors, as well as potential strategies that might be used to overcome them. The work described is not only important in providing leads for improvement in therapeutic outcome, but has also contributed substantially to knowledge about the biology of tumors in general, for example, in demonstrating tumor progression, heterogeneity of the properties of constituent cells, and mechanisms of gene regulation and amplification.

## 18.2 CAUSES OF CELLULAR DRUG RESISTANCE

### 18.2.1 Molecular Mechanisms of Drug Resistance

A wide range of biochemical properties of tumor cells may lead to drug resistance; some of the underlying mechanisms are summarized in Table 18.1. Alkylating agents and cisplatin cause cellular damage by binding to DNA, leading to crosslinkages and breaks in DNA strands (Chap. 16, Secs. 16.2 and 16.3). Cells may be resistant to these drugs through a number of mechanisms, including decreased cellular drug uptake (Sec. 18.2.2), enhanced efflux of drugs or their metabolites out of cells (Sec. 18.2.3), reduced drug activation or increased drug inactivation (Sec. 18.2.4), or increased repair of DNA damage caused by the cytotoxic agent (Sec. 18.2.7). Cross-resistance to chemically unrelated drugs has been observed for naturally occurring and semi-synthetic compounds such as doxorubicin, vincristine, and etoposide, owing to common mechanisms of enhanced drug efflux from cells (Sec. 18.2.3). Some of

these drugs exert their cytotoxicity through interaction with the nuclear enzymes topoisomerase I or II, which mediate conformational changes in DNA that are necessary for transcription of RNA and/or synthesis of DNA in preparation for cell division (Sec. 18.2.6). Thus, resistance to these drugs can occur when cells express decreased levels of topoisomerase I or II, or a mutant, catalytically active but cytoplasmic form of the type II enzyme.

It is well documented that multiple mechanisms of resistance may emerge in response to exposure to a single class of drugs. For example, resistance to antimetabolite drugs is known to result from impaired drug transport into cells, overproduction or reduced affinity of the drug target, upregulation of alternative biochemical pathways, impaired activation or increased inactivation of the drug, and increased drug efflux. The folic acid analog methotrexate is an excellent example of an antimetabolite drug that can be rendered ineffective by all of these mechanisms (Gorlick et al., 1996, Fig. 18.1). Because multiple mechanisms may contribute to resistance to every anticancer drug, it is not surprising that initial or acquired drug resistance is observed after treatment of most cell populations.

The following evidence indicates that many types of drug resistance are genetic in origin:

1. Characteristics of drug-resistant cells (i.e., their phenotypes) are often inherited in the absence of the selecting drug.
2. Drug-resistant cells are generated spontaneously at a rate that is consistent with known rates of genetic mutation. A fluctuation test has provided evidence for mutation and selection as a mechanism leading to resistance to a few anticancer drugs, including paclitaxel (Dumontet et al, 1996).

**Table 18.1.** General Mechanisms Associated with Resistance to Anticancer Drugs[a]

| Mechanism | Drugs |
| --- | --- |
| Decreased uptake | Methotrexate, nitrogen mustard, cisplatin, and other antimetabolites |
| Increased efflux | Anthracyclines, *Vinca* alkaloids, etoposide, taxanes, methotrexate |
| Decrease in drug activation | Many antimetabolites (e.g., 5-FU, araC) |
| Increase in drug catabolism | Many antimetabolites (e.g., 5-FU, araC) |
| Increase or decrease in levels of target enzyme | Methotrexate, topoisomerase inhibitors, 5-FU, imatinib |
| Alterations in target enzyme | Methotrexate, other antimetabolites, topoisomerase inhibitors, imatinib |
| Inactivation by binding to sulfhydryls (e.g., glutathione, metallothionein) | Alkylating agents, cisplatin |
| Increased DNA repair | Alkylating agents, cisplatin, anthracyclines, etoposide |
| Decreased ability to undergo apoptosis | Alkylating agents, cisplatin, anthracyclines, etoposide |

[a]Additional mechanisms are less well characterized, including some that lead to drug resistance that is expressed selectively in a solid-tumor environment (see Sec. 18.3).

5-FU, 5-fluorouracil; araC, cytosine arabinoside.

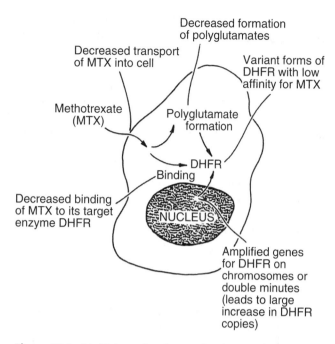

**Figure 18.1.** Multiple molecular mechanisms underlying cellular resistance to methotrexate. MTX, methotrexate; DHFR, dihydrofolate reductase.

3. Generation of drug-resistant cells is increased by exposure to compounds that cause mutations in genes or facilitate gene amplification (increased gene copy number). This property has been used to generate and select a large number of drug-resistant variant cells that have been used to study drug-resistant phenotypes. Because of the genomic instability of tumor cells, treatment may be expected to accelerate the development of drug resistance.

4. Defective proteins that are the products of mutated genes have been identified in some drug-resistant cells.

5. Many drug-resistant phenotypes have been transferred to drug-sensitive cells by transfer of genes, using techniques described in Chapter 4, Section 4.3.10.

The presence of drug-resistant cells among the cells in human tumors has implications for planning optimal chemotherapy. Goldie and Coldman (1984) have demonstrated that the probability of there being at least one drug-resistant cell in a tumor population is dependent on tumor size (Fig. 18.2). This probability increases from near zero to near unity over a small range of tumor sizes (six doublings), with the critical size depending on the rate of mutation to drug resistance. This effect implies a greater chance of cure if therapy is begun early, when only microscopic foci of tumor cells are present. The Goldie-Coldman model also predicts a better therapeutic effect when two equally effective and "non-cross-resistant" drugs are alternated rather than

given sequentially, because this minimizes the emergence of cell populations that are resistant to both drugs. However, it has been difficult to demonstrate the validity of this prediction in clinical trials.

Although drug-resistant phenotypes in many cultured tumor cell lines have been shown to be due to gene mutation or amplification, it is unclear how relevant these are to clinical drug treatments. One commonly used method to select drug-resistant cells has been to expose cells to mutagens, followed by selection in high concentrations of drug. This likely predisposes to selection of cells with genetically based drug resistance. However, exposure of cells to lower concentrations of drugs, without prior exposure to mutagens, can also lead to cells that show resistance that may be either stable or transient; transient resistance of some cells in the population may even occur spontaneously, without prior drug exposure.

Mechanisms underlying drug resistance that is unstable may include transient amplification of genes, changes in patterns of DNA methylation, and other factors that influence gene expression (these mechanisms are sometimes referred to as *epigenetic*). Methylation of cytosines located within CpG dinucleotides is the most common epigenetic modification in humans. CpG-rich regions (so-called CpG islands) are typically found in the promoter regions of genes and in normal cells are usually unmethylated. However, in tumor cells, such regions are often methylated and, consequently, transcription of the affected gene may be impaired. Gene inactivation by hypermethylation can affect virtually all

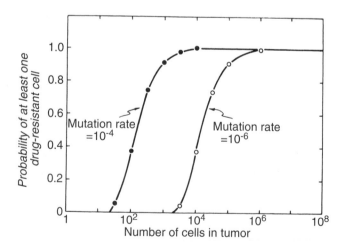

**Figure 18.2.** Probability that there will be at least one drug-resistant cell in a tumor containing varying numbers of cells, based on rates of mutation of $10^{-6}$ (*open symbols*) and $10^{-4}$ (*closed symbols*) per cell per generation. Note that this probability increases from low to high values over a relatively short period in the life history of the tumor and that drug-resistant cells are likely to be established prior to clinical detection. (Adapted from Goldie and Coldman, 1984.)

pathways in the cell. However, when genes encoding DNA repair enzymes (such as *MGMT* and *hMLH1*; Sec. 18.2.7, and Chap. 5, Sec. 5.3.2), drug transporters (such as the reduced folate carrier and the multidrug efflux pump *MDR1*; Secs. 18.2.2 and 18.2.3), or proteins that regulate the cell cycle (e.g., *p16INK^{4a}*, Chap. 9, Sec. 9.2.2) and apoptosis (Sec. 18.2.8) are hypermethylated, the response to antineoplastic agents can be markedly altered. Another epigenetic mechanism of gene regulation that can influence the drug sensitivity of tumor cells is that mediated by acetylation and deacetylation of histones, nuclear proteins closely associated with DNA. Hyperacetylated histones are associated with an open chromatin configuration and in this way, they permit transcription to occur. Tumor cell responses to drugs can be modulated if the gene affected is a known determinant of tumor cell drug sensitivity or resistance. For example, leukemic cells treated with a histone deacetylase inhibitor showed an increased expression of the nuclear drug target, topoisomerase II (Sec. 18.2.6) and an acquired hypersensitivity to etoposide (Kurz et al., 2001).

Clinically important drug resistance is probably due to both genetic and epigenetic mechanisms.

## 18.2.2 Resistance Due to Impaired Drug Uptake

Drug uptake into cells occurs by one of the following mechanisms: (1) passive diffusion, in which the drug enters the cell through the cell membrane by an energy- and temperature-independent process without interacting with specific sites on the membrane; (2) facilitated diffusion, in which the drug interacts in a chemically specific manner with a transport carrier on the cell membrane and is translocated into the cell in an energy- and temperature-independent process; and (3) active transport, in which the drug is actively transported by a carrier-mediated process that is both temperature- and energy-dependent. All three mechanisms allow for drug entry into cells down a concentration gradient, but the third mechanism can also lead to transport against a concentration gradient.

Impaired drug influx is a mechanism of resistance for several alkylating agents and cisplatin. For example, uptake of nitrogen mustard by mammalian cells is an active process. Resistance to nitrogen mustard is multifactorial, but one of the mechanisms leading to resistance is reduced binding affinity of the transport carrier for the drug and either a reduced number of transport sites and/or slower carrier mobility. Uptake of melphalan is also mediated by active transport and this drug may use one of two independent amino acid transport systems: (1) system ASC, which transports preferentially the amino acids alanine, serine, and cysteine, and (2) system L, the leucine-preferring carrier

(Goldenberg and Begleiter, 1984). Resistance to melphalan has been attributed to a specific mutation in the system L carrier leading to reduced binding affinity between the drug and this transport carrier.

Methotrexate is transported across cell membranes both by passive diffusion and by an energy-dependent active transport system, the reduced folate carrier. Drug-resistant cells may arise that have impaired transport of methotrexate into the cell, due to point mutations in the reduced folate carrier (Fig. 18.1; Drori et al., 2000); this appears to be a common mechanism of acquired resistance in patients with acute leukemia (Gorlick et al., 1996). Similarly, cellular uptake of nucleoside analogs such as fludarabine, gemcitabine, and cytarabine occurs primarily via nucleoside-specific membrane transport carriers (NT). Cells deficient in these carrier proteins are highly resistant to these drugs, at least in vitro. Moreover, nucleoside analog transport and sensitivity can be restored by transfection of a cDNA encoding a NT carrier protein (Galmarini et al., 2001; Lang et al., 2001).

## 18.2.3 Multiple Drug Resistance Due to Enhanced Drug Efflux

Many drugs that are either natural products or their derivatives (e.g., anthracyclines such as doxorubicin, *Vinca* alkaloids such as vincristine, etoposide, and the taxanes) may share common mechanisms of resistance. These drugs are often substrates for energy-dependent integral membrane transporter proteins that act to pump the drugs out of cells. The best characterized of these drug efflux pumps is P-glycoprotein (P=*pleiotropic*), which is encoded in humans by the multidrug–resistance (*MDR1*) gene (gene symbol *ABCB1*; for reviews see Endicott and Ling, 1989; Sharom, 1997; Ambudkar et al., 1999; http://nutrigene.4t.com/humanabc.htm). P-glycoprotein is now known to be a member of a superfamily of membrane proteins, known as the adenosine-triphosphate (ATP)–binding cassette (ABC) transporters, which use the energy from ATP-hydrolysis to move a very broad spectrum of molecules ranging from ions to sugars to small peptides across biological membranes (Fig. 18.3; Klein et al., 1999). This superfamily of approximately fifty human proteins is comprised of seven subfamilies (*A* through *G*) and contains several drug resistance proteins in addition to P-glycoprotein, including the multidrug-resistance protein 1 (MRP1; gene symbol *ABCC1*), and the breast cancer resistance protein, BCRP (gene symbol *ABCG2*; Cole et al., 1992; Doyle et al., 1998; Hipfner et al., 1999). A protein that does not belong to the ABC superfamily, known as the lung-resistance protein, LRP or MVP, encodes a major vault protein that is associated with drug resistance in clinical samples (Scheffer

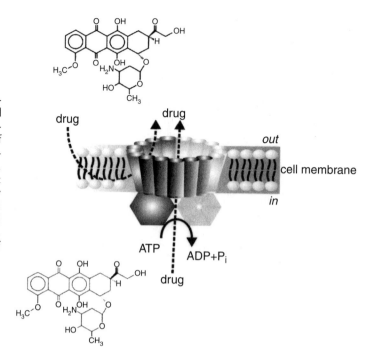

**Figure 18.3.** Transport of drug substrates by ABC efflux pumps is coupled to ATP hydrolysis. It is postulated that the transmembrane segments (here drawn as cylinders) are arranged to form a pore. Shown is a model of MRP1 with seventeen transmembrane segments (α-helices); P-glycoprotein has just twelve while BCRP has six. ATP-binding domains are localized to the cytoplasmic side of the membrane. Substrates which enter the cell by diffusion or active transport, or are formed inside the cell by conjugation, are thought to be exported from the cell either directly through the pore, or, in the case of hydrophobic drugs, are taken up from the inner leaflet of the membrane lipid bilayer.

et al., 1995; Izquierdo et al., 1996). However, the mechanistic role of LRP/MVP in conferring drug resistance is uncertain. Consequently, only multidrug resistance mediated by the better characterized ABC drug efflux transporters is described here. Alternative mechanisms that cause resistance to multiple drugs include changes in the activity of the enzyme topoisomerase II, changes in glutathione and other sulfhydryls, and increased DNA repair; these mechanisms are described in subsequent sections.

*P-Glycoprotein* The genes encoding P-glycoprotein have been cloned and sequenced from many different species (Endicott and Ling, 1989; Sharom, 1997; Ambudkar et al., 1999). In humans, two highly related

linked genes, *MDR1* (*ABCB1*) and *MDR2* (*ABCB3*), have been mapped to chromosome 7, but only *MDR1* confers drug resistance. P-glycoprotein is a phosphoglycoprotein of molecular weight 170 kiloDaltons, and contains two homologous halves, suggesting that it was derived by duplication of a smaller ancestral gene. Each half of P-glycoprotein is comprised of six transmembrane segments (α-helices) followed by a cytosolic ATP-binding site (or nucleotide binding domain). Thus, P-glycoprotein is a typical four-domain ABC transporter (Fig. 18.4) and all four domains are required for its full activity.

P-glycoprotein confers resistance against a wide spectrum of complex heterocyclic hydrophobic, natural product antineoplastic drugs that include the anthra-

P-glycoprotein (MDR1), MRP4, MRP5

MRP1, MRP2, MRP3

BCRP (MXR)

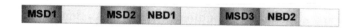

**Figure 18.4.** Domain organization of ATP-binding cassette (ABC) transmembrane transporter drug and conjugated drug metabolite efflux pumps. MSD, membrane spanning domain; NBD, nucleotide binding domain. There is strong evidence that each of the MSDs contains six transmembrane segments (α-helices) except for MSD1 of MRP1, 2, and 3, which contains just five.

cycline antibiotics, the *Vinca* alkaloids and the taxanes (Table 18.2). P-glycoprotein also transports other non-oncolytic drugs widely used in cancer chemotherapy such as the serotonin (5-hydroxytryptamine) receptor (5-HT$_3$) antagonist ondansetron, that is used to control emesis, and the opiate morphine that is used to control pain. Other fluorescent chemicals (e.g., rhodamine 123) or radiopharmaceuticals used in imaging (e.g., $^{99m}$Tc-sestamibi) are also known to be P-glycoprotein substrates and are being investigated for their ability to detect clinical drug resistance mediated by this and other transport proteins (Table 18.2). The remarkably broad substrate specificity of P-glycoprotein has intrigued scientists for years who have devoted considerable effort toward understanding how a single membrane protein can recognize so many structurally diverse chemical entities.

In addition to being frequently overexpressed in tumor cells, P-glycoprotein is also found in normal tissues. It is present at high levels in the normal human kidney and adrenal gland; at intermediate levels in lung, liver, colon, and rectum; and at low levels in most other tissues. P-glycoprotein is localized to the apical surface of cells that line tubules or ducts in these organs, suggesting that the protein provides such cells with a mechanism for extruding xenobiotic molecules, or for preventing uptake of these molecules. P-glycoprotein is also expressed in a polarized way on endothelial cells lining the blood-brain barrier, prompting the suggestion that it performs a related function in excluding toxic natural products from the central nervous system. Strong evidence for this function of P-glycoprotein comes from studies of mice in which these genes have been disrupted by homologous recombination. These mice display a marked increase in sensitivity to the neurotoxic side effects of several different drugs (Schinkel, 1997). Such animals also show enhanced oral absorption (bioavailability) of certain drugs such as paclitaxel. However, despite extensive knowledge of the pharmacological substrates of P-glycoprotein, the physiological substrates of this transporter remain uncertain.

Many investigators have measured levels of P-glycoprotein in human tumors, both before and after treatment with anticancer drugs. Elevated levels of P-glycoprotein have been found in untreated sarcomas and in cancers of the colon, adrenal gland, kidney, liver, and pancreas. All these tumors tend to be resistant to chemotherapy. Elevated levels of P-glycoprotein have also been detected following relapse after chemotherapy in more drug-sensitive tumors, including multiple myeloma and cancers of the breast and ovary. These findings suggest that P-glycoprotein may contribute to clinical drug resistance. Increased expression of P-glycoprotein has also been reported to correlate with a poor prognosis in children with neuroblastoma, rhabdomyosarcoma, and osteogenic sarcoma (Chan et al., 1991).

A variety of agents are known to inhibit the function of P-glycoprotein and to increase the sensitivity of drug-resistant tumor cells in culture (Sandor et al., 1998). Some of these agents appear themselves to be substrates for P-glycoprotein and competitively inhibit the efflux of anticancer drugs, but noncompetitive mechanisms have also been implicated. Multiple clinical trials have assessed the potential of P-glycoprotein antagonists to increase the sensitivity of human tumors to anticancer drugs such as doxorubicin. In many cases, the results have been inconclusive. In a few of these studies, some patients with hematologic malignancies that were drug resistant responded to the same anticancer drugs when an inhibitor of P-glycoprotein was added to the drug regimen. In general, however, the results of studies with solid tumors have been disappointing (Sandor et al., 1998). There are several possible reasons for the inconclusive outcomes of many of these clinical trials. These include poor trial design, resistance due to mechanisms in addition to, or other than, P-glycoprotein, and achievement of inadequate levels of the reversing agent in the tumor tissue. Several third-generation reversal agents with higher affinity and greater potency and specificity are under investigation in clinical trials.

**Table 18.2.** Substrates of P-glycoprotein Relevant to the Effectiveness of Cancer Chemotherapy and of Diagnostic Tests[a]

| | |
|---|---|
| Cytotoxic agents | Vinca alkaloids (vincristine, vinblastine)* |
| | Anthracyclines (doxorubicin, daunorubicin, epirubicin)* |
| | Epipodophyllotoxins (etoposide, teniposide)* |
| | Taxanes (paclitaxel, docetaxel) |
| | Actinomycin D |
| | Topotecan |
| | Methotrexate* |
| | Mitomycin C |
| Analgesics | Morphine |
| Antiemetics | Ondansetron |
| HIV protease inhibitors | Ritonavir |
| | Indinavir |
| | Saquinavir |
| Fluorescent compounds | Hoechst 33342 |
| | Rhodamine 123* |
| | Calcein-AM* |
| Other compounds | $^{99m}$Technetium-sestamibi* |

[a]Agents marked by an asterisk are also known to be transported by MRP1.

*Multidrug-Resistance Protein, MRP1* Like P-glycoprotein, the 190-kiloDalton multidrug-resistance protein, MRP1 (gene symbol *ABCC1*) is a member of the ABC

**Table 18.3.** Drug Substrates of MRP-related
ABC Transporters

| Transporter | Substrates |
|---|---|
| MRP1 | Anthracyclines, *Vincas*, etoposide, paclitaxel, SN-38, MTX (*short exposure*); conjugated organic anions (GS-, glucuronide, sulphate); oxyanions; flutamide |
| MRP2 | Cisplatin, *Vincas*, etoposide, mitoxantrone, doxorubicin, MTX; conjugated organic anions (GS-, glucuronide) |
| MRP3 | VP-16, cisplatin, vincristine, MTX; conjugated organic anions |
| MRP4 | MTX, PMEA, (*nucleoside phosphonates*) |
| MRP5 | 6-Mercaptopurine, thioguanine (*thiopurines*); PMEA |

MTX, methotrexate; PMEA, 9-(2-phosphonyl methoxyethyl) adenine; GS-, glutathione

superfamily of transmembrane transporter proteins. However, the two drug-resistant proteins share only 15 percent amino acid sequence identity (Hipfner et al., 1999; Leslie et al., 2001). MRP1 was originally identified on the basis of its elevated expression in multidrug resistant lung cancer cells which did not express P-glycoprotein and the *MRP1* gene has been mapped to chromosome 16 (Cole et al., 1992). The protein has seventeen transmembrane segments, five more than P-glycoprotein. These five extra transmembrane segments form a third NH$_2$-proximal membrane spanning domain with an extracytosolic NH$_2$-terminus (Fig. 18.4). The precise role of this NH$_2$-terminal hydrophobic extension has not yet been elucidated, but it may be im-

portant for the transport of some MRP1 substrates and has been implicated in protein folding and stabilization.

Increased expression of MRP1 leads to a net decrease in cellular accumulation of a variety of anticancer drugs including both natural products and the folic acid analog methotrexate (Table 18.3). The spectrum of oncolytic drug substrates is, however, slightly different from P-glycoprotein in that MRP1 confers, at most, low levels of resistance to paclitaxel and mitoxantrone. Furthermore, transport across membranes of some drugs (e.g., vincristine, daunorubicin) by MRP1 depends on the presence of reduced glutathione (GSH) or a tripeptide analog (Fig. 18.5). Precisely how GSH facilitates drug transport by MRP1 is not yet fully understood, but, at the very least, it serves to enhance the affinity of MRP1 for some of its substrates (Rappa et al., 1997; Loe et al., 1998; Leslie et al., 2001).

In addition to its ability to confer resistance to anticancer drugs, MRP1 is a primary active transporter of a broad spectrum of organic anions. Substrates include glutathione-, glucuronide-, and sulfate-conjugated metabolites of endo- and xenobiotics (Fig. 18.5). The highest affinity substrate identified so far is the cysteinyl leukotriene, LTC$_4$, a potent mediator of inflammation. Confirmation that this glutathionylated arachidonic acid derivative is a physiologically relevant MRP1 substrate was obtained by analysis of mice bearing a disrupted *Mrp1* gene which showed that these mice had an impaired response to pro-inflammatory stimuli (Wijnholds et al., 1997). Other potential physiological substrates of MRP1 include 17$\beta$-estradiol 17-$\beta$-(D-glucuronide), folic acid, estrone 3-sulfate, reduced and oxidized glutathione, as well as glutathione conjugates of prostaglandin A$_2$ and 4-hydroxy *trans*-2-nonenol, a toxic membrane lipid peroxidation product. MRP1 also

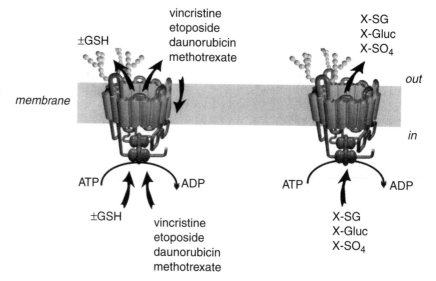

**Figure 18.5.** Transport of conjugated and unconjugated MRP1 substrates across cell membranes. Efflux of most unconjugated anticancer drugs from the cell is dependent on the presence of reduced glutathione. Methotrexate is an exception to this rule. However, MRP1 confers resistance to only short-term exposure to this drug. With some agents (e.g., vincristine, vinblastine, doxorubicin), GSH is cotransported with the drug. Glutathione (X-SG), glucuronide (X-Gluc), and sulphate (X-SO$_4$) conjugated organic anions are usually transported without the stimulation of GSH.

transports fluorescent organic anions such as calcein and fluo-3, which facilitates the measurement of the activity of this transport protein in clinical samples. Thus, the substrate specificity of MRP1 is even more diverse than that of P-glycoprotein (Leslie et al., 2001).

MRP1 has been detected in a wide variety of human tumors and normal tissues, where it is usually expressed at low levels (Nooter et al., 1995; Hipfner et al., 1999). Increased expression has been observed in several types of drug-resistant human tumors, such as lung cancer and some leukemias, and in many cell lines derived from human tumors. In children with neuroblastoma, expression of MRP1 was correlated with expression of the N-*myc* oncogene and predicted poor survival (Norris et al., 1996). Agents such as verapamil and cyclosporin A, which may reverse drug resistance due to P-glycoprotein in cell culture, have much less effect on drug resistance due to MRP1. A number of agents that antagonize the drug efflux activity of MRP1 are under development, and include drugs that act to deplete cellular GSH.

Since the discovery of MRP1 in 1992, four additional MRP-related proteins have been discovered that have been shown to confer some form of drug resistance, at least in vitro (Borst et al., 2000; Leslie et al., 2001). MRP2 (*ABCC2*) and MRP3 (*ABCC3*) are structurally the most similar to MRP1, but there are significant differences among the three proteins with respect to their substrate specificity, normal tissue distribution, and membrane localization in polarized cells. There are several studies suggesting that expression of MRP2 and MRP3 may be upregulated in several tumor types. These transporters may have an equally important influence on drug sensitivity and resistance through their roles in drug distribution and elimination in normal tissues. In particular, because MRP2 is expressed predominantly on apical membranes of the bile caniliculus, renal epithelium, and intestinal enterocytes, it is particularly well situated to play a role in the elimination, as well as oral bioavailability, of drugs and their metabolites that are substrates of this transport protein.

MRP4 (*ABCC4*) and MRP5 (*ABCC5*) are structurally quite different from MRP1–3 in that they lack the third NH2-terminal membrane spanning domain present in the latter three proteins (Fig. 18.4). In this way, the primary structures of MRP4 and MRP5 are more similar to P-glycoprotein. However, unlike P-glycoprotein and MRP1–3, MRP4 and MRP5 have been shown to transport nucleotide analogs such as 9-(2-phosphonyl methoxyethyl) adenine (PMEA), used to treat patients with human immunodeficiency virus infections, and MRP5 may confer resistance to the antimetabolites, 6-mercaptopurine and 6-thioguanine (Wijnholds et al., 2000; Table 18.4). There are as yet, few studies of MRP4

and MRP5 expression in human tumor samples so the clinical relevance of these transporters in drug-resistant malignancies is uncertain.

*Breast Cancer Related Protein*   A third ABC drug efflux pump that causes resistance to certain chemotherapeutic agents, called breast cancer related protein, BCRP (gene symbol *ABCG2*), was first cloned from a drug-resistant breast cancer cell line that expressed neither P-glycoprotein nor MRP1 (Doyle et al., 1998). The *BCRP* (*ABCG2*) gene is localized to human chromosome 4q22. The BCRP protein (also widely known as MXR) contains just 655 amino acids and is much smaller than P-glycoprotein and MRP1. Furthermore, because it is comprised of only a single membrane spanning domain and nucleotide binding domain, it is often referred to as a half-transporter. The structure of BCRP is also unusual for a human ABC protein in that its nucleotide binding domain precedes, rather than follows, its hydrophobic membrane spanning domain (Fig. 18.4).

When overexpressed, BCRP can render tumor cells resistant to mitoxantrone, doxorubicin, daunorubicin, topotecan (a camptothecin derivative), and SN-38, the active metabolite of irinotecan (Doyle et al., 1998; Honjo et al., 2001). Like P-glycoprotein and MRP1, BCRP also transports certain fluorescent molecules which should facilitate detection of this transporter in clinical samples. BCRP is expressed at low levels in normal tissues and, like P-glycoprotein and MRP2, is present on apical membranes of polarized cells. In a murine model system, BCRP has been shown to limit the bioavailability and fetal penetration of topotecan but the physiological substrates of this transporter are not yet known (Jonker et al., 2000).

*Physiological and Toxicological Roles of P-glycoprotein, MRP1, and BCRP*   As described earlier, P-glycoprotein, the MRPs, and BCRP are expressed in normal tissues and, according to their tissue distribution and membrane localization (basolateral vs. apical) in polarized cells, these transporters may contribute to drug absorption (bioavailability), distribution (access to so-called pharmacologic sanctuaries such as the brain and testes), and elimination (efflux into bile or urine; Fig. 18.6). Of additional interest are recent studies that have shown elevated BCRP expression in the so-called side population of bone marrow cells that are highly enriched for undifferentiated stem cells. It seems that BCRP expression is a conserved feature of stem cells from a wide variety of sources, which has prompted the speculation that this ABC transporter might serve to extrude a differentiating substance (Zhou et al., 2001). In vitro studies have shown that single amino acid substi-

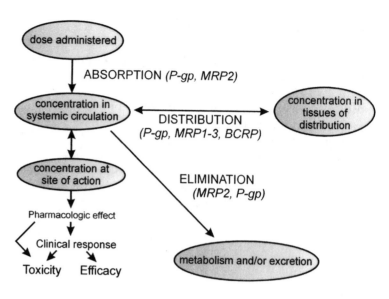

**Figure 18.6.** ABC transport proteins as determinants of drug efficacy and toxicity. ABC transporters may play a role in drug absorption (P-glycoprotein, MRP2) and distribution into various tissues (P-glycoprotein, MRP1–3, BCRP), as well as elimination of drugs and their conjugated metabolites from cells (P-glycoprotein, MRP2).

tutions can markedly alter the substrate specificity of these proteins (Ambudkar et al., 1999; Leslie et al., 2001). For example, mutation of $Gly^{185} \rightarrow Val$ in P-glycoprotein results in decreased resistance to vinblastine; substitution of $Trp^{1246}$ in MRP1 causes total loss of drug resistance; and differences in the amino acid at position 482 dramatically affect the substrate specificity of BCRP. Several naturally occurring polymorphisms of the *MDR1* gene have recently been described that affect the bioavailability and, hence, pharmacokinetics of digoxin. These and other mutations can be expected to affect the pharmacokinetics of other drug substrates important in the treatment and diagnosis of malignant disease (Table 18.3).

In summary, the ABC drug efflux pumps may influence the effectiveness of antineoplastic agents either by reducing drug accumulation in the tumor cells themselves or by affecting the pharmacokinetic properties of drugs that are substrates of these proteins. Pharmacological inhibition of P-glycoprotein (and other ABC transporters) is being explored as a means to improve oral absorption of drugs or enable better penetration of drugs into pharmacologic sanctuaries, tissues that are normally protected by these transporters (Leslie et al., 2001). Furthermore, the ability of these ABC proteins to confer drug resistance has led to the exploration of the use of gene therapy to deliver vectors encoding these transporters into bone marrow and other drug sensitive normal tissues to protect them from the toxic side effects of chemotherapy.

### 18.2.4 Resistance Due to Decreased Drug Activation or Increased Drug Inactivation

Many antimetabolite drugs are inactive in the form that they are administered to patients. Thus, these drugs

must first be taken up by cells and converted to an active form in order to exert their cytotoxic effects. Consequently, resistance to these agents can occur when there is a decrease in activity or levels of the activating enzyme(s), or an increase in the activity or levels of an enzyme that is responsible for detoxifying the active form of the drug. For example, drug-resistant leukemic cells may show a decrease in polyglutamation of intracellular methotrexate due to either decreased activity of the synthetic enzyme, folylpolyglutamate synthase, or increased activity of the catabolic enzyme, folylpolyglutamate hydrolase (Fig. 18.1; Gorlick et al., 1996). Resistance to the pyrimidine analog cytosine arabinoside may occur as a result of decreased activation by kinases, and/or enhanced inactivation by deaminases (Galmarini et al., 2001). Similarly, resistance to the fluoropyrimidine, 5-fluorouracil, is associated with alterations in the enzymes responsible for its activation and detoxification. There is some evidence that levels of dihydropyrimidine dehydrogenase, the first and rate-limiting 5-fluorouracil catabolic enzyme, may be an important predictor of intrinsic resistance to this drug in patients with colon cancer (Gorlick and Bertino, 1999; Chap. 16, Sec. 16.4.2).

Glutathione (GSH)-mediated detoxification pathways play a central role in the inactivation of certain antineoplastic agents and chemical carcinogens. Many of these compounds cause cellular damage by the production of reactive intermediates. Similar processes are involved during the interaction of ionizing radiation with tissue (Chap. 14, Sec. 14.2.3). One mechanism by which cells can protect themselves from damage caused by reactive agents is the synthesis of a high concentration of sulfhydryl containing molecules, especially the tripeptide GSH, which can react with reactive intermediates and render them nontoxic (Fig. 18.7). The im-

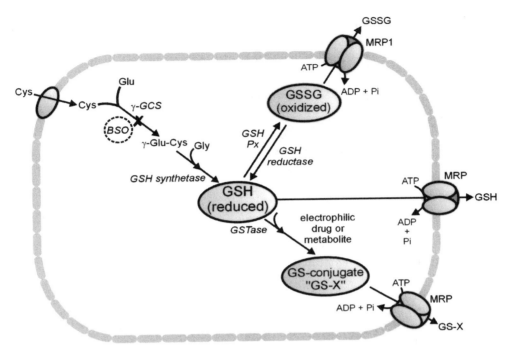

**Figure 18.7.** Cellular metabolism of glutathione. Reduced glutathione (GSH) can inactivate per-oxides and free radicals through reactions catalyzed by glutathione peroxidase (GSH Px) and a family of glutathione $S$-transferases (GSTs), respectively. The rate-limiting enzyme of GSH biosynthesis, $\gamma$-glutamyl cystine synthetase ($\gamma$-GCS), can be irreversibly inhibited by buthionine sulfoximine (BSO) causing cellular depletion of GSH. The ratio of reduced GSH to oxidized GSSG in the cell can be modulated by the activity of MRP1, which is an efficient transporter of GSSG. Cellular accumulation of GSH conjugated metabolites (GS-X) is also regulated by the activity of MRP1 (and MRP2). GSH also supports MRP1- and MRP2-mediated elimination of drugs and toxins from cells (see Fig. 18.5).

portance of GSH in the protection of normal cells is reflected in its widespread distribution and its relatively high intracellular concentration ($> 1$ mM). Reduced GSH can inactivate peroxides and free radicals, which may be produced by drugs such as doxorubicin. It can also react with positively charged electrophilic molecules, such as the active groups of alkylating agents (Chap. 16, Sec. 16.2), rendering them less toxic and more easily excreted. These reactions are catalyzed, respectively, by the enzymes glutathione peroxidase and GSH $S$-transferase (GST; Fig. 18.7).

By conjugating GSH to various drugs or their active metabolites, GSTs appear to play a role in the development of cellular resistance to some antineoplastic agents (Tew, 1994). The cytosolic GSTs are a multigene family of enzymes and are classified by their isoelectric points, as well as by their relative sequence homology, as basic ($\alpha$ class), neutral ($\mu$ class), and acidic ($\pi$ class). Each functional GST enzyme is a homo- or heterodimer made up of subunits encoded by gene loci from within a given class. Several lines of evidence support a role for GSTs in resistance to alkylating agents:

1. Nitrogen mustards can form GSH conjugates in reactions catalyzed by GSTs.

2. Human tumors and tumor cell lines often overexpress GST isozymes.

3. GST inhibitors can sometimes sensitize cultured tumor cells to alkylating agents.

4. Cell cycle–dependent sensitivity to melphalan correlates with the cell cycle–dependent expression of certain GSTs.

5. Transfection of cDNAs encoding certain GST isoforms can confer resistance to alkylating agents (Puchalski and Fahl, 1990).

6. Elevation of GST can occur within several days of exposure to chlorambucil as part of the normal cellular response.

In contrast, some cell lines selected for resistance to alkylating agents have shown no increase in GST protein levels or activity.

Drugs conjugated to GSH, glucuronide, or sulfate are negatively charged and these conjugated organic anions have long been known to be extruded from cells by an energy dependent process. So-called glutathione-conjugate export carriers (known variably as GS-X pumps or multispecific organic anion transporters) were known to be involved but only recently has it been appreciated that this export function is undertaken, in large part, by the MRP-related ABC transport proteins, particularly MRP1 and MRP2 (Konig et al., 1999; Leslie et al., 2001; Sec. 18.2.3). While conjugated metabolites are generally thought to be less reactive and detoxified already, their active efflux by the MRP-related transporters prevents their intracellular accumulation, thereby reducing the possibility of hydrolytic enzymes causing the regeneration of the active parent compound. In some instances, however, certain conjugated metabolites can be directly cytotoxic because of their ability to inhibit enzymes important for cell viability, as well as by product inhibition of the conjugating enzymes. Thus, elimination of conjugated metabolites from the cell can result in reduced cytotoxicity (Figs. 18.5 and 18.7).

Resistance to cisplatin and alkylating agents has also been associated with increased levels of metallothioneins, proteins rich in sulfhydryl-containing cysteine residues. The presumed mechanism is a neutralization of the toxic electrophilic drugs or their metabolites, by their interaction with these proteins. A cause-and-effect relationship has been suggested by development of resistance to cisplatin and alkylating agents in cells transfected with a human metallothionein gene (Kelley et al., 1988), and by increased sensitivity of cells that do not produce metallothionein (Kondo et al., 1995). Conversely, studies of cisplatin-resistant cells derived from human ovarian cancer did not show a correlation between resistance and metallothionein levels (Schilder et al., 1990). Multiple mechanisms are known to be involved in resistance to platinum-containing drugs (Table 18.1) and the relative contribution of enhanced detoxification by increased levels of metallothioneins is unclear.

## 18.2.5 Resistance Due to Increased Levels or Modification of the Drug Target

In order to exert their cytotoxicity, antimetabolites agents must interact with their intracellular protein targets. Changes may occur such that levels of the drug target protein are increased, thus requiring increased concentrations of drug to observe cytotoxicity. Alternatively, the levels of the drug target protein may remain the same but the gene encoding the protein can acquire a mutation that results in the production of a protein with normal metabolic activity but with a lower affinity for the drug. These resistance mechanisms have the potential to reduce the effectiveness of both conventional and novel therapeutic agents. For example, among the multiple mechanisms of resistance reported for 5-fluorouracil (5-FU), is the acquisition of mutations in its target enzyme, thymidylate synthase (Gorlick and Bertino, 1999; see also Chap. 16, Sec. 16.4.2). Clinical resistance to imatinib (Gleevec®), a recently developed

tyrosine kinase inhibitor, has also been shown to result from a point mutation that results in diminished interaction of this drug with its target, the p210 BCR-ABL protein. BCR-ABL is encoded by the Philadelphia chromosomal translocation found in chronic myeloid leukemia which fuses part of the BCR gene from chromosome 22 to part of the c-ABL gene on chromosome 9 (Chap. 7, Sec. 7.2.4). A single C → T change causes a threonine to isoleucine substitution at amino acid position 315, which disrupts a critical hydrogen bond between the drug target (BCR-ABL) and the drug imatinib (Gorre et al., 2001).

Methotrexate resistance may occur because of the production of variant forms of dihydrofolate reductase (DHFR), the target enzyme for this drug (Fig. 18.1; Gorlick et al., 1996). Variant enzymes have been found that retain adequate function for reduction of their normal substrate (dihydrofolate) but have decreased affinity for methotrexate.

Another common mechanism leading to methotrexate resistance in cell lines and experimental tumors exposed to increasing concentrations of this drug is elevated production of DHFR resulting from an increase in the number of copies of the DHFR gene (gene amplification; Schimke, 1984). High levels of methotrexate resistance in cultured cells have usually been observed after stepwise increases in the drug concentration in the medium, and this may lead to as many as 100 to 1000 copies of the DHFR gene. Amplification of DHFR has also been observed in human lung tumors from patients treated with methotrexate.

Although gene amplification has been studied most extensively in relation to methotrexate resistance, there is increasing evidence for the importance of this mechanism in determining resistance to several other drugs, including upregulation of the target enzymes for 5-FU (thymidylate synthase) and other antimetabolites. Amplification of genes encoding one of the integral membrane ABC drug efflux pumps (MDR1, MRP1, BCRP), can also lead to multiple drug-resistance phenotypes (Sec. 18.2.3; Fig. 18.8). Resistance to the kinase inhibitor imatinib in patients with chronic myeloid leukemia has also been associated with an increased copy number of the BCR-ABL fusion gene described earlier (Gorre et al., 2001).

Drug resistance due to gene amplification may be either stable or unstable when cells are grown in the absence of the drug. Stable amplification is typically associated with a chromosomal location of the amplified genes, often seen as homogeneously staining regions (HSRs) in stained chromosome preparations. Unstable amplification is usually associated with location of the genes in extrachromosomal chromatin structures known as double minutes (DMs). Both locations may be evident during selection for drug resistance (Fig. 18.8).

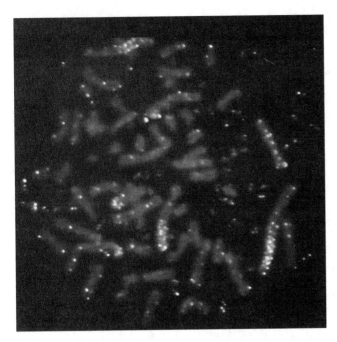

**Figure 18.8.** Fluorescent in situ hybridization analysis of *MRP1*. The normal cellular locus of the *MRP1 (ABCC1)* gene encoding the 190 kiloDalton ABC drug efflux pump, MRP1, is chromosome 16p13.1. However, in many drug-resistant cell lines, *MRP1* has been amplified. The figure shows a metaphase spread of a highly drug-resistant lung cancer cell which contains approximately 100 copies of *MRP1*. Note that the fluorescently labeled MRP1 probe has hybridized to several homogeneously staining regions (HSRS) and multiple double minute chromosomes (DMINS). (With permission from Slovak et al., 1993.) (See color plate.)

### 18.2.6 Topoisomerases and Drug Resistance

DNA topoisomerases are nuclear enzymes that catalyze topologic changes of DNA structure required for recombination and replication of DNA and for transcription of RNA. These enzymes also play a central role in chromosome structure, condensation/decondensation, and segregation (Li and Liu, 2001). Topoisomerases serve as cellular targets for several important antineoplastic agents.

Camptothecin and its close structural analogs topotecan and CPT-11 exert their anti-tumor activity by inhibiting DNA topoisomerase I (see Chap. 16, Sec. 16.5.1). The gene for human topoisomerase I is located on chromosome 20q12-13.2 and encodes a 100-kilo-Dalton monomeric protein. Under physiologic conditions, the enzyme produces transient single-strand breaks in DNA and binds covalently to the 3′-phosphoryl end of DNA at the break site through a tyrosine residue at position 723 in the COOH-terminus. It then facilitates passage of an intact DNA strand through the break site, followed by religation of the cleaved DNA. Camptothecin or its analogs form a reversible complex with topoisomerase I and DNA, which shifts the equilibrium reaction markedly in the direction of cleavage. This results in increased DNA damage and ultimately cell death. Downregulation and production of mutant forms of DNA topoisomerase I have been reported in cells resistant to these drugs (Pommier et al., 1999; Li and Liu, 2001; Urasaki et al., 2001). Point mutations involving amino acid residues 361 to 364 appear particularly critical for resistance to camptothecin and its derivatives. Recent analyses of the topoisomerase I crystal structure indicate that this region is important for hydrogen bonding to camptothecin and it is close to the catalytic tyrosine residue and the bound DNA (Urasaki et al., 2001).

Topoisomerase II is the intracellular target for a very different set of effective and clinically useful agents than topoisomerase I. All vertebrates have two forms of topoisomerase II termed topoisomerase IIα (170 kDa), encoded by the human *TOP2A* gene on chromosome 17q21-22 and topoisomerase IIβ (180 kDa), encoded by the *TOP2B* gene on chromosome 3p24 (Tan et al., 1992; Lang et al., 1998). Both enzymes function as homodimers and it is thought that their catalytic mechanisms are the same. The multiple steps of the catalytic cycle of topoisomerase II are illustrated schematically in Figure 18.9.

Drugs that target topoisomerase II may either convert topoisomerase II into a DNA damaging agent when it is bound to DNA or may act directly by inhibiting the enzyme: they may stabilize cleaved complexes and/or prevent DNA strand passage and/or inhibit the binding of topoisomerase II to DNA (Fig. 18.10). The drug-stabilized topoisomerase II-mediated DNA double-strand breaks, although often repaired, constitute a signal for programmed cell death (apoptosis) through a pathway that is still not completely understood. Resistance to etoposide, doxorubicin, mitoxantrone, and other drugs that exert their cytotoxicity through this enzyme can therefore result from any alterations that reduce the number of drug-stabilized topoisomerase II complexes formed.

Decreases in topoisomerase IIα levels caused by decreased protein synthesis or increased protein degradation, as well as a variety of point mutations and small deletions that alter the enzyme's ability to bind DNA and/or drug, have been associated with resistance in numerous cultured cell lines. Several of these mutations have also been observed in clinical samples. In almost all reports to date, topoisomerase II changes have involved the α isoenzyme, but decreases in topoisomerase IIβ levels have also been reported (Austin and Marsh, 1998; Lang et al., 1998).

Although closely related in amino acid sequence (homology >70%), topoisomerase II α and β differ in certain biochemical and biophysical characteristics as well as in their tissue specific expression, subcellular local-

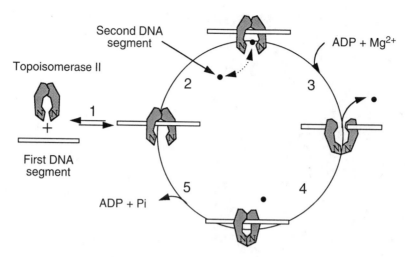

**Figure 18.9.** The catalytic cycle of topoisomerase II: the two-gate model. 1, DNA binding. In the absence of bound ATP, the enzyme is in the form of an open clamp and can bind to or dissociate from a segment of double-stranded DNA. The enzyme bound to the DNA creates a potential DNA gate. 2, Second DNA strand. A second DNA segment can enter and leave the DNA-bound enzyme as long as the gate remains open. 3, DNA cleavage and double-strand DNA passage. Binding of ATP to the enzyme closes the protein gate consisting of the N-terminal domain of each polypeptide in the homodimeric enzyme. A second gate on the opposite side to the N gate opens to allow exit to the second DNA segment from the interior of the enzyme. The opening of the second gate creates a transient double-stranded break in the DNA backbone. 4, Religation. The second gate closes, and the cleaved DNA is religated. 5, ATP hydrolysis and enzyme turnover. The enzyme returns to the open-clamp form bound to DNA following ATP hydrolysis. (Modified from Roca and Wang, 1994.)

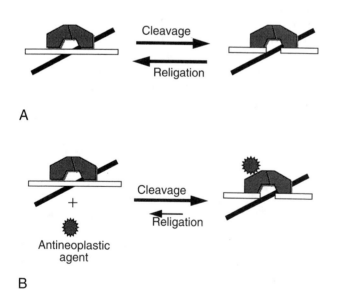

**Figure 18.10.** Interaction of certain antineoplastic agents with DNA topoisomerase II. (A) In the absence of drug, topo II binds to the DNA and establishes a DNA cleavage/religation equilibrium. (B) In the presence of drug, the antineoplastic agent binds to topo II, stabilizes the DNA-enzyme complex, and shifts the equilibrium markedly in the direction of DNA strand cleavage.

ization, cell cycle dependence, and sensitivity to some antineoplastic agents (Austin and Marsh, 1998). Thus, while it is clear that many drugs target both isoenzymes, there is also evidence that certain cytotoxic drugs prefer one or other protein. These observations have implications for the therapeutic potential of topoisomerase IIα-specific drugs in tumors, which have become resistant to topoisomerase IIβ-specific drugs and vice versa.

### 18.2.7 Drug Resistance and Repair of Drug-mediated DNA Damage

Tumor cells die because of the DNA damage caused by certain chemotherapeutic agents unless the damage is repaired. Conversely, resistance may occur because DNA repair processes in the tumor cells have become more efficient. DNA is constantly being subjected to damage by both exogenous and endogenous toxins. Consequently, it is not surprising that cells have developed multiple mechanisms of DNA repair, each of which corrects a different subset of lesions (Chap. 5, Sec. 5.3).

Alkylating agents and platinum-containing drugs exert their cytotoxicity, at least in part, by alkylation of guanine bases in DNA (Gerson and Willson, 1995; Chap. 16, Secs. 16.2 and 16.3). $O^6$-Alkylguanine DNA alkyltransferase ($O^6$-AGAT; also known as $O^6$-methyl-guanine-DNA methyltransferase, MGMT) is the predominant enzyme responsible for the repair of alkylated DNA. $O^6$-AGAT/ MGMT removes adducts from the $O^6$ position of guanine and transfers the alkyl group to a specific cysteine residue (acceptor site) on the enzyme itself (Fig. 18.11; see also Chap. 5, Sec. 5.3.1). Because this transfer and alkylation of $O^6$-AGAT/ MGMT renders the enzyme inactive, the enzyme is considered to act by a so-called suicide mechanism. Levels of $O^6$-AGAT/ MGMT or the methylation status of the *MGMT* promoter (which controls the expression of the gene) have been shown to be useful predictors of the responsiveness of certain tumors to alkylating agents (Esteller et al., 2000). Potential opportunities exist to circumvent drug resistance mediated by $O^6$-AGAT/ MGMT through the use of $O^6$-benzylguanine, a relatively nontoxic agent that can act as a noncompetitive substrate for $O^6$-AGAT/ MGMT, resulting in transfer of the benzyl group to the active site of the enzyme, causing irreversible inactivation. Resistance to nitrosoureas and cisplatin in human tumor cell lines has also been associated with elevated expression of several enzymes involved in nucleotide excision repair (Chap. 5, Sec. 5.3.4).

Alkylating agents, as well as other oncolytic drugs (including antimetabolites and topoisomerase I and II inhibitors), also cause the accumulation of double-stranded DNA breaks which leads to cell death unless the breaks are repaired. Repair of double-stranded DNA breaks can take place by either nonhomologous or homology-directed repair pathways, the relative contribution of which depends on a variety of different factors (Chap. 5, Secs. 5.3.5 and 5.3.6). Increased levels of the DNA-dependent protein kinase (DNA-PK), which is an essential component of nonhomologous DNA end-joining (NHEJ) repair of double-stranded DNA breaks, has been implicated in drug resistance in vitro. In con-

trast to NHEJ, homologous recombinational repair processes use the undamaged sister chromatid as a template and requires the concerted action of a relatively large number of proteins. Recently, resistance to melphalan in a panel of epithelial tumor cell lines was found to correlate with levels of one of these proteins, XRCC3 (Wang et al., 2001).

DNA damage caused by chemotherapeutic agents can also cause a delay in cell cycle progression until the damage is removed. Disruption of the so-called cell cycle checkpoints (Chap. 5, Sec. 5.4) interferes with homologous recombinational repair and consequently, inhibiting one or more of the proteins involved in checkpoint processes has been proposed as a means by which drug sensitivity can be increased. Indeed, there are some preliminary reports of kinase inhibitors that target the checkpoint proteins CHK1 and CHK2, causing an increase in the chemosensitivity of tumor cells in vitro (Sampath and Plunkett, 2001). However, it remains to be seen whether this is a viable strategy for circumventing drug resistance in vivo.

### 18.2.8 Resistance to Apoptosis

The mechanisms of drug resistance described in previous sections are those in which the interaction of the anticancer drug with its target has been modified such that the activation of the pathways that normally lead to tumor cell death may be diminished. However, differences in the sensitivity and resistance of tumor cells to anticancer drugs might also occur, because of cell-type specific differences in components of the pathways that mediate cell death. Following treatment with many anticancer drugs, apoptosis appears to be initiated by the mitochondrial cytochrome c/Apaf-1/caspase-9 pathway (Chap. 10, Sec. 10.2). Signaling through the death receptor pathway by drug-induced FasL upregulation seems less important, except possibly for 5-FU-induced cytotoxicity. Thus the pro-apoptotic and the anti-apoptotic members of the bcl-2 family, the kinases and phosphatases that regulate their activity and subcellular localization, the initiator and effector caspases, the various inhibitors of apoptosis proteins (IAPs), as well as the presence of wild-type or mutant p53, are all proteins that might affect the drug sensitivity of tumor cells. Cell death following treatment with other drugs, including cisplatin, may be mediated by the stress-activated protein kinase pathway, and mutations in this pathway might also lead to drug resistance (Zanke et al., 1996).

Laboratory studies provide evidence that in some cell types, drug sensitivity (as measured by a colony-forming assay or effects on growth of tumors), can be modulated by changing the expression levels and/or

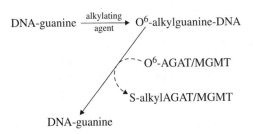

**Figure 18.11.** Repair of an alkylated guanine base by $O^6$-alkylguanine DNA alkyltransferase. The DNA repair enzyme ($O^6$-AGAT/MGMT) removes adducts from the $O^6$ position of guanine by transferring the alkyl group to a cysteine residue in the enzyme itself, resulting in auto-inactivation.

posttranslational modifications of proteins that are components of apoptotic signaling pathways. For example, in a human leukemia cell line, transfection of the *bcl-2* gene led to increased resistance to cytosine arabinoside (Hu et al., 1995). However, other investigators have found little or no effect on drug sensitivity from modulating pathways of apoptosis (e.g., Lock and Stribinskiene, 1996; Tannock and Lee, 2001) and the clinical relevance of apoptotic pathways in determing drug sensitivity is not clear. Markers of apoptosis (for example, an increase in TUNEL-positive cells; Chap. 10, Sec. 10.3) are observed commonly after treatment of malignant cells (or solid tumors) with anticancer drugs. A key determinant of whether the process of apoptosis might be modified to influence drug sensitivity is whether it is primary in converting damage into cellular lethality, or simply represents a pathway whereby cells that have already sustained lethal and nonrepairable damage undergo cellular lysis (Fig. 18.12; Brown and Wouters, 1999; Tannock and Lee, 2001). This probably depends on both the drugs used and the cell type that is treated.

The *p53* gene plays a role in apoptosis, and normal wild-type *p53* can stimulate apoptosis of cells that have sustained damage to DNA (Chap. 10, Sec. 10.2.4). Mutations in the *p53* gene, which are present in a substantial proportion of human cancers, may inhibit apoptosis. There is considerable evidence that the status of the p53 protein may influence response to anticancer drugs, and modification of apoptosis is probably one of several mechanisms of drug resistance that can be influenced (Ferreira et al., 1999). For example, in one study, transfection of wild-type *p53* into colon cancer cells that had an endogenous mutant p53 protein was found to increase sensitivity to 5-FU, camptothecin, and radiation (Yang et al., 1996). In another example, loss of p53 was reported to confer high-level multidrug resistance in neuroblastoma cells (Keshelava et al., 2001). There is evidence that hypoxia in solid tumors can lead to a selective growth advantage for cells that express a mutant *p53* gene, leading to a drug-resistant population (see Sec. 18.3.2 and Chap. 15, Sec. 15.4.2).

Apoptosis is a complex process that is regulated in a complex manner (see Chap. 10). A better understanding of the signaling pathways that lead to cell death in response to anticancer drugs and establishing the clinical relevance of these pathways is essential before effective strategies for their reversal can be implemented.

## 18.3 DRUG RESISTANCE IN VIVO

Many laboratory-based studies of the mechanisms that underlie drug resistance have followed an approach whereby cultured tumor cells at low density are exposed to repeated selection in increasing concentrations of the anticancer drug of interest. These studies have led to the characterization of the multiple mechanisms of drug resistance described in previous sections, many of which appear to be relevant to human cancer. However, several observations suggest that the selection of stable drug-resistant subpopulations, present because of spontaneous mutation or gene amplification, provides an incomplete model for the presence of drug resistance in human cancer. Drug resistance of human tumors often occurs without prior drug exposure or may emerge after brief exposure of solid tissue at high cell density to a relatively low concentration of drug or drugs achievable in plasma. Also, when human tumors relapse after initial chemotherapy, they may respond later to the same chemotherapy with a probability of response that is in the same range as would be expected for untreated tumors (Cara and Tannock, 2001), suggesting that the resistant phenotype may be transient. Clinical drug resistance, especially for solid tumors, may also occur as a result of mechanisms that depend on the in vivo environment. The cells in solid tumors have close cellular contact and a complex extracellular matrix (Chap. 11, Sec. 11.4). Tumors have a poorly formed vasculature, which leads to regions of hypoxia and extracellular acidity (Chap. 12, Sec. 12.3), and a requirement that anticancer drugs penetrate over relatively long intercapillary distances (as compared to those in normal tissues) to reach the target tumor cells. Variable concentration of nutrient metabolites in the extracellular environment, and other factors, lead to variable rates of cell proliferation before treatment, and of repopu-

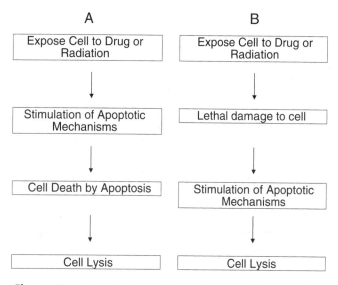

**Figure 18.12.** Apoptosis as (*A*) a primary or (*B*) secondary mechanism of cell lysis after drug treatment. (From Tannock and Lee, 2000.)

lation of surviving tumor cells after treatment, both of which influence drug sensitivity of experimental and clinical tumors.

The mechanisms of drug resistance in tumors that are discussed below have been observed using model systems that maintain cellular interactions with other cells and with the extracellular matrix to better reflect how tumors in patients undergoing chemotherapy are exposed to drugs. One commonly used model is provided by spheroids, in which malignant cells grow in contact with each other and with an extracellular matrix to form nodules in tissue culture (Sutherland, 1988; Durand, 1989; Fig. 18.13A). Alternatively, tumor cells can be grown on collagen-coated semiporous Teflon membranes to form multicellular layers to provide a useful model for studying drug penetration through tumor tissue (Hicks et al., 1997; Figs. 18.13B C; see Sec. 18.3.3).

## 18.3.1 Influence of Cell Contact and the Extracellular Matrix on Drug Resistance

Repeated treatment with chemotherapeutic agents of solid tissue, either in the form of spheroids or tumor-bearing mice, may lead to drug resistance that is expressed only when the cells are regrown in contact with one another as spheroids or tumors. The tumor cells do not display drug resistance when grown without cell-cell contact in dilute cell culture (Teicher et al., 1990; Kerbel et al., 1994; Oloumi et al., 2001). Further work has suggested that this type of drug resistance is correlated with the density of cell packing in spheroids and may be reversed by agents which inhibit adhesion between the cells (St. Croix et al., 1996; Shain and Dalton, 2001). Adherent drug-resistant cells in spheroids may express increased levels of the cell-cycle–inhibitory cyclin-dependent kinase, p27$^{KIP1}$ (Chap. 9, Sec. 9.2.2),

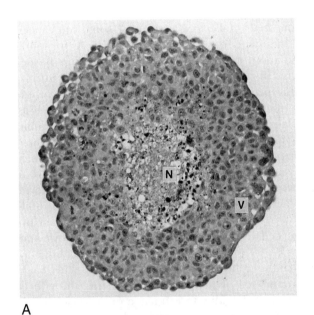

A

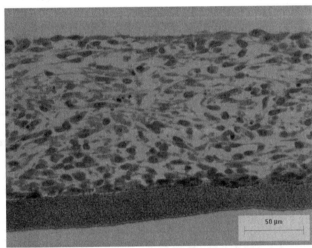

B

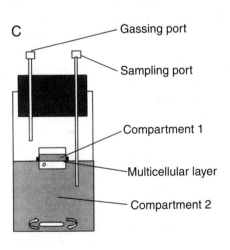

C

Gassing port

Sampling port

Compartment 1

Multicellular layer

Compartment 2

**Figure 18.13.** Models used for study of drug resistance that depends on the microenvironment found in solid tumors. (A) A spheroid. The distribution of fluorescent compunds may be imaged directly. (B) A multicellular layer (MCL). (C) An MCL grown on a collagen-coated Teflon membrane is floated on medium in a larger vessel. A drug is added to compartment 1 in dilute agar and sampled as a function of time in the stirred compartment 2, on the other side of the MCL.

so that these effects may be mediated in part by a low rate of cell proliferation in the solid tissue environment.

When drugs are tested against tumor cells in dilute tissue culture ($\sim 10^5$ cells/ml) there is an implicit assumption that relative cell kill will be similar at higher cell concentrations such as are found in solid tumors ($10^8$ to $10^9$ cells/mL). This assumption of first order kinetics is usually correct for drugs that are present in much higher concentration than their molecular targets, as is probably the case for most anticancer drugs that kill cells by depositing a limited amount of damage in DNA. This assumption may not be correct for agents that must inactivate a very large number of cellular targets in order to be effective. For example, agents such as verapamil or cyclosporin A, which reverse multiple drug resistance due to P-glycoprotein in dilute tissue culture, have been reported to lose their effect as the cell concentration in tissue culture increases (Tunggal et al., 1999). One can therefore predict lack of effectiveness of these inhibitors of P-glycoprotein at cell concentrations that are observed in solid tumors. Inactivity at high cell concentration could also be a problem for some other agents that are directed against targets on the cell surface, such as those that inhibit some growth factor receptors, if there are a large number of targets per cell.

In addition to the effects of high cellular concentration and cell-cell contact, the drug sensitivity of tumor cells can be modulated by direct contact with other components of the tumor cell environment. Thus, both in vitro and in vivo studies have shown that contact with the extracellular matrix can provide tumor cells with protection from drug-induced cell death. Resistance observed because of cell-cell interactions or because of the interaction of cancer cells with the extracellular matrix, has been described as cell-adhesion–mediated drug resistance (Shain and Dalton, 2001). Several strategies to circumvent this type of resistance have been proposed which target molecules in tumor cells and/or in the extracellular matrix that are required for cell adhesion. For example, increased drug sensitivity might be achieved by using synthetic peptides that block the binding of tumor cells to laminin, thus abrogating cellular adhesion.

## 18.3.2 Drug Resistance in Hypoxic Environments

Tumor vasculature is characterized by irregular blood flow and stasis, and by relatively large intercapillary distances as compared to those in normal tissues (Chap. 12, Sec. 12.3). This leads to regions in tumors that are hypoxic, and where the extracellular pH is relatively low due to the production of carbonic and lactic acids, and poor clearance of these and other acidic products of metabolism. Hypoxia is widely recognized as a major

factor leading to resistance of cells in solid tumors to radiotherapy (Chap. 15, Sec. 15.4), but several mechanisms may also cause cells in such regions to be resistant to anticancer drugs. Limited penetration of tissue by anticancer drugs may lead to low drug concentration in hypoxic regions of tumors as discussed in the following section; other potential mechanisms are reviewed below.

Not surprisingly, cells in nutrient-deprived regions of tumors tend to have a low rate of cell proliferation in comparison to that of cells situated close to functional blood vessels (Chap. 9, Sec. 9.4.5). Most of the available anticancer drugs have much greater toxicity for proliferating as compared to nonproliferating cells (Chap. 17, Sec. 17.2.4), so even if the drugs achieve potentially cytotoxic concentrations in these regions, the level of cell kill may be limited. Such cells may begin to proliferate more rapidly following loss of more sensitive cells closer to blood vessels, and may therefore allow regrowth of the tumor.

Hypoxia and extracellular acidity may have direct effects on the uptake and activity of some anticancer drugs, independent of proliferative status. As for ionizing radiation, the toxicity of some drugs may be dependent, in part, on the production of free radicals, and this process depends on availability of oxygen. Drugs that require active transport into cells, such as methotrexate, are dependent on ATP, and anaerobic metabolism is much less efficient than oxidative phosphorylation in producing ATP. Drugs that are weak bases, such as doxorubicin and mitoxantrone, have a greater proportion of molecules in the charged form under acidic conditions, and this decreases their ability to penetrate the cell membrane and be taken up into the cell, leading to decreased activity (Vukovic and Tannock, 1997). In contrast, extracellular acidity may enhance the uptake of drugs that are weak acids, such as chlorambucil or melphalan. In general, the effects of hypoxia and acidity to influence drug sensitivity directly are smaller than those for radiation.

Hypoxia may influence genetically based mechanisms of cellular drug resistance in at least two ways. Transient exposure to hypoxia, as may occur in tumors because of fluctuations in blood flow, may stimulate the amplification of genes, including those encoding DHFR which leads to resistance to methotrexate (Sec. 18.2.5), or P-glycoprotein (Rice et al., 1986). Also, cells in many tumors do not express wild-type *p53* (Chap. 7, Sec. 7.4.2). Hypoxia has been found to convey a selective survival and growth advantage for cells lacking wild-type *p53*, because such cells show a diminished rate of apoptosis under hypoxic conditions (Graeber et al., 1996; Fig. 18.14). This effect may explain why the presence of hypoxia in tumors is a poor prognostic factor after all types of management (including surgery as well as

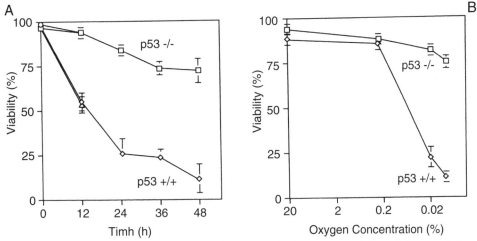

**Figure 18.14.** Selective outgrowth of p53$^{-/-}$ cells under hypoxic conditions. (*A*) Loss of viability due to apoptosis of p53$^{-/-}$ or p53$^{+/+}$ Rat I transformed cells under hypoxic conditions. (*B*) Loss of viability of the same cells following 24-hour exposure to different levels of oxygen (from Graeber et al., 1996).

radiotherapy; Chap. 15, Sec. 15.4). Following treatment with anticancer drugs that leads to selective killing of rapidly proliferating aerobic cells situated closer to tumor blood vessels, there may be selective repopulation of the tumor by *p53$^{-/-}$* cells, which have survived hypoxic conditions, and which may be resistant to many therapeutic agents. It has been found that the outgrowth of such *p53$^{-/-}$* cells can convey resistance to treatment directed against tumor blood vessels, as well as that with more conventional therapy (Yu et al., 2002).

### 18.3.3 Drug Access and Tumor Cell Resistance

Effective treatment of solid tumors requires both that the constituent cells be sensitive to the drug(s) that are used, and that the drugs achieve a sufficient concentration to exert lethal toxicity for all of the viable cells in the tumor. This depends on the efficient delivery of drugs through the vascular system of the tumor, and penetration of the drugs from tumor capillaries to reach tumor cells that are distant from them.

The distribution of fluorescent or radiolabeled drugs has been studied following their application to spheroids (Fig. 18.13*A*) and has indicated poor penetration within tissue of several drugs including doxorubicin and methotrexate. In another method, the vital fluorescent dye, Hoechst 33342, which binds to DNA, has been used to establish a gradient into tissue from the periphery of spheroids, or from tumor blood vessels following its injection into experimental animals. Following treatment with anticancer drugs, the tissue is dissociated, cells are separated on the basis of Hoechst fluorescence by cell sorting, and clonogenic cell survival is estimated as a function of distance into tissue. This method has confirmed that drug delivery is a major limitation for doxo-

rubicin, although not for 5-FU and several alkylating agents (Chaplin et al., 1985; Durand, 1989). Although the same factors that lead to slow drug penetration after acute administration may lead to longer drug retention after chronic exposure, most of the administered drug is likely to be metabolized and/or excreted before tissue penetration has occurred.

A conceptually simple technique has been established which allows direct assessment of tissue penetration by anticancer drugs (Hicks et al., 1997). Tumor cells are grown on a collagen-coated microporous Teflon membrane as a multicellular layer (MCL) that has similar characteristics to tumor tissue in vivo (Fig. 18.13*B*). These MCLs typically achieve a thickness of ~200 micrometer, similar to the maximum distance between blood vessels and necrosis in human tumors. Tumor cells within MCLs appear to have properties that reflect those in solid tumors, in that they have cellular contact with tight junctions between epithelial cells and develop an extracellular matrix (Tannock et al., 2002). Thus, MCLs provide a good model for studying drug penetration through solid tumor tissue that is likely to reflect drug penetration properties in vivo.

Several investigators have used MCLs to study drug penetration (e.g., Tannock et al., 2002). There are differences in the experimental systems used in different laboratories, but the essential features are that the drug of interest is added to one side of the MCL and is sampled from a second compartment on the other side of the MCL (Fig. 18.13*C*). The simplest experiments use radiolabeled drugs, although the radioactivity measured in the receiving compartment may, at least in part, be associated with drug metabolites and hence, represents an upper estimate of penetration of the parent drug. These studies are complemented by measur-

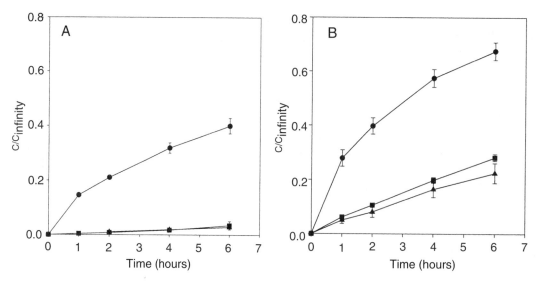

**Figure 18.15.** The time-dependent penetration of (A) doxorubicin and (B) 5-fluorouracil through multicellular layers (MCL) derived from human MCF-7 cells or murine EMT-6 cells. The concentration on the opposite side of the MCL to that where drugs are added is expressed as a ratio of the expected equilibrium concentration infinity. The upper curves represent drug penetration through the Teflon membrane in the absence of an MCL. *Note very poor tissue penetration, especially of doxorubicin.* (Adapted from Tunggal et al., 1999, with permission.)

ing the concentration of the drug and its metabolites by analytical methods such as HPLC. Representative curves describing penetration of some anticancer drugs that are used in the treatment of solid tumors are shown in Figure 18.15. The penetration of these drugs through MCLs is slow compared to that through the Teflon membrane alone and extremely poor for doxorubicin and mitoxantrone (Tunggal et al., 1999; Tannock et al., 2002). The slow establishment of equilibrium conditions in MCLs is likely to reflect the situation in solid tumors, where intermittent injections of relatively high doses of drugs is followed by a peak and rapid fall in serum concentration. Cells distal from blood vessels are then likely to experience only low concentrations of most drugs in their microenvironment. When solid tumors respond to anti-cancer agents, and particularly to doxorubicin and mitoxantrone, they may do so by repeated loss of cells close to blood vessels at the time of administration of successive courses of treatment, analogous to peeling an onion, or rather a series of inside-out onions.

The limited distribution of doxorubicin in relation to blood vessels of human breast cancer has also been demonstrated by comparing autofluorescence of the drug in tumor sections with that of a fluorescent marker to CD31 expressed on endothelial cells (Lankelma et al., 1999). This method can be extended to show also hypoxic regions of the tumor, using a fluorescent-tagged marker for hypoxic cells, such as EF-5 (Fig. 18.16).

It appears that the penetration of drugs through tissue is mainly through the extracellular matrix (ECM). The penetration of methotrexate through MCLs, for example, is increased in acidic conditions or in the presence of folic acid, both of which inhibit the uptake of methotrexate into cells. Also, the penetration of doxorubicin through MCLs composed of cells which express the drug efflux pump P-glycoprotein (Sec. 18.2.3) is enhanced compared with that through MCLs composed of cells of similar origin that do not express P-glycoprotein. Moreover, agents that inhibit the function of P-glycoprotein, such as verapamil, cause a decrease in tissue penetration of doxorubicin (Tunggal et al., 2000). These observations offer a partial explanation for the failure of strategies using small molecule inhibitors of P-glycoprotein to show therapeutic benefit for established solid tumors, as compared to isolated cells in culture.

Obtaining information about the factors which lead to limited penetration of anticancer drugs through tissue is important because it may provide approaches to improve tissue penetration. Because vascular access is far more limited in tumors than in normal tissues, strategies that improve tissue penetration have the potential to have a much greater impact on anti-tumor effects than on toxicity to normal tissues, and may thus be expected to improve the therapeutic index. Potential strategies that are under investigation include modification of the ECM and inhibition of the sequestra-

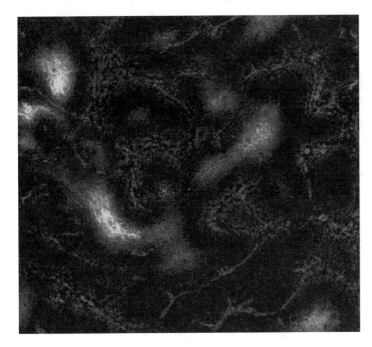

**Figure 18.16.** Three-color photomicrograph of a section of the 16C mouse mammary tumor generated with a Zeiss Axiovert fluorescent microscope showing immunostaining of blood vessels using anti-CD31 (red), hypoxic regions using anti-EF5 (green) and the distribution of fluorescent doxorubicin (blue) 20 minutes after intravenous injection. Bar = 100 $\mu$m. Unpublished data of Primeau and Tannock. (See color plate.)

tion of basic anticancer drugs (such as doxorubicin) in acidic compartments of cells.

## 18.3.4 Repopulation

The proliferation of surviving tumor cells between daily doses of fractionated radiotherapy is an important cause of failure to achieve local tumor control (Chap. 15, Sec. 15.6.2). There is evidence from several experimental systems that this process can accelerate with time, presumably as surviving cells are stimulated to divide by improving nutrition or by the action of growth factors. Studies of the relationship between the probability of tumor control and duration of fractionated radiotherapy suggest a similar acceleration of repopulation in human tumors undergoing treatment, and clinical trials have been designed to overcome this effect (Chap. 15, Sec. 15.6.2).

Radiotherapy is most often delivered as daily dose fractions. The process of repopulation is likely to be more important between courses of chemotherapy which are given typically at 3-week intervals. There have been a few studies of the rate of repopulation of tumor cells following treatment of experimental tumors or spheroids. In these studies, a higher rate of proliferation at some time after treatment of tumors by chemotherapy (i.e., of repopulation) than in untreated control tumors has been reported (reviewed in Davis and Tannock, 2000). Thus, accelerated repopulation may occur in experimental tumors following chemotherapy as well as during fractionated radiotherapy. The process of tumor recovery may be analogous to repopulation of the bone marrow from stem cells that are stim-

ulated to divide as a result of treatment. The therapeutic ratio for drug treatment may thus be dependent on relative rates of proliferation in the tumor and in critical normal tissues. These proliferative rates might change during treatment.

There are few relevant data on the rate of repopulation of human tumors following chemotherapy. It is not easy to study the proliferation of cells following tumor treatment, because at early intervals, it is difficult or impossible to distinguish true surviving cells from lethally damaged cells that have yet to undergo the morphological changes that will precede their ultimate lysis; however, this is less of a problem at longer intervals after drug treatment. In one study, tumor cell proliferation was assessed in patients with oropharyngeal cancer following induction chemotherapy (Bourhis et al., 1994); there was a higher rate of cell production in treated patients than in those that had not received chemotherapy, consistent with the notion of chemotherapy causing accelerated repopulation. The possible effects of repopulation following chemotherapy have been modeled and are illustrated in Figure 18.17 (Davis and Tannock, 2000). If the rate of repopulation is similar to the rate of proliferation of tumor cells prior to treatment, a human tumor may show net growth because of this process, even if each course of chemotherapy leads to killing of 70 percent of the viable tumor cells (Fig. 18.17A). Also a changing rate of repopulation can lead to regrowth following initial tumor shrinkage (Fig. 18.17B), in the absence of any change in the intrinsic drug sensitivity of the constituent cells, as is observed commonly in the treatment of sensitive human tumors. The process may be more complex than

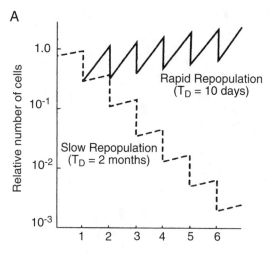

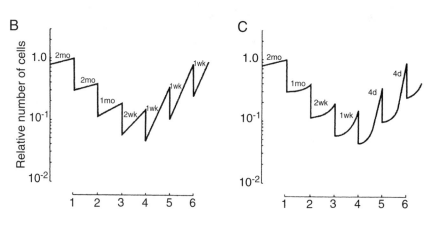

**Figure 18.17.** Models of cell killing and repopulation during chemotherapy. In (*A*) it is assumed that each 3-weekly course of treatment kills 70 percent of the tumor cells and repopulation is shown with a doubling time of 10 days (solid line) or 2 months (dashed line). In (*B*) the rate of repopulation increases between successive cycles of chemotherapy so that the doubling time of surviving cells decreases from 2 months to 1 week. In (*C*) the rate of repopulation also increases but the initial effect of chemotherapy to delay repopulation is illustrated. *Note that shrinkage and regrowth of tumors, observed commonly in the clinic, may occur due to accelerating repopulation and without any selection of drug-resistant cells.* (Adapted from Davis and Tannock, 2000, with permission.)

that illustrated by this simple modeling, because in addition to killing tumor cells, anticancer drugs may inhibit proliferation of surviving cells following their administration. However, this cytostatic effect is unlikely to last through the typical 3-week interval between cycles of treatment with chemotherapy. Including temporary cytostatic effects in the model does not substantially change the effect of accelerating repopulation to cause tumor shrinkage and regrowth (Fig. 18.17*C*).

As for radiotherapy, there are strategies that might be used to inhibit repopulation between courses of chemotherapy, and thereby to avoid the effective drug resistance that is observed. One method is to give drugs more frequently or continuously, and to stimulate recovery of bone marrow by using growth factors such as G-CSF (see Chap. 9, Sec. 9.4.3 and Chap. 17, Sec. 17.4.1). This strategy has led to apparent improvement in survival following adjuvant treatment for breast cancer using cycles of chemotherapy at 2-week intervals (Citron et al., 2003). Other approaches that are under investigation include the use of hormonal agents to

block proliferation between cycles of chemotherapy for hormone-sensitive tumors, or inhibition of receptors to growth factors that selectively stimulate tumor cell proliferation. Such agents will need to be short acting and discontinued just before the next cycle of chemotherapy because anticancer drugs are likely to be more effective in killing cycling tumor cells.

## 18.4 SUMMARY

The most important limitation to the therapeutic effects of chemotherapy is the presence of intrinsic or acquired resistance to drugs by tumor cell populations. Drug resistance occurs through a variety of mechanisms, the best studied of which are due to mutation or altered expression of genes. Some of these genetic changes lead to modification of the uptake, metabolism, or excretion of specific drugs. Mechanisms such as an increase in extrusion of drugs from cells by P-glycoprotein, MRP1, or BCRP, increased inactivation of drug, alterations in the drug target, increased potential for DNA repair, and inhibition of signaling pathways leading to cell death may lead to cross-resistance between chemically unrelated drugs. More transient changes in drug sensitivity of cells in human tumors probably occur by reversible mechanisms, including the methylation of regulatory regions of relevant genes.

Additional mechanisms of resistance may be due to the tumor cell environment. There is evidence that some types of drug resistance are expressed only when cells are in contact with one another, and the hypoxic microenvironment of solid tumors has been shown to favor the outgrowth of p53 mutant cells that may be resistant to several forms of therapy. A major problem in solid tumors is delivery of effective concentrations of drug to all of the tumor cells because penetration of tissue from sparsely distributed blood vessels is limiting for many anticancer drugs. Drug treatment of patients must also be scheduled to allow recovery of normal tissues such as bone marrow, but proliferation of surviving tumor cells between courses of treatment, known as repopulation, might lead to clinical resistance, especially if repopulation accelerates during successive courses of treatment. Each of these mechanisms might, in principle, be modified to lead to improvements in therapeutic outcome.

The emerging microarray technologies enabling the transcriptional and translational profiling of human tumors may be extremely valuable in characterizing causes of drug resistance in individual tumors. They may also facilitate the development of new agents or therapeutic strategies that enhance drug sensitivity.

# REFERENCES

Ambudkar SV, Dey S, Hrycyna CA, et al: Biochemical, cellular, and pharmacological aspects of the multidrug transporter. *Annu Rev Pharmacol Toxicol* 1999; 39:361–398.

Austin CA, Marsh KL: Eukaryotic DNA topoisomerase IIβ. *Bioessays* 1998; 20:215–226.

Borst P, Evers R, Kool M, Wijnholds J: A family of drug transporters: the multidrug resistance-associated proteins. *J Natl Cancer Inst* 2000; 92:1295–1302.

Bourhis J, Wilson G, Wibault P, et al: Rapid tumor cell proliferation after induction chemotherapy in oropharyngeal cancer. *Laryngoscope* 1994; 104:468–472.

Brown JM, Wouters BG: Apoptosis, p53 and tumor cell sensitivity to anticancer agents. *Cancer Res* 1999; 59:1391–1399.

Cara S, Tannock IF: Retreatment of patients with the same chemotherapy: implications for clinical mechanisms of drug resistance. *Ann Oncol* 2001; 12: 23–27.

Chan HSL, Haddad G, Thorner PS, et al: P-glycoprotein expression as a predictor of the outcome of therapy for neuroblastoma. *N Engl J Med* 1991; 325:1608–1616.

Chaplin DJ, Durand RE, Olive PL: Cell selection from a murine tumor using the fluorescent probe Hoechst 33342. *Br J Cancer* 1985; 51:569–572.

Citron ML, Berry DA, Cirrincione C, et al: Randomized trial of dose-dense versus conventionally scheduled and sequential versus concurrent combination chemotherapy as postoperative adjuvant treatment of node-positive primary breast cancer: first report of Intergroup Trial C9741/Cancer and Leukemia Group B Trial 9741. *J Clin Oncol* 2003; 21:1431–1439.

Cole SPC, Bhardwaj G, Gerlach JH, et al: Overexpression of a transporter gene in a multidrug-resistant human lung cancer cell line. *Science* 1992; 258:1650–1654.

Davis AJ, Tannock IF: Repopulation of tumor cells between cycles of chemotherapy: a neglected factor. *Lancet Oncol* 2000; 1:86–93.

Doyle LA, Yang W, Abruzzo LV, et al: A multidrug resistance transporter from human MCF-7 breast cancer cells. *Proc Natl Acad Sci USA* 1998; 95:15665–15670.

Drori S, Jansen G, Mauritz R, et al: Clustering of mutations in the first transmembrane domain of the human reduced folate carrier in GW1843U89–resistant leukemia cells with impaired antifolate transport and augmented folate uptake. *J Biol Chem* 2000; 275:30855–30863.

Dumontet C, Duran GE, Steger KA, et al: Resistance mechanisms in human sarcoma mutants derived by single-step exposure to paclitaxel (Taxol). *Cancer Res* 1996; 56: 1091–1097.

Durand RE: Distribution and activity of antineoplastic drugs in a tumor model. *J Natl Cancer Inst* 1989; 81:146–152.

Endicott JA, Ling V: The biochemistry of P-glycoprotein-mediated multidrug resistance. *Annu Rev Biochem* 1989; 58: 137–171.

Esteller M, Garcia-Foncillas J, Andion E, et al: Inactivation of the DNA repair gene MGMT and the clinical response of gliomas to alkylating agents. *N Engl J Med* 2000; 343:1350–1354.

Ferreira CG, Tolis C, Giaccone G: p53 and chemosensitivity. *Ann Oncol* 1999; 10:1011–1021.

Galmarini CM, Mackey JR, Dumontet C: Nucleoside analogues: mechanisms of drug resistance and reversal strategies. *Leukemia* 2001; 15:875–890.

Gerson SL, Willson JK: O6-alkylguanine-DNA alkyltransferase: a target for the modulation of drug resistance. *Hematol Oncol Clin North Am* 1995; 9:431–450.

Goldenberg GJ, Begleiter A: Alterations of drug transport. In Fox BW, Fox M, eds. *Handbook of Experimental Pharmacology*. Berlin: Springer-Verlag; 1984:241–298.

Goldie JH, Coldman AJ: The genetic origin of drug resistance in neoplasms: implications for systemic therapy. *Cancer Res* 1984; 44:3643–3653.

Gorlick R, Goker E, Trippett T, et al: Intrinsic and acquired resistance to methotrexate in acute leukemia. *N Engl J Med* 1996; 335:1041–1048.

Gorlick R, Bertino JR: Drug resistance in colon cancer. *Semin Oncol* 1999; 26:606–611.

Gorre ME, Mohammed M, Ellwood K, et al: Clinical resistance to STI-571 cancer therapy caused by BCR-ABL gene mutation or amplification. *Science* 2001; 293:876–880.

Graeber TG, Osmanian C, Jacks T, et al: Hypoxia-mediated selection of cells with diminished apoptotic potential in solid tumours. *Nature* 1996; 379:88–91.

Hicks KO, Ohms SJ, van Zijl PL, et al: An experimental and mathematical model for the extravascular transport of a DNA intercalator in tumours. *Br J Cancer* 1997; 76:894–903.

Hipfner DR, Deeley RG, Cole SPC: Structural, mechanistic and clinical aspects of MRP1. *Biochim Biophys Acta* 1999; 1461:359–376.

Honjo Y, Hrycyna CA, Yan QW, et al: Acquired mutations in the MXR/BCRP/ABCP gene alter substrate specificity in the MXR/BCRP/ABCP-overexpressing cells. *Cancer Res* 2001; 61:6635–6639.

Hu Z-B, Minden MD, McCulloch EA: Direct evidence for the participation of bcl-2 in the regulation of retinoic acid of the Ara-C sensitivity of leukemic stem cells. *Leukemia* 1995; 9:1667–1673.

Izquierdo MA, Scheffer GL, Flens MJ, et al: Major vault protein LRP-related multidrug resistance. *Eur J Cancer* 1996; 32A:979–984.

Jonker JW, Smit JW, Brinkhuis RF, et al: Role of breast cancer resistance protein in the bioavailability and fetal penetration of topotecan. *J Natl Cancer Inst* 2000; 92:1651–1656.

Kelley SL, Basu A, Teicher BA, et al: Overexpression of metallothionein confers resistance to anticancer drugs. *Science* 1988; 241:1813–1815.

Kerbel RS, Rak J, Kobayashi H, et al: Multicellular resistance: a new paradigm to explain aspects of acquired drug resistance of solid tumors. *Cold Spring Harbor Symp Quant Biol* 1994; 59:661–672.

Keshelava N, Zuo JJ, Chen P, et al: Loss of p53 function confers high-level multidrug resistance in neuroblastoma cell lines. *Cancer Res* 2001; 61:6185–6193.

Klein I, Sarkadi B, Varadi A: An inventory of the human ABC proteins. *Biochim Biophys Acta* 1999; 1461:237–262.

Kondo Y, Woo ES, Michalska AE, et al: Metallothionein null cells have increased sensitivity to anticancer drugs. *Cancer Res* 1995; 55:2021–2023.

Konig J, Nies AT, Cui Y, et al: Conjugate export pumps of the multidrug resistance protein (MRP) family: localization, substrate specificity and MRP2-mediated drug resistance. *Biochim Biophys Acta* 1999; 1461:377–394.

Kurz EU, Wilson SE, Leader KB, et al: The histone deacetylase inhibitor sodium butyrate induces DNA topoisomerase II α expression and confers hypersensitivity to etoposide in human leukemic cell lines. *Mol Cancer Ther* 2001; 1:121–131.

Lang AJ, Mirski SEL, Cummings HL, et al: Structural organization of the human *TOP2A* and *TOP2B* genes. *Gene* 1998; 221:255–266.

Lang TT, Selner M, Young JD, Cass CE: Acquisition of human concentrative nucleoside transporter 2 (hCNT2) activity by gene transfer confers sensitivity to fluoropyrimidine nucleosides in drug-resistant leukemia cells. *Molec Pharmacol* 2001; 60:1143–1152.

Lankelma J, Dekker H, Luque FR, et al: Doxorubicin gradients in human breast cancer. *Clin Cancer Res* 1999; 5:1703–1707.

Leslie EM, Deeley RG, Cole SPC: Toxicological relevance of the multidrug resistance protein 1, MRP1 (ABCC1), and related transporters. *Toxicology* 2001; 167:3–23.

Li TK, Liu LF: Tumor cell death induced by topoisomerase-targeting drugs. *Annu Rev Pharmacol Toxicol* 2001; 41:53–77.

Lock RB, Stribinskiene L: Dual modes of cell death induced by etoposide in human epithelial tumor cells allow Bcl-2 to inhibit apoptosis without affecting clonogenic survival. *Cancer Res* 1996; 56:4006–4012.

Loe DW, Deeley RG, Cole SPC: Characterization of vincristine transport by the 190 kDa multidrug resistance protein, MRP: evidence for co-transport with reduced glutathione. *Cancer Res* 1998; 58:5130–5136.

Nooter K, Westerman AM, Flens MJ, et al: Expression of the multidrug resistance-associate protein (MRP) gene in human cancers. *Clin Cancer Res* 1995; 1:1301–1310.

Norris MD, Bordow SB, Marshall GM, et al: Expression of the gene for multidrug-resistance-associated protein and outcome in patients with neuroblastoma. *N Engl J Med* 1996; 334:231–238.

Oloumi A, MacPhail SH, Johnston PJ, et al: Changes in subcellular distribution of the topoisomerase IIα correlate with etoposide resistance in multicell spheroids and xenograft tumors. *Cancer Res* 2001; 20:5747–5753.

Pommier Y, Pourquier P, Urasaki Y, et al: Topoisomerase I inhibitors: selectivity and cellular resistance. *Drug Resist Updat* 1999; 2:307–318.

Puchalski RB, Fahl WE: Expression of recombinant glutathione S-transferase π, Ya or Yb confers resistance to alkylating agents. *Proc Natl Acad Sci USA* 1990; 87:2443–2447.

Rappa G, Lorico A, Flavell RA, Sartorelli AC: Evidence that the multidrug resistance protein (MRP) functions as a cotransporter of glutathione and natural product toxins. *Cancer Res* 1997; 57:5232–5237.

Rice GC, Hoy C, Schimke RT: Transient hypoxia enhances the frequency of dihydrofolate reductase gene amplification in Chinese hamster ovary cells. *Proc Natl Acad Sci USA* 1986; 83:5978–5982.

Roca J, Wang JC: DNA transport by a type II DNA topoisomerase: evidence in favor of a two-gate mechanism. *Cell* 1994; 77:609–616.

Sampath D, Plunkett W: Design of new anticancer therapies targeting cell cycle checkpoint pathways. *Curr Opin Oncol* 2001; 13:484–490.

Sandor VA, Fojo T, Bates SE: Future perspectives for the development of P-glycoprotein modulators. *Drug Resist Updat* 1998; 1:190–200.

Scheffer GL, Wijngaard PLJ, Flens MJ, et al: The drug resistance-related protein LRP is the human major vault protein. *Nat Med* 1995; 1:578–582.

Schilder RJ, Hall L, Monks A: Metallothionein gene expression and resistance to cisplatin in human ovarian cancer. *Int J Cancer* 1990; 45:416–422.

Schimke RT: Gene amplification, drug resistance, and cancer. *Cancer Res* 1984; 44:1735–1742.

Schinkel AH: The physiological function of drug-transporting P-glycoproteins. *Semin Cancer Biol* 1997; 8:161–170.

Shain KH, Dalton WS: Cell adhesion is a key determinant in *de novo* multidrug resistance (MDR): new targets for the prevention of acquired MDR. *Molec Cancer Ther* 2001; 1:69–78.

Sharom FJ: The P-glycoprotein efflux pump: how does it transport drugs? *J Membrane Biol* 1997; 160:161–175.

Slovak ML, Ho JP, Bhardwaj G, et al: Localization of a novel multidrug resistance-associated gene in the HT1080/DR4 and H69AR human tumor cell lines. *Cancer Res* 1993; 53:3221–3225.

St. Croix B, Florenes VA, Rak JW, et al: Impact of the cyclin-dependent kinase inhibitor p27Kip1 on resistance of tumor cells to anticancer agents. *Nature Med* 1996; 2:1204–1210.

Sutherland RM: Cell and environment interactions in tumor microregions: the multicell spheroid model. *Science* 1988; 240:177–184.

Tan KB, Dorman TE, Falls KM, et al: Topoisomerase IIa and topoisomerase IIb genes: Characterization and mapping to human chromosomes 17 and 3, respectively. *Cancer Res* 1992; 52:231–234.

Tannock IF, Lee C: Evidence against apoptosis as a major mechanism for reproductive cell death following treatment of cell lines with anti-cancer drugs. *Br J Cancer* 2001; 84:100–105.

Tannock IF, Lee CM, Tunggal JK, et al: Limited penetration of anti-cancer drugs through tumor tissue: a potential cause of resistance of solid tumors to chemotherapy. *Clin Cancer Res* 2002; 8:878–884.

Teicher BA, Herman TS, Holden SA, et al: Tumor resistance to alkylating agents conferred by mechanisms operative only in vivo. *Science* 1990; 247:1457–1461.

Tew KD: Glutathione-associated enzymes in anticancer drug resistance. *Cancer Res* 1994; 54:4313–4320.

Tunggal JK, Ballinger JR, Tannock IF: Influence of cell concentration in limiting the therapeutic benefit of P-glycoprotein reversal agents. *Int J Cancer* 1999; 81:741–747.

Tunggal JK, Cowan DSM, Shaikh H, Tannock IF: Penetration of anticancer drugs through solid tissue: a factor that limits the effectiveness of chemotherapy for solid tumors. *Clin Cancer Res* 1999; 5:1583–1586.

Tunggal JK, Melo T, Ballinger JR, Tannock IF: The influence of expression of P-glycoprotein on the penetration of anticancer drugs through multicellular layers. *Int J Cancer* 2000; 86:101–107.

Urasaki Y, Laco GS, Pourquier P, et al: Characterization of a novel topoisomerase I mutation from a camptothecin-resistant human prostate cancer cell line. *Cancer Res* 2001; 61:1964–1969.

Vukovic V, Tannock IF: Influence of low pH on cytotoxicity of paclitaxel, mitoxantrone and topotecan. *Br J Cancer* 1997; 75:1167–1172.

Wang Z-M, Chen Z-P, Xu Z-Y, et al: *In vitro* evidence for homologous recombinational repair in resistance to melphalan. *J Natl Cancer Inst* 2001; 93:1473–1478.

Wijnholds J, Evers R, Van Leusden MR, et al: Increased sensitivity to anticancer drugs and decreased inflammatory response in mice lacking the multidrug resistance-associated protein. *Nat Med* 1997; 3:1275–1279.

Wijnholds J, Mol CAAM, van Deemter L, et al: Multidrug-resistance protein 5 is a multispecific organic anion transporter able to transport nucleotide analogs. *Proc Natl Acad Sci USA* 2000; 97:7476–7481.

Yang B, Eshlemen JR, Berger NA, et al: Wild-type p53 protein potentiates cytotoxicity of therapeutic agents in human colon cancer cells. *Clin Cancer Res* 1996; 2:1649–1657.

Yu JL, Rak JW, Coomber BL, et al: Effect of p53 status on tumor reponse to anti-angiogenic therapy. *Science* 2002; 295: 1526–1528.

Zanke BW, Boudreau K, Rubie E, et al: The stress-activated protein kinase (SAPK/JNK) pathway mediates cell death following cis-platinum or heat-induced injury. *Curr Biol* 1996; 6:606–613.

Zhou S, Schuetz JD, Bunting KD, et al: The ABC transporter Bcrp1/ABCG2 is expressed in a wide variety of stem cells and is a molecular determinant of the side-population phenotype. *Nat Med* 2001; 7:1028–1034.

# 19

# Hormones and Cancer

*Paul Rennie, Jason Read, and Leigh Murphy*

## 19.1 INTRODUCTION

Breast and prostate cancers are the most commonly occurring cancers in Western society, and are the second leading cause of cancer death (next to lung cancer) in women and men, respectively. Both of these cancers arise in tissues that require steroid sex hormones (estrogens and androgens) for their development, growth, and function. While human cancers occur in other hormone-dependent tissues, such as the uterus, ovary, and testis, this chapter will focus exclusively on breast and prostate cancer as models of hormone-dependent cancers.

The relationship between prostate enlargement and hormones produced by the testes has long been recognized. Although the chemical nature of androgens was not known, it was reported in 1895 that castration of elderly men with prostate enlargement, presumably due to benign prostatic hyperplasia, resulted in rapid atrophy of prostatic tissue. Early anecdotal evidence regarding the testicular (i.e., androgen) dependence of

the human prostate is also derived from studies involving eunuchs from the Ottoman and Chinese courts, which indicated that prostates did not develop in prepubertal castrates. Following the isolation of testosterone as the most potent androgenic compound in the testes in 1935, Huggins and Hodges demonstrated the efficacy of surgical orchiectomy for the treatment of metastatic prostate cancer—for which Huggins received the Nobel Prize for Medicine in 1966. Similarly, a link between estrogen and breast cancer growth was established at the end of the nineteenth century, when Beatson demonstrated that oophorectomy was useful in the treatment of metastatic breast cancer in some premenopausal women. However, a molecular basis for this observation was not forthcoming until the 1960s, with the discovery of the estrogen receptor, followed by the demonstrated expression of estrogen receptors in some human breast tumors.

Evidence for a direct link between the action of sex steroids and a causal role in the carcinogenic process leading to breast and prostate tumors was first provided by Robert Noble. He reported that prolonged exposure to estrogen, androgen, or combinations of the two led to breast and prostate cancers in rats. More recently, the successful use of the anti-estrogen, tamoxifen, in reducing the incidence of breast cancer in high-risk women supports a direct link between estrogen action and breast tumor formation. These hormones are fundamental not only to the development of normal prostate and mammary glands, but also to dysplastic and neoplastic processes that occur in these tissues.

In this chapter, relationships between hormones and cancers of the breast and prostate are explored in the context of basic mechanisms of hormone action, the natural history of the two diseases, and their treatment with hormonally based therapies.

## 19.2 BASIC MECHANISMS OF HORMONE ACTION

Hormones can be classified generally into two broad groups: (1) nonsteroidal (amino acids, peptides, and polypeptides), which usually require cell-membrane localized receptors that regulate second messenger molecules such as cAMP to mediate their action (see Chap. 8); and (2) steroidal, which bind directly to intracellular receptors to mediate their action. Because breast and prostate cancer are primarily dependent on steroid hormones for their growth and viability, this section will focus on the molecular mechanisms by which steroid hormones mediate their action at the target cell level. The steroid hormones of primary concern in breast and prostate cancer are estrogen and androgen, respectively. Other examples of steroid hormones include glucocorticoids, mineralocorticoids, and progestins.

### 19.2.1 Factors Affecting Bioavailability of Estrogens and Androgens

The bioavailability of steroid hormones at the site of action depends on several factors, including synthesis, transport via the blood, access to target tissue, metabolism of target tissue, and expression of receptors within the target cell.

*Synthesis and Metabolism of Estrogens* As indicated in Figure 19.1, all steroids are synthesized from the common precursor, cholesterol. The primary site of estrogen synthesis in premenopausal women is the parafollicular region of the ovary. Ovarian steroid synthesis in premenopausal women is cyclical and regulated via the gonad-hypothalamus-pituitary feedback axis as indicated in panel *A* of Figure 19.2. Other sites of estrogen biosynthesis include mesenchymal cells in adipose tissue and skin; these become major sources for estrogen synthesis in postmenopausal women where adrenal androgens, in particular, androstenedione, are converted

to estrone by aromatase cytochrome P450 (Simpson, 2000). Some estrone molecules can then be converted to estradiol-17$\beta$ by 17$\beta$-hydroxysteroid dehydrogenases (Miettinen et al., 2000). A large amount of estrone is converted by estrone sulfotransferase to estrone sulphate which has a longer half-life in blood, and therefore can act as an estrogen reservoir, being converted back to estrone by the action of sulfatases (Miettinen et al., 2000). Aromatase activity has been detected in normal human breast tissue and in more than 50 percent of human breast tumors (Sasano and Harada, 1998). Estrone sulfotransferase, sulfatase, and 17$\beta$-hydroxysteroid dehydrogenase type 1 have been detected in both normal and malignant human breast tissues (Miettinen et al., 2000), and the relative expression of these enzymes probably regulates the local availability of estrogen to target cells. Estrogen synthesis in postmenopausal women is not cyclical, but serum and local tissue levels can differ between individuals due to a variety of environmental and genetic factors such as obesity and genetic variation/polymorphism in steroid metabolizing (biosynthetic and degrading) enzymes (Thompson and Ambrosone, 2000).

*Synthesis and Metabolism of Androgens* The Leydig cells of the testes produce almost 90 percent of the body's androgens with the remainder being made mainly by the adrenal cortex. As illustrated in panel *B* of Figure 19.2, the testes make primarily testosterone, whereas the major adrenal androgens are dehydroepiandrosterone (DHEA) and its derived sulfate, which although weak androgens, can be converted in other tissues to testosterone. The principal circulating androgen in man is testosterone (Fig. 19.1). As with estrogen synthesis in the ovary, testosterone production in the testis is regulated by a negative feedback loop involving luteinizing hormone (LH) and luteinizing hormone-releasing hormone (LHRH) via the gonad-hypothalamus-pituitary feedback axis (Fig. 19.2*B*). While there are diurnal fluctuations of androgen secretion, their production does not follow a regular cyclical pattern. Also, there is no apparent equivalent to menopause in men, although there is a progressive decrease in testosterone levels with age, which is accompanied by some degree of testicular failure.

There are two principal pathways through which testosterone can undergo metabolic conversion to more potent forms (Fig. 19.1). The first involves the enzyme aromatase, which is present in many tissues (e.g., adipose tissue, testis, brain) and which can convert ~0.5 percent of the daily production of testosterone to estradiol. While this is a small proportion of the total amount, estradiol is a 200-fold more potent inhibitor of gonadotrophins than testosterone. The second major pathway is the conversion of testosterone to the more

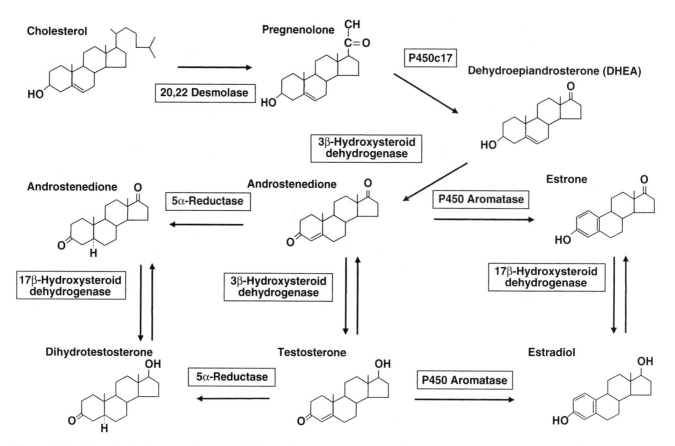

**Figure 19.1.** The principal mammalian steroid biosynthetic pathways for estradiol, testosterone, and dihydrotestosterone. The enzymes that catalyze the reactions are shown in the boxes. While the main sites for steroid synthesis are the gonads and the adrenals, metabolic interconversions and activations occur in sex-hormone target tissues, such as the prostate and breast, as well as other peripheral tissues, such as skin and adipose tissue.

potent androgen dihydrotestosterone (DHT) by the enzyme 5α-reductase, which is present in many androgen target tissues, such as the prostate and skin. There are two isoforms of 5α-reductase, each with different kinetic properties and sensitivity to inhibitors, with the Type II isoform predominating in human accessory sex tissue (Bruchovsky et al., 1988). There is evidence that DHT is three to four times more potent than testosterone with respect to inducing growth and maintenance of the prostate gland, whereas testosterone is more effective than DHT in regulating differentiation.

*Transport of Steroid Hormones in the Blood* As hydrophobic molecules in an aqueous environment, most steroid hormones are transported in the blood bound to proteins, predominantly sex hormone binding globulin (SHBG) and albumin (as shown in Fig. 19.3). Only about 2 percent are in an unbound form, which is thought to be the biologically active fraction. Recently, it has been shown that SHBG also plays a role in permitting certain steroid hormones to act without entering the cell. Estrogens and androgens bind with high affinity to SHBG, which in turn, interacts with a spe-

cific, high affinity receptor (SHBG-R) on cell membranes and transduces a signal via a G protein (Rosner et al., 1999). The steroid/SHBG-R/SHBG complex generates messages that have effects on the transcriptional activity of regular, intracellular receptors for steroid hormones. Clearly, factors that influence the levels of SHBG and albumin will affect the bioactivity of steroid hormones. For example, SHBG production is stimulated by both estrogens and by the anti-estrogen tamoxifen, whereas androgens and progestins have been shown to suppress it. Hence, SHBG not only modulates the amount of ligand available to bind to these steroid receptors, but may also modulate their activity through interaction with the cell membrane.

### 19.2.2 Steroid Hormone Receptors

A relatively simplistic overview of how steroid hormones regulate growth and differentiation of their target cells is shown in Figure 19.3. The majority of steroid hormone that enters the cell is derived from the small nonbound fraction in the circulation, which can enter by passive diffusion. Upon entry into the cell, the steroid

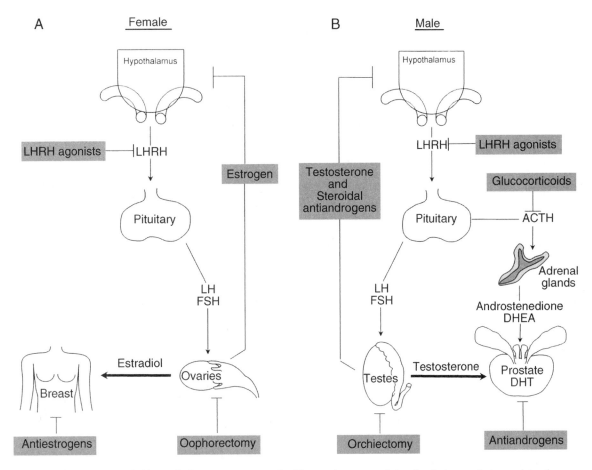

**Figure 19.2.** The gonadal-hypothalamic-pituitary axis. The pathways and feedback loops that regulate the production of estrogens in females (*A*) and androgens in males (*B*) and their target tissues are shown. The procedures and agents used for blocking the synthesis and activity of androgens and estrogens at the various steps in the pathway are highlighted.

or its metabolic derivative (e.g., DHT) binds directly to a predominantly cytoplasmic (androgen receptor) or nuclear (estrogen receptor) steroid-receptor protein. The steroid-receptor complex undergoes an activation step involving a conformational change and shedding of heat shock (including hsp70, hsp90, and hsp40) and other chaperone proteins, which are necessary to maintain the receptor in a competent ligand-binding state (Tsai and O'Malley, 1994). After homo- or heterodimerization, and nuclear transport in the case of the androgen receptor, the activated receptor dimer complex binds to specific palindromic DNA motifs called hormone responsive elements (HRE) found in the promoters of hormone-regulated genes (Tsai and O'Malley, 1994). The receptor-DNA complexes in turn associate dynamically with coactivators and basal transcriptional components to enhance the transcription of genes, whose mRNAs are translated into proteins that elicit specific biological responses. As indicated in Figure 19.4, it is likely that receptors that are not bound to their ligands, or those bound to antagonists, form complexes with corepressors to inhibit the transcription of specific genes (McKenna et al., 1999).

All steroid receptors are members of a so-called superfamily of more than 150 proteins. All are ligand-responsive transcription factors that share similarities with respect to their structural homology and functional properties. As shown in Figure 19.5, each member of the steroid receptor family possesses a modular structure composed of the following: (a) N-terminal region containing ligand-independent transcriptional activating functions (collectively referred to as *A*ctivating *F*unction-1 or AF-1); (b) a centrally located DNA binding domain of approximately sixty-five amino acids having two zinc fingers; (c) a hinge region which contains signal elements for nuclear localization; and (d) a ligand-binding domain in the C-terminal region of the protein containing a ligand-dependent transcriptional activating function (called AF-2).

AF1 and AF2 can function independently or synergistically depending on the gene promoter and/or the cell type (Tsai and O'Malley, 1994). Recently, a third

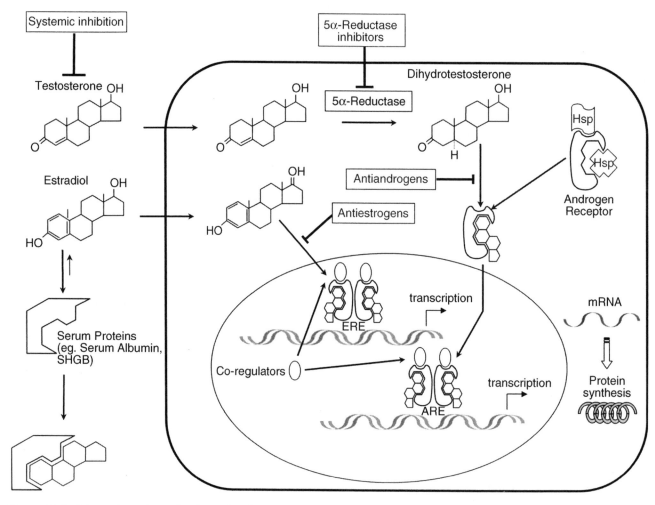

**Figure 19.3.** Schematic pathway for the molecular action of testosterone and estradiol in hormone target cells. A relatively simplistic overview of the key events in steroid hormone action with the sites at which the hormone signal can be inhibited are indicated. While the dynamics for estrogen and androgen action are similar, for full activity testosterone needs to be converted to dihydrotestosterone which binds to a cytoplasmic form of the androgen receptor and is translocated into the nucleus, whereas estradiol binds directly to its receptor in the cell nucleus (ERE, estrogen receptor element and ARE, androgen receptor element).

autonomous activation domain (AF2a) was identified spanning the end of the hinge region and the beginning of the ligand-binding domain (Norris et al., 1997). Between members of the family of steroid receptors, the N-terminal region has the highest degree of amino acid sequence variability, whereas the DNA binding domain has the most shared homology.

*Androgen Receptors*   The androgen receptor (AR) is encoded on the X chromosome. As a single allele gene in males, it is susceptible to genetic defects whose phenotypes can range from minor hypo-virilization to a complete female phenotype known as testicular feminization. The normal, wild-type AR has a molecular weight of ~110 kiloDaltons, although a second N-terminally truncated AR isoform (referred to as AR-A) has been observed in a variety of human normal and neoplastic tissues (Wilson and McPhaul, 1996). While

the biological significance of AR-A is unknown, when assays of AR function are performed under conditions in which levels of expression of the two isoforms are equivalent, the AR-A and the wild-type AR possess similar functional activities. In this chapter AR refers only to the wild-type, 110-kDa form.

Relative to many other steroid receptors, the AR has a large N-terminal domain, which occupies more than half of the molecule's primary sequence of 919 amino acids (Fig. 19.5). A unique feature of AR relative to other members of this family is the occurrence of several stretches of the same amino acids (termed *homopolymeric*) in the N-terminal domain. These include seventeen to twenty-nine repeating glutamine residues, starting approximately at amino acid 59, nine proline residues at amino acid 372, and a 24-residue polyglycine stretch beginning at amino acid 449. While the function of these repeating tracts is unknown, abnormal ex-

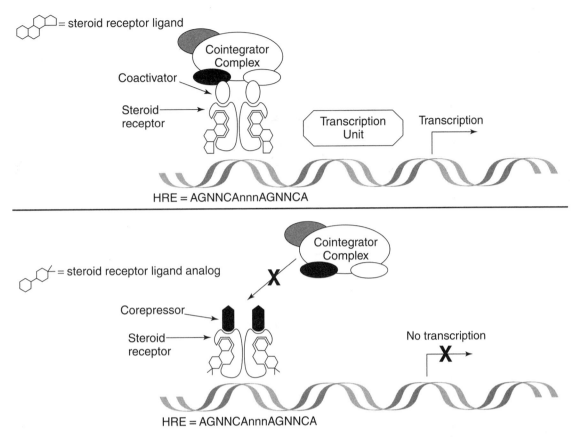

**Figure 19.4.** Illustration of the role of coactivators and corepressors in regulation of steroid receptor action. In the presence of agonistic ligands (e.g., estradiol for ER, DHT for AR), the steroid receptor/DNA complexes associate dynamically with coactivators, which in turn recruit other proteins, including cointegrator complexes, that contact and stabilize the basal transcription unit resulting in enhanced transcription of target genes. In the presence of antagonistic ligands (e.g., tamoxifen in the case of ER and flutamide for AR), the receptors are in a different conformational state and the receptor/DNA complexes dynamically associate with corepressors (Co-R) which destabilize basal transcription units and result in reduced transcription of target genes (HRE, hormone responsive element).

tension of the polyglutamine tract to forty or more residues is associated with X-linked spinal and bulbar muscular atrophy (La Spada et al., 1991). Also, a relationship between a decreased size of these homopolymers and development of prostate cancer has been reported (Giovannucci et al., 1997).

*Estrogen Receptors*   There are two estrogen receptors, ERα and ERβ, which unlike AR isoforms, are encoded by separate genes (Fig. 19.5). Several variant isoforms of each ER, generated by alternative RNA splicing, may also be expressed (Murphy et al., 1998). The centrally located DNA binding domain for ERα and ERβ (Fig. 19.5) is highly homologous (>95% identity) between the two ER forms. Their ligand-binding domains are about 60 percent identical. As with other steroid receptors, the ligand-binding domain contains a ligand-dependent dimerization function, and a ligand-dependent transactivation function, AF2. Similarly, a ligand

independent transactivation function, AF1, is present in the N-terminal domain. This latter domain is different between ERα and ERβ.

*Binding of Steroid Receptors to DNA*   As transcription factors, steroid receptors modulate gene expression by first binding to specific DNA sequences in the promoter regions of hormone-regulated genes (Fig. 19.4). The α-helix structure of the first zinc finger of the DNA binding domain of a receptor is the primary discriminator for binding to different DNA sequence motifs of hormone-response elements (HREs; Tsai and O'Malley, 1994). All members of the nuclear receptor family bind as dimers to pairs of a similar DNA sequence motif, AGNNCA (N, any nucleotide), which composes the HRE found in the promoters of steroid regulated genes (Glass, 1994). Nuclear receptors can be further subdivided on the basis of selection of the primary sequence of the core motif as either AGGTCA, for ER and thy-

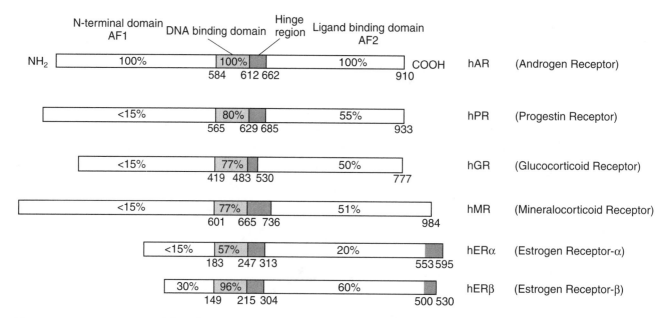

**Figure 19.5.** A comparison of the relative amino acid sequence homology within the functional domains of the principal members of the family of steroid hormone receptors. The relative amino acid sequence homology (represented by the percentages in the boxes) for hER-β is in reference to hER-α, whereas all the other receptors are relative to hAR. The numbers correspond to the amino acid positions from the N-terminus (NH₂), AF1 and AF2 refer to the transcriptional Activation Function 1 and 2 that reside in the N-terminal and ligand-binding domains, respectively.

roid receptor subfamily, or AGAACA for AR, glucocorticoid receptor (GR), or progestin receptor (PR). In general, two or more sets of interacting HREs in a gene promoter are required to elicit a steroid-mediated response (Rennie et al., 1993; Klinge, 1999). The very high sequence homology of HREs has raised the question as to how steroid receptors govern hormone-specific responses.

While there is no definitive mechanism to account for steroid receptor-specific gene regulation, at least five different mechanisms have been proposed:

1. *Availability of receptor and ligand.* This is probably not a major mechanism for receptor-specific responses in hormone target tissues, because in many cell types, two or more steroid receptors can coexist with access to their specific ligands.
2. *Activity of proximal transcription factors.* In a complex promoter other transcription factors bound proximal to the receptor-binding site may enhance the relative activity of one receptor more than another, although they have not been shown to regulate specificity.
3. *Cooperative binding of receptors to two or more DNA-binding sites.* This implies that particular configurations of binding sites act cooperatively for one specific type of receptor. While binding to multiple HREs has been demonstrated as noted above, in the case of the mouse mammary tumor virus promoter,

which is activated by GR, AR, and PR, the multiplicity of response elements in itself fails to discriminate between receptor types (Truss and Beato, 1993).

4. *DNA target motif recognition.* This implies that the natural genomic promoters, which are regulated specifically by one steroid receptor type, contain sequence variants from the corresponding HRE. Analysis of the role of individual nucleotide deviations within the DNA-binding sites for steroid receptors indicated that subtle changes do contribute somewhat to steroid-receptor specificity (Nelson et al., 1999).
5. *Interaction with unique combinations of coregulators.* This involves interaction with unique combinations of coregulators or other binding proteins, which may confer steroid-receptor specific gene regulation.

While all of the five mechanisms postulated above might contribute to steroid specificity, current research activities have focused largely on the involvement of coregulators.

*Interaction of Steroid Receptors with Coregulator Proteins* Important molecular mechanisms by which nuclear receptors regulate gene transcription involve not only direct interactions of steroid receptors with some of the basal transcription components, but also indirect interactions through recruitment of coregulator protein complexes to the promoters of target genes (McKenna et al., 1999; Fig. 19.4). Coregulators fall into two main classes, coactivators and corepressors, which enhance or repress transcription, respectively (as illustrated in Fig. 19.4). There are many genes that encode coactivators, but the *Steroid Receptor Co-activator* (SRC)/p160 family are relatively specific for nuclear receptors and are the best studied (Leo and Chen, 2000).

While the auxiliary molecular components involved and the dynamics of their interactions remain to be established, a general pattern is emerging. These coactivators and corepressors are important for mediating both AF2 and AF1 activities of steroid receptors. Their mechanism of transcriptional activation is thought to involve two stages. First, when recruited to the receptor by direct protein-protein binding, coregulators promote the local remodeling of chromatin structure through acetyltransferase or deacetylase activity and through their ability to recruit other proteins with chromatin remodeling activity (as outlined in Fig. 19.6). Second, the coactivators recruit and/or stabilize the basal transcription machinery by protein-protein interactions in order to enable efficient transcription of the target gene by RNA polymerase II (McKenna at al., 1999). The chromatin remodeling enables altered access of the promoter DNA to general transcription factors (Fig. 19.6).

The potential participation of many coactivators raises the question as to which are necessary or sufficient for transcriptional activation. While this remains largely unanswered, it has been shown in MCF-7 breast cancer cells that ER-α and a number of coactivators associate rapidly with target promoters in a dynamic, cyclic fashion, and that the p160 class of coactivators is sufficient for gene activation (Shang et al., 2000). It is likely that the relative availability of coregulators will vary in different tissues and may even be restricted to specific tissues. Similarly, while the occurrence of receptor-specific coregulators has not been confirmed, many coregulators bind preferentially to certain receptors (Leo and Chen, 2000). For example, a repressor of ER transcriptional activity, called *Repressor of Estrogen Receptor Activity* (REA) is active on ER-α or ER-β, but not other steroid receptors (Montano et al., 1999). Its mechanism of action involves a competition with coactivators such as SRC-1 for binding to the ligand binding domain of ER (Delage-Mourroux et al., 2000). Furthermore, a member of the SRC family, SRC-3 or *Amplified In Breast Cancer 1* (AIB1) may have a role in breast cancer, because it has been found to be amplified and overexpressed in some breast tumors (Anzick et al., 1997). ARA70 was believed originally to be an AR-specific coactivator, although recent reports have discounted its receptor specificity.

*Mechanisms for Transcriptional Regulation by Steroid Receptors* There are at least three different mechanisms by which steroid receptors regulate transcription of target genes: (1) ligand-dependent and requiring direct binding of steroid receptors to HREs in promoter

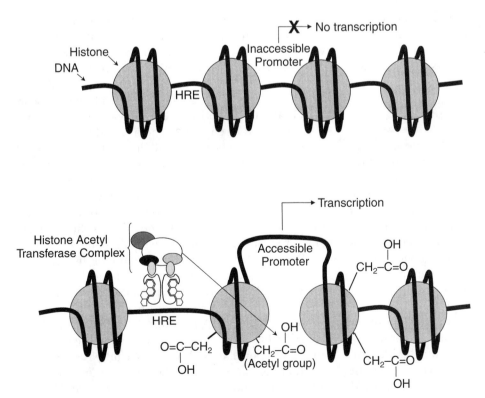

**Figure 19.6.** Remodeling of chromatin and activation of transcription by steroid hormone receptors. Steroid hormone receptors bind to hormone response elements (HRE) in the promoters of target genes and recruit coactivators (e.g., SRC-1) and cointegrators (e.g., CBP/p300), which have chromatin remodeling activity. Some coregulators and cointegrators have histone acetyltransferase (HAT) activity that results in dynamic nucleosomal histone acetylation and increased access of basal transcription units (which include RNA polymerase II) to the promoters of target genes.

DNA (as described above and illustrated in Figs. 19.3 and 19.4); (2) ligand-dependent but not requiring direct binding to DNA; (3) ligand-independent action.

Most hormone-regulated genes have ligand-dependent binding of receptors to HREs. Examples of target genes regulated in this fashion are prostate-specific antigen (*PSA*) and prostate-specific membrane antigen (*PSMA*). However, in some target genes, ligand-activated ER regulates transcription without directly contacting the DNA, but by direct protein-protein interaction with other transcription factors that are themselves in direct contact with DNA via their own specific response elements. For example, ER-$\alpha$ can bind to Sp1 and AP1 transcription factors and regulate transcription of some genes.

Ligand-independent activation of ER and AR can occur through crosstalk pathways with a variety of growth factors. Growth factors such as EGF and/or IGF-1 bind to their respective tyrosine kinase receptors located in the plasma membrane of target cells and activate signal transduction pathways involving activation of other kinases (Chap. 8, Sec. 8.2); these can lead to phosphorylation of steroid receptors. One enzyme activated by growth factor signaling that can directly phosphorylate both ERs as well as AR is *Mitogen Activated Protein Kinase* (MAPK; Abreu-Martin et al., 1999). Similarly, interleukin-6 and protein kinase A can directly activate AR and ER-$\alpha$ in the absence of the appropriate steroid ligand. Interleukin-6 may directly bind to and influence AR activity without specifically inducing phosphorylation of AR (Chen et al., 2000). Growth factor/phosphorylation pathways can also influence steroid hormone receptor pathways via their ability to modulate the activity of coactivators by phosphorylation (Lopez et al., 2001). These alternative pathways for regulation of ER and AR activity could have a profound influence on the emergence of hormone independence in tumors that have not lost their hormone receptors.

*Nontranscriptional Actions of Steroid Receptors*   There is increasing evidence that not all effects of steroid hormones are mediated via the regulation of genomic or transcriptional events (Kelly and Levin, 2001). Transcription-independent effects of estrogen manifest themselves as rapid responses in target cells in the order of seconds to a few minutes. For estrogen, examples of nongenomic effects include modulation of calcium ion flux, effects on membrane channels in the central nervous system and peripheral excitable cells, membrane-associated interactions with growth factor receptors, and interactions with survival/apoptosis pathways. There is good evidence that membrane associated ERs coupled to G proteins or nitric oxide generating systems mediate some of these actions. At least two categories of such receptors may exist: one related

to the classic intracellular ER-$\alpha$ or ER-$\beta$ (Kelly and Levin, 2001), and the other distinct from them (Nadal et al., 2000). There is evidence that other steroid hormones, such as progesterone and testosterone, may also have such actions (Kousteni et al., 2001). The importance of nontranscriptional actions of estrogen in breast cancer and in estrogen signaling is not known.

### 19.2.3 Quantification of Steroid Hormone Receptors

Estrogen receptors and PR are biomarkers in breast cancer. In particular they help to predict the likelihood of response to endocrine therapy. In an unselected group of breast cancer patients with advanced disease, 30 to 40 percent will respond to endocrine therapy. However, in patients selected for the presence of both ER and PR in their primary breast tumor, the response rate to endocrine therapy is 70 to 80 percent. In contrast, patients whose tumors are both ER and PR negative have <10 percent chance of responding to endocrine therapy.

Estrogen receptors and PR are now measured routinely in breast tumor biopsies using the methods outlined in Figure 19.7. In contrast, in prostate cancer, AR provides no prognostic or diagnostic value because both hormone dependent and independent tumors usually possess functioning AR. The most widely used assay, until recently, was the dextran-coated charcoal, ligand binding assay (Fig. 19.7A). In this assay radiolabeled steroid ligand was incubated with a soluble extract from tumor tissue that had been homogenized and ultracentrifuged. The unbound ligand was adsorbed to dextran-coated charcoal while the receptor-bound radiolabeled ligand remained in the supernatant/cytosol and was quantified (Fig. 19.7A). Estrogen-receptor- and/or PR-positivity were usually defined by a receptor content of greater than 10 femtomole of receptor per milligram of soluble protein. Originally, the ligand binding assay cutoff values were derived from clinical correlation with responsiveness to endocrine therapy, although variability in the cutoff value used by different laboratories could result in variable classification as receptor-positive or -negative and may explain why some receptor-negative tumors responded to hormonal therapy. This method required relatively large amounts of fresh or fresh-frozen tissue and could not identify the cellular origin of the receptors. False-negative results could occur due to dilution of tumor cells by nontumor tissue, occupancy of the receptor by estrogen or tamoxifen, or storage and technical artifacts due to denaturation of the receptor proteins. Also no distinction could be made between ER-$\alpha$ and ER-$\beta$ isoforms. However, ER determined by ligand binding assays in human breast tumors appears to correlate well with *ER-$\alpha$* mRNA levels measured in the same tissues. As well we now know that ER-$\alpha$ is markedly upregulated in breast cancer and ER-$\beta$ is

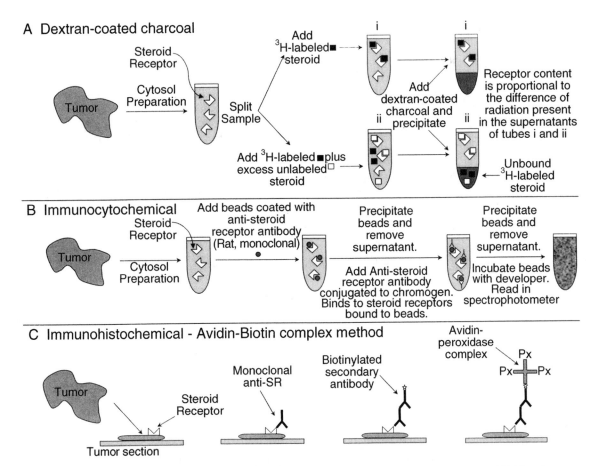

**Figure 19.7.** Methods for detection and quantification of steroid receptors in tumor tissue. (*A*) The dextran-coated charcoal method. Tumor tissue is homogenized and ultracentrifuged and the supernatant (cytosol) incubated with a known quantity of $^3$H-labeled steroid with or without excess unlabeled steroid. Dextran-coated charcoal is then added to adsorb unbound steroid. The receptor-bound $^3$H steroid remains in the supernatant and can be quantitated by the difference in $^3$H counts between the two tubes and expressed per milligram of cytosolic protein. (*B*) The immunocytochemical method. Tumor tissue is homogenized, ultracentrifuged, and the supernatant (cytosol) incubated with beads coated with monoclonal anti-steroid receptor antibody (anti-SR). Standards are also run containing known amounts of SR. Steroid receptor present in the sample binds to the beads and the supernatant is removed. Anti-SR, which is conjugated to a chromogen, is then added and binds to any SR present. Unbound conjugate is removed, the beads are incubated with a developing agent, and the intensity of color is read in a spectrophotometer. Color intensity is proportional to the concentration of SR in the sample. (*C*) The immunohistochemical avidin-biotin-peroxidase complex method. Thin sections of tumor are cut from formalin-fixed, paraffin-embedded biopsy specimens. The section is next exposed to a monoclonal antibody specific for the SR being assessed and binds to it. The section is then exposed to a second biotinylated antibody specific for the first antibody and binds to it. Finally, avidin-peroxidase complex is added, followed by a chromogen, and color appears where the SR is located.

usually downregulated in breast cancer, suggesting that most often ligand binding assays reflect ER-$\alpha$ expression.

Since the development of monoclonal antibodies to a number of steroid hormone receptors, immunochemical assays are now used in their routine quantification (Fig. 19.7*B* and *C*). Commercial kits are available for both immunohistochemical assays of tumor sections and for immunocytochemical (ER-ICA) assays, also called enzyme-linked immunosorbent assays (ELISA). These methods have several advantages over the radio-

ligand binding method (Table 19.1). They can be used on smaller tissue samples, are faster, and do not require the use of radiolabeled compounds. Also, false-negative results do not occur as a result of the receptor being occupied by tamoxifen or estrogen. Depending on the epitope (region of the protein) to which the antibody binds, immunochemical methods do not require a functional receptor. Although functionality (in particular ability to bind ligand) of the receptor and/or its alteration may be an inherent property of the receptor in the tumor, a major source of loss of function of recep-

**Table 19.1.** Advantages and Disadvantages of the Various Methods for Quantification of Estrogen and Progesterone Receptors in Human Breast Cancer Biopsy Samples

| Assay | Advantages | Disadvantages |
|---|---|---|
| Ligand binding assays (LBA) | Measures functional receptor protein | Requires large amounts of tissue<br>False negatives due to receptor occupancy with endogenous ligand |
| Immunocytochemical assay (ER-ICA) | Does not depend on functioning protein; detects protein with appropriate epitope<br>Faster than LBA<br>Avoids using radioisotopes<br>Avoids false negatives due to technical problems associated with denatured proteins<br>Avoids false negatives due to ligand occupied receptor | Requires less material than ligand binding but more than IHC<br>Homogenate required (see above)<br>Cannot distinguish between functional and nonfunctional protein |
| Immunohistochemical assay (IHC) | 5 $\mu$m tissue sections only required from formalin fixed-paraffin embedded blocks<br>Faster than LBA<br>Avoids using radioisotopes<br>Avoids false negatives due to technical problems associated with denatured protein<br>Avoids false negatives due to ligand occupied receptor | Semiquantifiable only<br>Antigen retrieval and suboptimal assay conditions<br>Cannot distinguish between functional and nonfunctional protein |

tors is technical due to suboptimal collection and handling of the biopsy specimen. The antibodies used are highly specific for ER-$\alpha$, do not cross-react with ER-$\beta$, and therefore another advantage of immunochemical-based assays is the lack of false-positives due to detection of the other ER.

Generally, results of immunochemical assays for ER and PR have been shown to correlate with the ligand binding methods. A disadvantage of the ELISA assays (Fig. 19.7$B$) is that a tissue homogenate is required, so that morphologic correlation with the presence of carcinoma cells is not possible. In contrast, immunohistochemical methods (Fig. 19.7$C$) can determine whether the detected receptor is within tumor cells, and can show receptor heterogeneity in tumor tissue. An example of ER heterogeneity within a breast tumor is shown in Figure 19.8. Heterogeneity refers to the observation that both ER$^+$ and ER$^-$ breast cancer cells can be present to varying degrees within any one human breast cancer biopsy sample, in addition to the presence of other types of cells (vascular cells, infiltrating cells of the immune system, normal stromal fibroblasts, normal breast adipocytes, and normal breast epithelial cells). Estrogen receptor immunohistochemical assay results are generally reported simply as positive or negative, although semiquantitative methods have been used. Positive results are generally reported when more than 10 percent of nuclei stain positively; this has been found to correlate with the threshold of

10 femtomole per milligram protein used for the dextran-coated charcoal method of receptor analysis. However, there is the need for some degree of quantification because there is a correlation between benefit and increasing receptor level, but results can vary among laboratories, especially in the low to middle range of the receptor spectrum. The major problem is associated with antigen retrieval and other assay conditions (Rhodes et al., 2000). Several approaches to quality control have been considered, and ER status determined by immunohistochemistry may be superior to the ligand binding assay in predicting endocrine responsiveness (Harvey et al., 1999).

## 19.3 NATURAL HISTORY OF BREAST AND PROSTATE CANCERS

### 19.3.1 Breast Cancer

*Risk Factors* Female gender and increasing age are the major risk factors for human breast cancer. Also, factors that increase the cumulative exposure and/or sensitivity of the breast epithelium to estrogen have been established as risk factors for breast cancer. For example, early menarche, late menopause, and obesity in postmenopausal women increase the cumulative exposure to estrogen and increase the risk of developing breast cancer. Factors that reduce the cumulative exposure to estrogens, such as early first pregnancy, multiple full-term pregnancies, ovariectomy in pre-

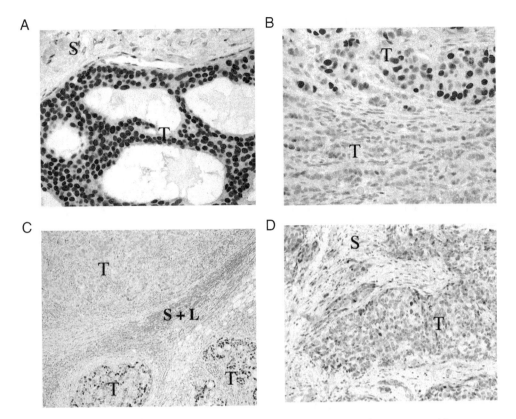

**Figure 19.8.** Immunohistograms illustrating heterogeneity of human breast cancer biopsy samples. Brown staining represents ER-α positivity. T, invasive breast cancer; S, stromal and connective tissue elements; L, lymphocytes. (A) Homogenous expression of ER-α within an invasive breast cancer, with negative adjacent vessels and stroma. (B) Moderate heterogeneity of expression of ER-α within an invasive breast cancer, with strong expression within solid nests of tumor cells in the upper field and weak or negative expression within less cohesive clusters of tumor cells in the lower field. Stromal and lymphocytic elements are negative for ER-α. (C) Marked heterogeneity of expression of ER-α within an invasive tumor metastatic to an axillary lymph node. In the upper part of the section one metastatic component is homogenously ER-α negative and in the lower section, the other component is moderate to high ER-α positive. These two different elements are separated in this field of view by a band of fibrous stroma and infiltrating lymphocytes. (D) Marked heterogeneity of ER-α expression within an invasive breast cancer with sporadic ER-α positive invasive breast cancer cells within a predominantly ER-α negative invasive tumor. (See color plate.)

menopausal women, and physical activity, are associated with a reduced risk of breast cancer. Consistent with these observations, increased serum levels of estrogen have been associated with postmenopausal breast cancer (Table 19.2).

Increased expression of ER in normal breast epithelium is probably a risk factor for breast cancer (Khan et al., 1998), as is increased mammographic breast density (Boyd et al., 2001) and increased circulating IGF-I levels (Hankinson et al., 1998). These latter two risk factors are correlated and may be functionally associated (Byrne et al., 2000). Estrogens have been shown to increase, and tamoxifen to decrease, mammographic density in women. The intimate association, and crosstalk of the IGF-I signaling pathway with the ER sig-

naling pathway in target cells may also play a role in the risk of breast cancer (Yee and Lee, 2000).

A family history of breast cancer is highly associated with the risk of breast cancer and two genes, *BRCA1* and *BRCA2*, have been identified which, when carrying a germline mutation, are associated with an inherited predisposition to breast cancer (Chap. 7, Sec. 7.4.5). Only 5 percent of all breast cancer incidence can be attributed to inherited mutations in these genes and <10 percent of all breast cancer incidence can be attributed to an inherited predisposition. Most breast cancers are sporadic, although polymorphisms in genes associated with the biosynthesis of estrogens (Thompson and Ambrosone, 2000) and factors that regulate ER activity, such as AR (Giguere et al., 2001), may influence breast

**Table 19.2.** Hormonally Related Epidemiologic Risk Factors for Breast Cancer

| Factor | Risk Group Low | Risk Group High | Relative Risk[a] |
|---|---|---|---|
| Sex | Male | Female | 183 |
| Oophorectomy | Age < 35 | No | 2.5 |
| Age at menarche | ≥14 y | ≤11 yr | 1.5 |
| Age at first birth | <20 y | ≥30 yr | 1.9 |
| Parity | ≥5 | Nulliparity | 1.4 |
| Age at natural menopause | <45 y | ≥55 y | 2.0 |
| Obesity (BMI)[b] | <22.9 | >30.7 | 1.6 |
| Oral contraceptive use | Never | Ever | 1.0 |
|  | Never | ≥4 y before First pregnancy | 1.7 |
| Estrogen replacement therapy | Never | Current | 1.4 |
|  | Never | >15 y | 1.3 |
| Dense mammogram[c] | None | ≥75% density | 5.3 |

[a]Using low-risk group as a reference.

[b]Body Mass Index (kg/m$^2$).

[c]Boyd et al., 2001.

*Source:* Adapted from Hulka et al. (1994).

cancer development. Breast cancer risk is complex, probably because of the influence of multiple genes with the environment.

The primary role of estrogen in breast cancer is thought to be due to its proliferative effect on breast epithelium. A complex interplay of steroid hormones, growth factors, extracellular matrix, and their respective receptors is likely involved.

*Development of Breast Cancer* Some of the cellular events associated with the natural history of breast cancer are illustrated in Figure 19.9*A*. Most invasive breast cancers arise from the epithelial cells of the terminal duct lobular unit (TDLU). Histopathological studies have identified a series of premalignant breast lesions referred to as hyperplasia without atypia/usual ductal hyperplasia (UDH), atypical hyperplasia (AH), and ductal carcinoma in situ (DCIS). Epidemiological evidence suggests that these lesions are associated with increasing risks of developing invasive breast cancer. For example, AH is associated with a five-fold increased risk, and DCIS is associated with a ten-fold increased risk (Page et al., 2000). Comparisons between premalignant and/or pre-invasive lesions in the same biopsy sample as invasive breast cancers have identified common genetic abnormalities, suggesting that the malignant lesions are clonally derived from the earlier lesions (Allred and Mohsin, 2000; Gong et al., 2001).

The normal development of the mammary gland is dependent on the presence of ER-α. Only a rudimentary ductal remnant is present in knockout mice that do not have the *ER-α* gene (Korach, 1994). The proliferative effects of estrogen in the normal mammary gland are indirect, likely mediated by paracrine effects because normal mammary epithelial cells that express ER-α are not the cells that are proliferating, as defined by the detection of markers of proliferation such as Ki-67. However, many ER-α expressing breast cancer cells are also proliferating, and addition of estrogen to ER-α positive breast cancer cells in culture causes them to grow (Anderson et al., 1998). Therefore, the effects of estrogen on ER-α positive breast cancer cells appear to be direct. Thus, an alteration in estrogen responsiveness and/or mechanism of estrogen action occurs during the development of breast cancer.

The expression of ER-α is low and infrequent in normal human breast epithelium and only 7 to 17 percent of normal breast epithelial cells express ER-α (Clarke et al., 1997), whereas greater than 70 percent of human breast tumors are ER-α$^+$. Often the level of ER-α expression in individual tumor cells is higher than that found in normal breast epithelial cells. A higher frequency of ER-α positive normal breast epithelial cells may be associated with increased risk of breast cancer (Khan et al., 1998). In general, therefore, the expression of ER-α increases during breast tumor develop-

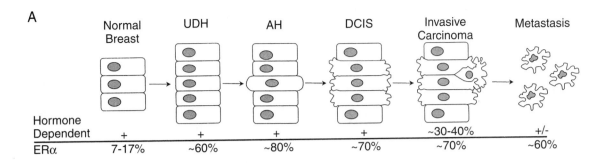

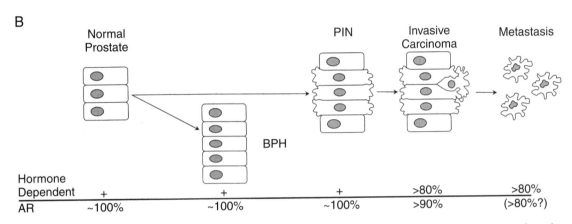

**Figure 19.9.** An overview of the natural history of cancers of the breast and the prostate indicating the relative hormonal dependency and receptor status. (*A*) Normal breast epithelium can undergo a stepwise transition from a series of premalignant breast lesions referred to as hyperplasia without atypia/usual ductal hyperplasia (UDH), atypical hyperplasia (AH), and ductal carcinoma in situ (DCIS), leading to invasive carcinoma. (*B*) Normal prostate epithelium can develop into benign prostatic hyperplasia (BPH), which is not a precursor to carcinoma, or can give rise to high-grade prostatic interstitial neoplasia (PIN), which can become invasive carcinoma. In each step, the relative hormone dependency and percent expressing ER-$\alpha$ or AR are indicated.

ment, and this occurs at an early stage. Most hyperplastic lesions, with or without atypia, show increased expression of ER-$\alpha$ and increased frequency of ER$^+$ cells compared to normal epithelium, while greater than 70 percent of CIS are ER-$\alpha^+$, similar to invasive breast cancer (Allred and Mohsin, 2000). In the normal breast, the frequency of ER-$\alpha^+$ cells increases with age, and this relationship remains in hyperplasia without atypia, but the age relationship is lost in AH and CIS (Shoker et al., 1999). Also, in normal breast epithelial cells ER-$\alpha$ and Ki-67, a marker of cell proliferation (see Chap. 9, Sec. 9.4.2), are rarely, if ever, co-expressed (Anderson et al., 1998), suggesting that either ER-$\alpha$ expressing cells are incapable of proliferating or that ER-$\alpha$ must be downregulated before normal breast epithelial cells can proliferate. This inverse relationship is maintained in UDH, but is lost in AH, CIS, and ER-$\alpha^+$ invasive breast cancer cells (Shoker et al., 1999).

ER-$\beta$ is also expressed in both normal and neoplastic human breast tissues (Leygue et al., 1998; Roger et al., 2001). Unlike ER-$\alpha$, this receptor does not play a pivotal role in development of the mammary gland because knockout mice for *ER-$\beta$* have normal development of the mammary gland (Couse and Korach, 1999). Expression of ER-$\beta$ is much more frequent than ER-$\alpha$ in normal human and rodent mammary glands, and its expression generally declines during breast cancer development (Leygue et al., 1998; Roger et al., 2001). Emerging data also support altered expression and possibly activity of some coregulators of ER during breast tumorigenesis (Murphy et al., 2000). As discussed earlier (Fig. 19.4), these coregulators are general for most steroid hormone receptors.

Growth suppression pathways associated with TGF-$\beta$ are also altered in some early lesions. For example, TGF-$\beta$ receptor type II is highly expressed in normal breast epithelium, but is downregulated in some UDH lesions and identifies a group of women at higher risk of developing breast cancer (Gobbi et al., 1999). Altered growth factor pathways that stimulate the cell cycle, for example, overexpression of HER2 (neu/erbB-2) and cyclin D1, and/or inactivation of tumor suppressor genes such as *p53*, can be detected in some premalignant lesions such as CIS (Allred and Mohsin, 2000).

*Progression of Invasive Breast Cancer* Amplification and upregulation of expression of several oncogenes, including those encoding growth factors such as EGF, TGF-$\alpha$, IGF, and their receptor tyrosine kinases, for example, EGFR, HER2, and IGF-R, together with inactivation or downregulation of tumor suppressor genes such as *p53*, *Rb*, or *BRCA1* have been associated with breast cancer progression. The introduction of comparative genomic hybridization (CGH), fluorescence in situ hybridization (FISH), spectral karyotyping (SKY) and DNA microarrays (Perou et al., 1999; Chap. 4, Sec. 4.4) is allowing a more global analysis of the molecular genetic alterations that occur during cancer progression.

Prognosis of patients with invasive breast cancer is related to lymph node involvement, tumor size, histological grade, and steroid receptor status. Approximately 70 percent of all primary invasive breast tumors are ER$^+$ and in general these tumors are more differentiated, less aggressive, and have lower levels of growth receptors compared to ER$^-$ tumors. In contrast, more consistent evidence has accumulated to show that young patients (<35 years) with ER$^+$ tumors have a worse prognosis than those with ER$^-$ tumors (Aebi et al., 2000). Estrogen receptor status not only is a prognostic factor but it is also a marker of response to treatment, as will be discussed subsequently. Whether ER$^+$ and ER$^-$ breast tumors are indicators of a different stage of the disease (i.e., ER$^-$ disease arises from an ER$^+$ precursor) or are different entities (i.e., arise from different breast epithelial cell types) has not been resolved. Because ER status only rarely changes during breast cancer progression (i.e., between primary and metastatic lesions in the same patient or in recurrent metastases after endocrine therapy; Robertson, 1996), and because tamoxifen has been found to reduce only the incidence of ER$^+$ breast cancer, it is likely that ER$^-$ breast cancer rarely develops from an ER$^+$ precursor. In the rare case where an ER$^-$ metastasis develops from an ER$^+$ primary tumor, it has not been possible to determine if ER expression was turned off in the metastatic cells or whether the original primary tumor was heterogeneous for ER status and the ER$^-$ cancer cells have a growth and survival advantage allowing them to metastasize.

There is evidence for the development of hormone independence with breast cancer progression (Fig. 19.9*A*). While approximately 70 percent of all primary breast tumors are ER-$\alpha^+$, only 50 percent of them will respond to endocrine therapy which is aimed at inhibiting the proliferative action of estrogen on ER$^+$ cells. Furthermore, of the ER$^+$ tumors that respond originally to endocrine therapies many will develop resistance despite still being ER$^+$. This is discussed below in the sections relating to hormonal treatment.

### 19.3.2 Prostate Cancer

*Risk Factors* Carcinogenesis of the prostate involves genetic and environmental influences with no obvious etiological agent. Risk factors include family history, age, and race (Gallagher and Fleshner, 1998). First-degree male relatives of prostate cancer patients have ~2.5-fold increase in risk, and the risk of prostate cancer appears to be higher for relatives of women with breast cancer. However, hereditary factors most commonly affect men with early onset disease and are responsible for relatively few cases (<10%).

Prostate cancer is a disease of the elderly, with more than 75 percent of cancers diagnosed in men over 65 years of age. However, microfoci of high-grade *p*rostatic *i*nterepithelial *n*eoplasia (PIN), the presumed precursor of the disease, can be found in men in their third and fourth decade. Most of the early tumors are microscopic, generally well to moderately differentiated, and tend to be multifocal. The frequency with which these neoplastic lesions are seen in autopsy material is similar among African Americans, white men, and Japanese men, but the incidence of clinical disease is much higher in African-American men and much lower in Japanese men. In Japanese immigrants, the incidence of prostate cancer rises to levels near those of white men within two generations, suggesting the involvement of environmental factors (Chap. 2, Sec. 2.3.1). Collectively, these observations suggest that the critical event in the natural history of prostate cancer is tumor promotion rather than tumor initiation and that promotion and progression of this cancer are strongly influenced by epigenetic or adaptive processes. Diet is probably important with the predominantly vegetarian diet of Asians providing a protective influence, whereas the intake of red meat associated with a typical American diet is associated with increased risk (Denis et al., 1999). In addition, fat soluble, environmental contaminants have been shown to influence endocrine pathways and may contribute to the association with diet (Kelce et al., 1998).

*Development of Prostate Cancer* Two pathological conditions that frequently coexist with latent and clinical prostate cancer are benign prostatic hyperplasia (BPH) and PIN (see Fig. 19.9*B*). Benign prostatic hyperplasia shares many biologic properties with prostate cancer, including androgen regulation of growth and increasing prevalence with advancing age. However, BPH is neither a premalignant lesion nor a precursor of invasive prostate cancer. A more likely candidate for this role is PIN, which is characterized by cytological atypia of proliferating luminal epithelium within pre-existing acini and ducts with no penetration of basement membrane, and is generally subdivided into low or high grade. Autopsy studies have revealed that high-grade PIN is found in association with cancer in 60 to 95 percent of malignant prostates and that a wide spectrum of molecular/genetic abnormalities are common to both high-grade PIN and prostate cancer (Sakr and Partin, 2001). Specific chromosomal alterations (e.g., loss of 8p, 10q, 16q, 18q, and gain of 7q31, 8q), amplification of the c-myc gene, along with changes in telomerase activity, cell cycle status, and proliferative indices suggest collectively that high-grade PIN is intermediate between benign epithelium and prostatic carcinoma (Sakr and Partin, 2001). A related staining profile for growth factors and for the AR has been demonstrated in the luminal epithelium of high-grade PIN and in carcinoma, with a tendency to higher expression of membrane EGFR, HER-2, and cytoplasmic TGF-$\alpha$, and lower levels of FGF-2, than in glands with low-grade PIN or BPH (Harper et al., 1998). In addition to being a precursor for prostate cancer, it is likely that PIN predates invasive cancer by at least a decade and thus may serve as a predictive marker for the disease.

*Progression of Invasive Prostate Cancer* When organ confined, prostate cancer is potentially curable by prostatectomy or radiation therapy. However, in locally advanced or metastatic disease treatment is largely palliative with androgen withdrawal as first-line treatment. The clinical approaches used for androgen withdrawal are described below. Despite high initial response rates of the order of 80 percent, patients will inevitably progress to hormone-independent disease in a manner analogous to that seen following hormonal therapy for metastatic breast cancer. Response to androgen ablation therapies depends on the degree of retention by the tumor of the capacity for activation of apoptosis after androgen withdrawal.

## 19.4 HORMONAL THERAPIES FOR BREAST AND PROSTATE CANCERS

### 19.4.1 Breast Cancer

*Hormonal Therapies* Endocrine therapies for patients with breast cancer are aimed at inhibiting the proliferative effect of estrogen on breast cancer cells. As outlined in Figure 19.2A, this is generally achieved in two ways: decreasing the level of circulating and/or local es-

trogen or blocking the action of estrogen on the target tissue. Only those breast tumors that express ER benefit from endocrine therapies.

**Reduction of estrogen levels.** Reduced levels of estrogen can be achieved both surgically, by oophorectomy, and pharmacologically. In premenopausal women, options are surgical or radiation-induced oophorectomy, or the use of LHRH agonists, which initially stimulate and then block the LHRH receptor in the pituitary gland. This leads to a reduction in levels of the gonadotropins which stimulate the ovary to synthesize estrogens.

In postmenopausal women, residual levels of estrogen can be reduced by selective aromatase inhibitors which inhibit the conversion of weak androgens to estrogens (see Fig 19.1). As shown in Figure 19.10, aromatase inhibitors fall into two main classes: the steroidal (type I, e.g., formestane and exemestane) and the nonsteroidal (type II, e.g., aminoglutethimide, fadrozole, anastrozole, or letrozole). The two classes differ in their mechanism of action. The steroidal inhibitors compete with endogenous substrates for the active site of the enzyme, and are processed to intermediates that bind irreversibly to the active site causing inhibition. The nonsteroidal inhibitors also compete with the endogenous substrates for the active site, but form a strong, although reversible, coordinate bond with the iron atom in heme, excluding endogenous substrates and oxygen from the enzyme. Removal of the nonsteroidal inhibitor results in reversal of enzyme inhibition. These agents may displace tamoxifen (see below) as the preferred first-line treatment of postmenopausal women, and may be used after oophorectomy or LHRH agonists have induced menopause in premenopausal women. Progestins such as megestrol acetate have been used often as second- or third-line endocrine therapies in breast cancer, and part of their mechanism of action could include the increased expression and/or activity of enzymes, which can metabolize strong estrogens into weaker compounds.

**Blocking estrogen action at the ER.** The nonsteroidal anti-estrogen tamoxifen has been the agent of choice for first-line endocrine therapy for the treatment of ER- and/or PR-positive breast cancer (Fig. 19.10). It leads to improved survival when used as adjuvant therapy for women with receptor-positive breast cancer of all ages, and may decrease the incidence of breast cancer in groups of women at high risk for the disease. Tamoxifen and its more active metabolite, 4-hydroxytamoxifen, competitively inhibit the binding of estradiol to the ligand binding site of the ER in a dose-dependent manner (Fig. 19.3). When tamoxifen or similar compounds bind to the receptor, they result in conformational changes of the ER that allows the inactive receptor to bind to DNA but not to activate transcription

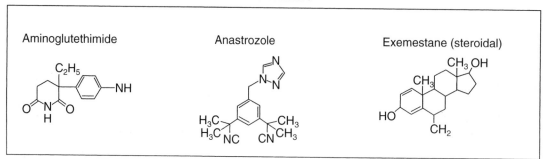

**Figure 19.10.** Structures of anti-estrogens and aromatase inhibitors. The anti-estrogens block estrogen binding to its receptor and the steroidal forms also increase turnover of the receptor protein. The aromatase inhibitors block the formation of estrogens from androgen precursors.

(Fig. 19.4). X-ray crystallography studies of the ER ligand domain bound to either estradiol or 4-hydroxytamoxifen show that estradiol binding causes formation of a hydrophobic cleft on the surface of this domain that serves as a docking site for coactivators. In contrast, anti-estrogens displace part of the receptor, blocking this site, and therefore blocking coactivator access (Shiau et al., 1998).

Compounds like tamoxifen have both estrogenic as well as anti-estrogenic properties, depending on the cell type or the promoter of any particular target gene. Tamoxifen has estrogenic effects in bone (which are desirable to prevent osteoporosis), in cardiovascular tissue, and in the uterus (which is undesirable as it may stimulate proliferation and lead to a low incidence of uterine cancer). Compounds with different selectivity in their estrogenic and anti-estrogenic properties are referred to collectively as *Selective Estrogen Receptor*

*Modulators* (SERMs). They induce slightly different conformational changes in the ER and therefore have differential abilities to interact with a variety of coregulators, whose expression and/or activation will vary between cell types and tissues, as illustrated in Figure 19.11 (McKenna and O'Malley, 2000). Because breast tumors often develop resistance to tamoxifen without loss of ER expression, and because tamoxifen has undesirable estrogenic properties in the uterus, other SERMs are being investigated for their usefulness in breast cancer treatment and prevention. For example, raloxifene is a SERM that has estrogenic effects on bone and the cardiovascular system, but is anti-estrogenic in the breast and uterus (Fig. 19.11; O'Regan and Jordan, 2001). A study (*Study of Tamoxifen and Raloxifene, STAR*) is under way to compare its efficacy with respect to tamoxifen in breast cancer prevention in high-risk women.

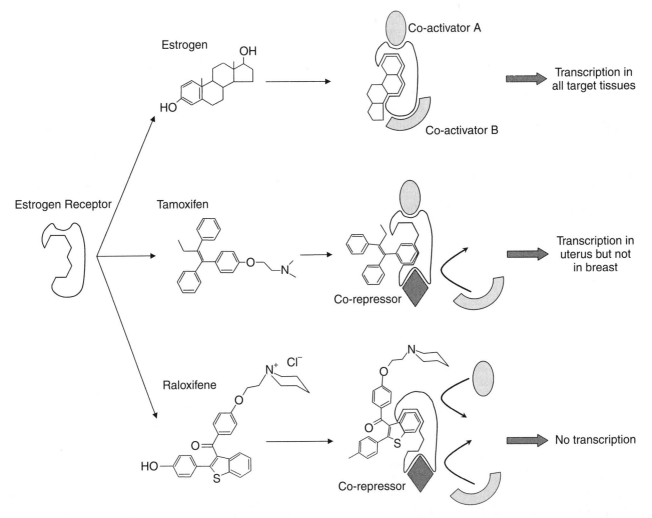

**Figure 19.11.** Schematic representation of conformational changes induced by different SERMs (estrogen, tamoxifen, and raloxifene) resulting in differential recruitment of coregulators and differential activity. Estrogen binds to the estrogen receptor (ER) causing a conformational change that leads to docking of appropriate coactivators (hypothetical coactivator *A* and coactivator *B*) with ER in all target tissues and results in enhanced transcription of target genes. Tamoxifen binds to ER giving rise to a different conformation such that it docks coactivator *A* and a hypothetical corepressor that in one tissue (breast) inhibits estrogen action but in another tissue partially activates estrogen action (uterus). Another SERM, called raloxifene, binds to ER resulting in another different conformation such that it only docks the corepressor and inhibits estrogen action in both target tissues.

Steroidal anti-estrogens such as fulvestrant (Fig. 19.10) that show little if any estrogenic activity (in particular in the uterus) retain activity in some women whose breast cancers have acquired resistance to tamoxifen. The mechanism of action of these pure anti-estrogens is distinct from the partial anti-estrogens such as tamoxifen, in that they downregulate ER expression by increasing its degradation, as well as inactivating the ER complex (O'Regan and Jordan, 2001). Such compounds have been named *Selective Estrogen Receptor Downregulators* (SERDs). Due to its steroidal nature, fulvestrant is not suitable for oral administration and is administered by intramuscular injection, which is a disadvantage. High-dose progestin treatment that is used as a second- or third-line endocrine treatment may also act partially by downregulating expression of the ER in breast tumors.

*Neoadjuvant and Adjuvant Hormonal Therapies* Systemic adjuvant therapy given after surgical removal of the primary tumor is aimed at eliminating subclinical, micrometastatic cancer cell deposits that have spread from the original tumor site (Chap. 11, Sec. 11.2.1). Adjuvant hormonal therapies, such as ovarian ablation in premenopausal women and tamoxifen (given for 5 y) in both premenopausal and postmenopausal women with breast cancer, have been shown to increase both relapse-free and overall survival of women with ER$^+$ early breast cancer. Further, the addition of tamoxifen to adjuvant chemotherapy further lowers the risk of recurrence of $ER^+$ breast cancer. The use of adjuvant aromatase inhibitors in postmenopausal women and LHRH agonists in premenopausal women is being investigated. The former has recently shown high clinical promise (Baum et al., 2002; Goss et al., 2003).

Neoadjuvant (preoperative) endocrine therapy (with or without chemotherapy) is also used in some patients to reduce the size of the primary breast cancer, thereby increasing the possibility of breast-conserving surgery and allowing assessment of response to treatment in primary tumors.

*Treatment of Advanced Disease*  Metastatic breast cancer is not curable, and the goals of therapy are to prolong survival and to maximize the quality of life of the patient. Tamoxifen therapy is beneficial in treating both pre- and postmenopausal $ER^+$ breast cancer patients. Ovarian ablation (surgical or medical, using LHRH agonists) is an option for initial treatment in premenopausal women, while recent data suggest that aromatase inhibitors may be superior to tamoxifen in the treatment of $ER^+$ breast cancer in postmenopausal women. Despite the initial responsiveness of advanced $ER^+$ breast cancer to first-line endocrine therapy, tumors eventually develop resistance to the treatment and progress. This occurs most often despite the continued expression of ER. Women who respond to initial endocrine treatment have about a 50 percent chance of responding to a second agent, and some will also respond to third-line agents such as megestrol acetate. However, breast cancer eventually becomes resistant to all forms of endocrine therapy (Fig. 19.12).

*Mechanisms Associated with the Development of Resistance to Hormonal Therapies*  Resistance to hormonal therapies is of two types, *de novo* and acquired. Resistance to tamoxifen has been studied most extensively. Tamoxifen used in treatment and prevention is useful only for $ER^+$ breast cancer; there is no effect of tamoxifen on the incidence of $ER^-$ breast cancers. However, only about 50 percent of patients with $ER^+$ breast tumors will respond to tamoxifen, with the remainder having intrinsic resistance. Patients whose disease responds initially to tamoxifen will develop acquired resistance over a time that ranges from several weeks to several years. Although acquired tamoxifen resistance may sometimes be due to loss of ER expression or the selection of an $ER^-$ tumor cell population from an originally heterogeneous tumor cell population, in most cases, the resistant recurrent tumors remain $ER^+$.

Mechanisms responsible for de novo and acquired tamoxifen resistance may differ because $ER^+$ breast tumors with de novo tamoxifen resistance are also generally resistant to other forms of endocrine therapy. In contrast, tumors with acquired tamoxifen resistance are

more likely to respond subsequently to second- and third-line endocrine therapy. No one mechanism has been shown to account for the majority of $ER^+$, tamoxifen-resistant, breast cancers in vivo, and multiple mechanisms may be involved in tamoxifen resistance. These mechanisms are explored in Section 19.5.

### 19.4.2 Prostate Cancer

*Androgen Withdrawal Therapies*  Approximately 80 percent of patients with metastatic prostate cancer will respond to androgen withdrawal therapy, as indicated by a fall in the serum marker of the disease, prostate-specific antigen (PSA), and by an improvement in symptoms (most often pain due to metastases in bone). Such treatment is associated with a median progression-free survival of 1 to 2 years and median overall survival of 2 to 4 years. The failure to eradicate the entire malignant population by androgen withdrawal results in progression to androgen independence (illustrated in Fig. 19.12), as manifested by a rising serum PSA and/or clinical signs and symptoms. The goal of any form of androgen withdrawal therapy is to activate apoptosis or block cell proliferation in prostate tumor cells by inhibiting the androgenic signal (Fig. 19.2B). There are several methods for achieving androgen withdrawal, by interfering either with the synthesis or metabolic conversion of androgens or with their ability to interact with the AR. However, because most androgen-independent prostate tumors have normal or elevated levels of AR (Fig. 19.9B), there is no prognostic value in measuring these receptors.

Bilateral orchiectomy (castration) is the most direct way to block androgen stimulation of the prostate and has the advantages of low morbidity, low cost, and

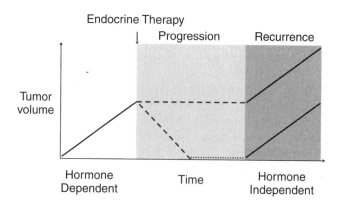

**Figure 19.12.** A schematic illustration of the effects of endocrine therapy, tumor regression, and hormone-independent recurrence on tumor volume. After blocking the activity of the appropriate steroid hormone, hormone-dependent or responsive tumors will regress or cease to grow respectively. After a variable time interval, tumor growth resumes and is hormone independent.

high compliance. However, the associated psychological problems have decreased its practice in favor of medical castration using LHRH agonists. LHRH agonists include goserelin, leuprolide, and buserelin which can be administered as long-acting (1 to 4 mo) depot formulations to block the secretion of LH by the pituitary gland and thereby inhibit the synthesis of testosterone by the testis (Fig. 19.2B). Initially, LHRH agonists cause a rise in LH and testosterone that is termed a *flare* response; this effect is avoided by temporary coadministration of an anti-androgen to inhibit AR signaling in the tumor cell. A rising serum PSA level is usually the earliest manifestation of progression following initial endocrine therapy, often predating clinical evidence of progression by more than 6 months.

Anti-androgens, some of which are shown in Figure 19.13, act competitively with testicular or adrenal an-

drogens to block AR activation within the prostate cell (Fig. 19.3), and apart from transient use to prevent the flare associated with LHRH agonists, are usually added as second-line hormonal therapy at time of progression. Nonsteroidal anti-androgens, such as flutamide or bicalutamide (Fig. 19.13), have no gonadotropic or hypothalamic feedback effect to suppress circulating levels of testosterone, whereas steroidal anti-androgens such as cyproterone acetate do possess this feedback activity (Fig. 19.2B). About 30 percent of patients who have responded and then progressed after initial hormone therapy will respond to the subsequent addition of an anti-androgen. At the time of progression following this treatment, discontinuation of the anti-androgen leads to further response in about 20 percent of patients. The underlying molecular mechanism responsible for the anti-androgen withdrawal syndrome

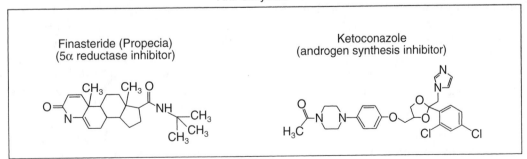

**Figure 19.13.** Structures of anti-androgens and anti-enzymes, which block androgen metabolism. The anti-androgens block androgen binding to its receptor and the steroidal forms also provide negative feedback to the hypothalamus. The anti-enzymes may in some cases inhibit the conversion of testosterone to the more active form dihydrotestosterone or alternatively may block androgen synthesis.

is not fully understood, but may relate to altered AR ligand specificity.

Other second- or third-line strategies include the use of ketoconazole (Fig. 19.13) to inhibit steroid synthesis in general (used more rarely because of toxicity to the liver), and glucocorticoids, such as prednisone or hydrocortisone, to inhibit production of ACTH, which leads to decreased production of weak androgens by the adrenal gland (Fig. 19.2*B*). Estrogens have also been used to suppress LH and FSH by feedback effects on the pituitary, but appear to have rare effects in patients who have already received several hormonal treatments and may have direct effects on prostate cancer cells, which express both ER-$\alpha$ and ER-$\beta$. Irrespective of the type of androgen withdrawal treatment used, the side effects can include hot flushes, loss of libido and sexual potency, gynecomastia, lethargy, depression, and loss of bone and muscle mass.

Many patients have received treatment with complete androgen blockade, which combines orchiectomy or an LHRH agonist with a nonsteroidal anti-androgen. However, a meta-analysis of several trials comparing complete androgen blockade with conventional medical or surgical castration showed no significant survival advantage (Prostate Cancer Trialists' Collaborative Group, 2000), and there is no basis for continuing to use this expensive treatment which also has more side effects than orchiectomy or an LHRH agonist alone.

*Neoadjuvant and Adjuvant Therapies*  As for the use of tamoxifen in breast cancer, hormone withdrawal therapies have been given before or after primary treatments such as prostatectomy or radiation therapy, or concurrent with radiation therapy. Initial hormone treatment can lead to a reduction in tumor size, but such therapy has not been shown to improve survival following radical surgery. It has been shown, however, to increase the effectiveness of radiation therapy for locally advanced prostate cancer, and combined hormonal and radiation therapy has become standard for such patients. There is supporting evidence from animal models that combined treatment with anti-androgen therapy and radiation may increase anti-tumor effects compared with either alone (Zietman, 2000).

## 19.5 MECHANISMS FOR PROGRESSION TO HORMONE INDEPENDENCE

Cancer progression involves a series of changes in the malignant cell whereby its appearance and behavior inevitably evolve toward a more aggressive and poorly differentiated phenotype (Chap. 11, Sec. 11.1.1; Fig. 19.9). In prostate cancer, the term *progression* is more commonly used in an endocrine sense to connote the process in which there is a change from androgen-dependent to androgen-independent disease, as shown in Figure 19.12. Similar progression from hormone dependence to independence occurs during progression of breast cancer.

### 19.5.1 Clonal Selection Versus Adaptation

Tumor progression is attributed usually to mutations, or to irreversible chromosomal rearrangements, losses, and duplications with selection of clones that have a growth or survival advantage (Chap. 11, Sec. 11.1.2). This widely accepted mechanism proposes that androgen- or estrogen-independent tumor cells are present initially and that hormonal therapy kills all but this population of cells, which subsequently becomes the dominant phenotype of the tumor. There is evidence to support this mechanism in some animal tumor models whose rapid regrowth after androgen withdrawal implies the pre-existence of androgen-independent clones (Gingrich et al., 1997). However, there also is evidence to support alternative mechanisms, including heritable perturbations in regulatory pathways that depend on interactions with inter- or intracellular factors, and which may be due in part to epigenetic/adaptive processes. The two mechanisms for progression are outlined in Figure 19.14.

There are many molecular processes linked to prostate cancer progression that imply an epigenetic mechanism (Rennie and Nelson, 1999). Early experiments by Noble (1980) demonstrated that chronic administration of combinations of testosterone and estradiol to Nb rats increased the incidence of prostate adenocarcinomas from less than 1 percent to >18 percent. Because neither estrogens nor androgens are mutagens, this suggests that prostate cancer can arise through an epigenetic mechanism. Furthermore, in this animal model, fractional replacement of estrogen by tamoxifen to keep the tumor in stasis (i.e., neither regressing nor growing), delayed or prevented progression to hormone independence, implying that progression was also driven by epigenetic processes.

For breast cancer, there are molecular data showing identical genetic abnormalities in synchronous premalignant, pre-invasive, and invasive breast cancer lesions that support clonal selection in breast cancer progression. However, unlike prostate cancer where the vast majority of invasive prostate cancers are AR$^+$, two biologically distinct groups of breast cancers exist, that is, ER$^+$ and ER$^-$ tumors. Rarely during progression does a tumor change its ER status, suggesting that the two tumor types are unlikely to be derived one from the other. Further, when it appears that ER status has changed during progression it has been impossible to distinguish between the possibility that ER expression

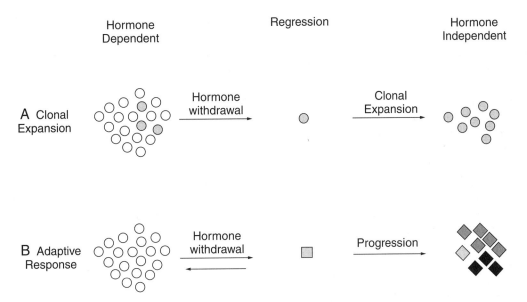

**Figure 19.14.** Clonal selection and epigenetic/adaptive mechanisms for emergence of hormone independence in tumors. (*A*) Upon hormone withdrawal, hormone-dependent cells are killed leaving behind preexisting hormone-independent clones (shaded) that re-populate the tumor. (*B*) Upon hormone withdrawal, most cells are killed except for those expressing critical cell survival genes. When re-exposed to hormone the pattern of gene expression reverts and the tumor regrows in response to hormone. However, through further adaptive changes in gene expression patterns, the cells no longer require hormone to sustain their growth.

was turned off, or that the original primary tumor was heterogeneous, containing both ER$^+$ and ER$^-$ breast cancer cells, with ER$^-$ cancer cells having a growth advantage. Most of the evidence suggests that progression to hormone independence and development of tamoxifen resistance in breast cancer is due to epigenetic and adaptive mechanisms.

The extent to which the development or progression of breast and prostate cancer are driven by epigenetic or genetic mechanisms is not trivial. If progression occurs primarily as a consequence of irreversible genetic changes, then options for prevention and treatment are limited. Conversely, if reversible adaptive or epigenetic processes are predominant, then breast and prostate cancer are potentially more amenable to therapeutic control.

### 19.5.2 Altered Pharmacology

A possible mechanism for tamoxifen resistance in breast cancer is altered uptake and metabolism of tamoxifen by the tumor leading to reduced intratumoral drug concentrations. Metabolism of tamoxifen to more estrogenic metabolites could also contribute to reduced efficacy, with tamoxifen being interpreted by the tumor cells as an estrogen, resulting in stimulation of tumor growth. Altered availability of tamoxifen to ER within the tumor may occur due to increased expression of binding proteins such as *Anti-Estrogen Binding Sites*

(AEBS), which do not bind estrogen but would sequester tamoxifen away from ER. Data consistent with each of these mechanisms have been described both in some human breast tumors and in a model of tamoxifen-resistant human breast cancer where breast cancer cell lines are grown as xenografts in athymic mice (Clarke et al., 2001).

Altered uptake and metabolism of anti-androgens have not been investigated sufficiently to assess their contribution to the androgen-independent phenotype. While the anti-androgen flutamide requires hydroxylation for activity in vivo, there are no reports linking altered pharmacology of this or other anti-androgens with prostate tumor progression.

### 19.5.3 Alternative Signal Transduction Pathways and the Importance of Stroma

There is substantial evidence that during progression to hormone independence, both autocrine and paracrine growth factor pathways are dysregulated and growth factors may replace estrogens or androgens as primary growth regulators. Epithelial cells, normal or neoplastic, do not exist in isolation within breast or prostatic tissue. They exist in a complex three-dimensional interaction with stromal cells (fibroblasts and adipocytes), blood vessels, and, often, immune cells within and surrounded by an extracellular matrix (ECM). Cell-cell interactions may be mediated by growth factors or through interactions with the ECM via adhesion molecules called integrins located on the cell surface (Chap. 11, Sec. 11.5.1). These interactions regulate signal transduction pathways and gene expression.

In prostate cancer, there is an increase in paracrine stimulation by growth factors produced in prostatic stroma with eventual autocrine production and stimulation by the prostate cancer epithelial cell (Rennie and Nelson, 1999). The EGFR/TGF-α system is a prime example of this trend. In benign prostatic hypertrophy (BPH), epithelial cells express EGFR but not its ligand TGF-α, whereas prostate stroma produces TGF-α but not EGFR. However, in many prostate epithelial tumor cells, co-expression of EGFR and TGF-α is observed, indicating a shift from paracrine to autocrine stimulation (Leav et al., 1998). Whether the molecular mechanisms responsible for the shift in this regulatory loop are due to mutational or adaptive processes is unknown. However, by simply adapting the amount of genistein in the diet, the expression of EGFR in the EGFR/TGF-α system can be manipulated (Dalu et al., 1998).

A similar shift from paracrine to autocrine regulation has been seen with the IGF system. In the normal prostate and in BPH, IGF-I and IGF-II are produced and secreted by the stroma, but exert their activities on prostate epithelia in a paracrine fashion through IGF-I and IGF-II receptors. However, in prostate cancers, production of both types of IGF occurs in the tumor cells, which results in an autocrine loop for androgen-independent growth stimulation (Wang and Wong, 1998). Overall, as prostate cancer progresses, the stromal component tends to become redundant for controlling prostate growth.

In breast cancer, ligand-independent activation of the ER has been demonstrated frequently, and although this can occur also in normal tissues, sustained upregulation of such pathways may lead to ligand independence of the ER in breast cancer and contribute to hormone independence and anti-estrogen resistance. Some of the more common alterations in breast tumors are upregulated and abnormally regulated growth factor pathways (EGFR, IGFR, HER2) and/or their intracellular signal transduction molecules (RAS, RAF, MAPK, PI-3K, AKT, Chap. 8, Sec. 8.2). It is known that growth factors such as IGF-I, heregulin, and EGF can activate ER in the absence or presence of estrogen through a mechanism involving phosphorylation of the ER (Ali and Coombes, 2000). Similar phosphorylation mechanisms are almost certainly operational for the ligand-independent activation of ER by protein kinase A, protein kinase C, pp90rsk1 and protein kinase B (Ali and Coombes, 2000; Clarke et al., 2001). The expression and/or activity of many of these kinases are often

increased in breast tumors compared to normal breast tissue, and specific phosphatases that deactivate these kinases have been shown to be expressed at higher levels in breast cancer cell lines with altered responses to estrogen. Thus, sustained and increased phosphorylation of the ER may underlie the progression to hormone independence and endocrine resistance. The ability of tamoxifen to effect ligand-independent activation of ER is variable, which suggests that other mechanisms participate in the development of anti-estrogen resistance (Clarke et al., 2001). For example, sustained activation of the PI-3K/AKT pathway (Chap. 8, Sec. 8.2.7), inducing a positive feedback loop whereby activated AKT activates ER-α in a ligand-independent fashion, and ER-α in the presence or absence of estrogen activates PI-3K, protects breast cancer cells against tamoxifen-induced apoptosis (Campbell et al., 2001; Sun et al., 2001). Because growth factors activate both the PI-3K and MAPK pathways and both can affect ER-α signaling, it seems that a marked amplification of ligand-independent ER signaling is inevitable. Furthermore, such amplified pathways can directly activate ER coactivators via phosphorylation (Font de Mora and Brown, 2000), further enhancing the ER signaling pathway to an extent that tamoxifen is unable to inactivate it, and indeed may alter coregulator profiles such that tamoxifen is seen as an estrogen. The relevance of this mechanism is underscored by the recent demonstration that high expression of the coactivator AIB1, in association with high expression of HER-2 in ER+ breast tumors, is linked to tamoxifen-resistance in vivo (Osborne et al., 2003).

Crosstalk between ER and other transcription factors or coregulator proteins may also play a role in progression to hormone independence. For example, crosstalk between ER and the transcription factor AP-1 takes several forms: estrogens can regulate the expression of the components of AP-1 transcription complexes, ER and AP-1 can directly interact by protein-protein interactions and regulate target gene expression, and activation of AP-1 complexes can downregulate ER expression (Clarke et al., 2001). Recent data, using a mouse model of tamoxifen-resistant breast cancer, also show an association of resistance with oxidative stress and increased AP-1 activity (Schiff et al., 2000). All of these mechanisms could influence the responsiveness of a breast cancer cell to tamoxifen, and there are some reports where altered AP-1 activity and/or levels of expression of AP-1 components can be correlated with acquired tamoxifen resistance. It is likely, therefore, that multiple alterations may be necessary for progression to hormone independence and the development of resistance to endocrine therapies.

## 19.5.4 Receptor Amplifications and Mutations

Unlike breast cancer, where *de novo* hormone independence is often associated with absence of ER, androgen-independent human prostate cancer is seldom associated with absence of AR. Immunohistochemical analysis of AR in biopsies from virtually every stage and grade of prostate cancer show that AR is retained regardless of hormone sensitivity. Only in some of the androgen-independent human prostate cancer cell lines, such as DU145 and PC3 cells, is there lack of detectable or functional AR. Because loss of AR expression is not normally associated with the malignant phenotype, attention has focused on more subtle mutational events in the AR gene that could give rise to alterations in AR activity.

There have been several reports of an increased risk of prostate cancer in men with a decrease in the number of polymorphic CAG nucleotide repeats, which encode the polyglutamine tracts found in the N-terminal domain of the AR protein, although other studies have failed to confirm this relationship. Furthermore, the mean lengths of polymorphic CAG repeats (as well as exons encoding other sequences in the AR) are similar in prostate tumors to those found in the normal population (Wallen et al., 1999). Paradoxically, there is one report that shorter CAG repeats in the AR gene found in breast cancer tissue are associated with more aggressive forms of the disease (Yu et al., 2000).

Estimates of the incidence of somatic point mutations in the AR gene range from 0 to 30 percent of patients with recurrent, hormone-refractory disease and there is a tendency for the incidence of AR mutations to occur more frequently in advanced or metastatic disease. Also, patients treated with anti-androgens are more likely to have AR mutations as compared to patients treated solely by surgical castration or LHRH agonists (Taplin et al., 1999). While few AR mutations have been functionally characterized, the mutation of threonine to alanine in the AR ligand binding domain of the LNCaP human prostate cancer cell line has been shown to alter androgen binding specificity such that it can be activated by high concentrations of virtually any steroid or anti-androgen (Culig et al., 1998). Similar types of mutations have been observed in some patients who manifest the anti-androgen withdrawal syndrome (Culig et al., 1998).

Amplification and overexpression of the wild-type *AR* gene is more common than mutation. Studies before and after androgen ablation have shown gene amplification of wild-type *AR* in about 30 percent of recurrent tumors. In *AR* gene-amplified tumors, PSA immunostaining appears to be about twice as high as in tumors with no amplification, indicating that *AR* gene amplification leads to upregulation of the *PSA* gene (and possibly other androgen-regulated genes). Thus, patients with *AR* gene amplification may have elevated serum PSA concentrations without a clear correlation with tumor burden (Koivisto and Helin, 1999).

A substantial proportion of ER$^+$ breast tumors are either de novo resistant to endocrine therapy or acquire resistance after treatment with endocrine therapies despite the continued expression of ER. The presence of *ER* mutations and/or amplifications in breast cancer is quite rare, but variant ERs generated by alternative RNA splicing of both *ER-α* and *ER-β* are common. Changes in expression of these variants have been documented in breast tumors, but no direct correlation with tamoxifen resistance has been reported.

## 19.5.5 Altered Receptor Structure and Function, Including Altered Coregulator Activity

The two ERs (α and β), although sharing some similarities structurally and functionally (Fig. 19.5), respond differentially to tamoxifen and other SERMs in a gene promoter specific fashion (Paech et al., 1997). Although the two ERs can be expressed separately in some target tissues, often they are co-expressed; therefore altered expression of ER-β or altered relative expression of the two ERs might change target-cell responsiveness to anti-estrogen, or even change responses from anti-estrogenic to estrogenic. Altered relative expression of the two ERs has been described in human breast cancer, which could underlie altered estrogen and anti-estrogen action (Leygue et al., 1998).

The ability to recruit coactivators and/or corepressors to a promoter plays an important role in transcriptional regulation by a steroid hormone (Fig. 19.4). Experimental alteration of the relative expression of coactivator to corepressor suggests that such a mechanism can influence how a target cell interprets tamoxifen, either as an anti-estrogen or an estrogen (McKenna and O'Malley, 1999). Alterations of specific coactivators and corepressors of ER have been described in human breast tumors, although correlations with resistance to tamoxifen have been documented only in an experimental model (Clarke et al., 2001).

Much attention has been given to the interaction between AR and coregulator proteins (Fig. 19.4), but there is little information linking altered activity or expression of coregulators with prostate cancer development or progression. Coactivators originally thought to be AR specific and candidates for modulators of AR activity in prostate cancers, such as ELE1/ARA70, have been shown subsequently to be weak coactivators with broad receptor specificity. However, a majority of recurrent prostate cancers express high levels of two coactivators, SRC-1 and TIF2 (Gregory et al., 2001). Over-expression of these coactivators might increase AR transactivation and thereby lower the ligand threshold such that physiological concentrations of adrenal androgens are adequate to drive androgen regulated responses, such as PSA expression.

### 19.5.6 Upregulation of Cell Survival Genes

The inappropriate upregulation of cell survival genes (see Chap. 10) is another potential mechanism whereby cancer cells become hormone refractory. Elevated expression of the anti-apoptotic gene bcl-2 is found in virtually all hormone refractory prostate cancers and overexpression confers resistance to androgen withdrawal by blocking the normal apoptotic signals (McDonnell et al., 1997). Another anti-apoptotic protein is clusterin (also known as TRPM-2 or SGP-2), which is upregulated during disease progression in prostate cancer leading to hormone resistance (Steinberg et al., 1997).

The bcl-2 family of genes has been implicated in progression of breast cancer and *BCL-2* is an estrogen inducible gene in ER$^+$ breast cancer cell lines. Other survival pathways, such as the AKT (protein kinase B) pathway, may also be important in progression of human breast cancer. As described above, AKT is activated by ligand-bound EGFR and IGFR, and can phosphorylate ER-$\alpha$ and activate it in a ligand-independent fashion. Furthermore, overexpression of AKT in breast cancer cell lines leads to upregulation of *BCL-2* and protects breast cancer cells from tamoxifen-induced apoptosis (Campbell et al., 2001). There appears to be a positive feedback loop involved in this pathway, whereby ER-$\alpha$ in the presence or absence of estrogen can activate the regulatory subunit of PI-3K, which in turn activates AKT.

Tumor suppressor genes, such as *Rb* and *p53*, are inactivated in many tumor types, including breast and the late stages of prostate cancer. E-cadherin and other cell adhesion genes, which have been characterized as suppressors of the metastatic phenotype (see Chap. 11, Sec. 11.5), are frequently inactivated or downregulated during progression to advanced prostate cancer and have been associated with poor clinical outcome (Bussemakers,1999).

The critical genetic events associated with progression of breast and prostate cancer are still poorly understood, but owing to the development of approaches like gene microarrays (see Chap. 4, Sec. 4.4.4), candidate genes are being discovered at an increasing rate. The current view is that the most likely mechanisms for progression of breast and prostate cancer involve ligand-independent activation of AR or ER via crosstalk with other transcription factors, signal transducers, and related pathways.

## 19.6 NEW APPROACHES TO THE APPLICATION OF HORMONAL THERAPIES

### 19.6.1 Breast Cancer

Proof of principle for the use of SERMs in breast cancer prevention and treatment has already been established, and newer SERMs are in clinical trials to establish their efficacy. An ideal SERM would have beneficial estrogen effects on bone and other tissues, but would be an anti-estrogen for the breast, uterus, and clotting system. Although the perfect SERM may not be achievable, the flexibility of tailoring treatment to an individual woman and avoiding the most important side effects for that individual has obvious advantages. Also, the efficacy of various combinations of SERMs (or SERDs) with either aromatase inhibitors or LHRH agonists is under investigation.

The fact that acquired tamoxifen resistance occurs in most cases without loss of ER expression suggests that the tumors may still require ER-dependent pathways for growth. Furthermore, tamoxifen-resistant human breast cancer is not always cross-resistant to steroidal anti-estrogens, such as fluvestrant, and these agents are being evaluated in acquired tamoxifen-resistant breast cancer. Fluvestrant is an example of a SERD because, in addition to competing for estrogen binding to ER and preventing its dimerization, it also results in a rapid degradation of the receptor protein.

The observation that different classes of ligands, when bound to the ER, result in different conformational structures that dictate differential cellular responses to SERMs, due to differential recruitment of coregulators, has led to two different approaches to therapy (Fig. 19.11). First, the use of different SERMs, such as raloxifene (Fig. 19.10), LY 353381, EM652, and GW5638, as new anti-estrogens in the treatment of tamoxifen-resistant breast cancer. Second, by using the ER ligand-binding domain bound with different ligands, peptides have been identified which interact exclusively with either the E-ER complex, or the Tam-ER complex. Such peptides, when expressed in appropriate target cells, will block the action of the appropriate ligand-bound ER complexes (Norris et al., 1999). These data suggest the possible use of designer peptides in the treatment of ER$^+$ breast cancer.

The use of agents that block specific kinases that can activate the ER in a ligand-independent fashion, either alone or with agents that inhibit growth factor receptor activation, may also be active in hormone refractory ER$^+$ breast cancer.

While several of these approaches have been developed, based upon hypotheses for the molecular mechanisms underlying acquired resistance, early and sustained activation of some of the pathways discussed above may also be involved in de novo resistance. Therefore, some of these approaches might have a role in treating de novo resistance. Analysis of the molecular profiles of human breast tumors using specific markers for activated pathways may lead to more accurate means of predicting treatment response, and thus improve choice of the most appropriate treatment regimen.

### 19.6.2 Prostate Cancer

*Intermittent Hormonal Therapy for Prostate Cancer* In addition to acting as mitogens to induce DNA synthesis and cell proliferation, estrogens and androgens are potent differentiating agents. In studies with castrated rodents, administration of small amounts of androgen was shown to induce markers of differentiation in the prostate without stimulating rounds of cell proliferation. This conditioning effect of androgens on surviving cells allowed them to retain desirable, hormone-regulated traits of differentiation—and the capacity to undergo apoptosis upon hormone withdrawal. Hence, periodic exposure to hormones might maintain hormone responsiveness of prostate tumors. An idealized representation of how intermittent hormone suppression might regulate tumor growth and be used in combination with cytotoxic drugs is shown in Figure 19.15.

The effectiveness of intermittent androgen suppression and replacement for delaying progression to androgen independence was first shown using the androgen-dependent Shionogi mouse mammary carcinoma (Akakura et al., 1993). With this tumor model, com-

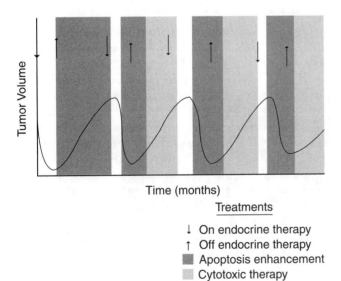

**Figure 19.15.** Theoretical overview of the repeated application of intermittent hormone suppression in combination with other nonendocrine therapies to control tumor volume. Optimal timing opportunities are indicated for treatments that enhance apoptosis (e.g., antisense knockout of cell survival genes such as *BCL-2*) or are cytotoxic to hormone-stimulated, proliferating cells (e.g., docetaxel).

plete remissions are observed after androgen withdrawal, but invariably the disease recurs and is refractory to further hormonal manipulations. This tumor consists mainly of differentiated cells, but a small number of stem cells, which are responsible for eventual regrowth, are initially androgen dependent but progress, presumably through an unknown adaptive mechanism, to an androgen-independent state. Because progression to androgen independence was linked to the cessation of androgen-induced differentiation of these stem cells, the effect of replacement of androgens at the end of a period of regression was tested by transplantation into noncastrated males (Akakura et al., 1993). This cycle of transplantation and castration-induced apoptosis was repeated four times before growth became androgen-independent during the fifth cycle. Relative to one-time castration, intermittent androgen suppression approximately tripled the time to androgen independence. Also, the proportion of total stem cells in the tumor was constant during the first three cycles but increased fifteen-fold between the third and fourth cycles. While the transplantation procedure itself may have slowed cell proliferation, there were no differences in tumor doubling times during successive cycles.

Analogous results were obtained using the LNCaP human prostate cancer tumor model to compare the effects of continuous versus intermittent androgen suppression (Sato et al., 1996). In this system, serum PSA levels were measured in tumor-bearing athymic mice that were castrated and then subjected to cycles of implantation or removal of a testosterone pellet. It was found that intermittent androgen suppression could delay the onset of androgen-independent PSA gene regulation approximately three-fold longer than continuous androgen suppression. These animal models provided the proof of principle necessary for testing the intermittent protocol in patients with prostate cancer. An example of a 47-year-old patient treated for over 7 years with intermittent androgen suppression is shown in Figure 19.16.

Prospective phase II trials have evaluated intermittent hormonal therapy and have found no obvious negative impact on patient outcomes. There is reduced treatment-related toxicity and cost, and quality of life is improved when the patient is off therapy. Several randomized phase III trials comparing intermittent androgen suppression to continuous androgen withdrawal in men with metastatic or recurrent disease are ongoing.

*New Hormone-Biologic Therapies* There is interest in the development of hormonal therapies with fewer side effects, which might preserve a higher quality of life. Therapy with a single nonsteroidal anti-androgen like bicalutamide has been evaluated, and gives only a small decrement in survival as compared to use of orchiec-

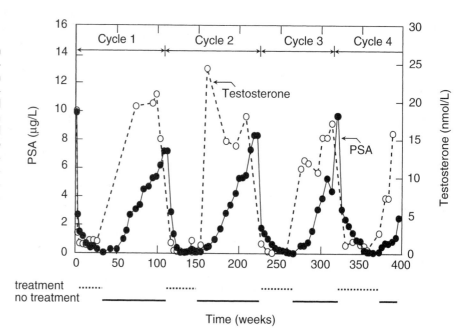

**Figure 19.16.** Intermittent androgen suppression. Approximately 8 years after radical prostatectomy and radiation treatment for positive surgical resection margins, the patient was started on a regimen of intermittent androgen suppression when his serum PSA had increased from a nadir of 0.6 $\mu$g/L to 10.4 $\mu$g/L. He was treated with a combination of anti-androgen (cyproterone acetate) and LHRH agonist (leuprolide acetate). The patient has undergone four cycles of androgen withdrawal and replacement over a period of >7 years. Open circles indicate serum testosterone values (nmol/L) and closed circles are serum levels of PSA ($\mu$g/L). (With permission from Dr. N. Bruchovsky.)

tomy or LHRH agonists. Because serum testosterone levels are not reduced with nonsteroidal anti-androgens, some of the usual side effects of androgen ablation are avoided, and men may retain potency.

Microarray analysis is demonstrating that many genes become upregulated during the early stages of progression of prostate cancer to androgen independence. It is likely that targeting those genes with an established role in cell survival (e.g., *TRPM-2, BCL-2, IGFBP-5,* etc.), will enhance apoptotic cell kill more than androgen withdrawal alone and also may delay time to recurrence and emergence of androgen independence. Several preclinical studies using androgen-regulated tumor models have demonstrated proof of principle that administration of antisense oligodeoxynucleotides is a viable approach to accomplishing this goal. For example, overexpression of bcl-2 frequently occurs in prostate carcinomas and is associated with resistance to both hormone therapy and chemotherapy. Treatment of LNCaP and Shionogi tumors with bcl-2 antisense oligodeoxynucleotides enhanced their chemosensitiv-ity to paclitaxel or mitoxantrone by at least ten-fold (Miyake et al., 2000). Furthermore, antisense treatments of androgen-dependent Shionogi tumors after castration resulted in more rapid regression and a significant delay in recurrence of androgen-independent tumors. Targeting cell survival genes in combination with androgen withdrawal and/or chemotherapy may enhance tumor cell kill.

*Hormone and Chemoprevention Strategies*  Epidemiological studies of prostate cancer suggest that diet and life style probably contribute more to prostate carcino-genesis than racial or familial factors. The observation that premalignant prostatic lesions (PIN) occur with almost equal frequency in different racial populations with both high or low risk of prostate cancer implies that a limiting step is progression from subclinical to locally invasive carcinoma. Also, there is considerable evidence that androgen stimulation over a long period of time is a necessary prerequisite for prostate cancer and therefore an obvious target in any chemoprevention strategy.

Clinical trials using tamoxifen as a chemopreventive agent for breast cancer in high-risk groups of women have provided a paradigm for using drugs that block androgen action and thereby prevent the emergence of prostate cancer. Two drugs that show promise are the anti-androgen bicalutamide and the 5$\alpha$-reductase inhibitor finasteride (Fig. 19.13), which blocks the intracellular metabolism of testosterone to the more potent DHT (Fig. 19.3). The toxicity of anti-androgens such as bicalutamide (gynecomastia, gastrointestinal toxicity, etc.) poses concerns for application in prevention studies, but the toxicity profile of finasteride is more favorable. An ongoing phase III trial of 18,000 men over 50 years of age has completed accrual and will evaluate whether a standard dose of finasteride (vs. placebo) will prevent the development of prostate cancer.

There are several, nonhormone related drugs and dietary supplements under investigation as chemopreventatives for prostate cancer. For example, vitamin D and vitamin A analogs, phenylbutyrate, polyamine inhibitors, and nonsteroidal anti-inflammatory agents (cyclooxygenase-2 inhibitors) are under evaluation as antiproliferative or differentiating agents for arresting the growth of prostate tumors. Epidemiological and laboratory studies also suggest that individuals with high selenium and vitamin E intake may have a lower risk of prostate cancer. This is the basis for a large selenium and vitamin E cancer prevention trial (SELECT).

## 19.7 SUMMARY

Breast and prostate cancer share many common epidemiological and biological features. While many factors contribute to their etiology, a Western-type diet appears to be a major factor associated with high incidence. Both prostate and breast cancer require long-term exposure to sex-steroid hormones in order to develop. A direct causal link to overstimulation with androgens and estrogens has been demonstrated in animal tumor models, and conversely, a protective effect has been observed from treatments that block the action of these hormones (e.g., prepubertal castration or administration of anti-hormonal drugs).

Estrogens and androgens share many features in their mechanism of action: both are synthesized from common precursors (e.g., cholesterol), both are carried mainly by the same protein in the blood (i.e., SHGB), and both bind to structurally related intracellular receptors. Both types of hormone-receptor complexes in turn bind to comparable regulatory DNA sequences in the promoters of genes and interact with similar sets of coregulator proteins to activate or repress gene expression.

About 70 percent of breast carcinomas are ER$^+$ and about 50 percent of these will respond to endocrine therapy, giving an overall response rate of ~35 to 40 percent. By comparison, most prostate cancers are AR$^+$ and most (>80%) respond to hormonal therapy. Therefore, ER assays are performed routinely and only ER$^+$ tumors are treated hormonally, whereas no receptor-based selection process is applied to prostate tumors. The treatment modalities used to kill hormone-dependent breast or prostate tumor cells are based on the same principles of either blocking the synthesis of the steroid hormone or blocking their activity in the target cell. Unfortunately, endocrine therapy for locally advanced or metastatic disease is not curative as the tumors progress from hormone dependence to hormone independence.

Potential mechanisms leading to hormone independence include ascendancy of alternative signal transduction pathways, receptor gene mutations or amplifications, ligand-independent receptor crosstalk with growth factors or kinases, and upregulation of cell survival genes. Whether the hormone-independent phenotype is due to the outgrowth of pre-existing clones with these genetic abnormalities or due to adaptive/epigenetic changes is unknown. This is important because abnormal adaptive responses may be reversible, whereas mutational events are more difficult to alter or correct.

There are no proven treatments to delay or prevent progression to hormone independence in either prostate or breast cancer. However, there are several ongoing prospective clinical trials to test the efficacy of intermittent androgen suppression on delay of progression and survival of patient with prostate cancer. Hormonal approaches to *primary* prevention are under study with anti-hormone agents such as tamoxifen or finasteride. Anti-hormone drugs with minimal side effects are likely to become an integral part of any chemoprevention strategy for people at high risk for either disease.

Increased understanding of steroid hormone action and improved drug design, together with the use of DNA and protein microarrays allow for the development of biomarkers for the prediction of treatment response and prognosis. The identification of these new targets for treatment and prevention of breast and prostate cancer are likely to lead to new treatment strategies to improve patient outcome.

## REFERENCES

Abreu-Martin MT, Chari A, Palladino AA, et al: Mitogen-activated protein kinase 1 activates androgen receptor-dependent transcription and apoptosis in prostate cancer. *Mol Cell Biol* 1999; 19:5143–5154.

Aebi S, Gelber S, Castiglione-Gertsch M, et al: Is chemotherapy alone adequate for young women with oestrogen receptor-positive breast cancer? *Lancet* 2000; 355:1869–1874.

Akakura K, Bruchovsky N, Goldenberg SL, et al: Effects of intermittent androgen suppression on androgen-dependent tumors. Apoptosis and serum prostate-specific antigen. *Cancer* 1993; 71:2782–2790.

Ali S, Coombes RC: Estrogen receptor alpha in human breast cancer: occurrence and significance. *J Mammary Gland Biol Neoplasia* 2000; 5:217–281.

Allred DC, Mohsin SK: Biological feastures of premalignant disease in the human breast. *J Mammary Gland Biol Neoplasia* 2000; 5:351–364.

Anderson E, Clarke RB, Howell A: Estrogen responsiveness and control of normal human breast proliferation. *J Mammary Gland Biol Neoplasia* 1998; 3:23–35.

Anzick SL, Kononen J, Walker RL, et al: AIB1, a steroid receptor coactivator amplified in breast and ovarian cancer. *Science* 1997; 277:965–968.

Baum M, Buzdar AU, Cuzick J et al: Anastrazole alone or in combination with tamoxifen versus tamoxifen alone for adjuvant treatment of postmenopausal women with early breast cancer: first results of the ATAC randomized trial. *Lancet* 2002; 359:2131–2139.

Boyd NF, Martin LJ, Stone J, et al: Mammographic densities as a marker of human breast cancer risk and their use in chemoprevention. *Curr Oncol Rep* 2001; 3:314–321.

Bruchovsky N, Rennie PS, Batzold FH, et al: Kinetic parameters of 5 alpha-reductase activity in stroma and epithelium of normal, hyperplastic, and carcinomatous human prostates. *J Clin Endocrinol Metab* 1988; 67:806–816.

Bussemakers MJ: Changes in gene expression and targets for therapy. *Eur Urol* 1999; 35:408–412.

Byrne C, Colditz GA, Willett WC, et al: Plasma insulin-like growth factor (IGF) I, IGF-binding protein 3, and mammographic density. *Cancer Res* 2000; 60:3744–3748.

Campbell RA, Bhat-Nakshatri P, Patel NM, et al: Phosphatidylinositol 3-kinase/AKT mediated activation of estrogen receptor alpha: a new model for anti-estrogen resistance. *J Biol Chem* 2001; 276:9817–9824.

Chen T, Wang LH, Farrar WL: Interleukin 6 activates androgen receptor-mediated gene expression through a signal transducer and activator of transcription 3-dependent pathway in LNCaP prostate cancer cells. *Cancer Res* 2000; 60:2132–2135.

Clarke R, Leonessa F, Welch J, Shaar T: Cellular and molecular pharmacology of anti-estrogen action and resistance. *Pharmacol Rev* 2001; 53:25–71.

Clarke RB, Howell A, Potten CS, et al: Dissociation between steroid receptor expression and cell proliferation in the human breast. *Cancer Res* 1997; 57:4987–4991.

Couse JF, Korach KS: Estrogen receptor null mice: what have we learned and where will they lead us? *Endocr Rev* 1999; 20:358–417.

Culig Z, Hobisch A, Hittmair A, et al: Expression, structure, and function of androgen receptor in advanced prostatic carcinoma. *Prostate* 1998; 35:63–70.

Dalu A, Haskell JF, Coward L, et al: Genistein, a component of soy, inhibits the expression of the EGF and ErbB2/Neu receptors in the rat dorsolateral prostate. *Prostate* 1998; 37:36–43.

Delage-Mourroux R, Martini PG, Choi I, et al: Analysis of estrogen receptor interaction with a repressor of estrogen receptor activity (REA) and the regulation of estrogen receptor transcriptional activity by REA. *J Biol Chem* 2000; 275:35848–35856.

Denis L, Morton MS, Griffiths K: Diet and its preventive role in prostatic disease. *Eur Urol* 1999; 35:377–387.

Font de Mora J, Brown M: AIB1 is a conduit for kinase-mediated growth factor signaling to the estrogen receptor. *Mol Cell Biol* 2000; 20:5041–5047.

Gallagher RP, Fleshner N: Prostate cancer: 3. Individual risk factors. *CMAJ* 1998; 159:807–813.

Giguere Y, Dewailly E, Brisson J, et al: Short polyglutamine tracts in the androgen receptor are protective against breast cancer in the general population. *Cancer Res* 2001; 61:5869–5874.

Gingrich JR, Barrios RJ, Kattan MW, et al: Androgen-independent prostate cancer progression in the TRAMP model. *Cancer Res* 1997; 57:4687–4691.

Giovannucci E, Stampfer MJ, Krithivas K, et al: The CAG repeat within the androgen receptor gene and its relationship to prostate cancer. *Proc Natl Acad Sci USA* 1997; 94:3320–3323.

Glass CK: Differential recognition of target genes by nuclear receptor monomers, dimers, and heterodimers. *Endocr Rev* 1994; 15:391–407.

Gobbi H, Dupont WD, Simpson JF, et al: Transforming growth factor-$\beta$ and breast cancer risk in women with mammary epithelial hyperplasia. *J Natl Cancer Inst* 1999; 91:2096–2101.

Gong G, DeVries S, Chew K, et al: Genetic changes in paired atypical and usual ductal hyperplasia of the breast by comparative genomic hybridization. *Clin Cancer Res* 2001; 7:2410–2414.

Goss PE, Ingle JN, Martino S, et al: A randomized trial of letrozole in postmenopausal women after five years of tamoxifen therapy for early-stage breast cancer. *N Engl J Med* 2003; 349:1793–1802.

Gregory CW, He B, Johnson RT, et al: A mechanism for androgen receptor-mediated prostate cancer recurrence after androgen deprivation therapy. *Cancer Res* 2001; 61:4315–4319.

Hankinson SE, Willett WC, Colditz GA, et al: Circulating concentrations of insulin-like growth factor-I and risk of breast cancer. *Lancet* 1998; 351:1393–1396.

Harper ME, Glynne-Jones E, Goddard L, et al: Expression of androgen receptor and growth factors in premalignant lesions of the prostate. *J Pathol* 1998; 186:169–177.

Harvey JM, Clark GM, Osborne CK, et al: Estrogen receptor status by immunohistochemistry is superior to the ligand-binding assays for predicting response to adjuvant therapy in breast cancer. *J Clin Oncol* 1999; 17:1474–1485.

Hulka BS, Edison LT, Lininger RA: Steroid hormones and risk of breast cancer. *Cancer* 1994; 74:1111–1124.

Kelce WR, Gray LE, Wilson EM: Antiandrogens as environmental endocrine disruptors. *Reprod Fertil Dev* 1998; 10:105–111.

Kelly M, Levin E: Rapid actions of plasma membrane estrogen receptors. *Trends Endocrinol Metab* 2001; 12:152–156.

Khan S, Rogers M, Khurana K, et al: Estrogen receptor expression in benign epithelium and breast cancer risk. *J Natl Cancer Inst* 1998; 90:37–42.

Klinge CM: Estrogen receptor binding to estrogen response elements slows ligand dissociation and synergistically activates reporter gene expression. *Mol Cell Endocrinol* 1999; 150:99–111.

Koivisto PA, Helin HJ: Androgen receptor gene amplification increases tissue PSA protein expression in hormone-refractory prostate carcinoma. *J Pathol* 1999; 189:219–223.

Korach KS: Insights from the study of animals lacking functional estrogen receptor. *Science* 1994; 266:1524–1527.

Kousteni S, Bellido T, Plotkin L, et al: Non genomic, sex-nonspecific signaling through the estrogen or androgen receptors: dissociation from transcriptional activity. *Cell* 2001; 104:719–730.

La Spada AR, Wilson EM, Lubahn DB, et al: Androgen receptor gene mutations in X-linked spinal and bulbar muscular atrophy. *Nature* 1991; 352:77–79.

Leav I, McNeal JE, Ziar J, et al: The localization of transforming growth factor alpha and epidermal growth factor receptor in stromal and epithelial compartments of developing human prostate and hyperplastic, dysplastic, and carcinomatous lesions. *Hum Pathol* 1998; 29:668–675.

Leo C, Chen JD: The SRC family of nuclear receptor coactivators. *Gene* 2000; 245:1–11.

Leygue E, Dotzlaw H, Watson PH, et al: Altered estrogen receptor alpha and beta mRNA expression during human breast tumorigenesis. *Cancer Res* 1998; 58:3197–3201.

Lopez GN, Turck CW, Schaufele F, et al: Growth factors signal to steroid receptors through mitogen-activated protein kinase regulation of p160 coactivator activity. *J Biol Chem* 2001; 276:22177–22178.

McDonnell TJ, Navone NM, Troncoso P, et al: Expression of bcl-2 oncoprotein and p53 protein accumulation in bone marrow metastases of androgen independent prostate cancer. *J Urol* 1997; 157:569–574.

McKenna NJ, Lanz RB, O'Malley BW: Nuclear receptor coregulators: cellular and molecular biology. *Endocr Rev* 1999; 20:321–344.

McKenna NJ, O'Malley BW: An issue of tissues: divining the split personalities of selective estrogen receptor modulators. *Nat Med* 2000; 6:960–962.

Miettinen M, Isomaa V, Peltoketo H, et al: Estrogen metabolism as a regulator of estrogen action in the mammary gland. *J Mammary Gland Biol Neoplasia* 2000; 5:259–270.

Miyake H, Tolcher A, Gleave ME: Chemosensitization and delayed androgen-independent recurrence of prostate cancer with the use of antisense bcl-2 oligodeoxynucleotides. *J Natl Cancer Inst* 2000; 92:34–41.

Montano MM, Ekena K, Delage-Mourroux R, et al: An estrogen receptor-selective coregulator that potentiates the effectiveness of anti-estrogens and represses the activity of estrogens. *Proc Natl Acad Sci USA* 1999; 96:6947–6952.

Murphy LC, Dotzlaw H, Leygue E, et al: The pathophysiological role of estrogen receptor variants in human breast cancer. *J Steroid Biochem Mol Biol* 1998; 65:175–180.

Murphy LC, Simon SL, Parkes A, et al: Altered expression of estrogen receptor coregulators during human breast tumorigenesis. *Cancer Res* 2000; 60:6266–6271.

Nadal A, Ropero A, Laribi O, et al: Nongenomic actions of estrogens and xenoestrogens by binding at a plasma membrane receptor unrelated to estrogen receptor α and estrogen receptor β. *Proc Natl Acad Sci USA* 2000; 97:11603–11608.

Nelson CC, Hendy SC, Shukin RJ, et al: Determinants of DNA sequence specificity of the androgen, progesterone, and glucocorticoid receptors: evidence for differential steroid receptor response elements. *Mol Endocrinol* 1999; 13:2090–2107.

Noble RL: Production of Nb rat carcinoma of the dorsal prostate and response of estrogen-dependent transplants to sex hormones and tamoxifen. *Cancer Res* 1980; 40:3547–3550.

Norris J, Paige L, Christensen D, et al: Peptide antagonists of the human estrogen receptor. *Science* 1999; 285: 744–746.

Norris JD, Fan D, Kerner SA, et al: Identification of a third autonomous activation domain within the human estrogen receptor. *Mol Endocrinol* 1997; 11:747–754.

O'Regan R, Jordan VC: Tamoxifen to raloxifene and beyond. *Semin Oncol* 2001; 28:260–273.

Osborne CK, Bardou V, Hopp TA, et al: Role of the estrogen receptor coactivator AIB1 (SRC-3) and HER-2/neu in tamoxifen resistance in breast cancer. *J Natl Cancer Inst* 2003; 95:353–361.

Paech K, Webb P, Kuiper GG et al: Differential ligand activation of estrogen receptors ERalpha and ERbeta at AP1 sites. *Science* 1997;277: 1508–1510.

Page Dl, Jensen RA, Simpson J, et al: Historical and epidemiological background of human premalignant breast disease. *J Mammary Gland Biol Neoplasia* 2000; 5:341–349.

Perou CM, Jeffrey SS, van de Rijn M, et al: Distinctive gene expression patterns in human mammary epithelial cells and breast cancers. *Proc Natl Acad Sci USA* 1999; 96:9212–9217.

Prostate Cancer Trialists' Collaborative Group: Maximum androgen blockade in advanced prostate cancer: an overview of the randomised trials. *Lancet* 2000; 355:1491–1498.

Rennie PS, Bruchovsky N, Leco KJ, et al: Characterization of two cis-acting DNA elements involved in the androgen regulation of the probasin gene. *Mol Endocrinol* 1993; 7:23–36.

Rennie PS, Nelson CC: Epigenetic mechanisms for progression of prostate cancer. *Cancer Metastasis Rev* 1999; 17: 401–409.

Rhodes A, Jasani B, Balaton AJ, et al: Immunohistochemical demonstration of oestrogen and progesterone receptors: correlation of standards achieved on in house tumours with that achieved on external quality assessment material in over 150 laboratories from 26 countries. *J Clin Pathol* 2000; 53:292–301.

Robertson JF: Oestrogen receptor: a stable phenotype in breast cancer. *Br J Cancer* 1996; 73:5–12.

Roger P, Sahla ME, Makela S, et al: Decreased expression of estrogen receptor beta protein in proliferative preinvasive mammary tumors. *Cancer Res* 2001; 61:2537–2541.

Rosner W, Hryb DJ, Khan MS, et al: Sex hormone-binding globulin mediates steroid hormone signal transduction at the plasma membrane. *J Steroid Biochem Mol Biol* 1999; 69:481–485.

Sakr WA, Partin AW: Histological markers of risk and the role of high-grade prostatic intraepithelial neoplasia. *Urology* 2001; 57(Suppl 1):115–120.

Sasano H, Harada N: Intratumoral aromatase in human breast, endometrial and ovarian malignancies. *Endocr Rev* 1998; 19:593–607.

Sato N, Gleave ME, Bruchovsky N, et al: Intermittent androgen suppression delays progression to androgen-independent regulation of prostate-specific antigen gene in the LNCaP prostate tumour model. *J Steroid Biochem Mol Biol* 1996; 58:139–146.

Schiff R, Reddy P, Ahotupa M, et al: Oxidative stress and AP-1 in tamoxifen resistant breast tumors *in vivo*. *J Natl Cancer Inst* 2000; 92:1926–1934.

Shang Y, Hu X, DiRenzo J, et al: Cofactor dynamics and sufficiency in estrogen receptor-regulated transcription. *Cell* 2000; 103:843–852.

Shiau AK, Barstad D, Loria PM, et al: The structural basis of estrogen receptor/coactivator recognition and the antagonism of this interaction by tamoxifen. *Cell* 1998; 95:927–937.

Shoker B, Jarvis C, Sibson D, et al: Oestrogen receptor expression in the normal and pre-cancerous breast. *J Pathol* 1999; 188:237–244.

Simpson ER: Biology of aromatase in the mammary gland. *J Mammary Gland Biol Neoplasia* 2000; 5:251–258.

Steinberg J, Oyasu R, Lang S, et al: Intracellular levels of SGP-2 (Clusterin) correlate with tumor grade in prostate cancer. *Clin Cancer Res* 1997; 3:1707–1711.

Sun M, Paciga J, Feldman R, et al: Phosphatidyl-3–OH kinase (PI3K)/AKT2, activated in breast cancer, regulates and is induced by estrogen recepter alpha via interaction between ER alpha and PI3K. *Cancer Res* 2001; 61:5985–5991.

Taplin ME, Bubley GJ, Ko YJ, et al: Selection for androgen receptor mutations in prostate cancers treated with androgen antagonist. *Cancer Res* 1999; 59:2511–2515.

Thompson PA, Ambrosone C: Molecular epidemiology of genetic polymorphisms in estrogen metabolizing enzymes in human breast cancer. *J Natl Cancer Inst Monogr* 2000; 27: 125–134.

Truss M, Beato M: Steroid hormone receptors: interaction with deoxyribonucleic acid and transcription factors. *Endocr Rev* 1993; 14:459–479.

Tsai MJ, O'Malley BW: Molecular mechanisms of action of steroid/thyroid receptor superfamily members. *Annu Rev Biochem* 1994; 63:451–486.

Wallen MJ, Linja M, Kaartinen K, et al: Androgen receptor gene mutations in hormone-refractory prostate cancer. *J Pathol* 1999; 189:559–563.

Wang YZ, Wong YC: Sex hormone-induced prostatic carcinogenesis in the Noble rat: the role of insulin-like growth factor-I (IGF-I) and vascular endothelial growth factor (VEGF) in the development of prostate cancer. *Prostate* 1998; 35:165–177.

Wilson CM, McPhaul MJ: A and B forms of the androgen receptor are expressed in a variety of human tissues. *Mol Cell Endocrinol* 1996; 120:51–57.

Yee D, Lee AV: Crosstalk between the insulin-like growth factors and estrogens in breast cancer. *J Mammary Gland Biol Neoplasia* 2000; 5:107–115.

Yu H, Bharaj B, Vassilikos EJ, et al: Shorter CAG repeat length in the androgen receptor gene is associated with more aggressive forms of breast cancer. *Breast Cancer Res Treat* 2000; 59:153–161.

Zietman, AL: The case for neoadjuvant androgen suppression before radiation therapy. *Mol Urol.* 2000; 4:203–208; discussion 215.

# 20

# Cancer and the Immune System

*Nancy N. Berg-Brown, Linh T. Nguyen, and Pamela S. Ohashi*

## 20.1 INTRODUCTION

The immune system is a sophisticated network of cells that communicate and collaborate in order to recognize and mount an effective response against foreign pathogens, resulting in their eradication. *Antigens* are substances, usually foreign, that are specifically recognized by receptors on the cells of the immune system. *Adaptive immunity* is the antigen-specific host defense that is mounted following exposure to antigen involving lymphocytes and their products. Adaptive immunity is intertwined with *innate immunity*, which results from a collection of cells and factors that constitute the early host defense system.

A new immune response is induced upon encounter with each different foreign antigen as each immune response is extremely specific. Therefore, the immune system must be diverse in its capacity to recognize and respond to foreign substances. Importantly, the immune system has the ability to mount a rapid response upon subsequent exposure to the same antigen. This is called immunological memory and it protects the host from recurrent infections with the same pathogen. Therefore, the immune system has the remarkable properties of specificity, diversity, and memory.

Another feature of the immune system is its ability to respond to foreign antigen and to not respond to self-antigen. This is often referred to as *self/nonself-discrimination* or *self-tolerance*. This is essential because an immune response against self-antigen would result in tissue damage or autoimmunity. Immunological self-tolerance is achieved by a combination of *central tolerance*, which is learned during lymphocyte development in the thymus (Sec. 20.3.2), and *peripheral tolerance* (Sec. 20.3.3). The mechanisms that ensure protection against self-reactivity were traditionally believed to be an impediment against the immune system being able to eliminate tumors. However, recent data have demonstrated that the immune system can be directed against tumors.

## 20.2 BIOLOGY OF THE IMMUNE RESPONSE

### 20.2.1 Adaptive Immunity

The adaptive immune system is responsible for the induction of immunity and immunological memory upon exposure to foreign antigens. T and B lymphocytes, which are an integral part of the adaptive immune system, are responsible for the specificity and diversity that are defining features of the immune system. Lymphocytes have exquisite specificity for recognizing antigens. The antigen receptors on lymphocytes recognize small parts of proteins or peptides called *epitopes*. Each antigen receptor is specific for a particular epitope.

The immune system must be prepared to mount an immune response against the world of foreign antigens, therefore, the diversity of the lymphocyte receptors must be enormous. The receptors are present on the lymphocyte surface prior to exposure to antigen: the T-cell receptor (TCR) on T lymphocytes and the immunoglobulin molecule or B-cell receptor (BCR) on B lymphocytes. It is estimated that the lymphocyte repertoire collectively has specificity for at least $10^{15}$ different antigens. This immense diversity is generated through a mechanism of gene rearrangement during lymphocyte development (Sec. 20.2.4).

B and T lymphocyte activation is triggered by different forms of the antigen (Fig. 20.1). Intact protein interacting with membrane-bound immunoglobulin molecules (BCR) is the antigen-specific stimulus for B lymphocytes. The T-cell receptor (TCR) on T lymphocytes is triggered by interacting with a small peptide presented by self major histocompatibility complex (MHC) molecules on an antigen presenting cell (APC) or target cell.

Recognition of antigen initiates an immune response. Activated B lymphocytes proliferate and differentiate into plasma cells that secrete soluble immunoglobulin (antibody) molecules responsible for humoral (antibody-mediated) immunity. Activated T lymphocytes are responsible for cell-mediated immunity. One effector cell is the cytotoxic T lymphocyte (CTL) whose primary function is the lysis of target cells. Both humoral and cell-mediated immune responses are mounted in cooperation with T helper ($T_h$) lymphocytes. Strategies for immunotherapy of cancer are directed most often to the activation of CTLs, and the T lymphocytes are therefore the focus of this chapter.

### 20.2.2 The Major Histocompatibility Complex

The major histocompatibility complex (MHC) is a collection of genes within a continuous DNA region that encode many proteins including the MHC molecules. T lymphocytes recognize peptide antigens bound to

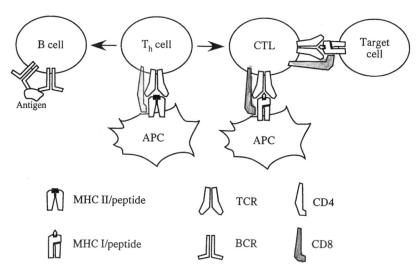

**Figure 20.1.** Antigen recognition by T and B lymphocytes. B cells are triggered by membrane-bound immunoglobulin molecules (B-cell receptor; BCR) interacting with intact protein antigen. The T-cell receptor (TCR) on T cells recognizes antigen in the form of a peptide presented by self major histocompatibility complex (MHC) molecules. The TCRs on T helper ($T_h$) cells, together with CD4, recognize peptide presented by MHC class II molecules on antigen presenting cells (APCs), whereas the TCRs on cytotoxic T lymphocytes (CTLs), together with CD8, recognize peptide presented by MHC class I molecules on APCs or target cells. $T_h$ cells cooperate with both B cells and CTLs in order to mount effective immune responses.

MHC molecules on the surface of antigen presenting cells (APCs) or target cells (Fig. 20.1).

The genes encoding the MHC molecules are grouped into three different classes. Class I MHC molecules are expressed on virtually all cells, whereas the expression of class II molecules is generally limited to APCs. Class I and II MHC molecules are transmembrane glycoproteins. Class III MHC proteins include components of the complement system and some cytokines such as tumor necrosis factor (TNF)-$\alpha$ and TNF-$\beta$.

In the mouse the MHC is referred to as the H-2 complex. It has three MHC class I proteins, H-2D, H-2K, and H-2L (referred to as D, K, and L), and two MHC class II proteins, I-A and I-E. The human MHC region is referred to as the HLA (human leukocyte antigen) complex and it consists of three MHC class I proteins, HLA-A, HLA-B, and HLA-C, and three MHC class II proteins, HLA-DQ, HLA-DR, and HLA-DP.

Major histocompatibility complex class I proteins are composed of a transmembrane heavy chain noncovalently associated with a light chain, $\beta_2$ microglobulin ($\beta_2$m). The heavy chain contains three domains: $\alpha$1, $\alpha$2, and $\alpha$3. The MHC class II proteins are composed of two transmembrane heavy chains ($\alpha$ and $\beta$), each containing two domains: $\alpha1/\alpha2$ and $\beta1/\beta2$ (Fig. 20.2).

Each of the loci within the MHC has several different alleles. Therefore, the MHC molecules exhibit allelic polymorphism within a population. These polymorphisms can be homozygous, but normally two different alleles are expressed from the two chromosomes of an individual.

The peptide-binding cleft is comprised of the membrane distal domains of the MHC molecules—$\alpha$1 and $\alpha$2 in class I and $\alpha$1 and $\beta$1 in class II. Its general structure is two $\alpha$-helices and a $\beta$-pleated sheet forming the sides and the floor of the cleft, respectively. The amino acid residues that form the peptide-binding cleft display the most polymorphism among the various MHC alleles.

Major histocompatibility complex class I molecules bind peptides of eight to eleven amino acids, whereas MHC class II molecules bind peptides of fifteen to eighteen amino acids (Bjorkman, 1997). Each MHC allele has the ability to bind to many different peptides. This is necessary to enable the limited number of MHC molecules to bind a large number of peptides.

The T-cell receptor (TCR) recognizes both the antigen bound to the peptide-binding cleft of the MHC molecule and the MHC molecule (Fig. 20.1). T cells recognize and respond to foreign antigen only when the antigen is presented in the context of a self MHC molecule. T cells from one individual recognize foreign antigen presented by self MHC molecules and not by other allelic variants of the MHC molecules.

Major histocompatibility complex class I and II molecules generally bind peptides by two different pathways, the endogenous and the exogenous, respectively (Fig. 20.3). Endogenous intracellular proteins are degraded by a multisubunit protease called the proteasome. Under normal, healthy conditions the endogenous proteins are self-proteins including housekeeping, metabolic, and misfolded proteins. During a viral infection, these proteins will include foreign viral proteins. The peptides, self-proteins, or foreign viral proteins are transported into the endoplasmic reticulum (ER) by the transporter associated with antigen processing (TAP). Major histocompatibility complex class I molecules are translocated into the ER as they are synthesized and associate with ER molecular chaperones to facilitate peptide binding. Following peptide binding, the MHC class I molecules are transported to the Golgi complex where they undergo glycosylation before being transported to the plasma membrane. Therefore, the endogenous pathway of antigen presentation displays a sampling of the intracellular contents of a cell to the immune system. When the MHC class I/peptide complex is detected as foreign, the cell will become a target for cytotoxic T lymphocyte (CTL)-mediated lysis (Pamer and Cresswell, 1998).

In the exogenous pathway, APCs take up extracellular proteins into endosomes by the process of endocytosis. The proteins are then degraded through a series of compartments with decreasing pH that contain various enzymes. The MHC class II molecules are synthesized in the ER, where they associate with a molecule known as the invariant chain (Fig. 20.3). Part of the invariant chain binds to the peptide-binding cleft. From

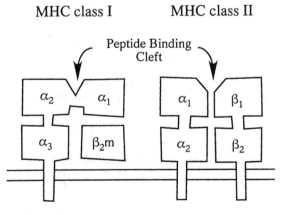

**Figure 20.2.** Basic structure of MHC class I and class II molecules. MHC class I molecules are composed of a transmembrane heavy chain ($\alpha$1, $\alpha$2, and $\alpha$3 domains) noncovalently associated with a light chain, $\beta_2$ microglobulin ($\beta_2$m). MHC class II molecules are composed of two transmembrane heavy chains each containing two domains: $\alpha1/\alpha2$ and $\beta1/\beta2$.

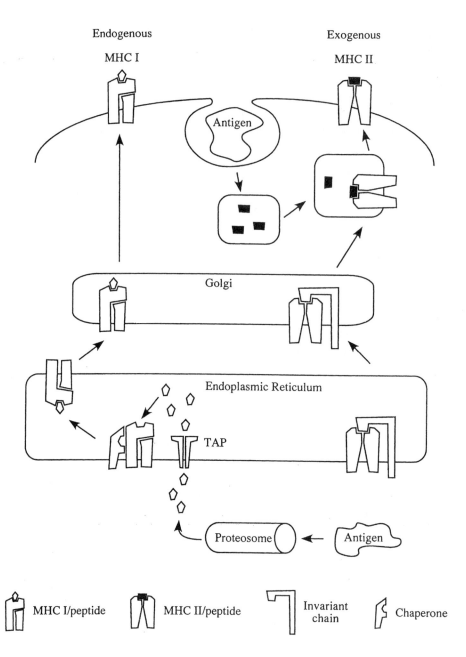

**Figure 20.3.** Antigen processing and presentation by MHC class I and class II molecules. Endogenous antigen is degraded by the cytosolic proteasome and the resulting peptides are transported into the endoplasmic reticulum (ER) by the transporter associated with antigen processing (TAP). MHC class I molecules are translocated into the ER and peptide binding occurs in the ER with the help of molecular chaperones. Following binding of peptide, the MHC class I molecules are transported to the cell surface via the Golgi. Exogenous antigen is endocytosed and degraded into peptides in a series of endocytic compartments. MHC class II molecules are synthesized in the ER and translocated to the endocytic compartment with the assistance of the invariant chain. Following the degradation of the invariant chain, MHC class II molecules bind peptide antigen and are transported to the plasma membrane.

the ER, the MHC class II molecules enter the Golgi complex for modification by glycosylation and then enter the endocytic compartment. Following degradation of the invariant chain (assisted by chaperone-like molecules), the MHC class II molecules bind peptide and are transported to the plasma membrane (Watts, 1997). When the MHC class II/peptide complex expressed by APCs is recognized as foreign by antigen-specific T$_h$ cells, an immune response will be initiated.

The association of endogenous antigen processing with MHC class I presentation and exogenous antigen processing with MHC class II presentation is not absolutely strict. A mechanism called *cross-presentation* occurs wherein extracellular soluble antigens can be presented by MHC class I molecules and this process is

critical for the initiation of cell-mediated immune responses and peripheral tolerance (Sec. 20.2.6).

### 20.2.3 T Lymphocytes

T cells are divided into two subsets with distinct effector functions. Cytotoxic T lymphocytes (CTLs) function primarily to eliminate virally infected cells and potentially play a role in the elimination of tumor cells. Cytotoxic T lymphocytes express the coreceptor CD8 and recognize peptide antigen presented by MHC class I molecules (Fig. 20.1). Following activation and conjugate formation with its target cell, the CTL secretes a pore-forming protein, perforin, into the junctional space between the two cells. Perforin polymerizes, forming polyperforin pores in the target cell membrane which facilitate the delivery of enzymes to the target cell. The enzymes activate an endogenous pathway in the target cell that results in DNA fragmentation and ultimately cell death (Kagi et al., 1996). For anti-tumor immunity, a CTL response is desired as most tumors express MHC class I molecules on their surface.

T helper cells express the coreceptor CD4 and recognize peptide antigen presented by MHC class II molecules (Fig. 20.1). T helper cells function primarily to regulate other cells of the immune system by secreting a range of cytokines. Cytokines are soluble mediators produced by hematopoietic cells that stimulate other hematopoietic cells. The cytokines act as growth factors for the proliferation and differentiation of antigen-triggered CD8$^+$ and CD4$^+$ T cells and B cells. The T$_h$ cells are further subdivided into three general categories based on their pattern of cytokine secretion. T$_h$1 cells secrete interleukin (IL)-2, interferon-$\gamma$ (IFN$\gamma$), and granulocyte macrophage colony-stimulating factor (GM-CSF). These cytokines are involved in the cell-mediated branch of the immune response. T$_h$2 cells secrete IL-4, IL-5, IL-10, IL-13, and GM-CSF and are involved in the activation of B cells and the humoral (antibody-mediated) arm of the immune response. T$_h$3 cells secrete predominantly transforming growth factor (TGF)-$\beta$ or IL-10 and are believed to assist in regulating immune responses (O'Garra and Arai, 2000). There are many examples where there is overlap in the cytokines secreted by these categories of T$_h$ cells.

### 20.2.4 T-cell Receptor and T-cell Recognition

Interactions between T cells and APCs or target cells involve the ligation of adhesion molecules on opposing cells. For example, intercellular adhesion molecule (ICAM)-1 binds its ligand, leukocyte function-associated antigen (LFA)-1, promoting cell-cell adhesion (Dustin and Chan, 2000). This cell-cell contact facilitates the engagement of the TCR with MHC/peptide complexes on APCs or target cells. The TCR signal, together with signals generated from several other receptor/ligand interactions, generate intracellular signaling cascades resulting in T-cell activation and effector function. These events are essential for the induction of an effective immune response.

The TCR is composed of either an $\alpha$ and a $\beta$ chain ($\alpha\beta$TCR) or a $\gamma$ and a $\delta$ chain ($\gamma\delta$TCR). Approximately $10^5$ TCRs are expressed at the T-cell membrane as transmembrane proteins. The two chains of the TCR are coupled by an interchain disulfide bond near the plasma membrane. TCRs with $\alpha\beta$ chains are on 90 to 95 percent of the T cells found in the blood, thymus, lymph nodes, and spleen, whereas T cells expressing the $\gamma\delta$TCR are scarce in the circulation and in lymphoid

organs, but are present in high numbers in the skin and intestinal epithelium. T cells expressing the $\alpha\beta$ TCR (TCR henceforth) are primarily responsible for the antigen-specific immune response.

Each TCR chain has two immunoglobulin domains that are formed by an intrachain disulfide bond followed by a transmembrane region and a very short cytoplasmic tail (5 to 12 amino acids; Fig. 20.4A). The membrane distal domain has tremendous sequence diversity and is termed the variable (V) domain, whereas the membrane proximal domain is conserved in its sequence and is termed the constant (C) domain. Between the V and C domains, the $\beta$ chain also has a diversity (D) and a joining (J) region while the $\alpha$ chain has a J region. These domains are encoded by corresponding gene segments that undergo rearrangement during lymphocyte development to generate the complete $\alpha$ and $\beta$ chains (Fig. 20.4B). The process of gene rearrangement is responsible for generating the enormous diversity in antigen specificity of the TCRs. Additional diversity is generated by mechanisms including addition and deletion of nucleotides during recombination, the combination of multiple genes for V-J or V-D-J joining, flexibility in joining the gene segments during rearrangement, and combinatorial association of $\alpha$ and $\beta$ chains.

The TCR has three hypervariable regions referred to as the *complementarity determining regions* (CDR). The CDRs are important for antigen recognition as they primarily contact the peptide antigen. For both the $\alpha$ and $\beta$ chain, CDR1 and 2 are encoded by the V gene and CDR3 occurs at the V-(D)-J junction (Bjorkman, 1997).

Within the membrane, the TCR is associated with a group of nonpolymorphic transmembrane proteins (Fig. 20.4A). They are the CD3$\delta$, CD3$\gamma$, CD3$\epsilon$, TCR$\zeta$, and TCR$\eta$ chains. These chains are paired in dimers of CD3$\delta\epsilon$, CD3$\gamma\epsilon$, and TCR$\zeta\zeta$ (including a minor population of TCR$\zeta\eta$ and together with the $\alpha\beta$ TCR comprise the TCR complex (Wange and Samelson, 1996). The intracellular tails of the CD3 and TCR$\zeta$ chains are considerably longer than the TCR $\alpha$ and $\beta$ chains and each chain has one or more regions referred to as the *immunoreceptor tyrosine-based activation motif* (ITAM). The ITAM regions contain tyrosine residues that play a critical role in signal transduction following the antigen-specific engagement of the TCR. Therefore, the CD3 and TCR$\zeta$ proteins function as the intracellular signaling component of the TCR complex (Samelson, 2002).

The TCR complex is also associated with the nonpolymorphic transmembrane proteins CD4 or CD8. CD4 and CD8 distinguish the two T-cell populations; CD4 is primarily expressed on T$_h$ lymphocytes, whereas CD8 is primarily expressed on CTLs (Fig. 20.1). T-cell receptor recognition of antigen on an APC or target cell is facilitated by CD4 or CD8 binding to the membrane

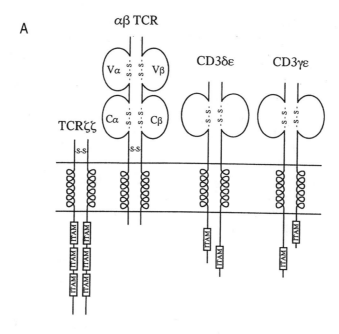

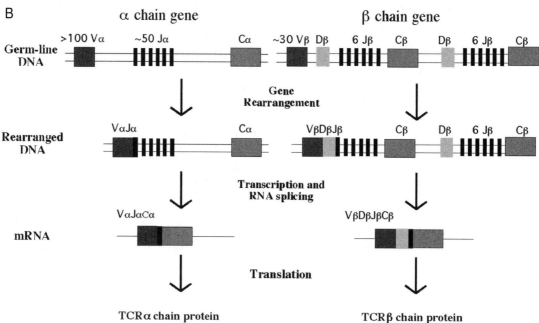

**Figure 20.4.** The T-cell receptor (TCR). (*A*) The TCR is composed of two chains, α and β, each containing two immunoglobulin domains formed by an intrachain disulfide bond. The TCR is associated with the dimeric proteins CD3δε, CD3γε, and TCRζζ and, together with the αβTCR, they comprise the TCR complex. ITAM, immunoreceptor tyrosine-based activation motifs. (*B*) The variable (V), diversity (D), joining (J), and constant (C) domains of the TCR are encoded by corresponding gene segments that undergo somatic rearrangement to generate the αβTCR heterodimer. In the mouse, the α chain consists of over 100 V, approximately 50 J and 1 C gene segments. The β chain consists of approximately thirty V regions and two clusters each of one D, six J, and one C gene segments. Following V(D)J gene rearrangement and transcription, the RNA is spliced to the C gene segment. The resulting mRNA encodes the TCR chains that dimerize to form the complete TCR protein.

proximal region of the same MHC molecule that is interacting with the TCR. CD4 binds the β2 region of MHC class II molecules and CD8 binds the α3 region of MHC class I molecules. CD4 and CD8 are referred to as *coreceptors* as they function to increase the overall avidity of the interaction between the T cell and the APC or target cell and/or contribute to signaling following antigen recognition. The cytoplasmic tails of

CD4 and CD8 molecules associate with intracellular signal transduction molecules (Zamoyska, 1994).

### 20.2.5 Overview of the Immune Response

An immune response is mounted following a foreign assault such as a viral infection. The immune response directed toward tumor antigens will be addressed in Section 20.4. Initially following infection the antigen load accumulates (such as during viral replication) until sufficient antigen is present to trigger the antigen-specific lymphocytes. This requires the presentation of antigen by mature professional APCs (macrophages, dendritic cells, and activated B cells) resulting in activation of T and B cells. Some of the unique properties of *professional* APCs are their ability to capture and present antigens and the ability to express costimulatory molecules. Lymphocyte proliferation and expansion gives rise to a clonal population from the single activated cell. This selective expansion is critical for host defense. A foreign entity such as a virus will contain several different antigenic peptides recognized by several antigen-specific lymphocytes. The immune response that ensues will consist of a cohort of expanded clonal populations.

Activated lymphocytes differentiate into *effector* and *memory* cells. Effector cells execute the immune function. For example, activated B cells produce antibodies and CTLs eliminate target cells such as virally infected or tumor cells. During the effector phase of the immune response the antigen is cleared, thus eliminating the source of lymphocyte activation. At this stage, a large number of effector cells are no longer required and many lymphocytes die by *programmed cell death* (see Chap. 10). This is a highly regulated process in which the cell plays an active role in bringing about its own death. As a result of an immune response, long-lived cells responsible for immunological memory are generated such that upon subsequent exposure to the same antigen a rapid immune response is mounted. The mechanism by which some lymphocytes develop into memory cells and survive for long periods of time in the periphery is unknown.

### 20.2.6 Overview of Lymphocyte Activation

The initiation of lymphocyte activation and an immune response is spatially quite challenging. Antigens from infected cells and tumor-associated antigens can be found essentially anywhere in the body, whereas T lymphocytes are found primarily in the secondary lymphoid tissues (spleen and lymph nodes) and in the circulation. T cells do not normally enter nonlymphoid tissue; however, they must locate and recognize antigen situated in these peripheral locations. In addition, the cells bearing the foreign antigen (such as virally infected cells or tumor cells) often cannot activate naive lymphocytes as they do not provide costimulatory signals. Lymphocyte activation in response to tumor growth is addressed in Section 20.5.

Antigen-presenting cells, in particular dendritic cells, overcome these geographical boundaries and are the cells that initiate an immune response. Dendritic cells (DCs) are a heterogeneous group of cells including Langerhans cells, interstitial DCs (heart, kidney, gut, lung), interdigitating DCs, follicular DCs, lymphoid tissue DCs, and veiled DCs. They do not express T cell, B cell, or natural killer (NK) cell markers, but they express MHC class I and II molecules important for activating T lymphocytes and for adhesion and costimulation of the immune response. Immature dendritic cells reside in most tissues where they are proficient at capturing and processing antigens from the peripheral tissues and forming MHC/peptide complexes. Stimuli, such as infectious agents, induce maturation and mobilization of dendritic cells. They continue to process antigen as they migrate to the lymphoid organs such as the spleen and lymph nodes. During the maturation process, they downregulate their antigen capture functions and upregulate the expression of MHC and costimulatory molecules. These attributes enable dendritic cells to interact with and activate naive T lymphocytes (Steinman et al., 2003). Dendritic cells attract T cells and B cells to the T-cell areas of the lymphoid organs, creating a microenvironment where lymphocyte activation and an immune response can be generated.

Effective activation of lymphocytes requires a molecular dialogue between a variety of receptors and ligands expressed by lymphocytes and dendritic cells. Adhesion molecules expressed by dendritic cells include ICAM-1 that binds its ligand LFA-1 on lymphocytes, thereby promoting cell adhesion. Dendritic cells upregulate B7-1 (CD80) and B7-2 (CD86), both of which bind to CD28, an important costimulatory molecule constitutively expressed on T cells (Caux et al., 1994; Lenschow et al., 1996). Another member of the immunoglobulin superfamily is ICOS (inducible costimulatory molecule). The ligand for ICOS is expressed on APCs and interacts with ICOS on activated and memory T cells (Hurwitz et al., 2000). CD40 is a member of the TNF receptor superfamily and is expressed on dendritic cells. It binds to its ligand that is expressed mainly by activated $T_h$ cells (Grewal and Flavell, 1998).

Naive $CD4^+$ T cells are triggered by MHC class II/peptide complexes expressed on dendritic cells following processing of exogenous proteins (Sec. 20.2.2; Fig. 20.5). Naive $CD8^+$ T cells are triggered by MHC class I/peptide complexes if the dendritic cell itself is infected followed by processing and presentation of the foreign endogenous protein. However when cells other than dendritic cells are infected, then the dendritic cell endocytoses and processes the exogenous antigen shed from the infected cell by the process of *crosspresentation*.

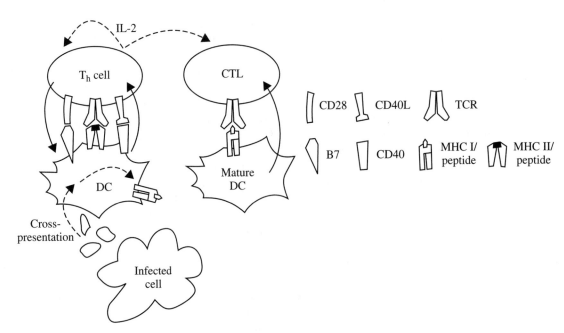

**Figure 20.5.** An overview of lymphocyte activation. Immature dendritic cells (DCs) acquire antigen, process it through various pathways and present peptide antigen to $T_h$ and CTLs in the context of MHC class II and I molecules, respectively. Receptor/ligand interactions between $T_h$ cells and dendritic cells lead to $T_h$ cell activation and DC maturation. Following activation, $T_h$ cells secrete various cytokines including IL-2 that serves as a growth factor for $T_h$ cells and CTLs.

The result is MHC-class I–restricted presentation of exogenous antigen (Carbone et al., 1998).

Antigen-triggered $T_h$ cells upregulate the expression of CD40 ligand (CD40L), which then interacts with CD40 on the dendritic cell (Fig. 20.5). CD40 ligation leads to the maturation of the dendritic cell resulting in the upregulation of costimulatory molecules and cytokine secretion (Steinman et al., 2003). Increased expression of the costimulatory molecule B7-1 provides a ligand for CD28 on the $T_h$ cells leading to complete $T_h$ cell activation. Stimuli such as infectious agents also induce dendritic cell maturation.

The maturation of dendritic cells as a result of CD40 ligation by $T_h$ cells enables the dendritic cell to efficiently activate naive CD8$^+$ T cells (Bennett et al., 1998; Ridge et al., 1998; Schoenberger et al., 1998). The interaction with functional mature dendritic cells facilitates naive CD8$^+$ T-cell activation as the dendritic cell can provide signals including TCR-specific and costimulatory signals. Following activation, CTLs carry out their effector function to achieve the clearance of antigen. Activated $T_h$ cells produce the cytokine IL-2 and express receptors for growth factors including IL-2 leading to autocrine growth. Interleukin-2 also promotes proliferation of CD8$^+$ T-cells.

The antigen-specific signal for B lymphocytes is delivered through its membrane immunoglobulin molecule interacting with an antigenic site of on intact protein. Subsequently, B cells can endocytose antigen, process it and present it on the cell surface complexed with MHC class II molecules (Sec. 20.2.2). The development of an effective antibody response also requires CD4$^+$ T-cell help in the form of costimulation. Current models suggest that costimulation is provided by the ligation of CD40 on B cells by CD40 ligand (CD40L) expressed on activated $T_h$ cells that are recognizing MHC class II/peptide complexes. The dendritic cell microenvironment facilitates B-cell activation both by activating $T_h$ cells and by secreting cytokines such as IL-12 which B cells require for antibody production (Banchereau and Steinman, 1998). Additional cytokines produced in the microenvironment facilitate the differentiation of immune effector cells.

In addition to dendritic cells, other antigen presenting cells such as macrophages and activated B cells can stimulate naive T cells; however, they are less potent. For example, dendritic cells have a 10- to 100-fold greater number of MHC/peptide complexes on their cell surface, they produce greater quantities of IL-12, and they express costimulatory molecules and adhesion receptors at higher levels (Guery and Adorini, 1995).

After activation, T and B cells leave the lymphoid tissue. T cells enter the blood and then exit the circulation and accumulate at the site of antigen deposition. In this manner, the T-cell response is limited to the site of infection or cancer growth.

## 20.3 TOLERANCE AND THE IMMUNE SYSTEM

### 20.3.1 T-cell Development

T cells develop and mature in the thymus from immature T cells called *thymocytes*. The stages of thymocyte development can be marked by the expression of the T-cell coreceptors, CD4 and CD8 (Fig. 20.6). Double negative (CD4⁻CD8⁻) thymocytes that do not express the TCR enter the thymus and undergo initial proliferation. They then express the TCRβ chain. Signals from the pre-TCR permit progression to the CD4⁺CD8⁺ (double positive) stage. Following rearrangement and the expression of the TCRα chain, the αβTCR complex on immature thymocytes can interact with thymic stromal cells expressing self MHC/self peptide complexes. Thymocytes that express a TCR that is capable of interacting weakly with self MHC molecules are chosen to differentiate and survive through a process called *positive selection*. Thymocytes that are positively selected by recognizing MHC class II/peptide complexes will downregulate CD8 to become CD4⁺ thymocytes, whereas thymocytes that recognize MHC class I/peptide complexes will downregulate CD4 and be positively selected to the CD8⁺ thymocyte subset. After further maturation, thymocytes leave the thymus and populate the periphery as naive resting T lymphocytes (Sebzda et al., 1999). Therefore, positive selection results in a mature peripheral T-cell population whose TCRs can interact with self MHC molecules.

Because random gene rearrangements occur to generate TCR diversity, the TCR repertoire expressed by immature thymocytes will have specificity for both self and foreign protein antigens. During maturation, thymocytes that express a TCR that is capable of interacting strongly with self MHC/self peptides complexes are eliminated by a process called *negative selection*. Negative selection eliminates thymocytes that express a TCR with high affinity for self MHC or self MHC complexed with self peptides. This is one stage where tolerance to self-antigens is established.

Therefore, the fate of the developing thymocyte is determined by TCR interactions. According to the *quantitative-avidity model* of thymocyte selection, it is the overall avidity of interaction between the T-cell receptors on immature thymocytes and MHC/peptide complexes on thymic stromal cells and the subsequent signaling that is important (Fig. 20.7). The avidity is determined by both the quantity and the affinity of the interaction. The model predicts that no interaction or a very low avidity interaction will lead to death-by-neglect for the thymocyte. An intermediate avidity interaction will lead to positive selection and thymocyte survival, whereas a high avidity interaction will lead to negative selection and thymocyte programmed cell death (Sebzda et al., 1999). The strength or duration of TCR triggering is somehow interpreted by the cell to determine the thymocyte fate (survival or deletion).

### 20.3.2 Central Tolerance

The first demonstration that clonal deletion of immature thymocytes contributes to the elimination of self-reactive thymocytes and therefore central tolerance was in 1987. The fate of a subset of T cells specific for a defined protein was followed using an antibody specific for the T-cell population. Cells that were specific for the defined protein were absent from the mature thymocyte and peripheral T-cell pools of mice expressing the defined protein. This indicated that they were deleted during development thereby contributing to central tolerance (Kappler et al., 1987). Many other studies have confirmed the elimination of self-reactive

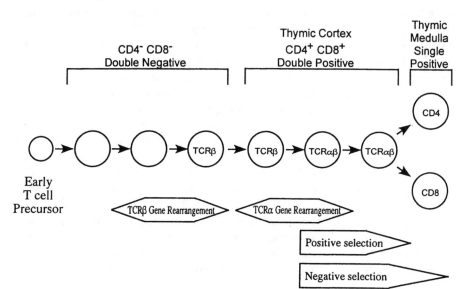

**Figure 20.6.** Basic stages of thymocyte development. The expression of cell surface markers (CD4 and CD8) and the T-cell receptor (TCR) chains are shown corresponding to the various stages of thymocyte development. In addition, the stage of development during which thymocyte selection occurs is shown.

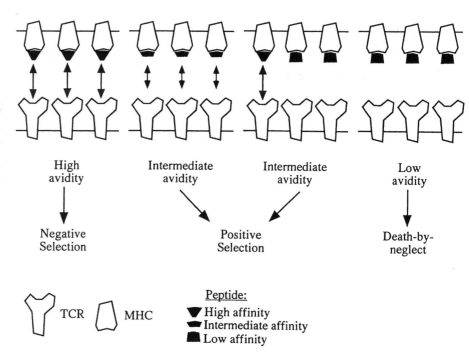

**Figure 20.7.** The affinity/avidity between thymocytes (lower row of four) and thymic stromal cells (upper row of four) determines the fate of immature thymocytes. The model predicts that no interaction or a very low avidity interaction leads to death-by-neglect. An intermediate avidity interaction leads to positive selection and thymocyte survival, whereas a high avidity interaction leads to negative selection and thymocyte death.

thymocytes during development (e.g., Kappler et al., 1988; Kisielow et al., 1988).

In addition to deletion of self-reactive thymocytes, clonal inactivation is also a mechanism of central tolerance. Induction of anergy or unresponsiveness in the thymus was first shown using bone marrow chimeric mice made by transferring bone marrow cells from one mouse (donor) into a second irradiated mouse (host). Radiation destroys the bone marrow cells of the host allowing the donor bone marrow to populate and develop in the host thymus. Using this experimental system it was shown that donor bone marrow that developed in the host thymus generated peripheral T cells that were tolerant to a defined self antigen expressed only on the stromal cells of the host thymus. The mature T cells, specific for this defined self-antigen, were present but were unresponsive. The expression of the self antigen thus induced anergy (Ramsdell et al., 1989). Therefore, both clonal deletion and clonal inactivation contribute to central tolerance.

### 20.3.3 Peripheral Tolerance

A few decades ago it was believed that under normal conditions all self-reactive lymphocytes were eliminated during development. However, it is now clear that the lymphocyte repertoire in a normal, healthy individual includes B and T lymphocytes specific for self antigens that escape tolerance mechanisms. Self-reactive thymocytes can escape thymic deletion as there are proteins expressed in peripheral tissues that will not be present

in the thymus during thymocyte selection. Moreover, some proteins are expressed in the thymus at a level that is insufficient for the deletion of all self-reactive lymphocytes. Consequently, central tolerance generated during development is imperfect. Several mechanisms exist to keep self-reactive mature lymphocytes in check in the periphery following development and this is collectively referred to as *peripheral tolerance*. Peripheral tolerance is defined as the induction and maintenance of unresponsiveness in mature T cells to self-antigens encountered in extrathymic compartments (Garza et al., 2000). Understanding the mechanisms of peripheral tolerance will greatly enhance the design of effective treatment strategies against autoimmune disease and cancer. The mechanisms of peripheral tolerance are summarized in Figure 20.8.

Two important immunological tools that facilitate the study of peripheral tolerance are monoclonal antibodies and transgenic mice. Because monoclonal antibodies recognize a single, specific epitope, they are ideally suited for following the localization, activation, and fate of a specific T-cell population in an experimental animal model. Transgenic mice that are designed to express a model self-antigen or to express a transgenic TCR are valuable model systems in which to study peripheral tolerance. Mice that express a transgenic tissue-specific antigen will bear the antigen as self. The transgenic TCR dictates that the majority of T cells in the mouse will have a defined antigenic specificity and therefore this makes it possible to observe antigen-specific or self antigen-specific T cells in vivo.

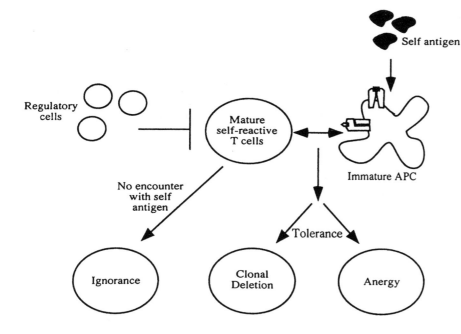

**Figure 20.8.** Mechanisms of peripheral tolerance. Mature self-reactive T cells that escape central tolerance populate the periphery. If these T cells encounter sufficient levels of self antigen in the periphery in the context of an immature antigen presenting cell (APC) then they will become tolerant through deletion or the induction of anergy. However, if the self-reactive T cells do not encounter or encounter insufficient levels of self antigen, then they remain ignorant or unaware of their self antigen. Regulatory T cells contribute to peripheral tolerance by regulating mature self-reactive T cells.

*Clonal Deletion of Mature T cells* A number of experimental systems have shown that mature T cells can be deleted upon encounter with tolerizing antigens. The first demonstration used a system of injecting a defined antigen into thymectomized mice that do not express the antigen. Therefore the T-cell repertoire of the host will include T cells that are reactive to the defined antigen. Tolerance to the antigen was induced in the host by the elimination of the reactive CD4$^+$ T cells. Prior to their deletion, there was a marked activation and expansion of the CD4$^+$ T cells. This study not only shows that self tolerance can be achieved by the elimination of mature T cells, but also that extrathymic clonal deletion and tolerance can result after the antigen-specific expansion of T cells (Webb et al., 1990).

Experimental models have also demonstrated deletion of self-reactive mature CD8$^+$ T cells. CD8$^+$ T cells specific for a defined antigen were adoptively transferred into transgenic mice expressing the same antigen specifically in the $\beta$ cells of the pancreas and the kidney (Fig. 20.9). Therefore, the transferred T cells were specific for the self antigen expressed in the pancreas and kidney. The antigen-specific T cells expressed activation markers and proliferated only in the pancreatic and kidney (draining lymph nodes). Bone marrow derived cells were required for this activation indicating that the tissue-specific self antigen is cross-presented by antigen presenting cells (Sec. 20.2.6). The adoptively transferred T cells were deleted from the peripheral pool following activation (Kurts et al., 1997). Therefore self antigens can be taken up by antigen presenting cells, processed, and presented in the context of MHC class I molecules. This can lead to the deletion of mature CD8$^+$ T lymphocytes and peripheral tolerance.

*Induction of Anergy* T-cell anergy is a mechanism of peripheral tolerance wherein self-reactive T cells are present, but are rendered inactive. A lymphocyte is called anergized when it is unresponsive to antigen stimulation under optimal conditions as measured by the lack of proliferation and IL-2 production.

Anergy was originally identified in vitro by a series of experiments by Schwartz and his collaborators (Mueller et al., 1989). Anergy, as a mechanism of peripheral tolerance, was first demonstrated in vivo by injecting cells expressing a defined antigen into mice that do not express the defined antigen. Initially the population of antigen-reactive CD4$^+$ T cells expands and then undergoes clonal deletion, as described above. However, there is a population of antigen-specific T cells that remain and these cells are anergic as indicated by their inability to respond to the defined antigen in a subsequent challenge (Rammensee et al., 1989). Generally, in response to a tolerogenic antigen, specific T cells expand, followed by deletion. The remaining antigen-specific cells are unresponsive to restimulation with antigen (Blackman et al., 1990).

*Ignorance* Clonal deletion and clonal anergy contribute to tolerance of T cells to self antigens in the periphery. However, some T cells simply remain ignorant or unaware of their self antigen. Immunological ignorance to extrathymic proteins was shown in a double

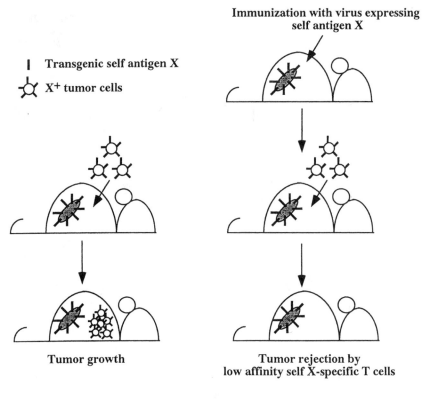

**Figure 20.9.** Low affinity T cells specific for tumor-associated antigen can be elicited in tumor bearing mice. Mice expressing a transgenic tissue-specific self antigen (X) were injected with tumor cells expressing the same antigen and progressive tumor growth occurred. Transgenic mice that were immunized with a recombinant virus expressing the self antigen prior to the injection of tumor cells were able to reject the tumor. In this model, functional low affinity cytotoxic T lymphocytes (CTLs) were stimulated and activated by the prior immunization and mediated the tumor rejection.

transgenic mouse that expressed (1) a viral glycoprotein in the pancreatic $\beta$ cells under the control of the rat insulin promoter (RIP) and (2) a TCR that was specific for the viral glycoprotein epitope (Fig. 20.10A). Despite having the self-antigen and the self-reactive T cells, there was no spontaneous immune response mounted against the pancreatic $\beta$ cells. However, virus-specific T cells isolated from the mice were functional, demonstrating that tolerance by neither deletion nor anergy occurred. Moreover, when the mice were infected with live virus, effector CTLs were generated and the mice developed severe infiltration of the pancreas with activated lymphocytes, hyperglycemia (increase in blood glucose levels), and diabetes due to the destruction of pancreatic islet cells (Ohashi et al., 1991; Oldstone et al., 1991). Therefore, the glycoprotein-specific T cells were neither actively deleted nor anergized, but were ignorant or unaware of their self antigen. This model demonstrates that not all tissue-specific antigens are seen by the immune system, either by direct tissue recognition or by efficient crosspresentation. Therefore, T cells specific for some tissue antigens remain in the functional mature T-cell repertoire. This must be considered during the development of strategies to boost anti-tumor immunity (Sec. 20.5.2).

*Regulation of Self-reactive T cells by Other Cells: Immunoregulation* The induction of regulatory T cells is a mechanism that maintains peripheral tolerance. In the early 1970s a population of lymphocytes was defined as suppressor cells by their ability to inhibit the function of other immune cells. Recently, there is a renewed interest in these cells as many models have rediscovered regulatory cell populations.

Collectively, experiments have shown that the depletion of T-cell subpopulations can render model animals more susceptible to spontaneous autoimmunity. This suggests that there is a population of regulatory T cells that plays a role in suppressing the activation of self-reactive T cells in the normal immune system, consequently contributing to peripheral tolerance. Different regulatory T-cell populations are still not definitively characterized. One population contains CD4[+] cells, which express additional cell surface markers including CD25 (IL-2 receptor $\alpha$ chain). However these markers are not specific to regulatory T cells as they are also expressed by other cell populations. The regulatory T cells develop in the thymus through a selection process. Controversial data suggest that they have TCRs that are specific for the same antigen as the cells they are regulating (Sakaguchi, 2000; Jordan et al., 2001).

Both the target cell and the mechanism by which regulatory T cells exert their immunosuppressive effect are unknown. Two mechanisms are considered possible. First, the suppression may be ascribed to the pattern of cytokines secreted by these regulatory T cells. The secretion of immunosuppressive cytokines will influence the generation of an immune response. Alternatively,

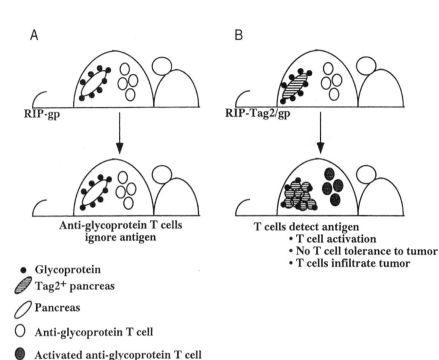

A
RIP-gp

Anti-glycoprotein T cells
ignore antigen

B
RIP-Tag2/gp

T cells detect antigen
• T cell activation
• No T cell tolerance to tumor
• T cells infiltrate tumor

● Glycoprotein
▨ Tag2⁺ pancreas
� Pancreas
○ Anti-glycoprotein T cell
◍ Activated anti-glycoprotein T cell

**Figure 20.10.** Tumor growth can lead to limited T-cell activation in the absence of tolerance. (*A*). T cells expressing a T-cell receptor (TCR) specific for a viral glycoprotein (gp) expressed in the β cells of the pancreas [rat insulin promoter (RIP-gp)] do not exhibit glycoprotein-specific T-cell activation. (*B*). Mice that express both the viral glycoprotein and the SV40 large-T antigen in the β cells of the pancreas (RIP-Tag2/gp) provide a model to monitor the specific T-cell response (anti-glycoprotein T cells) to a tumor-associated antigen (viral glycoprotein) in a naturally arising tumor (insulinoma). Tumor growth in the triple transgenic mice promoted the activation of the tumor-specific T cells in the absence of T-cell tolerance to tumor.

other systems have demonstrated a requirement for cell contact between the regulatory T cell and their target cell in the absence of immunosuppressive cytokines (Shevach, 2000). Depletion of regulatory T cells is a potential strategy in the design of immunotherapy to boost the anti-tumor immune response (Shimizu et al., 1999; Sec. 20.5.3).

### 20.3.4 Factors That Influence the Induction of Tolerance

There are several factors that influence the response of the immune system to a self-antigen in the thymus or the periphery. In the thymus, it is evident that a threshold exists where a low level of self-antigen expression is insufficient to induce central tolerance. Some T cells can escape negative selection if the expression of self-antigen is limiting (Oehen et al., 1994).

It appears that the density of self-peptides influences whether peripheral tolerance will be induced with high antigen expression levels leading to clonal deletion and low antigen expression levels leading to ignorance (Kurts et al., 1999; Morgan et al., 1999). Evidence suggests that the determining factor between peripheral tolerance and ignorance is the amount of cross-presented tissue-specific self-peptide that is available in the lymph nodes that drain a particular organ.

The accessibility of self-peptides to self-reactive lymphocytes will also influence the induction of tolerance. Proteins found in the circulation will be presented to T cells by APCs in the thymus and spleen and induce tolerance (Zal et al., 1994). Mature self-reactive T cells

specific for peripheral tissue peptides may not encounter their ligand as naive T cells do not usually circulate through nonlymphoid tissues. The result is self-reactive T cells that are not rendered tolerant, but instead remain ignorant of their self-peptides.

### 20.3.5 Induction of Tolerance Versus Immunity

The induction of tolerance requires a self-peptide-specific signal through the TCR. However, the induction of an immune response also involves an antigen-specific signal through the TCR. How does the T cell discriminate between a signal leading to tolerance and an activation signal? Bretscher and Cohn (1970) proposed a "two signal model of lymphocyte activation" in which recognition of one antigenic determinant leads to "paralysis," whereas recognition of two antigenic determinants leads to "induction" of B cells and antibody production. Later studies proposed that costimulatory signals, such as those mediated by a T cell specific molecule, CD28, were important for "signal 2" (Schwartz, 1992). This model has been updated and extended to encompass "costimulation" as a collection of signals that are required, in addition to an antigen-specific signal, for the induction of immunity.

More recently, it has been appreciated that dendritic cells are a focal point in the control of induction of tolerance versus immunity. As dendritic cells mature, they acquire the ability to communicate with lymphocytes in a manner that fosters the full activation of lymphocytes as well as migration and inflammation through a variety of cell surface costimulatory molecules and secreted cytokines and chemokines (Steinman et al., 2003). This includes the upregulation or induction of molecules such as B7-1 and CD40 (Fig. 20.5). Therefore, the current models speculate that when T cells interact with resting immature APCs expressing sufficient levels of a given antigen, T-cell tolerance will be induced by deletion or anergy. Whereas, when T cells interact with mature APCs expressing sufficient levels of a given antigen and costimulatory molecules, T-cell activation and induction of an efficient immune response will occur.

## 20.4 TUMOR IMMUNOLOGY

### 20.4.1 Innate Anti-tumor Response

The primary focus of this chapter is the *adaptive* immune response and its relationship to tumor immunity. However, the *innate* arm of the immune system may also be important for the defense against the initiation of tumor growth, and tumor cells can be targeted by innate effector cells (Bendalac and Medzhitov, 2002). The cells responsible for innate immunity include the granulocytes (neutrophils, eosinophils, and basophils), mast cells, natural killer (NK) cells, a subset of T cells called NKT cells, dendritic cells, and macrophages. During the initiation of an immune response, dendritic cells promote NK cell activation, whereas NK cells influence dendritic cell maturation. This bidirectional crosstalk among innate effector cells may be important in generating an immune response against tumor growth (Zitvogel, 2002).

Natural killer cells recognize their target cells in a different way compared to T cells. NK cells are able to detect changes in the expression level of MHC molecules on the cell surface of potential target cells. A reduction of certain MHC class I molecules leads to NK cell-mediated destruction. Therefore, tumor cells that have downregulated their surface MHC class I molecules are targets for NK cell lysis. The mechanism of NK cell cytotoxicity is similar to that of CTLs (Sec. 20.2.3). NK cells secrete a number of different cytokines following target cell recognition and are themselves responsive to cytokines for their anti-tumor cytolytic function. In addition, there is a subset of T-cells called NKT cells which have a very limited TCR repertoire, express some NK cell markers, and regulate both CTL and NK cell anti-tumor activity through cytokine secretion.

The activity of NK and NKT cells is controlled by inhibitory and stimulatory receptors and a balance of positive and negative signals from the various receptors determines their activity. The inhibitory receptors on NK cells are specific for MHC class I molecules and their interaction inhibits target cell lysis. Evidence suggests that tumors express ligands for stimulatory receptors on NK and NKT cells that trigger anti-tumor activity. NK

T cells have been shown to have a role in anti-tumor immunity and therefore tumor regression, but these cells can also suppress an anti-tumor response (Smyth et al., 2001).

### 20.4.2 Immunosurveillance

The theory of "immunosurveillance" was originally coined in the 1950s and describes an individual's natural immunological resistance to the development of cancer. Essentially, if tumors express tumor-associated antigens (TAA) that can be presented to T cells then an immune response should be mounted and the tumor eradicated. However, the role of immunosurveillance is still controversial. Arguments against the theory stem primarily from the fact that mice that lack a thymus, and therefore have limited T-cell–mediated immunity, do not have an increased frequency of induced cancers (Dunn et al., 2002).

Recent studies have indicated that a modified interpretation of immunosurveillance may be necessary. The observation that there is enhanced tumor development in the absence of the cytokine IFNγ suggests that IFNγ acts as a tumor surveillance system and protects against the development of chemically induced and spontaneously arising tumors (Kaplan et al., 1998). In addition, mouse tumor models have revealed a role for innate effector cells in immunosurveillance of tumors with NK and NKT cells being involved in tumor rejection (Smyth et al., 2000).

The frequency of both spontaneous and carcinogen-induced cancers was examined in mice that were deficient in recombination-activating gene-2 (RAG-2) and/or signal transducer and activator of transcription (Stat)-1. RAG-2 is a lymphocyte-specific enzyme that catalyzes the rearrangement of gene segments necessary to generate functional TCR and immunoglobulin proteins. RAG-2 is responsible for the expression of diverse antigen receptors on lymphocytes and therefore adaptive immunity. Stat-1 is the transcription factor involved in mediating signals from the IFN receptors and is therefore important in innate immunity. The cancer incidence for both single gene-deficient and double gene-deficient mice was found to be higher than for wild-type mice. These data support the concept of immunosurveillance and that lymphocytes and IFNγ collaborate in their function to suppress cancer development. It appears that the mechanisms of RAG-2–mediated and Stat-1–mediated tumor surveillance overlap. RAG-2–deficient mice had cancer of the epithelial tissue in the intestine, whereas the RAG-2/Stat-1–deficient mice had these cancers in addition to mammary gland carcinomas. This observation suggests that different arms of the immune system protect against the development of cancers in distinct locations (Shankaran et al., 2001).

## 20.4.3 Tumor Antigens

Most antigens expressed by tumors are derived from self-molecules (see also Chap. 21, Sec. 21.1.1). Tumor-associated antigens (TAA) may be encoded by mutant cellular genes that consequently encode mutated self-proteins that are involved in the genetic transformation events of tumor progression. Examples of proteins from which the mutant antigenic peptides originate include kinases, helicases, GTPases, and tumor suppressor proteins. Another class of TAA arises following gene overexpression leading to protein overexpression (Boon et al., 1997).

At least some TAA appear to be encoded by normal genes that are either expressed at undetectable levels in normal cells or normally expressed at distinct stages in development such as embryonic or fetal antigens. These antigens can be inappropriately expressed and detected as a result of malignant transformation or tumor progression. Numerous TAA have been identified and are being investigated for their use as targets for tumor immunotherapy (Chap. 21, Secs. 21.3 and 21.4).

## 20.5 INDUCTION OF TUMOR IMMUNITY

### 20.5.1 Tumors and Tolerance

Despite the fact that TAA have been identified, many researchers have remained skeptical about tumor immunotherapy because it was widely believed that the immune system is tolerant toward self-peptides, including tumor antigens. The normal exposure of tumor antigens to the immune system may induce tolerance through the mechanisms of deletion, anergy, or regulatory cell-mediated suppression. The induction of tolerance, however, does not apply to all self/tumor peptides as demonstrated by the accumulating evidence from different tumor models (Pardoll, 2003).

Many models for studying tumor immunity rely on transplantation of tumors or tumor cells. Models employing transplanted tumors are designed such that the genetic background of the tumor donor and the tumor host are identical. That is, the mouse strain from which the tumor originally arose and the host mouse strain are the same. However, tumor cells that are grown in culture may be subject to modification that results in small antigenic differences prior to their use in the animal model. Therefore, concerns are raised against the possibility that the immunogenicity of a particular cultured tumor is associated with mutations that have arisen during culture. In addition, the manipulation of injecting cultured cells may be perceived by the host as immunogenic or even tolerogenic and may induce a very different immune response compared to naturally arising tumors. All transplantation tumor models are, of course, models and the results must be critically evaluated. A few examples are given below to describe the variable responses of T cells specific for tumor antigens.

Several models suggest that CD4+ T cells become tolerant in response to tumor antigen. In one model, mice were coinjected with tumor cells expressing an influenza hemagglutinin (HA) epitope and with T cells expressing an HA-specific TCR. Therefore, the T cells are specific for the tumor-associated antigen. Although the T cells expanded initially, this was followed by a decline in cell number with the remaining cells being nonresponsive when challenged in vitro. Tumor growth was normal (no rejection) with or without coinjection of tumor antigen-specific T cells. These results suggest that tumor antigen-specific T-cell deletion and anergy is an early event in tumor progression (Staveley-O'Carroll et al., 1998).

Another study examined tumor growth following injection of tumor cells into transgenic mice expressing a tumor antigen-specific TCR. Despite the fact that tumor antigen-specific CD8+ T cells were present, tumors grew. However, a skin allograft expressing tumor antigen was rejected indicating that systemic T-cell deletion or anergy was not the cause of tumor growth (Wick et al., 1997). Thus, even in the presence of large numbers of CTLs, the spontaneous anti-tumor response was minimal. Together these two studies suggest that immunosurveillance, while providing a small window of protection, is not sufficient to engage a repertoire of effective anti-tumor specific CTL. It has been shown that cross-presentation (Sec. 20.2.6) of exogenous tumor antigen by bone-marrow–derived cells is necessary for presentation of MHC-class-I–restricted tumor antigens and activation of CTLs against tumor antigens (Huang et al., 1994). Therefore, the ineffective anti-tumor responses described may be due to limited crosspresentation of tumor antigen and limited activation of sufficient numbers of CTLs in the draining lymph nodes (Wick et al., 1997; Nguyen et al., 2002).

Other models demonstrate that high affinity T-cells specific for a self-peptide are rendered tolerant while low affinity, but functionally competent T-cells, remain. Mice expressing a transgenic tissue-specific antigen were injected with tumor cells bearing the same antigen and progressive tumor growth occurred (Fig. 20.9). This was due to tolerance to the antigen. However, if the transgenic mice were immunized with a recombinant virus expressing the self-antigen prior to the injection of tumor cells, the mice rejected the tumor. This rejection was mediated by functional low affinity CTLs that were present, but required stimulation to be activated (Morgan et al., 1998). This study and others provide evidence that functional T cells specific for a tumor-associated antigen remain in the repertoire and that a functional anti-tumor response can be induced (Speiser et al., 1997).

Other models demonstrate that tumor growth can break immunological ignorance and tolerance. The T-cell response to tumor growth and its relation to tolerance was evaluated (Fig. 20.10). In the model, double transgenic mice express a viral glycoprotein (gp) under the control of the rat insulin promoter (RIP) targeting its expression to the β cells of the pancreas and a transgenic TCR specific for the viral glycoprotein peptide. There was no activation of the antigen-specific T cells in response to the viral glycoprotein self-antigen. Hence, the T cells are ignorant of the self-antigen (Fig. 20.10A; Sec. 20.3.3) (Ohashi et al., 1991). Transgenic mice that express the SV40 large-T antigen (Tag2) in the pancreatic β cells (RIP-Tag2) develop tumors (insulinomas) and the insulin secretion by the tumor cells causes a decrease in blood glucose levels providing a way to monitor tumor growth. The RIP-Tag2 mice were crossed to the double transgenic mice generating mice that express a defined TAA, the viral glycoprotein, expressed on the pancreatic β cells (Nguyen et al., 2002). These triple transgenic mice therefore provide a system to examine TAA-specific T cells (anti-viral glycoprotein) in the presence of a TAA-expressing, naturally arising tumor (RIP-Tag2/gp insulinoma; Fig. 20.10B). They also provide a way to monitor the efficiency of immunosurveillance. In the triple transgenic mice tumor growth promotes the activation of the tumor-specific T cells as the T cells display increased expression of activation markers in the pancreatic draining lymph nodes compared to tumor-free mice. Further experiments showed that the majority of TAA-specific T cells were neither deleted nor rendered anergic. These data suggest that the tumor naturally provides an inflammatory microenvironment wherein T-cell tolerance does not occur. The studies found that tumor-specific T cells proliferated in the regional lymph nodes and subsequently infiltrated the tumor (Nguyen et al., 2002). Further studies with this model demonstrated that a tumor-specific response could be efficiently induced in these mice using multiple approaches (Speiser et al., 1997; Nguyen et al., 2002).

The T-cell response to tumors will be different in different circumstances and it remains unclear which situations lead to tolerance to tumor antigens and which situations lead to activation and immunosurveillance (Fig. 20.11). In models where the immune system is exposed to a sufficiently high load of tumor antigen, such as by intravenous or intraperitoneal injection of cultured tumor cells, immunological tolerance may occur by deletion or anergy. However, in models in which TAA are expressed at lower levels, two outcomes may occur. First, effective activation of the immune response will occur if a critical balance is achieved with a sufficient level of TAA to generate antigen-specific stimulation of T cells, together with pro-inflammatory stimuli which would promote the maturation of APCs. Tissue disruption as a result of tumor invasion may potentially generate the pro-inflammatory signal. This activation of tumor-specific T cells can occur by tumors localized in secondary lymphoid tissues or through the activated APCs cross-presenting tumor-specific antigen to T cells in the lymph nodes. Alternatively, this low level expression of the TAA may not be sufficient for activation or tolerance, thus leaving TAA-specific T cells ignorant. The situation where lower levels of TAA result in immune activation or ignorance is the ideal situation for tumor immunotherapy. It is likely that some TAA are expressed at the appropriate level to qualify as targets for immunotherapy.

As discussed, the mechanisms of peripheral tolerance (Sec. 20.3.3) influence the induction of immunity directed against tumors. Figure 20.12 illustrates several avenues of potential immunotherapy to combat the mechanisms of peripheral tolerance and boost anti-tumor immune responses.

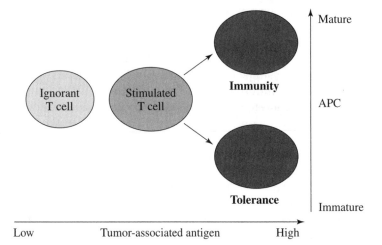

**Figure 20.11.** A model for the induction of tolerance or immunity to tumor antigens. This model suggests that immunological tolerance may result from a high load of tumor-associated antigen (TAA) in the absence of mature antigen presenting cells (APCs). If a balance is attained with sufficient TAA to generate stimulation of TAA-specific T cells, together with pro-inflammatory stimuli, which would promote the maturation of APCs then an anti-tumor immune response could occur. Lower levels of TAA may not be sufficient for activation or the induction of tolerance leaving TAA-specific T cells ignorant.

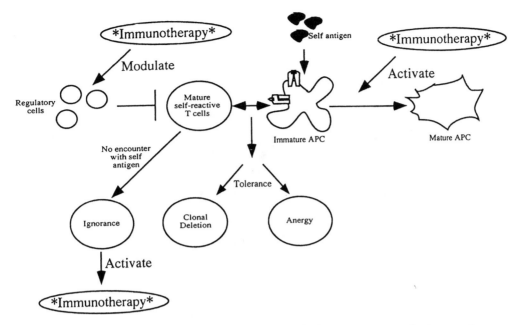

**Figure 20.12.** Overcoming the mechanisms of peripheral tolerance as a target for immunotherapy. Several potential routes for inducing an anti-tumor immune response focus on diverting the immunoregulation mediated by regulatory T-cell subpopulations. Likewise, the activation of ignorant tumor-associated antigen (TAA)-specific T cells is an ideal target. Current models speculate that the interaction of T cells specific for TAA with resting immature antigen presenting cells (APCs) leads to T-cell tolerance through deletion or induction of anergy. Immunotherapy that results in the maturation of APCs will promote T-cell activation and induction of an efficient anti-tumor immune response.

### 20.5.2 Boosting the Immune System: Modulating Costimulation and Dendritic Cells

It is apparent from the incidence of cancer that many tumor components do not elicit an effective antigen-specific T-cell response. This may be due to a lack of costimulation at the site of tumor growth, which prevents the generation of an immune response. Nonhematopoietic cells do not express costimulatory molecules. A lack of costimulation could also lead to anergy. More specifically, the failure of the immune system to reject a tumor has been attributed to the absence of functional dendritic cells in tumors. There is evidence that the maturational state of the APC is a determining factor in whether tolerance or induction of T cells occurs and this is possibly related to the costimulatory molecules expressed or the cytokines secreted by the APC (Banchereau and Steinman, 1998). Therefore, effective tumor destruction might be achieved through the provision of costimulation and/or activation of APCs that have captured or express tumor-associated antigens. Several approaches have focused upon activating APCs as a way to help elicit an anti-tumor response.

The ligation of CD40 on APCs, particularly dendritic cells, results in expression of costimulatory molecules and production of cytokines, both of which are required for initiating an immune response. Evidence from several mouse models supports the need for CD40 ligation on dendritic cells for the development of an anti-tumor immune response (Fig. 20.13). For example, CD40-deficient mice immunized with irradiated tumor cells and challenged with live tumor cells succumb to tumor. However, if the mice are also immunized with CD40$^+$ dendritic cells, the mice are protected from tumor challenge. Therefore, CD40 expression on dendritic cells is required for their function in an anti-tumor response (Mackey et al., 1998). Likewise, vaccination of mice with a plasmid expressing a trimer of CD40 ligand boosted CTL responses and prevented the development of metastatic tumor growth following a lethal challenge with tumor cells (Gurunathan et al., 1998).

Tumor-bearing mice were also treated with tumor-specific T cells and anti-CD40 antibody. Antibody to CD40 serves to experimentally activate APCs. This treatment resulted in tumor rejection. Treatment with anti-CD40 antibody alone showed activation of endogenous antigen-specific T cells in lymph nodes, suggesting both that APCs are continuously migrating to lymph nodes with tumor antigen and that they are capable of triggering tumor-specific T cells (Levitsky, 2000).

Other approaches that have been taken to induce anti-tumor immunity help to activate the T cell itself.

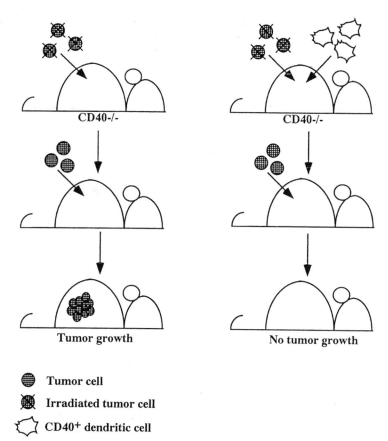

**Figure 20.13.** CD40 ligation on dendritic cells is required for the development of an anti-tumor immune response. CD40–deficient mice were immunized with irradiated tumor cells alone or along with CD40⁺ dendritic cells. Immunization in the absence of the CD40⁺ dendritic cells led to progressive tumor growth following tumor challenge, whereas immunization with CD40⁺ dendritic cells protected the mice from tumor growth following tumor challenge.

T cells express a plethora of costimulatory molecules including members of the immunoglobulin superfamily CD28, and ICOS and members of the TNF/TNF receptor superfamily 4-1BB, OX40, and CD40L, while APCs express the counterreceptors. Activation of T cells likely involves composite costimulatory signals with contributions from multiple receptors (Hurwitz et al., 2000). There is evidence to indicate that modulating costimulatory signals on T cells with or without other treatment has the potential to stimulate anti-tumor immunity.

Modulation of costimulatory signals through CD28 on T cells has been examined by the expression of its ligand, B7, on tumor cells (Fig. 20.14). Mice injected with tumor cells modified to express B7 rejected the tumor cells while unmanipulated tumor cells grew progressively. B7⁺ tumor cells also mediated rejection of wild-type tumors at distant sites and had some effect against established tumors (Chen et al., 1992). These studies were followed by the demonstration that antibody-mediated blocking of another receptor for B7, CTLA-4, enhanced anti-tumor immunity to both B7-expressing and wild-type tumor cells. CTLA-4 serves to negatively regulate T-cell activation; therefore prevention of the interaction of CTLA-4 with B7 promotes T-cell activation and enhances anti-tumor immunity (Leach et al., 1996).

T-cell stimulation via 4-1BB has also been examined as a way to enhance an anti-tumor T-cell response. Treatment of mice, bearing established, large tumors, with activating anti-4-1BB monoclonal antibody resulted in the eradication of tumors that killed untreated mice. The protection appeared to be long-lasting and was due, in part, to increased anti-tumor cytotoxicity. 4-1BB is expressed on activated T cells and antibody treatment likely amplifies the immune response (Melero et al., 1997). In related studies, inoculation of mice with tumor cells that express 4-1BB ligand (4-1BBL) resulted in tumor cell rejection while unmanipulated tumor cells grew. However, injection of 4-1BBL⁺ tumors had little effect on established wild-type tumors (Melero et al., 1998). In general, immunotherapy is a race between the tumor and the repetitive induction of an efficient immune response. Limited induction of anti-tumor immunity will not provide sufficient therapeutic help in the correct time frame.

Additional experimental strategies to boost anti-tumor immune responses include treatment with cancer-cell–derived heat shock protein/peptide complexes (Tamura et al., 1997) and vaccination with tumor cells genetically engineered to express cytokines or chemokines such as IL-12 and GM-CSF (Mach and Dranoff, 2000). The anti-tumor effect of IL-12 likely encompasses both innate and adaptive immunity in addi-

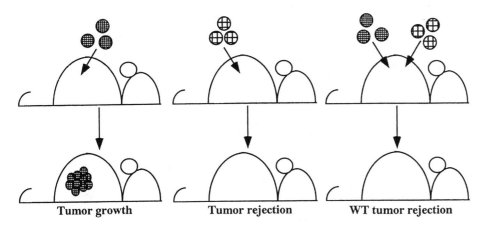

**Figure 20.14.** Modulating costimulatory signals on T cells has the potential to stimulate anti-tumor immunity. Mice were inoculated with either wild-type (WT) or B7– expressing tumor cells. Only the B7–expressing tumor cells were rejected. However, injection of B7+ tumor cells immediately before injection of wild-type tumor cells led to rejection of both tumor cells.

⊕ **Tumor cell**

⊕ **B7+ tumor cell**

tion to promoting the destruction of tumor vasculature and inhibiting angiogenesis. Granulocyte macrophage colony-stimulating factor is particularly important for the recruitment and maturation of dendritic cells which promotes an anti-tumor immune response. Other cytokines being investigated include IL-2, 4, 6, 7, and IFNγ, TNF, and granulocyte colony-stimulating factor (G-CSF). An immunotherapy strategy of modulating T-cell costimulatory signals in combination with either GM-CSF or anti-CD40 antibody treatment has shown some positive results for fostering anti-tumor immunity (Hurwitz et al., 2000). Such strategies have the advantage of targeting two different aspects of the immune response.

### 20.5.3 Evasion of Immunity by Tumors

Tumor cells acquire characteristics that allow them to evade T-cell recognition. For example, tumor cells have been shown to downregulate the expression of MHC class I molecules. This is attributed to mutations in components of the antigen processing and presentation machinery such as the transporter associated with antigen processing (TAP) and $\beta_2$ microglobulin ($\beta_2$m). An effective attack by effector CTLs requires an antigenic target which is presented together with MHC molecules. These tumor cells may become better targets for NK cell cytotoxicity (Sec. 20.4.1; Gilboa, 1999). Strategies to increase immunogenicity of tumor cells include transfection with MHC class I or class II molecules. Moreover, some antigenic epitopes are lost as the tumor progresses (Schreiber, 1999).

Tumors may also secrete immunosuppressive cytokines such as TGF-$\beta$ and IL-10, which can cause a local downregulation of the immune response (Smyth et al., 2001). Transforming growth factor $\beta$ promotes a T helper 2 (T$_h$2) pattern of cytokine secretion (Sec.

20.2.3), which is associated with antibody-mediated immune responses. This diverts the immune response from a cell-mediated immune response which is required for anti-tumor immunity.

Data also suggest that the tumor itself may develop the ability to terminate the anti-tumor response by directly killing the CTLs that are attacking it. Evidence indicates that tumor-facilitated killing of CTLs occurs by the expression of Fas ligand (CD95L) on tumor cells interacting with Fas (CD95), the apoptosis-inducing receptor, on activated CTLs. The resulting elimination of CTLs would prevent an effective anti-tumor immune response.

Regulatory T cells are involved in the maintenance of peripheral tolerance and may, therefore, form an obstacle to mounting an anti-tumor immune response. CD4+CD25+ regulatory T cells appear to suppress the activation of CD4+ and CD8+ T cells. Therefore, the modulation of these regulatory cell populations may be a way to induce an immune response against tumor antigens (Fig. 20.12). Inoculation of mice with radiation-induced leukemia cells followed by in vivo treatment with anti-CD4 monoclonal antibody resulted in regression of the tumors that grew progressively in untreated mice (Matsuo et al., 1999). Moreover, in another mouse model, in vivo administration of anti-CD25 monoclonal antibody caused a decrease in the number of CD4+CD25+ T cells in peripheral lymphoid tissue and a regression of tumor growth that otherwise killed untreated animals (Onizuka et al., 1999).

### 20.5.4 Vaccination with Dendritic Cells

Vaccination with dendritic cells is being examined as a tool to stimulate anti-tumor immunity in vivo, and a review of some of the clinical results is provided in Chapter 21. Such a strategy ensures that tumor antigens are presented in the context of costimulatory molecules. Briefly, inoculation with dendritic cells exposed to tumor antigens can lead to tumor-specific protection in naive animals in several different experimental systems. Early studies have also shown some regression of established tumors using tumor antigen-pulsed dendritic cells. Therefore, dendritic cells can prime anti-tumor T cells in vivo and induce effective anti-tumor CTL responses. Other ways in which dendritic cells are being manipulated for immunotherapy include genetically engineering them to express tumor antigens or cytokines such as IL-12 and GM-CSF (Dallal and Lotze, 2000). Vaccination with dendritic cells is being examined for the treatment of patients and some specific anti-tumor responses have been induced (Dallal and Lotze, 2000; Nestle at al., 2001). However, many issues remain unresolved concerning the design of the most effective vaccines.

## 20.6 SUMMARY

Tumor-specific T cells are present in the T-cell repertoire. Many may be specific for tissue-specific antigens that are expressed at low levels. Activation of these T cells has the potential to combat tumors. Successful strategies for the induction of an effective anti-tumor response will encompass several areas of immunology. First, sufficient numbers of different tissue-specific TAA must be identified that are expressed at levels that do not induce T-cell tolerance. Second, optimal strategies to induce a specific anti-tumor response will have to be defined that include either dendritic cell vaccination or agents that induce antigen-presenting cell maturation and migration in vivo. Third, the various ways that the tumors regulate the anti-tumor response by mechanisms of immune evasion have to be overcome. Understanding several aspects of immunology, including T-cell activation, tolerance, migration, and regulation, are critical to the generation of optimal tumor vaccines.

Strategies for the induction of an effective anti-tumor response focus on boosting the immune system. This includes approaches aimed at modulating costimulation, survival, and maturation of dendritic cells with an emphasis on combinatorial strategies. Dendritic cell vaccination, as well as dendritic cell tumor immunotherapy, are also predicted to be promising avenues for cancer therapy.

## REFERENCES

Bendelac A, Medzhitov R: Adjuvants of immunity: harnessing innate immunity to promote adaptive immunity. *J Exp Med* 2002; 195:F19–F23.

Bennett SRM, Carbone FR, Karamalis F, et al: Help for cytotoxic-T-cell responses is mediated by CD40 signalling. *Nature* 1998; 393:478–480.

Bjorkman PJ: MHC restriction in three dimensions: a view of T cell receptor/ligand interactions. *Cell* 1997; 89:167–170.

Blackman MA, Gerhard-Burgert H, Woodland DL, et al: A role for clonal inactivation in T cell tolerance to Mls-1ᵃ. *Nature* 1990; 345:540–542.

Boon T, Coulie PG, Van den Eynde B: Tumor antigens recognized by T cells. *Immunol Today* 1997; 18:267–268.

Bretscher P, Cohn M: A theory of self-nonself discrimination. *Science* 1970; 169:1042–1049.

Carbone FR, Kurts C, Bennett SRM, et al: Cross-presentation: a general mechanism for CTL immunity and tolerance. *Immunol Today* 1998; 19:368–373.

Caux C, Massacrier C, Vanbervliet B, et al: Activation of human dendritic cells through CD40 cross-linking. *J Exp Med* 1994; 180:1263–1272.

Chen L, Ashe S, Brady WA, et al: Costimulation of antitumor immunity by the B7 counterreceptor for the T lymphocyte molecules CD28 and CTLA-4. *Cell* 1992; 71:1093–1102.

Dallal RM, Lotze M: The dendritic cell and human cancer vaccines. *Curr Opin Immunol* 2000; 12:583–588.

Dunn GP, Bruce AT, Ikeda H, et al: Cancer immunoediting: from immunosurveillance to tumor escape. *Nat Immunol* 2002; 3:991–998.

Dustin ML, Chan AC: Signaling takes shape in the immune system. *Cell* 2000; 103:283–294.

Garza KM, Chan VSF, Ohashi PS: T cell tolerance and autoimmunity. *Rev Immunogenet* 2000; 2:2–17.

Gilboa E: How tumors escape immune destruction and what we can do about it. *Cancer Immunol Immunother* 1999; 48:382–385.

Grewal IS, Flavell RA: CD40 and CD154 in cell-mediated immunity. *Annu Rev Immunol* 1998; 16:111–135.

Guery J-C, Adorini L: Dendritic cells are the most efficient in presenting endogenous naturally processed self-epitopes to class II-restricted T cells. *J Immunol* 1995; 154:536–544.

Gurunathan S, Irvine KR, Wu C-Y, et al: CD40 ligand/trimer DNA enhances both humoral and cellular immune responses and induces protective immunity to infectious and tumor challenge. *J Immunol* 1998; 161:4563–4571.

Hahne M, Rimoldi D, Schröter M, et al: Melanoma cell expression of Fas(Apo-1/CD95) Ligand: implications for tumor immune escape. *Science* 1996; 274:1363–1366.

Huang AYC, Golumek P, Ahmadzadeh M, et al: Role of bone marrow-derived cells in presenting MHC class I-restricted tumor antigens. *Science* 1994; 264:961–965.

Hurwitz AA, Kwon ED, van Elsas A: Costimulatory wars: the tumor menace. *Curr Opin Immunol* 2000; 12:589–596.

Jordan MS, Boesteanu A, Reed AJ, et al: Thymic selection of CD4+CD25+ regulatory T cells induced by an agonist self-peptide. *Nat Immunol* 2001; 2:301–306.

Kagi D, Ledermann B, Burki K, et al: Molecular mechanisms of lymphocyte-mediated cytotoxicity and their role in immunological protection and pathogenesis in vivo. *Annu Rev Immunol* 1996; 14:207–232.

Kaplan DH, Shandaran V, Dighe AS, et al: Demonstration of an interferon γ-dependent tumor surveillance system in immunocompetent mice. *Proc Natl Acad Sci USA* 1998; 95:7556–7561.

Kappler JW, Roehm N, Marrack P: T cell tolerance by clonal elimination in the thymus. *Cell* 1987; 49:273–280.

Kappler JW, Staerz U, White J, Marrack PC: Self-tolerance eliminates T cells specific for Mls-modified products of the major histocompatibility complex. *Nature* 1988; 332:35–40.

Kisielow P, Bluthmann H, Staerz UD, et al: Tolerance in T-cell-receptor transgenic mice involves deletion of non-mature CD4$^+$8$^+$ thymocytes. *Nature* 1988; 333:742–746.

Kurts C, Kosaka H, Carbone FR, et al: Class I-restricted cross-presentation of exogenous self-antigens leads to deletion of autoreactive CD8$^+$ T cells. *J Exp Med* 1997; 186:239–245.

Kurts C, Sutherland RM, Davey G, et al: CD8 T cell ignorance or tolerance to islet antigens depends on antigen dose. *Proc Natl Acad Sci USA* 1999; 96:12703–12707.

Leach DR, Krummel MF, Allison JP: Enhancement of anti-tumor immunity by CTLA-4 blockade. *Science* 1996; 271: 1734–1736.

Lenschow DJ, Walunas TL, Bluestone JA: CD28/B7 system of T cell costimulation. *Annu Rev Immunol* 1996; 14:233–258.

Levitsky HI: Augmentation of host immune responses to cancer: overcoming the barrier of tumor antigen-specific T cell tolerance. *Cancer J Sci Am* 2000; 6:S281–S290.

Mach N, Dranoff G: Cytokine-secreting tumor cell vaccines. *Curr Opin Immunol* 2000; 12:571–575.

Mackey MF, Gunn JR, Maliszewski C, et al: Dendritic cells require maturation via CD40 to generate protective antitumor immunity. *J Immunol* 1998; 161:2094–2098.

Marsden VS, Strasser A: Control of apoptosis in the immune system: Bcl-2, BH-3-only proteins and more. *Annu Rev Immunol* 2003; 21:71–105.

Matsuo M, Wada H, Honda S, et al: Expression of multiple unique rejection antigens on murine leukemia BALB/c RL1♂1 and the role of dominant Akt antigen for tumor escape. *J Immunol* 1999; 162:6420–6425.

Melero I, Bach N, Hellstrom KE, et al: Amplification of tumor immunity by gene transfer of the co-stimulatory 4–1BB ligand: synergy with the CD28 co-stimulatory pathway. *Eur J Immunol* 1998; 28:1116–1121.

Melero I, Shuford WW, Newby SA, et al: Monoclonal antibodies against the 4–1BB T-cell activation molecule eradicate established tumors. *Nat Med* 1997; 3:682–685.

Morgan DJ, Kreuwel HTC, Fleck S, et al: Activation of low avidity CTL specific for a self epitope results in tumor rejection but not autoimmunity. *J Immunol* 1998; 160:643–651.

Morgan DJ, Kreuwel HTC, Sherman LA: Antigen concentration and precursor frequency determine the rate of CD8+ T cell tolerance to peripherally expressed antigens. *J Immunol* 1999; 163:723–727.

Mueller DL, Jenkins MK, Schwartz RH: Clonal expansion versus functional clonal inactivation: A costimulatory signalling pathway determines the outcome of T cell antigen receptor occupancy. *Annu Rev Immunol* 1989; 7:445–480.

Nestle FO, Banchereau J, Hart D: Dendritic cells: On the move from bench to bedside. *Nat Med* 2001; 7:761–765.

Nguyen LT, Elford AE, Murakami K, et al: Tumor growth enhances cross-presentation leading to limited T cell activation without tolerance. *J Exp Med* 2002; 195:423–435.

Oehen SU, Ohashi PS, Burki K, et al: Escape of thymocytes and mature T cells from clonal deletion due to limiting tolerogen expression levels. *Cell Immunol* 1994; 158:342–352.

O'Garra A, Arai N: The molecular basis of T helper 1 and T helper 2 cell differentiation. *Trends Cell Biol* 2000; 10:542–550.

Ohashi PS, Oehen S, Buerki K, et al: Ablation of "tolerance" and induction of diabetes by virus infection in viral antigen transgenic mice. *Cell* 1991; 65:305–317.

Oldstone MB, Nerenberg M, Southern P, et al: Virus infection triggers insulin-dependent diabetes mellitus in a transgenic model: role of anti-self (virus) immune response. *Cell* 1991; 65:319–331.

Onizuka S, Tawara I, Shimizu J, et al: Tumor rejection by *in vivo* administration of anti-CD25 (interleukin-2 receptor $\alpha$) monoclonal antibody. *Cancer Res* 1999; 59:3128–3133.

Pamer E, Cresswell P: Mechanisms of MHC class I-restricted antigen processing. *Annu Rev Immunol* 1998; 16:323–358.

Pardoll D: Does the immune system see tumors as foreign or self? *Annu Rev Immunol* 2003; 21:807–839.

Rammensee H-G, Kroschewski R, Frangoulis B: Clonal anergy induced in mature V$\beta$6$^+$ T lymphocytes on immunizing Mls-1B mice with Mls-1C expressing cells. *Nature* 1989; 339: 541–544.

Ramsdell F, Lantz T, Fowlkes BJ: A nondeletional mechanism of thymic self tolerance. *Science* 1989; 246:1038–1041.

Ridge JP, Di Rosa F, Matzinger P: A conditioned dendritic cell can be a temporal bridge between a CD4$^+$ T-helper and a T-killer cell. *Nature* 1998; 393:474–478.

Sakaguchi S: Regulatory T cells: key controllers of immunologic self-tolerance. *Cell* 2000; 101:455–458.

Samelson LE: Signal transduction mediated by the T cell antigen receptor: The role of adapter proteins. *Annu Rev Immunol* 2002; 20:371.

Schoenberger SP, Toes REM, van der Voort EIH, et al: T-cell help for cytotoxic T lymphocytes is mediated by CD40–CD40L interactions. *Nature* 1998; 393:480–483.

Schreiber H: Tumor immunology. In Paul WE, ed. *Fundamental Immunology*, 4th ed. Philadelphia: Lippincott-Raven; 1999:1237–1270.

Schwartz RH: Costimulation of T lymphocytes: the role of CD28, CTLA-4, and B7/BB1 in interleukin-2 production and immunotherapy. *Cell* 1992; 71:1065–1068.

Sebzda E, Mariathasan S, Ohteki T, et al: Selection of the T cell repertoire. *Annu Rev Immunol* 1999; 17:829–874.

Shankaran V, Ikeda H, Bruce AT, et al: IFN$\gamma$ and lymphocytes prevent primary tumour development and shape tumour immunogenicity. *Nature* 2001; 410:1107–1111.

Shevach EM: Regulatory T cells in autoimmunity. *Annu Rev Immunol* 2000; 18:423–449.

Shimizu J, Yamazaki S, Sakaguchi S: Induction of tumor immunity by removing CD25$^+$CD4$^+$ T cells: a common basis between tumor immunity and autoimmunity. *J Immunol* 1999; 163:5211–5218.

Smyth MJ, Godfrey DI, Trapani JA: A fresh look at tumor immunosurveillance and immunotherapy. *Nat Immunol* 2001; 2:293–299.

Smyth MJ, Thia KYT, Street SEA, et al: Differential tumor surveillance by natural killer (NK) and NKT cells. *J Exp Med* 2000; 191:661–668.

Speiser DE, Miranda R, Zakarian A, et al: Self antigens expressed by solid tumors do not efficiently stimulate naive or activated T cells: implications for immunotherapy. *J Exp Med* 1997; 186:645–653.

Staveley-O'Carroll K, Sotomayer E, Montgomery J, et al: Induction of antigen-specific T cell anergy: an early event in the course of tumor progression. *Proc Natl Acad Sci USA* 1998; 95:1178–1183.

Steinman RM, Hawiger D, Nussenzweig MC: Tolerogenic dendritic cells. *Annu Rev Immunol* 2003; 21:685–711.

Tamura Y, Peng P, Liu K, et al: Immunotherapy of tumors with autologous tumor-derived heat shock protein preparations. *Science* 1997; 278:117–120.

Wange RL, Samelson LE: Complex complexes: Signaling at the TCR. *Immunity* 1996; 5:197–205.

Watts C: Capture and processing of exogenous antigens for presentation on MHC molecules. *Annu Rev Immunol* 1997; 15:821–850.

Webb S, Morris C, Sprent J: Extrathymic tolerance of mature T cells: clonal elimination as a consequence of immunity. *Cell* 1990; 63:1249–1256.

Wick M, Dubey P, Koeppen H, et al: Antigenic cancer cells grow progressively in immune hosts without evidence for T cell exhaustion or systemic anergy. *J Exp Med* 1997; 186:229–238.

Zal T, Volkmann A, Stockinger B: Mechanisms of tolerance induction in major histocompatibility complex class II-restricted T cells specific for a blood-borne self-antigen. *J Exp Med* 1994; 180:2089–2099.

Zamoyska R: The CD8 coreceptor revisited: one chain good, two chains better. *Immunity* 1994; 1:243–246.

Zitvogel L: Dendritic and natural killer cells cooperate in the control/switch of innate immunity. *J Exp Med* 2002; 195: F9–F14.

# 21

# Biological Therapy of Cancer

*Neil L. Berinstein*

## 21.1 INTRODUCTION

Recent advances in the understanding of both the genetic alterations that contribute to the pathogenesis of cancers and of the immune response to cancer have led to the development of biologically-based approaches to anti-cancer treatment. These new strategies exploit expanding insights into the nature of tumor antigens, the molecular and cellular requirements for immune activation, the role of cytokines in amplifying the immune response, and the evolution of recombinant DNA approaches to introduce genetic material into eukaryotic cells.

### 21.1.1 Tumor-Associated Antigens

The existence of tumor antigens that can be recognized by the immune system is critical for the generation of an immune response against the tumor. Such antigens may either be expressed on the cell surface, where they are available for recognition by antibodies, or they may be intracellular antigens, which can be presented by molecules of the major histocompatibility complex (MHC) to T cells (see Chap. 20, Sec. 20.2.2). These antigens may be tumor specific, such as unique products of mutated or activated oncogenes, or they may be antigens such as oncofetal or differentiation proteins, which are not usually expressed in normal tissues of the adult.

The existence of tumor-associated antigens (TAAs) was suggested about 40 years ago by the demonstration that mice injected with syngeneic tumor cells (i.e., those derived from the same inbred strain of mice) induced by the carcinogen methylcholanthrene developed a cellular immune response that could protect against subsequent challenge with the same tumor cells, but not with other tumor cells. Numerous experiments have since demonstrated TAAs expressed by a variety of murine tumors induced by chemicals, ultraviolet (UV) radiation, and several oncogenic viruses. These TAAs can stimulate cytotoxic T lymphocytes (CTLs), which express CD8 on their cell surface.

A number of different TAAs that can be recognized by human T cells have been identified. These antigens have been grouped in several different ways and one classification is shown in Table 21.1. There is evidence that these TAAs are processed and presented both on antigen presenting cells and cancer cells. For many antigens, the parts (known as epitopes) that are presented on MHC molecules have also been defined. These epitopes can be recognized by and can activate human T cells. These observations are of fundamental importance in both understanding the immune response to cancer and in eventually trying to manipulate this response.

Cancer-testis antigens are for the most part limited in expression to tumors, spermatocytes or spermatogo-

**Table 21.1.** Classification of Tumor-associated Antigen

| Tumor Antigen | Normal Tissue Expression | Tumor Expression |
|---|---|---|
| **Cancer testis** | | |
| MAGE 1 | | Melanoma, breast, lung, sarcoma, thyroid, colon |
| MAGE 3 | | Melanoma, lung, gastric, head + neck, esophageal |
| MAGE 6 | Testis | Melanoma, lung, colon |
| BAGE | | Melanoma |
| GAGE | | Melanoma, breast, ovary |
| NYESO-1 | | Melanoma, sarcoma, liver, bladder, lung, ovary, breast |
| **Differentiation antigens** | | |
| MART 1/Melan A | | Melanoma |
| MC1R | | Melanoma |
| GP100 | | Melanoma |
| Tyrosinase | Melanoma, skin, retina, ganglia | Melanoma |
| TRP-1 | | Melanoma |
| TRP-2 | | Melanoma |
| PSA | Prostate | Prostate |
| **Widely expressed antigens** | | |
| CEA | Liver, colon | Colon, pancreas, gastric, breast, renal |
| Cyp-B | All at low levels | Lung, breast, ovary, esophageal |
| Her2/neu | Epithelial | Melanoma, ovary, breast |
| hTERT | Hematopoietic stem cells, germinal center cells, keratinocytes, gonadal cells | Lung, ovary, melanoma, leukemia, non-Hodgkin's lymphoma |
| MUC1 | None | Breast, ovary |
| PRAME | Testis, endometrium, ovary, adrenals, kidney, breast, skin | Melanoma, head + neck, lung, small-cell lung, renal, sarcoma |
| WT1 | Kidney, ovary, testis, spleen | Gastric, colon, lung, breast, ovary, uterine, liver |
| **Tumor specific antigens** | | |
| Immunogobulin idiotype | B-cells | NHL, myeloma |
| RAS | None | Pancreas, colon, gastric |
| CDK-4 | None | Melanoma |
| MUM-1 | None | Melanoma |
| β-catenin | None | Melanoma |
| **Fusion proteins** | | |
| BCR-ABL | None | CML, AML |
| ETV6/AML | None | ALL |
| PML/RAR2 | None | APL |
| TEL/AML1 | None | AML |
| **Viral proteins** | | |
| HPV16-E7 | None | Cervical, anal |
| Epstein-Barr Virus | Lymphoma B-cells | NHL, head + neck, liver |
| Human T cell lymphotropic virus | None | Acute T-Cell Leukemia |
| Hepatitis B and C | Liver | Liver, NHL |
| Human herpes virus type 8 | Neurons | Kaposi's sarcoma |

CML = Chronic Myelogenous Leukemia; AML = Acute Myelogenous Leukemia; ALL = Acute Lymphocytic Leukemia; APL = Acute Promyelocytic Leukemia; NHL = Non-Hodgkin's Lymphoma.

nia of the testis, and, occasionally, to the placenta. Examples of these include the MAGE, BAGE, and GAGE antigens identified by Boon and colleagues (1994). A second group of well-characterized TAAs includes differentiation antigens and specifically melanocyte differentiation antigens: their expression is limited to melanomas and to melanocytes in normal skin. Differentiation antigens from tissues other than skin, such as PSA in prostate cancer and the lymphoid differentiation antigens (i.e., CD10, CD5, CD20), have also been identified. A third group includes the widely expressed antigens, such as carcinoembryonic antigen (CEA), PRAME, MUC1, WT1, and many more. These TAAs may be expressed at various levels in some normal tissues. A fourth group includes the tumor-specific antigens. These may arise from point mutations of genes that are involved in the process of transformation and are not usually found in normal tissues: examples include ras and $\beta$-catenin. A fifth group of tumor-specific antigens includes fusion proteins such as BCR-ABL in chronic myelogenous leukemia (Chap. 7, Sec. 7.3). Finally, viral antigens can be associated with various tumors, such as the E7 protein of human papillomavirus (HPV) in human cervical cancer and various Epstein-Barr virus proteins in hepatoma and Burkitt's lymphoma (Chap. 6, Sec. 6.2). These are often restricted in expression to the tumor and to normal cells from which the tumor arose.

Tumor-specific CTLs (Chap. 20, Sec. 20.5.2) have been a powerful tool for the identification of TAAs. For example, the methylcholanthrene-induced P815 mastocytoma cell line was mutagenized to obtain variant subclones that, unlike the parental cell clone, were unable to form tumors in syngeneic mice and were recognized by specific CTLs (Boon et al., 1994). These variants, called *tum⁻*, were used to prepare a library of total genomic DNA cloned into cosmid expression vectors, which was introduced into the parental clone (Chap. 4, Sec. 4.3.3). Parental clones activating CTLs that recognized the *tum⁻* variant were isolated, and the responsible genes sequenced. A single point mutation in a protein known as P91A was found to be responsible for the ability of the *tum⁻* variants to activate CTLs, thus demonstrating the power of this approach to isolate TAAs. Subsequently, Boon and others have employed similar approaches to isolate a number of TAAs from human tumors, including the MAGE series of antigens and tyrosinase from human melanoma (Boon et al., 1994). These antigens all correspond to non-mutated non-oncogenic proteins that either are developmental antigens re-expressed as a result of transformation (e.g., MAGE) or differentiation antigens that are lineage-specific (e.g., tyrosinase) (Table 21.1).

An alternative method for detection and isolation of TAAs is to acid-elute peptides from MHC molecules and then separate them into fractions by reverse phase high-performance liquid chromatography (Pardoll, 1994). Tumor-specific CTLs are used subsequently to detect biologically-active fractions by adding the protein fractions to antigen-processing mutant cells that express MHC class I molecules (Chap. 20, Sec. 20.5.2). With this approach, a glycoprotein, gp100, was identified as a human melanoma TAA. Cytotoxic T-lymphocytes obtained from four different patients with melanoma recognized gp100, thus illustrating the potential of this approach to identify and isolate common shared antigens. The gp100 antigen is also expressed on normal melanocytes, but not in other normal tissues.

Several other approaches used for the identification of TAAs do not rely on identification by T cells, but rather on molecular methods. For example, expressed proteins from the cancer cell may be compared to those expressed by the normal cells/tissue from which the cancer arose. The differentially expressed proteins can be eluted from a gel and sequenced by mass spectroscopy. Using a similar strategy, microarray technologies can be used to obtain profiles of expressed RNAs from the cancer of interest and to compare the overexpressed RNAs to the corresponding normal tissue and to other normal tissues (Chap. 4, Sec. 4.4.4). Other molecular approaches, such as subtractive hybridization and serial analysis of gene expression (SAGE) can be employed to identify novel proteins in tumors in comparison to normal tissues (Velculescu et al., 1995). Finally, TAAs can be identified by a technique called serological analysis of recombinant complementary DNA (cDNA) expression libraries (SEREX). In this method, serum from a patient is used to screen cDNA libraries made from the patient's tumor to identify proteins that are recognized by the patient's serum (Scanlan et al., 1998).

### 21.1.2 Molecular and Cellular Requirements for Immune Activation

As reviewed in Chapter 20, the first step in lymphocyte activation is recognition of a tumor antigen. Unfortunately, the failure of CTLs to eradicate the cancers to which they are sensitized indicates that tolerance or anergy to these TAAs has developed, just as tolerance/anergy may develop to other self-antigens (see Chap. 20, Sec. 20.3). Consequently, many biological approaches to cancer therapy are directed at strategies to augment T-cell activation by TAAs and to reverse this tolerance. Such strategies must take into account the complexity of T-cell activation. This requires that the antigen be presented on appropriate cells in association with molecules of the MHC, as well as accessory signals in addition to those generated through the T-cell receptor (see Chap. 20, Sec. 20.2, and Sec. 21.4). It also depends on the pattern of lymphokine release, which further amplifies the immune response. The remainder of this chapter will describe various approaches to the biological treatment of cancer, many of which attempt to activate or augment immunological responses against tumor antigens.

## 21.2 GENE THERAPY

### 21.2.1 Approaches to Gene Therapy

Strategies for gene therapy of cancer (Fig. 21.1) include:

1. Reversing genetic alterations associated with the cancer cell by transfer of antisense constructs to inhibit expression of oncogenes, or by transfer of wild-type tumor suppressor genes such as *p53*.

2. Transfer of genes that cause death of the cell.
3. Enhancing the activity of immune effector cells by the transfer of genes encoding cytokines such as interferon or interleukin 2 (IL-2).
4. Increasing the drug resistance of hematopoietic stem cells by transfer of genes that encode proteins that cause drug resistance.
5. Enhancing the immunogenicity of the cancer cell itself by the transfer of genes encoding cytokines or costimulatory molecules.

Promising results in animal models have been obtained using several of these strategies, and clinical trials of gene therapy are evaluating the safety and efficacy of these approaches in patients with cancer (see Sec. 21.2.5). Gene transfer may be performed in vitro (e.g., enhancing immune effector cells with cytokine

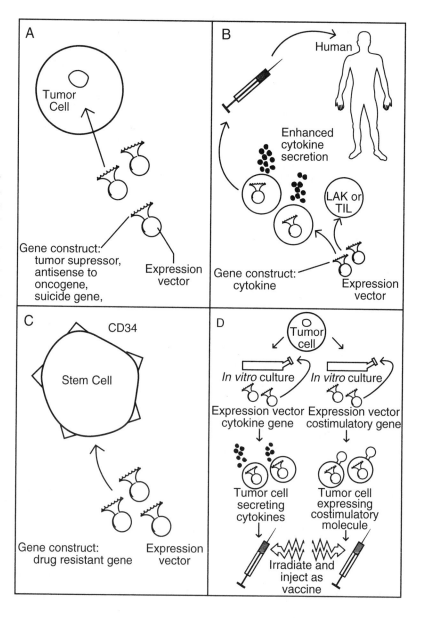

**Figure 21.1.** Approaches to gene therapy for cancer. (*A*) Expression vectors containing gene constructs for tumor suppressor genes, antisense to oncogenes, or suicide genes can be introduced in vivo into tumor cells. (*B*) Expression vectors containing genes for various cytokines can be introduced into tumor-infiltrating lymphocytes (TIL) or lymphokine-activated killer (LAK) cells that have been expanded in vitro. (*C*) Expression vectors containing genes for drug-resistance proteins can be introduced into hematopoietic stem cells (CD34+) that have been cultured in vitro. (*D*) Expression vectors containing genes for cytokines or costimulatory molecules can be introduced either in vitro or in vivo into tumor cells. In vitro gene-modified tumor cells (shown in figure) are irradiated and then injected with an immune adjuvant back into the patient as a therapeutic anticancer vaccine.

genes or increasing drug resistance of hematopoietic stem cells) or in vivo (e.g., reversing the genetic alteration of cancer cells or transfer of suicide genes). Because current gene transfer technologies do not permit transfer of the therapeutic gene to every cancer cell, strategies for in vivo gene therapy generally aim to augment other therapies.

Genetic material can be introduced into cells by physical methods or by infection with viruses. Because physical methods are characterized by a 100- to 1000-fold lower efficiency of gene transfer and because some cell types are fragile or resistant to these methods (see Chap. 4, Sec. 4.3.10), most investigators have focused on viral approaches for gene transfer, referred to as *transduction* (for review, see Crystal, 1995).

## 21.2.2 Viral Methods for Gene Transfer

*Retroviruses* Retroviruses contain a diploid RNA genome that is converted into a DNA intermediate by the retrovirally-encoded enzyme reverse transcriptase upon entry into the cytoplasm of a cell. The DNA is then transported to the nucleus, where it integrates randomly into the genome. The viral genetic material contains information for the three protein regions of the virus: *gag* (structural proteins), *pol* (RNA-dependent DNA polymerase/reverse transcriptase), and *env* (surface or envelope proteins). The linear double-stranded viral DNA is flanked by long terminal repeats (LTR) and has an RNA polymerase II promoter in the 5′LTR. In addition, the DNA contains motifs to allow efficient encapsidation and DNA priming. Once the DNA has integrated into the cellular genome, it is transcribed, processed, and translated into proteins. These proteins subsequently assemble into virions, which encapsidate two copies of viral RNA, leave the cell, and infect other cells to complete the viral life cycle (Chap. 6, Sec. 6.3).

The use of retroviruses for gene transfer requires a two-component approach. The first involves the replacement of the genetic material encoding the gag, pol, and env proteins with the DNA to be transferred. This DNA is expressed under the control of the promoter elements in the 5′LTR. Strategies have been developed to insert more than one gene into this region and can include alternative splicing of LTR-initiated transcripts, the use of multiple internal promoters, or the use of specific regions of DNA (IRES or internal ribosome entry sites) that can initiate internal translation of the tandemly-linked mRNA (Hawley et al., 1994). The second component involves the introduction of this DNA into a retroviral packaging cell line to produce viruses able to infect the appropriate host species. This cell line contains a replication-defective helper retrovirus that will provide the gag, pol, and env pro-

teins and an encapsidation signal for efficient viral packaging. Several generations of such packaging lines/helper viruses have been developed to reduce the likelihood of replication-competent retroviruses being generated through random recombination events between the genetically-modified retrovirus and the helper virus. The envelope proteins of such helper viruses can be modified to alter the host range of infectivity of the virus and to target retroviruses specifically to a cell of interest for the purposes of gene therapy.

Although retroviruses can infect cells and transfer the gene of interest at a relatively high efficiency (usually leading to infection of more than 10% of cells), there are some disadvantages associated with their use (Table 21.2). First, retroviruses transfer the gene of interest permanently into the genome of the target cell, which could result in chronic overexpression of the inserted gene or to mutation of a gene into which they are inserted. In addition, retroviruses only infect proliferating cells, which will decrease their usefulness for gene transfer into stem cells, which are largely noncycling. Retroviruses can accommodate less than 9 kilobases of foreign genetic information. Finally, retroviruses are associated with numerous technical problems related to recombination, rearrangement, and low viral titers.

*Adenoviral Vectors* Adenoviruses are DNA viruses with a 36-kilobase genome that encode four early proteins (E1 to E4) and five late proteins (L1 to L5). Because replication is controlled by E1, it is usually deleted in adenoviral vectors used for gene therapy and replaced by the gene to be transferred. The resultant recombinant adenovirus is replication incompetent. This recombinant adenoviral DNA is then transferred into a complementing cell line containing E1 sequences in its genome (but lacking other sequences required for replication) to generate viral particles that are infectious but replication defective. Adenoviruses enter a cell by means of two receptors that interact with the adenovirus fiber and penton proteins. After binding, the virus is internalized into a cytoplasmic endosome; it then enters the cytoplasm and subsequently the nucleus, where its double-stranded DNA is transcribed episomally without integrating into the cell's genome (Chap. 6, Sec. 6.2.2).

Adenoviruses have certain advantages over retroviruses for gene therapy (Table 21.2). They can be produced in high titer ($>10^{13}$ viral particles/mL) and can transfer genes efficiently into both replicating and nonreplicating cells. As the transferred genetic material exists episomally, the risks of permanently altering the genetic material of the cell and of insertional mutagenesis are avoided. A disadvantage of adenoviral vectors is that the viral proteins are immunogenic and can induce nonspecific inflammation and specific cellular re-

**Table 21.2.** Advantages and Disadvantages of Vectors for Gene Therapy

|  | Advantages | Disadvantages |
| --- | --- | --- |
| Retroviruses | Moderate gene transfer efficiency; long-term expression | Recombination; low titer; insertional mutagenesis; infect replicating cells only; accommodate less than 9 kbp of foreign DNA |
| Adenoviruses | High gene transfer efficiency; infect replicating and nonreplicating cells; high titer | Transient expression; immunogenic; accommodate less than 7 kbp of foreign DNA |
| Adeno-associated viruses | High gene transfer efficiency; infect replicating and nonreplicating cells, long-term expression | Insertional mutagenesis; often low titer; contamination with helper virus |
| Plasmid liposomes | Nonreplicating | Low gene transfer efficiency |
| DNA complexes | Accommodate large therapeutic genes | No specific target-cell population; naked DNA |
| Oncolytic adenovirus | Replicate in tumor tissues—more efficient gene transfer | Minimal clinical experience |
| Poxviruses | Infect all mammalian cells; nonreplicating; accommodate large inserts | Low yield production |
| Alphaviruses | Infect multiple cell types; high level of gene expression | Strategies to limit replication need further development |

sponses to viral proteins. Only approximately 7 kilobases of foreign DNA can be accommodated. Also, episomes tend to be lost from infected cells within 2 to 4 weeks, so that repeated administration may be necessary. Immune responses directed against the virus may, however, limit the effectiveness of repeated treatments.

Recently tumor-selective oncolytic adenoviruses have been engineered (Kirn, 2000). The objective has been to develop adenoviruses that will replicate in tumor tissues and not normal tissues. This strategy exploits the concept that tumor tissues and adenoviruses inactivate similar proteins in the same critical proliferative pathways (i.e., Rb and p53 pathways). Viral proteins necessary to inactivate these proteins (that could otherwise inhibit the successful replication of the virus) will not be necessary because the tumor has already inactivated the proteins (through mutations that commonly occur in *p53* or in *Rb*). Thus, these oncolytic viruses are engineered with deletions of such viral proteins.

The most studied of these approaches involves an adenovirus (dl1520, also known as Onyx-015) engineered with a deletion of the E1B gene (McCormick, 2000). The E1B gene product has been shown to neutralize p53 and prevent p53-induced apoptosis. Thus, the adenovirus will be able to replicate and spread in cancer cells with a deficiency in p53 function, whereas infected normal cells (with a normal p53 pathway) will undergo apoptosis, thus limiting the extent of replication and the ability of the adenovirus to infect and kill adjacent normal cells. This adenovirus has shown activity in clinical trials, but is limited because it requires direct in-

jection into the tumor. Although the virus may replicate in tumor cells with wild-type p53 it is postulated that these tumor cells may have disturbances in the p53 pathway through other mechanisms.

*Adeno-associated Viruses (AAV)*   Adeno-associated viruses are parvoviruses that are not pathogenic in humans. Unlike adenoviruses, AAV may integrate into the host genome and do so at preferred locations—in particular, at one site on chromosome 19. Thus, long-term expression is more stable than with adenoviruses. Recombinant AAV vectors used for gene transfer contain a 145-base-pair terminal repeat sequence, and a polyadenylation site; they have had most of the viral genome deleted and replaced with DNA encoding the therapeutic gene. Because few viral proteins are expressed, these viruses induce less of an immune response than adenoviruses. Like adenoviruses, AAV vectors do not require cell replication for integration, but high AAV titers are often difficult to achieve. Also, because the production of infectious AAV requires the use of an adenoviral helper virus, contamination of the AAV with adenovirus is a concern.

*Other Viral Vectors*   Several members of the herpesvirus family are of interest because they infect specific cell types. Herpes simplex virus is specific for neurons, while human herpes virus 7 infects T lymphocytes. Recombinant vaccinia and poxviruses (such as the canary pox virus) can accommodate large foreign therapeutic genes, do not induce significant immune neutralizing response against viral proteins, and do not integrate into the genome (Perkus et al., 1995). Multiple genes (as many as seven to date) can be engineered into these vectors, but expression is transient and decreases over weeks. These viral vectors have proven to be safe in initial clinical studies.

Reoviruses have recently been shown to have oncolytic capabilities. These are double-stranded RNA viruses that can preferentially infect and kill cells with an activated RAS signaling pathway. At least 50 percent of malignancies have alterations of these pathways at some level. In preclinical studies, these viruses have been shown to be selective for tumor cells and not to kill normal cells from which the tumors were derived (Norman et al., 2002). Clinical trials with intratumoral injection of these viruses are in progress.

Alphaviruses are single-stranded RNA viruses that are attractive vectors for gene therapy because of their ability to infect many cell types and because of their high level of replication and gene expression (Polo et al., 2000). The foreign gene of interest is substituted for the structural genes, and four viral proteins forming the viral replicon mediate cytoplasmic replication of these viruses. By retaining the genes encoding these proteins, the vector RNA, including the foreign gene of interest, self-amplifies. The infected vector RNA can be used for gene transfer or alternatively can be packaged into viral-like particles that retain the tropism of the wild-type alphaviruses. These particles contain the replicon and two defective helper RNAs encoding the structural proteins. In animal models very high levels of gene expression can be obtained. These viruses will be tested in the clinic.

## 21.2.3 Physical Methods for Gene Transfer

DNA on a plasmid can be introduced into cells by physical strategies. It can be injected directly into smooth muscle, or a gene gun can be used to bombard skin or subcutaneous tissue with microparticles coated with DNA (see Sec. 21.4.4). Another approach involves encapsulation of plasmid DNA containing the therapeutic gene into lipid complexes called *liposomes* (Farhood et al., 1994). These complexes fuse with the plasma membrane, their contents enter the cell, and the plasmid DNA is expressed extrachromosomally. In vivo electroporation has also been tested in animal models: in this method naked plasmid DNA encoding the therapeutic protein is injected into tumors followed by a series of electric pulses that induce pore formation in the cell membrane, which augments the uptake of DNA into the cells. In a CT26 colon carcinoma model, enhanced expression of interferon γ, infiltration with CD8$^+$ T lymphocytes, and tumor regression were documented after intratumoral in vivo electroporation of the IL-12 gene (Tamura et al., 2001).

There are many potential advantages of using physical methods for gene transfer: (1) expression cassettes containing the therapeutic foreign DNA can be of almost any size, (2) liposomes and naked plasmid DNA are noninfectious and cannot replicate, and (3) liposomes do not express foreign proteins and hence, will not elicit an inflammatory response. The disadvantages of plasmid-liposome vectors are primarily related to their inefficiency of gene transfer and their inability to target tumors specifically.

## 21.2.4 Antisense Therapy of Cancer

There has been increasing interest in the therapeutic use of exogenously administered antisense oligonucleotides to interfere with the expression of genes thought to be involved in the pathogenesis of certain cancers (for review, see Jansen and Zangemeister-Wittke, 2002). These oligonucleotides have sequences that are complementary to regions of specific strands of RNA. Upon entry into the cell the oligonucleotide will bind to its specific RNA and eliminate expression of the related protein through mechanisms that include prevention of RNA transport, abrogation of RNA splicing, and arrest of protein translation. Arrest of translation is mediated by RNAase-mediated DNA cleavage (RNAase mediates cleavage of RNA in DNA/RNA hybrids), inhibition of the initiation of translation and/or inhibition of ribosome movement. Mechanisms, not related to antisense activity, such as immune activation by CpG motifs within the oligonucleotide, may also play a role.

There are several requirements for optimizing this technology. First, the antisense oligonucleotide must enter the cell and the nucleus. Intracellular penetration may occur through an energy-dependent endocytosis mechanism or through a mechanism involving direct penetration into the cell. Because oligonucleotides are hydrophilic with an anionic backbone, membrane permeation is low. To enhance intracellular transport, lipophilic transfection has been studied but has not been shown to be of value in the clinic. It is also important to use the optimal antisense sequence for the RNA of interest. The AUG start site has often been chosen for antisense targeting because RNAs are single stranded at this site to facilitate ribosomal entry, so that this site should be accessible for oligonucleotide hybridization. Other experimental and computational (based on predicting mRNA secondary structure and folding patterns) approaches to identify target sites for antisense action are being evaluated.

The sensitivity of antisense oligonucleotides to cellular degradation by nucleases may limit the usefulness of antisense therapy, and modifications to the sugar, base, and phosphodiester backbone have been evaluated to improve stability. Improvements in stability have been obtained by replacement of an oxygen atom with sulphur resulting in phosphorothioate antisense oligonucleotides, which are being evaluated in clinical trials. Additional modifications such as 2′ modification with an electronegative molecule such as 2′-O-methyl or 2′-O-ethyl groups, which may enhance affinity of the oligonucleotide, are also under evaluation.

The choice of target gene for the antisense approach is of critical importance. Ideally the gene must be differentially expressed in the cancer and must play a role in the oncogenic process. The list of such genes is growing, and includes those involved in cell proliferation, apoptosis, angiogenesis, and metastases (Table 21.3). Toxicity related to nonspecific hybridization to unrelated targets with homologous sequences, or interference with loss of the function of the targeted gene in normal cells will be very dependent on the choice of target.

### 21.2.5 Clinical Studies of Gene Therapy

Despite enthusiasm for applying gene therapy to the treatment of cancer, this therapeutic strategy has developed slowly for several reasons. First, there has been only modest success in initial trials of gene therapy, perhaps due to the difficulty in achieving gene expression in a high percentage of the cancer cells in vivo. Strategies to combine gene therapy with other modalities such as irradiation and cytotoxic therapy may be more promising. Second, there has been unexpected toxicity associated with gene therapy and the death of a patient

**Table 21.3.** Targets for Antisense Therapy

| Target | Function |
|---|---|
| BCL-2 | Inhibitor of apoptosis |
| PKC α | G-protein coupled phosphorylation—regulates cell growth |
| cRAF | Serine-threonine kinase associated with RAS—regulates cell proliferation |
| Ha-Ras | Associated with transformed phenotype |
| Clusterin | Promotes cell survival |
| PKA-R1-α | Regulates cell proliferation |
| C-MYB | Regulates proliferation |
| Ribonucleotide reductase | DNA synthesis/cell proliferation |
| DNA methyltransferase | Gene inactivation |
| p53/MDM-2 | Regulation of apoptosis |
| BCR-ABL | Tyrosine kinase associated with transformation |
| Insulin-like growth factor (IGF1) | Mitogenic/Inhibitor of apoptosis |

in 1999 who was included in a gene therapy trial has resulted in the implementation of much stricter regulatory requirements. Third, many tumors are not amenable to local gene therapy because of difficulties with access and inoculation. This has resulted in interest in vectors with the potential to replicate in a controlled fashion (e.g., reoviruses and oncolytic adenoviruses) which might infect a large number of tumor cells (Kruyt and Curiel, 2002).

Many strategies of gene therapy seek to induce or augment an immune rejection response against tumor cells; these methods are described in Section 21.4. Strategies for gene therapy that do not depend on immunologic mechanisms and will be or are being tested clinically include the following.

*Tumor Suppressor/Antisense*  In this approach, expression vectors containing tumor suppressor genes such as *P53* or antisense constructs for oncogenes such as *BCR-ABL* (in chronic myelogenous leukemia), *C-MYB* (in acute and chronic myelogeneous leukemia), or *C-FOS* (in breast cancer) are introduced in vivo. There have been documented anti-tumor responses after treatment of head and neck patients with adeno-*P53* gene therapy in combination with involved-field irradiation. Several clinical trials are under way or have been completed with various antisense reagents directed to different targets in different types of tumor. Antisense constructs have been delivered as retroviruses, adenoviruses, or oligonucleotides. Except for the anti-BCL-2 reagent G3139 and the anti-protein kinase C reagent ISIS 3521, most of these are being tested in early trials. Some of these trials are evaluating the antisense reagent as monotherapy and some are evaluating them in combination with cytotoxic drugs. Continuous subcutaneous infusion of G3139 resulted in reduction in expression of the anti-apoptotic BCL-2 protein in nine of twenty-one patients with non-Hodgkin's lymphoma (Waters et al., 2000) and in serial tumor biopsies from patients with melanoma (Jansen et al., 2000). A few objective tumor responses were seen when the G3139 was given with the cytotoxic drug DTIC (Chap. 16, Sec. 16.2) in patients with melanoma leading to the initiation of a randomized phase III trial. Similarly, a phase III trial with ISIS 3521 has been organized, based on promising results when this reagent was given with carboplatin and paclitaxel to patients with non–small-cell lung cancer (Yuen et al., 2000). Dose-limiting thrombocytopenia and fatigue were the major toxicities in these initial trials.

*Drug Sensitivity*  A number of clinical trials are testing the efficacy of gene transfer of the herpes simplex virus thymidine kinase (HSV-TK) gene in sensitizing various cancer cells to the drug gancyclovir. Gancyclovir, which is nontoxic in eukaryotic cells, is metabolized to the cytotoxic gancyclovir triphosphate in cells expressing HSV-TK. In animal models, a bystander effect occurs where neighboring cells that have not been transduced are also lysed. This may be mediated by transfer of toxic metabolites through gap junctions or by phagocytosis by live tumor cells. The clinical trials mostly involve in vivo gene transfer, usually by retroviruses, and are directed at glioblastomas, ovarian cancers, and melanomas. In patients with prostate cancer, adenoviral delivery of the herpes simplex virus thymidine kinase gene with gancyclovir treatment resulted in an increase in the mean doubling time of serum PSA values from 16 to 42.5 months; with decrease in PSA levels in 28 percent of patients (Miles et al., 2001). Vector DNA was detectable by the polymerase chain reaction (PCR) in most serum samples.

*Drug Resistance* These studies have involved transferring genes that mediate drug resistance, such as multidrug resistance-1 (*MDR-1*), into hematopoietic stem cells ex vivo and the transfected cells are then infused to enhance bone marrow protection during chemotherapy. Most of these studies use retroviruses to mediate gene transfer. It remains to be determined whether there will be sufficient bone marrow protection to allow high enough increases in the intensity of chemotherapy to enhance therapeutic outcome.

## 21.3 PASSIVE IMMUNOTHERAPY

The biological treatment of cancer includes both active and passive immunotherapy. Passive immunotherapy includes the use of anti-tumor reagents that have been generated in vitro, such as monoclonal antibodies (MAbs) or cytokines, or the use of expanded effector cells such as lymphokine-activated killer (LAK) cells or tumor-infiltrating lymphocytes (TILs) in adoptive cellular therapy.

### 21.3.1 Cytokines

Many cytokines have been evaluated in animal models and in clinical trials for their anti-tumor activity. These molecules have been chosen because they are known to regulate various aspects of the immune response. Most of these molecules are produced by recombinant genetic techniques and hence are available in large quantities as highly purified products. Several of these cytokines are known to mediate anti-tumor activity in animal models and their clinical activity is being evaluated.

The *interferons* (IFN) have been studied most extensively. Interferons inhibit cell proliferation, increase gene expression, and augment the proliferation and cytotoxicity of CTLs and natural killer (NK) cells (see Chap. 20, Sec. 20.5.2). Interferon-α induces responses in over 90 percent of patients with hairy cell leukemia, although most patients will relapse within 2 years. Interferon-α may also prolong remissions obtained with chemotherapy in patients with chronic myelogeneous leukemia, and it has some anti-tumor activity against myeloma, low-grade non-Hodgkin's lymphoma, metastatic renal carcinoma, and Kaposi's sarcoma related to acquired immunodeficiency syndrome (AIDS). Recent results have shown that IFN-α may reduce the likelihood of recurrence in patients with high-risk stage II or III melanoma (Kirkwood et al., 2001).

*Interleukin 2* (IL-2) stimulates the proliferation of T lymphocytes, NK cells, LAK cells, and TILs. Interleukin 2 has been approved by the U.S. Food and Drug Administration (FDA) for the treatment of renal cell carcinoma and malignant melanoma based on an approximate 15 to 20 percent partial response rate for these cancers. A major limiting feature of IL-2 treatment is toxicity, and particularly the capillary-leak syndrome which results in hypotension, weight gain, and peripheral and pulmonary edema. Toxicity is lower with lower-dose subcutaneous injection, but so is efficacy.

Factors secreted by tumors may suppress intracellular signaling in lymphocytes by downregulating components of the T-cell receptor such as the zeta chain (see Chap. 20, Sec. 20.2.4). This prevents T cells from becoming fully activated to the tumor cells. Macrophage-derived reactive oxygen intermediates may also have a similar effect. Histamine may protect NK cells and T lymphocytes from the toxic effects of reactive oxygen species that may mediate the down modulation of CD3 zeta chain signaling. Preclinical studies have shown that histamine may augment the effects of IL-2 in preclinical models of melanoma. Based upon this observation, a randomized clinical trial comparing low-dose IL-2 with low-dose IL-2 and histamine was carried out in patients with metastatic melanoma. A statistically significant prolongation of survival was seen with the IL-2/histamine combination (Agarwala et al., 2002).

*Interleukin 4* (IL-4) enhances proliferation of B and T lymphocytes, facilitates immunoglobulin class switching to IgG and IgE from IgM, and has multiple other pleiotrophic effects on the immune system. Interleukin 4 along with IL-2 can increase the expansion of TILs. Infusion of IL-4 has been ineffective against solid tumors but has induced occasional anti-tumor responses in several hematologic malignancies. Interleukin 4 is not being developed as a single agent for the therapy of cancer.

*Tumor necrosis factor* (TNF-α) is produced by macrophages and is available by recombinant technology. Tumor necrosis factor is cytostatic or cytolytic for many human tumor cells in culture and has been shown to induce necrosis of transplanted tumors (including human xenografts) in mice. Unfortunately, TNF-α has proven to be toxic (septic shock-like syndrome) when administered systemically with only minimal activity in the clinic. For this reason isolated limb perfusion has been used to administer TNF-α locally into the limbs of patients requiring surgery for soft-tissue sarcoma. In one study in which TNF-α was administered concomitantly with melphalan, more than 90 percent of patients experienced objective responses and complete responses occurred in thirteen of thirty-five patients; twenty-nine of thirty-four patients were spared amputation or extensive surgical procedures (Gutman et al., 1997). It was possible to administer approximately ten times more TNF-α than could be tolerated systemically. As well as directly inducing apoptosis of the cancer cells, TNF-α might damage the tumor capillary network leading to increased retention of melphalan locally. A similar approach has been applied to unresectable bone sarcomas.

*Interleukin 12* (IL-12) has been shown to mediate promising anti-tumor activity in animal models. This cytokine—secreted primarily by macrophages, monocytes, and B lymphocytes—is a heterodimer consisting of 35- and 40-kDa subunits; it can be synthesized by recombinant DNA technology. Interleukin 12 is an essential factor for the generation of T helper cells, and it stimulates the proliferation of activated T lymphocytes and NK cells. It synergizes with the costimulatory molecule B7-1 in the activation of T-cell proliferation (Chap. 20, Sec. 20.5.2) and produces dramatic increases in the secretion of IFN-α and other cytokines from T and NK cells. In animal models, IL-12 injected systemically or locally into tumors, or secreted locally by fibroblasts, resulted in marked antitumor activity. Both T and NK cells may play important roles in this antitumor activity. Escalating doses of IL-12 have been administered to fifty-one patients with renal cell cancer, and resulted in increased systemic levels of IFN-γ: only modest therapeutic activity was observed (Motzer et al., 1998).

Several other cytokines including IL-15 and IL-18 are being evaluated in the clinic. Interleukin 15 may be of interest in cancer therapy because although it shares many functions with IL-2 (growth factor for lymphocytes) it does not lead to apoptosis of activated T cells. Memory T cells may also be induced with IL-15.

### 21.3.2 Adoptive Cellular Therapy

The immune rejection of cancers in animal models can be mediated by the *adoptive transfer* of sensitized lymphocytes. Studies of adoptive cellular therapy in murine models have established that (1) efficacy is dependent on the number of immune cells infused, (2) both fresh and cultured immune lymphocytes can mediate the effect, and (3) concomitant administration of IL-2 can

enhance the in vivo activity of adoptive cellular therapy (for review, see Ettinghausen and Rosenberg, 1995).

Lymphokine-activated killer cells, which are generated by culturing lymphocytes in IL-2 do not express B- or T-cell markers, but have been found to lyse nonspecifically autologous and allogeneic tumor cells but not normal untransformed cells. In vivo administration of LAK cells with IL-2 has reduced micrometastatic tumor burden in murine models of pulmonary metastases. These results prompted the assessment of adoptive immunotherapy with LAK cells and IL-2 in patients with cancer. Responses have been observed in patients with renal cell cancer or melanoma, and the overall results of studies involving more than 500 highly selected patients from eight phase II clinical trials show a response rate of approximately 22 percent in patients with metastatic renal cell cancer (for review, see Hoffman et al., 2000). Although the infusions of LAK cells were well tolerated, the systemic administration of high doses of IL-2 produced major toxicity, predominantly related to the development of a capillary leak syndrome. There have been three randomized trials comparing IL-2/LAK with IL-2 alone. The pooled results suggest that IL-2/LAK is no more effective therapeutically than IL-2 infusions alone.

Lymphocytes from tumors can be isolated by culturing dissociated tumor biopsies in IL-2. These tumor infiltrating lymphocytes TILs express CD3 and CD8 and lyse specifically cells in the tumor from which they are derived in an MHC-restricted fashion. They do not lyse cells from tumors in other patients. Studies in mice showed that TILs were approximately 50 to 100 times more effective than LAK cells in treating pulmonary micrometastases, and the combination of cyclophosphamide, TILs, and IL-2 could effectively treat macroscopic pulmonary metastases. Based on these results, TILs and IL-2 have been evaluated in patients with metastases from various cancers. The treatment may cause tumor regression, especially in patients with melanoma or renal cancer, and in single institution trials, response rates of up to 35 percent have been reported in patients with renal cell carcinoma (for review, see Hoffman et al., 2000).

### 21.3.3 Production of Monoclonal Antibodies

Kohler and colleagues (1976) showed that it was possible to stimulate hybridization between malignant plasma cells maintained in continuous culture and immune lymphoid cells. Hybrid cells that grew in culture and produced antibodies with the single defined specificity of the immune lymphoid cell could then be selected by cloning. The basic technique for production of such MAbs is shown in Figure 21.2. Spleen cells from an animal that has been immunized with foreign anti-

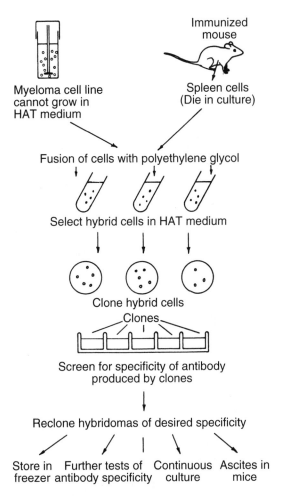

**Figure 21.2.** Schematic diagram indicating major steps in the production of monoclonal antibodies by hybridoma technology.

Monoclonal antibodies that recognize antigenic determinants on cells of human tumors of a given histologic type (e.g., melanoma-associated antigens) are now available for many types of tumors (see Table 21.1). These antibodies may react with the cells of normal tissues if these tissues also express these antigens. Monoclonal antibodies are important for diagnostic tests in cancer and recently have been used for cancer treatment.

Most MAbs have been made using rodent cell lines. This is a problem when they are used for treatment of human cancer because they are recognized as foreign proteins and elicit an immune response that leads to their rapid clearance and loss of activity or to anaphylactic reactions. This response is due to human antimouse antibodies (HAMA) and is referred to as the *HAMA response*. The strength of such a reaction might be decreased or even eliminated by using MAbs of human origin. Attempts to obtain stable hybridoma cultures by fusion of human lymphoid and mouse myeloma cells have been frustrated by selective loss of human chromosomes from the hybrid cells, with consequent failure to continue secretion of antibody. Problems have also been encountered in attempts to fuse human lymphoid cells with human myeloma cell lines. Future work in this area is required before human MAbs become a clinical entity.

Strategies which utilize molecular genetic techniques have been developed to produce human MAbs (Fig. 21.3). The first such approach involved generation of *chimeric antibodies* that have a constant region of human origin and a variable region of murine origin. These can be generated by molecular cloning of the hybridoma's heavy- and light-chain immunoglobulin genes and linking the variable region components to human heavy- and light-chain constant regions. Alternatively, utilizing the process of homologous recombination, the human heavy- and light-chain constant regions can be introduced into the hybridoma cells to replace the murine constant region. Another approach, termed *CDR engraftment*, involves cloning only the variable regions of the murine heavy and light chains that bind to antigen (the CDR 1, 2, and 3 regions) and replacing the corresponding human regions with these. A third strategy for producing human MAbs involves *phage display*, in which random recombinations of independently cloned heavy- and light-chain human immunoglobulin genes are expressed in λ or filamentous phage systems. These are then screened for binding to the target antigen, and selected phage can be expanded. Mice that contain large regions of unrearranged human immunoglobulin genes have also been generated by transgenic technology (Chap. 4, Sec. 4.3.12), while the endogenous murine heavy- and light-chain immunoglobulin loci were disrupted. Immunization and subsequent hybridoma generation produce hy-

gens are placed in culture with a continuously-growing myeloma cell line in the presence of polyethylene glycol to stimulate cell fusion. The myeloma line used in the experiments is a mutant that does not secrete immunoglobulin and has been selected for an enzyme deficiency that prevents its growth in medium containing hypoxanthine, aminopterin, and thymidine (HAT medium). The normal spleen cells cannot grow in culture; thus, only hybrid cells, formed by fusion, will grow in HAT medium because the missing enzyme is provided by the fused lymphoid spleen cell. After selection in HAT medium, hybrid cells are cloned by placing individual cells into single wells of a multiwell tissue-culture plate. Antibodies secreted by each clone of hybrid cells (known as a *hybridoma*) can then be tested for specificity—for example, by reactivity to cells expressing the antigens used for immunization but not to non-antigen expressing cells. Large quantities of MAbs may be obtained from supernatants of hybridoma cell cultures or by growing the hybridoma as an ascites tumor in mice. Hybrid cells can also be frozen and stored.

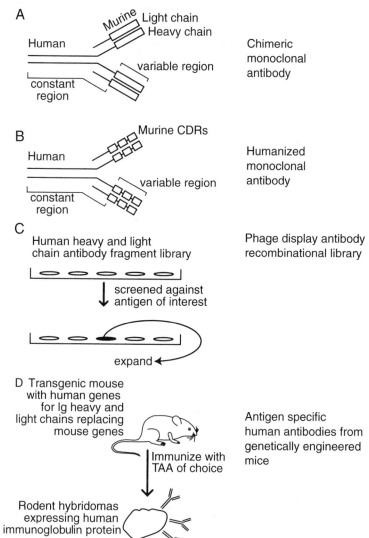

**Figure 21.3.** Strategies to generate human monoclonal antibodies. (*A*) Chimeric antibodies can be generated by recombinant genetic techniques where the gene fragments for the murine heavy- and light-chain immunoglobulin constant regions are replaced by the equivalent human gene fragments. (*B*) Humanized monoclonal antibodies can be generated by using recombinant genetic techniques to replace the regions for the human heavy- and light-chain CDR regions (which bind to antigen) with the corresponding murine CDR regions specific for a particular monoclonal antibody. (*C*) Recombinatorial phage display libraries for human heavy- and light-chain immunoglobulin proteins can be generated and screened for reactivity to a particular antigen. (*D*) Transgenic mice generated by deleting the endogenous heavy- and light-chain genes, and by introducing genomic material for human immunoglobulin heavy- and light-chain genes can be immunized to a particular tumor-associated antigen (TAA). Hybridomas can be generated by standard techniques and screened for reactivity to the antigen used for immunization.

bridomas secreting human immunoglobulin genes of the desired specificity (for review, see Morrison, 1994).

### 21.3.4 Immunotherapy with Monoclonal Antibodies

Monoclonal antibodies against tumor antigens can bind to their specific targets and mediate lysis of tumor cells either through complement-mediated lysis or antibody-dependent cellular cytotoxicity (ADCC). In ADCC, Fc-receptor–bearing effector cells such as NK cells, macrophages, or polymorphonuclear cells bind to the Fc part of the targeting MAb and lyse the tumor cell to which the antibody is bound. Monoclonal antibodies may also elicit anti-tumor activity by blocking a receptor for a growth factor that the cell depends upon for proliferation or by inducing apoptosis through direct intracellular signaling (Fig. 21.4).

Monoclonal antibodies recognizing surface determinants expressed on human cancer cells have been

tested for their therapeutic value in patients. A number of factors have been shown to limit the therapeutic effectiveness of MAbs in patients. These include tumor cell heterogeneity, antigenic cross-reactivity, antigenic modulation and shedding, ineffective tumor penetration, immune responses to the rodent protein, and defects in the host immune system (see Table 21.4).

The following approaches have been proposed to address some of the above problems and to enhance the therapeutic effectiveness of MAbs.

*Chimeric or Humanized Monoclonal Antibodies* Rodent-derived MAbs are less efficient than human MAbs in interacting with human effector cells and human complement. Also, rodent MAbs can trigger a HAMA response. To circumvent these problems, MAbs have been genetically engineered to contain either human constant regions (chimeric antibodies) or to be almost

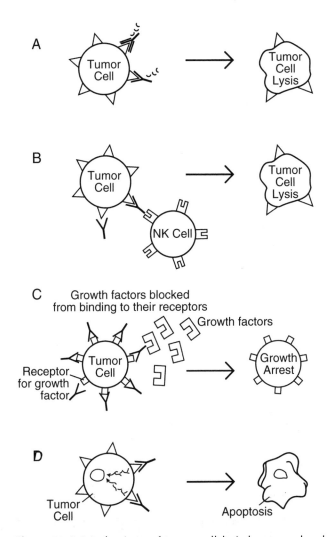

**Figure 21.4.** Mechanisms of tumor-cell lysis by monoclonal antibodies. Monoclonal antibodies can mediate tumor cell lysis by binding to their tumor target through the Fab part of the molecule and (A) activating the complement cascade through interactions mediated by the Fc regions of certain antibody isotypes, (B) interacting with the Fc receptors expressed on certain host effector cells (macrophages, natural killer cells, and polymorphonuclear leukocytes), (C) blocking the binding of certain important growth factors to their receptors expressed on some tumor types, and (D) generating an intracellular signal that activates a pathway to programmed cell death.

entirely human, containing only the murine variable region that recognizes the tumor antigen, as described in Section 21.3.3. Some of these chimeric or humanized antibodies have been or are being tested in phase I, II or III clinical studies, and results for some of the more promising monoclonal antibodies are described below.

*Rituximab* is a chimeric MAb directed against CD20 that is expressed at high levels on nearly all B-cell non-Hodgkin's lymphomas. It is not toxic to T cells, stem cells, or nonhematopoietic cells because they do not ex-

press CD20, and has a favorable toxicity profile. In a non-randomized clinical trial involving 166 patients with recurrent refractory low-grade non-Hodgkin's lymphoma, the overall response rate was 48 percent, with 6 percent complete responses with a median duration of about 12 months (McLaughlin et al., 1998). Serum levels of rituximab increased during the four infusions and could be detected up to 6 months posttreatment; there was an association between serum rituximab levels and response (Berinstein et al., 1998).

The therapeutic mechanisms of rituximab activity include ADCC, complement-mediated lysis, and direct effects on intracellular signaling. An association between FcR polymorphisms and response has been found. These polymorphisms result in different binding affinities of these receptors for the Fc region of IgG on macrophages and NK cells, which in turn alter the level of ADCC mediated by these cells. Loss of therapeutic activity has been documented in mice with deletion of the FcR where the ability to mediate ADCC was eliminated (Clynes et al., 2000). Evidence for direct effects of rituximab has been obtained using in vitro models where immunologic mechanisms have been eliminated. Also, in a randomized clinical trial where rituximab was combined with cytotoxic chemotherapy, about 15 percent improvement in overall survival was found at 2 years compared to the chemotherapy combination alone (Coiffier et al., 2002).

Studies with the *CAMPATH 1H* humanized monoclonal antibody, which recognizes the CDW52 antigen expressed on both B and T lymphocytes, have demonstrated activity in patients with chronic lymphocytic leukemia (CLL) and prolymphocytic leukemia (Dyer, 1999). However, the CAMPATH antibody produced prolonged lymphopenia, due to its effects on both B and T lymphocytes and was associated with a relatively high frequency of viral and opportunistic infections. There was also infusion-related toxicity associated with release of several cytokines, including IL-6, TNF-$\alpha$, and IFN-$\gamma$. Large trials are under way to evaluate the value of CAMPATH 1H in CLL and low-grade non-Hodgkin's lymphoma.

*Bevacizumab* is a humanized monoclonal antibody against vascular endothelial growth factor (VEGF), which targets the vasculature in human tumors (Chap. 12, Sec. 12.1.1). The agent has activity in preclinical models, and a randomized clinical trial has shown improved survival when used with chemotherapy to treat metastatic colorectal cancer (Hurwitz et al., 2004).

*Trastuzumab* is a humanized monoclonal antibody that recognizes the HER2/NEU protein (also known as ERB-B2), which is expressed on tumor cells of about 25 percent of patients with metastatic breast cancer, and also on those of some other epithelial tumors. When used alone trastuzumab leads to responses in about

**Table 21.4.** Strategies to Enhance the Efficacy of Therapy With Monoclonal Antibodies

| Factors Limiting the Efficacy of Monoclonal Antibody Therapy | Approach to Enhance Efficacy |
| --- | --- |
| Specificity of tumor antigen Tumor-cell heterogenicity | Identification of tumor-specific antigens Radiolabeled MAb |
| Antigenic cross-reactivity | Antibody specificity |
| Antigenic modulation and shedding | Antibody specificity |
| Tumor penetration | Radiolabeled MAb Cytokine enhancement |
| Immune response (HAMA) to rodent antibody | Chimeric/humanized MAb |
| Defects in the host immune system | Chimeric/humanized MAb Radiolabeled MAb Immunotoxins Cytokine enhancement Bispecific MAb |

15 percent of patients with breast cancer whose tumors express HER2/NEU. A randomized clinical trial has shown that this agent can lead to an increase in duration of survival when it is used with chemotherapy, as compared to the same type of chemotherapy used alone, although it may add cardiac toxicity (Slamon et al., 2001). Trastuzumab has been licensed for use in patients with metastatic breast cancer whose tumors overexpress the HER2/NEU protein.

*Cetuximab (C225, Erbitux)* The epidermal growth factor receptor (EGFR, also known as ERB-B1) is expressed on a wide variety of human epithelial tumors. Cetuximab, a chimeric antibody to EGFR, has shown antitumor activity in patients with a variety of EGFR–expressing solid cancers including lung, gastrointestinal, head and neck and colorectal cancers (Robert et al., 2001; Cunningham et al., 2004). As for molecules that inhibit signaling from the EGFR receptor, the major toxicity from IMC-C225 was a skin rash, presumably because of activity against EGFR expressed in the skin. Phase III trials evaluating IMC-C225 in combination with radiation therapy and chemotherapy are in progress.

*Edrecdomab* a monoclonal antibody recognizes the EP-CAM-1 (or KSA) cell surface adhesion molecule expressed at relatively high levels on most gastrointestinal cancers. This moncolonal antibody was associated with significant reductions in overall mortality and recurrence rate in a randomized clinical trial involving 189 patients with Dukes C colon carcinoma treated postoperatively (Riethmuller et al., 1998). Confirmatory trials are in progress.

*Radiolabeled Monoclonal Antibodies* Radioisotopes have been attached to MAbs for the targeted delivery of radiation to cancer cells (Fig. 21.5A). Antibody coupling has most frequently involved the use of long-range $\gamma$-emitting radioisotopes or $\beta$-emitters, such as iodine 131 ($^{131}$I), yttrium 90 ($^{90}$Y), and rhenium 186 ($^{186}$Re). Iodine 131 is both a $\beta$- and $\gamma$-emitter with a half-life of 8.1 days and a path length of 0.8 millimeters. Yttrium 90 is a pure $\beta$-emitter with a shorter half-life of 2.5 days but a longer path length of 5.3 millimeters. The shorter half-life and absence of $\gamma$-emission with $^{90}$Y permit use in outpatients because there is no exposure to others from the electrons emitted. With radiolabeled antibodies, the problems of tumor penetration, uneven tumor-cell binding, and host effector cell dysfunction are reduced, as cancer cells are killed by the radiation and not by the immune system. However, normal cells adjacent to tumor cells that have bound the antibody may be killed, as well as cells in sites of nonspecific MAb uptake (e.g., liver, bone marrow), and toxicities include myelosuppression. In addition, human anti-mouse antibody responses may also occur if Mabs are of murine origin, and thyroid toxicity can occur with radiolabeled iodine conjugates. Animal studies have shown that the dose of radiation delivered to tumor cells by a specific radiolabeled MAb is higher than that delivered by a nonspecific MAb.

In general, myeloablative or nonmyeloablative doses of the radiolabeled monoclonal antibodies may be administered. When myeloablative doses are administered as with $^{131}$I anti-B1 (B1 is expressed on mature B-cells) autologous stem cells must be administered to reconstitute bone marrow function because of nonspe-

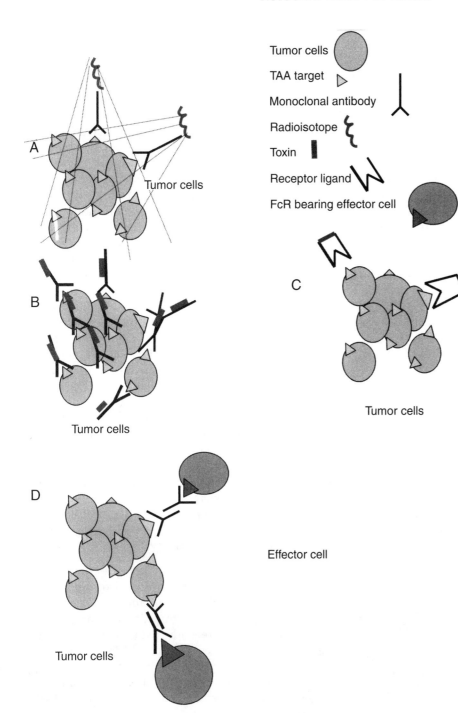

Tumor cells

TAA target

Monoclonal antibody

Radioisotope

Toxin

Receptor ligand

FcR bearing effector cell

A

Tumor cells

B

Tumor cells

C

Tumor cells

D

Effector cell

Tumor cells

**Figure 21.5.** Approaches to therapy using conjugated antibodies. (*A*) Radiolabeled monoclonal antibodies can induce cytolysis of cells that have not bound to the monoclonal antibody but that are within the path length of the radiation emitted. (*B* and *C*.) Immunotoxins must bind to the cell and be internalized to induce cytotoxicity. Toxins can be bound to either (*B*) a monoclonal antibody or (*C*) to a ligand that is internalized after binding to its receptor. (*D*) Bispecific antibodies consist of two antibodies or fragments of antibodies that are linked together by chemical or recombinant techniques. These bispecific antibodies can bind to both an effector cell that may mediate cytotoxicity and the specific target on a tumor cell.

cific toxicity to marrow. In contrast, bone marrow dysfunction is transient with nonmyeloablative doses of $^{90}$Y anti-CD20 (ibitumomab) or with $^{131}$I anti-B1 (tositumomab). High response rates with moderately durable remissions have been seen with nonmyeloablative doses of these agents (for review, see Dillman, 2002). With nonmyeloablative doses of $^{90}$Y anti-CEA, used to treat colorectal cancer, reversible thrombocytopenia and leukopenia were dose limiting and prevented the de-

livery of doses necessary to achieve a substantial frequency of objective tumor regressions.

*Immunotoxins* Immunoconjugates can selectively deliver various toxic agents to cancer cells (for review, see Kreitman, 1999). Cytotoxic drugs, such as doxorubicin, or plant or animal toxins, such as diptheria toxin or ricin, have been used (Fig. 21.5*B*). Toxins have binding domains, which allow binding to the target cell, followed by internalization, translocation to the cytosol, and subsequent catalytic inhibition of protein synthesis. When used as an immunoconjugate, the binding domain is usually removed or mutated so that nonspecific binding to cells other than the cancer cell will be prevented. The conjugation process is critical to prevent release of the cytotoxic molecule into the serum, which would result in nonspecific toxicity. Nonspecific uptake of the immunoconjugate may occur in normal tissues, such as the reticuloendothelial system, which can bind antibodies nonspecifically through their Fc receptors.

The choice of monoclonal antibody for immunoconjugates is important and must target specific cell surface antigens that internalize upon binding. As an alternative to monoclonal antibodies, ligands specific for receptors on cancer cells can be utilized (see Fig. 21.5C). Thus, IL-2 has been used to target malignancies of T cells that express the IL-2 receptor, and epidermal growth factor (EGF) to target the EGFR that is overexpressed in many types of cancer. DAB389 IL2 (Oncotac) consisting of IL-2 fused to the first 388 amino acids of diptheria toxin is the first immunotoxin approved by the U.S. Food and Drug Administration and is used for the treatment of recurrent cutaneous T-cell lymphoma. At the preclinical level, highly specific isoforms to VEGF have been utilized to target tumor vasculature (Wild et al., 2000).

*Enhancement of Effector Function of Monoclonal Antibodies With Cytokines or Other Immunologic Reagents* Studies in animals have shown that concomitant infusions of cytokines, such as IFN-$\alpha$, IL-2, or GM-CSF can increase the effectiveness of treatment with MAbs. These cytokines increase the number and activity of effector cells, including NK cells, and enhance their ability to mediate antibody-dependent cellular cytotoxicity. A recent phase II clinical trial suggested that IFN-$\alpha$ could increase the duration of responses seen with the anti-CD20 monoclonal antibody rituximab. Preclinical results have shown that hypomethylated bacterial derived CpG sequences can also enhance the therapeutic activity of monoclonal antibodies. CpGs are DNA sequences randomly found unmethylated in the genome of bacteria, which have been shown to activate the innate arm of the immune system by binding to the Toll-like receptor 9 expressed on dendritic cells and other cells, such as NK cells. Clinical trials to evaluate the combination of CpGs and rituximab are in progress.

*Bispecific Monoclonal Antibodies* Two antibodies that recognize different specificities can be linked together by chemical or recombinant genetic techniques (Fig. 21.5D). Thus, it is possible to link an antibody recognizing a TAA to an antibody that can target or activate a particular subset of effector cells. Although chemical conjugation was used initially, this approach resulted in unstable reagents. Genetic engineering overcomes these problems and can result in high yields of bispecific antibodies (for review, see Kriangkum et al., 2001).

Use of bispecific antibodies may help to overcome cancer-related immunosuppression and can target specific effector cells to the tumor. Such approaches have been shown to be both effective and specific in vitro and in mice. For example, bispecific antibodies made up of an anti-IL-2 receptor MAb linked to an anti-CD3 antibody can bind to peripheral blood mononuclear T cells and lyse specifically tumor cells expressing the IL-2 receptor (Xiong et al., 2002). Several other bispecific antibodies have been evaluated in preclinical studies, including an anti-CD20 x anti-CD3, and a series of recombinant bispecific antibodies with anti-CD3 linked to the HER-2/NEU receptor (Maletz et al., 2001). These studies have shown specific lysis of various epithelial tumor lines using peripheral blood mononuclear cells or bone marrow derived mononucleur cells as effectors.

Bispecific antibodies are being tested in clinical trials. In a phase II trial, twenty-five patients with HER2/NEU positive advanced prostate cancer were treated with the MDX-210 antibody, which consists of an anti-HER2/NEU antibody chemically conjugated to anti-CD64 (high affinity type 1 Fc-$\gamma$ receptor). Patients also received recombinant subcutaneous GM-CSF to enhance monocyte- and granulocyte-mediated antibody-dependent cellular cytotoxicity, and PSA responses and reduction in bone pain were reported (James et al., 2001).

## 21.4 ACTIVE IMMUNOTHERAPY

Active immunotherapy involves strategies designed to generate an anti-tumor response in vivo. The earliest approaches included immunization with lethally-damaged tumor cells or with protein or peptide epitopes of TAAs. More recently, plasmid DNA or viruses encoding TAAs have been employed for active immunization. Other strategies have included gene therapy to enhance the immunogenicity of the tumor or the use of antigen-presenting cells, such as dendritic cells, to present TAAs to the host immune system.

### 21.4.1 Generation of an Immune Response Against Tumors

Most tumor cells do not have all of the required characteristics to be able to stimulate a primary immune response. In order to prime an immune response, TAAs from the tumor cell must be presented on either MHC class I or class II complexes on formal antigen presenting cells (APCs; see Fig. 20.3) as described in Chapter 20, Section 20.5.1 (for review, see Thery and Amigorena, 2001). In contrast, secreted products from tumor cells will enter the cell through endosomes and eventually be processed and presented on MHC class II molecules. Processed antigens presented on class I MHC will be recognized by CD8$^+$ cytotoxic T lymphocytes and those presented on MHC class II will be recognized by CD4$^+$ T helper lymphocytes. These T helper lymphocytes can differentiate into either a TH1 or TH2 phenotype with the TH1 phenotype secreting cytokines (IL-2 and IFN-$\gamma$) that will promote CTL activity, whereas the TH2 phenotype will secrete cytokines (IL-4 and IL-10) that will support B-cell class switching and a humoral response. Whereas CD8$^+$ CTLs may have a direct cytotoxic effect on the tumor cells, the CD4 cells may both enhance the CD8 response and facilitate the development of a humoral response to surface antigens expressed on the tumor cell. For these priming responses to occur, the antigen-presenting cells must provide second signals to the T cells mediated by the B7 family of costimulatory molecules. In addition, these responses may be damped by various degrees of tolerance that may be induced to many TAAs, which are mostly auto-antigens that may become dysregulated through the transformation process (see Chap. 20, Secs. 20.2, 20.3, and 20.4).

Both CD4$^+$ and CD8$^+$ T-cells, and B cells, can be activated in the immune response against a tumor, and all of these cells may play important roles in the anti-tumor response. Immunoglobulins secreted by plasma cells derived from B lymphocytes have been shown to bind to many antigens expressed on tumor cells. These antibodies, like monoclonal antibodies directed at various cell surface antigens, can mediate anti-tumor activity in preclinical and clinical studies. They use a variety of effector mechanisms, including complement-mediated lysis, antibody-dependent cellular cytotoxicity, direct induction of apoptotic pathways, and interference with autocrine signaling pathways that mediate cell proliferation. However, antibodies can only be effective in anti-tumor immunity by binding to antigens expressed on the cell surface, which limits their anti-tumor activity.

In many preclinical studies, the induction of CTLs recognizing processed and presented antigenic epitopes from tumor cells is associated with anti-tumor activity. Human CD8$^+$ T cells have also been shown to recognize processed and presented MHC class I epitopes from many different TAAs. Further induction of human CD8$^+$ T cells by various different anticancer active vaccination strategies has been associated with anti-tumor activity in several clinical trials (e.g., Nestle et al., 1998; Rosenberg et al., 1998). Thus, there is evidence that CD8$^+$ T cells play a role in mediating anti-tumor activity in humans.

CD4$^+$ T helper cells are also important in the immune response to cancer (Hung et al., 1998; Wang, 2001). These cells may optimize the CTL response by secreting important immune-modulatory cytokines and may also optimize signaling through antigen-presenting cells. They may provide memory responses and extend the CD8$^+$ response. Results from a B16 melanoma model have shown that tumor rejection requires CD4$^+$ T lymphocytes at the effector stage of the rejection (Hung et al., 1998; Wang 2001). There are preclinical data in several different models where anti-tumor immune responses are mediated primarily by these cells. The role of T helper cells in the anti-tumor response in humans has not yet been defined, although there is increasing evidence that some of the cytokines secreted by these cells (i.e., IL-2) may be required to maintain effective anti-tumor memory and cytotoxic responses.

In summary, for intracellular TAAs CD8$^+$ CTLs are probably the primary immune effector cells but the activity and longevity of these cells can be enhanced by CD4$^+$ T helper cell activation. For cell surface TAAs, both CTL and humoral responses may mediate anti-tumor activity, since CD8$^+$ CTLs and the CD4$^+$ T helper cells are required to promote the generation of an effective humoral response.

### 21.4.2 Monitoring the T-Cell Response

Although methods for quantitating humoral responses to various antigens are well established, only recently have quantitative assays been established for measuring the T-cell response to an antigen (Table 21.5). These approaches include in vivo and in vitro methods and the latter involve both phenotypic and functional assays (for review, see Clay et al., 2001).

The most frequently utilized in vivo approach is delayed-type hypersensitivity (DTH) skin testing. This involves injecting soluble antigen intradermally and measuring the diameter of the erythema and induration 48 to 72 hours later. Delayed-type hypersensitivity testing is easy to perform and is useful as a general screen of immune responsiveness. There is some correlation between the DTH response and clinical outcome. It is important to supplement the results of DTH testing with more detailed and specific immunologic analysis.

Phenotypic in vitro assessments include T-cell receptor (TCR) V gene utilization (see Chap. 20, Sec. 20.2.4) and tetramer analysis. T-cell receptor V gene utilization refers to the analysis of the TCR $\beta$ or $\alpha$ genes selected by T-cell clones that respond and expand in response to the developing tumor. Limited repertoires of these gene segments may be selected for rearrangement of the antigen receptor in the responding T lymphocytes and these may be documented by flow cytometry (Chap. 9, Sec. 9.4.2) or by the polymerase chain reaction (Chap. 4, Sec. 4.3.5). The analysis of TCR V gene uti-

**Table 21.5.** In Vitro Assays to Monitor T-cell Activation

|            |                         | In Vitro Culture | T-cell Assessed  |
|------------|-------------------------|------------------|------------------|
| Phenotype  | V gene utilization      | No               | CD4, CD8         |
|            | Tetramers               | No               | CD8 (some CD4)   |
| Functional | Lymphocyte proliferation| +++              | CD4, CD8         |
|            | Bulk cytokine           | +++              | CD4, CD8         |
|            | Intracellular cytokine  | Overnight        | CD4, CD8         |
|            | ELISPOT                 | +/++             | CD4, CD8         |

+, ++, +++: Variable lengths of culture required.

lization has several limitations because the immune response to an antigen or to multiple antigens may involve several clones of T cells and for most tumors, TCRs involved in the response have not been characterized. Also, monoclonal antibodies that recognize many specific forms of the TCR are not yet available.

Tetramers are reagents that are designed to quantitate the frequency of T cells that express a receptor (TCR) that can bind a particular MHC-peptide complex and thus provide a very specific assessment of the potential T-cell response to a TAA. They are fluorophor-conjugated complexes involving four MHC class I heavy/light chain molecules and a class I binding peptide of choice (Altman et al., 1996; Fig. 21.6). Tetramers can be analyzed by flow cytometry and, with multiparameter analyses, the phenotypic profile and state of activation of the antigen-specific T cells can be determined. A limitation is that the function of the im-

**Figure 21.6.** Use of tetrameric MHC class I molecules to quantitate T cells that recognize processed and presented tumor-associated antigens. (*A*) Tetramers consist of complexes of a heavy chain of MHC class I molecules, β2 microglobulin, and MHC I binding peptide epitopes derived from particular tumor-associated antigens. These complexes are biotinylated and four such molecules combine to form tetrameric molecules by binding to avidin. These complexes can be linked to a fluorochrome. A complex consisting of four β2 microglobulin, heavy-chain, and peptide fragments linked to the fluorochrome will bind to T cells with the appropriate T-cell receptor for the class I/peptide complex. Tetramers can be quantitated by flow cytometry to measure the frequency of T cells responsive to a particular tumor-associated antigen. (*B*) Flow cytometry profiles showing the increase in frequency of CD8+ T cells recognizing tetramers containing a gp100 class I binding epitope (inset box). Gp 100 is a tumor-associated antigen in a high percentage of malignant melanomas. A significant increase in such T cells was seen after administration of a vaccine containing gp100 in patients with melanoma.

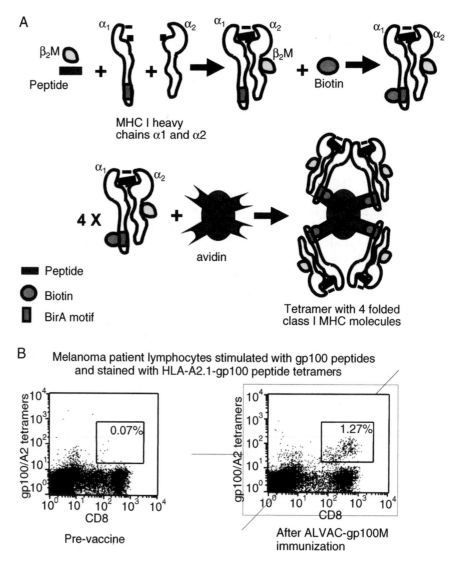

mune effector cells is not assessed and there have been examples where tetramer-positive cells are unable to lyse the cells bearing the target antigen. However, tetramer-positive cells can be sorted and analyzed further in functional assays.

There are four major types of functional assays that have been utilized for immune monitoring in cancer trials. Lymphocyte proliferation assays usually measure the CD4$^+$ T helper response. In these assays, purified T cells or peripheral blood mononuclear cells (PBMC) are incubated with the protein form of the target antigen and proliferation is assessed after different periods of incubation. The assay is relatively direct and the cells do not need to be incubated in vitro for prolonged periods with the antigen. However, measurement of proliferation of helper T cells may not have direct relevance to an anti-tumor effect and this assay may not correlate with the frequency of functionally-activated T lymphocytes. A variation on the lymphocyte proliferation assay involves harvesting the supernatant rather than the cells after the incubation period. This supernatant can then be assessed by ELISA (enzyme-linked immunoadsorbant) assays for the levels of various cytokines. This method is of limited value because it does not quantitate the number of responsive T cells nor does it define the in vivo cytokine profile of the cells because of the in vitro incubation period.

Intracellular cytokine measurements can be undertaken by multi-parameter flow cytometry following a brief in vitro incubation period (4 to 6 h) in the presence of antigen, where brefeldin A is added during the last 3 to 4 hours to prevent secretion of the cytokines (Picker et al., 1995). Information on the subset of T helper cells can be obtained from their cytokine expression profile. Serial analyses have been undertaken in a few clinical studies and have shown a correlation with clinical outcome. Samples for analysis can be obtained from multiple sites including tumor, lymph node, and/or peripheral blood. The major limitation of this approach is that the cells are no longer viable because they are permeabilized, and cannot be used for functional analyses. Newer modifications of this approach may allow preservation of the viability of the cells.

The gold standard for functional detection of T-cell activation is the ELISPOT (enzyme-linked immunospot) assay (Schmittel et al., 2000; Whiteside, 2000). In this assay, a microtiter plate is coated with an antibody to a cytokine of choice (e.g., IFN-γ; Fig. 21.7). Stimulator APC exposed to or expressing the antigen/epitope of choice are then added. Peripheral blood mononuclear cells are incubated with these cells on the plate. After varying lengths of time the plate is developed by washing the cells and adding a labeled second antibody to detect the antibody-cytokine complex. The length of in-

cubation is an important variable and serves to amplify the response to weakly immunogenic epitopes. Each spot represents one cytokine-secreting T cell, and their frequency can be determined by dividing the number of spots by the number of cells in each well. This assay is quantitative and results correlate with the function of cytotoxic T cells.

There have been reports of a correlation between the ELISPOT assay and clinical outcome. For example, in a trial of a polyvalent cellular melanoma vaccine, an improvement in recurrence-free survival was documented in patients who had increases in ELISPOT reactivity post immunization (Reynolds et al., 1997). However, increases in ELISPOT activity are not always associated with improved outcome (e.g., Marchand et al., 1999; Nielsen and Marincola, 2000).

A possible reason for the variability in results is that the threshold level of T cells required to mount an immune rejection response is not known. In a murine tumor cell model, infusion of $1 \times 10^4$ T cells specific for a target on the tumor cells (representing up to 0.5% of the circulating T cells) was required to mediate rejection of an established sarcoma (Hanson et al., 2000). Infusion of $10^7$ ml CD8$^+$ T cells specific for Epstein-Barr virus (representing 1% of the circulating T lymphocytes) could reduce the viral load by two to three logs and eradicate EBV$^+$ lymphoproliferation in patients (Rooney et al., 1998). Prospective trials will be required to determine whether a level of threshold reactivity in ELISPOT assays correlates with clinical outcome.

### 21.4.3 Protein and Peptide Immunogens

Tumor-associated antigens (TAAs) may be used in a variety of strategies as relatively specific protein immunogens for anti-tumor vaccines (Fig. 21.8). Effective and specific anti-tumor responses can be induced in animals. For example, injection of the purified immunoglobulin idiotype protein expressed on murine B-cell lymphomas was able to induce protection of animals from subsequent challenge with tumor and some animals with pre-existing tumors could be cured (Campbell et al., 1989; George and Stevenson, 1989). The activity of these vaccines has been associated with the development of high titers of anti-idiotype antibodies, and idiotype-specific CD4$^+$ T cells have also been detected. In these experiments, the idiotype protein was administered with an immune adjuvant and was often coupled to a carrier protein to enhance its immunogenicity.

Protein TAAs can be prepared in several ways for use in patients (Fig. 21.8). Supernatants containing antigen shed from the tumor cells have been used in patients with melanoma and have resulted in the induction of

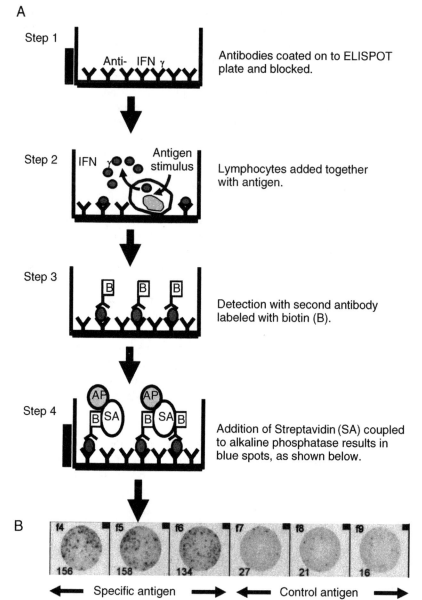

**Figure 21.7.** ELISPOT assays are used to quantitate the frequency of T cells that recognize a particular tumor-associated antigen MHC class I binding epitope. (*A*) In this assay, a polystyramine plate is coated with antibodies that bind to a cytokine such as interferon γ (IFN-γ). Antigen-presenting cells, of a particular MHC type, are loaded on to the plate along with a peptide epitope for that particular MHC type. Subsequently, T cells are added to the plates and after addition of a biotinylated antibody to IFN-γ, spots are formed where T cells recognizing the MHC/peptide epitope were located. (*B*) Quantitation. The spots can be counted and the frequency of T cells recognizing a particular MHC/peptide epitope can be quantitated.

both cellular and humoral responses. Tumor-cell lysates, purified proteins, or glycoproteins have been used as immunogens. Often, as with the polyvalent ganglioside vaccines for melanoma, multiple TAAs are included in the vaccine preparation. Conjugation to a carrier, such as keyhole limpet hemocyanin (KLH), or addition of an adjuvant, such as bacillus Calmette-Guérin (BCG), may enhance the activity of the vaccine. Recombinant genetic techniques have been used to synthesize TAAs. For example, a fusion protein between the idiotype protein of B-cell lymphomas and GM-CSF generated an anti-idiotype humoral response and protection against tumor challenge without the need for carrier proteins or adjuvant (Tao and Levy, 1993).

Immune responses and prolonged remission have been documented in patients with B-cell lymphoma treated with idiotype protein conjugated to KLH generated by either hybridoma fusion or recombinant methodologies (Hsu et al., 1997; Bendandi et al., 1999). High titer humoral responses occurred only if the protein was first coupled to the immunogenic carrier KLH. Two multicenter phase III trials have been initiated to determine whether idiotype vaccination can enhance survival in patients with indolent lymphoma after responding to first-line combination chemotherapy.

In another approach, antibodies (called Ab1s) generated to a particular antigen can induce the generation of another set of antibodies (Ab2s) that may struc-

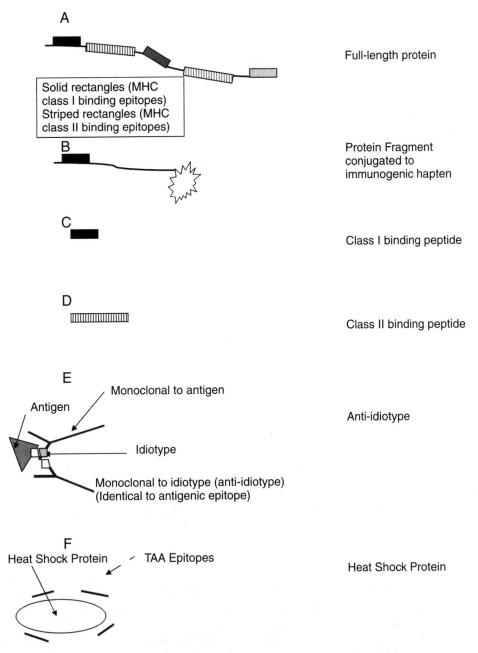

**Figure 21.8.** Different approaches to utilize protein immunogens for cancer therapy. (*A* and *B*) Whole proteins or fragments of proteins can be used to vaccinate against TAAs. These soluble proteins will be taken up by the endosome and processed through the MHC class II pathway and result in T helper cell activation. Immunogenicity can be enhanced by linking the fragment to an immunogenic hapten such as KLH. (*C*) MHC Class I binding epitopes can be generated from a tumor associated antigen and used to activate a CD8+ CTL response. (*D*) MHC Class II binding epitopes can be synthesized from a TAA and used to facilitate the activation of a CD4+ T helper cell response. (*E*) Anti-idiotype proteins are mirror images of the antigen-binding end of an antibody to the antigen and can be used to generate antibodies that bind to the initial TAA as described in the text. (*F*) Heat shock proteins are complexes containing tumor associated antigen epitopes that are effective in accessing an MHC class I pathway and activating CD8+ CTL responses.

turally resemble the antibody-binding component of the original antigen (Chatterjee et al., 1994). These anti-idiotype antibodies, in turn, can induce a third set of antibodies (called Ab3s), which may bind to the original antigen and mediate an anti-tumor response. Thus, Ab2 antibodies can be used for vaccination purposes. In mice, humoral and cellular anti-tumor activity has been induced by this technique against established sarcomas and L1210 murine leukemia cells. Early studies have demonstrated specificity and immunogenicity using Ab2s to the Gp37 antigen on acute lymphoblastic leukemias and cutaneous T-cell lymphomas, to CEA on colon carcinomas, to melanoma-associated proteoglycan (MPG), and to several other TAAs expressed on solid tumors. A phase III clinical trial is in progress with the Ab2 to CEA, and preliminary results have demonstrated the induction of anti-tumor Ab3 and proliferative T-cell responses (for review, see Foon and Bhattacharya-Chatterjee, 2001).

Another approach to tumor vaccination makes use of the observation that tumor-derived heat-shock proteins (HSPs) could induce specific immunity directed at the tumor from which they were isolated (Srivastava, 2002). Heat-shock proteins, such as HSPgp96 or HSP70, bind a broad array of peptides derived from several hundred cellular proteins, and anti-tumor immunity elicited by HSPs is lost when these peptides are eluted from the HSP. The mechanism of the anti-tumor response involves macrophages and CD8$^+$ CTLs, because depletion of these subsets in the priming phase abrogates the anti-tumor response elicited by HSPgp96. T-cells may recognize the peptide fragments of TAAs presented on surface-expressed HSPs. Approaches using HSPs to elicit anti-tumor immunity might involve immunization with tumor-derived HSPs or immunization with an HSP mixed with peptides generated from a common TAA, such as MAGE1 (Moroi et al., 2000).

It is possible to predict the peptide sequences (or epitopes) from protein TAAs that are expected to bind to certain MHC class I or II complexes. Also, using mass spectrographic approaches, processed peptides can be eluted from these complexes. These epitopes can be sequenced and subsequently synthesized and used in therapeutic cancer vaccines. When injected, these epitopes are expected to bind to MHC complexes on APCs and stimulate the activation of T cells that recognize the TAA from which they were derived.

Boon and his colleagues have synthesized nonamer peptides from the MAGE 1 and 3 antigens, shown to bind to HLA A1, and these have been injected into patients with metastatic melanoma. Although they were unable to document increases in T cells recognizing MAGE 1 or 3 in the peripheral blood of these patients, objective clinical responses were seen in some patients (Marchand et al., 1999). Rosenberg and colleagues syn-thesized nonamer peptides from the GP100 antigen expressed in melanomas and these were further modified by changing the amino acid sequence to enhance binding to HLA A2. These modified peptides were better able to activate specific T cells than the nonmodified peptides. In combination with infusion of IL-2, these peptide vaccines mediated clinical regressions of approximately 40 percent of patients with melanoma (Rosenberg et al., 1998). Similarly, longer peptides able to bind to MHC class II complex have been shown to increase T helper cell responses to HER2/NEU in patients with breast cancer (Disis and Schiffman, 2001).

## 21.4.4 DNA and Viral Immunogens

The ability to introduce DNA into cells in vivo has prompted the development of immunization approaches using purified plasmid DNA (for review, see Haupt et al., 2002). DNA can be introduced into muscle, epithelial or other cells by injection or bombardment with microparticles, often gold, coated with DNA (Fig. 21.9). The particles and DNA enter the cytosol and cells that have taken up these microparticles express the genetic material encoded on the plasmid. DNA not taken up by cells is degraded by nucleases present in serum and tissue fluids. In muscle cells, expression of the plasmid DNA has been documented for up to 1 year. In studies using DNA encoding for influenza A hemagglutinin, both humoral and cell-mediated responses comparable to the responses seen after influenza A virus infection can be generated (Ulmer et al., 1993).

The direct injection of plasmid DNA encoding HIV Gp160 induced protective anti-tumor responses against a murine myeloma cell line that had been transfected with this antigen (Wang et al., 1993). Humoral responses were generated and were thought to mediate the anti-tumor response. Anti-tumor responses against established adenocarcinomas expressing the $\beta$-gal TAA have been elicited by gold-coated plasmid DNA encoding $\beta$-gal administered intradermally. Splenocytes from immunized mice were able to produce an anti-tumor effect after transfer to other syngeneic mice (Irvine et al., 1996). Co-administration of cytokines (particularly IL-12) enhanced the anti-tumor activity. However, activity in clinical trials has been minimal.

Peripheral T-cell tolerance to carcino-embryonic antigen (CEA) can be broken in CEA transgenic mice by immunization with an oral DNA vector that was derivied from *Salmonella typhimurium* encoding CEA (Xiang et al., 2001). In these mice the CEA is expressed throughout embryonic development and thus immunologic tolerance to CEA is induced (Chap. 20, Sec. 20.5.1). Such mice may provide conditions relevant to

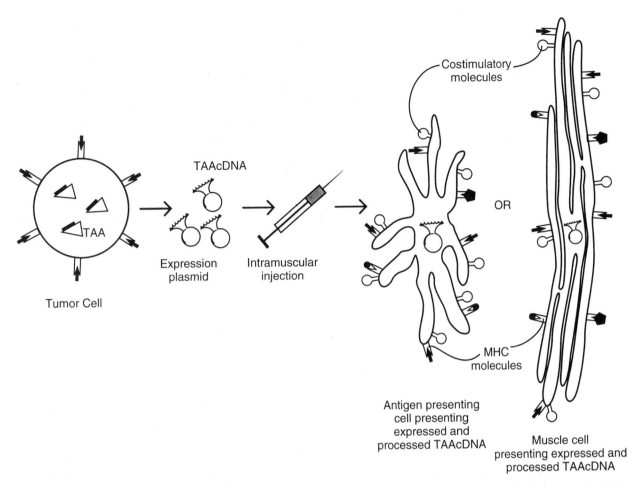

**Figure 21.9.** Active immunotherapy with DNA immunogens derived from TAAs. The cDNA encoding a particular TAA, isolated by recombinant techniques, or the cDNA encoding a known common TAA, is cloned into an expression plasmid. This is then injected intramuscularly or subcutaneously into the patient without the requirement for an adjuvant. The cDNA is taken up by muscle or antigen-presenting cells and the encoded protein is processed and presented on MHC molecules for T-cell activation.

spontaneous tumors where most TAAs are self-antigens and some degree of tolerance has been induced. The protective effect was mediated by CD8[+] T cells. Similarly, CTL were induced with a salmonella DNA vector encoding hGp100 and protective immunity was found against B16 murine melanoma cells expressing human Gp100 (Cochlovius et al., 2002).

The type of immune response to a DNA vaccine can be modulated by the inclusion of genes that encode cytokines. A DNA-based vaccine encoding PSA induced both a cellular and a humoral response when innoculated into macaques. When inoculated together with a cDNA construct that encoded IL-2, the humoral response to PSA was augmented and when inoculated together with IL-12, the humoral response was reduced (Kim et al., 2001). Proliferation of T helper cells in mice was stimulated by coadministration of plasmids containing IL-2, IL-12, and IL-20.

DNA might be valuable in inducing immune responses to viral proteins expressed in virally induced tumors such as HPV-associated cervical cancer or dysplasia. These lesions are associated with HPV types, such as 16 and 18, and express the viral E6 and E7 transforming proteins (Chap. 6, Sec. 6.2.3). In animal models vaccination with a DNA vaccine encoding E7 fused to sequences for the lysosome-associated membrane protein (thus targeting the E7 to the lysosome for degradation) was effective in controlling liver and lung metastases (Chen et al., 2000). Various DNA vaccines against HPV are being evaluated in clinical trials.

Viruses have also been used to introduce TAAs for the purposes of vaccination. Probably the most studied vector system for this purpose has been the canary-pox virus Alvac, which can accommodate large and multiple inserts (see Sec. 21.2.2). The virus cannot replicate in humans and thus has a very high safety profile. Several phase I trials using the canary-pox vector engineered to express CEA with or without the costimulatory molecule B7.1 have been reported. These trials have shown that the vaccine is safe and can induce increased frequency of specific T cells recognizing CEA in the majority of patients receiving the vaccine (Horig et al., 2000; von Mehren et al., 2000). Randomized trials are required to document the therapeutic activity of these vaccines.

### 21.4.5 Immunization with Tumor Cells

Immunization with autologous or allogeneic tumor cells (which have usually received a lethal dose of radiation), either with or without a nonspecific adjuvant, has been used to elicit an enhanced immune response against tumors. Many such experiments have been performed in animal models and clinical trials have been conducted in cancer patients, especially those with melanoma and renal cancer. Because autologous tumor cells share the same MHC complexes as the cells of the patient's immune system, they may act as APCs. However, with allogeneic tumor cell vaccines, the tumor cells are not likely to share the same MHC haplotypes as the patient so this rarely occurs. Two mechanisms could explain T-cell activation by these allogeneic tumor cells. First, tumor cells might activate T cells by behaving as APCs and presenting TAAs on any shared histocompatibility complexes that may be present. Second, the allogeneic cells could either be broken down in vivo, or secrete TAAs on components known as exosomes, and the TAAs could then be processed and presented on self-MHC molecules after phagocytosis by host antigen-presenting cells. This mechanism is termed cross-priming and is probably the most important explanation for the immunogenicity of allogenic cellular

vaccines. Cross-priming is dependent on a functional TAP transporter system to mediate antigen processing and presentation (Huang et al., 1996; Fig. 21.10; see also Chap. 20, Sec. 20.2.6).

The use of a common allogeneic vaccine (e.g., pooled melanoma cells) has the advantage that it can be mass produced and made easily available (for review, see Safa and Foon, 2001). A major disadvantage is that the vaccine may not contain TAAs expressed on the recipient patient's melanoma. A large number of patients with melanoma has been treated with an irradiated melanoma cell vaccine derived from three melanoma cell lines. The polyvalent melanoma cell vaccine (PMCV) contains a number of melanoma antigens including the gangliosides GM2, GD2, and Gd3, MAGE 1, MAGE 3, MART 1, tyrosinase, gp100, and gp75 and HLA types that would cover more than 95 percent of the population (Chan and Morton, 1998). The vaccine was injected intradermally (initially with BCG) and induced delayed-type hypersensitivity and IgM responses. Some tumor responses were reported, as well as unexpectedly long survival in some patients, but randomized clinical trials are required to document the therapeutic efficacy of the vaccine.

A randomized clinical trial in patients has been completed with another type of allogeneic cellular melanoma lysate vaccine containing the antigens, tyrosinase, gp100 and MART-1, but not Mage-1. In this trial, the vaccine combined with cyclophosphamide was compared to combination chemotherapy including dacarbazine, cisplatin, carmustine, and tamoxifen. No significant differences in response rates or survival were seen although there were fewer side effects in the vaccine arm (Mitchell, 1998).

To increase the immunogenicity of allogeneic cellular vaccines, nucleus-free cell lysates were made of four

**Figure 21.10.** T-cell activation by cross-presentation. Allogeneic tumor cells can activate T cells by two different pathways. (*A*) In the first pathway the allogeneic tumor cell undergoes apoptosis and the apoptotic bodies are processed and presented by the host antigen-presenting cells. This will result in cross-presentation of the processed TAA on the MHC proteins of the host. (*B*) In the second pathway, exosomes secreted by the foreign allogeneic tumor cells will be taken up by host antigen-presenting cells, processed and presented through a predominantly class II pathway and activate host cytotoxic T cells.

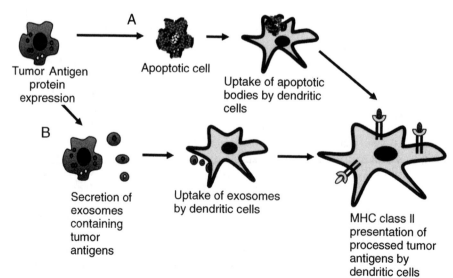

vaccinia virus infected cell lines and used as a vaccine—termed *vaccinia melanoma oncolysate* (VMO). Although an initial phase II trial showed responses, a subsequent double-blind randomized phase III trial of 217 stage III melanoma patients treated with either VMO or vaccinia alone showed no improvement in disease-free or overall survival (Wallack et al., 1998).

Autologous cellular vaccines (i.e., those prepared from the patient's own tumor cells) may have advantages over allogeneic vaccines. These vaccines will contain all of the TAAs found in the patient's tumors and these vaccines will express the patient's own MHC types to allow presentation of processed TAAs to the immune system. However, it is difficult to make clinical-grade vaccines individually for each patient. Also, unless modified or injected with an adjuvant, these vaccines may not be able to overcome tolerance which has developed to the patient's own tumor cells. Autologous vaccines have been studied as adjuvant treatments following surgery in stage II and III colorectal cancer. Three randomized trials have been completed using an autologous vaccine administered with BCG as an adjuvant. In a trial involving 412 patients with stage II and III colon cancer, no significant differences in survival were found, although better disease-free survival and overall survival was seen in patients found to have an increased DTH response to the vaccine (Harris et al., 2000). In another phase III trial, improvements in disease-free survival but not overall survival were seen in patients with stage II colon cancer (Vermorken et al., 1999).

Active immunotherapy has led to tumor responses in many transplantable animal tumors, usually when immunization is applied either before tumor transplantation or when the tumor burden is low. Unfortunately, the results of tumor-cell vaccination seen in preclinical animal models have not translated into effective clinical treatments. The animal tumors may not be ideal models for human cancer for the following reasons: (1) genetic drift of the cell lines, and of the animals into which they are implanted, may lead to effects that are due to transplantation antigens rather than to TAAs; (2) prevention of tumor outgrowth by vaccination in an animal model is not analogous to inducing regression of established tumors in patients; (3) the immune system of a patient with an extensive and progressive cancer (and after immunosuppressive chemo- and radiation therapies) may not be as responsive to active immunotherapeutic approaches as that of a healthy murine immune system. The strategies used in patients may not be sufficient to reverse the tolerance that has been induced by the tumor. Because tumor cell lysates include the entire repertoire of antigens expressed by the cell, there may be competition between different TAAs and self-antigens, which may dilute the required immune response. Future trials should integrate vaccine therapy with other therapies shown to be effective in the mangement of the cancer and/or be evaluated as adjuvant therapy in patients with minimal disease.

### 21.4.6 Genetically-Modified Tumor Cells

The introduction of cytokine genes into tumor cells that possess TAAs will result in the local secretion of specific cytokines; this should enhance the activation of immunoreactive lymphocytes, and this activation might be sufficient to eliminate unmodified tumor cells (Fig. 21.11). Moreover, the local delivery of a cytokine should eliminate the common major toxicities associated with the high systemic doses of cytokines that are often required to mediate immune activation.

Many experimental studies have evaluated the anti-tumor effects of various cytokines introduced into tumor cells. Genetically modified tumor cells, often irradiated, are introduced into syngeneic mice to determine whether the expressed cytokine gene can induce an anti-tumor immune response against the unmodified tumor cells. Experiments to identify the cell types that mediate the anti-tumor response may include deletion of various host effector-cell subsets to test their importance, or in vitro assessments of lymphocyte proliferation or cytotoxic T lymphocyte activity. Anti-tumor activity has been documented in murine models evaluating tumor cells genetically modified with a variety of cytokines including IL-2 and GM-CSF. Granulocyte colony-stimulating factor (GSF) and GM-CSF promote differentiation of the myeloid lineage, including macrophages and dendritic cells (Chap. 8, Sec. 8.2). Transduction of a murine adenocarcinoma cell line with a cDNA expressing GM-CSF decreased the ability of that cell line to produce tumors even in mice that lacked T cells or NK cells, suggesting that anti-tumor enhancement was being mediated by granulocytes or macrophages. Macrophages treated with GM-CSF demonstrate enhanced antibody-dependent cellular cytotoxicity, as well as enhanced phagocytosis and antigen presentation. Dranoff and colleagues (1993) showed that irradiated B16 murine melanoma cells expressing GM-CSF induced long-lasting and specific anti-tumor immunity that was dependent on both CD4[+] and CD8[+] T cells. These authors also compared the relative efficacy of ten different cytokines used for tumor-cell transduction and anti-tumor immunity using the same syngeneic tumor model. Live and irradiated transduced tumor cells were assessed. They found that (1) irradiation of tumor cells appeared to enhance their immunogenicity, (2) IL-2 transduced cells could produce local but not systemic protection, and (3) GM-CSF was the most effective of the cytokines in inducing specific and systemic anti-tumor protection.

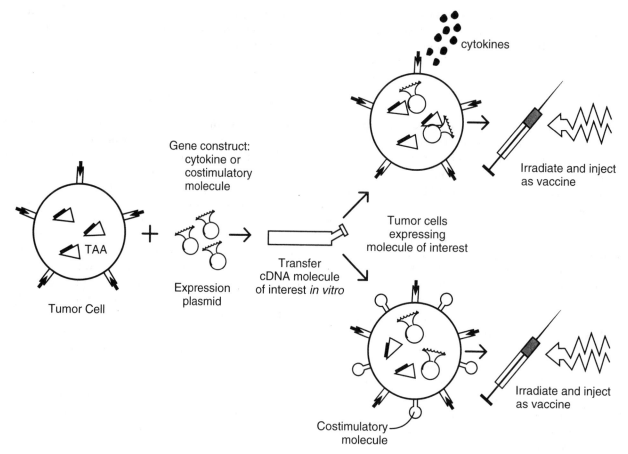

**Figure 21.11.** Active immunotherapy with genetically-modified tumor cells. Expression vectors containing genes for co-stimulatory molecules or cytokines are introduced in vitro into cells obtained from a tumor biopsy. The tumor cells, now expressing the introduced gene, are irradiated and injected subcutaneously or intramuscularly into the patient in an attempt to enhance the activation of tumor-specific T cells.

Early clinical studies to evaluate active immunotherapy with GM-CSF-transduced tumor cells have shown interesting results. A phase I trial of GM-CSF-transduced irradiated autologous melanoma cells in twenty-one patients showed that the immunization sites were densely infiltrated with T lymphocytes, dendritic cells, macrophages, and eosinophils in all patients (Soiffer et al., 1998). Resected metastatic sites had similar infiltrations and there was evidence of tumor cell destruction in most patients studied, but there were infrequent reductions in tumor volume. Eleven immunocompetent patients with prostate cancer were immunized with irradiated autologous prostate cancer cells that were transduced with GM-CSF (Simons et al., 1999). Intense infiltrates were seen at the vaccination site of all patients, and several developed DTH responses to untransduced autologous tumor cells, as well as antibodies to prostate cancer cells. Finally, in a trial in which GM-CSF-transduced allogeneic tumor cells were used to vaccinate fourteen patients with resected pancreatic carcinoma, DTH responses to autologous tumor cells were seen in patients receiving greater than $10^7$ tumor cells in their vaccine (Jaffee et al., 2001).

The B7-1 and B7-2 costimulatory molecules provide the second signal required to activate T lymphocytes after engagement of their antigen receptor and the immune response to autologous or syngeneic tumors can be modulated by manipulation of B7-1 expression (see Chap. 20, Secs. 20.2 and 20.5). Resected tumors from fifteen patients with metastatic renal cell carcinoma were cultured and transduced with a replication defective adenoviral vector encoding B7.1. Increasing doses were administered to cohorts of five patients every 4 weeks for three injections and IL-2 was given after the vaccination. Perivascular T-cell infiltrates developed at tumor sites in three patients, and there was some evidence of anti-tumor activity. In another trial, thirty patients were enrolled in a clinical trial to evaluate two different doses of a B7.1 modified allogeneic cell line administered with or without GM-CSF or BCG as an adjuvant (Schoof et al., 1998). The cell line was known to express HER-2/NEU as a TAA. The treatment was well tolerated, DTH sites revealed extensive infiltration with eosinophils and T-cells, and some patients developed increased levels of HER-2/NEU specific antibodies.

In general, preclinical and early clinical results suggest that tumor cell vaccines modified with various genes may have biologic activity, but the therapeutic anticancer activity of these vaccines remains to be demonstrated.

### 21.4.7 Antigen-Pulsed Dendritic Cells

Dendritic cells are bone-marrow–derived APCs that express relatively high cell-surface levels of critical costimulatory and adhesive molecules such as B7-1, B7-2, ICAM-1, and ICAM-3, as well as MHC class I and class II molecules (for review, see Gunzer and Grabbe, 2001; see also Chap. 20, Sec. 20.5.4). They are able to internalize, process, and present soluble antigen and have been shown to prime class I and class II restricted T cells in vivo. Dendritic cells can be purified from mouse bone marrow or from the peripheral blood of humans. A number of cytokines, including GM-CSF, IL-4, steel factor, CD40 ligand, TNF-$\alpha$, and Flt-3 ligand, have been shown to induce proliferation of dendritic cells, thus providing adequate numbers of dendritic cells for possible anti-tumor therapy.

The rationale for employing dendritic cells as anticancer vaccines has been established in pre-clinical studies. Small numbers of dendritic cells, incubated or pulsed with an ovalbumin peptide, protected mice against challenge with thymoma or melanoma tumor cells transfected with the peptide (Fig. 21.12; Celluzzi et al., 1996). This protection was mediated by CD8[+] T cells. Mice that were protected against transfected tumor cells were also protected against subsequent challenge with the nontransfected tumor cells. The limitation of adding a purified known TAA to the dendritic cells may be eliminated by using peptides that are acideluted from MHC molecules on various tumor cells. When incubated with dendritic cells, these peptides are able to induce immunity against subsequent challenge with the tumor cells from which they had been eluted and this immunization mediated regression of established tumors (Zitvogel et al., 1996). The anti-tumor response was found to be dependent on both CD4[+] and CD8[+] T cells, while neutralizing antibodies to IL-12, TNF-$\alpha$, IFN-$\gamma$, and the B7 pathway blocked the response.

Dendritic cells obtained from the peripheral blood of thirty-five patients with B-cell lymphoma were pulsed with purified immunoglobulin idiotype proteins expressed on the surface of the patient's lymphoma cells

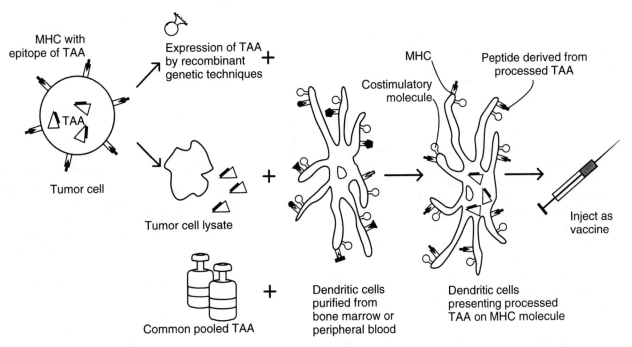

**Figure 21.12.** Active immunotherapy with antigen pulsed dendritic cells. Dendritic cells are purified from the peripheral blood of a patient and may be expanded in vitro by culture with various growth factors. These dendritic cells are incubated with a source of TAA extracted from lysates of the patient's tumor cells or generated by recombinant genetic techniques. Protein formulations of common TAAs may also be commercially available. The dendritic cells will process and present the TAA on MHC molecules and, in the context of other costimulatory molecules endogenously expressed on dendritic cells, will activate tumor-specific T cells.

(Timmerman et al., 2002). Idiotype protein was coupled to keyhole limpet hemocyanin (KLH) for twelve patients. Cellular and humoral responses specific for the patient's idiotype protein were induced in a majority of patients although high titer anti-idiotype IgG responses required coupling to KLH. Cytotoxic T-cell lytic activity against the patients' tumor cells could also be demonstrated in vitro and anti-tumor responses were seen in a few patients. Idiotype vaccination using dendritic cells has also been studied after autologous peripheral blood progenitor stem-cell transplantation for treatment of multiple myeloma or lymphoma. Strong humoral responses to KLH were seen in all lymphoma patients and ten of twelve patients mounted idiotype-specific humoral responses, with a smaller number developing idiotype-specific cellular responses (Liso et al., 2000; Davis et al., 2001).

Encouraging clinical results have also been obtained in one trial where dendritic cells pulsed with tumor cell lysates or melanoma TAAs were injected into lymph odes of sixteen patients with melanoma; KLH was added as a nonspecific cell adjuvant (Nestle et al., 1998). Delayed-type hypersensitivity responses to peptide-pulsed dendritic cells occurred in eleven of the sixteen patients and peptide specific CTLs were also demonstrated at the DTH challenge site. Objective clinical responses were documented, including regression of distant metastases.

In order to increase the presentation of TAA-specific epitopes to the immune system, dendritic cells have been pulsed with two HLA-specific epitopes of prostate-specific membrane antigen (PSMA; Murphy et al., 1999). These epitopes were designed to bind to HLA-A2 MHC molecules. Thirty-three HLA-A2$^+$ and A2$^-$ patients with hormone refractory prostate cancer were treated. Eight of twenty-five patients evaluated for response had a documented clinical response and three of these patients were A2$^-$. The authors suggested this unexpected finding might be a result of the dendritic cells capturing other TAAs and activating the immune system to antigen presented on endogenous MHC molecules. Another strategy to augment immunogenicity involved pulsing the dendritic cells with a fusion protein consisting of prostatic acid phosphatase (PAP) and GM-CSF. The GM-CSF was used to enhance antigen presentation and preclinical experiments showed that this fusion protein induced the strongest cellular and clinical responses (Small et al., 2000).

Dendritic cells have also been pulsed with peptide epitopes to CEA which had been modified to enhance binding to the T-cell receptors of responding lymphocytes (Fong et al. 2001; Foon and Bhattacharya-Chatterjee, 2001).

Other strategies to enhance dendritic cell approaches include their transfection with DNA or RNA encoding TAAs, cytokines, or CD40 ligand (for review, see Gunzer and Grabbe, 2001).

## 21.5 SUMMARY

The development of biologically-based therapies for cancer has been facilitated by the identification of many TAAs, by elucidation of the roles of cellular subsets that comprise the immune system, their requirements for activation, and the importance of various cytokine mediators.

Of the biologically based treatments, monoclonal antibodies have had the greatest impact on clinical practice. The ability to humanize or chimerize monoclonal antibodies provides several important advantages and proof of principle that such MAbs can mediate clinical activity. The power of these therapeutic agents has been shown by the positive results found when MAbs, such as rituximab or trastuzumab, are combined with cytotoxic drugs. Technologies to enhance these reagents, such as conjugation to radiolabels or toxins, will expand this area.

Immune-based therapies include passive immunotherapy with cytokines or infusions of different effector lymphocyte subsets (LAK cells and TILs). Some therapeutic activity has been obtained with high doses of IL-2 in renal cell carcinoma and melanoma, and with IFN-$\alpha$ in melanoma and some hematologic malignancies, but systemic infusion of cytokines has been limited by serious adverse events. Infusion of LAK cells with IL-2 has proven no more effective than infusions of the cytokine itself. Limb infusion of TNF-$\alpha$, together with chemotherapy, has resulted in limb preservation in patients with sarcomas.

The challenge of active vaccination will be to induce immune responses that will overcome both the intrinisic immune tolerance to self-TAAs and immune suppressive properties mediated by the cancer. Genetic modification of tumor cells and the ability of allogeneic cells to activate the immune system through cross-priming hold promise. Various protein immunogens can reverse tolerance and induce humoral responses while viral approaches have been successful in eliciting cellular and, specifically, MHC class I CD8$^+$ responses. Reinfusion of the patient's own dendritic cells that present TAAs has generated high levels of lymphocyte activation and evidence of objective clinical responses, but logistical problems may limit this approach. Promising biologic activity is being shown for several strategies in early phase clinical trials, but randomized phase III trials are required to establish therapeutic efficacy.

# REFERENCES

Agarwala S, Glaspy J, O'Day SJ, et al: Results from a randomized phase III study comparing combined treatment with histamine dihydrochloride plus interleukin-2 versus interleukin-2 alone in patients with metastatic melanoma. *J Clin Oncol* 2002; 20:125–133.

Altman J, Moss P, Goulder PJ, et al: Phenotypic analysis of antigen-specific T lymphocytes. *Science* 1996; 274:94–96.

Bendandi M, Gocke C, Kobrin CB, et al: Complete molecular remissions induced by patient-specific vaccination plus granulocyte-monocyte colony-stimulating factor against lymphoma. *Nat Med* 1999; 5:1171.

Berinstein N, Grillo-Lopez A, White CA, et al: Association of serum rituximab (IDEC-C2B8) concentration and anti-tumour response in the treatment of recurrent low-grade or follicular non-Hodgkin's lymphoma. *Ann Oncol* 1998; 9:995–1001.

Boon T, Cerottini JC, Van den Eynde B, et al: Tumour antigens recognized by T lymphocytes. *Ann Rev Immunol* 1994; 12:337–365.

Campbell M, Esserman L, Byars NE, et al: Development of new therapeutic approach to B cell malignancy: the induction of immunity by the host against cell surface receptor on the tumour. *Int Rev Immunol* 1989; 4:251–270.

Celluzzi C, Mayordomo J, Storkus WJ, et al: Peptide-pulsed dendritic cells induced antigen-specific, CTL-mediated protective tumour immunity. *J Exp Med* 1996; 183:283–287.

Chan A, Morton D: Active immunotherapy with allogeneic tumour cell vaccines: present status. *Sem Oncol* 1998; 25:611–622.

Chang LJ, He J: Retroviral vectors for gene therapy of AIDS and cancer. *Curr Opin Mol Ther* 2001; 3(5):468–475.

Chatterjee M, Foon K, Kohler H: Idiotypic antibody immunotherapy of cancer. *Cancer Immunol Immunother* 1994; 38:75–82.

Chen C, Wang T, Hung CF, et al: Boosting with recombinant vaccinia increases HPV-16 E7–specific T cell precursor frequencies of HPV-16 E7–expressing DNA vaccines. *Vaccine* 2000; 18:2015–2022.

Chopra R, Pu QQ, Elefanty AG: Biology of BCR-ABL. *Blood Rev* 1999; 13(4):211–229.

Clay TA, Hobeika A, Mosca PJ, et al: Assays for monitoring cellular immune responses to active immunotherapy of cancer. *Clin Cancer Res* 2001; 7:1127–1135.

Clynes R, Towers T, Presta LG, Ravetch JV: Inhibitory Fc receptors modulate in vivo cytotoxicity against tumour targets. *Nat Med* 2000; 6:373–374.

Cochlovius B, Stassar M, Schreurs MW, et al: Oral DNA vaccination: antigen uptake and presentation by dendritic cells elicits protective immunity. *Immunol Lett* 2002; 80:89–96.

Coiffier B, Lepage E, Briere J, et al: CHOP chemotherapy plus rituximab compared with CHOP alone in elderly patients with diffuse large-B-cell lymphoma. *N Eng J Med* 2002; 346:235–242.

Crystal R: Transfer of genes to humans: early lessons and obstacles to success. *Science* 1995; 270:404–410.

Cunningham D, Humblet Y, Siena S, et al: Cetuximab monotherapy and cetuximab plus irinotecan in irinotecan-refractory metastatic colorectal cancer. *N Engl J Med* 2004; 351(4):337–345.

Davis T, Hsu F, Casper CB et al: Idiotype vaccination following ABMT can stimulate specific anti-idiotype immune responses in patients with B-cell lymphoma. *Biol Blood Marrow Transplant* 2001; 7:517–522.

Dillman R: Radiolabeled anti-CD20 monoclonal antibodies for the treatment of B-cell lymphoma. *J Clin Oncol* 2002; 15:3545–3557.

Disis M, Schiffman K: Cancer vaccines targeting the HER2/neu oncogenic protein. *Semin Oncol* 2001; 28(Suppl 18): 12–20.

Dranoff G, Jaffee E, Lazenby A, et al: Vaccination with irradiated tumor cells engineered to secrete murine granulocyte-macrophage colony-stimulating factor stimulates potent, specific, and long-lasting anti-tumor immunity. *Proc Natl Acad Sci USA* 1993; 90:3539–3543.

Dyer MJ: The role of CAMPATH-1 antibodies in the treatment of lymphoid malignancies. *Semin Oncol* 1999; 26:52–57.

Ettinghausen S, Rosenberg S: Immunotherapy and gene therapy of cancer. *Adv Surg* 1995; 28:223–254.

Farhood H, Gao X, Son K, et al: Cationic liposomes for direct gene transfer in therapy of cancer and other disease. *Ann NY Acad Sci* 1994; 716:23–34.

Feltkamp MC, Smits HL, Vierboom MP, et al: Vaccination with cytotoxic T lymphocyte epitope-containing peptide protects against a tumor induced by human papillomavirus type 16-transformed cells. *Eur J Immunol* 1993; 23(9):2242–2249.

Fong L, Hou Y, Rivas A, et al: Altered peptide ligand vaccination with Flt3 ligand expanded dendritic cells for tumor immunotherapy. *Proc Nat Acad Sci USA* 2001; 10:1073–1078.

Foon K, Bhattacharya-Chatterjee M: Are solid tumor anti-idiotype vaccines ready for prime time. *Clin Cancer Res* 2001; 7:1112–1115.

George A, Stevenson F: Prospects for the treatment of B cell tumours using idiotypic vaccination. *Int Rev Immunol* 1989; 4:271–310.

Gunzer M, Grabbe S: Dendritic cells in cancer immunotherapy. *Crit Rev Immunol* 2001; 21:133–145.

Gutman M, Inbar M, Lev-Shlush D, et al: High dose tumor necrosis factor-α and melphalan administered via isolated limb perfusion for advanced limb soft tissue sarcoma results in a >90% response rate and limb preservation. *Cancer* 1997; 79:1129–1137.

Hanson H, Donermeyer D, Ikeda H, et al: Eradication of established tumours by CD8+ T cell adoptive immunotherapy. *Immunity* 2000; 13:265–276.

Harris JE, Ryan L, Hoover HC Jr, et al: Adjuvant active specific immunotherapy for stage II and III colon cancer with an autologous tumor cell vaccine: Eastern Cooperative Oncology Group Study E5283. *J Clin Oncol* 2000; 18:148–157.

Haupt K, Roggendorf M, Mann K: The potential of DNA vaccination against tumour-associated antigens for antitumour therapy. *Exp Biol Med* 2002; 227:227–237.

Hawley R, Lieu F, Fong AZ, Hawley TS: Versatile retroviral vectors for potential use in gene therapy. *Gene Therapy* 1994; 1:136–138.

Hoffman D, Gitlitz B, Belldegrun A, et al: Adoptive cellular therapy. *Sem Oncol* 2000; 27:221–233.

Horig H, Lee D, Conkright W, et al: Phase I clinical trial of a recombinant canarypoxvirus (ALVAC) vaccine expressing human carcinoembryonic antigen and the B7.1 costimulatory molecule. *Cancer Immunol Immunother* 2000; 49:504–514.

Hsu F, Caspar C, Czerwinski D, et al: Tumor-specific idiotype vaccines in the treatment of patients with B-cell lymphoma—long-term results of a clinical trial. *Blood* 1997; 89:3129–3135.

Huang A, Bruce A, Pardoll DM, Levitsky HI: In vivo cross-priming of MHC class I-restricted antigens requires the TAP transporter. *Immunity* 1996; VV:349–355.

Hung K, Hayashi R, Lafond-Walker A, et al: The central role of CD4+T cells in the antitumour immune response. *J Exp Med* 1998; 188:2357–2368.

Hurwitz H, Fehrenbacher L, Novotny W, et al: Bevacizumab plus irinotecan, fluorouracil, and leucovorin for metastatic colorectal cancer. *N Engl J Med* 2004; 350(23):2335–2342.

Irvine KR, Rao JB, Rosenberg SA, Restifo NP: Cytokine enhancement of DNA immunization leads to effective treatment of established pulmonary metastases. *J Immunol* 1996; 156:238–245.

Jaffee E, Hruban R, Biedrzycki B, et al: Novel allogeneic granulocyte-macrophage colony-stimulating factor-secreting tumor vaccine for pancreatic cancer: a phase I trial of safety and immune activation. *J Clin Oncol* 2001; 19:145–156.

James N, Atherton P, Jones J, et al: A phase II study of the bispecific antibody MDX-H210 (anti-HER2 X CD64) with GM-CSF in HER2+ advanced prostate cancer. *Br J Cancer* 2001; 85:152–156.

Jansen B, Wacheck V, Heere-Ress E, et al: Chemosensitisation of malignant melanoma by BCL-2 antisense therapy. *Lancet* 2000; 356:1728–1733.

Jansen B, Zangemeister-Wittke U: Antisense therapy for cancer—the time of truth. *Lancet* 2002; 3:672–683.

Kim J, Yang J, Dang K, et al: Engineering enhancement of immune responses to DNA-based vaccines in a prostate cancer model in rhesus macaques through the use of cytokine gene adjuvants. *Clin Cancer Res* 2001; 7:882s–889s.

Kirkwood J, Ibrahim J, Sosman JA, et al: High-dose interferon alfa-2b significantly prolongs relapse-free and overall survival compared with the GM2-KLH/QS021 vaccine in patients with resected stage IIB-III melanoma: results of intergroup trial E1694/S9512/C509801. *J Clin Oncol* 2001; 19:2370–2380.

Kirn D: Replication-selective oncolytic adenoviruses: virotherapy aimed at genetic targets in cancer. *Oncogene* 2000; 19:6660–6669.

Kohler G, Howe S, Milstein C: Fusion between immunoglobulin-secreting and non-secreting myeloma cell lines. *Eur J Immunol* 1976; 6:292–295.

Kourilsky P, Bousso P, Calbo S, Gapin L: Immunological issues in vaccine trials: T-cell responses. *Dev Biol Stand* 1998; 95:117–124.

Kreitman R: Immunotoxins in cancer therapy. *Curr Opin Immunol* 1999; 11:570–578.

Kriangkum J, Xu B, Nagata LP, et al: Bispecific and bifunctional single chain recombinant antibodies. *Biomol Eng* 2001; 18:31–40.

Kruyt F, Curiel D: Toward a new generation of conditionally replicating adenoviruses: pairing tumor selectivity with maximal oncolysis. *Hum Gene Ther* 2002; 13:485–495.

Liso A, Stockerl-Goldstein K, Auffermann-Gretzinger S, et al: Idiotype vaccination using dendritic cells after autologous peripheral blood progenitor cell transplantation for multiple myeloma. *Biol Blood Marrow Transplant* 2000; 6:621–7.

Little M, Kipriyanov SM, Le Gall F, et al: Of mice and men: hybridoma and recombinant antibodies. *Immunol Today* 2000; 21(8):364–370.

Maletz K, Kufer P, Mack M, et al: Bispecific single-chain antibodies as effective tools for eliminating epithelial cancer cells from human stem cell preparations by redirected cell cytotoxicity. *Int J Cancer* 2001; 93:409–416.

Marchand M, van Baren N, Weynants P, et al: Tumour regressions observed in patients with metastatic melanoma treated with an antigenic peptide encoded by gene MAGE-3 and presented by HLA-A1. *Int J Cancer* 1999; 80:219–230.

McCormick F: Interactions between adenovirus proteins and the p53 pathway: the development of ONYX-015. *Cancer Biol* 2000; 10:453–459.

McLaughlin P, Grillo-Lopez A, Link BK, et al: Rituximab chimeric anti-CD20 monoclonal antibody therapy for relapsed indolent lymphoma: half of patients respond to a four-dose treatment program. *J Clin Oncol* 1998; 16: 2825–2833.

Miles B, Shalev M, Aguilar-Cordova E, et al: Prostate-specific antigen response and systemic T cell activation after *in situ* gene therapy in prostate cancer patients failing radiotherapy. *Hum Gene Ther* 2001; 12:1955–1967.

Mitchell M: Perspective on allogeneic melanoma lysates in active specific immunotherapy. *Semin Oncol* 1998; 25(6):623–635.

Moroi Y, Mayhew M, Trcka J, et al: Induction of cellular immunity by immunization with novel hybrid peptides complexed to heat shock protein 70. *Proc Natl Acad Sci USA* 2000; 97:3485–3490.

Morrison S: Success in specification. *Nature* 1994; 368:812–813.

Motzer R, Rakhit A, Schwartz LH, et al: Phase I trial of subcutaneous recombinant human interleukin-12 in patients with advanced renal cell carcinoma. *Clin Cancer Res* 1998; 4:1183–1191.

Murphy G, Tjoa B, Simmons SJ, et al: Infusion of dendritic cells pulsed with HLA-A2-specific prostate-specific membrane antigen peptides: a phase II prostate cancer vaccine trial involving patients with hormone-refractory metastatic disease. *Prostate* 1999; 38:73–78.

Murray RJ, Kurilla MG, Brooks JM, et al: Identification of target antigens for the human cytotoxic T cell response to Epstein-Barr virus (EBV): implications for the immune control of EBV-positive malignancies. *J Exp Med* 1992; 176:157–168.

Nestle F, Alijagic S, Gilliet M, et al: Vaccination of melanoma patients with peptide or tumor lysate-pulsed dendritic cells. *Nat Med* 1998; 4:328–332.

Nielsen M, Marincola M: Melanoma vaccines: the paradox of T cell activation without clinical response. *Cancer Chemother Pharmacol* 2000; 46:62–66.

Norman K, Coffey M, Hirasawa K, et al: Reovirus oncolysis of human breast cancer. *Hum Gene Ther* 2002; 13:641–652.

Pardoll D: Tumour antigens: a new look for the 1990s. *Nature* 1994; 369:357–358.

Perkus M, Tartaglia J, Paoletta E: Poxvirus-based vaccine candidates for cancer, AIDS, and other infectious diseases. *J Leuk Biol* 1995; 58:1–13.

Picker L, Singh M, Zdraveski Z, et al: Direct demonstration of cytokine synthesis heterogeneity among human memory/effector T cells by flow cytometry. *Blood* 1995; 86:1408.

Polo J, Gardner J, Ji Y, et al: Alphavirus DNA and particle replicons for vaccines and gene therapy. *Dev Biol (Basel)* 2000; 104:181–185.

Reynolds S, Oratz R, Shapiro RL, et al: Stimulation of CD8+ T cell responses to MAGE-3 and melan A/MART-1 by immunization to a polyvalent melanoma vaccine. *Int J Cancer* 1997; 72:972–976.

Riethmuller G, Holz E, Schlimok G, et al: Monoclonal antibody therapy for resected Dukes' C colorectal cancer: seven-year outcome of a multicentre randomized trial. *J Clin Oncol* 1998; 16:1788–1794.

Robert F, Ezekiel M, Spencer SA, et al: Phase I study of anti-epidermal growth factor receptor antibody Rituximab in combination with radiation therapy in patients with advanced head and neck cancer. *J Clin Oncol* 2001; 19:3234–3243.

Rooney C, Roskrow M, Suzuki N, et al: Treatment of relapsed Hodgkin's disease using EBV-specific cytotoxic T cells. *Ann Oncol* 1998; 9:129–132.

Rosenberg S, Yang J, Schwartzentruber DJ, et al: Immunologic and therapeutic evaluation of a synthetic peptide vaccine for the treatment of patients with metastatic melanoma. *Nat Med* 1998; 4:321–327.

Safa M, Foon K: Adjuvant immunotherapy for melanoma and colorectal cancers. *Semin Oncol* 2001; 28:68–92.

Scanlan M, Chen Y, Williamson B, et al: Characterization of human colon cancer antigens recognized by autologous antibodies. *Int J Cancer* 1998; 76:652–658.

Schmittel A, Keilholz U, Thiel E, Scheibenbogen C: Quantification of tumour-specific T lymphocytes with the ELISPOT assay. *J Immunother* 2000; 23:289–295.

Schoof D, Smith JW, Disis ML, et al: Immunization of metastatic breast cancer patients with CD80–modified breast cancer cells and GM-CSF. *Adv Exp Med Biol* 1998; 451:511–518.

Shinoura N, Hamada H: Gene therapy using an adenovirus vector for apoptosis-related genes is a highly effective therapeutic modality for killing glioma cells. *Curr Gene Ther* 2003; 3:147–153.

Sievers EL, Linenberger M: Mylotarg: antibody-targeted chemotherapy comes of age. *Curr Opin Oncol* 2001; 13:522–527.

Simons J, Mikhak B, Chang JF, et al: Induction of immunity of prostate cancer antigens: results of a clinical trial of vaccination with irradiated autologous prostate tumor cells engineered to secrete granulocyte-macrophage colony-stimulating factor using *ex vivo* gene transfer. *Cancer Res* 1999; 59:5160–5168.

Slamon D, Leyland-Jones B, Shak S, et al: Use of chemotherapy plus a monoclonal antibody against HER2 for metastatic breast cancer that overexpresses HER2. *N Engl J Med* 2001; 344:783–792.

Small E, Fratesi P, Reese DM, et al: Immunotherapy of hormone-refractory prostate cancer with antigen-loaded dendritic cells. *J Clin Oncol* 2000; 18:3894–3903.

Soiffer R, Lynch T, Mihm M, et al: Vaccination with irradiated autologous melanoma cells engineered to secrete human granulocyte-macrophage colony-stimulating factor generates potent antitumor immunity in patients with metastatic melanoma. *Proc Nat Acad Sci USA* 1998; 95:13141–13146.

Sorrentino BP: Gene therapy to protect haematopoietic cells from cytotoxic cancer drugs. *Nat Rev Cancer* 2002; 2:431–441.

Srivastava P: Roles of heat-shock proteins in innate and adaptive immunity. *Nat Rev Immunol* 2002; 2:185–194.

Tamura T, Nishi T, Goto T, et al: Intratumoral delivery of interleukin 12 expression plasmids with *in vivo* electroporation is effective for colon and renal cancer. *Hum Gene Ther* 2001; 12:1265–1276.

Tao M, Levy R: Idiotype/granulocyte-macrophage colony-stimulating factor fusion protein as a vaccine for B cell lymphoma. *Nature* 1993; 362:755–758.

Thery C, Amigorena S: The cell biology of antigen presentation in dendritic cells. *Curr Opin Immunol* 2001; 13:45–51.

Timmerman J, Czerwinski D, Davis TA, et al: Idiotypic-pulsed dendritic cell vaccination for B-cell lymphoma: clinical and immune responses in 35 patients. *Blood* 2002; 99:1517–1526.

Ulmer JB, Donnelly JJ, Parker SE, et al: Heterologous protection against influenza by injection of DNA encoding a viral protein. *Science* 1993; 259:1745–1749.

Velculescu V, Zhang L, Vogelstein B, Kinzler KW: Serial analysis of gene expression. *Science* 1995; 270:484–487.

Vermorken J, Claessen A, van Tinteren H, et al: Active specific immunotherapy for stage II and stage III human colon cancer: a randomised trial. *Lancet* 1999; 353:345–350.

von Mehren M, Arlen P, Tsang KY, et al: Pilot study of a dual gene recombinant avipox vaccine containing both carcinoembryonic antigen (CEA) and B7.1 transgenes in patients with recurrent CEA-expressing adenocarcinomas. *Clin Cancer Res* 2000; 6:2219–2228.

Wallack M, Sivanandham M, Balch CM, et al: Surgical adjuvant active specific immunotherapy for patients with stage III melanoma: the final analysis of data from a phase III, randomized, double-blind, multicenter vaccinia melanoma oncolysate trial. *J Am Coll Surg* 1998; 187:69–79.

Wang B, Ugen K, Srikantan V, et al: Gene inoculation generates immune responses against human immunodeficiency virus type I. *Proc Natl Acad Sci USA* 1993; 90:4156–4160.

Wang R: The role of MHC class II-restricted tumour antigens and CD4+T cells in antitumour immunity. *Trends Immunol* 2001; 22:269–276.

Waters J, Webb A, Cunningham D, et al: Phase I clinical and pharmacokinetic study of bcl-2 antisense oligonucleotide therapy in patients with non-Hodgkin's lymphoma. *J Clin Oncol* 2000; 18:1812–1823.

Whiteside T: Immunologic monitoring of clinical trials in patients with cancer: technology versus common sense. *Immunol Invest* 2000; 29:149–162.

Wild R, Dhanabal M, Olson TA, Ramakrishnan S: Inhibition of angiogenesis and tumour growth by VEGF121–toxin conjugate: differential effect on proliferating endothelial cells. *Br J Cancer* 2000; 83:1077–1083.

Wlazlo AP, Deng H, Giles-Davis W, Ertl HC: DNA vaccines against the human papillomavirus type 16 E6 or E7 oncoproteins. *Cancer Gene Ther* 2004; 11:457–464.

Xiang R, Silletti S, Lode HN, et al: Protective immunity against human carcinoembryonic antigen (CEA) induced by an oral DNA vaccine in CEA-transgenic mice. *Clin Cancer Res* 2001; 7:856s–864s.

Xiong D, Xu Y, Liu H, et al: Efficient inhibition of human B-cell lymphoma xenografts with an anti-CD20 x anti-CD3 bispecific diabody. *Cancer Lett* 2002; 177:29–39.

Yuen A, Halsey J, Lum B, et al: Phase I/II trial of ISIS 3521, an antisense inhibitor of PKC, with carboplatin and paclitaxel in non-small cell lung cancer. *Clin Cancer Res* 2000; 6(Suppl):4572s.

Zhang L, Zhou W, Velculescu VE, et al: Gene expression profiles in normal and cancer cells. *Science* 1997; 276:1268–1272.

Zitvogel L, Mayordomo J, Tjandrawan T, et al: Therapy of murine tumours with tumour peptide-pulsed dendritic cells: dependence on T-cells, B7 costimulation, and T helper cell 1-associated cytokines. *J Exp Med* 1996; 183:87–97.

# 22

# Guide to Studies of Diagnostic Tests, Prognostic Factors, and Treatments

*David C. Hodgson and Ian F. Tannock*

---

---

## 22.1 INTRODUCTION

Clinical oncologists must be experts in the application of diagnostic tests, the estimation of prognosis, and the selection of therapy for people with cancer. They must be able to select, evaluate, and interpret relevant clinical studies from the burgeoning literature of medical research. This chapter provides a critical overview of methods used in clinical research and of the interpretation of clinical data.

## 22.2 DIAGNOSIS

Diagnostic tests are used to screen for cancer among people who are symptom free, to establish the existence or extent of disease among people suspected of having cancer, and to follow changes in the extent and severity of the disease during therapy. The evaluation of di-

agnostic tests usually focuses on aspects of test performance—that is, the ability of the test to detect disease reliably. Although test performance is important, the usefulness of a test must be gauged by its impact on the lives of those being tested. The application of a test may influence both duration and quality of life. Unfortunately, these crucial outcomes are rarely evaluated.

### 22.2.1 Diagnostic Tests as Discriminators

Diagnostic tests are used to distinguish between people with a particular cancer and those without it. Test results may be expressed quantitatively on a continuous scale or qualitatively on a categorical scale. The results of serum tumor marker tests, such as prostate-specific antigen (PSA), are usually expressed quantitatively as a concentration, whereas the results of imaging tests, such as a computed tomography (CT) scan, are usually expressed qualitatively as normal or abnormal. To assess how well a diagnostic test discriminates between those with and without disease, it is necessary to have an independent means of classifying those with and without disease—a gold standard. This might be the findings of surgery, the results of a biopsy, or the clinical outcome of patients after prolonged follow-up. If direct confirmation of the presence of disease is not possible, the results of a different diagnostic test may be the best standard available.

Simultaneously classifying the subjects into diseased (D+) and nondiseased (D−) according to the gold-standard test and positive (T+) or negative (T−) according to the diagnostic test being assessed defines four subpopulations (Fig. 22.1). These are true-positives (TP, people with the disease in whom the test is positive), true-negatives (TN, people without the disease in whom the test is negative), false-positives (FP, people without the disease in whom the test is positive), and false-negatives (FN, people with the disease in whom the test is negative). The proportion of people with disease is referred to as the *prevalence of disease.*

Test performance can be described by indices calculated from the $2 \times 2$ table shown in Figure 22.1. Vertical indices are calculated from the columns of the table and describe the frequency with which the test is positive or negative in people whose disease status is known. These indices include sensitivity (the proportion of people with disease who test positive) and specificity (the proportion of people without disease who test negative). These indices are characteristic of the particular test and do not depend on the prevalence of disease in the population being tested. The sensitivity and speci-

ficity of a test can be applied directly to populations with differing prevalence of disease.

Horizontal indices are calculated from the rows of the table and describe the frequency of disease in individuals whose test status is known. These indices indicate the predictive value of a test—for example, the probability that a person with a positive test has the disease (positive predictive value) or the probability that a person with a negative test does not have the disease (negative predictive value). These indices depend on characteristics of both the test (sensitivity and specificity) and the population being tested (prevalence of disease). The predictive value of a test cannot be applied directly to populations with differing prevalence of disease.

Figure 22.2 illustrates the influence of disease prevalence on the performance of a hypothetical test assessed in populations with high, intermediate, and low prevalence of disease. Sensitivity and specificity are constant because they are independent of prevalence. As the prevalence of disease declines, the positive predictive value of the test declines. This occurs because, although the *proportions* of TP results among diseased subjects and FP results among nondiseased subjects remain the same, the *absolute numbers* of TP and FP results differ. In the high-prevalence population, the absolute number of false-positives (10) is small in comparison with the absolute number of true-positives (80): a positive result is eight times more likely to come from a subject with disease than a subject without disease, and the positive predictive value of the test is relatively high. In the low-prevalence population, the absolute number of false-positives (1000) is large in comparison with the absolute number of true-positives (80): a positive result

**Disease Status**

| Test Result | | Disease present (D+) | Disease absent (D−) |
|---|---|---|---|
| | Test positive (T+) | True positive (TP)<br>T+D+ | False positive (FP)<br>T+D− |
| | Test negative (T+) | False negative (FN)<br>T−D+ | True negative (TN)<br>T−D− |

**Figure 22.1.** Selection of a cut-off point for a diagnostic test defines four subpopulations as shown. Predictive values (but not sensitivity and specificity) depend on the prevalence of disease in the population tested.

*"Vertical properties"* calculated from columns:

$$\text{Sensitivity} = \text{TP}/(\text{TP}+\text{FN})$$
$$\text{Specificity} = \text{TN}/(\text{TN}+\text{FP})$$
$$\text{False-negative rate} = \text{FN}/(\text{FN}+\text{TP})$$
$$\text{False-positive rate} = \text{FP}/(\text{FP}+\text{TN})$$

*"Horizontal properties"* calculated from rows:

$$\text{Prior probability (prevalence)} = (\text{TP}+\text{FN})/(\text{TP}+\text{FN}+\text{FP}+\text{TN})$$
$$\text{Posterior probability (positive predictive value)} = \text{TP}/(\text{TP}+\text{FP})$$
$$\text{Negative predictive value} = \text{TN}/(\text{TN}+\text{FN})$$

**High Prevalence (50%)**

|       | D+  | D−  |                     |     |
|-------|-----|-----|---------------------|-----|
| T+    | 80  | 10  | Sensitivity         | 80% |
|       |     |     | Specificity         | 90% |
| T−    | 20  | 90  | Predictive Value (+)| 89% |

**Intermediate Prevalence (~9%)**

|       | D+  | D−  |                     |     |
|-------|-----|-----|---------------------|-----|
| T+    | 80  | 100 | Sensitivity         | 80% |
|       |     |     | Specificity         | 90% |
| T−    | 20  | 900 | Predictive Value (+)| 44% |

**Low Prevalence (~1%)**

|       | D+  | D−   |                     |      |
|-------|-----|------|---------------------|------|
| T+    | 80  | 1000 | Sensitivity         | 80%  |
|       |     |      | Specificity         | 90%  |
| T−    | 20  | 9000 | Predictive Value (+)| 7.4% |

**Figure 22.2.** Test properties and disease prevalence. Examples of application of a diagnostic test (T) to populations in which disease (D) has high, intermediate, or low prevalence. The predictive value of the test decreases when there is a low prevalence of disease.

is 12.5 times more likely to come from a subject without disease, and the positive predictive value is relatively low. For this reason, diagnostic tests that may be useful in patients where there is already suspicion of disease (high-prevalence situation) may not be of value as screening tests in a less selected population (low-prevalence situation; see Sec. 22.2.4).

If a quantitative test is to be used to distinguish subjects with or without cancer, then a cut-off point must be selected that distinguishes positive results from negative results. Quantitative test results are often reported with a normal or reference range. This is the range of values obtained from some arbitrary proportion, usually 95 percent, of apparently healthy individuals; the corollary is that 5 percent of apparently healthy people will have values outside this range.

The effects of choosing different cutoff points for a diagnostic test are shown in Figure 22.3. A cut-off point at level A provides some separation of subjects with and without cancer, but because of overlap, there is always some misclassification. If the cut-off point is increased to level C, fewer subjects without cancer are wrongly

classified (i.e., the specificity increases) but more people with cancer fall below the cut-off and will be incorrectly classified (i.e., the sensitivity decreases). A lower cut-off point at level B has the opposite effect: more subjects with cancer are correctly classified (sensitivity increases), but at the cost of incorrectly classifying larger numbers of people without cancer (specificity decreases). This trade-off between sensitivity and specificity is a feature of all diagnostic tests.

The test for serum levels of PSA provides a useful example. The reported normal range for serum PSA level is less than 4 nanograms per milliliter, a definition based on the distribution of PSA levels in apparently healthy men. Lowering the cut-off point to 3 nanograms per milliliter will increase its sensitivity for detecting prostate cancer (increases the number of true positives—men with prostate cancer and with a PSA level above the cut-off) but will decrease its specificity (increases the number of false-positives—men without prostate cancer but with a PSA level above the cut-off).

The $2 \times 2$ table and the indices derived from it (Fig. 22.1) provide a simple and convenient method for describing test performance at a single cut-off point, but they give no indication of the effect of using different cut-off points. The receiver-operating-characteristic (ROC) curve provides a method for summarizing the effects of different cut-off points on sensitivity, specificity, and test performance. Examples of ROC curves are shown in Figure 22.4. The ROC curve plots the true-positive rate (TPR, which equals sensitivity) against the false-positive rate (FPR, which equals 1 − specificity) for different cutoff values. The best cut-off point is the one that offers the best compromise between TP and FP rates. This is represented by the point on the ROC curve closest to the upper-left-hand corner. The performance of a test across the range of cut-off points is summarized by the area under the ROC curve: the greater the area under the curve, the better the test. A worthless

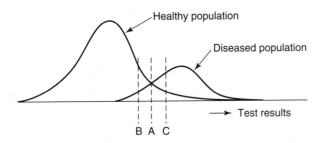

**Figure 22.3.** Interpretation of a diagnostic test (e.g., PSA for prostate cancer) requires the selection of a cut-off point that separates negative from positive results. The position of the cut-off point (which might be set at A, B, or C) influences the proportion of patients who are incorrectly classified as being healthy or having disease.

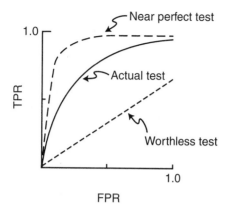

**Figure 22.4.** Curves showing receiver-operating characteristics (ROCs) in which the true-positive rate (TPR) is plotted against the false-positive rate (FPR) of a diagnostic test as the cut-off point is varied. The performance of the test is indicated by the shape of the curve, as shown.

test, equivalent to tossing a coin, has an area under the curve of 0.5; a perfect test has an area under the curve of unity.

### 22.2.2 Sources of Bias in Evaluation of Tests

The performance of a diagnostic test is usually evaluated in a research study to estimate its usefulness in clinical practice. Differences between the conditions under which a test is evaluated and the conditions under which it will be used may produce misleading results. Important factors relating both to the people being tested and the methods being used are summarized in Table 22.1 (see also Jaeschke et al., 1994). If a test is to be used to identify patients with colon cancer, then the study sample should include people with both localized and advanced disease (a wide clinical spectrum). The

**Table 22.1.** Factors That May Distort the Estimated Performance of a Diagnostic Test

Spectrum of patients for evaluation of the test
  Clinical spectrum: Should include patients with a wide range of features of the disease
  Comorbid spectrum: Should include patients with a wide range of other diseases
  Pathologic spectrum: Should include patients with a range of histological types of disease

Potential sources of bias in test evaluation
  Exclusion of equivocal cases
  Workup bias: Results of the test influence the choice of subsequent tests that confirm or refute diagnosis
  Test review bias: Results of the test influence the interpretation of subsequent tests to establish diagnosis
  Diagnostic review bias: Knowledge of the disease influences the interpretation of the test
  Incorporation bias: Test information is used as a criterion to establish diagnosis

sample should also include people with other clinical conditions that might be mistaken for colon cancer (e.g., diverticular disease) in order to evaluate the ability of the test to distinguish between these conditions, or to detect colon cancer in its presence (comorbidity). If there are different histologic types of a cancer, then the test should be evaluated in a sample of patients that have these different histologic types.

The evaluation of diagnostic test performance requires subjects to be classified by both disease status (diseased or nondiseased) and test status (positive or negative). For the evaluation to be valid, the two acts of classification must be independent. If either the classification of disease status is influenced by the test result (*incorporation bias*) or the interpretation of the test result is influenced by disease status (*diagnostic review bias*), then there will be an inappropriate and optimistic estimate of test performance (see Table 22.1).

*Workup bias* arises if the results of the diagnostic test under evaluation influence the choice of other tests used to determine the subject's disease status. For example, suppose that the performance of a positron emission tomography (PET) scan is to be evaluated as an indicator of regional spread of lung cancer by comparing it with the results of mediastinal lymph node biopsy. Work-up bias will occur if only patients with abnormal PET scans are selected for mediastinoscopy because regional spread in patients with normal PET scans will remain undetected. This leads to an exaggerated estimate of the predictive value of PET scanning.

*Test-review bias* occurs when the subjective interpretation of one test is influenced by knowledge of the result of another test. For example, a radiologist's interpretation of a PET scan might be influenced by knowledge of the results of a patient's CT scan. Using the CT scan to help interpret the results of an ambiguous PET scan may lead to a systematic overestimation of the ability of a PET scan to identify active tumor. The most obvious violation of independence of the test and the method used to establish diagnosis arises when the test being evaluated is itself incorporated into the classification of disease status (*incorporation bias*).

### 22.2.3 Bayes' Theorem and Likelihood Ratios

The results of diagnostic tests are rarely conclusive about the presence or absence of disease; rather, they raise or lower the probability that disease is present (Jaeschke et al., 1994). This concept is embodied in *Bayes' theorem*. This theorem allows an initial estimate of the probability that a disease is present to be adjusted to take account of new information from a diagnostic test, thus producing a revised estimate of the probability that the disease is present. Bayes' theorem applies also to clinical trials (Sec. 22.4) where the prior probability that a new treatment is better than a standard treatment is adjusted according to the results of a clinical trial to give a revised estimate of probability that the new treatment is superior. The initial estimate is referred to as the *prior* or *pretest probability*; the revised estimate is the *posterior* or *posttest probability*.

For example, the pretest probability of breast cancer in a 45-year-old American woman presenting for screening mammography is about 3 in 1000 (the prevalence of disease in women of this age). If her mammogram is reported as suspicious for malignancy, then her posttest probability of having breast cancer rises to about 300 in 1000; whereas if the mammogram is reported as normal, then her posttest probability of having breast cancer falls to about 0.4 in 1000 (Kerlikowske et al., 1996).

*Bayes' theorem* describes the mathematical relationship between the posttest probability, the prior probability (i.e., the prevalence of disease in the tested population), and the additional information provided by the diagnostic test (or clinical trial). This relationship can be expressed with two formulas that look different but are logically equivalent. For a diagnostic test with the characteristics defined in Figure 22.1, *the probability form of Bayes' theorem* can be expressed as

Posttest probability =

$$\frac{\text{true-positive rate}}{\text{true-positive rate} + \text{false-positive rate}}$$

$$\frac{\text{sensitivity} \times \text{prevalence}}{(\text{sensitivity} \times \text{prevalence}) + (1 - \text{specificity})(1 - \text{prevalence})}$$

The alternative form of Bayes' theorem is expressed in terms of a likelihood ratio and is much easier to use. The *likelihood ratio* is a useful concept that for any test result represents the ratio of the probability that disease is present to the probability that it is absent. For a positive diagnostic test, the likelihood ratio is the likelihood that the positive test represents a true-positive rather than a false-positive:

Likelihood ratio of a positive test result
= true-positive rate/false-positive rate
= sensitivity/(1 − specificity)

For a negative diagnostic test, the likelihood ratio is the likelihood that the negative result represents a false-negative rather than a true-negative (i.e., false-negative rate/true-negative rate). A good diagnostic test has a high likelihood ratio for a positive test (ideally greater than 10) and a low likelihood ratio for a negative test (ideally less than 0.1). A nomogram which allows estimation of the probability of disease, based on the likelihood ratio, is shown in Figure 22.5.

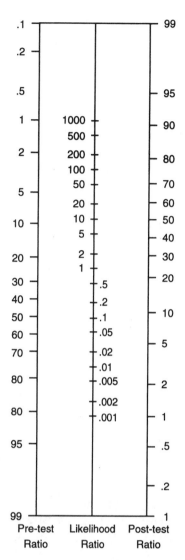

**Figure 22.5.** Nomogram for interpreting results of diagnostic tests, using the likelihood ratio (From Jaeschke et al., 1994, with permission.) The post-test ratio (the ratio of probability that disease is present to the probability that disease is absent) can be estimated by extrapolating a straight line joining the pre-test probability and the likelihood ratio of the test (see text).

### 22.2.4 Diagnostic Tests for Screening of Disease

Diagnostic tests are often used to screen an asymptomatic population to detect precancerous lesions or early cancers that are more amenable to treatment than cancers detected without screening. There are factors that influence the value of a screening program other than the sensitivity and specificity of the screening test. First, the cancer must pass through a pre-clinical phase that can be detected by the screening test. Slowly growing tumors are more likely to meet this criterion. Second, treatment must be more effective for screen-detected patients than for those treated after symptoms develop:

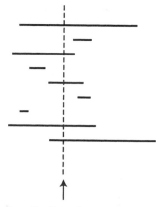

Point of application of screening test

**Figure 22.6.** Illustration of length-time bias in a screening test. The test is more likely to detect disease that is present for a long time (i.e., slowly growing disease). Horizontal lines represent the length of time that disease is present prior to the death of the patient.

if the outcome of treatment is uniformly good or bad regardless of the time of detection, then screening will be of no benefit. Third, the prevalence of disease in the population must be sufficient to warrant the cost of a screening program. Fourth, the screening test must be acceptable to the target population: painful and inconvenient tests are unlikely to be accepted as screening tools by asymptomatic individuals.

The primary goal of a screening program is to reduce *disease-specific mortality*, that is, the proportion of people in a population who die of a given cancer in a specified time. For disease-specific mortality, the denominator is the whole population; it is therefore independent of factors that influence the time of diagnosis of disease. Other endpoints often reported in screening studies include stage of diagnosis and *case fatality rate* (the proportion of patients with the disease who die in a specified period). However, these intermediate endpoints are affected by several types of bias, particularly length-time bias and lead-time bias.

*Length-time bias* is illustrated in Figure 22.6. The horizontal lines in the figure represent the length of time from the inception of disease to the death of the patient. Long lines indicate slowly progressing disease and short lines indicate rapidly progressing disease. A single examination, such as screening for breast cancer with mammography (represented in the figure by the dashed vertical line), will intersect (detect) a larger number of long lines (people with indolent disease) than short lines (people with aggressive disease). Thus, a screening examination will selectively identify those people with slowly progressing disease.

*Lead-time bias* is illustrated in Figure 22.7. The purpose of many diagnostic tests, and of all tests that are used to screen healthy people, is to allow clinicians to

identify disease at an earlier stage in its clinical course than would be possible without the test. Four critical time points in the clinical course of the disease are indicated in Figure 22.7: the time of disease inception (0), the time at which the disease becomes incurable (1), the time of diagnosis under ordinary circumstances (2), and the time of death (3). Many patients with common cancers are incurable by the time that their disease is diagnosed, and the aim of a screening test is to advance the time of diagnosis to a point where the disease is curable. Even if the cancer is incurable despite the earlier time of diagnosis, survival will appear to be prolonged by early detection because of the additional time (the lead-time) that the disease is known to be present (Fig. 22.7). In screening for breast cancer with mammography, the lead-time is estimated to be about 2 years. Advancing the date of diagnosis may be beneficial if it increases the chance of cure. However, if it does not increase the chance of cure, then advancing the date of diagnosis may be detrimental, because patients spend a longer time with the knowledge that they have incurable disease.

The strongest study design for evaluating the impact of a diagnostic or screening test involves the randomization of people to have the test or to be followed in the usual way without having the test. The most important outcome measures that are assessed in such

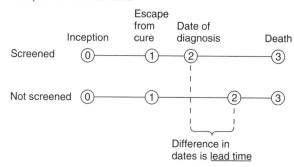

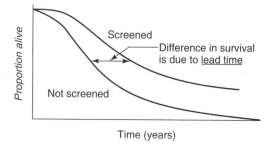

**Figure 22.7.** Illustration of lead-time bias. (*A*) Application of a test may lead to earlier diagnosis without changing the course of disease. (*B*) There is an improvement in survival when measured from time of diagnosis.

a trial include overall survival, disease-specific survival, and quality of life. Randomized trials have demonstrated reductions in mortality rates associated with mammographic screening for breast cancer in postmenopausal women (Kerlikowske et al., 1995; Bjurstam et al., 2003; Duffy et al., 2003) and with fecal occult blood testing for colorectal carcinoma (Hardcastle et al., 1996; Kronberg et al., 1996; Zheng et al., 2003). However, an overview of the quality of trials of screening mammography has questioned whether there is a true reduction in mortality (Olsen and Gotzsche, 2001). Also, there has been a decrease in disease-specific mortality, but an increase in death rate due to all causes in some trials (Black et al., 2002). Thus, some screening procedures might be harmful in that they lead to investigations with some associated morbidity and mortality. Randomized trials have failed to demonstrate any benefit associated with screening for lung cancer, and those assessing the value of PSA screening for prostate cancer are in progress.

## 22.2.5 Diagnostic Tests During Follow-Up of Treated Tumors

Among patients who have had a complete response to treatment, most follow-up tests can be viewed as a form of screening for local or metastatic recurrence. Consequently, many of the requirements for an effective screening test described above also apply to follow-up tests. Because most recurrent cancers are not curable (particularly metastatic recurrences), it is uncommon that early intervention to treat asymptomatic recurrence will produce a true improvement in disease mortality. Studies of follow-up tests that report improvement in case-fatality rates usually suffer from lead-time bias. As with screening studies, randomized trials provide the best methodology to compare the utility of alternative approaches to follow-up. Two studies have compared the effects of two policies of follow-up on overall survival and quality of life following treatment for early breast cancer: intensive follow-up testing with routine x-rays, bone scans, and serum biochemistry versus less intensive follow-up with testing only when the patient develops symptoms. Neither study reported an advantage for more intensive follow-up testing (GIVIO Investigators, 1994; Rosseli Del Turco et al., 1994). These findings demonstrate that for follow-up tests to improve survival, they must detect recurrences for which effective treatment is available; unfortunately, for most common tumors in adults such treatment is rarely available.

## 22.3 PROGNOSIS

A prognosis is a forecast of expected course and outcome for a patient with a particular stage of disease. It may apply to the unique circumstances of an individual or to the general circumstances of a group of individuals. People with apparently similar types of cancer live for different lengths of time, have different patterns of progression, and respond differently to the same treatments. Variables associated with the outcome of a disease that can account for some of this heterogeneity are known as *prognostic factors*, and they may relate to the tumor, the host, or the environment. An increasing number of tumor-related factors, such as degree of tumor hypoxia (Chap. 15, Sec. 15.4.2) or p53 status (Chap. 7, Sec. 7.4.2), have been found to convey prognostic information.

Differences in prognostic characteristics may account for larger differences in outcome than do differences in treatment. For example, in women after surgical removal of their primary breast cancer, differences in survival according to lymph node status are much greater than differences in survival according to subsequent treatment. Imbalances in the distribution of such important prognostic factors in clinical trials, which compare different treatments, may produce biased results by either obscuring true differences or creating spurious ones. Furthermore, the effects of treatment may be different in patients with differing prognostic characteristics.

## 22.3.1 Methods for Identifying Prognostic Factors

Two stages are often used in the characterization of prognostic factors. In an initial exploratory analysis, apparent patterns and relationships are examined, and are used to generate hypotheses. In a confirmatory analysis, the level of support for a prespecified hypothesis is examined critically using a different set of data. Most studies evaluate a number of candidate prognostic factors with varying levels of prior support.

In univariate analysis, the strength of association between each candidate prognostic factor and the outcome is assessed separately. Univariate analyses are simple to perform, but they do not indicate whether different prognostic factors are providing the same or different information. For example, in women with breast cancer, lymph node status and hormone receptor status are both found to be associated with survival duration in univariate analysis; however, they are also found to be associated with one another. Univariate analysis will not provide a clear indication as to whether measuring both factors provides more prognostic information than measuring either factor alone. Multivariate analyses are more difficult to perform, but adjust for the simultaneous effects of several variables on the outcome of interest. Variables that are significant when included together in a multivariate model provide independent prognostic information.

*Cox proportional hazards regression* is a commonly used form of multivariate modeling of potential prognostic factors. Cox regression can be used to model time-to-relapse or time-to-death in a cohort of patients who have been followed for different lengths of time. The method models the hazard function of the event, which is defined as the rate at which the event (e.g., relapse) occurs. The effect of the prognostic factor on the event rate, called the *hazard ratio* or *relative risk*, represents the change in risk due to the presence or absence of the prognostic factor. For example, if the outcome of interest is tumor recurrence, a hazard ratio of 2 represents a two-fold increase in the risk of recurrence due to the presence of the prognostic factor. A hazard ratio of 1 implies that the prognostic factor does not have an effect. The farther the hazard ratio is from 1 the larger the effect.

The Cox proportional hazards method assumes that the relative effect of a given prognostic factor compared to the baseline is constant throughout the patient's follow-up period (i.e., there is a constant proportional hazard). For many factors of clinical interest, this assumption may be incorrect, and a Cox model may provide misleading estimates of prognostic value. For example, one may wish to investigate whether high-dose chemotherapy with stem cell transplantation influences prognosis of patients with a certain type of cancer as compared to historic controls receiving less intensive treatment. Compared to conservative treatment, stem cell transplantation might increase the rate of early death due to toxicity, but subsequently reduce the hazard of death among those able to complete treatment. Therefore, using stem cell transplantation as a factor in a Cox model may violate the assumption of proportional hazards, and the model may produce an inaccurate estimate of the influence of intensive treatment on survival.

A Cox model may also assume linearity, meaning that a given absolute increase in the level of a factor is assumed to have the same prognostic significance throughout the range of its measured values. For example, if PSA is modeled as a continuous linear variable (as is often done) when studying the association between pretreatment PSA level and relapse rate, an increase from 5 nanograms per milliliter to 15 nanograms per milliliter is assumed to have the same prognostic significance as an increase from 105 nanograms per milliliter to 115 nanograms per milliliter. Because tumors tend to grow exponentially (Chap. 9, Sec. 9.4.1) this is not likely to be correct; adjustment of the model can be undertaken to account for a nonlinear association between PSA on outcome (e.g., by using $ln$(PSA) in the model). Finally, variables may interact with each other biologically, and such interaction will not be accounted for in a Cox model unless a specific interaction term is included. For example, the relationship between prostate tumor grade and serum PSA level is complex because some high-grade prostate tumors may not produce elevated levels of PSA. Consequently, a Cox model will more accurately indicate the relationship between PSA, grade, and outcome if it includes an interaction term between grade and PSA.

*Recursive partitioning* is a tree-based form of modeling that can be used to group patients with similar prognosis according to different levels of the prognostic factors of interest. The outcome of interest may be measured on a binary (e.g., relapse/no relapse), ordinal, or continuous scale. Recursive partitioning has several advantages. The method more easily accounts for interaction between prognostic variables, without the necessity of explicit inclusion of interaction terms, as is required for Cox models. This is especially advantageous when analyzing complex data with substantial interaction between prognostic variables (e.g., performance status, age, and mental status among patients with malignant glioma). Also, recursive partitioning yields transparent and easily interpretable clinical categories that can be used to predict prognosis. The major disadvantage of recursive partitioning is overfitting of the data, such that small changes in the characteristics of the patients used to create the tree may create substantial changes in the results. This can reduce the predictive power of the recursive partitioning tree if it is not pruned by excluding some variables and then tested in a confirmatory study on a cohort of patients different from that used to create the tree. Also, an important prognostic variable may be excluded from the tree if it is highly correlated with other variables in the tree, thereby masking its significance (Breiman et al., 1984.)

### 22.3.2 Evaluation of Studies of Prognostic Factors

The quality of studies of prognostic factors is variable, and several factors may diminish the validity of studies that report the discovery of a significant prognostic factor. Prognostic studies usually report outcomes for patients who are referred to academic centers and/or who participate in clinical studies. These patients may differ systematically from patients in the community with the same type of malignancy, leading to *referral bias*. Also, there is some, albeit imperfect, evidence that patients who participate in clinical trials have better outcomes than those who do not participate in clinical trials, even if they receive similar treatment (Peppercorn et al., 2004). Thus, population-based data—for example, data from cancer registries—may provide more relevant information regarding overall prognosis than data from highly selected patients referred to academic centers or enrolled in clinical trials. However, the *relative* influence of a prognostic factor is less likely to be affected by referral bias than the *absolute* influence on prognosis for that disease. For example, if hormone-receptor status influences survival, it is likely to do so within each center, even if the absolute survival of patients differs between centers. Ideally, a prognostic study should include all identified cases within a large, geographically defined area.

Objective criteria, independent of knowledge of the patients' initial prognostic characteristics, must be used to assess the relevant outcomes such as disease recurrence or cause of death in studies of prognosis. *Work-up bias*, *test-review bias*, and *diagnostic-review bias*, discussed in Section 22.2.2, have their counterparts in studies of prognosis. For example, a follow-up bone scan, in a patient with breast cancer, that is equivocal may be more likely to be read as positive (i.e., indicating recurrence of disease) if it is known that the patient initially had extensive lymph node involvement or that she subsequently developed proven bone metastases. To avoid these biases, all patients should be assessed with the same frequency, using the same tests, interpreted with the same explicit criteria, and without knowledge of the patient's initial characteristics or subsequent course.

Several deficiencies in statistical analysis are common in studies of prognostic factors. Typically, a large number of candidate prognostic factors are assessed in univariate analyses, and those factors exhibiting some degree of association, often defined in terms of a $p$ value less than 0.05, are included in a starting set of variables for the multivariate analysis. The final multivariate model reported usually contains only the subset of these variables that remain significant when simultaneously included in the same model. Consequently, a multivariate model reported in a study that contains ten prognostic variables may be the result of hundreds of different statistical comparisons. Because the probability of detecting spurious associations due to chance increases dramatically with the number of comparisons, the conventional interpretation of a $p$ value, as the probability of detecting an association if none existed, is inappropriate in this setting. Using a multivariate model that is prespecified before the analysis avoids the problem that the large number of comparisons may make the calculated $p$ values invalid. Similarly, for a factor that is measured on a continuous or ordinal scale, it is not valid to identify an optimal cut-point using the study cohort, and then demonstrate that the factor is associated with prognosis in the same cohort. Cut-points should be defined prior to analysis and ideally the prognostic model should be developed in a training set of patients, with the robustness of the results tested in a separate confirmatory set.

Many prognostic factor studies are based on a sample of patients treated at a single institution. Frequently, these cohorts are too small to allow detection of potentially significant prognostic factors. A rough but widely accepted guideline is that a minimum of ten outcome events should have occurred for each prognostic factor assessed. Thus, in a study assessing prognostic factors for survival in 200 patients of whom 100 have died, no more than ten candidate prognostic factors should be assessed.

Studies of new biological markers often correlate the presence of the marker with known prognostic factors (e.g., tumor grade). While this might provide insight into biology of the tumor, it does not indicate the prognostic value of the marker. Further, even if a multivariate analysis adds the new marker preferentially into a prognostic model and excludes a recognized prognostic factor, this does not necessarily indicate the superior prognostic value of the marker in clinical practice. This is because the analysis of models that are used to include and exclude variables that are associated with each other will depend on the data set used; the results may not give the same preference between the two markers for other cohorts of patients with minor differences in outcome. Also, because conventional prognostic factors are generally easier to measure than novel biologic markers, the practical question is whether the new marker provides clinically important *additional* prognostic information after controlling for known prognostic factors, rather than whether the new marker can replace an old one. However, molecular markers are important because they can ultimately give more fundamental information about factors that cause the cancer and influence its progression.

## 22.3.3 Uses and Limitations of Prognostic Information

Methods of classifying cancer are based on factors known to influence prognosis, such as anatomic extent and histology of the tumor. The widely used TNM system for staging cancers is based on the extent of the primary tumor (T), the presence or absence of regional lymph node involvement (N), and the presence or absence of distant metastases (M). Other attributes of the tumor that have an influence on outcome, such as the estrogen-receptor concentration in breast cancer, are also included as prognostic factors in the analysis and reporting of therapeutic trials. The identification of novel prognostic factors using the methods of molecular biology is an area of active investigation. Guidelines for selecting useful prognostic factors have been suggested by Levine and colleagues (1991).

Prognostic classifications based solely on attributes of the tumor ignore patient-based factors known to affect prognosis, such as performance status, quality of life, and the presence of other illnesses (comorbidity). Performance status, a measure of an individual's physical functional capacity, is one of the most powerful and consistent predictors of prognosis across the spectrum of malignant disease (Weeks, 1992). Studies in breast cancer (Coates et al., 1992), melanoma (Coates et al., 1993), lung cancer (Ganz et al., 1991), and prostate cancer (Tannock et al., 1996) have consistently demonstrated strong, independent associations between simple measures of quality of life, obtained by patients completing validated questionnaires (see Sec. 22.4.8), and survival. Incorporation of these measures into clinical studies will reduce the heterogeneity that remains after accounting for attributes of the tumor.

The utility of a prognostic factor depends on the accuracy with which it can be measured. For example, the size and extent of the primary tumor are important prognostic factors in men with early prostate cancer, but there is substantial variability between observers in assessing these attributes (Smith and Catalona, 1995). This variation between observers contributes to the variability in outcome among patients assigned to the same prognostic category by different observers.

### 22.3.4 Analysis of DNA Microarrays

The development of DNA microarray technology holds promise for utilizing data about the selective expression of large numbers of genes in tumors to improve diagnosis, prognosis, and tailoring of treatment. The technical aspects of creating gene expression profiles are described in Chapter 4, Section 4.4.4. *Cluster analysis* is performed to identify genes with similar expression patterns, which are grouped together using either *supervised* or *unsupervised analysis.* Supervised analysis involves using samples with two or more known characteristics (e.g., malignant or benign cells) and developing a gene-expression classification scheme to identify these characteristics. For example, Golub and colleagues (1999), created a classification scheme that was able to distinguish acute myelogenous leukemia from acute lymphoid leukemia based on the expression of fifty genes in thirty-eight samples. This classification method was subsequently able to categorize correctly twenty-nine of thirty-four test samples. Several alternative methods of classification have been described, including logistic regression, neural networks, and linear discriminant analysis (see Brazma and Vilo, 2000, for explanation of these methods).

In unsupervised analysis genes and/or samples with similar properties are clustered together, without reference to predefined sample characteristics. Again, several different algorithms have been developed to perform such cluster analysis. For example, a hierarchical algorithm has been used to cluster different samples of diffuse large B-cell lymphoma with similar gene expression profiles. They were able to identify two distinct forms with gene expression profiles indicative of different phases of B-cell development. These different clusters could not be identified on the basis of tradi-

tional histologic features, but the two different clusters identified patients that differed in prognosis (Alizadeh et al., 2000).

The analysis of gene expression profiles is evolving rapidly, and several methodologic issues surrounding the use of microarrays in prognostic or other studies must yet be resolved.

1. There is minimal standardization of methods for preparing DNA microarrays and it will be important to demonstrate reproducibility of expression profiles among laboratories.
2. There is little information about the reliability of gene expression levels in microarray experiments. Every measurement has a margin of error. Most clinicians are familiar with the concept of the confidence interval, which is used to quantify the uncertainty with which different estimates (e.g., of 5-year survival) are made. There are data suggesting that false-positive overexpression, or false-negative underexpression of genes may occur if microarray experiments are not replicated (Lee et al., 2000).
3. The optimal statistical method for measuring the similarity between the level of expression of different genes is unknown.
4. DNA microarrays allow one to assess the association between prognosis and the expression of thousands of different genes. The vast amount of DNA expression data obtained from tumor samples from a series of cancer patients virtually ensures that some constellation of gene expression can be found to be associated with prognosis, if that is the goal. Consequently, it is vital that a prognostic gene expression profile developed on a training set of tumor samples be tested on a separate confirmatory set of samples to ensure reproducibility of the results.

## 22.4 TREATMENT

### 22.4.1 Purpose of Clinical Trials

Clinical trials are designed to assess the effects of interventions on the health of human beings. Possible interventions include treatment with drugs, radiation, or surgery; modification of diet, behavior, or environment; and surveillance with physical examination, blood tests, or imaging tests. This section focuses on trials of treatment.

Clinical trials may be separated conceptually into *explanatory* trials, designed to evaluate the biological effects of treatment, and *pragmatic* trials, designed to evaluate the practical effects of treatment (Schwartz et al., 1980). This distinction is crucial, because treatments that have desirable biological effects may not lead to improvement in duration or quality of life. The major

**Table 22.2.** Classification of Clinical Trials

| Characteristic | Explanatory | Pragmatic |
|---|---|---|
| Purpose | The results will be used to guide further research and not to formulate treatment policy; the purpose of the work is to contribute new knowledge | The results will be used to select future treatment policy |
| Treatment | Choose treatment most likely to demonstrate the phenomenon under study | Choose treatment appropriate for the target population |
| Assessment criteria | Choose criteria that give biological information such as tumor response | Choose information of practical importance such as functional capacity or survival |
|  | Use single or a small number of criteria | Take account of all practically important criteria, but require a *single* decision about adoption of a new treatment or not |
| Choice of patients | Choose patients most likely to demonstrate an effect | Choose patients who are representative of the population to whom the results of the research will be applied |
|  | Patients are used as a "means to an end" in the research | The effect of treatment on patients is the end product of the research |
|  | Idealized conditions | "Real-life" conditions |

differences between explanatory and pragmatic trials are listed in Table 22.2.

The evaluation of new cancer treatments usually involves progression through a series of clinical trials. Phase I trials are designed to evaluate the relationship between dose and toxicity and aim to establish a tolerable schedule of administration. Phase II trials are designed to screen treatments for their anti-tumor effects in order to identify those worthy of further evaluation. Phase I and II trials are explanatory—they assess the biological effects of treatment on host and tumor in small numbers of subjects to guide decisions about further research. Phase III trials are designed to determine the usefulness of treatments in the management of patients, and are therefore pragmatic.

Phase I trials are designed to assess the safety of a new treatment. They are used commonly to define the maximum tolerable dose of a new drug, with a focus on the relationship between dosage and toxicity and on pharmacokinetics (Chap. 16, Sec. 16.1.1). Small numbers of patients are treated at successively higher doses until the maximum acceptable degree of toxicity is reached. Many variations have been used; a typical design is to use a low initial dose, unlikely to cause severe side effects, based on tolerance in animals. A *modified Fibonacci sequence* is then used to determine dose escalations: using this method, the second dose level is 100 percent higher than the first, the third is 67 percent higher than the second, the fourth is 50 percent higher than the third, the fifth is 40 percent higher than the fourth, and all subsequent levels are 33 percent higher

than the preceding levels. Three patients are treated at each level in the absence of dose-limiting toxicity. Six patients are treated at any dose where dose-limiting toxicity is encountered. The maximum tolerated dose (MTD) may be defined as the maximum dose at which dose-limiting toxicity occurs in less than one-third of the patients tested. This design is based on the experience that few patients have life-threatening toxicity and on the assumption that the MTD is also the most effective anticancer dose. It has been criticized because most patients receive doses that are well below the MTD and are therefore participating in a study where they have little chance of therapeutic response. This design may also not be appropriate for molecular targeted agents (Chap. 16, Sec. 16.8 and Chap. 17, Sec. 17.6.2). Such agents may inhibit their target maximally at doses below the MTD and biological assays should be included to evaluate this (Parulekar and Eisenhauer, 2004).

Phase II trials are designed to determine whether a new treatment has sufficient activity to justify further evaluation. They usually include highly selected patients with a given type of cancer, exclude those with nonevaluable disease, and use tumor response rate as the primary measure of outcome. Their sample size is calculated to distinguish active from inactive therapies according to whether the response rate is greater or less than some arbitrary level, often 20 percent. The resulting sample size is inadequate to provide a precise estimate of activity. For example, a phase II trial with twenty-four patients and an observed response rate of 33 percent has a 95 percent confidence interval of 16 percent to 55 percent. While tumor response rate is a reasonable endpoint for assessing the anticancer activity of a cytotoxic drug, time to progression may be a better endpoint for molecular targeted agents which are generally cytostatic. Neither is an adequate surrogate for patient benefit. Phase II trials are suitable for guiding decisions about further research but are rarely suitable for making decisions about patient management. The literature is confusing, however, because phase II trials are often reported and interpreted as if they did provide answers to questions about patient management (Tannock and Warr, 1988).

Phase III trials are designed to answer questions about the usefulness of treatments in patient management. Their endpoints should reflect patient benefit, such as duration and quality of survival. Questions about patient management tend to be comparative because they involve choices between alternatives—that is, an experimental versus the current standard of management. The current standard may include other anticancer treatments or may be best supportive care without specific anticancer therapy. The aim of a phase III trial is to estimate the difference in outcome associated with a difference in treatment, sometimes referred to as the *treatment effect*. Ideally, alternative treatments are compared by administering them to groups of patients that are equivalent in all other respects. Randomized controlled phase III trials are the best and often only reliable means of determining the usefulness of treatments in patient management. The following discussion focuses on randomized controlled phase III trials.

## 22.4.2 Sources of Bias in Clinical Trials

Important characteristics of the patients enrolled in a clinical trial include demographic data (e.g., age and gender), clinical characteristics (the stage and pathologic type of disease), the performance status of the patients, and other prognostic factors. The selection of subjects, inclusion criteria, and exclusion criteria must be described in sufficient detail for clinicians to judge the degree of similarity between the patients in a trial and the patients in their practice. Treatments must be described in sufficient detail to be replicated. This applies equally to treatment with drugs, radiation, or surgery. Differences between the treatment specified in the protocol and the treatment actually received by the patients should be reported clearly. For unknown reasons, patients enrolled in clinical trials may have better outcomes (even if receiving standard treatment) than patients who are seen in routine practice (Peppercorn et al., 2004). While patients in randomized trials may differ from those in clinical practice, this difference does not usually detract from the primary conclusion of a randomized trial. Randomized trials

are designed to estimate differences between treatments rather than the absolute effect of individual treatments.

The outcomes of treatment for people with cancer depend on their initial prognostic characteristics, and imbalances in prognostic factors can have profound effects on the results of a trial. The reports of most randomized clinical trials include a table of baseline prognostic characteristics for patients assigned to each arm. The $p$ values often reported in these tables are misleading because any differences between the groups, other than the treatment assigned, *are known* to have arisen by chance. The important question as to whether any such imbalances influence the estimate of treatment effect is best answered by an analysis that is adjusted for any imbalance in prognostic factors (see Sec. 22.4.5).

*Compliance* refers to the extent to which a treatment is delivered as intended. It depends on the willingness of physicians to prescribe treatment as specified in the protocol and the willingness of patients to take treatment as prescribed by the physician. Patient compliance with oral medication is variable and may be a major barrier to the delivery of efficacious treatments.

*Contamination* occurs when people in one arm of a trial receive the treatment intended for those in another arm of the trial. This may occur if people allocated to placebo obtain active drug from elsewhere, as has occurred in trials of treatments for human immunodeficiency virus (HIV) infection. This type of contamination is rare in trials of anticancer drugs but common in trials of dietary treatments, vitamin supplements, or other widely available agents. The effect of contamination is to blur distinctions between the treatment arms.

*Crossover* is a related problem that influences the interpretation of trials assessing survival duration. It occurs when people allocated to one treatment subsequently receive the alternative treatment when their disease progresses. While defensible from pragmatic and ethical viewpoints, crossover changes the nature of the question being asked about survival duration. In a two-arm trial without crossover, the comparison is of treatment A versus treatment B, whereas with crossover, the comparison is of treatment A followed by treatment B versus treatment B followed by treatment A.

*Co-intervention* occurs when treatments are administered that may influence outcome but are not specified in the trial protocol. Examples are blood products and antibiotics in drug trials for acute leukemia, or radiation therapy in trials of systemic adjuvant therapy for breast cancer. Because co-interventions are not allocated randomly, they may be distributed unequally between the groups being compared and can contribute to differences in outcome.

## 22.4.3  Importance of Randomization

The ideal comparison of treatments comes from observing their effects in groups that are otherwise equivalent, and randomization is the only effective means of achieving this. Comparisons between historical controls, between concurrent but nonrandomized controls, or between groups that are allocated to different treatments by clinical judgment are almost certain to generate groups that differ systematically in their baseline prognostic characteristics. Important factors that are measurable can be accounted for in the analysis; however, important factors that are poorly specified—such as comorbidity, a history of complications with other treatments, the ability to comply with treatment, or family history—cannot. Comparisons based on historical controls are particularly prone to bias due to changes over time in factors other than treatment, including altered referral patterns, different criteria for selection of patients, and improvements in supportive care. These changes over time are difficult to assess and therefore difficult to adjust for in analysis. Such differences tend to favor the most recently treated group and therefore to exaggerate the apparent benefits of new treatments.

*Stage migration* (see Fig. 22.8) occurs when patients are assigned to different clinical stages because of differences in the precision of staging rather than differences in the true extent of disease. This can occur if patients staged very thoroughly as part of a research protocol are compared with patients staged less thoroughly in the course of routine clinical practice, or if patients staged with newer more accurate tests are compared with historical controls staged with older, less accurate tests. Stage migration is important because the introduction of new and more sensitive diagnostic tests produces apparent improvements in outcome for each anatomically defined category of disease in the absence of any real improvement in outcome for the overall population of patients (Feinstein et al., 1985). This paradox arises because, in general, the patients with the worst prognosis in each category are reclassified as having more advanced disease. As illustrated in Figure 22.8, a proportion of those patients initially classified as having localized disease (stage I) will be found to have regional spread, and a proportion of those initially classified as having only regional spread (stage II) will be found to have systemic spread. The patients moving from the localized to the regional category will have a worse prognosis than the group they are leaving and a better prognosis than the group they are joining. The same applies for patients moving from the regional to the systemic category (stage III).

The major benefit of randomization is the unbiased distribution of *unknown* and *unmeasured* prognostic factors between treatment groups. However, it is only ethical to allocate patients to treatments randomly when there is uncertainty about which treatment is best. The difficulty for individual clinicians is that this ambivalence, known as equipoise, usually resides among physicians collectively rather than within them individually (Freedman, 1987).

Random allocation of treatment does not ensure that treatment groups are equivalent, but it does ensure that any differences in baseline characteristics are due to chance. Differences in outcome, therefore, must be due to either chance or treatment. Standard statistical tests estimate the probability ($p$ value) that differences in outcome, as observed, might be due to chance alone. The lower the $p$ value, the less plausible the *null hypothesis* that the observed difference is due to chance, and the more plausible the *alternate hypothesis* that the difference is due to treatment.

Randomization can be stratified and blocked to reduce imbalances in known prognostic factors. *Stratification* refers to the grouping of patients with similar prognostic characteristics. For example, in a trial of adjuvant hormone therapy for breast cancer, patients might be stratified according to the presence or absence of lymph node involvement, hormone receptor levels, and menopausal status. *Blocking* ensures that treatment

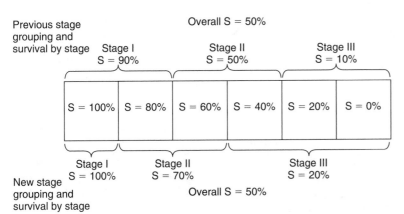

**Figure 22.8.** Stage migration. The diagram illustrates that a change in staging investigations may lead to the apparent improvement of results within each stage without changing the overall results. In the hypothetical example, patients are divided into six equal groups, each with the indicated survival. Introduction of more sensitive staging investigations moves patients into higher-stage groups, as shown. There is an apparent improvement in outcome for each stage of disease with the new grouping but the overall survival of 50 percent remains unchanged. (From Tannock, 1989, with permission; adapted from Bush, 1979.)

allocation is balanced for every few patients within each stratum. This is practical only for a small number of strata. Randomization in multicenter trials is often blocked and stratified by treatment center to account for differences between centers; however, this carries the risk that when there is almost complete accrual within a block the physicians may know the arm to which the next patient(s) will be assigned. Multivariate statistical methods can also be used to adjust for imbalances in prognostic factors.

If feasible, it is preferable that both physicians and patients be unaware of which treatment is being administered. This optimal double-blind design prevents bias. Evidence for bias in nonblinded randomized trials comes from the observation that they lead more often to apparent improvements in outcome from experimental treatment than blinded trials and that assignment sequences in randomized trials have sometimes been deciphered (Chalmers et al., 1983; Shulz, 1995).

### 22.4.4 Choice and Assessment of Outcomes

The measures used to assess a treatment should reflect the goals of that treatment. Much treatment for advanced cancer is given with palliative intent—to reduce symptoms or prolong survival without realistic expectation of cure. Survival duration has the advantage of being an unequivocal endpoint that can be unambiguously measured, but if a major aim of treatment is to improve quality of life or symptoms, then this should be measured (Sec. 22.4.8). Anticancer treatments may prolong survival through toxic effects on the cancer or may shorten survival through toxic effects on the host. Similarly, anticancer treatments may improve quality of life by reducing cancer-related symptoms or may worsen quality of life by adding toxicity due to treatment. Patient benefit depends on the trade-off between these positive and negative effects, which can be assessed only by measuring duration of survival and quality of life directly.

Surrogate or indirect measures of patient benefit, such as tumor shrinkage or disease-free survival, can sometimes provide an early indication of efficacy, but they are not substitutes for more direct measures of patient benefit. For example, the use of disease-free survival rather than overall survival in studies of adjuvant treatment requires fewer subjects and shorter follow-up but ignores what happens following the recurrence of disease. Higher tumor response rates or advantages in disease-free survival do not always translate into longer overall survival or better quality of life. Changes in the concentrations of tumor markers in serum, such as PSA for prostate cancer, have been used as outcome measures in several types of cancer. Levels of these mark-

ers may reflect tumor burden in general, but the relationship is quite variable; there are individuals with extensive disease who have low levels of a tumor marker in serum. The relationship between serum levels of a tumor marker and outcome is also variable. In men who have received local treatment for early-stage prostate cancer, the reappearance of PSA in the serum indicates disease recurrence. In men with advanced prostate cancer, however, baseline levels of serum PSA may not be associated with duration of survival, and changes in PSA following treatment are not related consistently to changes in symptoms (Tannock et al., 1996).

It is essential to assess outcomes for all patients who enter a clinical trial. It is common in cancer trials to exclude patients from the analysis on the grounds that they are not evaluable. Reasons for nonevaluability vary, but may include death soon after treatment was started or failure to receive the full course of treatment. It may be permissible to exclude patients from analysis in explanatory phase II trials that are seeking to describe the biological effects of treatment; these trials indicate the effect of treatment in those who were able to complete it. It is seldom appropriate to exclude patients in randomized phase III trials, which should reflect the conditions under which the treatment will be applied in practice. Such trials test a policy of treatment, and the appropriate analysis for a pragmatic trial is by intention to treat: patients should be included in the arm to which they were allocated regardless of their subsequent course.

For some events (e.g., death) there is no doubt as to whether the event has occurred, but assignment of a particular cause of death (e.g., whether it was cancer related) is a subjective matter, as is the assessment of tumor response, recognition of tumor recurrence, and, therefore, determination of disease-free survival. The compared groups should be followed with similar types of evaluation so that they are equally susceptible to the detection of outcome events such as recurrence of disease. Whenever the assessment of an outcome is subjective, variation between observers should be examined. Variable criteria of tumor response and imprecise tumor measurement have been documented as causes of variability when this endpoint is used in clinical trials (Warr et al., 1984; Tonkin et al., 1985).

### 22.4.5 Survival Curves and Their Comparison

Subjects may be recruited to clinical trials over several years, and followed for an additional period to determine their time of death or other outcome measure. Subjects enrolled early in a trial are observed for a longer time than subjects enrolled later and are more likely to have died by the time the trial is analyzed. For this reason, the distribution of survival times is the preferred outcome measure for assessing the influence of treatment on survival. Survival duration is defined as the interval from some convenient zero time, usually the date of enrollment in a study, to the time of death. Subjects who have died provide actual observations of survival duration. Subjects who were alive at last follow-up provide *censored* (incomplete) observations of survival duration: their eventual survival duration will be at least as long as the time to their last follow-up. Most cancer trials are analyzed before all subjects have died, so a method of analysis that accounts for censored observations is required.

Actuarial survival curves provide an estimate of the eventual distribution of survival duration (when everyone has died) based on the observed survival duration of those who have died and the censored observations of those still living. Actuarial survival curves are preferred to simple cross-sectional measures of survival because they incorporate and describe all of the available information. The *life-table method* for construction of an actuarial survival curve is illustrated in Table 22.3. The period of follow-up after treatment is divided into convenient short intervals—for example, weeks or months. The probability of dying in a particular interval is estimated by dividing the number of people who died during that interval by the number of people who were known to be alive at its beginning ($E = C/B$ in Table 22.3). The probability of surviving a particular interval, having survived to its beginning, is the complement of the probability of dying in it ($F = 1 - E$). The actuar-

ial estimate of the probability of surviving for a given time is calculated by cumulative multiplication of the probabilities of surviving each interval until that time.

The *Kaplan-Meier method*, also known as the product limit method, is identical except that the calculations are performed at each death rather than at fixed intervals. The Kaplan-Meier survival curve is depicted graphically by a step function with the probability of survival on the y-axis and time on the x-axis: vertical drops occur at each death. The latter part of a survival curve is often the focus of most interest because it estimates the probability of long-term survival; however, it is also the least reliable part of the curve because it is based on the fewest observations. The validity of all actuarial methods depends on the time of censoring being independent of the time of death—that is, those who have been followed for a short period of time or who are lost to follow-up are assumed to have similar probability of survival as those who have been followed longer. The most obvious violation of this assumption occurs if subjects are lost to follow-up because they have died or are too sick to attend clinics.

Overall survival curves do not take into account the cause of death. Cause-specific survival curves are constructed by considering only death from specified causes; patients dying from other causes are treated as censored observations at the time of their death. The advantage of cause-specific survival curves is that they focus on deaths due to the cause of interest. However, they may be influenced by uncertainty about the in-

**Table 22.3.** Calculation of Actuarial Survival

| Follow-up Interval (A) | Number at Risk (B) | Number Dying (C) | Number Withdrawn Alive (D) | Probability of Dying During Interval (E) | Probability of Surviving During Interval (F) | Overall Probability of Survival (G) |
|---|---|---|---|---|---|---|
| 0 | 100 | — | — | — | — | 1 |
| 1 | 100 | 8 | 2 | 0.080 | 0.920 | 0.920 |
| 2 | 90 | 3 | 2 | 0.033 | 0.967 | 0.890 |
| 3 | 85 | 1 | 0 | 0.012 | 0.988 | 0.879 |
| 4 | 84 | 3 | 1 | 0.036 | 0.964 | 0.847 |
| 5 | 80 | 7 | 3 | 0.088 | 0.912 | 0.773 |
| 6 | 70 | 6 | 4 | 0.086 | 0.914 | 0.706 |
| 7 | 60 | 5 | 5 | 0.083 | 0.917 | 0.648 |
| 8 | 50 | 1 | 4 | 0.020 | 0.980 | 0.635 |
| 9 | 45 | 1 | 2 | 0.022 | 0978 | 0.621 |
| 10 | 42 | 1 | 1 | 0.024 | 0.976 | 0.606 |

Note: *A*. Follow-up intervals may be of any convenient size; usually days, weeks, or months. *B*. Number at risk means number of patients alive at the start of the interval. *C*. Number dying is number of patients dying during each interval. *D*. Number withdrawn alive refers to patients alive who have not been followed longer than the interval after randomization. *E*. Probability of dying during each interval is number of patients dying (*C*) divided by the number at risk (*B*). *F*. Probability of survival during each interval is the complement (1 − *E*) of the probability of dying. *G*. Overall probability of survival is the cumulative product of the probabilities in (*F*). The numbers in this column may be plotted against time as an actuarial survival curve.

fluence of cancer or its treatment on death due to apparently unrelated causes. Deaths due to cardiovascular incidents, accidents, or suicides, for example, may all occur as an indirect consequence of cancer or its treatment.

The first step in comparing survival distributions is visual inspection of the survival curves. Ideally, there will be indications of both the number of censored observations and the number of people at risk at representative time points, often indicated beneath the curve (Fig. 22.9). Curves that cross are difficult to interpret because this means that short-term survival is better in one arm, while long-term survival is better in the other. Two questions must be asked of any observed difference in survival curves: (1) whether it is likely to have arisen by chance and (2) whether it is clinically important. The first is a question of statistical significance that depends on the size of the difference and the sample size of the trial. The second is a value judgment that will be based on factors such as toxicity, baseline risk, and cost.

The *statistical significance* of a difference in survival distributions is expressed by a *p* value, which is the probability that a difference as large as or larger than that observed would have arisen by chance alone. Several statistical tests are available for calculating the *p* value for differences in survival distributions. The log-rank test (which has several different names) and the Wilcoxon test are the most commonly used methods for analyzing differences in survival curves. Both methods quantify the difference between survival curves by comparing the difference between the observed number of deaths and the number expected if the curves were equivalent. The Wilcoxon test gives more weight to early

follow-up times when the number of patients is greater, and consequently it is less sensitive than the log-rank test to differences between survival curves that occur later in follow-up.

The precision of an estimate of survival is conveniently described by its *95 percent confidence interval*. Confidence intervals are closely related to *p* values: a 95 percent confidence interval that excludes a treatment effect of 0 indicates a *p* value of less than 0.05. The usual interpretation of the 95 percent confidence interval is that there is a 95 percent probability that the true value in the population (mean, proportion, odds ratio, etc.) lies within the interval.

Survival analyses can be adjusted, in principle, for any number of prognostic variables. For example, a trial comparing the effects of two regimens of adjuvant chemotherapy on the survival of women with early-stage breast cancer might include women with or without spread to axillary lymph nodes and with or without hormone-receptor expression. An unadjusted analysis would compare the survivals of the two treatment groups directly. The estimate of the treatment effect can be adjusted for any imbalances in these prognostic factors by including them in the analysis. The log-rank test allows adjustment for prognostic variables that are categorical (e.g., presence or absence of involved lymph nodes). The more complex Cox's proportional hazards model allows adjustment for continuous and time-dependent variables as well (Tibshirani, 1982). In large randomized trials, such adjustments rarely affect the conclusions because the likelihood of major imbalances is small.

Differences in the distribution of survival times for two treatments compared in a randomized trial may

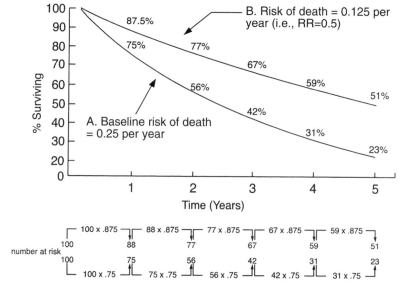

**Figure 22.9.** Hypothetical actuarial survival curves for two patient groups. In a one-year interval, patients in group A have a 0.25 probability of dying, while those in group B have a 0.125 probability of dying (i.e., *RR* = 0.5). Calculation of actuarial survival is indicated in the lower part of the figure (see also text). At the end of 5 years, 77 percent of patients in group A have died (survival rate = 23%). Note that although the hazard rate of death in group B = 0.5, by the end of 5 years, the cumulative risk of death is 49 percent, not 0.5 × 77% (= 38.5%).

be summarized in several ways: (1) the absolute difference in the proportion of patients that are expected to be alive at a specified time after treatment (e.g., at 5 or 10 years). (2) The hazard ratio, or the ratio of the time-specific mortality rate for the two arms. (3) The odds ratio, or reduction in the odds of death, which is defined for each arm as the probability of dying in a given period divided by the probability of surviving in that period. In practice, the odds ratio (applied to short time intervals) will be almost identical to the hazard ratio. (4) The number of patients who would need to be treated for a given period of time to save one life.

Differences in data presentation may create substantially different impressions of the clinical benefit derived from a new treatment. For example, a substantial reduction in hazard ratio may correspond to only a small improvement in absolute survival and a large number of patients who would need to be treated to save one life. These values depend on the expected level of survival in the control group. For example, a 25 percent reduction in the annual odds of death has been found for use of adjuvant combination chemotherapy in younger women with breast cancer (Early Breast Cancer Trialists Collaborative Group, 1992). If this treatment effect is applied to node-positive women with a control survival at 10 years of less than 50 percent, it will lead to an absolute increase in survival of about 10 percent (Gelber et al., 1993); between five and eight women would need to be treated to save one life over that 10-year period (Chatellier et al., 1996). The same 25 percent reduction in hazard ratio would lead to about a 7 percent increase in absolute survival at 10 years for poor-risk node-negative women (e.g., from about 65 to 72 percent), and about a 3 percent gain for good-risk node-negative women (e.g., from about 87 to 90 percent; Gelber et al., 1993). Corresponding numbers of women that need to be treated to save one life over 10 years are about fourteen and thirty (Chatellier et al., 1996). When presented with different summaries of trials, physicians may select the experimental treatment on the basis of what appears to be a substantial reduction in hazard or odds ratio but reject treatment on the basis of a smaller increase in absolute survival or a large number of patients that need to be treated to save one life, even though these represent different expressions of the same effect (Naylor et al., 1992; Chao et al., 2003). Note also that over a long time interval, the cumulative risk of death in one group cannot be determined simply by multiplying the hazard ratio by the cumulative risk of death in the baseline group. Because the number of patients at risk changes with time, the absolute gain in survival does not equal the product of this calculation (Fig. 22.9).

### 22.4.6 Statistical Issues

The number of subjects required for a randomized clinical trial where the primary endpoint is duration of survival depends on several factors:

1. The minimum difference in survival rates that is considered clinically important: the smaller the difference, the larger the number of subjects required.
2. The number of deaths expected with the standard treatment used in the control arm: the larger the number of deaths, the smaller the number of subjects required. Because more patients will have died during longer follow-up, fewer subjects are required for trials with longer follow-up.
3. The probability of (willingness to accept) a false-positive result ($\alpha$, or type I error): the lower the probability, the larger the number of subjects required.
4. The probability of (willingness to accept) a false-negative result ($\beta$, or type II error): the lower the probability, the larger the number of subjects required.

The minimum difference that is clinically important is the smallest difference that would lead to the adoption of a new treatment. This judgment will depend on the severity of the condition being treated and the feasibility, toxicity, and cost of the treatment(s). Methods are available to help quantify such judgments. For example, the practitioners who will be expected to make decisions about treatment based on the results of the trial can be asked what magnitude of improvement would be sufficient for them to change their practice by adopting the new treatment. Based on such information, the required number of patients to be entered into a trial can be estimated from tables similar to Table 22.4. The acceptable values for the error probabilities are matters of judgment. Values of 0.05 for $\alpha$ (false-positive error) and 0.1 or 0.2 for $\beta$ (false-negative error) are well entrenched. There are good arguments for using lower (more stringent) values, although perhaps even more important is that important trials should be repeated by independent investigators before their results are used to change clinical practice.

In a trial assessing survival duration, it is the number of deaths, not the number of subjects, that determines the reliability of its conclusions. For example, a trial with 1000 subjects and 200 deaths will be more reliable than a trial with 2000 subjects and 150 deaths. From a statistical point of view, this means that it is more efficient to perform trials in subjects at a higher risk of death than at a lower risk of death. It also explains the value of prolonged follow-up—longer follow-up means more deaths, which produce more reliable conclusions.

**Table 22.4.** Total Number of Patients Required to Detect or Exclude an Improvement in Survival in a Two-arm Trial[a]

| | | Expected Survival in Experimental Group | | | | | | | | | | |
|---|---|---|---|---|---|---|---|---|---|---|---|---|
| | | 0 | 0.1 | 0.2 | 0.3 | 0.4 | 0.5 | 0.6 | 0.7 | 0.8 | 0.9 | 1.0 |
| | 0 | | 150 | 75 | 50 | 35 | 30 | 25 | 20 | 15 | 15 | 10 |
| | 0.1 | | | 430 | 140 | 75 | 50 | 35 | 25 | 20 | 15 | 15 |
| | 0.2 | | | | 625 | 185 | 90 | 55 | 40 | 30 | 20 | 15 |
| Expected | 0.3 | | | | | 755 | 210 | 100 | 60 | 40 | 25 | 20 |
| survival in | 0.4 | | | | | | 815 | 215 | 100 | 55 | 35 | 25 |
| control | 0.5 | | | | | | | 815 | 210 | 90 | 50 | 30 |
| group | 0.6 | | | | | | | | 755 | 185 | 75 | 35 |
| | 0.7 | | | | | | | | | 625 | 140 | 50 |
| | 0.8 | | | | | | | | | | 430 | 75 |
| | 0.9 | | | | | | | | | | | 150 |
| | 1.0 | | | | | | | | | | | |

[a]$\alpha = 0.05$; power, $1 - \beta = 0.90$.

Source: Adapted from Walter (1979).

*Power* The power of a trial refers to its ability to detect a difference between treatments when in fact they do differ. The power of a trial is the complement of $\beta$, the type II error (power $= 1 - \beta$). The relationship between expected difference between treatments and the number of patients required is shown in Table 22.4. A randomized clinical trial that seeks to detect an absolute improvement in survival of 20 percent, compared with a control group receiving standard treatment whose expected survival is 40 percent, will require about 108 patients in each arm at $\alpha = 0.05$ and a power of 0.9. This means that a clinical trial of this size has a 90 percent chance of detecting an improvement in survival of this magnitude. Detection of a smaller difference between treatments—for example, a 10 percent absolute increase in survival—would require about 408 patients in each arm. A substantial proportion of published clinical trials is too small to detect clinically important differences reliably. This may lead to important deficiencies in the translation of clinical research into practice. If an underpowered study finds no statistically significant difference associated with the use of a given treatment, the results may mask a clinically significant therapeutic gain that the trial was unable to detect. If there are insufficient patients to have an 80 to 90 percent chance of detecting a worthwhile difference in survival, then the trial should probably not be undertaken.

*False-positive and False-negative Trials* Clinical trials are analogous to diagnostic tests (Sec. 22.2.1): they generate both false-positives (positive trial despite no true advance) and false-negatives (negative trial despite a true advance), as well as true-positives and true-negatives. The positive predictive value of a clinical trial—that is, the probability of a true advance given a positive trial—will depend not only on the nature of the trial (sensitivity and specificity) but also on the background prevalence of true advances. If the prevalence of true gains in survival is as low as has been found generally for new treatments of a cancer such as breast cancer (Chlebowski and Lillington, 1994), then apparently positive trials will often be false-positives.

The probability of a false-positive result increases with the number of different endpoints (outcomes) assessed. The usual interpretation of a $p$ value is predicated on the performance of a single statistical test per study. The probability of detecting a difference at the .05 level in the absence of a true difference is 5 percent for a single test, 10 percent for two tests, 23 percent for five tests, and 40 percent for ten tests, assuming that the tests are independent. A single trial might assess overall survival, disease-specific survival, progression-free survival, tumor response rate, various measures of treatment toxicity, and multiple dimensions of quality of life. The number of tests increases further if interim analyses are performed during the course of a trial, which might be used for early stopping and analysis. The number of statistical comparisons reported in a typical cancer clinical trial is large and many more tests are performed than are reported (Tannock, 1996). Ideally, a single primary endpoint and time of analysis should be specified in a trial protocol and identified in the final report. Other comparisons (e.g., analysis of subgroups) may be important in generating new hypotheses but should not be regarded as giving definitive information.

*P* values should not be interpreted as dichotomous criteria for acceptance ($p > .05$) or rejection ($p < .05$) of a null hypothesis, nor should they be interpreted as indicating the chance that a null hypothesis is true; *p* values are best interpreted as indicators of support for the competing hypotheses. The lower the *p* value, the less the support for the null hypothesis and the greater the support for the alternative hypothesis that an observed difference between treatments is real.

### 22.4.7 Meta-analysis

Meta-analysis is a method by which data from individual randomized clinical trials that assess similar treatments (e.g., adjuvant chemotherapy for breast cancer vs. no chemotherapy) are combined to give an overall estimate of treatment effect. Meta-analysis can be useful because (1) the results of individual trials are subject to random error and may give misleading results, and (2) a small effect of a treatment (e.g., about 5 percent improvement in absolute survival for node-negative breast cancer from use of adjuvant chemotherapy) may be difficult to detect in individual trials. Detection of such a small difference will require several thousand patients to be randomized, yet is of sufficient importance to recommend adoption of the new treatment as standard.

Meta-analysis requires the extraction and combination of data from trials addressing the question of interest. The preferred method involves collection of data on individual patients (date of randomization, date of death, or date last seen if alive) that were entered in individual trials. The trials will, in general, compare related strategies of treatment to standard management (e.g., radiotherapy with or without chemotherapy for stage III non–small-cell lung cancer) but will not be identical (e.g., different types of chemotherapy might be used). Composite actuarial survival curves for experimental and control groups are derived and treatment effect is estimated usually by the odds ratio and its 95 percent confidence interval (see Sec. 22.4.5). Data are presented typically as in Figure 22.10, which illustrates the comparison of a strategy (in this example, ovarian ablation as adjuvant therapy for breast cancer) used alone versus no such treatment (upper part of figure) and a related comparison where patients in both arms also received chemotherapy (lower part of figure). Here, each trial included in the meta-analysis is represented by a symbol, proportional in area to the number of patients on the trial, and by a horizontal line representing its confidence interval. A vertical line represents the null effect, and a diamond beneath the in-

dividual trials represents the overall treatment effect and confidence interval. If this diamond symbol does not intersect the vertical line representing the null effect, a significant result is declared.

Meta-analysis is an expensive and time-consuming procedure. Important considerations are as follows:

1. The question addressed must be of sufficient importance to influence fundamental decisions about treatment.
2. The included trials must be of high quality. Bias in individual trials will influence the results of a meta-analysis, although the relative influence of such trials may be smaller.
3. Attempts should be made to include the latest results of all trials; unpublished trials should be included to avoid publication bias (i.e., the bias to publish the results of trials with positive results compared to those with negative results, which applies even to large randomized trials (Krzyzanowska et al., 2003).
4. Because of publication bias and other reasons, meta-analyses obtained from reviews of the literature tend to overestimate the effect of experimental treatment as compared with a meta-analysis based on data for individual patients obtained from the investigators (Stewart and Parmar, 1993).
5. Since meta-analysis may combine trials with related but different treatments (e.g., less effective and more effective chemotherapy) the results may underestimate the effects of treatment that could be obtained under optimal conditions.

There is extensive debate in the literature about the merits and problems of meta-analyses and their advantages and disadvantages as compared with a single large well-designed trial (Eysenck, 1994; Cappelleri et al., 1996; Parmar et al., 1996). However, a well-performed meta-analysis uses all the available data, recognizes that false-negative and false-positive trials are likely to be common, and may limit the inappropriate influence of individual trials on practice.

### 22.4.8 Assessment of Quality of Life

Quality of life is an abstract, multidimensional concept reflecting physical, psychological, and social aspects of life that includes, but is not limited to, the concept of health. It reflects an individual's perception of and response to his or her unique circumstances. This definition gives primacy to the individual's views and identifies self-assessment as essential. *Instruments* (questionnaires) addressing differing aspects of quality of life from a variety of perspectives are now available. Questionnaires range from generic instruments designed for heterogenous populations typical of health services re-

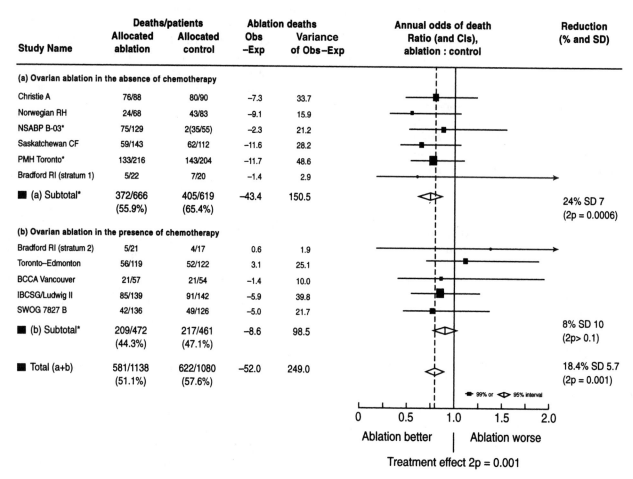

**Figure 22.10.** Typical presentation of results of a meta-analysis. Each trial (identified at right) is represented by a square symbol, whose area is proportional to the number of patients entered, and by a horizontal line. These represent the mean and 95 percent confidence interval (CI) for the ratio of annual odds of death in the experimental and standard arms. A vertical line drawn through the odds ratio 1.0 represents no effect. The trials are separated into those asking a simple question (in this example: ovarian ablation vs. no adjuvant treatment for early breast cancer) and a related but more complex question (ovarian ablation plus chemotherapy vs. chemotherapy alone). Diamonds represent overall mean odds ratios and their 95 percent confidence intervals for the two subsets of trials and for overall effect. (Percent reduction in odds of death, with its standard deviation (SD) and p-value are indicated at right.) The vertical dashed line represents mean reduction in annual odds of death for all trials. Obs = observed; Exp = expected. (Adapted from Early Breast Cancer Trialists Collaborative Group, 1996.)

search to instruments designed for patients with a specific type and stage of cancer.

Examples, from the most generic through increasing degrees of specificity, include the Medical Outcomes Study Short Form 36 (MOS SF-36; Ware et al., 1993); the Functional Assessment of Cancer Therapy—General (FACT-G), developed for people receiving cancer treatments (Cella et al., 1993); the European Organisation for Research and Treatment of Cancer Core Quality of Life Questionnaire (EORTC QLQ-C30), developed for people with cancer participating in international clinical trials (Aaronson et al., 1993); and the Prostate Cancer Specific Quality-of-Life Instrument (PROSQOLI), developed for men receiving treatment for advanced prostate cancer (Tannock et al., 1996).

The EORTC and FACT questionnaires are now used most commonly; each of these instruments combines a core questionnaire relevant to most patients with cancer, as well as subscales that include additional disease or symptom-specific items.

The *validity* of an instrument refers to the extent to which it measures what it is supposed to measure. The validity of a quality-of-life instrument is always open to question because there is no objective, external gold standard for comparison. Instead, a variety of indirect methods are used to gauge the validity of quality-of-life instruments (Aaronson et al., 1993). Examples include *convergent validity*, the degree of correlation between instruments or scales purporting to measure similar attributes; and *discriminant validity* or the degree to which an instrument can detect differences between different aspects of quality of life. *Face validity* and *content validity* refer to the extent to which an instrument addresses the issues that are important. *Responsiveness* refers to the detection of changes in quality of life with time, such as those due to effective treatment, while *predictive validity* refers to the prognostic information of a quality-of-life scale in predicting an outcome such as duration of survival. Validated quality-of-life scales are often strong predictors of survival (see Sec. 22.3.3).

Validity is *conditional*—it cannot be judged without specifying for what and for whom it is to be used. The context may be very narrow, as is the case of the Prostate Cancer Specific Quality-of-Life Instrument, or very broad, as is the case of the Medical Outcomes Study Short Form 36. Good validity in symptomatic men with advanced hormone-resistant prostate cancer does not guarantee good validity in men with earlier-stage prostate cancer, for whom pain might be less important and sexual function more important. Even within the same population of subjects, differences between interventions, such as toxicity profiles, might influence validity. For example, nausea and vomiting might be important in a trial of cisplatin-based chemotherapy, whereas sexual function might be more important in a trial of hormonal therapy. The context in which an instrument is to be used and the context(s) in which its validity was assessed must be re-examined for each application. Quality of life also changes over time, often dramatically in people with cancer. The pace and magnitude of these changes are highly variable and there may be changes in a patient's frame of reference as to what is considered normal quality of life (Sprangers, 1996).

## 22.5 SUMMARY

Advances in oncology depend on rigorous evaluation of new diagnostic tests, screening programs, prognostic markers and new treatments.

The methodologic principles that define valid high-quality studies have been established but many studies are subject to various types of bias. For example, numerous studies of PET scanning suffer from test-review and selection bias, and such studies can impede the appropriate use of this imaging modality.

As our understanding of tumor biology improves, so too will our ability to predict tumor response and patient outcome based on biological parameters. The large amount of biological data becoming available will lead to the development and refinement of new methods for recognizing and analyzing prognostic information from the expression profiles of thousands of genes.

The evaluation of new treatments in clinical trials remains the backbone of clinical research in oncology.

The language of clinical trial design and evaluation has become commonplace. However, the role of trials in setting the standards of oncology care can expand: only a small proportion of the interventions provided to cancer patients have been tested in phase III trials. Further, the continued publication of underpowered trials provides an ongoing need for meta-analyses to detect clinically meaningful outcomes.

Although tumor relapse and duration of survival are important outcomes and are easily measured in trials, they are often not the most relevant measures of treatment success. In many cases, treatment is offered to reduce symptoms, or one may have a choice between different treatments with apparently equivalent anti-tumor activity. In such cases quality of life or symptom control is important. Clinicians will need to have increasing familiarity with methods for evaluating quality of life: these methods will be used more widely to measure the benefits of palliative treatment and to indicate the better of two treatments which otherwise produce equivalent disease control.

## REFERENCES

Aaronson NK, Ahmedzai S, Bergman B, et al: The European Organisation for Research and Treatment of Cancer QLQ-C30: a quality of life instrument for use in international clinical trials in oncology. *J Natl Cancer Inst* 1993; 85:365–376.

Alizadeh AA, Eisen MB, Davis RE, et al: Distinct types of diffuse large B-cell lymphoma identified by gene expression profiling. *Nature* 2000; 403:503–511.

Bjurstam N, Bjorneld L, Warwick J, et al: The Gothenburg Breast Screening Trial. *Cancer* 2003; 97:2387–2396.

Black WC, Haggstrom DA, Welch HG: All-cause mortality in randomized trials of cancer screening. *J Natl Cancer Inst* 2002; 94:167–173.

Bush RS: Cancer of the ovary: natural history. In Peckham MJ, Carter RL, eds. *Malignancies of the Ovary, Uterus and Cervix: The Management of Maligant Disease*, Series #2. London: Edward Arnold; 1979:26–37.

Brazma A, Vilo J: Gene expression data analysis. *FEBS Lett* 2000; 480:17–24.

Breiman L, Friedman JH, Olshen RA, Stone CJ: *Classification and Regression Trees*. Belmont, CA: Wadsworth; 1984.

Cappelleri JC, Ioannidis JPA, Schmid CH, et al: Large trials vs meta-analysis of smaller trials: How do their results compare? *JAMA* 1996; 276:1332–1338.

Cella DF, Tulsky DS, Gray G, et al: The Functional Assessment of Cancer Therapy scale: development and validation of the general measure. *J Clin Oncol* 1993; 11:570–579.

Chalmers TC, Celano P, Sacks HS, Smith H Jr: Bias in treatment assignment in controlled clinical trials. *N Engl J Med* 1983; 309:1358–1361.

Chao C, Studts JL, Abell T, et al: Adjuvant chemotherapy for breast cancer: how presentation of recurrence risk influences decision-making. *J Clin Oncol* 2003; 21:4299–4305.

Chatellier G, Zapletal E, Lemaitre D, et al: The number needed to treat: a clinically useful nomogram in its proper context. *Br Med J* 1996; 312:426–429.

Chlebowski RT, Lillington LM: A decade of breast cancer clinical investigation: results as reported in the Program/ Proceedings of the American Society of Clinical Oncology. *J Clin Oncol* 1994; 12:1789–1795.

Coates A, Gebski V, Murray P, et al: Prognostic value of quality of life scores during chemotherapy for advanced breast cancer. *J Clin Oncol* 1992; 10:1833–1838.

Coates A, Thompson D, McLeod GRM, et al: Prognostic value of quality of life scores in a trial of chemotherapy with or without interferon in patients with metastatic malignant melanoma. *Eur J Cancer* 1993; 29A:1731–1734.

De Haes JCJM, Zittoun RA: Quality of life. In Peckham M, Pinedo HM, Veronesi V, eds. *Oxford Textbook of Oncology.* Oxford: Oxford University Press; 1995:2400–2408.

Detsky AS, Naglie IG: A clinicians guide to cost-effectiveness analysis. *Ann Intern Med* 1990; 113:147–154.

Dillman RO, Herndon J, Seagreen SL, et al: Improved survival in stage III non-small cell lung cancer: seven-year follow-up of Cancer and Leukemia Group B (CALGB) 8433 trial. *J Natl Cancer Inst* 1996; 88:1210–1215.

Doyle C, Stockler M, Pintilie M, et al: Resource implications of palliative chemotherapy for ovarian cancer. *J Clin Oncol* 1997; 15:1000–1007.

Duffy SW, Tabar L, Vitak B, et al: The Swedish Two-County Trial of mammographic screening: cluster randomisation and end point evaluation. *Ann Oncol* 2003; 14:1196–1198.

Early Breast Cancer Trialists' Collaborative Group: Systemic treatment of early breast cancer by hormonal, cytotoxic or immune therapy: 133 randomized trials involving 31000 recurrences and 24000 deaths among 75000 women. *Lancet* 1992; 339:1–5, 71–85.

Early Breast Cancer Trialists' Collaborative Group: Ovarian ablation in early breast cancer: overview of the randomised trials. *Lancet* 1996; 348:1189–1196.

Eysenck HJ: Meta-analysis and its problems. *Br Med J* 1994; 309:789–792.

Feinstein AR: *Clinical Epidemiology: The Architecture of Clinical Research.* Philadelphia: Saunders; 1985.

Feinstein AR, Sosin DM, Wells CK: The Will Rogers phenomenon: stage migration and new diagnostic techniques as a source of misleading statistics for survival in cancer. *N Engl J Med* 1985; 312:1604–1608.

Freedman B: Equipoise and the ethics of clinical research. *N Engl J Med* 1987; 317:141–145.

Freedman LS: Tables of the number of patients required in clinical trials using the log rank test. *Stat Med* 1982; 1:121–129.

Ganz PA, Lee JJ, Siau J: Quality of life assessment: an independent prognostic variable for survival in lung cancer. *Cancer* 1991; 67: 3131–3135.

Gelber RD, Goldhirsch A, Coates AS, for the International Breast Cancer Study Group: Adjuvant therapy for breast cancer: understanding the overview. *J Clin Oncol* 1993; 11:580–585.

GIVIO Investigators: Impact of follow-up testing on survival and health-related quality of life in breast cancer patients:

a multicenter randomized controlled trial. *JAMA* 1994; 271:1587–1592.

Golub TR, Slonim DK, Tamayo P, et al: Molecular classification of cancer: class discovery and class prediction by gene expression monitoring. *Science* 1999; 286:531–537.

Hardcastle JD, Chamberlain JO, Robinson MHE, et al: Randomized controlled trial of faecal-occult-blood screening for colorectal cancer. *Lancet* 1996; 348:1472–1477.

Hillner BE, Smith TJ: Efficacy and cost-effectiveness of adjuvant chemotherapy in women with node-negative breast cancer: a decision analysis model. *N Engl J Med* 1991; 324:160–168.

Jaeschke R, Guyatt GH, Sackett DL, for the Evidence-Based Medicine Working Group: Users' guides to the medical literature: III. How to use an article about a diagnostic test. *JAMA* 1994; 271:389–391, 703–707.

Kerlikowske K, Grady D, Barclay J, et al: Likelihood ratios for modern screening mammography: Risk of breast cancer based on age and mammographic interpretation. *JAMA* 1996; 276:39–43.

Kerlikowske K, Grady D, Rubin SM, et al: Efficacy of screening mammography: a meta-analysis. *JAMA* 1995; 273:149–154.

Kronberg O, Fenger C, Olsen J, et al: Randomized study of screening for colorectal cancer with faecal-occult-blood test. *Lancet* 1996; 348:1467–1471.

Krzyzanowska MK, Pintillie M, Tannock IF: Factors associated with failure to publish large randomized trials presented at an oncology meeting. *JAMA* 2003; 290:495–501.

Laupacis A, Wells G, Richardson S, et al, for the Evidence-Based Medicine Working Group: Users' guides to the medical literature: V. How to use an article about prognosis. *JAMA* 1994; 272:234–237.

Lee M-LT, Kuo FC, Whitmore GA, Sklar J: Importance of replication in microarray gene expression studies: Statistical methods and evidence from repetitive cDNA hybridizations. *Proc Natl Acad Sci U S A* 2000; 97:9834–9839.

Levine MN, Browman GP, Gent M, et al: When is a prognostic factor useful? A guide for the perplexed. *J Clin Oncol* 1991; 9:348–356.

Mason J, Drummond M, Torrance G: Some guidelines on the use of cost-effectiveness league tables. *Br Med J* 1993; 306:570–572.

Moore MJ, O'Sullivan B, Tannock IF: How expert physicians would wish to be treated if they had genitourinary cancer. *J Clin Oncol* 1988; 6:1736–1745.

Naylor CD, Chen E, Strauss B: Measured enthusiasm: does the method of reporting trial results alter perceptions of therapeutic effectiveness? *Ann Intern Med* 1992; 117:916–921.

Olsen O, Gotzsche PC: Cochrane review on screening for breast cancer with mammography. *Lancet* 2001; 358:1340–1342

Parmar MKB, Stewart LA, Altman DG: Meta-analyses of randomised trials: when the whole is more than just the sum of the parts. *Br J Cancer* 1996; 74:496–501.

Parulekar WR, Eisenhauer EA: Phase I trial design for solid tumor studies of targeted, non-cytotoxic agents: theory and practice. *J Natl Cancer Inst* 2004; 96:990–997.

Peppercorn JM, Weeks, JC, Cook, EF, Joffe S: Comparison of outcomes in cancer patients treated within and outside clinical trials: conceptual framework and structured review. *Lancet* 2004; 363:263–270.

Rosseli Del Turco M, Palli D, Cariddi A, et al: Intensive diagnostic follow-up after treatment of primary breast cancer: a randomized trial. *JAMA* 1994; 271:1593–1597.

Schwartz D, Flamant R, Lellouch J: *Clinical Trials.* London: Academic Press; 1980.

Shulz KF: Subverting randomization in controlled trials. *JAMA* 1995; 274:1456–1458.

Slevin ML, Stubbs L, Plant HJ, et al: Attitudes to chemotherapy: comparing views of patients with cancer and those of doctors, nurses, and general public. *Br Med J* 1990; 300:1458–1460.

Smith DS, Catalona WJ: Interexaminer variability of digital rectal examination in detecting prostate cancer. *Urology* 1995; 45:70–74.

Sprangers MAG: Response-shift bias: a challenge to the assessment of patients' quality of life in cancer clinical trials. *Cancer Treat Rev* 1996; 22(Suppl A):55–62.

Stewart LA, Parmar MKB: Meta-analysis of the literature or of individual patient data: Is there a difference? *Lancet* 1993; 341:418–422.

Tannock IF: Combined modality treatment with radiotherapy and chemotherapy. *Radiother Oncol* 1989; 16:83–101.

Tannock IF: False positive results in clinical trials: multiple significance tests and the problem of unreported comparisons. *J Natl Cancer Inst* 1996; 88:206–207.

Tannock IF, Osoba D, Stockler MR, et al: Chemotherapy with mitoxantrone plus prednisone or prednisone alone for symptomatic hormone-resistant prostate cancer: a Canadian randomized trial with palliative endpoints. *J Clin Oncol* 1996; 14:1756–1764.

Tannock I, Warr D: Non-randomized trials of cancer chemotherapy: Phase II or III? *J Natl Cancer Inst* 1988; 80:800–801.

Tibshirani R: A plain man's guide to the proportional hazards model. *Clin Invest Med* 1982; 5:63–68.

Tonkin K, Tritchler D, Tannock I: Criteria of tumor response used in clinical trials of chemotherapy. *J Clin Oncol* 1985; 3:870–875.

Torrance GW: Utility approach to measuring health-related quality of life. *J Chronic Dis* 1987; 40:593–600.

Walter S: In defense of the arcsine approximation. *Statistician* 1979; 28:219–222.

Ware JE Jr, Snow KK, Kosinski M, Gandek B: *SF-36 Health Survey: Manual and Interpretation Guide.* Boston: The Health Institute, New England Medical Center; 1993.

Warr D, McKinney S, Tannock I: Influence of measurement error on assessment of response to anticancer chemotherapy: proposal for new criteria of tumor response. *J Clin Oncol* 1984; 2:1040–1046.

Weeks J: Performance status upstaged? *J Clin Oncol* 1992; 10:1827–1829.

Zheng S, Chen K, Liu X, et al: Cluster randomization trial of sequence mass screening for colorectal cancer. *Dis Colon Rectum* 2003; 46:51–58.

## BIBLIOGRAPHY

Crowley J: *Handbook of Statistics in Clinical Oncology.* New York: Dekker, 2001.

Green S, Benedetti J, Crowley J: *Clinical Trials in Oncology.* New York: Chapman & Hall; 1997.

Hennekens CM, Buring JE: *Epidemiology in Medicine.* Boston: Little, Brown; 1987.

Morrison AS: *Screening in Chronic Disease.* New York: Oxford University Press; 1986.

Piantadosi S: *Clinical Trials: A Methodologic Approach.* New York: Wiley, 1997.

Sackett DL, Haynes RB, Guyatt GH, Tugwell P: *Clinical Epidemiology: A Basic Science for Clinical Medicine.* Boston: Little, Brown; 1991.

Sackett DL, Richardson WS, Rosenberg W, Haynes RB: *Evidence Based Medicine: How to Practice and Teach EBM.* London: Churchill Livingstone; 1997.

# Glossary

**Accelerated fractionation:** A schedule used in radiation therapy whereby the total treatment time is reduced to less than the conventional time (5 to 6 weeks), usually by giving more than one radiation fraction per day. (See Chap. 15, Sec. 15.7.4.)

**Active immunotherapy:** A treatment strategy that attempts to generate or stimulate an antitumor response by the host's own immune system. (See Chap. 21, Sec. 21.4.)

**Active transport:** The transport of molecules into a cell by an energy-dependent process. This process can transport molecules against a concentration gradient.

**Acute transforming virus:** A virus that contains an **oncogene** and, following integration into the host-cell DNA, can cause malignant **transformation** of normal cells quite rapidly. (See Chap. 6, Sec. 6.3.2 and Chap. 7, Sec. 7.2.1.)

**Adaptor protein:** A protein that may act in **signal transduction** in cells by facilitating the association between other molecular components of signaling pathways. The protein often lacks an intrinsic catalytic activity (e.g. kinase activity), and possesses distinct protein- or phosphoprotein-binding domains, thus bridging proteins with catalytic activity (See Chap. 8, Sec. 8.2.4.)

**Additivity:** The range of effects that might be expected when two or more cytotoxic agents are used in combination for treatment of cells or tumors when there is no specific interaction between them. This range of additivity can be defined from dose-response curves for the individual agents. (See Chap. 17, Sec. 17.5.2.)

**Adjuvant:** A substance that will enhance an immunologic response. An example is bacille Calmette-Guerin (BCG). A probable mechanism is stimulation of the secretion of **cytokines** that aid in the activation of an acquired immune response. (See Chap. 21, Sec. 21.4.3.)

**Adjuvant chemotherapy or hormone therapy:** Treatment given to patients following surgical removal of their primary tumor and/or radiotherapy, when there is known to be a high risk of occult micrometastases but no clinical or radiological evidence of metastatic disease. If chemotherapy is given prior to treatment of the primary tumor, this therapy is referred to as "neoadjuvant chemotherapy." (See Chap. 17, Sec. 17.3.3 and Chap. 19, Sec. 19.4.)

**Adoptive immune therapy:** A treatment strategy in which active immune cells are transferred to a tumor-bearing host; these cells have the capacity for stimulating tumor rejection. (See Chap. 21, Sec. 21.3.2.)

**Alkylating agent:** A compound that has positively charged (i.e., electron-deficient) groups or that may be metabolized to form such groups. These reactive (**"electrophilic"**) groups can form covalent linkages with negatively charged chemical groups on biologic molecules such as those on the bases of DNA. A monofunctional alkylating agent can form a single adduct, whereas bifunctional alkylating agents can form two adducts, leading to inter- or intrastrand DNA–DNA **cross-links** or to DNA-protein cross-links. Alkylating agents include commonly used anticancer drugs such as cyclophosphamide. They may also have **mutagenic** and **carcinogenic** properties. (See Chap. 3, Sec. 3.2 and Chap. 16, Sec. 16.2.)

**Alleles:** The genetic (DNA) sequences that represent the same genetic locus (**gene**) on homologous **chromosomes.**

**Allograft:** Tissue that is transplanted between genetically different individuals of the same species.

**Alpha error:** Another term for **type I error** in statistical analysis. (See Chap. 22, Sec. 22.4.6.)

**Ames assay:** A widely used short-term assay for detecting substances that are mutagenic. It uses a mutant bacterial strain *Salmonella typhimurium*, which is unable to synthesize the essential amino acid histidine. The assay detects revertant colonies that can grow because of **mutations** rendering them independent of histidine. (See Chap. 3, Fig 3.11.)

**Anaphase bridge:** Improper segregation of chromosomal DNA that leads to the formation of a DNA bridge between two cells in the latter stages of mitosis (during **anaphase**, when sister chromatids normally separate).

**Anaplasia:** Histopathologic appearance of a tumor that lacks features allowing easy identification with the tissue of origin. Anaplastic tumors are usually rapidly growing and have a large number of cells in mitosis. (A synonym is "undifferentiated").

**Anchorage-independence:** A property of most cells that have undergone malignant transformation and of normal hematopoietic cells. These cells can proliferate in semisolid media such as agarose or methylcellulose without adherence to glass or specially coated plastic tissue-culture plates.

**Androgens:** Steroid sex hormones (e.g. testosterone) that cause masculine features. Androgens stimulate the growth of prostatic cancers. (See Chap. 19, Sec. 19.2.1.)

**Androgen Receptor:** Intracellular receptor which binds to **androgens**. (See Chap. 19, Sec. 19.2.2.)

**Anergy:** A state of non-responsiveness to **immunogenic** stimuli. (See Chap. 20, Sec. 20.3.3.)

**Angiogenesis:** Formation of new blood vessels. This process is essential for tumor growth and appears to be stimulated by endothelial cell **growth factor(s).** (See Chap. 12.)

**Angiopoietins:** Ligands that bind to the **Tie** family of **receptor tyrosine kinases** on endothelial cells. The four members of the family have either agonistic or antagonistic effects on endothelial cell proliferation. (See Chap. 12, Sec. 12.2.3.)

**Angiostatin:** Proteolytic fragment of the **extracellular matrix** protein plasminogen, that inhibits the proliferation of endothelial cells. (See Chap. 12, Sec. 12.4.1.)

**Anthracyclines:** A family of multi-ringed planar anticancer drugs that includes daunorubicin, doxorubicin, and epirubicin. (See Chap. 16, Sec. 16.5.3.)

**Antibody:** A soluble protein molecule produced by plasma cells in response to an **antigen** and capable of specifically binding to that antigen. (See Chap. 20, Sec. 20.2.)

**Antigen:** An agent that is foreign (i.e., "nonself") to an animal and that is recognized by the immune system. (See Chap. 20, Sec. 20.1.)

**Antigen-presenting cell (APC):** A cell that can present peptide antigens on its cell surface in association with molecules of the **major histocompatibility complex.** "Professional APCs" include **dendritic cells,** Langerhans cells in the skin, macrophages, and activated **B lymphocytes;** these cells are capable of fully activating lymphocytes and inducing an immune response. (See Chap. 20, Sec. 20.2 and Chap. 21, Sec. 21.4.7.)

**Antimetabolite:** A type of anticancer drug that is an analog of a normal metabolite. Antimetabolites may inhibit metabolic pathways or may be mistaken for normal metabolites during the synthesis of macromolecules such as DNA or RNA. Examples are methotrexate and 5-fluorouracil, which are analogues of folic acid and thymine (or uracil), respectively. (See Chap. 16, Sec. 16.4.)

**Antisense RNA:** An RNA molecule with a sequence that is complementary to the mRNA sequences expressed from a target **gene.** The resultant double-stranded RNA molecule inhibits the translation of the target protein. (See Chap. 4, Sec. 4.3.11.)

**Antisense therapy:** Anticancer therapy that uses an antisense RNA molecule to inhibit the synthesis of a protein – most often a protein that facilitates tumor growth. (See Chap. 21, Sec. 21.2.4.)

**Apoptosis:** A process resulting in cell death due to the activation of a genetic program that causes cells to lose viability before they lose membrane integrity. The process involves **endonuclease**-mediated cleavage of the DNA into fragments of specific lengths, leading to a **"DNA ladder"** when it is subjected to gel **electrophoresis.** Apoptosis is also called **programmed cell death** and is important in maintaining tissue **homeostasis;** it may be important in the response of tumor and normal tissue cells to therapeutic agents. (See Chap. 10.)

**Area under the curve (AUC):** A measure of the total exposure of blood or tissue to a chemical agent such as a toxin or anticancer agent. The AUC is obtained by plotting the concentration of the agent as a function of time and obtaining the AUC by integration. (See Chap. 16, Sec. 16.1.2.)

**Ataxia telangiectasia (AT):** A clinical syndrome in which patients have a variety of symptoms including ataxia (unstable gait) and telangiectasia (prominent and tortuous blood vessels). Cells from such individuals are sensitive to ionizing radiation and defective in **repair of DNA** damage. The AT patients have a high incidence of lymphoma. (See Chap. 5, Sec. 5.2.2.)

**ATP-binding cassette (ABC) transporters:** Membrane-based proteins that transport various molecules across the cell membrane. Examples include **P-glycoprotein** and **multiple drug resistance-associated protein,** whose expression causes resistance to multiple anticancer drugs. (See Chap. 18, Sec. 18.2.3.)

**Autocrine:** Refers to the production of substances (i.e., **growth factors** or hormones) that can influence the metabolism of the cell producing them.

**Autonomous:** A cellular process that is self-contained. For example, cell-autonomy refers to a property that is inherent to the cell, and not influenced by surrounding cells.

**Autoradiography:** A technique to identify where a radioactive isotope is localized in cells or subcellular components. The process involves covering biological material with photographic film or emulsion or placing it on a radiation detector. The radioactivity produced by the isotope then causes local exposure of the overlying film, emulsion, (or detector) which, upon development (or digitally), can be detected as dark grains (or bright spots) close to the location of the isotope. (See Chap. 9, Sec. 9.4.2.)

**Autosome:** Any **chromosome** other than the sex chromosomes.

**B cell (or B lymphocyte):** A lymphocyte that is a precursor of antibody-producing plasma cells and expresses a specific **antibody** molecule (an **immunoglobulin** or B-cell receptor) on its cell surface. (See Chap. 20, Sec. 20.2.1.)

**Bacteriophage:** A virus that infects bacteria. Bacteriophage are commonly used as carriers of **cloned genes.**

**Base excision repair:** A mechanism of **DNA repair** whereby one damaged base is removed from the DNA. (See Chap. 5, Sec. 5.3.3.)

**Basement membrane:** A membranous tissue that surrounds nests of epithelial or endothelial cells and provides a structural framework for their organization. A basement membrane may also surround certain types of mesenchymal cells.

**Bayes' theorem:** Bayes' theorem is used in the interpretation of diagnostic tests to estimate the probability that disease may be present, based on previous knowledge of the probability that such disease is present and the new information gained in the diagnostic test. (See Chap. 22, Sec. 22.2.3.)

***BCL-2/BAX:*** Members of a family of **genes** involved in the control of **apoptosis.** Their products form **dimers,** and increased *bcl-2* expression is associated with inhibition of apoptosis, whereas increased expression of *bax* is associated with stimulation of apoptosis. *bcl-2* may act as an **oncogene.** (See Chap. 10, Sec. 10.2.1.)

***BCR/ABL:*** A fusion **gene** formed by the **translocation** of the *c-abl* sequences on chromosome 9 next to the *bcr* (break-point cluster region) gene on chromosome 22. This **reciprocal translocation,** which gives rise to the characteristic **Philadelphia chromosome,** occurs in chronic myelogenous leukemia. (See Chap. 7, Sec. 7.2.4.)

**Beta error:** Another term for **type II error** in statistical analysis. (See Chap. 22, Sec. 22.4.6.)

**Bias:** Systematic departure from the true state (as compared to error, which is random departure from the true state). Faulty design may lead to the presence of many types of bias in trials of cancer causation and cancer treatment. (See Chap. 2, Sec. 2.2.7 and Chap. 22, Sec. 22.4.2.)

**Bioassay:** Quantitation of an agent by measuring the extent of its interaction with living organisms whose dose response has been predetermined. Examples are the assessment of the quantity of active metabolites of a drug in human serum by the toxicity of that serum for cells of known sensitivity, or the assessment of the level of a **growth factor** by measuring the stimulation of growth of sensitive cells.

**Bioavailability:** The proportion of an administered drug that is delivered to its site of action. For most agents, this is the proportion of drug entering the circulation. Bioavailability may be low if a drug is given orally. (See Chap. 16, Sec. 16.1.1.)

**Biomarker:** A substance produced by tumor cells and released into the blood such that the concentration in blood may be related to the bulk of tumor present in the individual.

**Brachytherapy:** A form of radiotherapy in which tissue receives radiation from a radioactive isotope that is implanted or inserted into a body cavity. (See Chap. 15, Sec. 15.2.3.)

**BRCA1 and BRCA2:** **Tumor suppressor genes** in which **mutations** are associated with a high incidence of breast and ovarian cancer. Their protein products appear to be involved in DNA repair. (See Chap. 7, Sec. 7.4.5.)

**Bystander effect:** An effect whereby therapeutic agents that target specific types of cells may influence the viability or other properties of non-targeted neighboring cells. (See Chap. 14, Sec. 14.2.4.)

**Cadherins:** Membrane proteins that can interact to allow cell-cell adhesion. Cadherins can also play a role in **signal transduction.** (See Chap. 11, Sec. 11.5.2.)

**Carcinoembryonic antigen (CEA):** A **glycoprotein** produced in the embryo and in lower concentrations in the adult colon. It may also be produced in higher concentrations by certain types of tumor cells, such as those originating in the colon or rectum. CEA is one example of substances that are known generally as **oncofetal antigens** and are used as tumor **markers.**

**Carcinogen:** A substance that causes cancer. Some chemical carcinogens can act directly, but others require metabolism in vivo before becoming effective. Most carcinogens are **mutagens.** (See Chap. 3.)

**Carcinoma:** Type of cancer arising in epithelial tissue (i.e., tissue lining internal or external organs, or glandular tissue). Most human cancers are carcinomas.

**Carcinoma in situ:** A pathologic description of tissue that has undergone changes in cellular features characteristic of malignant **transformation** but without invasion through the epithelial **basement membrane.**

**Case-control study:** An epidemiologic study in which individuals with disease (cases) are matched with those who are not diseased (controls), followed by assessment of these individuals for their previous exposure to putative causative agents such as **carcinogens.** (See Chap. 2, Sec. 2.2.4.)

**Caspases:** A family of proteases that effect **programmed cell death** or apoptosis. Also known as ICE proteases. (See Chap. 10, Sec. 10.2.3.)

**cDNA:** A DNA copy complementary to mRNA sequences transcribed from a given **gene** or genes. cDNA therefore will **hybridize** with the DNA of the nontranscribed strand of these genes and, if radiolabeled, will allow their detection in **chromosomes ("in situ hybridization")** or in DNA or mRNA extracted from cells and separated by **electrophoresis** (in **Southern** or **northern blots,** respectively). (See Chap. 4, Sec. 4.3.3.)

**Cell adhesion molecules (CAMs):** Molecules that are expressed on the surface of cells and that mediate the attachment of cells to the extracellular matrix and/or to other cells. Such molecules may be attached to the **cytoskeleton** and may also be involved in **signal transduction** pathways. (See Chap. 11, Sec. 11.5.)

**Cell cycle time:** The time taken for cells to complete one cell cycle, i.e. to progress from one mitosis to the next. There will be a range of cell cycle times for cells in any given tissue. (See Chap. 9, Sec. 9.4.2.)

**Cell differentiation (CD) antigens:** A classification for **antigens** expressed on the surface of different types of cells. The identification of CD antigens (usually with **monoclonal antibodies**) provides information about the nature and function of a particular cell. This classification has been particularly useful in differentiating the function of various hematologic precursor cells and of cells involved in the immune response.

**Cell-mediated immunity:** Immunologic defense against foreign agents that is mediated by cells (e.g., various types of lymphocytes) rather than by **antibodies.** (See Chap. 20, Sec. 20.2.)

**Cell survival:** A major determinant of the efficacy of anticancer drugs or radiation. Cell survival is determined by the ability of treated cells to proliferate to form a colony or **clone.** A **cell-survival curve** relates cell survival (usually plotted on a logarithmic scale) to dose of radiation or anticancer drug. (See Chap. 14, Secs. 14.3.1 and Chap. 17, Sec. 17.2.3.)

**Centromere:** The region of the **chromosome** at which the two identical components after DNA replication (known as **chromatids**) are held together, prior to their separation at mitosis. (See Chap. 4, Sec. 4.2.)

**Chaperone protein:** A protein that binds to other proteins and assists their correct folding during and after their translation. Such proteins may also play a role in directing the new protein to the correct location in the cell.

**Chimeric antibody:** A **monoclonal antibody** that is genetically engineered so that the variable region that recognizes the antigen is of mouse origin but the rest of the molecule is of human origin (also called a humanized antibody). This minimizes the chance of rejection of the molecule by the **human antimouse antibody (HAMA)** response when used in immunotherapy. (See Chap. 21, Sec. 21.3.4.)

**Chromatin:** The DNA and associated proteins seen in the nucleus of cells in **interphase.**

**Chromosome:** The structural unit containing the genetic material (DNA) and associated proteins within a cell. Human cells usually have 46 chromosomes consisting of 22 pairs of **autosomes** plus the sex chromosomes (XX in females, XY in males). Different chromosomes may be recognized in metaphase cells by their shape and by the application of various stains that lead to the production of characteristic **bands.** After DNA replication, each chromosome contains a pair of **chromatids** joined at the **centromere.** Alterations in the structure of chromosomes are known as aberrations. They are common in cancer cells. (See Chap. 4, Sec. 4.2.)

**Chromosome banding/G-banding:** A method of staining **chromosomes** from metaphase cells to facilitate their recognition. G-banding is obtained by application of the Giemsa stain to metaphase chromosomes that have been treated briefly with the proteolytic enzyme trypsin. (See Chap. 4, Sec. 4.2.)

**Chronic Tumor Virus:** A virus that can cause malignant **transformation** in target cells through integration into the host-cell DNA and the aberrant activation of adjacent cellular **genes.** In contrast to an **acute transforming virus,** a chronic tumor virus does not contain an **oncogene** and transformation takes place more slowly. (See Chap. 6, Sec. 6.3.3.)

**Clonal evolution/Clonal selection:** There is evidence that most tumors originate from a single cell (i.e., are clonal), but ongoing genetic changes during tumor growth lead to the generation of different subclones. "Clonal evolution/selection" refers to the growth advantage of certain **clones** within

the tumor, generally those expressing more malignant properties. (See Chap. 11, Sec. 11.1.1.)

**Clone:** A family of cells all derived from one parent cell. A clonal marker (e.g., an abnormal **chromosome** or protein product) may identify all of the cells within a given clone. Most human tumors appear to arise from a single cell and hence are clonal.

**Cloned gene:** A **gene** that has been isolated and inserted into a "vector," such as a **plasmid** or **bacteriophage.** The vector containing the gene can be produced in large amounts, thereby providing many copies of the gene suitable for assays and studies of its function. Cloned genes can be used to produce large quantities of pure protein products of cells (e.g., insulin, **interferons**). (See Chap. 4, Sec. 4.3.3.)

**Clonogenic assay:** An experimental method that assesses the probability of survival of colony-forming (i.e., **clonogenic**) cells after some form of treatment, as with radiation or anticancer drugs. (See Chap. 14, Sec. 14.3 and Chap. 17, Sec. 17.2.3.)

**Clonogenic cell:** A cell that has the ability to generate progeny that form a colony of predetermined minimum size when plated in appropriate growth conditions. Such a cell is also referred to as a colony-forming unit (CFU). Clonogenic cells may be identified in assays of **cell survival.** The term "CFU" is most often applied to progenitor cells in the bone marrow that may produce **clones** of cells in one or more pathways of **differentiation.**

**Cluster analysis:** A method for analyzing the similarity of increased or decreased expression of **genes** in **microarrays.** In *supervised* cluster analyses, tissues with known characteristics (such as malignant versus normal tissue) are compared. In *unsupervised* cluster analyses, genes are clustered together without reference to predefined characteristics. (See Chap. 22, Sec. 22.3.4.)

**Coding region:** The coding region is that part of a gene which codes for a protein. The part of the DNA molecule that is initially transcribed into messenger RNA (mRNA) contains both **introns** and **exons.** The **introns** are regions of mRNA that are **spliced** out during posttranscriptional processing. The **exon** regions in the mRNA comprise the processed message; they contain the coding regions and therefore are the "expressed" portion of the **gene.** The processed mRNA usually contains (untranslated) regions both 5' and 3' to the coding region that are not translated into protein; these untranslated regions contain important regulatory signals.

**Codon:** A group of three DNA or mRNA bases that code for a given amino acid. Codons thus form the "words" of the genetic code.

**Cohort study:** An epidemiologic study whereby subsets of a given population are defined on the basis of exposure or nonexposure to a factor suspected of increasing the risk of developing a disease (such as cancer) and then followed forward in time to observe the development of the disease. (See Chap. 2, Sec. 2.2.3.)

**Co-intervention:** An intervention, not specified in the protocol of a clinical trial, which may influence the treatment outcome and hence confound the results of the trial. (See Chap. 22, Sec. 22.4.2.)

**Colony-forming assay:** Another term for **clonogenic assay.**

**Colony-stimulating factor:** A **growth factor** that stimulates the formation of colonies of progeny from certain types of cell. The term is used most commonly to describe growth factors that act on precursors of hematopoiesis. (See Chap. 9, Sec. 9.4.3.)

**Comparative genomic hybridization (CGH):** A method that allows detection of amplified or deleted segments of DNA. In this technique, DNA from two different types of cells is labeled with two different fluorochromes (e.g red and green) and then **hybridized** simultaneously to normal chromosomal metaphase spreads. Regions of gain or loss of DNA sequences in one cell as compared with the other are seen as changes in the ratio of the intensities of the red or green fluorescence along the target chromosome. (See Chap. 4, Sec. 4.4.2.)

**Complementation:** A technique that can assist in identifying a defective **gene.** Two types of cell containing different genetic defects are **fused** and complementation is said to occur if the hybrid cell lacks these genetic defects. This result indicates that the genes are located at a distinct chromosomal locus, so that the normal chromosomal component provided by one cell complements the defect in the other. In yeast, complementation also refers to the ability of a given gene, when expressed from an exogenous source such as a plasmid, to rescue the phenotype associated with a particular endogenous mutation or gene deletion.

**Compliance:** The extent to which treatment is delivered as intended. Low compliance is a particular problem with oral medications that cause toxicity. (See Chap. 22, Sec. 22.4.2.)

**Computed tomography (CT) scanning:** An imaging procedure that uses a thin beam of X-rays and a detector placed on the other side of the patient that are rotated together through 360° and then uses computer methods to construct images of cross-sections of the body. (See Chap. 13, Sec. 13.2.1.)

**Contamination:** The extent to which patients in one arm of a clinical trial receive treatment that is intended for those in the other arm. (See Chap. 22, Sec. 22.4.2.)

**Cosmid:** A circular piece of DNA that has properties similar to those of a **plasmid.** It is larger than a plasmid and may contain different regulatory elements.

**Costimulatory molecule:** A molecule expressed on the surface of **antigen-presenting cells** that provides a second signal (augmenting the primary signal initiated by the binding of the **antigenic** peptide presented by a **major histocompatibility molecule** to the **T cell receptor**) for stimulation of a cell-mediated immune response. (See Chap. 20, Sec. 20.5.2.)

**Cross-links:** Abnormal bonding between (interstrand) or within (intrastrand) DNA strands or between DNA strands

and proteins (DNA-protein) that can be induced by radiation or anticancer drugs.

**Cyclin/cyclin-dependent kinase:** Cyclins are proteins whose activity varies around the cell cycle. Cyclins bind to cyclin-dependent kinases (CDKs), which are small serine/threonine kinases expressed at relatively constant levels through the cell cycle. Activation of cyclins in these complexes is associated with progression of cells from one cell cycle phase to the next. Different cyclins and CDKs are involved in different phases of the cell cycle. (See Chap. 9, Sec. 9.2.1.)

**Cyclin-dependent kinase (CDK) inhibitor:** A protein that inhibits the function of **cyclin–dependent kinases** and thereby inhibits cell cycle progression. CDK inhibitors are members of two families known as the KIP (*K*inase *I*nhibitor *P*rotein) family and the INK-4 (*In*hibitor of CD*K-4*) family. (See Chap. 9, Sec. 9.2.2.)

**Cytochrome P-450:** A large family of drug metabolizing enzymes that are important in the activation of **carcinogens.** (See Chap. 3, Sec. 3.2.2.)

**Cytokine:** A protein molecule that is secreted by cells and acts to modify the proliferation, **differentiation,** or function of other cells that express specific **receptors.** Cytokines are particularly important in the generation and control of immune responses. (See Chap. 21, Sec. 21.3.1.)

**Cytoskeleton:** The group of molecules that provides physical structure and defines the form and shape of cells.

**Cytotoxic T lymphocytes:** Activated T lymphocytes responsible for the killing of target cells during a cell-mediated immune response. (See Chap. 20, Secs. 20.2.3 and 20.5.2.)

**Death receptor:** **Receptors** on cells, that when bound by **ligands,** stimulate signaling pathways that initiate **apoptosis** and lead to their death. Death receptors include Fas (CD95), Tumor Necrosis Factor (TNF) receptor type 1 (TNFR-1) and TNF-related apoptosis-inducing ligand (Trail). (See Chap. 10, Sec. 10.2.6.)

**Deletion:** Loss of DNA. Deletions can be small, affecting only a small part of a single **gene,** or large—for example, a **chromosomal** deletion involving many genes.

**Dendritic cell:** A cell derived from the bone marrow that expresses high cell surface levels of critical **major histocompatibility antigens** as well as **costimulatory** and adhesive molecules that render it an efficient **antigen-presenting cell.** Purified dendritic cells are being used in approaches to immunotherapy. (See Chap. 20, Sec. 20.5 and Chap. 21, Sec. 21.4.7.)

**Dicentric chromosome:** An abnormal chromosome that contains two **centromeres.**

**Differentiation:** The development by cells of specific characteristics that allow the normal function of tissues. Tumors may show varying degrees of differentiation, depending on their similarity to the structure of the organ from which the tumor was derived. **Terminal differentiation** is said to occur when cells form progeny that are no longer capable of division.

**Dimer:** A complex formed by the joining of two molecules. In a homodimer, the constituent molecules are identical; in a heterodimer, they are different.

**Diurnal rhythm:** Variation in the biological properties of an organism throughout the day. Many properties—such as the concentration of hormones or the activity of certain enzymes—may show diurnal variation.

**DNA adduct:** A chemical group bound to DNA that will usually interfere with DNA replication and/or transcription. (See Chap. 3, Sec. 3.2.4.)

**DNA damage checkpoint:** Phases of the cell cycle in which cells arrest in response to DNA damage. These checkpoints may allow for **DNA repair** prior to the cell entering the subsequent cell cycle phase (e.g. G1 arrest prior to S-phase and DNA replication or G2 arrest prior to mitosis. (See Chap. 5, Sec. 5.4.)

**DNA ladder:** A pattern seen in **electrophoresis** of DNA from apoptotic cells. **Endonucleases** induced during **apoptosis** cut DNA into fragments that are multiples of about 180 base pairs. When the DNA of such cells is subjected to gel **electrophoresis,** a characteristic ladder-like pattern of DNA fragments is produced. (See Chap. 10, Sec. 10.3.4.)

**DNA methylation:** Bases in DNA, particularly cytosine, may become methylated. This can modify or inhibit the transcription of a gene. Such methylations are potentially reversible and are often referred to as "**epigenetic** changes" to distinguish them from **mutations** involving changes in DNA bases.

**DNA microarray:** A matrix of a large number of known DNA molecules (or parts of DNA molecules) attached to an inert substrate. Such matrices can be **hybridized** with unknown mixtures of mRNAs or DNAs to identify those **genes** that are being expressed or are the subject of genomic imbalance in the cells from which the mixtures were derived. (See Chap. 4, Sec. 4.4.4 and Chap. 22, Sec. 22.3.4)

**DNA repair:** The process whereby damaged DNA acts as a substrate for enzymes that attempt to restore its normal structure and the original base sequence. It is a complex process involving many enzymes and may lead to repair of damage in one or both strands. Repair may lead to complete restoration of the DNA (error-free repair) or may result in alteration or deletion of bases (error-prone repair). (See Chap. 5, Sec. 5.3.)

**Double minute:** A small amount of genetic material seen in some cells as a paired body resembling a very small **chromosome** without a **centromere.** Because they lack a centromere, double minutes distribute themselves randomly at mitosis and are easily lost during cell growth. Double minutes have been shown to contain amplified **genes.** (See Chap. 4, Fig. 4.14 and Chap. 18, Sec. 18.2.5.)

**Double-strand break (DSB):** A lesion causing interruption of both strands (sugar-phosphate "backbone") of a DNA molecule. Such DSBs are believed responsible for the cytotoxic effects of ionizing radiation. (See Chap. 5, Secs. 5.3.5 and 5.3.6 and Chap. 14, Sec. 14.2.3.)

**Doubling time:** The time taken for an exponentially growing tumor (or cell population) to double its volume (or number of cells). (See Chap. 9, Sec. 9.4.1.)

**Dysplasia:** Abnormal morphologic changes in the cells of a tissue involving their nuclei, organization, and maturation.

**Electrophile:** A molecule or chemical group that is positively charged and attracts electrons. Electrophiles interact with negatively charged electron-rich groups on biological molecules such as DNA. The active forms of many **carcinogens** are electrophiles and therefore they can bind to DNA. (See Chap. 3, Sec. 3.2.)

**Electrophoresis:** The separation of molecular components (peptides, proteins, or pieces of DNA or RNA) by their different rates of migration in an electric field. **Gel electrophoresis** refers to electrophoresis through an agarose or polyacrylamide gel and is used commonly in molecular technology. Molecules of lower molecular weight usually migrate more rapidly under electrophoresis. (See Chap. 4, Sec. 4.3.4.).

**End-to-end fusions:** Loss of telomere function can lead to covalent ligation (fusion) of two chromosomes at their ends, creating a **dicentric chromosome**.

**Endogenous:** A property intrinsic to the cell, for example, referring to a gene or protein that normally resides in the cell and has not been introduced or expressed from an exogenous source.

**Endonuclease:** An enzyme that can cut an intact strand of DNA or RNA at some point in the strand other than at an end. Endonucleases are important in **DNA repair** (see Chap. 5, Sec. 5.3) and are responsible for cutting of DNA during **apoptosis.** (See Chap. 10, Sec. 10.3.4.)

**Endostatin:** Proteolytic fragment of the **extracellular matrix** protein collagen XVIII, that inhibits the proliferation of endothelial cells. (See Chap. 12, Sec. 12.4.1.)

**Enhancer:** A DNA sequence that increases the activity of **promotor** sequences or initiators of mRNA transcription. Enhancers can be located anywhere in the noncoding regions of a gene.

**Enzyme-linked immunoadsorbent assay (ELISA):** A sensitive method for measuring the amount of a substance. The method requires the availability of an **antibody** to the substance and depends on measuring the activity of an enzyme (e.g., alkaline phosphatase) bound to the antibody.

**Ephrins:** A large family of **ligands** that are tethered to the cell membrane and which bind to Eph receptors to stimulate intracellular signaling pathways that are involved in **angiogenesis.** (See Chap. 12, Sec. 12.2.4.)

**Epidermal growth factor (EGF):** A **growth factor** that binds to a specific **receptor** (EGFR) that can initiate **signal transduction** in target cells of the epidermis and other normal or malignant epithelial tissues. (See Chap. 8, Sec. 8.2.1.)

**Epigenetic:** Epigenetic changes alter the expression of **genes** without causing permanent base damage. **DNA methylation**

**or histone acetylation** represent forms of epigenetic change in DNA.

**Episome:** A circular form of DNA that replicates in cells independent of the **chromosomes.** Viral DNA may form episomes in cells. **Plasmids** used for gene cloning grow as episomes in bacteria.

**Epitope:** A small part of a protein molecule that can be recognized by antibodies or **antigen receptors** on lymphocytes and which elicits an immune response against that molecule. (See Chap. 20, Sec. 20.2.1.)

**Epstein-Barr virus:** A DNA virus associated with Burkitt's lymphoma, nasopharyngeal cancer, and Hodgkin's disease. (See Chap. 6, Sec. 6.2.4.)

**Erythropoietin:** A hormone produced by the kidney that stimulates the proliferation of red cell precursors in the bone marrow. It is now being used to treat anemia. (See Chap. 9, Sec. 9.4.3.)

**Estrogens:** Steroid sex hormones (e.g. estradiol) that cause female features. Estrogens stimulate the growth of some breast cancers. (See Chap. 19, Sec. 19.2.1.)

**Estrogen receptor:** Intracellular receptor which binds to **estrogens.** (See Chap. 19, Sec. 19.2.2.)

**Exons:** The regions of a **gene** that contain the DNA sequences necessary to direct translation of the polypeptide gene product from the transcribed mRNA. These sequences include the **coding region,** and the 5′ and 3′ untranslated regions.

**Exonuclease:** An enzyme that catalyzes the base-by-base destruction of DNA or RNA starting at one end of a strand.

**Experimental metastasis assay:** A technique for studying the ability of cells to form **metastases** in experimental animals after injection into a blood vessel. (See Chap. 11, Sec. 11.2.2.)

**Extracellular matrix (ECM):** The complex group of molecules that exist in tissue outside the cells and provide an adhesive environment for the cells and other molecules such as growth factors. (See Chap. 11, Sec. 11.4.)

**Extrachromosomal DNA:** DNA fragments or circles not contained within the normal chromosomes; e.g. artificially introduced, or generated by aberrant recombinational events.

**Facilitated diffusion:** A process in which the diffusion of certain substances into cells is enhanced. Specific molecules in the cell membrane (permeases) bind to the substance and assist its diffusion through the membrane down a concentration gradient from outside to inside the cell.

**Fluorescence-in-situ hybridization (FISH):** A technique in which a fluorescently-labeled DNA probe binds to the **complementary gene** segment in **chromosomes** of metaphase spreads. FISH, therefore, allows the localization of genes to specific chromosomes. The technique can also be used in interphase cells to determine the number of copies of the gene that the cells contain. Using chromosome-specific probes the technique can identify chromosome aberrations, particularly **translocations.** (See Chap. 4, Sec. 4.4.1.)

**Flow cytometry:** A technique in which cells are tagged with a fluorescent dye and then directed in single file through a laser beam. The intensity of fluorescence induced by the laser light is detected and the number of cells exhibiting different levels of fluorescence is recorded. The method is used frequently to study cell-cycle properties, since several dyes are available, whose binding in cells—and hence fluorescence intensity—is proportional to DNA content. It is also used to measure the proportion of cells in a population expressing a specific cell surface marker. Cells may also be separated according to the intensity of their fluorescence in a process known as fluorescence-activated cell sorting (FACS). (See Chap. 9, Sec. 9.4.2.)

**Frameshift mutation:** A DNA mutation that leads to a change in the initiation point of translation of the mRNA transcript, such that the normal reading frame for the **codons,** which define the amino acid sequence of the protein product, is shifted by one or two bases, resulting in a different amino acid sequence, or in many cases a premature stop codon (PTC).

**Free radical:** An unstable chemical species that is highly reactive due to the presence of an unpaired electron. It may be formed when drugs or radiation interact with tissue. Free radicals may be responsible for much of the biological damage that occurs after such interactions.

**Functional imaging:** Imaging that demonstrates tissue function (such as blood flow or biochemical processes). (See Chap. 13, Sec. 13.3.)

**Fusion protein:** A protein formed by transcription from fused genetic segments of two or more **genes.** Fusion proteins may occur naturally (for example, the *BCR/ABL* protein formed by **translocation** in chronic myelogenous leukemia) or may be genetically engineered to produce a protein of desired characteristics (for example, a protein that is fused from components that are (1) toxic and (2) bind to a **receptor** on a tumor cell). (See Chap. 7, Sec. 7.2.4 and Chap. 21, Sec. 21.3.4.)

**Gap junctions:** Junctions between neighboring cells, formed by connexin proteins that allow the passage of molecules between cells. (See Chap. 11, Sec. 11.5.6.)

**Gene:** A sequence of DNA that codes for a single polypeptide or protein. This sequence includes **coding** and noncoding regions as well as regulatory regions. Genes may sometimes be overlapping, so that the same sequence contributes to two different proteins.

**Gene amplification:** Amplification may occur through multiplication of the DNA sequences of the **gene;** a large amount of amplification can often be recognized by the presence of either **homogeneously staining regions** (HSRs) on **chromosomes** or by the presence of **double minutes.** (See Chap. 4, Fig. 4.14 and Chap. 18, Sec. 18.2.5.)

**Gene targeting:** The process by which an endogenous gene sequence is altered by introduction of an altered gene sequence via site-specific **homologous recombination.**

**Genetic (or molecular) epidemiology:** Study of the distribution among populations of various genetic defects such as those predisposing to various types of cancer (e.g., *BRCA-1* or retinoblastoma gene mutations). (See Chap. 2, Sec. 2.3.3)

**Genetic instability:** Increased propensity for a cell to undergo genetic alterations. Often such cells do not exhibit the normal complement of 46 chromosomes, and contains evidence of chromosomal aberrations or other intrinsic mutations.

**Genome:** Refers to the normal complement of DNA for a given organism. In humans, the genome is comprised of 46 chromosomes within the nucleus (the DNA within the mitochondria is usually considered separately).

**Glutathione:** A small molecule composed of three amino acids (glycine, cysteine, glutamate) that is prevalent within cells and can bind to reactive compounds and aid in their excretion. (See Chap. 18, Sec. 18.2.4.)

**Glycoprotein:** A protein to which various types of sugar molecule have been attached. Glycoproteins are important components of the cell surface.

**Grade:** The histopathologic appearance of a tumor in terms of its degree of **differentiation**. A low-grade tumor is well differentiated and a high-grade tumor tends to be **anaplastic.**

**Gray:** The unit of radiation dose. It is defined by the energy absorbed per unit mass (1 Gray is equivalent to 1 Joule/kg). (See Chap. 14, Sec. 14.2.1.)

**Green fluorescent protein (GFP):** The **gene** encoding GFP is often **transfected** in association with other genes or fused to specific proteins and, when expressed, causes green coloration, hence marking the tissue or intracellular expression of the associated genes. (See Chap. 11, Sec. 11.3.2.)

**Growth factor:** A polypeptide produced by cells that stimulates or inhibits proliferation by either the same cell or other cells. Several types of growth factor have been isolated and some of these may be associated with abnormal regulation of growth in **transformed** cells. Growth factors interact with cells through specific **receptors** in the cell membrane. (See Chap. 7, Sec. 7.3.1 and Chap. 8, Sec. 8.2.)

**Growth fraction:** The proportion of cells within a tumor that are actively proliferating (i.e., progressing through the cell cycle). (See Chap. 9, Sec. 9.4.2.)

**Half-life (plasma):** The plasma clearance curve describes the concentration of a drug in plasma as a function of time after administration, and frequently has components that are approximately exponential. Plasma half-lives characterize the exponentially decreasing components of these clearance curves and represent the time for drug concentration to decrease by 50 percent. (See Chap. 16, Sec. 16.1.2.)

**Half-life (radioactivity):** Radioactive isotopes decay randomly, so that on average there is a constant time for the activity to decay to half of its starting value. This time is the half-life.

**Heat-shock proteins:** A family of stress proteins whose synthesis is stimulated by the exposure of cells to heat or various other stimuli, including hypoxia and hypoglycemia. Heat-shock proteins have diverse functions; for example, some

heat-shock proteins bind to steroid hormone receptors and play a part in regulating their function, while other HSPs may act as **chaperone proteins** that bind to and assist other proteins to fold correctly. (See Chap. 19, Sec. 19.2.2.)

**Hedgehog signaling:** A signaling pathway important in embryonic development. Abnormal activation of the pathway has been associated with the development of sporadic cancers. (See Chap. 8, Sec. 8.4.3.)

**Heterogeneity:** Variability in the properties of cells within an individual tumor. Wide heterogeneity of many properties is found among cancer cells. (See Chap. 11, Sec. 11.1.)

**Heterozygosity:** The presence of different **alleles** of a **gene** on the two copies of the same chromosome.

**Histocompatibility antigen:** Rejection of foreign tissue is determined by differences in histocompatibility antigens on cells of the donor and host tissues. One locus (which includes several **genes**) is associated with strong rejection and is known as the **major histocompatibility complex** (MHC). MHC molecules present peptide fragments from degraded molecules as antigens on the surface of **antigen-presenting cells.** Class I MHC molecules present peptide fragments from degraded intracellular molecules, whereas class II MHC molecules present fragments of extracellular peptides that have been endocytosed into the cell. (See Chap. 20, Sec. 20.2.2.)

**Histone deacetylase (HDAC):** HDACs remove acetyl groups from core nucleosomal proteins (histones) and thereby inhibit the **transcription** of **genes.** Inhibitors of this activity are being evaluated as anticancer agents in clinical trials. (See Chap. 7, Sec. 7.3.4 and Chap. 17, Sec. 17.6.2.)

**Homeostasis:** The maintenance of a normal physiologic state. Homeostasis is often maintained through feedback systems employing signals (e.g., hormones or **growth factors**) that have opposing effects.

**Homogeneously staining region (HSR):** A region appearing uniform on **chromosomes** that have been stained to examine their banding pattern. It often represents amplification of **genes.** HSRs tend to be stably inherited by daughter cells. (See Chap. 4, Fig. 4.14 and Chap. 18, Sec. 18.2.5.)

**Homologous recombination:** The crossing over and rejoining of corresponding (homologous) regions of DNA on opposite **chromosomes** that occur normally during meiosis. A similar process can occur between a segment of DNA introduced into a cell and the homologous region on one of the chromosomes, or during **repair of DNA** damage. (See Chap. 5, Sec. 5.3.5.)

**Homology:** Correspondence of the sequence of bases on different strands of DNA or RNA such that either strand will **hybridize to** complementary sequences.

**Homozygosity (homozygous):** When the two **alleles** of a **gene** on the two copies of the same **chromosome** in a cell are identical.

**Hormone response element:** A palindromic DNA sequences found in the **promoter** regions of hormone-responsive **genes**

that binds to an activated hormone **receptor** dimer complex. (See Chap. 19, Sec. 19.2.2.)

**Human antimouse antibody (HAMA) response:** The rejection response that can occur when **monoclonal antibodies** derived from murine cells are injected into humans for immunotherapy or immunodiagnosis. (See Chap. 21, Sec. 21.3.4.)

**Humoral immunity:** The part of the immune response mediated by **antibodies.** (See Chap. 20, Sec. 20.2.1.)

**Hybridization:** (1) The fusion of two somatic cells to form a single cell. (2) The binding of complementary sequences of DNA or RNA. Such complementary binding may take place under different conditions (degrees of stringency) that dictate the extent of complementarity required for binding to occur. Radiolabeled pieces of DNA or RNA can be used as **probes** to identify the presence of specific DNA sequences by hybridization. The technique may also localize **genes** to specific **chromosomes** in a process known as "**fluorescence in situ hybridization (FISH).**" (See Chap. 4, Sec. 4.3.1.)

**Hybridoma:** The term is used most commonly to describe a population of hybrid cells that produces **monoclonal antibodies.** Such a cell is produced by fusing an antibody-producing normal cell and a non-antibody-secreting myeloma cell. (See Chap. 21, Sec. 21.3.3.)

**Hydrophilic:** A molecule or chemical group that has high solubility in water primarily because of its polarity.

**Hydrophobic:** A molecule or chemical group that has low solubility in water, usually because it is nonpolar. Such molecules usually have higher solubility in lipids.

**Hyperfractionation:** A schedule used in radiation therapy where multiple (two or three) small dose fractions are given each day. (See Chap. 15, Sec. 15.7.4.)

**Hyperplasia:** An increase in the number of normal cells in a tissue. Hyperplasia can be either a normal (physiologic) or an abnormal (pathologic) process.

**Hyperthermia:** The use of elevated temperature as an anticancer treatment.

**Hypoxia inducible factor-1 (HIF-1):** A **transcription factor** that stimulates the expression of certain **genes** in response to a hypoxic microenvironment. (See Chap. 15, Sec. 15.4.2.)

**Hypoxic cell:** A cell, often within a tumor, that lacks oxygen. Such cells are important because they are resistant to the effects of radiation therapy and are usually in regions with poor vascular supply. (See Chap. 15, Sec. 15.4.)

**Idiotype:** The variable (V) region of an **antibody** or **T cell receptor.** The idiotype is, itself, **antigenic,** and anti-idiotype responses have been used in the treatment of lymphomas. (See Chap. 21, Sec. 21.4.3.)

**Immortalization:** The process that allows cells to form a cell line (i.e., to be able to proliferate indefinitely) in culture. Normal cells will proliferate for only a limited number of passages in culture before they undergo **senescence** or die. Immortal-

ization appears to be a necessary but not sufficient step for **transformation** to a **malignant** state.

**Immunogen:** Any molecule that can elicit an immune response. (See Chaps. 20 and 21.)

**Immunoglobulin:** An **antibody** molecule. In general, immunoglobulins consist of two heavy chains and two light chains linked by disulfide bonds (IgM-class immuno-globulins have 10 heavy and 10 light chains). The **immunoglobulin superfamily** consists of molecules with related structure and sequence that are found as components of a number of protein molecules, including those involved in cellular interactions with the **extracellular matrix.** (See Chap. 11, Sec. 11.5.3 and Chap. 20, Sec. 20.2.1.)

**Immunohistochemistry:** A histologic process whereby a colored stain is linked to an **antibody** (usually a **monoclonal antibody**) that is used on tissue sections to recognize cells that express specific **proteins** that bind the **antibody.**

**Immunosuppression:** A state in which immune responses are impaired. This may occur in patients with some types of cancer, following treatment with drugs and radiation, or following treatment given as part of the preparation for organ transplantation. Certain inbred strains of mice may be immunosuppressed (or immune-deprived) by virtue of **mutations** that they carry in their genome [e.g., **nude** mice or mice with severe combined immunodeficiency (**SCID**)].

**Immunosurveillance:** A proposed mechanism whereby the immune response recognizes the development of **malignant** cells at an early stage and inactivates them before they can develop into tumors. (See Chap. 20, Sec. 20.4.2.)

**Immunotoxin:** A molecule that recognizes and binds to target cells by immune-mediated mechanisms and which has a toxic component that can inactivate target cells. The term is used most commonly to describe a hybrid molecule consisting of a **monoclonal antibody** that is conjugated or fused to a toxin. (See Chap. 21, Sec. 21.3.4.)

**Imprinting:** A process whereby a specific **gene** or **allele** is silenced (prevented from producing a product), usually by **methylation** of cytosine bases. This usually occurs in the embryo and is often tissue-specific.

**Incidence:** A term used in epidemiology to describe the number of new cases (e.g., of cancer) observed in a population in a given unit of time, usually one year. (See Chap. 2, Sec. 2.2.1.)

**Initiation:** The first stage in the classic process of carcinogenesis. It involves interaction of the **carcinogen** with the DNA of the target cells to produce, after DNA replication, a permanent lesion. Subsequent steps include **promotion** and **progression.** (See Chap. 3, Sec. 3.2.1.)

**Innate immunity:** A component of the immune system that is nonspecific and present at all times in normal individuals. It depends on a group of cells and released factors that provide natural resistance as the first-line of defense against invading pathogens. (See Chap. 20, Sec. 20.2.1.)

**Insertional mutagenesis:** The process in which there is a change (or loss) of function of a **gene** as a result of the incorporation of a piece of exogenous DNA (often from a virus or **plasmid** introduced into the cell) into the DNA of that gene, thereby disrupting its normal transcription and translation or the control of these processes.

**Integration:** The process by which viral or **plasmid** DNA, or DNA copies of the RNA of a **retrovirus,** are incorporated into the chromosomal DNA of a cell.

**Integrins:** A family of membrane **glycoproteins** that can bind to a range of molecules present in the **extracellular matrix** and that can mediate adhesion between a cell and the extracellular matrix. Integrins can also initiate **signal transduction.** (See Chap. 8, Sec. 8.3.3 and Chap. 11, Sec. 11.5.1.)

**Interferon:** A protein produced by cells in response to viral infection. Several types of interferon have been identified and they have multiple effects on the host immune response as well as more general effects on cell growth and **differentiation.**

**Interleukins:** A family of molecules that are secreted, most often by lymphocytes, and which regulate the proliferation, **differentiation,** or function of hematopoietic cells or cells of the immune system. (See Chap. 21, Sec. 21.3.1.)

**Intravital videomicroscopy:** A technique for studying dynamic events in a living organism. (See Chap. 11, Sec. 11.3.2.)

**Intron:** A noncoding region in the internal portion of a **gene.** Sequences transcribed from these regions are **spliced** out during processing of the initial mRNA transcript.

**Invasion:** Infiltration by cancer cells into neighboring normal tissues. It is one of the distinguishing features of malignancy.

**Ionizing radiation:** Radiation (e.g., X- or γ-rays) that is sufficiently energetic for its interactions with matter (tissue) to cause the formation of ions. (See Chap. 14, Sec. 14.2.1.)

**Isobologram:** A diagram in the format of a graph whose axes represent doses of two cytotoxic agents A and B. The isobologram joins points at which the combination of different doses of A and B produce an equal level of biological damage. The diagram is useful in determining whether the effects of two agents may be **additive,** subadditive (or antagonistic), or supraadditive (or **synergistic**). (See Chap. 17, Sec. 17.5.2.)

**Isoeffect curve:** An isoeffect curve indicates graphically the relationship between different dose schedules of a treatment that produce the same biological effect. The curve is used mainly to represent the effects of radiation treatments given as different numbers of fractions or in different overall times. The total radiation dose is plotted as a function of the fraction number, fraction size, or treatment time. (See Chap. 15, Sec. 15.7.2.)

**Isomer:** One structural form of a chemical compound that can occur naturally in a number of different structural forms. An example is diammine dichloroplatinum II, in which a different arrangement of the attachment of the amine and chloride groups to the platinum atom gives rise to the *cis-* and *trans-*isomers, which have very different biological activities.

**Isozyme (isoenzyme):** One of several chemical forms of an enzyme that have the same biological function. Tumor cells often produce one particular isozyme, frequently that associated with fetal tissue.

**Kaposi's sarcoma:** A vascular skin tumor that is observed commonly in subjects with the acquired immunodeficiency syndrome (AIDS). (See Chap. 6, Sec. 6.2.6.)

**Karyotype:** The **chromosome** content of a particular cell. The karyotype is usually displayed by imaging the chromosomes in a metaphase cell and ordering them according to a standard notation. (See Chap. 4, Sec. 4.2.)

**Knockout mouse:** A mouse derived from an embryonic stem (ES) cell that has been manipulated to cause a dysfunctional (knockout) mutation in a specific **gene.** (See Chap. 4, Sec. 4.3.12.)

**Knudson's hypothesis:** The hypothesis that at least two genetic events are required in order to transform a normal cell into a **malignant** cell. It was postulated originally by Knudson to explain the inheritance pattern of retinoblastoma, a rare childhood malignancy.

**Labeling index:** The proportion of cells in any tissue that are synthesizing DNA and that, therefore, can be recognized as labeled by uptake of DNA precursors such as $^3$H-thymidine or bromodeoxyuridine (BrdUrd). (See Chap. 9, Sec. 9.4.2.)

**Late effects (late tissue responses):** Toxicity to normal tissues that becomes apparent at a time long after (months to years) the application of radiation therapy. Late effects usually limit the dose of radiation that can be given. (See Chap. 15, Sec. 15.5.3.)

**Lead-time bias:** A type of **bias** that can confound the interpretation of screening studies. Screening is designed to detect disease at an earlier stage than would normally occur, and survival from the time of diagnosis will therefore be increased by the lead time that is gained by the screening assay. This is independent of any change in survival due to earlier initiation of therapy. (See Chap. 2, Sec. 2.2.7 and Chap. 22, Sec. 22.2.4.)

**Lectins:** Naturally occurring proteins that can bind to specific oligosaccharide structures on cell-surface **glycoproteins** and glycolipids. They may have two or more binding sites and hence can cause cell agglutination.

**Length-time bias:** A type of **bias** in screening studies that arises because a test performed at fixed intervals is more likely to detect slower-growing disease (that which is present for a longer time) than rapidly progressive disease. Thus, patients whose disease is detected by such a screening test may have a better prognosis. (See Chap. 22, Sec. 22.2.4.)

**Lethal dose 50 percent (LD$_{50}$):** The dose of radiation or of a drug that will, on average, cause 50 percent of animals receiving it to die.

**Ligand:** A molecule that binds to a **receptor.**

**Likelihood ratio:** The ratio of the probability that disease is present and the probability that it is absent following application of a diagnostic test. (See Chap. 22, Sec. 22.2.3.)

**Linear energy transfer (LET):** A measure of the density of energy deposition along the track of a given type of **ionizing radiation** in matter. The deposition of energy in matter by ionizing radiation occurs randomly along the particle track and in different amounts, hence LET is a quantity usually averaged over segments of the track length (track-averaged LET). (See Chap. 14, Sec. 14.2.2 and Chap. 15, Sec. 15.2.4.)

**Linear quadratic equation:** An equation describing biological effect as a function of dose of a cytotoxic agent, such as radiation, which contains both linear and quadratic (squared) terms of dose with constants $\alpha$ and $\beta$ respectively. It provides a useful model for describing the shape of radiation **survival curves** and for comparing **isoeffective** radiation treatments. (See Chap. 14, App. 14.1 and Chap. 15, Sec. 15.7.3.)

**Linkage:** A measure of the proximity of two **genes** on a **chromosome.** The more closely linked the two genes the less likely they are to be separated by crossing over of chromosomes during meiosis and hence the more likely they are to be inherited together. (See Chap. 2, Sec. 2.3.3.)

**Lipophilic:** A substance that is lipid-soluble. Lipophilic substances penetrate readily into cells, since they are soluble in the cell membrane.

**Liposome:** A small vesicle containing fluid surrounded by a lipid membrane. Liposomes may be constructed to have varying lipid content in their membranes and to contain various types of drugs or other molecules. They may be used to introduce **genes** into cells. (See Chap. 17, Sec. 17.6.3 and Chap. 21, Sec. 21.2.3.)

**Loss of heterozygosity (LOH):** An individual with two different **alleles** of a **gene** is said to be **heterozygous** for that gene. Loss of heterozygosity signifies loss of one of the alleles. This may occur by simple loss of an allele or by replacement of one allele with a duplicated copy of the other allele. In a tumor cell, LOH may indicate that the tumor suppressor properties of the product of a normal allele has been replaced by a mutant allele which has lost these properties. (See Chap. 7, Sec. 7.4.1.)

**Magnetic resonance imaging (MRI):** An imaging technique that depends on the magnetization of tissue when a patient is placed in a strong externally-applied magnetic field. The magnetic field results in the alignment of proton spins; an alignment that can be perturbed by an electromagnetic pulse. The different rates of realignment of such proton spins (relaxation) in different tissues allows an image to be generated. (See Chap. 13, Sec. 13.2.4.)

**Magnetic resonance spectroscopy (MRS):** A variant of MRI that allows study of the biochemical processes in tissue by virtue of measuring the different absorption energy of different biochemical species (chemical shift spectra). (See Chap. 4, Sec. 4.5.3 and Chap. 13, Sec. 13.2.4.)

**Major histocompatibility complex (MHC):** The complex locus of **genes** transcribed into proteins (**histocompatibility antigens**) that are expressed on cells and are responsible for the rejection of foreign tissue. Class I MHC molecules are expressed on almost all cells and generally bind to peptides derived from endogenous intracellular proteins. Class II MHC molecules are expressed primarily on **antigen-presenting cells** and bind to peptides derived from exogenous proteins. (See Chap. 20, Sec. 20.2.2.)

**Malignancy:** The essential property of cancer cells that is demonstrated by their ability to proliferate indefinitely, to invade surrounding tissue, and to **metastasize** to other organs.

**Mass spectroscopy:** A process used for very precise measurement of the mass of components of proteins and other biological molecules. (See Chap. 4, Sec. 4.5.1.)

**Meta-analysis:** A statistical technique for combining the results of clinical trials evaluating similar strategies. The technique facilitates the detection of small but clinically important differences between experimental and standard therapies. (See Chap. 22, Sec. 22.4.7.)

**Metalloproteinases:** Proteolytic enzymes secreted by cells that may cause degradation of components of **the extracellular matrix.** These enzymes may be involved in the process of **metastasis.** (See Chap. 11, Sec. 11.6.)

**Metastasis:** The spread of cells from a primary tumor to a noncontiguous site, usually via the bloodstream or lymphatics, and the establishment of a secondary growth. (See Chap. 11.)

**Microenvironment:** The environment surrounding cells in solid tissue. The microenvironment may change quite markedly over short distances with respect to metabolic factors such as level of oxygen and pH as well as in the consistency of the **extracellular matrix.** (See Chap. 11, Sec. 11.4.)

**Microsatellite instability:** Microsatellites are short repetitive DNA sequences scattered throughout the genome. Instability in these sequences is associated with many sporadic and familial cancers and related to mutations in **mismatch repair** genes. (See Chap. 4, Sec. 4.3.9 and Chap. 5, Sec 5.3.2)

**Microtubule:** Intracellular structures containing the protein tubulin that form the mitotic spindle allowing separation of daughter cells and which provide structure and function to nerves. Some anticancer drugs, including **taxanes** and **vinca alkaloids,** bind to tubulin and inhibit the function of microtubules. (See Chap. 16, Sec. 16.6.)

**Mismatch repair:** A mechanism for **repair of DNA** that contains single-base mispairs or small insertions or **deletions.** Defects in mismatch repair **genes** may predispose to cancer and to progressive genetic changes in malignant cells. (See Chap. 2, Sec. 2.3.3 and Chap. 5, Sec. 5.3.2.)

**Mitochondria:** Cellular organelles that are responsible for the production of energy or ATP, via a complex chain of electron transfers within the mitochondrial membranes. A mitochondrial membrane transition refers to the loss of electrostatic potential within the membrane that often occurs during **apoptosis.**

**Mitogen:** A substance that stimulates the proliferation of cells.

**Mitogen-activated protein kinase (MAPK) pathway:** A signaling pathway that transmits signals imparted by **growth factors** or other **mitogens** at the cell surface to influence proliferation-related **genes** in the cell nucleus. (See Chap. 8, Sec. 8.2.6.)

**Mitotic death (mitotic catastrophe):** The degradation and lysis of cells in mitosis. This is observed frequently following radiation. (See Chap. 14, Sec. 14.3.2.)

**Mitotic delay:** Delay in the passage of a cell through its growth cycle (particularly mitosis) that is induced by radiation and some anticancer drugs. (See Chap. 14, Sec. 14.4.2.)

**Mitotic index:** The proportion of cells in a tissue that are in mitosis at any given time.

**Molecular imaging:** Imaging that can detect molecular or biochemical changes in tissue. (See Chap. 13, Sec. 13.3.)

**Molecular targeted therapy:** Therapy with agents that are designed to inhibit a specific biological target or pathway. (See Chap. 16, Sec. 16.8 and Chap. 17, Sec. 17.6.2.)

**Monoclonal antibody:** An **antibody** of a single defined specificity, most commonly obtained from a single clone of antibody-producing cells or **hybridoma.** A monoclonal antibody binds to a specific **epitope** of the foreign protein it recognizes. (See Chap. 21, Sec. 21.3.3.)

**Mucositis:** Inflammation of the mucous membranes, especially in the mouth, which may occur after treatment with radiation or anticancer drugs.

**Multicellular layer:** An in vitro model used for studying drug penetration through tumor tissue. Tumor cells grow to form a multicellular layer after plating on a semiporous collagen coated Teflon membrane. (See Chap. 18, Fig. 18.13.)

**Multiple drug resistance:** Resistance to a group of chemically unrelated drugs that develops in cells and may be induced or selected for by exposure of the cells to any one of the drugs. One form of multiple drug resistance is caused by expression of **P-glycoprotein** on the cell surface, which is encoded by *mdr* **genes.** (See Chap. 18, Sec. 18.2.3.)

**Multiple drug resistance–associated protein (MRP):** A protein expressed on the surface of some drug-resistant cells that facilitates the excretion of certain anticancer drugs, either alone or in association with glutathione, thereby increasing the dose of the drug required for toxicity. Expression of MRP is one cause of **multiple drug resistance.** (See Chap. 18, Sec. 18.2.3.)

**Multivariate (multivariable) analysis:** A statistical method that allows analysis of the influence of several factors on prognosis or outcome after treatment to determine which factors may be independently predictive of that outcome. (See Chap. 22, Sec. 22.3.2.)

**Mutation:** A change in one or more of the DNA bases in a **gene.** Changes can include insertion of extra bases or **deletion** of a base or bases. Mutations in coding **exons** may lead to altered protein products; mutations in noncoding regions can lead to altered amounts of protein. **Missense mutation:** A mutation that leads to a nonfunctioning protein or to nonproduction of protein. **Germline mutation:** A mutation in the germline cells that is, therefore, inherited.

**Mutation hot spot:** A region of a **gene** where mutations are found more frequently than in the rest of the gene.

*MYC* **gene:** An oncogene that encodes a transcription factor, and which is frequently over-expressed in human cancer. (See Chap. 7, Sec. 7.2.)

**Myelosuppression:** A reduction in mature blood cells in the peripheral circulation, particularly granulocytes, that may occur after treatment with anticancer drugs. (See Chap. 17, Sec. 17.4.1.)

**Natural killer cell:** A lymphocyte (part of the **innate immune system**) that can kill certain types of malignant cells without prior specific sensitization. (See Chap. 20, Sec. 20.4.1.)

**Necrosis:** Death of cells. It often occurs in solid tumors, leading to areas containing degenerating or pyknotic cells.

**Neoplasm:** Literally, a new growth or tumor. Often used to describe a **malignant** tumor or cancer.

**Northern blot analysis:** A technique for determining the presence of specific mRNA sequences in cells. Messenger RNA molecules are separated by **electrophoresis** and then blotted onto nitrocellulose paper. A labeled **probe,** containing DNA sequences (**cDNA**) complementary to the mRNA that is to be detected, is applied to the blot and allowed to **hybridize.** The labeled cDNA is then detected by a technique such as **autoradiography,** phosphoimaging, or chemiluminescence. (See Chap. 4, Sec. 4.3.4.)

**Notch receptor signaling:** A signaling pathway important in embryonic development. Abnormal activation of the pathway has been associated with the development of sporadic cancers. (See Chap. 8, Sec. 8.4.2.)

**Nucleophile:** A substance that can interact with negatively charged molecules such as DNA. (See also **electrophile.)**

**Nucleotide excision repair (NER):** A **DNA repair** process that involves excision of a group of nucleotides containing damaged or altered base(s) in one strand of a DNA molecule and its replacement by synthesis of new DNA using the opposite strand as a template. (See Chap. 5, Sec. 5.3.4.)

**Nude mouse:** A mouse that congenitally lacks a thymus and hence has no mature **T cells. Xenografts** of human tumors will often grow in such immune-deficient animals. These mice are also hairless, hence the term "nude." (See Chap. 17, Sec. 17.3.1.)

**Null hypothesis:** A statistical term used in testing the significance of a difference between two samples. The null hypothesis assumes that the two samples are drawn at random from the same population. The null hypothesis is rejected if the probability that a difference of the magnitude observed could arise by chance is very low, usually less than 5 percent (1 in 20). (See Chap. 22, Sec. 22.4.6.)

**Nullizygosity:** When both alleles of a given gene are disrupted; synonymous with **homozygosity** for a null mutation (a mutation which completely disrupts gene function) or targeted gene disruption.

**Oligonucleotide:** A short piece of DNA or RNA usually containing a defined sequence of bases.

**Oligomer:** A molecular complex made up of a number of copies of the same molecule (e.g., the form of **p53** that binds to DNA is a tetramer of four p53 protein molecules).

**Oncofetal antigen:** A protein produced by fetal tissue that is usually present at very low levels in the adult. Many tumors produce oncofetal antigens (e.g., **carcinoembryonic antigen**), which have been used as **markers** of tumor bulk and may be suitable as targets (**tumor associated antigens**) for immunotherapy. (See Chap. 21, Sec. 21.1.1.)

**Oncogene:** A **gene** whose protein product may be involved in processes leading to **transformation** of a normal cell to a **malignant** state. The gene may be known as a **viral oncogene** if it was detected in a transforming virus. (See Chap. 7, Sec. 7.2.)

**Open reading frame (ORF):** The sequence of DNA that contains the protein-coding sequence for a given gene, from the initial amino acid (usually a methionine) to the stop codon in the mRNA transcript.

**Orthotopic:** Literally, of the same type. Tumor cells are said to be transplanted orthotopically if they are inoculated into an organ of the same tissue type (e.g., breast carcinoma cells transplanted into a mammary gland).

**Oxygen enhancement ratio:** The ratio of the radiation dose given in the absence of oxygen required to produce a given level of cell killing or tissue damage divided by the dose required to give the same level of killing or damage in the presence of oxygen. (See Chap. 15, Sec. 15.4.1.)

**Oxygen radical:** An oxygen molecule that is highly reactive with other biological molecules because it has an unpaired electron.

***P53* gene:** A **tumor suppressor gene,** so named because of the molecular weight of the corresponding protein ($\sim$53 kDa). The p53 protein is involved in control of the progression of cells through the cell cycle, particularly, the transition from G1 phase to S phase. It appears to be active in preventing cells with DNA damage from progressing into S phase. (See Chap. 7, Sec. 7.4.2.)

**Papillomavirus:** A family of DNA-containing viruses, some of which are capable of inducing **malignant transformation** of cells. Some papillomaviruses are implicated in causing human cervical and anal cancers. (See Chap. 6, Sec. 6.2.3.)

**Paracrine:** Refers to the production of substances (usually hormones or **growth factors**) produced by one cell and secreted to act on a neighboring cell.

**Parenchyma:** The cells of a tissue that are responsible for its various functions, as distinct from **stroma,** which refers to blood vessels and connective tissue.

**Passive diffusion:** A process by which substances enter or leave cells as a result of a concentration gradient into or out of the cells.

**Passive immunotherapy:** Nonspecific stimulation of the host immune system to induce an immune reaction against a tumor, or transfer into the body of **antibodies** or immune cells, reactive against the tumor, that were created outside the body. (See Chap. 21, Sec. 21.3.)

**P-glycoprotein:** A membrane protein of molecular weight 180 kDa that has been implicated in the development of **multiple drug resistance** of tumor cells. High levels of P-glycoprotein are effective in pumping cytotoxic drugs and other foreign substances out of the cells. (See Chap. 18, Sec. 18.2.3.)

**Pharmacodynamics:** The effects of a drug within the body. (See Chap. 16, Sec. 16.1.3.)

**Pharmacokinetics:** The time course of drug absorption, distribution, metabolism, and excretion within the body. (See Chap. 16, Sec. 16.1.1.)

**Phase I, phase II, and phase III trials:** Designation of different types of clinical trials according to their purpose. **Phase I trials** seek to determine the maximum tolerated dose and an appropriate schedule for administration of a new drug. **Phase II trials** seek evidence of biological effect. **Phase III trials** evaluate benefit to patients, usually by comparing experimental and standard therapy in a randomized trial. (See Chap. 22, Sec. 22.4.1.)

**Phenotype:** Characteristics of a cell or tissue resulting from the expression of specific **genes.**

**Philadelphia chromosome:** A characteristically altered copy of chromosome 22 that is found in chronic myelogenous leukemia cells and is the result of a specific **chromosome translocation** involving chromosomes 9 and 22. The translocation provides a **fusion** between the *bcr* and *abl* genes. (See Chap. 7, Sec. 7.2.4.)

**Phosphoinositides:** A family of molecules involved in intracellular signaling. (See Chap. 8, Sec. 8.2.7.)

**Plasmid:** A circular piece of DNA that may reproduce separately from chromosomal DNA within cells, bacteria, or other organisms.

**Plating efficiency:** The fraction of **clonogenic** cells in a population.

**Ploidy:** A description of the **chromosome** content of the cell. Normal mammalian cells contain two copies of each chromosome (except for the sex chromosomes in males) and are diploid. Germ cells contain only one copy of each chromosome and are haploid. Cells in tumors often have missing or additional chromosomes (aneuploidy) and/or may have one or more **chromosome aberrations.** (See Chap. 4, Sec. 4.2.)

**Polymerase chain reaction (PCR):** A method by which a given segment of DNA is amplified multiple times by the synthesis of complementary strands. **RT-PCR** is a method for amplifying mRNA, that involves an initial **reverse transcription** of the mRNA to **cDNA** before amplification by PCR. (See Chap. 4, Secs. 4.3.5 and 4.3.6.)

**Polymorphism:** An altered DNA base sequence in a gene, either between the two alleles in one individual or between different individuals, that occurs naturally in the population with a frequency greater than 1%. and usually leads to little or no changes in the function of the coded protein.

**Positron emission tomography (PET) scan:** An imaging technique that is based on the injection of a radioactive tracer that emits a positron (positive electron). When the positron is emitted it rapidly interacts with an electron causing the creation of two 511kev $\gamma$-rays that are emitted at 180° to each other and are detected by a ring detector. The image is created by back projection using a technique similar to that used in **CT scanners** (See Chap. 13, Sec. 13.2.3.)

**Potential doubling time ($T_{pot}$):** The predicted doubling time of a population of cells (usually a tumor) calculated from measured parameters such as the labeling index (LI) and the length of S phase ($T_S$) and based on the assumption that no cells are lost from the growing population. (See Chap. 9, Secs. 9.4.2 and 9.4.5.)

**Potentially lethal damage:** Damage to a cell that may be caused by radiation or drugs and that may or may not be repaired depending on the environment of the cell following treatment. (See Chap. 14, Sec. 14.3.3.)

**Power:** The probability that a clinical trial will be able to detect a real difference between two treatments. The power of a study depends strongly on its sample size. (See Chap. 22, Sec. 22.4.6.)

**Predictive assay:** An assay that measures a specific biological parameter, the value of which is expected to be predictive for the outcome of treatment. (See Chap. 15, Sec. 15.3.2 and 15.5.6 and Chap. 17, Sec. 17.2.)

**Prevalence:** The frequency of disease in a population at a given time. (See Chap. 2, Sec. 2.2.1.)

**Probe:** A **cloned gene** or fragment of a cloned gene that can be labeled and used to detect **homologous** DNA (**Southern blot** or in situ hybridization) or RNA (**northern blot or in situ hybridization**). (See Chap. 4, Sec. 4.3.3.)

**Procarcinogen:** A chemical that can be metabolized in the body to form a **carcinogenic** compound. (See Chap. 3, Sec. 3.2.2.)

**Prognosis:** The expected outcome (e.g., chance of survival) for a patient with a particular type and stage of disease. (See Chap. 22, Sec. 22.3.)

**Prognostic factor:** A detectable feature of a cancer or patient that can be used to predict the likely outcome of treatment of the cancer. (See Chap. 22, Sec. 22.3.)

**Programmed cell death:** An orderly process by which cells die. Also known as **apoptosis.** (See Chap. 10.)

**Progression:** The tendency of tumors to become more **malignant** as they grow. (See Chap. 11, Sec. 11.1.)

**Proliferation-dependent antigen:** A molecule that is expressed selectively in actively cycling cells. (See Chap. 9, Sec. 9.4.2.)

**Promoter (or promotor):** (1) A DNA sequence involved in the initiation of transcription. Promoters, in contrast to **enhancers,** have direction and are always located near the beginning of the first **exon.** (2) A compound that may not itself be **carcinogenic** but that stimulates the proliferation of **initiated** cells to form a cancer. Promotion is reversible and is normally a slow process. (See Chap. 3, Sec. 3.2.1.)

**Prostate specific antigen (PSA):** A peptide molecule that is released by prostatic cells. A raised level of PSA may indicate the presence of a prostatic cancer. In this case, the serum level of PSA is useful as a **biomarker,** as it relates to the volume of prostatic tumor that is present in the body.

**Protein denaturation:** Destruction, usually by heating, of the three-dimensional structure of a protein required for its function.

**Protein kinase:** An enzyme that catalyzes the phosphorylation of proteins. Phosphorylation and dephosphorylation of proteins are major mechanisms controlling their function. Many **oncogenes** code for protein kinases.

**Protein truncation test:** A technique used to detect **mutations** in a **gene** that lead to the production of a truncated or smaller-than-normal protein. (See Chap. 4, Sec. 4.3.9.)

**Proteolytic enzyme:** An enzyme that can catalyze the breakdown of other proteins.

**Proteomics:** Study of the structure and function of proteins. (See Chap. 4, Sec. 4.5.)

**Proteosome:** A protein complex in cells that is responsible for degrading unneeded or defective (e.g improperly folded) proteins usually after they have been polyubiquitinated. (see Chap. 9, Fig. 9.4)

**Protooncogene:** A **gene,** in a normal cell, **homologous** to a viral transforming gene. Some proto-oncogenes encode proteins that influence the control of cellular proliferation and **differentiation. Mutations, amplifications, rearrangements,** etc., of protooncogenes may allow them to function as **oncogenes,** i.e., genes whose products are involved in cell **transformation.** (See Chap. 6, Sec. 6.1.)

**Provirus:** A DNA copy of the RNA of a **retrovirus,** which is integrated into the chromosomal DNA of a cell. (See Chap. 7, Sec. 7.2.2.)

***PTEN* gene:** A **tumor suppressor gene** that is frequently mutated in human cancer. (See Chap. 7, Sec. 7.4.3.)

**Pyrimidine dimer:** The formation of chemical bonds between two adjacent pyrimidine bases (thymine or cytosine) in DNA results in a pyrimidine dimer. This can be caused by exposure to ultraviolet light. (See Chap. 14, Sec. 14.2.5.)

**Q-FISH:** A method of quantitation of the copy number of a specific DNA sequence using FISH; e.g the quantification of telomere signal intensity at telomeres, by hybridizing a telomere-specific fluorescent probe to a metaphase spread, and measuring the intensity of fluorescent telomere signal at each chromosome end. (See Chap. 4, Sec. 4.4.1)

**Quality of life:** A measure of the overall health of a patient during and after treatment that addresses symptoms and function rather than just the state of the disease being treated. (See Chap. 22, Sec. 22.4.8.)

**Radioimmunoassay (RIA):** A sensitive method that may be used for the quantitation of any substance recognizable by an **antibody.** It depends on the binding of radiolabeled antibodies to the substance.

**Radioimmunotherapy:** A therapeutic technique in which a radioisotope is linked to an **antibody** or other **ligand** that binds to **receptors** on cancer cells, thereby delivering selective radiation to such cells. (See Chap. 15, Sec. 15.2.3.)

**Radioprotection:** Use of agents that protect cells or tissues from radiation damage. (See Chap. 15, Sec. 15.5.8.)

**Radiosensitizer:** A compound that increases the sensitivity of cells to ionizing radiation. (See Chap. 15, Sec. 15.4.5.)

**Randomization:** A process by which patients (or other experimental subjects) are assigned to treatment groups on the basis of random selection, so that the selection is not subject to **bias** by any unknown variables. This process is part of **phase III clinical trials.** (See Chap. 22, Sec. 22.4.3.)

*Ras* **gene:** A gene involved in signal transduction pathways that can induce cell proliferation. It is an oncogene that is commonly mutated in human cancers. (See Chap. 7, Sec. 7.3.2 and Chap. 8, Sec. 8.2.5.)

**Rearrangement:** Changes in the sequence of **genes** or of DNA sequences within genes that lead to alteration in their protein products. Rearrangement of genes is important in such processes as the generation of diversity of **antibody** molecules. Abnormal rearrangements between different genes appear to be important in **malignant transformation**.

**Receiver-operating-characteristics (ROC) curve:** A technique for assessing the efficacy of a diagnostic test based on knowledge of the true-positive and false-positive rates for the test in question. (See Chap. 22, Sec. 22.2.1.)

**Receptor:** A molecule inside or on the surface of cells that recognizes a specific hormone, **growth factor,** or other biologically active molecule. The receptor also mediates transfer of signals within the cell. Many receptors are **Protein kinases**.

**Reciprocal translocation:** A **chromosomal** aberration that involves the reciprocal exchange of parts of two chromosomes without loss of genetic material.

**Recombination (DNA):** A process that results in exchange of segments between two DNA molecules. **Homologous recombination** occurs when the segments have matching (homologous) sequences over at least part of the segment (usually at both ends). **Nonhomologous recombination** is said to occur when there is little or no homology between the exchanged segments. This latter process is believed to occur when a **provirus** is integrated into the cellular DNA.

**Redistribution:** When treatment (with radiation or drugs) is differentially toxic to cells in different parts of the cell cycle, the treatment will cause partial synchrony of the cells surviving the treatment. Between treatments, these surviving cells will redistribute around the cell cycle. (See Chap. 15, Sec. 15.6.3.)

**Regional chemotherapy:** Treatment with chemotherapy in which the drug is introduced directly into the tumor-bearing region of the body by, for example, intra-arterial infusion or intra-thecal injection. (See Chap. 16, Sec. 16.1.5.)

**Relative biological effectiveness (RBE):** A measure of the relative effectiveness of a given type of radiation. RBE is defined as the ratio of the dose of a commonly used type of radiation (e.g., $^{60}$Co $\gamma$-rays) to the dose of the test radiation that gives the same biological effect. (See Chap. 14, Sec. 14.3.1.)

**Relative risk:** The ratio of disease frequency in exposed and unexposed members of a population. (Exposure implies any attribute, personal, environmental, or genetic, that may cause or protect against disease). (See Chap. 2, Sec. 2.2.1.)

**Remission:** Decrease in tumor volume (or cell number) following treatment. Complete remission indicates that disease cannot be detected by physical examination or clinical tests but does not necessarily imply that the disease has been cured. Partial remission is usually defined as shrinkage by at least 50 percent of the cross-sectional area of measurable tumors.

**Reoxygenation:** A process by which cells in a tumor that are at low oxygen levels because of poor blood supply, and hence are resistant to radiation, gain access to oxygen following a treatment so that they become more sensitive to a subsequent radiation treatment. (See Chap. 15, Sec. 15.6.4.)

**Repopulation:** Proliferation of surviving cells in a tumor (or normal tissue) during or following cytotoxic treatment. Repopulation during a course of fractionated therapy (radiation or chemotherapy) may lead to a requirement for an increased total dose to eradicate the tumor. (See Chap. 15, Sec. 15.6.2 and Chap. 18, Sec. 18.3.4.)

**Restriction enzymes:** Enzymes obtained from bacteria that make cuts at specific sequences of four to eight bases in double-stranded DNA. (See Chap. 4, Sec. 4.3.2.)

**Restriction-fragment-length polymorphism (RFLP) analysis:** A method, based on **Southern blot analysis** of DNA cut by one or more **restriction enzymes,** that may be used to identify unique DNA sequences within a cell. (See Chap. 4, Fig. 4.6.)

**Retinoblastoma (Rb) gene:** A **tumor suppressor gene** that was identified initially because it was **mutated** in inherited cases of retinoblastoma (a childhood eye tumor). The gene is now known to be involved in controlling the movement of cells through the cell cycle, in particular the transition from the G1 phase to S phase. (See Chap. 7, Sec. 7.4.4.)

**Retrovirus:** A virus in which the genome comprises RNA. (See Chap. 6, Sec. 6.3.)

**Reverse transcriptase:** An enzyme, found mostly in **retroviruses,** that catalyzes the production of a complementary DNA (**cDNA**) strand from an RNA strand. (See Chap. 6, Sec. 6.3.1.)

**Sarcoma:** A **malignant** tumor derived from mesenchymal cells (e.g., connective tissue, vascular tissue, bone).

**SCID mouse:** A mouse that has severe combined immunodeficiency by virtue of having no functioning **T** or **B lymphocytes** because of a **mutation** that prevents effective **rearrangement** of the **immunoglobulin and T-cell receptor genes.** Such mice will allow the growth of human tumor **xenografts** because of their immunodeficiency. (See Chap. 17, Sec. 17.3.1.)

**Screening:** (1) The application of a test (e.g., mammography) that may detect disease in a population of individuals having no symptoms of the disease. (See Chap. 22, Sec. 22.2.4.) (2) The use of assays for detecting antitumor activity of compounds. (See Chap. 17, Sec. 17.6.1.)

**Second messenger:** A substance involved in transmission of information (i.e., **signal transduction**) between the surface of the cell and its interior, often leading to changes in the expression of specific **genes.** Nonsteroidal hormones stimulate second messengers such as cyclic AMP or phosphoinositides to influence the behavior of cells.

**Selectins:** Small **lectin-**like adhesion receptors. They are upregulated on endothelial cells and platelets during an inflammatory response and may play a role in metastasis. (See Chap. 11, Sec. 11.5.4.)

**Selective Estrogen Receptor Modulator (SERM):** Compounds with different selectivity in causing **estrogenic** and antiestrogenic responses. They are used in the treatment of breast cancer. (See Chap. 19, Sec. 19.4.1.)

**Self-renewal:** Proliferation of a cell to produce two daughter cells, at least one of which retains the properties of the original cell. Usually applied to **stem cells.**

**Senescence (Terminal Growth Arrest):** The slow loss of proliferative potential and eventual cell arrest that occurs when normal cells are grown over periods of time in culture. Immortalized cells have overcome this effect and can grow indefinitely in culture. Senescence is believed to be associated with the shortening of **telomeres** during multiple rounds of proliferation; immortalized cells have upregulated **telomerase** activity, which can prevent telomere attrition from occurring. (See Chap. 5, Sec. 5.5.2 and Chap. 9, Sec. 9.2.6 and Chap. 14, Sec 14.3.2.)

**Sensitivity:** The probability that a diagnostic test will identify those patients who have a given disease or attribute. (See Chap. 22, Sec. 22.2.1.)

**SH2 and SH3 domains:** The *Src-H*omology domains are homologous to regions in src family protein kinases. They are present in many proteins involved in signal transduction and give the proteins the ability to bind to other proteins in a manner facilitating **signal transduction.** (See Chap. 8, Secs. 8.2.3 and 8.2.4.)

**Signal transduction:** A process by which information is transmitted from the surface of the cell to the nucleus. It involves a series of molecular components (proteins), that activate subsequent members of the cascade (usually by phosphorylation), resulting in activation of **transcription factors.** (See Chap. 8.)

**Single nucleotide polymorphism (SNP):** Difference in DNA sequence at a single nucleotide in the genome. (See Chap. 4, Sec. 4.3.7.)

**Single photon emission computed tomography (SPECT):** An imaging technique that combines injection of a radioisotope with detection of the radioactive emissions using a ring detector. An image of the radioisotopes distribution in the body is then created using computer-generated reconstruction algorithms similar to those used in **computed tomographic (CT)** scanning. (See Chap. 13, Sec. 13.2.2.)

**Single-strand break:** A break in one of the sugar-phosphate backbones of a double-stranded DNA molecule.

**Single-strand conformation polymorphism (SSCP):** A technique for detecting **mutations** in **genes** by virtue of changes in the migration of the DNA using **gel electrophoresis.** (See Chap. 4, Sec. 4.3.9.)

**Site-directed mutagenesis:** A technique for introducing a change in DNA sequence at a given site in DNA. (See Chap. 4, Sec. 4.3.11.)

**Somatic cell hybrid:** The fusion of two somatic (nongerm) cells to produce a **hybrid** cell that retains all (or some selected fraction) of the DNA of both of the parent cells. Such cells can be used in genetic studies, particularly those involving **complementation** analysis.

**Southern blot analysis:** A technique used for detecting specific DNA sequences in cells. DNA is extracted from cells and cut with one or more **restriction enzymes.** The DNA fragments are separated by gel **electrophoresis** and blotted onto nitrocellulose paper or a nylon membrane. The DNA is then **hybridized** using a labeled DNA **probe** with a sequence complementary to the specific sequence to be detected. The DNA fragments that hybridize with the probe can be detected by techniques such as **autoradiography,** phosphoimaging, or chemiluminescence. (See Chap. 4, Sec. 4.3.4.)

**Specificity:** The probability that a negative diagnostic test will correctly identify those patients who do not have a given disease or attribute. (See Chap. 22, Sec. 22.2.1.)

**Spectral karyotyping (SKY):** A technique that allows identification of **chromosomes** by application of fluorescent chromosome-specific paints. (See Chap. 4, Sec. 4.4.3.)

**S-phase:** The discrete phase of the cell cycle in which DNA is synthesized. (See Chap. 9, Sec. 9.4.2.)

**Spheroid:** A spherical aggregation of cells that can be grown in tissue culture and provides a useful model for studying the properties of solid tumors. (See Chap. 18, Fig. 18.13.)

**Splicing (RNA):** The process in which the initial RNA copy made from DNA during transcription is modified to remove certain sections (such as **introns**) prior to use as a template for translation. Many **genes** can undergo **alternative splicing,** which can remove some **exons** (as well as the **introns**), resulting in mRNAs of different length that may be translated to produce proteins of different sizes.

**Stage migration:** The application of more sensitive diagnostic techniques can lead to the identification of a greater extent of disease, and consequent upstaging, of some patients. Stage migration confounds the comparison of a current series of patients with historical controls. (See Chap. 22, Sec. 22.4.3.)

**Stem cell:** A cell that has the capacity to repopulate functional units within a tissue. The term is most aptly applied to renewal tissues such as the bone marrow, where it is possible to demonstrate the presence of a cell that can regenerate all the various **differentiated** cells in blood. The term is also used to describe a cell in a tumor that can produce a very large number of progeny and which, if it survives, can regenerate the tumor after treatment.

**Stem-cell transplantation:** Injection of (bone marrow) stem cells into the circulation of an animal or human in order to replace **stem cells** killed by cytotoxic treatment. (See Chap. 16, Sec. 16.1.6 and Chap. 17, Sec. 17.4.2.)

**Stress-activated protein kinase (SAPK):** A protein kinase that is part of the signal transduction pathway of the same name. This pathway is activated by exposure of the cell to stress, such as that caused by cytotoxic agents, heat, or hypoxia. (See Chap. 8, Sec. 8.2.6.)

**Stroma:** The part of tissue that provides the supporting structure for the **parenchymal** (functional) cells of that tissue. Stroma includes blood vessels, connective tissue such as fibroblasts, and the **extracellular matrix** (ECM).

**Sublethal damage:** Damage to a cell that may be caused by radiation or drugs and that can be repaired within a few hours after the treatment. Classically, repair of sublethal damage is revealed by giving two treatments separated by a variable time interval. (See Chap. 14, Sec. 14.3.3.)

**Survival curve:** (1) See **cell survival curve.** (2) A graph indicating the proportion of patients who are alive at different times after treatment (or diagnosis). (See Chap. 22, Sec. 22.4.5.)

**Surviving fraction:** The fraction of cells that retain long-term proliferative potential (i.e., usually **clonogenic** cells) following treatment with a cytotoxic agent. (See Chap. 14, Sec. 14.3.1 and Chap. 17, Sec. 17.2.3.)

**Synchronized cells:** A population of cells most of which are at a given stage of the growth cycle at any one time and that move through the cell cycle as a cohort. Drugs that kill cells at a given phase of the cell cycle cause partial synchrony among the survivors.

**Synergy:** An interaction between two agents that is greater than would be predicted from the activity of either alone. This word is commonly misused in describing the interaction between drugs or between drugs and radiation, since there is a range of effects that would be predicted as being **additive.** (See Chap. 17, Sec. 17.5.2.)

**T cell (or T lymphocyte):** A lymphocyte that has been processed by the thymus and may have cytotoxic or regulatory functions in the immune response. T cells express the **T-cell receptor** on their surface. (See Chap. 20, Sec. 20.2.3.)

**T-cell receptor:** A receptor on the surface of **T cells** that is required for them to recognize **antigens** presented on the surface of **antigen-presenting cells** and to interact with other cells of the immune system. (See Chap. 20, Sec. 20.2.4.)

**T-helper cells:** A subset of T lymphocytes that can be activated to secrete **cytokines,** which stimulate other cells of the immune system to mount an immune response. (See Chap. 20, Sec. 20.2.3.)

**Taq polymerase:** A DNA polymerase, isolated from a thermoresistant bacterium (*Thermus aquaticus*), which is thermostable at the high temperatures (~90°C) used in PCR to denature the double strands of DNA. (See Chap. 4, Sec. 4.3.5.)

**Taxane:** A type of anticancer drug that kills cells through interaction with the microtubules. Family members include docetaxel and paclitaxel. (See Chap. 16, Sec. 16.6.2.)

**Telomerase:** An enzyme complex comprised of essential RNA (telomerase RNA) and protein (**TERT**) constituents, that is responsible for the de novo addition of telomere DNA, one nucleotide at a time, to chromosome ends. The enzyme may be upregulated in tumors and prevent the **senescence** observed in normal cells. (See Chap. 5, Sec. 5.5.1.).

**Telomerase reverse transcriptase (TERT):** An element of the enzyme **telomerase** which prevents the erosion of **telomeres** during cell division. (See Chap. 5, Sec. 5.5.1.)

**Telomere:** The ends of **chromosomes** that contain multiple repeats of specific DNA sequences and associated proteins. The DNA replication machinery in most normal cells has difficulty replicating these ends completely. Shortening of the telomeres may lead eventually to **senescence** and cell death. (See Chap. 5, Sec. 5.5.)

**Therapeutic index (therapeutic ratio):** The dose of a therapeutic agent required to produce a given level of damage to a critical normal tissue divided by the dose of the agent required to produce a defined level of antitumor effect. Therapeutic index is therefore a measure of the relative efficacy of therapy against tumors as compared with the normal tissue damage caused. (See Chap. 15, Sec. 15.5.7 and Chap. 17, Sec. 17.3.5.)

**Thrombospondin-1:** An **extracellular matrix glycoprotein** that is an endogenous inhibitor of angiogenesis. (See Chap. 12, Sec. 12.4.1.)

**Tie receptors: Receptor tyrosine kinases,** expressed on endothelial cells, that bind **angiopoietins**. Stimulation of receptors may have either agonistic or antagonistic effects on **angiogenesis**. (See Chap. 12, Sec. 12.2.3)

**Tissue inhibitors of metalloproteinases (TIMPS):** Proteins that can bind to and inhibit the proteolytic action of **metalloproteinases**. (See Chap. 11, Sec. 11.6.)

**Tolerance:** A term used in immunology to indicate the process whereby specific **antigens** fail to elicit an immunologic response. Tolerance is required to prevent a response against "self-antigens"; it can also be induced against foreign antigens. (See Chap. 20, Sec. 20.3.)

**Topoisomerases:** Enzymes that allow breakage of one or both DNA strands, unwinding of DNA, and resealing of the strands. The enzymes are required for DNA and RNA synthesis and are important for the action of some anticancer drugs. Decreased activity of topoisomerases is a cause of **multiple drug resistance**. (See Chap. 18, Sec. 18.2.6.)

**Transactivation:** The process by which the transcription of a gene is increased by proteins that interact with the **promoter** DNA of the transcribed gene.

**Transcription factors:** Proteins that can bind to DNA (often after their association to form **dimers**) and that control the **transcription** of genes. (See Chap. 7, Sec. 7.3.4. and Chap. 8, Sec. 8.2.8.)

**Transduction:** The process by which the behavior of a cell is modified by introduction of foreign DNA via a retrovirus or phage. (See Chap. 6, Sec. 6.1.)

**Transfection:** The direct transfer of DNA molecules into a cell. Transfection of specific **genes** is a powerful tool for determining their function. (See Chap. 4, Sec. 4.3.10.)

**Transformation:** Commonly used to describe the conversion of normal cells to those with abnormalities in cellular appearance and growth regulation in tissue culture (morphologic transformation). **Malignant transformation** indicates that the cells can produce a tumor in an appropriate animal. (See Chap. 3, Sec. 3.3.1.)

**Transforming growth factors $\alpha$ and $\beta$ (TGF-$\alpha$, and TGF-$\beta$):** Growth factors that were originally isolated from tumor cells and believed to be responsible for their growth, hence their name as **transforming** growth factors. TGF-$\alpha$ is now known to be related to **epidermal growth factor** (EGF) and to bind to and stimulate its **receptor** (EGFR) on cells. TGF-$\beta$ is a multi-

functional growth factor that can both inhibit and stimulate the growth of different cell types and can induce **differentiated** functions in cells, such as the production of collagen by fibroblasts. (See Chap. 8, Sec. 8.4.4.)

**Transgenic mouse:** A mouse produced from a germline cell into which a specific **gene** has been introduced. All cells of such mice carry this gene, including the germline. (See Chap. 4, Sec. 4.3.12.)

**Translocation:** The displacement of one part of a **chromosome** to a different chromosome or to a different part of the same chromosome. An example is the translocation between chromosomes 9 and 22, which leads to the appearance of the **Philadelphia chromosome** in chronic myelogenous leukemia. (See Chap. 7, Sec. 7.2.4.)

**Tumor-associated antigen:** An antigenic determinant on the surface of a tumor cell that is not usually expressed by normal cells of the same histopathologic type. Such antigens may or may not be **immunogenic**. (See Chap. 20, Sec. 20.4.3 and Chap. 21, Sec. 21.1.1.)

**Tumor suppressor gene:** A gene whose mutation or loss may lead to cellular **transformation** and to the development of cancer. (See Chap. 7, Sec. 7.4.)

**TUNEL assay:** A technique (*T*erminal deoxynucleotidyl transferase d*U*DP *N*ick *E*nd *L*abeling) widely used to detect cells that are undergoing **apoptosis**. (See Chap. 10, Sec. 10.3.4.)

**Type I and type II error:** Types of error associated with assessing the statistical significance of a clinical trial (or a set of experimental observations). Type I error (also known as the **alpha error**) relates to the probability that different outcomes between two different treatment arms in a clinical trial (or in an experimental study) could arise by chance. If this probability ($p$ value) is less than 5 percent (i.e., less than 1 in 20 that the result could have occurred by chance), the result is usually regarded as statistically significant, although the cutoff value for statistical significance may have to be reduced if multiple comparisons are being made. Type II error (also known as the **beta error**) relates to the probability that, by chance, the trial will fail to demonstrate a statistically significant difference even though a real difference between the two treatment arms actually exists. (See Chap. 22, Sec. 22.4.6.)

**Tyrosine kinase:** An enzyme that has the ability to phosphorylate proteins on the amino acid tyrosine. The phosphorylation is often highly specific for individual tyrosine residues, depending on the amino acids surrounding the tyrosine in the protein. Tyrosine kinases comprise intracellular components of many **receptors** for **growth factors** and function also in intracellular signaling (See Chap. 8, Sec. 8.2.2.)

**Ultrasound:** The reflection of ultrasound from tissue interfaces is useful in imaging of organs and in determining blood flow. (See Chap. 13, Sec. 13.2.5.)

**Uncapping:** Refers to the loss of **telomere** integrity that often leads to **end-to-end fusions,** which can occur through loss of essential telomere binding regulatory factors, or via the gradual loss of telomere DNA in the absence of telomere replenishment by **telomerase.**

**Vascular endothelial growth factor (VEGF):** A **growth factor** that acts on endothelial cells to promote their proliferation as part of new vessel formation (**angiogenesis**). This factor induces increased vascular permeability and is also known as "vascular permeability factor" (VPF). (See Chap. 12, Sec. 12.2.1.)

**Vector:** A short piece of DNA or RNA, such as a DNA **plasmid** or RNA virus, into which genetic material of interest is incorporated and which is used to transfer this genetic material into a cell for either transient or long-term expression. (See Chap. 4, Sec. 4.3.10.)

**Vinca alkaloid:** A type of anticancer drug that kills cells through interaction with the microtubules. Family members include vinblastine and vincristine. (See Chap. 16, Sec. 16.6.1.)

**Western blot analysis:** A procedure analogous to **Southern** and **northern blot** analyses that allows the detection of specific proteins. Proteins are separated by **electrophoresis** and transferred onto a membrane. They are usually detected following binding with labeled antibodies. (See Chap. 4, Sec. 4.3.4.)

**Wild type:** The usual or normal configuration of a **gene** or protein (as compared with a mutant form).

**Wnt signaling:** A signaling pathway important in embryonic development. Abnormal activation of the pathway has been associated with the development of sporadic cancers, most likely mediated by $\beta$-catenin. (See Chap. 8, Sec. 8.4.1.)

**Xenobiotic:** A substance (usually a chemical) that is foreign to the body.

**Xenograft:** Tissue that is transplanted from one species of animal into another. Most commonly this refers to the transplantation of a human tumor into an immune-deficient mouse (e.g., a **nude mouse** or **SCID mouse**). (See Chap. 17, Sec. 17.3.1.)

**Xeroderma pigmentosum:** A human genetic disease characterized by extreme sensitivity to sunlight and the early onset of skin cancers. The genetic defect lies in the inability of the individual's cells to **repair DNA** damage (by NER) caused by ultraviolet light. (See Chap. 5, Secs. 5.2.2 and 5.3.4.)

**X-ray crystallography:** A technique for imaging the three-dimensional structure of molecules. The substance is allowed to form a crystal in which the molecules have a repeating alignment. The crystal is then exposed to x-rays and the diffraction pattern of the crystal is used to deduce the structure. (See Chap. 4, Sec. 4.5.2.)

**Zinc-finger domain:** The region of a protein that is formed into a finger-like projection by binding of some of the amino acids (cysteines or histidines) to a zinc ion. This configuration usually provides a DNA-binding region and is often found in **transcription factors.** (See Chap. 8, Sec. 8.2.8.)

# Index